Neurologic Rehabilitation: Neuroscience and Neuroplasticity in Physical Therapy Practice

Edited by

Deborah S. Nichols-Larsen, PT, PhD, FASAHP
Professor and Director, School of
Health & Rehabilitation Sciences
Associate Dean, College of Medicine
Associate Vice President, Health Sciences
Columbus, Ohio

Deborah A. Kegelmeyer, PT, DPT, MS, GCS
Associate Professor Clinical Health
and Rehabilitation Sciences
Physical Therapy Division
The Ohio State University
Columbus, Ohio

John A. Buford, PT, PhD
Associate Professor and Director
Division of Physical Therapy
School of Health and Rehabilitation Sciences
The Ohio State University
Columbus, Ohio

Anne D. Kloos, PT, PhD, NCS
Professor Clinical Health and Rehabilitation Sciences
Division of Physical Therapy
School of Health and Rehabilitation Sciences
The Ohio State University
Columbus, Ohio

Jill C. Heathcock, MPT, PhD
Assistant Professor
Division of Physical Therapy
School of Health and Rehabilitation Sciences
The Ohio State University
Columbus, Ohio

D. Michele Basso, EdD, PT
Professor, Associate Director
School of Health and Rehabilitation Sciences
The Ohio State University
Columbus, Ohio

McGraw Hill Education

New York Chicago San Francisco Athens London Madrid Mexico City

Milan New Delhi Singapore Sydney Toronto

Neurologic Rehabilitation: Neuroscience and Neuroplasticity in Physical Therapy Practice

1 2 3 4 5 6 7 8 9 0   DSS/DSS   20 19 18 17 16
MHID 0-07-180715-2
ISBN 978-0-07-180715-9

Notice

Medicine is an ever-changing science. As new research and clinical experience broaden our knowledge, changes in treatment and drug therapy are required. The authors and the publisher of this work have checked with sources believed to be reliable in their efforts to provide information that is complete and generally in accord with the standards accepted at the time of publication. However, in view of the possibility of human error or changes in medical sciences, neither the authors nor the publisher nor any other party who has been involved in the preparation or publication of this work warrants that the information contained herein is in every respect accurate or complete, and they disclaim all responsibility for any errors or omissions or for the results obtained from use of the information contained in this work. Readers are encouraged to confirm the information contained herein with other sources. For example and in particular, readers are advised to check the product information sheet included in the package of each drug they plan to administer to be certain that the information contained in this work is accurate and that changes have not been made in the recommended dose or in the contraindications for administration. This recommendation is of particular importance in connection with new or infrequently used drugs.

This book was set in Minion Pro 10/12 by MPS Limited.
The editors were Michael Weitz and Christie Naglieri.
The production supervisor was Catherine Saggese.
Project Management was provided by Asheesh Ratra, MPS Limited.
RR Donnelley/China was printer and binder.

This book is printed on acid-free paper.

Library of Congress Cataloging-in-Publication Data
Neurologic rehabilitation : neuroscience and neuroplasticity in physical
therapy practice / edited by Deborah S. Larsen [and 5 others].
     p. ; cm.
  Includes index.
  ISBN 978-0-07-180715-9 (hardcover : alk. paper) — ISBN 0-07-180715-2
I. Larsen, Deborah S., editor.
[DNLM: 1. Nervous System Diseases—rehabilitation. 2. Nervous System—anatomy & histology. 3. Nervous System Physiological Processes. 4. Physical Therapy Modalities. WL 140]
RC349.8
616.8'046—dc23
                                                  2015015572

This book is dedicated to the physical therapy students over the years, who have challenged us to keep it relevant; the MS and PhD students, who have challenged us to keep it fresh; our colleagues, who have helped us think more clearly; our friends and families, who have allowed us the time and space to write; and most especially, our patients who have allowed us to see the miracle of the nervous system in action as we helped guide their recovery.

Contents

Contents

Preface

The practice of neurologic physical therapy relies on the growing body of evidence from the field of neuroscience. This text uniquely brings the fields of neuroscience and neurologic physical therapy practice together in a single volume that explores neurologic pathologies and their management across the lifespan. This field is crucial to our understanding of neurologic function, the effects of neurologic damage, and the plasticity of the nervous system as it responds to development, aging, damage, and activity. Therapists need a strong foundation in neuroscience to maximize their treatment methods and efficacy, so this text includes seven introductory chapters that provide a neuroscience foundation along with an introduction to the concepts of neuroplasticity in Chapter 8. Chapter 9 is an overview of the neurologic physical therapy evaluation that affords a foundation for disease-specific assessment, which is incorporated into the remaining 11 chapters. These 11 chapters delineate common neurologic disease and injury processes and the targeted physical therapy evaluation and treatment for each, examining the emerging evidence of how physical therapy can influence neuroplasticity. Each chapter is anchored by clinical cases, following a patient through the diagnostic process, physical therapy assessment, and potential treatment options across stages of the condition. Cases progress from acute care through inpatient and outpatient rehabilitation for conditions such as stroke or spinal cord injury, from infancy through adolescence for developmental disorders, or from early diagnosis through disease progression for conditions such as Parkinson's disease or multiple sclerosis. In addition, this text includes a lifespan approach encompassing changes associated with aging (Chapter 17) and three chapters on common pediatric conditions that effect the nervous system (Chapters 18–20), including myelomeningocele, cerebral palsy, intellectual developmental disability, autism spectrum disorder, and others. Ultimately, this text unites the fields of neuroscience, neurologic rehabilitation, and neuroplasticity to guide the physical therapy student into their career as evidence-based practitioners.

INTRODUCTION TO THE NEUROSCIENCE OF PHYSICAL THERAPY

SECTION

INTRODUCTION TO THE
NEUROSCIENCE OF
PHYSICAL THERAPY

Introduction to Neuroanatomy

John A. Buford

● INTRODUCTION TO NEUROANATOMY

The brain is a fascinating structure. From the brain to the spinal cord, white matter to gray, axons to synapses, and at countless other levels, understanding neuroanatomy is a prerequisite to understanding brain function. In this chapter, the reader is introduced to the major parts of the nervous system with relevance for the rehabilitation professional. For this purpose, the focus will be on sensory and motor systems. Structures associated with the special senses, learning, memory and cognition, language, and other systems with strong relevance to physical rehabilitation will be addressed in some detail. However, details of systems in neuroscience such as vision, hormonal regulation,

and others, are not covered in detail here. For a broader coverage of neuroscience across all systems, the reader is referred to *Principles of Neural Science*.

Directions and Planes in the Nervous System

In musculoskeletal anatomy, the cardinal plane directions are anterior–posterior, superior–inferior, and medial–lateral. In the nervous system, we can use these same directions. However, because of the way the nervous system curves around from the front of the skull to the back and then turns to descend into the spine, a direction system relative to the nervous system itself, independent of the cardinal planes, is often more useful. Rather than anterior–posterior, it is often more useful to refer to ventral–dorsal directions (Figure 1-1). For a person standing up, in the spinal cord, anterior and ventral are equivalent, as are dorsal and posterior. However, in the brain, the top surface of the brain would still be the **dorsal** side, but this would be **superior** in the anatomical planes. Likewise, the lower, undersurface of the brain is **ventral**, but also **inferior**. Dorsal and ventral are more consistent across regions of the nervous system and are typically used rather than the cardinal planes. Likewise, the front of the brain right behind the forehead is **anterior**, and the back of the brain, **posterior**. However, the brainstem and spinal cord curve downward as they form and emerge from the foramen magnum, so anterior–posterior no longer describes the direction we would move in going from the brain to the spinal cord. Instead, we use the terms rostral and caudal. **Rostral** means toward the nose, whereas **caudal** means toward the tail (or in the human, toward the coccygeal segments). In this frame of reference, the brain is always rostral to the spinal cord, no matter what posture the person adopts. The relative directional terms dorsal–ventral and rostral–caudal are useful at any stage of embryologic development, and in any vertebrate species, when studying the nervous system.

Gray Matter and White Matter

The first distinction we make in examining tissues in the nervous system is whether we are looking at gray matter or white matter (Figure 1-2). Gray matter is composed of a variety of structures including: (1) neurons – the active, information processing cells of the nervous system with both the cell bodies of large projecting neurons and entire smaller interneurons; (2) glial cells – cells that provide immune, metabolic, and structural support to neurons; (3) axons and their synapses (connections)

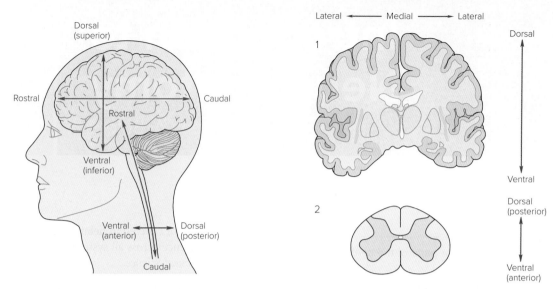

FIGURE 1-1 The directions used in the nervous system. The rostral direction is toward the nose and caudal is toward the tail. In the head of a person standing, rostral and anterior are roughly the same direction, and caudal and posterior are the same for the cerebral cortex. However, as the brainstem forms and descends into the spinal cord, the meaning of rostral and caudal shifts. In the brainstem, rostral would be closer to the cerebrum and caudal would be closer to the spinal cord. Within the spinal cord, rostral would be toward the brainstem and caudal would be toward the coccygeal segments. In the person standing, for the spinal cord, rostral and superior are the same, and caudal and inferior are the same. The other directions used in the nervous system are dorsal, toward the back, and ventral, toward the front. The ventral side of the nervous system is the anterior part of the brainstem and spinal cord and the inferior part of the cerebrum. The dorsal part is the superior part of the cerebrum and the posterior part of the brainstem and spinal cord. Medial and lateral directions in the nervous system have the same meaning as in the regular cardinal planes. (Adapted with permission from Kandel ER, Schwartz JH, Jessell TM, et al. *Principles of Neural Science*, 5th ed. New York, NY: McGraw-Hill; 2013.)

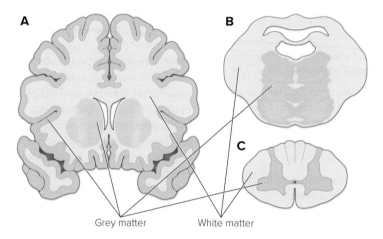

FIGURE 1-2 Brain, brainstem, and spinal cord sections showing gray and white matter. All levels of the central nervous system have a combination of gray matter and white matter. Gray matter is composed of the neurons and the supporting cells, along with the connections between neurons. The gray matter is where the information processing of the brain occurs. White matter is composed of axons carrying information between parts of the nervous system. In the cerebral hemispheres, there is white matter in the middle forming connections, and gray matter at the surface and in nuclei within the brain. In the brainstem and spinal cord, there is white matter on the outside, and gray matter within. (Part B: Used with permission of John A. Buford, PT, PhD. Part C: Adapted with permission, from Kandel ER, Schwartz JH, Jessell TM, Siegelbaum SA, Hudspeth AJ. *Principles of Neural Science*, 5th ed. New York, NY: McGraw-Hill; 2013, Fig 16-1, Pg 357.)

coming into the tissues; and (4) the axons leaving the tissues. White matter, in contrast, is composed of axons and the fatty substance called myelin that insulates them, along with the glial cells that produce and sustain the myelin. Hence, white matter is relatively uniform in its appearance throughout the nervous system; although, the physical structure of large groups of axons that might take a straight path versus a curved or crossing path does provide some variation in the gross appearance of certain sections of white matter. Gray matter, in contrast, is quite variable in appearance, just as the sizes and shapes of neurons and the patterns of incoming and outgoing axons are quite variable in the various regions of the nervous system.

TABLE 1-1	Common Terms in Neuroscience
TERM	**GENERAL USAGE**
Nucleus	A group of neurons in a gray matter structure that is anatomically relatively distinct from the surrounding tissue. A sub-nucleus would be a small nucleus that is a relatively distinct part of a larger nucleus
Ganglion	Typically a nucleus located around the origin of a nerve; occasionally used instead of nucleus
Cortex	The outer layer of the brain of both the cerebrum and the cerebellum, composed of gray matter
Peduncle	A large bundle of axons that physically connects one structure to another
Commissure	A group of axons travelling together to cross the midline
Tract	A bundle of axons having a common origin, destination, and function
Pathway	A route through which information travels, usually involving connections among multiple neurons. For example, there is a pathway from the cerebral cortex to the cerebellum that involves a connection with neurons in the brainstem. If the axons traveled directly from the cortex to the cerebellum, it would be called a tract, but because there is a connection to a neuron in the brainstem along the way, it is a pathway
Lamina	A thin layer of white matter separating nuclei or sub-nuclei in gray matter
Mesial	An inner surface formed by the apposition of two structures; in the nervous system, most commonly used along the midline where left and right parts of the brain are touching each other

Key Terms

Understanding how structures relate to each other and work together for function is the really interesting part about understanding the brain. As is often the case in science, however, there is a large amount of nomenclature to be learned first. Fortunately, there are some key terms that are used repeatedly in neuroscience, and these are provided in Table 1-1.

● PARTS OF THE BRAIN

Cerebral Hemispheres

The **cerebral hemispheres** are the large structures at the most rostral end of the nervous system (Figure 1-3). They are bilateral, with a **left** and a **right** hemisphere. The cerebral hemispheres contain the structures that provide for consciousness, voluntary actions, intelligence, memory, movement, sensation, feelings and emotions, and more. When we think of things we need our "brain" to accomplish, we are usually thinking of something that happens in the cerebral hemispheres. Another term used for both hemispheres together is the cerebrum. In general, the structure of the hemispheres is characterized by an external layer of gray matter called the **cerebral cortex**. In shorthand parlance, rather than saying "the cerebral cortex," people often simply say, "the cortex." While the outer layer of the cerebral hemispheres is the cell-rich cortex, they also contain many **deep nuclei**, including the basal ganglia, and are filled with **white matter** connecting the various components of the hemispheres and other brain regions.

Cerebellum

The cerebellum is within the cranial cavity, posterior and inferior to the cerebrum (Figure 1-3). Literally, cerebellum means little brain. The cerebellum is primarily associated with motor function and motor learning. Newer evidence shows it may also play a role in the imagination of movements. The cerebellum connects to the rest of the nervous system through the brainstem and has pathways connecting it with the spinal cord, brainstem, and cerebrum. Like the cerebrum, the cerebellum has an outer layer of gray matter called the **cortex**, **inner nuclei**, and **white matter** for connections. Even though the cerebellum also has a cortex, it is generally understood that when people say, "the cortex," they mean "the cerebral cortex." To refer to the cortical tissue of the cerebellum, one should always say, "the cerebellar cortex."

Brainstem

The brainstem is the physical connection between the cerebral hemispheres, the spinal cord, and the cerebellum (Figure 1-3A). It is also home to a wide variety of complex nuclei and circuits for functions such as hearing, respiration, arousal, posture and locomotion, chewing, and many others. In addition, there are 12 cranial nerves that together make connections with the face, mouth, and throat, the nose, eyes, and ears, and the balance organs. Most of these cranial nerves have nuclei in the brainstem, and nerves that exit or enter the brainstem.

Spinal Cord

The spinal cord is the final source of direct connections between the brain and the body (Figure 1-3A). A large portion of the physical structure of the spinal cord is dedicated to these connections. Spinal nerves projecting from the left and right sides of each vertebral segment allow connection with peripheral muscles and sensory receptors; long fiber tracts within the cord convey information between the brain and the spinal cord. Functionally, however, the spinal cord is much more than this set of physical connections. The spinal cord contains complex neural circuits within its central gray matter that can coordinate complex behaviors like withdrawing a limb from a painful stimulus, reflexive control of bowel and bladder function, and even the rudimental elements for the neural control of walking (discussed in detail in Chapter 2).

FIGURE 1-3 Gross anatomical divisions of the CNS. The cerebral hemispheres are found at the rostral end of the nervous system. The basal ganglia are contained within the cerebrum. The midbrain, pons, and medulla oblongata together are called the brainstem, and caudal to that is the spinal cord. Rostral to the midbrain is the diencephalon, the thalamus, and hypothalamus, which together with the cerebrum is called the forebrain. In this scheme (forebrain, midbrain, and hindbrain), the midbrain is itself, and the hindbrain is the pons, medulla, and cerebellum. (Adapted with permission, from Kandel ER, Schwartz JH, Jessell TM, Siegelbaum SA, Hudspeth AJ. *Principles of Neural Science*, 5th ed. New York, NY: McGraw-Hill; 2013, Box 1-1, Pg 9.)

● THE MENINGES

The central nervous system is encased in bone, so the outermost protective structure is bone, either of the skull or of the vertebral column. The meninges are a multilayered set of membranes that enclose the nervous system and separate it from the protective bony structures. If a window in the bone is opened to reveal the central nervous system, the outermost structure seen will be the **dura mater** (Figure 1-4A). The dura mater is a tough, relatively inelastic tissue that is several layers thick. In addition to surrounding the brain, there are some large infoldings of the dura mater to further protect and stabilize certain brain structures.

FIGURE 1-4 The meninges. A and **B**. This image of a brain shows layers of meninges removed, revealing the tough dura matter and the thinner arachnoid. The pia is continuous with the brain surface and cannot be distinguished without a microscope. **C**. The falx cerebri is a dura mater structure that separates the two cerebral hemispheres. (Part C: Reproduced with permission from Martin JH. *Neuroanatomy Text and Atlas*, 4th ed. New York, NY: McGraw-Hill; 2012, Figure 1-6B, pg. 25.)

For example, in between the two cerebral hemispheres is the **falx cerebri** (Figure 1-4B, C). Lying over the top of the cerebellum is the **cerebellar tentorium** (Figure 1-4C). The dura mater also surrounds and protects several large venous sinuses that collect blood from the brain to return it to the venous circulation. The dura mater forms a seal around the outside of the brain through which fluid will not pass, except through blood vessels.

The innermost layer of the meninges is the **pia mater**. The pia is very thin and adheres directly to the underlying nervous tissue, even in its deeper enfolding on the cerebral cortex. It takes a microscope to view the pia. In a gross dissection, the pia matter would appear to be the surface of the brain. The pia also seals the brain as a part of the blood–brain barrier.

In between the dura mater and the pia mater is the **arachnoid mater** (Figure 1-4B). The arachnoid is a loose layer of tissue immediately below the dura. It does not extend to all brain surfaces like the pia mater does and more closely parallels the dura mater. Underneath the arachnoid and above the pia is where the cerebrospinal fluid (CSF) is found. Arteries along the surface of the nervous system travel through the space between the arachnoid and the pia. The arachnoid forms into small tubes called **villi** that conduct CSF out of the subarachnoid space and into the dural sinuses, where the CSF eventually mixes with the venous blood to return to the circulation (see discussion in Chapter 18).

When the meninges become infected, the result is called meningitis. This can be life threatening because the inflammation within the enclosed cranial cavity puts pressure on the brain, and if pressure is high enough, brain damage and even death can occur. There are both viral and bacterial forms of meningitis. If the pathogen gets through the pia mater and infects the brain tissue directly, this is called encephalitis.

● LOBES OF THE BRAIN

The cerebral hemispheres are divided into lobes. Modern nomenclature indicates four lobes, the frontal, parietal, occipital, and temporal. There are two other regions which were once considered lobes, the insular region and the limbic region. These are indicated in Figure 1-5.

Frontal

The frontal lobe is associated with thoughts, planning, decisions, and actions. It is also considered the home to what we think of as the personality. The frontal lobe is relatively large in humans and other animals we would consider intelligent. The frontal lobe begins at the **central sulcus**, such that everything rostral to the central sulcus is frontal lobe.

Parietal

The parietal lobe is associated with sensation and perception. It is the primary location for the initial sensations coming in from the somatosensory system (skin, muscles, joints, etc.) but not the special senses (vision, hearing, etc.). The parietal lobe does integrate somatosensory sensation with information from the special senses to form an overall perception. Hence, although initial hearing and seeing occurs in other lobes, the parietal lobe is where we would perceive where a sound came from, or where an object was seen, in relation to the position of our body. Higher order sensory experiences like music appreciation also occur in the parietal lobe. The rostral boundary of the parietal lobe is the central sulcus, and the caudal boundary is the parietal–occipital sulcus, which is most prominent on the mesial surface of the brain. An imaginary line separates parietal and occipital lobes on the lateral aspect of the brain.

Occipital

The occipital lobe is dedicated to vision. There are a variety of stations in the processing of visual information, including the initial perception, the elucidation of color, the recognition of motion, distinguishing objects from the background, and so on. Coming from the occipital lobe, visual information takes two

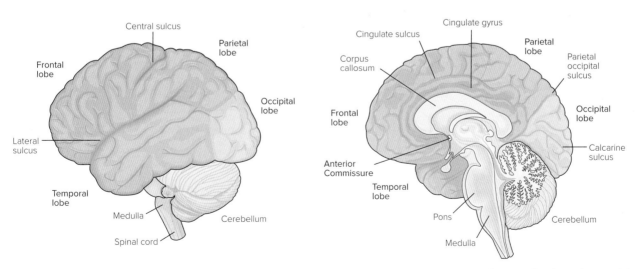

FIGURE 1-5 Lobes of the cerebral cortex and the landmarks structures that form their boundaries. On the left, a lateral view of the brain shows the four major lobes. The central sulcus and the lateral sulcus are visible here. On the right, the medial view of the brain is shown, with the brain split in the sagittal plane, along the midline. The parietal–occipital sulcus is visible here, along with the cingulate gyrus. (Adapted with permission from Martin JH. *Neuroanatomy Text and Atlas*, 3rd ed. New York, NY: McGraw-Hill; 2003. Fig 1-9, Pg 14.)

major routes. The dorsal visual stream provides information for the parietal lobe to use in locating objects and integrating vision into perception. The ventral visual stream leads to the temporal lobe for the recognition and naming of objects, such as faces, food, predators and prey, tools, etc. The occipital lobe is bounded by the temporal lobe laterally and the parietal lobe medially.

Temporal

The temporal lobe is associated with auditory processing, especially language, as well as memory and the identification of objects. The temporal lobe is separated from the parietal and frontal lobes by the lateral sulcus; however, there is no clear demarcation between the temporal and occipital lobes.

Special Regions of the Cortex

Insular Cortex

The insular cortex is no longer considered a lobe, but rather, a region (Figure 1-6A, B). It is found deep in the lateral sulcus, in between the temporal and parietal lobes. Cortical tissue here is associated with eating and digestive functions, autonomic function, and feelings such as pain or pleasure, especially when associated with sensory experiences.

Cingulate Cortex

The cingulate cortex (Figure 1-5, right) is associated with basic drives and motivations such as hunger, emotions, and initiation. Once thought of as a part of a lobe called the limbic lobe, the

FIGURE 1-6 Internal structures in the cerebral cortex. The lateral view at the top right shows where each section was made. (Reproduced with permission from Nieuwenhuys, Voogd, and van Huijzen. *The Human Central Nervous System: A Synopsis and Atlas*, 3rd edition. New York: Springer-Verlag; 1988.)

cingulate cortex, like insular cortex, is now considered a region. The cingulate can be found superior to the corpus callosum.

SUBCORTICAL STRUCTURES

Within the cerebral hemispheres are a variety of important white and gray matter structures. Those most relevant to this text are listed below.

Thalamus

The thalamus is a major nucleus that receives and processes information that will be sent to the cerebral cortex (Figure 1-6C). Almost all information that comes into the brain must eventually reach the thalamus and synapse on a neuron there. The thalamic neuron will then bring the information to the cortex. The thalamus is comprised of a number of nuclei that serve as relay stations for specific motor and sensory projections.

Basal Ganglia

The basal ganglia are a set of nuclei within the cerebral hemispheres that process cortical information and send it back to the cortex by way of the thalamus (Figures 1-3A, 1-6A–C). There are some direct outputs from the basal ganglia to the oculomotor and postural control system, but most basal ganglia output goes back to the cortex. The specific nuclei included in the basal ganglia are the **caudate** and **putamen** (together called the **striatum**), the **globus pallidus**, the **subthalamic nucleus**, and the **substantia nigra**. The latter is located in the dorsal midbrain rather than within the cerebral hemispheres, and the subthalamic nucleus sits just below the thalamus within the portion of the brain, known as the diencephalon (e.g., thalamus, hypothalamus, epithalamus, and subthalamus). The caudate borders and follows the lateral ventricles and can be divided into the **head** (anterior portion within the frontal lobes), the **body** (extending back through the parietal lobe), and the **tail** (extending down into the temporal lobe). The globus pallidus and putamen appear as a single nucleus, referred to as the **lenticular nucleus**, just medial to the insular region.

Hypothalamus

The hypothalamus is the region inferior to the thalamus (Figure 1-6B). This is where hormones are regulated by the brain, thirst and hunger are detected based on physiologic signals, sleep–wake cycles are determined, and many other basic physiological functions for homeostasis are regulated. This region has connections to and from many other parts of the brain allowing it to cross reference many sources of information.

Hippocampal Formation

This region of cortex is in the medial part of the temporal lobe, on the inferior surface of the brain (Figure 1-6C). It is specifically associated with the formation of declarative memory, the ability to memorize information and experiences (see Chapter 7).

Amygdala

The amygdala is a nucleus in the temporal lobe that can be found at the rostral end of the hippocampal formation. The amygdala works with the hippocampal formation in the generation of memories, especially those associated with intense emotional states such as fear and anger.

Corpus Callosum

The corpus callosum is the major structure connecting the left and right cerebral hemispheres (Figures 1-5, 1-6A–C). It is comprised entirely of axons passing between the left and right cerebral hemispheres, principally the frontal and parietal lobes.

Anterior Commissure

The anterior commissure is like the corpus callosum, but is mainly comprised of axons crossing between the left and right temporal lobes. Because of its regular appearance and location (Figure 1-5), it is often used as a point of reference in brain imaging studies to allow for alignment of the images from an individual at various points in time as well as to align an individual brain with images from brain atlases.

Internal Capsule

The internal capsule is a white matter pathway with axons going up to and coming down from the cerebral cortex (Figure 1-6). Its **anterior limb** becomes evident at the beginning of the separation of the caudate and putamen in the frontal lobe (Figure 1-6A, B). Its **posterior limb** separates the thalamus from the basal ganglia (Figure 1-6C). Axons from neurons of the cerebral cortex pass through the internal capsule on their way to the brainstem and spinal cord. Axons of the sensory systems coming into the brain pass through the internal capsule on the way to thalamus, and thalamic fibers projecting to the cortex are also found in the internal capsule. Lesions in the internal capsule can have severe sensory and motor consequences (see Chapter 10, Stroke).

Corona Radiata

There is a great deal of white matter underneath the cerebral cortex that is not part of the internal capsule. This is not labeled specifically in the diagrams above because that would be impracticable: it comprises the bulk of the subcortical white matter. Most of this is formed by axons from cortical neurons that are projecting from one part of the cortex to another. These cortico-cortical connections do not need to pass through the thalamus, they project straight to the cortex. Projections from cortical tissue to subcortical structures such as the caudate and putamen are also found in this white matter. Compared to these cortical-cortical connections, a relatively small number of axons actually leave the cerebral hemispheres to influence other parts of the nervous system.

VENTRICULAR SYSTEM

As noted above, the brain is surrounded by meninges, and within the meninges, there is CSF. Just as CSF surrounds the brain, it can also be found inside the brain in cavities called the ventricles. The ventricular system includes the ventricles, passageways between the ventricles, the tissue that secretes the CSF, and the system for collecting the fluid to return it to the circulation. In Chapter 18, there are illustrations of the ventricular system, additional discussion of the flow of CSF, and examples of disorders of this flow that result in hydrocephalus. The names of these structures are provided here.

Within the cerebral hemispheres are two large ventricles called the lateral ventricles, one on the left and one on the right. Neither is formally labeled the first or second, but since there are two, the next one is called the third ventricle, and after that comes the fourth. The third ventricle is a midline structure located around the level of midbrain, and the fourth ventricle is also a midline structure located in between the brainstem and the cerebellum. CSF is secreted within the ventricular system by a type of tissue called the **choroid plexus**. Choroid plexus is found within the lateral ventricles and the fourth ventricle, but usually not in the third. The passage of fluid between the lateral ventricle and the third ventricle on each side occurs through an opening called the **interventricular foramen**. The third and fourth ventricles are connected by the **cerebral aqueduct**.

CSF exits the ventricular system through one of three openings. The largest is the median aperture, also called the **foramen of Magendie**. This is a midline opening from the fourth ventricle to the posterior aspect of the medulla in the brainstem. The space here where CSF collects under the cerebellum and behind the brainstem is called the **cisterna magna**. There are also two lateral apertures, a left and right, coming out from each side of the fourth ventricle in the space between the cerebellum and pons. The lateral apertures are also called the **foramina of Luschka**. The place where CSF collects here anterior and lateral to the cerebellum is called the **cerebello pontine angle cistern**. The central canal of the spinal cord, forming in the caudal medulla, is also a place for CSF to leave the fourth ventricle, but it is quite small compared to the other foramina.

Once outside the ventricular system, CSF is contained within the meninges so that the brain has a cushion of fluid on the inside and the outside, keeping it essentially floating within the CSF. The subarachnoid space holds the CSF in between the arachnoid mater and the pia mater. Venous sinuses are formed within the dura mater, and protrusions from the arachnoid into these sinuses, called **arachnoid villi**, allow the CSF to leak slowly into the venous blood, returning the fluid to the circulation.

● THE CEREBELLUM

The cerebellum, like the cerebrum, has external layer of gray matter called the cortex, nuclei of gray matter deep within, and white matter structures providing the connections (Figure 1-6D). The best single word to describe cerebellar function is coordination. Literally, this word means to co-ordinate, to control two or more things at once. The connections and circuitry of the cerebellum serve this purpose in many ways. When a pitcher throws a baseball, (s)he must coordinate anticipatory postural adjustments with the leg and trunk motions of the windup, and the visual scene in the batter's box with the throwing motion of the arm. Speech requires coordination of the muscles of the throat and vocal cords with the movements of the tongue and lips and respiratory muscles for controlled exhalation. Motor learning requires coordination of the experience from past trials with plans for the next attempt. Further details of cerebellar function are provided in Chapter 5. Here, we focus on the anatomy.

Cortex

Cerebellar cortex is simpler and more uniform in structure than cerebral cortex. There are three layers: a parallel fiber layer, a Purkinje layer, and a granular layer, each named for the predominant structural feature. **Granule cells** in that layer receive the information coming into the cerebellum. The axons of granule cells project to the cerebellar cortex and split in two, running along the surface of the cortex in parallel with the folia, the small enfoldings of tissue evident on the surface of the cerebellar cortex. These parallel fibers synapse in the synaptic tree of the Purkinje cells. The Purkinje cells make axons that project to the nuclei within the cerebellum, often referred to as the deep cerebellar nuclei.

Deep Cerebellar Nuclei (DCN)

The DCN are a group of gray matter structures located inside the cerebellum. In a general sense, all neurons in the DCN are the same kind of cell. The fact that we can observe apparently distinct cerebellar nuclei is simply a consequence of the way the white matter structures pass among these neurons, dividing them into anatomically distinct entities. From a functional standpoint, each of the DCN tends to connect consistently with a certain part of the cerebellar cortex, and to the extent that there is differentiation of the function in parts of the cerebellar cortex, there is also differentiation in function among the DCN. However, this differentiation is a consequence of the connections, not any difference in the neurons themselves. In the human, we can observe four distinct DCN: the **fastigial** nucleus, the **globose** and **emboliform** nuclei, and the **dentate** nucleus. In other animals, these nuclei may be combined in different ways with different names, but the essential function of the deep cerebellar nucleus neurons is the same.

Lobes/Regions of Cerebellum

The cerebellum can be divided according to two schemes, lobes and functional divisions. There are three lobes. The **anterior lobe** is the part underneath the occipital lobe, rostral to a cerebellar cortex structure called the **primary fissure**. The **posterior cerebellum** is everything else, with the exception of a small structure called the **flocculonodular lobe**, which is at the opposite end of the cerebellum from the anterior lobe and can be found on the anterior surface, apposed to the fourth ventricle (Figure 1-7A, B).

The functional divisions are more often useful to the rehabilitation professional. These are the vestibulocerebellum, the spinocerebellum, and the cerebrocerebellum (Figure 1-7C). The flocculonodular lobe is identical to the **vestibulocerebellum**. The other two include both anterior and posterior cerebellum, but the functional divisions are divided along a mediolateral axis. The **spinocerebellum** includes the midline cerebellar tissue called the vermis, as well as the medial parts of each cerebellar hemisphere, called the paravermis. The **cerebrocerebellum** is the remainder of the cerebellar hemispheres.

Each of the DCN is connected mainly with a certain function division of the cerebellum. The **vestibulocerebellum** is connected to the fastigial nucleus (and also has some direct connections to the vestibular nuclei); thus, its function relates to vestibular control of eye movement, posture, and balance. The spinocerebellum is connected to the fastigial, globose, and

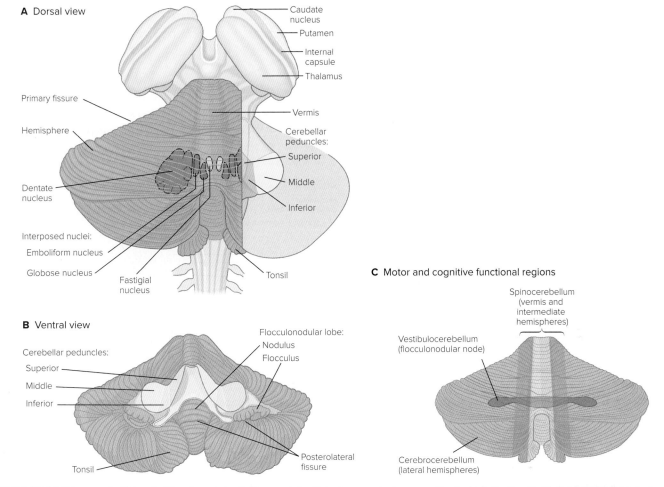

FIGURE 1-7 The cerebellum. A. The deep cerebellar nuclei within the cerebellum are illustrated. On the right, the cerebellum has been removed to show how the cerebellar peduncles come from the brainstem. **B.** This is the view of the cerebellum that would be seen from the front if it was removed from the brainstem. **C.** The functional regions of the cerebellum are shown. (Reproduced with permission from Nieuwenhuys R: *Chemoarchitecture of the Brain.* New York: Springer-Verlag, 1985.)

emboliform nuclei, receiving postural sensory information via the spinocerebellar tracts and projecting to the medial descending system (rubrospinal, vestibulospinal, and reticulospinal tracts) to control postural stability. The cerebrocerebellum is connected to the dentate nucleus, sending efferents via the thalamus to the motor cortex and other cortical areas to participate in motor planning and motor control (see Chapter 5).

Cerebellar Peduncles

On each side, there are three cerebellar peduncles, the white matter connections between the cerebellum and the brainstem; these are the inferior, middle, and superior cerebellar peduncles (Figure 1-7B). The **inferior cerebellar peduncle** contains axons carrying information from the spinal cord with highly detailed sensory information about the body and its position and movements. It also carries information in from a nucleus in the brainstem called the **inferior olivary complex** to convey indications of errors that require improved coordination. The **middle cerebellar peduncle** carries information from nuclei in the pons to the cerebellum. These pontine nuclei are the targets of axons from the cerebral cortex, so the middle cerebellar peduncle is the second leg of the pathway from cortex to cerebellum, which

is called the **cortico-ponto-cerebellar** pathway. The **superior cerebellar peduncle** is mainly comprised of axons exiting the cerebellum from the DCN to project to brainstem and cortical structures for motor control. There are also certain kinds of information from the spinal cord entering through the superior cerebellar peduncle. More information about the cerebellum is provided in Chapter 5.

● THE BRAINSTEM

The brainstem (Figure 1-8) has a wide variety of important structures involved in all types of neural function, including sensory, motor, autonomic, and integrative. Basic functions for taste and eating, hearing, balance, and vision are found here, as are systems for the control of posture and locomotion, perception and modulation of pain, regulation of cardiorespiratory function, and arousal. In addition, all white matter connections between the brain and spinal cord must pass through the brainstem. Any serious injury to the brainstem is usually fatal.

Certain structures span much of the rostro–caudal length of the brainstem and are not confined to any particular region. One

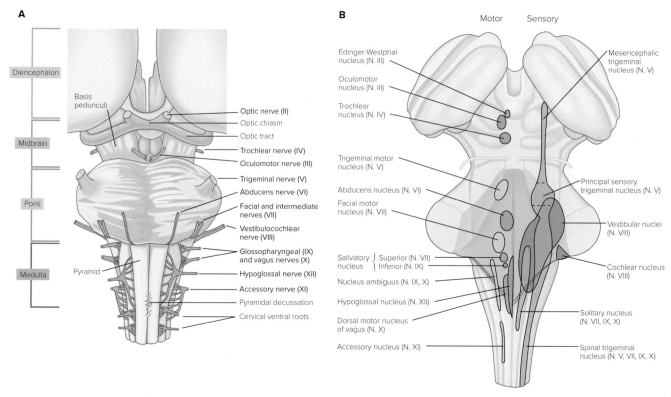

FIGURE 1-8 The cranial nerves. On the left (**A**), a ventral view of the brainstem and diencephalon shows where each of the cranial nerves exits the brainstem. On the right (**B**), a dorsal view shows where the cranial nerve nuclei are located for motor outputs and sensory inputs. (Modified with permission from Kandel ER, Schwartz JH, Jessell TM, Siegelbaum SA, Hudspeth AJ. *Principles of Neural Science*, 5th ed. New York, NY: McGraw-Hill; 2013, Figures 45-1 and 45-5, Pgs 1020 & 1025.)

is the **trigeminal nucleus**, which spans from the midbrain to the medulla. Different regions have different specializations in the trigeminal complex, but overall, this is a very long structure serving all sensory and motor functions of the trigeminal nerve. Another is called the **reticular formation**. This is a long column of gray matter found ventrolateral to the cerebral aqueduct and fourth ventricle extending from the midbrain to the medulla. The reticular formation has a variety of functions. Those of most importance in rehabilitation are the pathways from the brainstem to spinal cord, the **reticulospinal tracts**, which are key sources for the regulation of posture, locomotion, and gross limb movements. Medial and somewhat ventral to the reticular formation in the caudal pons and rostral medulla are the **raphe nuclei**. These have a variety of functions that regulate the state of other parts of the nervous system, including arousal, the spinal cord circuits for control of walking, and the transmission and modulation of pain.

Midbrain

The midbrain is the most rostral level of the brainstem. The most prominent white matter features at this level are the **cerebral peduncles**, containing all axons coming from the cerebrum and projecting to brainstem and spinal cord structures below. Within the midbrain, we find several key nuclei. The **substantia nigra**, part of the basal ganglia, is located at the midbrain level. The **periaqueductal gray**, a central structure involved in pain regulation, is also a midbrain structure. A key motor nucleus involved in coordination between the cerebrum and cerebellum

is called the **red nucleus**, which is a prominent spherical nucleus in the midbrain and origin of the rubrospinal tract. On the posterior aspect of the midbrain we find two dome-like protrusions on each side, the superior colliculus and the inferior colliculus. The **superior colliculus** is for visual function, and the **inferior** is auditory. In addition, certain cranial nerve nuclei are found at this level, including the oculomotor nucleus (CN III) and the trochlear nucleus (CN IV). The **pedunculopontine nucleus** is a specialized structure in the brainstem that plays a critical role in the initiation of locomotion and the release of acetylcholine in selected brain areas. The **locus coeruleus** projects widely throughout the CNS, releasing a neuromodulator called norepinephrine that regulates overall excitability. Finally, the **ventral tegmental area** is associated with dopamine projections for regulating reward and pleasure and projects through the basal ganglia to the frontal lobe.

Pons and Medulla

The pons and medulla are mainly distinguished from each other by the middle cerebellar peduncle, which is the prominent white matter feature on the anterior aspect of the pons formed by axons exiting the pons to wrap around caudally toward the cerebellum. Within the pons, the ventral region contains the **pontine nuclei**, where corticopontine projections synapse en route to the cerebellum. In the dorsal pons we find the **trigeminal nucleus** for the fifth cranial nerve (CN V), the nucleus for the sixth cranial nerve, abducens (CN VI), and the nucleus for the seventh cranial nerve, the facial nerve (CN VII). The **vestibular nuclei** are in the pons slightly lateral to midline and just ventral to the fourth ventricle. They receive afferents from the vestibular system and interconnect the vestibulocerebellum with the control of head, neck, and eye movements, as well as postural responses to head movements and position. The **cochlear nucleus** receives incoming auditory information from the cochlea, and the superior olivary complex contains neural circuits used for the initial localization of sound. Special senses, including hearing and the vestibular system, are discussed in Chapter 6.

The **medulla** emerges as the most caudal part of the brainstem, beneath the pons. The most prominent surface features of the medulla anteriorly are the **medullary pyramids** and the **inferior olives**. The pyramids are formed by the axons of the corticospinal tract, fibers for motor control running from the cerebral cortex to the spinal cord. The olives surround an internal structure called the **inferior olivary complex**, a source of information about errors to be sent up into the cerebellum. On the dorsal aspect of the brainstem, we see the continuation of two ascending fiber bundles rising from the spinal cord on each side. Along the midline is the **fasciculus gracilis** carrying ascending sensory information from the legs and lower trunk, and lateral to that is the **fasciculus cuneatus** carrying ascending sensory information from the upper trunk and arms. These tracts together are called the dorsal columns, and at the top are found the dorsal column nuclei (cuneatus and gracilis). The dorsal column nuclei contain the second sensory neuron in the pathway from the spinal cord to the brain (see Chapter 3).

Within the medulla there are many important nuclei, including the cranial nerve nuclei for nerves IX–XII (glossopharyngeal, vagus, spinal accessory, and hypoglossal). In addition, the cardiorespiratory regulation centers are in the medulla.

Cranial Nerves

The first cranial nerve is the **olfactory nerve**. This is somewhat unique among the cranial nerves in that the sensory neurons project to the olfactory bulb, and from there second-order sensory neurons project directly to cerebral cortex. The second cranial nerve is the **optic nerve** from the eyes. This nerve carries the visual information into the brain, and the axons synapse in a structure called the lateral geniculate nucleus, which can be thought of as a part of the thalamus. Some visual fibers also project to midbrain structures, such as the superior colliculus and third cranial nerve nucleus, for subconscious reactions to light such as orienting to a bright light, controlling pupillary constriction, photoregulation of the sleep–wake cycle, etc. The third cranial nerve is the **oculomotor nerve**. This carries motor axons to four of the six extra-ocular muscles (all except lateral rectus and trochlear mm.). The third cranial nerve also carries the autonomic nervous system fibers for control of the pupil and lens of the eye, which originate in the nucleus of **Edinger–Westphal**, located in the midbrain near the oculomotor nucleus (N. III) (Figure 1-8). The fourth cranial nerve is the **trochlear nerve**, carrying the motor axons to the trochlear muscle of the eye and originating from the trochlear nucleus in the midbrain (N. IV).

The fifth cranial nerve is the **trigeminal nerve**, which serves sensory and motor functions for much of the face and head. The motor fibers innervate key muscle of mastication, including temporalis, the pterygoids, and the masseter. These come from the trigeminal motor nucleus in the lower mesencephalon. The sensory fibers divide into ophthalmic branches innervating skin and structures of the forehead as well as the nose, maxillary branch for the cheek and upper lip, and the mandibular branch for the jaw and chin. The discriminative touch conveyed by the trigeminal nerve comes into the principal sensory nucleus, whereas information on pain and temperature comes into the spinal nucleus of the fifth cranial nerve.

The sixth cranial nerve is **abducens**, and this carries the motor axons to the lateral rectus muscle of the eye, originating in the abducens nucleus (N. VI) in the pons. The seventh is the **facial nerve**, which projects to all facial muscles not controlled by the trigeminal, focused on facial expressions, and also receives taste from the anterior part of the tongue. The seventh cranial nerve also innervates the lacrimal and salivary glands for tears and saliva. The seventh cranial nerve's motor fibers for the facial muscles originate in the facial nucleus in the pons (N. VII); efferents to the salivary glands projecting through VII come from the **salivatory nucleus**. Afferents for taste project through CN VII to the **solitary nucleus**, and some pain afferents project through CN VII to the spinal trigeminal nucleus in the medulla. The eighth cranial nerve is the **vestibulocochlear** nerve. This carries all the information for the cochlea and from the vestibular apparatus in the inner ear to the corresponding nuclei in the brainstem. The ninth cranial nerve is the **glossopharyngeal nerve**, which receives taste from the posterior tongue and sensation from soft palate and the pharynx. The motor fibers come from nucleus ambiguous and innervate pharyngeal muscles and the parotid salivary gland. The taste fibers project to the solitary nucleus. Some pain fibers traveling in CN IX reach the spinal trigeminal nucleus in the medulla. The 10th cranial nerve is the **vagus**, which projects from the brainstem to the pharynx and into the thoracic and abdominal cavities. In the pharynx, the vagus controls many of the muscles involved in swallowing, as well as the gag reflex (in response to glossopharyngeal afferents). The motor fibers come from the nucleus ambiguous and the dorsal motor nucleus of the vagus, both in the medulla. Some taste and pain fibers come in through the vagus to reach the solitary nucleus and the spinal trigeminal nucleus, respectively. The vagus reaches the thoracic and upper abdominal cavities for parasympathetic nervous system control of the cardiorespiratory and upper digestive systems. The 11th cranial nerve is the **spinal accessory nerve**, which carries motor axons to the upper trapezius muscle and to the sternocleidomastoid muscle. Its origin is the accessory nucleus, located in the upper few cervical segments. The 12th cranial nerve is the **hypoglossal**, which provides efferent motor control to the tongue. Its motor fibers come from the hypoglossal nucleus in the medulla.

Major Fiber Tracts

As noted above, major fiber tracts evident on the surface of the brainstem include the cerebral and cerebellar peduncles, the medullary pyramids, and the dorsal columns. There are also certain internal white matter tracts of importance in rehabilitation (Figure 1-9). The **medial lemniscus** is the bundle of axons

FIGURE 1-9 Selected fiber tracts in the brainstem. The medial lemniscus and spinothalamic tracts carry sensory information upward toward the brain. The medial longitudinal fasciculus carries oculomotor control signals as well as commands for head and neck movements.

ascending from the dorsal column nuclei to carry sensory information to the thalamus (see Chapter 3). A bundle of fibers along the midline on each side is called the **medial longitudinal fasciculus**. The ascending fibers of the MLF connect the vestibular nuclei with cranial nerve nuclei and other structures for control of eye movement (see Chapter 6). The descending fibers of the MLF project to the upper parts of the spinal cord to control head and neck movements, and this part of the system is commonly called the medial vestibulospinal tract.

● THE SPINAL CORD

Gross Anatomical Features

The spinal cord (Figure 1-10) is surrounded by meninges, including dura, arachnoid, and pia mater layers just like the rest of the CNS. Unique to the spinal cord, small extensions of pia mater extend laterally at each level of spinal cord to form **denticulate**

ligaments to attach the spinal cord to the dura mater, keeping the cord stable within the spinal column. There is also an extension of pia surrounded by dura at the caudal end of the spinal cord, which is called the **filum terminale**, and tethers the caudal end of the spinal cord to the lower end of the vertebral canal.

Viewing the spinal cord as a whole, the dorsal aspect reveals the dorsal columns, containing sensory fibers ascending toward the medulla. There is a median fissure evident throughout the rostro–caudal length of the spinal cord. In the upper thoracic and cervical portions of the spinal cord, both gracile (medial) and cuneate (lateral) fasciculi can be appreciated in the dorsal columns. In lower thoracic and lumbosacral spinal cord, there is only a gracile fasciculus.

The dorsal roots are formed by sensory fibers entering the spinal cord, and the dorsal root entry zone forms the lateral border of the dorsal columns. The white matter on the lateral aspect of the spinal cord is called the lateral funiculus. The ventral roots are formed by the efferent axons of motor and autonomic effects projecting from the spinal cord to the body. The white matter on the surface of spinal cord, ventral and medial to the ventral roots, is called the ventral (or anterior) funiculus.

Segmental Organization

The spinal cord is organized into segments named for the vertebral bone that formed alongside that segment during embryological development. At each segment of the spinal cord, a spinal nerve is formed by the combination of the dorsal and ventral roots. The first spinal nerve exits through the intervertebral foramen above the first cervical vertebra, and the eighth spinal nerve exits below the seventh cervical vertebra (above T1). These first eight segments are called the cervical segments, so although there are only seven cervical vertebrae, there are eight cervical spinal segments. From there on, the spinal segment is named by the vertebra above the exit of its spinal nerve. Hence, the first thoracic segment has a spinal nerve that exits below the first thoracic vertebra. The third lumbar segment has a nerve that exits below the third lumbar vertebra, and so on. With the convention, there are 8 cervical spinal segments, 12 thoracic, 5 lumbar, 5 sacral, and 1 coccygeal segmental levels in the human spinal cord, and an equal number of spinal nerves on each side.

In each segment, the organization is consistent. As noted above, sensory fibers ascend in the dorsal columns. There are also some ascending fibers in the lateral funiculus, some destined for the cerebellum and others for the brainstem and thalamus. Descending fibers from the cortex and brainstem are found in the lateral and ventral funiculus. Some of these descending fibers are for direct motor control, and others are for modulation of spinal cord neurons and circuits. The gray matter is located in the center of the spinal cord. The dorsal horn is dedicated to sensory processing, and the ventral horn is dedicated to motor outputs. In the cervical and lumbosacral regions, the lateral expansion of the ventral horns is where limb muscle motoneurons are located. Throughout the spinal cord, muscles of the vertebral column and trunk have their motoneurons located medially. The organization and function of the spinal cord are discussed in detail in Chapter 2.

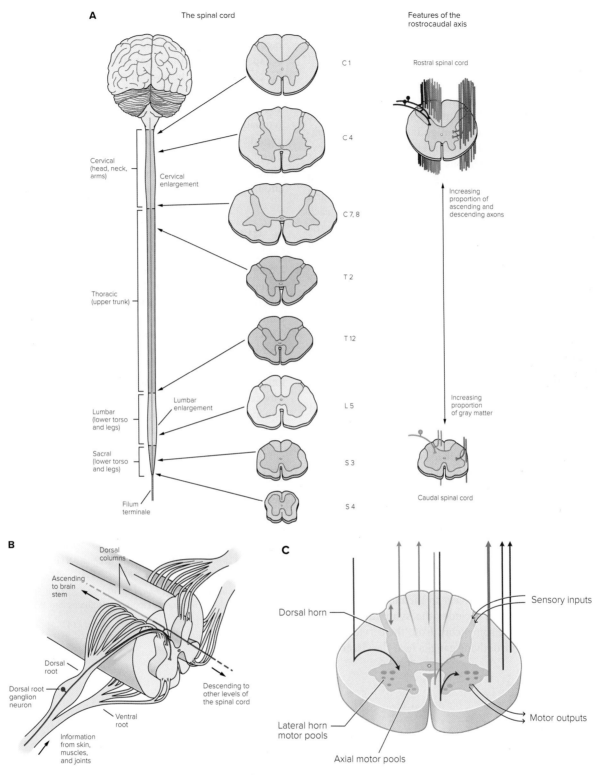

A. The spinal cord

Features of the rostrocaudal axis

FIGURE 1-10 The spinal cord. A. The spinal cord carries all information between the brain and the body except that carried by the cranial nerves. There are enlargements at the cervical and lumbosacral levels to contain the extra gray and white matter for the arms and legs. Cross sections representative of each segmental level are illustrated. Note how the relative proportion of white matter decreases at lower levels; few sensory axons have accumulated from below, and most motor axons have already terminated at levels above. **B.** The organization of a typical spinal segment is shown, including the dorsal roots, ventral roots, dorsal root ganglion, and spinal nerve. **C.** The general organization of information moving up and down the spinal cord is shown. Descending fibers (red) can travel in the lateral or ventral funiculus. Ascending fibers travel in the lateral and dorsal funiculus, some bound for the brain (green) and some for the cerebellum (purple). Special systems also descend to release neuromodulators that regulate spinal cord circuits (orange). (A: Reproduced permission from Kandel ER, Schwartz JH, Jessell TM, Siegelbaum SA, Hudspeth AJ. *Principles of Neural Science*, 5th ed. New York, NY: McGraw-Hill; 2013, Fig 16-2, Pg 359.) (B: Reproduced permission from Kandel ER, Schwartz JH, Jessell TM, Siegelbaum SA, Hudspeth AJ. *Principles of Neural Science*, 5th ed. New York, NY: McGraw-Hill; 2013, Fig 16-3 Pg 360.)

THE PERIPHERAL NERVOUS SYSTEM

The peripheral nervous system is formed by the motor and sensory axons coming from and heading into the central nervous system. An important difference in these two parts of the nervous system is the type of cell that makes myelin. In the central nervous system, myelin is made by **oligodendrocytes**. Each oligodendrocyte will form a part of the myelin sheath around several axons. In the peripheral nervous system, there are **Schwann cells**, instead. Each Schwann cell wraps around a segment of only one axon. In the upper cervical, thoracic, lower sacral, and the coccygeal segments, the spinal nerves are individual, each innervating a defined segment of the body. However, in the lower cervical segments, including T1, and in the lumbosacral segments, the spinal nerves blend and merge into nerve plexuses on the way to the arms and legs. Specific peripheral nerves emerge from these plexuses to innervate the muscles, skin, and other structures.

THE AUTONOMIC NERVOUS SYSTEM

The autonomic nervous system consists of sympathetic and parasympathetic divisions that regulate the visceral organs, vasculature, and glands. In general, the **sympathetic nervous system** is associated with arousal, often referred to as our fight or flight system, and the **parasympathetic** division is associated with relaxation. Arousal would occur, for example, during exercise or in response to fear. Relaxation would be associated with increased digestive function, voiding of excretions, and rest. The parasympathetic parts of the autonomic nervous system are in the cranial nerves and their associated nuclei, along with specialized structures in the sacral spinal cord. Preganglionic neurons exit these areas and project to target ganglia in the periphery; then, postganglionic neurons project to the target organs. The sympathetic nervous system includes the **sympathetic chain ganglia** that run along the spinal cord from the cervical to the coccygeal segments, some outlying ganglia near the viscera, and specific regions in gray matter of the thoracic and upper lumbar spinal cord that govern these structures. Efferents from the thoracolumbar regions exit the cord with other motor efferents but synapse in a sympathetic ganglion, traveling up or down within the chain to a specific level where they synapse on second-order fibers. Then, the second-order neurons project to target organs. These two systems function in harmony such that an increase in sympathetic activity is associated with a concomitant decrease in parasympathetic activity. For example, when we exercise, our digestive system's activity is diminished while our heart and respiration rates increase, thus targeting blood flow to our heart and muscles rather than our stomach.

SUMMARY

Understanding of the nervous system requires a combined understanding of the anatomical structures along with their functions. This includes understanding how the structures are connected with each other, what kinds of neurons and neural circuits exist within the structure, and how neurotransmitters and neuromodulators function in the structure. From this knowledge, we can understand the alterations in brain structure and function associated with pathologies, and we can see how and why certain approaches to treatment with physical therapy will be beneficial. Overall, the goal of this text is to help the reader see these connections and apply them to practice to help the patient.

SUGGESTED READINGS

Kandel S, Schwartz JH, Jessell TM, Siegelbaum SA, Hudspeth AJ. *Principles of Neural Science*. 5th ed. New York: McGraw-Hill; 2013.

Vanderah T, Gould D. *Nolte's The Human Brain*. 7th ed. Philadelphia: Elsevier; 2015. ISBN-10: 1455728594.

Parent A, Carpenter MB. *Carpenter's Human Neuroanatomy*. Baltimore: Williams and Wilkins; 1996. ISBN 0683067524.

Haines D. *Neuroanatomy in Clinical Context: An Atlas of Structures, Sections, and Systems*. 9th ed. Baltimore: Lippincott Williams and Wilkins; 2015. ISBN 1451186258.

Martin JH. *Neuroanatomy Text and Atlas*. 4th ed. New York: McGraw-Hill; 2012.

Review Questions

1. **In a person standing, what two directions are roughly equivalent in the cerebral hemispheres?**
   A. Anterior–ventral
   B. Inferior–dorsal
   C. Anterior–rostral
   D. Posterior–dorsal

2. **What kind of neural structure can be found in gray matter and in white matter?**
   A. Neuronal cell bodies
   B. Axons
   C. Dendrites of neurons
   D. Synapses

3. **How is a ganglion different from a nucleus**
   A. A ganglion has neuronal cell bodies
   B. A ganglion is outside the CNS
   C. A ganglion has incoming and outgoing connections
   D. A ganglion is for sensory neurons

4. **The cerebellum is physically connected to the rest of the nervous system at the level of the**
   A. Cerebrum
   B. Brainstem
   C. Spinal cord
   D. All of the above

5. **Which part of the meninges is toughest and thickest?**
   A. The dura mater
   B. The arachnoid mater
   C. The subarachnoid space
   D. The pia mater

6. **Match the lobe of the cerebral hemisphere with the functions listed**
   A. Frontal   Sensations and perception   B
   B. Parietal   Forming memories   D
   C. Occipital   Making decisions   A
   D. Temporal   Vision   C

7. **Which of the following structures is most prominent on the mesial surface of the cerebral cortex along the midline?**
   A. Lateral sulcus
   B. Central sulcus
   C. Parietal occipital sulcus
   D. Insular cortex

8. **Which part of the basal ganglia is found immediately lateral to the lateral ventricle?**
   A. Caudate nucleus
   B. Putamen
   C. Globus pallidus
   D. Substantia nigra

9. **What structure would not contain any corticospinal fibers passing from the cortex to the spinal cord?**
   A. The internal capsule
   B. The corpus callosum
   C. The cerebral peduncle
   D. The medullary pyramid

10. **What structure is associated with the brain's regulation of hormones in the bloodstream?**
    A. The amygdala
    B. The hypothalamus

C. The subthalamic nucleus
D. The nucleus of Edinger–Westphal

11. **What is the name of the tissue that secretes cerebrospinal fluid?**
    A. Ventricular tissue
    B. Choroid plexus
    C. Pia mater
    D. Dural sinus

12. **What is the name of the passageway between the third and fourth ventricles?**
    A. The foramen of Magendie
    B. The interventricular foramen
    C. The cerebral aqueduct
    D. The central canal

13. **Which of the deep cerebellar nuclei is principally connected through the thalamus to the cerebral cortex?**
    A. Fastigial
    B. Globose
    C. Emboliform
    D. Dentate

14. **The vermis is considered part of which functional division of the cerebellum?**
    A. Cerebrocerebellum
    B. Vestibulocerebellum
    C. Spinocerebellum
    D. Paleocerebellum

15. **Which part of the basal ganglia is in the midbrain?**
    A. Caudate
    B. Putamen
    C. Globus pallidus
    D. Substantia nigra

16. **Where are the dorsal column nuclei found?**
    A. Midbrain
    B. Pons
    C. Medulla
    D. Spinal cord

17. **Which cranial nerve carries motor effects to extraocular muscles and autonomic efferents to the muscles of the pupil and lens?**
    A. Optic nerve (II)
    B. Oculomotor nerve (III)
    C. Trochlear nerve (IV)
    D. Abducens nerve (VI)

18. **Which cranial nerve has a long series of nuclei reaching from the midbrain to the medulla?**
   A. Trigeminal (V)
   B. Facial (VII)
   C. Vestibulocochlear (VIII)
   D. Glossopharyngeal (IX)

19. **Which part of the spinal cord has more spinal cord segments than there are actual vertebral bones for that region?**
   A. Cervical
   B. Thoracic
   C. Lumbar
   D. Sacral

20. **Which structure in the thoracic and abdominal cavities is the initial target for neurons of the autonomic nervous system?**
   A. The cephalic ganglion
   B. The dorsal root ganglion
   C. The sympathetic chain ganglion
   D. The epigastric ganglion

Answers

1. C	**2.** B	**3.** B	**4.** B	**5.** A
6. A	**7.** C	**8.** A	**9.** B	**10.** B
11. B	**12.** C	**13.** D	**14.** C	**15.** D
16. C	**17.** B	**18.** A	**19.** A	**20.** C

TABLE	Major structures and landmarks in the nervous system, with emphasis on function in sensory and motor systems	
STRUCTURE	**FUNCTIONS**
Meninges	Protect the brain and spinal cord
Lobes of the Cerebrum	
Frontal	Motor planning and initiation, language output, personality, problem solving, insight, and foresight
Parietal	Sensory perception and integration, visual location, auditory location, music appreciation
Occipital	Vision (primary visual cortex and visual association cortex)
Temporal	Auditory processing, especially language, identification of objects, learning and memory
Insular	Gustatory (taste) perception
Limbic	Emotional responses, drive-related behavior, and emotional memory
Major Cortical Landmarks	
Central Sulcus	Divides frontal and parietal lobes
Parieto–Occipital Sulcus	Divides parietal and occipital lobes
Lateral Sulcus	Superior border of temporal lobe
Cingulate Sulcus	Superior border of limbic lobe
Precentral Gyrus	Primary motor cortex
Postcentral Gyrus	Primary sensory cortex
Posterior Parietal Association Area	Integration of body awareness with visual perception

(Continued)

TABLE	Major structures and landmarks in the nervous system, with emphasis on function in sensory and motor systems (*Continued*)	
STRUCTURE	**FUNCTIONS**	
Subcortical Structures		
Lateral ventricle	C-shaped chambers in each cerebral hemisphere where most of the cerebrospinal fluid (CSF) is made; communicate with the third ventricle via the two interventricular foramen	
Third ventricle	Midline cavity in diencephalon that connects with the fourth ventricle via the cerebral aqueduct	
Fourth ventricle	Tent-like cavity between the cerebellum posteriorly and the pons and rostral medulla anteriorly that communicates with subarachnoid space	
Choroid Plexus	Vascularized tissue that secretes CSF	
Cerebral Aqueduct	Narrow channel through the midbrain that connects the third and fourth ventricles	
Foramen of Magendie	Median aperture (opening) of fourth ventricle through which CSF flows into the subarachnoid space	
Foramina of Luschka	Two lateral apertures of fourth ventricle through which CSF flows into the subarachnoid space	
Basal Ganglia	Initiation and selection of thoughts and especially actions	
Caudate Nucleus	Receives information primarily from association areas of the cerebral cortex; important for cognitive functions of the basal ganglia	
Head	Rostral – Main target for prefrontal cortex	
Body	Superior – parietal areas	
Tail	Wraps around into the temporal lobe – temporal areas	
Putamen	Functionally and cellularly just like the Caudate, but anatomically separated from Caudate by fibers of the internal capsule. Receives information primarily from motor and somatosensory areas of the cerebral cortex; important for motor functions of the basal ganglia	
Striatum	A name used to refer to the caudate and putamen in combination	
Globus pallidus – external segment (GPe)	One target of output from Striatum. Involved in intermediate stage of basal ganglia processing	
Globus pallidus – internal segment (GPi)	Final output nucleus targeted by GPe and STN – has neurons with axons leaving basal ganglia to go to the thalamus and thereby influence cortex and the control of movement	
Subthalamic nucleus	Works with GPe for intermediate steps in basal ganglia processing	
Substantia nigra	The largest nucleus in the midbrain	
Pars compacta (SNpc)	Location of dopamine producing cells that project into the striatum (caudate and putamen) to control movement	
Pars reticulata (SNpr)	Just like cells in GPi but SNpr cells control eye movements, while GPi cells are for the rest of the body	
Internal Capsule	Funnel-shaped region separating the thalamus from the basal ganglia; contains fiber tracts that relay almost all of the information going to and from the cerebral cortex and other (non-cortical) parts of the brain	
Hippocampus	Memory formation (declarative)	
Amygdala	Emotions, learning whether something is "good" or "bad," aggression	
Thalamus	Receives, filters, and distributes information bound for the cerebral cortex	
Hypothalamus	Autonomic functions, drives, hormones	

(*Continued*)

TABLE	Major structures and landmarks in the nervous system, with emphasis on function in sensory and motor systems (*Continued*)	
STRUCTURE	**FUNCTIONS**	
Cerebellum	Receives information from sensory systems, the cerebral cortex and other sites, and participates in the planning and coordination of movement	
Cerebellar Cortex	Three-layered structure that receives cerebellar inputs and projects them to the deep cerebellar nuclei	
Folia	Repeated horizontal folds or gyri of the cerebellum	
Vermis	Midline lobe of the cerebellum important for cerebellar control of body and posture	
Flocculonodular lobe	Cerebellar control for vestibular responses and eye movements	
Spinocerebellum	Consists of the vermis and medial parts of the lateral cerebellar hemispheres that receive spinal inputs; involved with regulation of posture and coordination of limb movements	
Lateral cerebellar hemispheres	Main lobes of the cerebellum on each side of the vermis; medial part is part of spinocerebellum as stated above; lateral parts are part of the cerebrocerebellum, a functional division that communicates with the cerebral cortex for the coordination of motor planning and to some extent the coordination of higher order thought processes	
Deep cerebellar nuclei	Location for cells send axons projecting out of the cerebellum to affect other parts of the nervous systems, especially the brainstem and (via the thalamus) the cortex	
Brainstem	Consists of the midbrain, pons, and medulla	
Midbrain	The most rostral of the three subdivisions of the brainstem	
Cerebral peduncles	Two large cylindrical masses on ventral surface of midbrain containing descending motor fibers from the cortex	
Red nucleus	Involved in cerebellar circuitry and in control of limb movements, especially shaping the hand during reaching	
Cerebral aqueduct – PAG	Site of origin of a descending pain-control pathway	
Superior colliculi	Involved in directing visual attention and controlling eye movements	
Inferior colliculi	Major link in the auditory system	
Pons	The second of the three parts of the brainstem, continuous rostrally with the midbrain and caudally with the medulla	
Pontine nuclei	Nuclei in the basal pons that receive inputs from the cerebral cortex and project to contralateral cerebellum	
Cerebellar peduncles	Three paired fiber bundles connecting the cerebellum and brainstem via cerebellar afferents and efferents	
Vestibular nuclei	Involved in regulating posture and coordinating eye and head movements	
Reticular formation	Complex network of nuclei involved in integrative functions such as control of complex movements, transmission of pain information, vital functions, and arousal and consciousness	

(Continued)

TABLE	Major structures and landmarks in the nervous system, with emphasis on function in sensory and motor systems (*Continued*)	
STRUCTURE	**FUNCTIONS**	
Medulla	The most caudal of the three subdivisions of the brainstem	
Pyramids	Two rounded masses on the ventral surface of the medulla containing motor fibers	
Inferior olivary complex	Origin of "climbing fibers" to cerebellum that are involved in motor learning	
Dorsal column nuclei	Nuclei for relay of proprioceptive and discriminative touch for dorsal column-medial lemniscus system	
Vestibular nuclei	Involved in regulating posture and coordinating eye and head movements	
Reticular formation	Complex network of nuclei involved in integrative functions such as control of complex movements, transmission of pain information, vital functions, and arousal and consciousness	
Spinal Cord	Conducts sensory/motor information to/from the brain; contains central pattern generators for control of walking	
White matter	Fiber tracts (i.e., myelinated axons) that carry information up and down	
Gray matter	Contains neuronal cell bodies and reflex circuits	
Cervical enlargement (C5–T1)	Expanded gray matter to control the arms, and expanded white matter for incoming and outgoing information	
Lumbar enlargement (L2–S3)	Expanded gray area to control the legs, and expanded white matter for incoming and outgoing information	
Dorsal roots	Incoming (sensory) information	
Ventral roots	Outgoing (motor) commands	
Spinal nerves	Where dorsal and ventral roots fuse before exiting the intervertebral foramina	
Cauda equina	Spinal nerves in lower vertebral column on their way to their original foramina (vertebral column longer than spinal cord in adults)	
Sympathetic chain	Series of interconnected ganglia that lie ventral and lateral to the vertebral column that contain cell bodies of postganglionic neurons in the sympathetic nervous system	
Corpus Callosum	White matter fiber tracts connecting left and right cerebral hemispheres	

Neuronal Structure and Function

John A. Buford and D. Michele Basso

2

● INTRODUCTION

In a multicellular organism, cells communicate with each other. This is true of all cells, and the broad name used in biology to describe this phenomenon is **cellular signaling**. Neurons are cells specialized for cellular signaling so that information can be received, processed, transmitted, stored, and retrieved.

As described in Chapter 3, neurons receive information from receptors in the body. These can be sensitive to internal signals (interoceptors) or external signals (exteroceptors). As described in Chapter 4, sensory neurons that receive certain kinds of input will transmit that information to the spinal cord where it can be processed to produce an outgoing neural command for a reflexive response. And for the reader of this chapter, it is hoped that some of the information can be stored and later retrieved from the brain.

How do neurons do this? This chapter will explain basic mechanisms of neural structure and function. In addition, the structure and function of the glial cells, cells in the nervous system that support the functions of neurons, will also be described.

A Typical Neuron

A typical neuron has five main parts. First, there is the **dendritic tree**. This is a structure of processes resembling the arbor of a tree that emanates from the cell body of the neuron. The dendritic tree is typically where information from other neurons is received (Figure 2-1, A, C; blue). Next is the **soma**, the main part

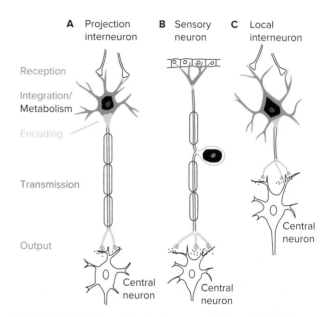

FIGURE 2-1 Picture of typical neuron with parts labeled by function. A shows a projection interneuron. This is the kind of cell that sends information over a relatively long distance in the nervous system. For example, there are projection neurons with their cell bodies in the cerebral cortex that reach the spinal cord with their axons. There are projection neurons in the deep cerebellar nuclei that reach the brainstem, etc. A projection neuron receives information through its dendrites and also on its cell body, the soma. The soma of this type of cell integrates the electrical information and also provides metabolic support for the cell as a whole. The place where the axon comes out of the soma is called the axon hillock, and this is where the information is encoded into action potentials, as explained later in this chapter. A projection neuron sends its output to other neurons. A sensory neuron (**B**) has a different structure. There is a distal projection of the axon to a peripheral receptor (or a free nerve ending), and a central projection into the spinal cord or brainstem. The cell body of a sensory neuron is located in a ganglion outside the central nervous system, and provides metabolic support, but typically does not serve as a point of connection among neurons. The distal part of the sensory axon is where information is integrated and encoded into action potentials, which travel into the nervous system to affect other cells. Local interneurons (**C**) are like projection interneurons, but much smaller. Their axons travel short distances and do not leave their local structure. The axons of these cells are not myelinated. For each type of cell, the function served by each part is color coded. (Adapted with permission from Kandel et al. *Principles of Neural Science*, New York, NY: McGraw-Hill; 2013. Fig 2-9, pg. 30.)

of the neuron's cell body (Figure 2-1, black). As with any cell, a neuron has a cell nucleus and the usual complement of intracellular organelles. These are contained in the soma, so from a biological perspective, the soma is the metabolic center of the cell. In terms of information processing, the soma is thought of as an integrator for most neurons (Figure 2-1, A, C, green). From a certain point of view, all the information coming into the cell, at any point in time, is ultimately represented as one number: the voltage level of the cell membrane at the soma. So, the soma integrates all that input to form one result. The next part of the neuron is called the **axon hillock** (Figure 2-1, gold), which is where the axon comes out of the soma, and ultimately, it can be thought of as the place where the action potential, the electrical event representing excitation of the neuron, is initiated. The next structure is the **axon**, a tubular process coming out of the soma (Figure 2-1, orange). It is the axon that allows for information to be transmitted from one place to another. Finally, there is the **axon terminal**, where packets of neurotransmitter are stored in vesicles that are ready to be released (Figure 2-1, pink). This neurotransmitter release is the typical means by which information from one neuron can be transmitted to another.

Sensory neurons have a slight variation in these parts (Figure 2-1, B). The sensory receptor leads to a trigger zone near the end of the axon, so reception, integration, and encoding all occur within this distal region. The soma of a sensory neuron provides metabolic support but does not serve as an integrator of electrical information. But as with other kinds of cells, the sensory neuron will have an axon to transmit information and axon terminals for output.

Overview of Neural Function

The Action Potential

Referring back to the parts of the neuron, we can begin to understand its functions. Let us start with the dendrites. For this example, some other neuron in the nervous system will release a neurotransmitter upon the dendrites. The place where this information exchange occurs is called a **synapse**. At the synapse, the neurotransmitter binds to receptor proteins in the cell membrane of the dendrite. These receptor proteins respond to the neurotransmitter, and thereby, have an effect on the cell. In the typical example, this effect would be to open a pore in the cell membrane that allows increased permeability to a certain species of ion, such as sodium, at an active synapse.

At rest, due to metabolic processes and intracellular contents specific to neurons, there will be an electrical potential present between the inside and outside of the neuron. Typically, the inside of the cell is resting with a voltage level of about −65 mV compared to the outside. If sodium is allowed to flow into the cell at an active synapse, this will reduce the relatively negative potential inside the cell. Because the cell was negatively polarized before this event and becomes less negative once sodium starts coming in, this positive deflection of the cell's internal voltage potential is called **depolarization** of the cell.

A single synapse in reality would have an almost imperceptible effect. Real neurons have thousands, even millions, of incoming synapses. But for the sake of this example, we will think of this one synapse as representing the concerted effort of many.

The depolarization of the dendrites causes a voltage change in the soma and, in turn, at the axon hillock as the electrical potential spreads passively along the membrane of the cell. At the axon hillock, there is a strong concentration of special kinds of proteins in the cell membrane. These are called **voltage-gated sodium channels**. This is a type of protein that changes its shape, depending on the voltage potential of the cell membrane where it is located. At the relatively negative resting membrane potential, the voltage-gated sodium channel is closed, but when the membrane potential depolarizes past a certain level, called the **threshold**, the voltage-gated sodium channel snaps open and allows sodium to rush into the cell. This of course makes the cell depolarize even more, and sets off a brief period where there is a positive feedback loop: the rising voltage potential opens more voltage-gated sodium channels, causing an even further rise in potential. During this phase of the action potential, the neuron's membrane potential rises rapidly. At this point, we would say that the **action potential** has been initiated.

As this voltage begins to rise, a second type of voltage-gated channel opens, the **voltage-gated potassium channel**. Unlike sodium, which is at a relatively low concentration inside the cell, potassium is at a relatively high concentration inside the cell (a cellular process called the **sodium potassium pump** maintains this concentration gradient). Potassium, therefore, rushes out of the cell, and as this positive charge is lost, the cell's membrane potential is pulled back down toward the resting membrane potential. At the same time, the voltage-gated sodium channels enter a special state called **inactive**. In the inactive state, caused by the very high membrane potential at the peak of the action potential, the sodium channels close and are temporarily stuck that way. In a typical cell, they will stay closed and inactive for about a millisecond. During this time, the potassium rushing out of the cell is able to return the membrane potential to a level at or below its resting potential. Because the voltage-gated sodium channels are inactive, it is impossible for the cell to make another action potential during this time. We call this the **absolute refractory period.** Then, the voltage-gated potassium channels begin closing, the voltage-gated sodium channels come out of their inactive state, and the sodium potassium pump works to restore the preexisting concentration gradients. At this point, the action potential is over, and the cell is ready to respond again. For a time, it is still relatively difficult to make a new action potential while the cell reestablishes equilibrium, and this period is called the **relative refractory period** (Figure 2-2).

One thing to bear in mind is that very little actual flow of sodium and potassium ions is required to make the action potential. Remembering from basic physics, voltage (V) is the product of current (I) and resistance (R): $V = I \times R$. The resistance of a cell membrane is very, very high. Therefore, it doesn't require very much current to get V to change. This means that the actual concentrations of sodium and potassium inside and outside of the cell have not changed dramatically, during the action potential. There is not much work for the sodium potassium pump to do in order to restore the resting state.

Propagation of Action Potentials

Once an action potential is initiated, it will spread like a wave along the length of the axon. In some neurons, part of the cell

A Action potential voltage and currents

B Voltage-gated sodium channel states

Closed, active   Open, active   Open, Inactive

FIGURE 2-2 Explaining the action potential with channels, ions, and voltages. In (**A**), the voltage that would be recorded between the inside and outside of a single neuron during an action potential is illustrated in black. The green curve indicates how easily Na+ can flow through the cell membrane (i.e., Na+ conductance) during the action potential, and the blue curve shows K+ conductance. Threshold is the voltage level required for an action potential. Once the membrane potential exceeds the threshold, and action potential will definitely occur. RMP stands for resting membrane potential. E_K is the voltage the membrane would reach if potassium channels were open and stayed open (called the reversal potential), and E_{NA} is the reversal potential for sodium. ARP stands for absolute refractory period, the time when a new action potential cannot begin. RRP stands for relative refractory period, the time when it is relatively difficult to make a new action potential. In (**B**), the three possible states for voltage-gated sodium channels are illustrated. Sodium can flow only during the open, active state. (Adapted with permission from Kandel et al. *Principles of Neural Science*, New York, NY: McGraw-Hill; 2013. Figure 7-13 on page 163.)

body and even the most proximal parts of the dendrites also have the appropriate complement of ion channels to create and propagate action potentials. For the purpose of this explanation, we will only consider propagation along an axon.

As explained above, when enough current enters the cell at a synapse to bring the membrane potential above threshold, an action potential is initiated. We can think of the current flowing into the cell through the voltage-gated sodium channels at the initiation of the action potential in the same way. Once membrane potential rises, in the part of the membrane, where threshold has been reached, the voltage is also felt in the surrounding membrane. However, the farther away we are along the membrane, the more the voltage has decayed. In a healthy axon, the voltage-gated sodium channels are close enough together that, as long as one segment of membrane has reached threshold, there definitely will be enough voltage present at the location of the next voltage-gated sodium channel to bring it above threshold, as well. Hence, if the axon is healthy, once an action potential is initiated, it will propagate all the way to the end of the axon.

In a myelinated axon, special glial cells called Schwann cells (explained later) provide an insulating layer around the axon. This helps prevent the passive decay of the potential so that the

voltage-gated sodium channels can be spaced farther apart. While it is true that the voltage-gated sodium channels open very quickly once threshold is reached, there is definitely time required for the protein shape to change and the pore to open. The illustration in Figure 2-3 explains how myelin allows for faster propagation of the action potential. The second major factor determining conduction velocity of a nerve is its diameter. Increased diameter of a nerve also allows greater spacing between ion channels, and therefore, also increases conduction velocity. Myelin is much more effective at increasing conduction velocity than size, so myelination allows axons to be both small and fast.

Synaptic Function

When the action potential reaches the end of the axon, its electrical potential arrives at the synaptic terminals. Here, instead of voltage-gated sodium channels, there are **voltage-gated calcium channels**. When these open, the influx of calcium activates a system that transports synaptic vesicles full of neurotransmitter to the edge of the synaptic membrane. The vesicles release the neurotransmitter into the gap, called the **synaptic cleft**, between the synaptic terminal and the next neuron. In describing the function of a synapse, we call the cell releasing

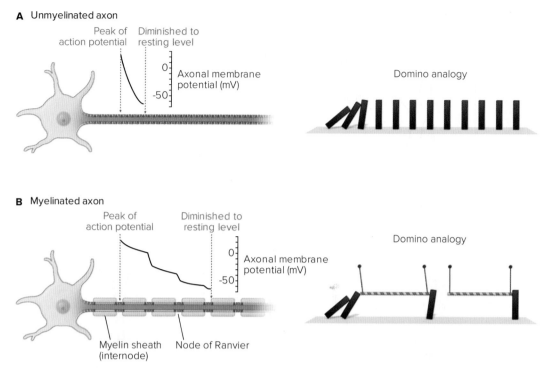

FIGURE 2-3 Propagation of an action potential along an axon, including the function of myelin. In (**A**), the function of an unmyelinated axon in propagating an action potential is shown. Blue indicates resting potential (negative), and red indicates depolarization, which is excitatory and relatively positive. If the cell is excited enough to pass threshold at the axon hillock, the action potential occurs there. At the point of the red arrow, we can imagine this is the peak voltage of the action potential. As we proceed farther down the axon, we see this voltage decrease due to passive decay. However, the voltage-gated sodium channels are spaced closely enough so that the voltage is still above threshold and the next voltage-gated sodium channel opens, allowing the action potential to propagate. Because myelin reduces leakage, the voltage-gated sodium channels can be farther away in the myelinated axon (**B**). At each node of Ranvier (the gaps between myelin), there is more leakage and voltage is lost. But in a healthy neuron, there is enough preservation of voltage to surpass threshold two or three nodes away from the peak of the action potential. In the domino analogy, we can see how this allows the action potential to spread faster. The voltage itself is a physical phenomenon. Although it loses energy over distance, it is present instantly. Likewise, the contact between the dominos is a physical force. With voltage-gated sodium channels close together in the unmyelinated axon, the time required for each channel to open and generate voltage via current flow is analogous to the time required for one domino to tip far enough to hit the next. But with myelin, the distance between channels can be greater. Like the straw transmitting force between the dominos in the lower figure, the myelin allows the voltage to travel farther, so fewer voltage-gated sodium channels are needed. Hence, the last domino will tip over sooner in the lower example, just as the action potential will reach the end of the axon sooner in the myelinated axon. (Used with permission of John A. Buford, PT, PhD.)

the neurotransmitter the **presynaptic neuron**, and the cell being affected the **postsynaptic neuron**. The neurotransmitter diffuses to bind with receptors on the postsynaptic neuron, and this allows the postsynaptic cell to receive the information.

The receptor in the membrane of the postsynaptic neuron will have a part outside the membrane, which is the part where the chemical binding occurs with the neurotransmitter, and a part that spans the cell membrane and reaches inside the cell. As shown in Figure 2-4, these are called the extracellular domain and the intracellular domain. Some receptors serve as ion channels, such that when the neurotransmitter binds to the receptor, the ion channel opens and current flows to change the membrane potential of the postsynaptic neuron. These are called **ionotropic receptors**. Other kinds of receptors, called **metabotropic receptors**, have an intracellular domain that influences the postsynaptic neuron. Metabotropic receptors could act on ion channels from the inside of the cell to influence their permeability or could influence cellular processes through biochemical pathways. In most cases, the effects of

metabotropic receptors are longer lasting than those of ionotropic receptors. When we think of the rapid transmission of information from one neuron to the next, we are usually thinking of functions dominated by ionotropic receptors. When we are thinking of longer term processes like sleep–wake cycles or learning, these are typically dominated by metabotropic receptor functions.

To this point, we have focused on the ability of the postsynaptic neuron to respond to the presynaptic neuron. It is just as necessary for this response to come to an end. Otherwise, a synapse could be activated only once, and no new information could ever be received. There are two basic processes that lead to the end of the synaptic response. The first is simple **diffusion**. Like any chemical reaction, the binding between the neurotransmitter and the receptor depends on a concentration gradient. The neurotransmitter will not stay bound forever. As time passes, the neurotransmitter molecules diffuse out of the synaptic cleft and can no longer bind with the receptors. The second is **enzymatic degradation**. Enzymes, produced either

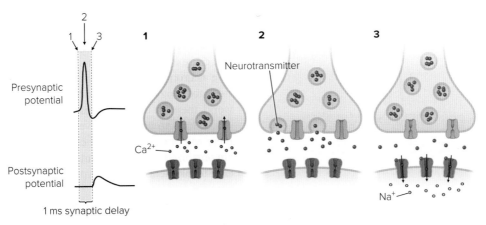

FIGURE 2-4 Synaptic function. In 1, the synapse is shown just before an action potential arrives. The voltage is just about to rise in the presynaptic terminal. Synaptic vesicles have neurotransmitter (blue dots) ready to release, and Ca^{2+} is present in the extracellular space. At the time point labeled 2, the action potential has arrived, voltage-gated calcium channel are open, and Ca^{2+} is entering the presynaptic terminal. This causes exocytosis of the neurotransmitter into the synaptic cleft. There is a time delay for diffusion and the binding of the neurotransmitter to the postsynaptic cell's receptors, before any sodium can enter the postsynaptic cell at time 3 to produce a voltage change in the postsynaptic cell. This time lag is called the synaptic delay. (Adapted with permission from Kandel et al. *Principles of Neural Science*, New York, NY: McGraw-Hill; 2013. Fig 8-8 on page 185.)

by neurons or glia, are present in the extracellular space around neurons, and these cleave neurotransmitter molecules into constituent parts, which also lowers the concentration of neurotransmitter. Not every neurotransmitter is subjected to enzymatic degradation. For very small neurotransmitter molecules, diffusion may be sufficient.

In addition to diffusion and enzymatic degradation, the presynaptic neuron will often have a **reuptake** process. Whole or broken down neurotransmitter will be actively resorbed into the presynaptic terminal and repackaged into vesicles. This saves the cell energy compared to reassembling the molecule from scratch. Some neurotransmitters can be reassembled quickly at the terminal of the presynaptic neuron, whereas others must be transported back to the soma by a process called **retrograde axonal transport**. There is also a system that carries proteins from the soma to the terminals, and this is called **anterograde axonal transport**. In this way, the metabolic machinery required for the synapse to function is kept in good working order, and ready supply of neurotransmitter is maintained.

Non-synaptic Communication between Neurons

At some locations in the nervous system, there are connections between dendrites of neurons called gap junctions where the electrical potential of one cell directly affects the other without the need for a chemical synapse. There are also receptors on neurons that are not at synapses. These would be sensitive to hormones and neuromodulators. Neuromodulators are like neurotransmitters, but their action is indirect. A neuromodulator can bind to metabotropic receptors to modify the effectiveness of a neurotransmitter. There are neurons in the CNS that release neuromodulators in a relatively nonspecific manner into the space around a group of neurons, providing a concentration of the neuromodulator through the local tissue, affecting many neurons in the region simultaneously. In a sense, this allows for a local concentration of a hormone-like substance to regulate a group of cells.

BOX 2-1 **Understanding Pharmacology and Tract Tracing Based on Synaptic Function**

As explained in this section, there are receptors in postsynaptic neurons, and neurotransmitters are chemicals that bind to these receptors. For synaptic function to succeed, there is either an active reuptake process or an enzymatic degradation process so that the action of a neurotransmitter can be short lived. Many of the medicines that act on the nervous system do so by affecting synaptic function. Some medicines bind to the receptors in a more durable way than the natural neurotransmitter and are harder for the enzymatic degradation systems to break down. They act like super potent neurotransmitters. Neurotoxins would be the extreme case where potency is so high, the synapse is irreversibly blocked. Another type of medicine will affect the reuptake process, allowing longer lasting effects from the naturally present neurotransmitters. These **reuptake inhibitors** have the advantage that the presence of the neurotransmitter at any given synapse is natural.

The ability of neuroscientists to trace tracts in the nervous system also stems from what we just learned. Through experimentation, compounds have been discovered that have a part of their molecular structure shaped just right to make the presynaptic neuron absorb and transport the compound back to the soma as if it was needed by the cell. Typically, these compounds are inert and have no effect on neural function, but because they are not natural, histological processing of the tissue followed by microscopic analysis can show which neurons have the compound. This is called **retrograde tracing**. Likewise, there are compounds that are absorbed by the soma and will be carried through the anterograde axonal transport system, allowing **anterograde tracing**. Through these experimental approaches, scientists have traced many of the pathways in the brain, and this monumental effort continues.

The Integrative Functions of Neurons

As described earlier, the postsynaptic neuron responds because it has a receptor. The action of the receptor on the postsynaptic cell is what determines the response. If the receptor allows

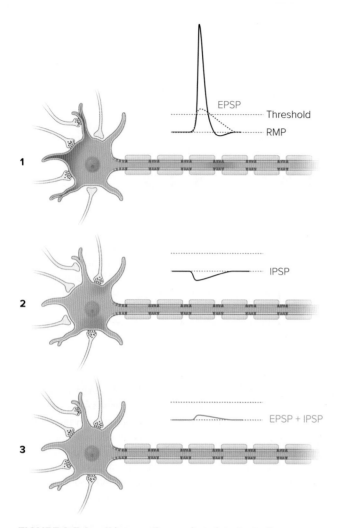

FIGURE 2-5 A cell integrating various inputs. In the upper panel, a cell being excited by multiple excitatory synapses is shown. The EPSP is large and triggers an action potential. In the middle panel, the cell is affected by a pair of inhibitory synapses, and it makes an IPSP. In 3, both sets of synapses are active. Because the inhibitory synapses are closer to the axon hillock and because they increase the conductance of the cell, the EPSP is substantially reduced in amplitude and does not produce an action potential. With the ion channels on the soma opened by the inhibitory synapses, passive potentials from the dendrites are not transmitted very well to the axon hillock. Hence, inhibition tends to override excitation.

positive current to flow into the cell, then it depolarizes the postsynaptic neuron, which is called **excitation**. However, if activating the receptor allows current flow to make the inside of the cell even more negative (hyperpolarized), we call this **inhibition**. The potential recorded in the postsynaptic neuron is, therefore, given one of two names, either an **excitatory postsynaptic potential** (EPSP) or an **inhibitory postsynaptic potential** (IPSP).

As we look at the organization of synaptic inputs on a typical neuron, we notice a consistent pattern. Synapses that produce EPSPs tend to be on the dendritic tree but can also be on the soma. However, the synapses that produce IPSPs consistently

tend to be on or near the soma. This leads to what is referred to as the **integrative property of neurons**. It takes a concerted effort to generate enough EPSPs to depolarize a neuron above threshold and cause it to generate an action potential. However, inhibition of a neuron can be effective quickly and can efficiently override incoming excitation. Once we take an action on the outside world, there are consequences, and if the action was a mistake, it can be hard to undo. However, if we choose not to take action, there will often be a second chance. Synaptic inputs to neurons are organized in such a manner that there must be strong influence to take action and "no votes" seem to take priority.

Transduction and Encoding of Information by Neurons

Membrane Potential

The ultimate result of the integration of EPSPs and IPSPs by a neuron is the generation of a membrane potential at the axon hillock (Figure 2-5). For a typical neuron within the central nervous system, synaptic inputs are the influences that determine fluctuations in membrane potential. However, there are other means by which the membrane potential can change. Indeed, in some neurons, synaptically driven EPSPs and IPSPs do not even occur. One example is in sensory receptors. For these cells, the adequate stimulus is what creates a change in membrane potential. For a sensory receptor in the skin, mechanical deformation of the receptor channels is what opens the ion channel, allowing sodium to flow in. In this case, the initiation of the action potential actually starts at the end of the axon and proceeds towards the cell body, as explained in Chapter 3. In the vestibular system, hair cells create membrane potential changes in a different manner. Despite these variations, one common principle applies: the more depolarized the cell membrane is, the more excited the cell is, and the nervous system must have a way to transfer that level of excitement from one neuron to the next.

Rate Coding

Rate coding is the principal means by which the excitement level of one neuron is transferred to the next. At a synapse, when action potentials arrive in rapid succession, the concentration of neurotransmitter in the synaptic cleft rises and a higher proportion of the receptors are activated for a greater proportion of the time. This translates into larger EPSPs and a greater depolarization of the postsynaptic cell. In this way, the higher level of excitement is transferred from one cell to the next. Likewise, in sensory receptors, when the stimulus is stronger, more receptor channels are open for a longer time, and the generator potential is stronger (Figure 2-6).

How, then, does this higher level of excitement transfer again to the next cell? The greater the level of depolarization at the axon hillock (or for a sensory neuron, at the initial segment), the more rapidly action potentials are created. If the membrane potential is just barely above threshold, then, after the action potential occurs, there will be a relatively weak electrical current flowing to push the membrane potential back over threshold, and the next action potential will not occur right away. However, if the membrane potential is substantially above threshold due to strong excitation, then, there will be a strong

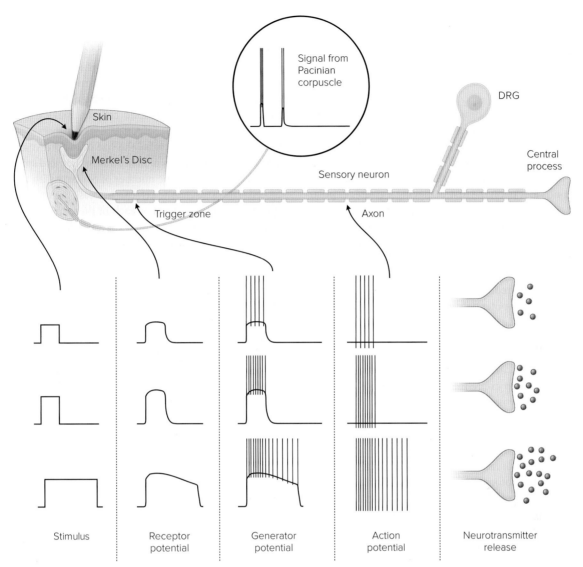

FIGURE 2-6 Rate coding and temporal coding. The encoding of information by a sensory receptor is illustrated. Imagine a pencil touches the skin for a fixed duration, gently in the upper panel, moderately in the middle, and moderately and for a longer duration on the bottom. The receptor potential in the sensory receptor (e.g., Merkel's disc) is proportional in size and duration to the actual stimulus. At the trigger zone, this is translated into a burst of action potentials with a rate that is proportional to the size of the receptor potential. By the time the burst of action potentials is propagated along the axon, the voltage from the receptor potential has passively decayed, but the information about the stimulus is preserved in the rate of action potentials. When this reaches the axon terminal, higher rate and longer burst durations results in higher amounts of neurotransmitter release. This in turn affects EPSP size in the postsynaptic membrane as information is transferred to the next cell. The relationship between stimulus amplitude and the rate of action potentials is called rate coding. The relationship between the onset and offset of the stimulus and the beginning and end of the burst of action potentials is called temporal coding. There is a second aspect to temporal coding, shown by the Pacinian corpuscle (green). These receptors fire rapidly at the beginning and end of the stimulus, providing increase accuracy in detecting the onset and offset of the stimulus. (Adapted with permission from Kandel et al. *Principles of Neural Science*, New York, NY: McGraw-Hill; 2013. Fig. 10-11 on page 223.)

electrical current, and the cell will rapidly exceed threshold and fire again. Of course, the relative refractory period will tend to limit the firing rate once very high rates are reached, and the absolute refractory period places an upper limit on firing rate.

Temporal Coding

Temporal coding, in the simplest sense, means that when the stimulus or neural drive begins, this is signaled by an increase (or decrease) in the firing rate, and the change occurs back to the baseline condition, when the stimulus or period of central drive is finished. In addition, the nervous system frequently uses a secondary means of temporal coding. Some neurons have a rapid burst (or sudden dropout) of activity at the beginning or end of an event. This helps accentuate the beginning and end of a command from one part of the nervous system to the other. In sensory systems, we call these rapidly adapting cells. Within the nervous system, cells that respond like this are often called **phasic neurons**. Other kinds of neurons have more steady responses, continue to make action potentials at a consistent rate as long as the stimulus is present or the command is ongoing. In sensory systems, these are called **slowly adapting cells**. Within the CNS, we call these **tonic neurons**.

Temporal Summation

As described above for rate coding, when multiple EPSPs arrive in rapid succession, the response of the postsynaptic cell is stronger. In part, this is because the synapse is fully activated. But another factor is that the membrane potential caused by the first EPSP may still be present when the second EPSP occurs. The voltage from the second rides upon the first, achieving a greater depolarization than either alone could have achieved. This is called temporal summation and will be discussed further in Chapter 4. It can occur for IPSPs as well as for EPSPs. For most central nervous system pathways, arrival of one EPSP on the postsynaptic cell will not be sufficient to generate an action potential. Temporal summation is usually required. The presynaptic neuron might need to send a dozen action potentials in rapid succession to get the postsynaptic cell to make just a few action potentials.

Spatial Summation

Spatial summation occurs when multiple different incoming sources are all trying to excite the cell. For example, your balance control system, your reflexes, and your voluntary effort might all be trying to produce the same response at the same time. In this case, the motoneurons for the relevant muscle will be receiving EPSPs from three separate pathways all at the same time. These synaptic contacts would all be landing on slightly different parts of the motoneuron, so the voltage from these different spatial locations on the cell would all combine to produce a substantial depolarization. This is spatial summation.

Storage of Information: Neural Plasticity

Changes in Synaptic Strengths and Connections between Neurons

Synapses can change over time to become stronger or weaker.[1] The presence of an action potential in a neuron is not only an electrical event, but it is also a metabolic event. Through receptors and biochemical pathways that are sensitive to the intracellular consequences of the action potential, long-term changes in the cell can occur. This can occur through the growth of dendritic spines, such that the postsynaptic cell develops a small outgrowth to make closer contact with the presynaptic terminal. It can also involve expansion of the postsynaptic membrane's receptor zone under the synapse. The postsynaptic cell can make a larger number of receptors so that the response at its synapses is stronger. The presynaptic cell can increase the size of the presynaptic terminal, release higher quantities of neurotransmitter, and sprout new axon terminals to increase the number of contacts with the postsynaptic cell. The postsynaptic cell can increase the number and size of synaptic receptor zones. For each of these instances above, there can be a decrease, instead, and these kinds of changes can occur for synapses that make EPSPs or IPSPs. As noted in the section on non-synaptic communication between neurons, neuromodulators can regulate the effectiveness of neurotransmitters. In addition to this short-term effect, they can also stimulate the long-term changes in synaptic function described above (Figure 2-7).

There is also a phenomenon known as a **silent synapse.**[2,3] There are potential connections between neurons in the nervous system that are not functioning because the postsynaptic cell does not have the proper complement of receptors. If a new behavioral pattern develops (e.g., lots of practice of a new skill) such that the activity of the two cells is correlated and they are firing together, the silent synapses can become active. For this to occur, the postsynaptic cell activates metabolic pathways to make receptors and insert them in the postsynaptic membrane to make that synapse active and able to respond to the presynaptic cell.

In sum, connections between neurons change with experience and practice. As an analogy, if you find that every time you take advice from a certain friend, you succeed, you will pay more and more attention to that friend. If activity between a presynaptic and postsynaptic neuron is correlated with success, the connection will become stronger. Synapses that do not become stronger through this process will become weaker in comparison. A common saying that comes from this phenomenon is, "Neurons that fire together wire together," based on the work published by Hebb in 1949 and since confirmed through more basic studies.

FIGURE 2-7 Changes in synapses and sprouting. In (**A**), increased effectiveness of a synapse is illustrated by an increased number of postsynaptic receptors. In (**B**), the development of a synaptic spine is shown, such that the size of the synaptic cleft is reduced, making the synapse more efficient. In (**C**), an axon collateral sprouts to connect to a nearby cell that was previously not connected. In (**D**), the axon sprouts a new branch to increase the number of connections to the postsynaptic cell. (Used with permission of John A. Buford, PT, PhD.)

● GLIAL CELLS

Glia of the Nervous System

The most predominant cells in the central nervous system are not neurons but rather glia – small cells having multiple processes but no axons or dendrites. Their prevalence and size suggested to early scientists that they functioned as "glue" to hold the nervous system together and were given the name for glue in Greek – glia. While there is little evidence that glia work as glue, recent findings are showing that they play important roles in maintaining normal homeostasis within the CNS. In fact, some scientists are beginning to explore whether dysfunction of glia alone can create clinical impairments. There are three types of glia or neuroglia, as they are also called – astrocytes, microglia, and oligodendrocytes.

Astrocytes

Astrocytes are named because of their star-like shape and radial projections. They can be divided into two types, based on differences in shape and location. Protoplasmic astrocytes occupy gray matter regions in the brain and spinal cord and have many main projections with uniform small branches, forming a dense globoid structure (Figure 2-8). Fibrous astrocytes are found in white matter regions and have long, thin fibers. Both of these types of astrocytes place end feet onto blood vessels which allows them to monitor changes in the vasculature. This tight relationship means that astrocytes detect and respond to blood vessel dilation, movement of cells across the vessel wall, and CNS edema. Astrocytes also make contact with neural synapses, in the gray matter, and with nodes of Ranvier, in the white

matter. Thus, each astrocyte extends end feet to both vessels and neural structures, comprising the neurovascular unit. In some regions of the brain, a single astrocyte covers more than 100,000 synapses from many different neurons.[4] Astrocytes also extend processes to neighboring astrocytes. In this way, they form a tile-like pattern with astrocytic processes touching, but not overlapping each other, and covering the entire nervous system.

Historically, neuroglia were considered only as structural support for neurons and axons. However, with scientific and technological advances, it is now clear that the structural organization of astrocytes allows them to influence or control a wide number of functions in the CNS. The large number of contacts on both blood vessels and synapses enables them to control blood flow in the brain and spinal cord to match the needs of neural regions with high activity.[5] Greater synaptic activity produces higher calcium levels in the astrocyte that translate into the release of compounds that increase blood vessel dilation to produce greater blood flow in an activity-dependent manner. Astrocytes also release compounds that induce vasoconstriction and appear to finely regulate regional blood flow in the CNS.

Astrocytes play a fundamental role in metabolic and trophic support to neurons. Glycogen storage occurs primarily in astrocytes, and the highest concentrations are found in brain regions with the highest neural activity, and therefore, the greatest metabolic need.[6] Neurotransmitters like glutamate, released during neural firing, modulate glycogen. Astrocytes break down glycogen, producing the metabolite lactate, which is critical for maintaining synapses and promoting new synaptic growth. The synaptic strength needed for learning and memory depends on astrocytic metabolic support.[7] The metabolites are transferred

FIGURE 2-8 Microscopic images of oligodendrocytes, astrocytes, and microglia. The oligodendrocyte cell body is centrally located and surrounded by numerous delicate protrusions. Note the different morphology of the fibrous and protoplasmic astrocytes which are located in the white and gray matter, respectively. The tile-like relationship of the protoplasmic astrocytes is clear, with only the end feet in close proximity. Microglia are shown in three states – resting, bushy profile and activated. The activation of microglia includes thickening of the ramifications which presents as a bushy morphology. When they are fully activated, the cell body greatly enlarges and the arms are retracted. Oligodendrocytes and astrocytes were labeled with a green fluorescent protein while the microglia were labeled with a brown chromagen. (Used with permission of D. McTigue and DM Basso, The Ohio State University).

to both neurons and axons, where they are used for aerobic metabolism when other sources of energy are low.

One of the most important roles of astrocytes is to maintain normal, nontoxic ionic, fluid, and neurotransmitter levels. Astrocytes shuttle ions like potassium from the extracellular space through transporters on their surface.[6] To control interstitial fluids, water channels, called aquaporin 4, are highly concentrated on astrocytic end feet on blood vessels and reduce fluids. Astrocytes buffer the neurotoxic effects of high levels of neurotransmitters, especially glutamate. Excessive glutamate, as occurs after brain or spinal cord injury, induces pronounced cell death in the CNS and must be quickly and carefully buffered. Astrocytes play a primary role in removing excess glutamate from the extracellular space via transporters that move glutamate into the astrocyte, where it is converted into its precursor, and then, released back into the synaptic space for future use. These homeostatic mechanisms are often overwhelmed in acute CNS trauma and lead to lesion expansion beyond the initial insult. Extensive research is directed toward improving these homeostatic mechanisms in an effort to enhance ion, fluid, and glutamate clearance.

Astrocytes respond to a variety of molecules, including growth factors, inflammatory substances, degeneration substrates, like Abeta, and cell death factors, like free radicals. Two important responses emerge in reaction to these events: (1) calcium signaling to neurons and other astrocytes and (2) astrogliosis. By regulating internal calcium concentrations, oscillations develop within the astrocyte that trigger neurotransmitter release that likely changes synaptic activity directly.[6] The internal calcium influx also moves in waves to the neighboring astrocytes through gap junctions and can convey cellular changes over great distances from one part of the nervous system to another. The calcium waves enable signaling in both astrocytes and neurons under normal conditions and during disease or trauma. In times of disease or damage, the astrocytes change their shape, function, and number. The astrocytes closest to the site of injury or disease have the greatest response, and it gradually decreases the farther away from the site. Here, the astrocytes adopt a reactive phenotype with enlarged cell bodies and processes and increase in number by migrating to the site or through proliferation. Unlike in the normal state, reactive astrocytes overlap extensively, which has important implication for neuropathology of spinal cord injury which will be discussed in Chapter 12. Taken together, these complex changes are called **astrogliosis**. High levels of astrogliosis produce glial scarring, which can be neuroprotective by limiting the spread of toxins, inflammation, and infection. Glial scarring can also be disruptive by preventing axonal growth or synaptic plasticity, producing inflammation, releasing toxic substances, like glutamate, and causing edema.

Microglia

Microglia, under normal conditions, are tiny cells with many, finely ramified processes. Like astrocytes, they are widely distributed, without overlapping, throughout the gray and white matter in the brain and spinal cord. Microglia are the resident immune cells in the CNS and protect the nervous system from infection, disease, and the consequences of injury. In their finely ramified state, they are considered to be "resting microglia" (see Figure 2-8) but routinely perform surprisingly fast movements. The fine microglial endings repeatedly extend to the nearby cells, interstitial fluid, and neuropil to survey for unusual changes. Scientists have been able to label brain microglia, allowing them to capture microglial surveillance movements under normal conditions. These movies are fascinating in how active and expansive the resting microglia movements are.[8]

As resident immune cells, a variety of microbes and substances can activate microglia, and in response, they adopt different shapes along a continuum. From the resting, finely ramified state (Figure 2-8), microglia partially retract their processes becoming thicker and bushy while the cell body enlarges (Figure 2-8). With greater exposure to the signals, microglia become fully activated with fewer protrusions and even larger cell bodies (Figure 2-8). In the final stage, the microglia assume a round, amoeboid shape without any protrusion. In this form, they are called macrophages that phagocytose debris and damaged cells. Interestingly, monocytes from the blood also cross the vasculature into the parenchyma and become macrophages. Resident and blood-borne macrophages are indistinguishable from each other.

Activated microglia and macrophages restore homeostasis not only by engulfing damaged cells but also by modulating excitotoxicity and promoting neuroplasticity. Injured neurons emit toxic factors such as excessive glutamate and free radicals, which recruit activated microglia to surround the toxic neuron.[9] This synaptic stripping reduces the toxic cascade and may support neural regeneration. Additionally, at least one important signal comes from the neuron and binds to a receptor on the activated microglia/macrophage which is thought to protect the neuron from phagocytosis.[9] Activated microglia also participate in neuroplasticity by pruning synapses or secreting enzymes that open space in the neuropil for new growth. The microglia also appear to preferentially encircle synapses that are highly active, suggesting a role in experience-dependent plasticity.

Microglia defend the CNS against frank disruption from trauma, disease, or infection while also putting mechanisms in place to restore homeostasis. They mediate the immune response in the CNS by presenting antigen-initiating microglial activation and recruiting other cells to the threatened region.[10] Microglia express many substances or receptors in response to changes in homeostasis. These factors are called cytokines and chemokines. **Cytokines** determine the state of activation of microglia and function by activating not only the cell that expresses them but also neighboring microglial. This means they exert autocrine and paracrine effects. Cytokines fall into two broad categories and define microglial function as anti-inflammatory or pro-inflammatory. Microglia also produce **chemokines**, which microglia use to move to areas where the neural tissue is threatened by infection, disease, or injury.[10] Microglia also use chemokines to recruit lymphocytes, monocytes, and neutrophils into the brain and spinal cord to help restore homeostasis. Once these peripheral, blood-borne cells enter the CNS, microglia signal them through cytokines and antigen presentation to determine their role and use chemokines to distribute them anywhere in the nervous system. Once the threat to the CNS has been contained or cleared away, activated microglia return to a resting state and most phagocytic macrophages undergo cell death, thereby, restoring homeostasis.

Oligodendrocytes

Oligodendrocytes (oligos) are the only cells in the CNS that myelinate neurons. Their equivalent partners in the periphery are Schwann Cells. Oligos are primarily located within the white matter of the CNS and have a small, centralized cell body with multitudes of radial extensions (Figure 2-8). Each extension ensheaths a different axon, thus, allowing a single oligo to myelinate many neural axons. Oligos myelinate axons of specific sizes. As in the periphery, small diameter axons are typically unmyelinated. Oligos myelinate axons that are 0.2 μm or larger.[11] While it is unclear what signals the oligos use to identify axons of specific sizes, it is clear that axonal activity is an important but indirect regulator. The action potential, traveling down the axon, releases molecules that target astrocytes. In response, the astrocytes express a factor that induces myelin formation around the axon. This close relationship indicates that changes in astrocytes, especially during development or after injury, can cause problems in myelination.

Myelination is very important to the structure and function of the neuron–axon unit. Myelin is mostly comprised of lipid, which serves as an insulator of the axon, enabling the action potential to continue to the terminal. The oligo ensheaths segments of the axon, leaving gaps between myelinated areas.[12] Within these gaps, sodium channels cluster and are called nodes of Ranvier. These myelinated segments, separated by nodes of Ranvier, allow the action potential to move down the axon by jumping from one node to the next. This type of progression is called **saltatory conduction** and facilitates much faster axonal conduction. In addition to conduction, myelin also supports axonal transport, which is important for moving proteins, transmitters, and growth factors from the neuronal cell body to the axon terminal. The myelin sheath also provides trophic support to the underlying axon and the neuron by secreting several different types of growth factors.

There is a large demand placed on oligos as they wrap axons in myelin. At least 50 axons are myelinated by a single oligo, which represents a membrane load that is 100 times its cell body weight.[12] This means the oligos have a high metabolic rate and consume high levels of oxygen and ATP for energy, which can create toxic byproducts, called reactive oxygen species. Unfortunately, oligos have very low levels of antioxidants that buffer this toxicity. Thus, oligos are quite vulnerable to shifts in homeostasis, and toxic damage can result in oligo cell death. This type of damage and oligo cell death occurs in multiple sclerosis, injury, and ischemia. Additionally, exposure to inflammation, inflammatory cytokines, or cytotoxic T lymphocytes put oligos at risk for demyelination or cell death.[12]

The central nervous system retains the ability to remyelinate, or restore, myelin to axons that have been demyelinated. Oligodendrocyte precursor cells (OPCs), immature cells found in different regions of the adult brain and spinal cord, receive signals from microglia and astrocytes that cause the OPCs to migrate to affected areas and to increase in number.[12] Once they arrive in the demyelinated zone, the OPCs develop into mature oligos and begin the remyelination process. One consequence of remyelination is that fewer wraps are made around the axons, so they are only thinly myelinated. This difference in thickness slows axonal conduction and may allow the action potential to dwindle away. Over time, the CNS is unable to mount a remyelination response, but it is unclear what factors are responsible.

Oligodendrocytes are the only glial cell to receive neural input. There is mounting evidence that increased neural activity, as occurs during skill learning or adaptation after CNS injury, induces greater myelination.[13] The greater neural drive appears to add internodal segments of myelin to the axon. Not all axons in the adult nervous system are fully myelinated from the neuronal cell body to the axon terminal. In fact, the length of cortical neurons is only intermittently myelinated.[14] One method to enhance learning and neuroplasticity is to add myelin internodes to axons that are only partially myelinated.[13] By adding internodes, the conduction of the action potential increases and the risk of it decaying before it reaches the terminal is reduced. By ensuring synaptic activity and increasing postsynaptic firing, stronger relationships between the cells (neuron-to-neuron or neuron-to-OPC) can occur, in an activity-dependent manner. This synaptic strengthening has important implications for motor learning and recovery after CNS impairment. A recent study shows, for the first time, that learning a complex wheel running task increases the number of OPCs in the brain, in mice.[15] To prove that these OPCs were necessary to learn the complex task, the scientists blocked specific genes that allowed maturation. When OPCs were retained in their precursor form and could not mature into myelinating oligos, the mice could not learn the task. This is strong evidence that learning a new skill or relearning functions, during rehabilitation, will be dependent on generating OPCs and converting them into myelinating cells.

In summary, all glia of the nervous system play a crucial role in maintaining a healthy microenvironment so that the neurons can function properly. Under challenging conditions, astrocytes and microglia become activated while OPCs increase in number. These different forms of glia help buffer toxicity, bolster repair processes, and facilitate learning and plasticity.

REFERENCES

1. Merzenich MM, Van Vleet TM, Nahum M. Brain plasticity-based therapeutics. *Front Hum Neurosci.* 2014;8:385.

2. Buno W, Cabezas C, Fernandez de SD. Presynaptic muscarinic control of glutamatergic synaptic transmission. *J Mol Neurosci.* 2006;30(1-2):161-164.

3. Kasten MR, Fan Y, Schulz PE. Activation of silent synapses with sustained but not decremental long-term potentiation. *Neurosci Lett.* 2007;417(1):84-89.

4. Bushong EA, Martone MA, Jones YZ, Ellisman MH. Protoplasmic astrocytes in CA1 stratum radiatum occupy separate anatomical domains. *J Neurosci.* 2002;22:183-192.

5. Howarth C. The contribution of astrocytes to the regulation of cerebral blood flow. *Front Neurosci.* 2014;8(103):1-9.

6. Sofroniew MV, Vinters HV. Astrocytes: biology and pathology. *Acta Neuropathol.* 2010;119:7-35.

7. Suzuki A, Stern SA, Bozdagi O, Aberini CM. Astrocyte-neuron lactate transport is required for long-term memory formation. *Cell.* 2011;144:810-823.

8. Davalos D, Grutzendler J, Yang G, Kim JV, Zuo Y, Jung S, Littman DR, Dustin ML, Gan WB. ATP mediate rapid microglial response to local brain injury in vivo. *Nat Neurosci.* 2005;8(6):752-758.

9. Ziebell JM, Adelson PD, Lifshitz J. Microglia: dismantling and rebuilding circuits after acute neurological injury. *Metab Brain Dis.* 2014; April; doi:10.1007/s11011-014-9539-y

10. Rock RB, Gekker G, Hu S, Sheng WS, Cheeran M, Lokensgard JR, Peterson PK. Role of microglia in central nervous system infections. *Clin Microbiol Rev.* 2004;October:942-964.

11. Simons M, Trajkovic K. Neuron-glia communication in the control of oligodendrocyte function and myelin biogenesis. *J Cell Biochem.* 2006;119:4381-4389.

12. Bradl M, Lassmann H. Oligodendrocytes: biology and pathology *Acta Neuropathol.* 2010;119(1):37-53.

13. O'Rourke M, Gasperini R, Young K. Adult myelination: wrapping up neuronal plasticity. *Neural Regen Res.* 2014;9:1261.

14. Tomassy GS, Berger DR, Chen HH, et al. Distinct profiles of myelin distribution along single axons of pyramidal neurons in the neocortex. *Science.* 2014;344:319-324.

15. McKenzie IA, Ohayon D, Li H, Paes de Faria J, Emery B, Tohyama K, Richardson WD. Motor skill learning requires active central myelination. *Science.* 2014;346(6207):318-322.

Review Questions

1. **What is the name of the fatty substance the covers axons to improve their ability to conduct action potentials?**

   A. Adipose tissue

   B. Extracellular matrix

   C. Myelin

   D. Neurolemma

2. **For the type of axon noted above, what is the name of the gap not covered by fatty substance?**

   A. Internode

   B. Voltage-gated sodium channel

   C. Axon hillock

   D. Node of Ranvier

3. **What is the name of the force that determines which way ions will flow across the neural cell membrane when a certain ion pore opens?**

   A. Electrical gradient

   B. Electromechanical gradient

   C. Electrochemical gradient

   D. Concentration gradient

4. **What kind of ion channel must be opened to initiate an action potential at the axon hillock of a projection interneuron?**

   A. Voltage-gated potassium channel

   B. Voltage-gated sodium channel

   C. Voltage-gated calcium channel

   D. Metabotropic receptors

5. **Assuming other characteristics are equal, the neuron with the fastest conduction velocity would be the one with the …**

   A. Largest diameter axon

   B. Longest axon

   C. Highest number of voltage–gated sodium channels

   D. Smallest number of inhibitory synapses

6. **What is different about the axon membrane at the nodes of Ranvier than in the axon where it is wrapped with the substance produced by Schwann cells?**

   A. There is a high degree of membrane resistance

   B. There is a high concentration of voltage-gated sodium channels

   C. There is no passive decay of the membrane potential

   D. Ligand-gated receptors are present to respond to neurotransmitters

7. **Which one of these processes can NOT contribute to the removal of the neurotransmitter so the synapses can recover to normal?**

   A. Diffusion

   B. Enzyme degradation

   C. Reuptake into the presynaptic terminal

   D. Glial cells scavenging up the breakdown products

   E. Absorption of the neurotransmitter into the postsynaptic cell

8. **When a neuron is active, the number of action potentials it makes per second should be proportional to the membrane potential at the trigger zone of the cell. What is the name for this relationship?**

   A. Temporal coding

   B. Population coding

   C. Rate coding

   D. Amplitude coding

9. **Which of these cells would not be found inside the cerebral cortex?**

   A. Astrocytes

   B. Schwann Cells

   C. Oligodendrocytes

   D. Microglia

10. **In learning a new motor skill, what oligodendrocyte changes would be expected?**

    A. Increased myelination and a decreased number of internodal segments

    B. Decreased myelination and an increased number of internodal segments

    C. Increased myelination and an increased number of internodal segments

    D. Decreased myelination and a decreased number of internodal segments

11. **How do astrocytes react in the presence of injury?**

    A. They adsorb glutamate to prevent neuronal death

    B. They induce excitotoxicity

    C. They become enlarged and more widely spaced

    D. They enhance axonal regeneration through the formation of a glial scar

12. **Which of the following correctly describes the activity of cytokines and chemokines, during neural injury?**

    A. Chemokines determine the state of activation of microglia

    B. Cytokines activate microglia in both an autocrine and paracrine manner

    C. Cytokines recruit lymphocytes and monocytes to areas of damage

    D. Both cytokines and chemokines stimulate free radical release to repair damaged neurons.

Answers

1. C	2. D	3. C	4. B	5. A
6. B	7. E	8. C	9. B	10. C
11. A	12. B			

Somatosensory Pathways and Perception

Deborah S. Nichols-Larsen

3

OBJECTIVES

1) Differentiate the neuroanatomical structures that support sensory perception and discrimination

2) Differentiate the concepts of perception, discrimination, and haptics

3) Introduce methods of testing sensation

4) Discuss how sensory information contributes to reflexes and function

● INTRODUCTION

Human somatosensation is supported by complex networks, allowing the perception of touch, joint pressure and motion, muscle stretch and tension, pain, pressure, temperature, vibration, and itch. From these simple modalities, the human sensory system can characterize the location of touch, the magnitude of the stimulus, the orientation of the body or limb in space, and the identification of object properties such as texture, roughness, weight, shape, and identity. This chapter will focus on the neural processing of somatosensory sensations and how that processed information is used. We will also address how common tests of sensation can be used to elucidate different sensory abilities.

● SENSATION

To say that sensation is complex, is at best an incredible understatement. Think of some of the sensations that you have experienced such as the tickle of hair as the hairdresser cuts your bangs or the feel of an ice cube melting in your hand. Imagine the feel of cool crisp sheets as you climb into bed at night or the rumpled warmth of those same sheets the next morning. Feel the golf club in your hand as you take a long back swing and then swing forward to hit the ball from the tee, immediately sensing whether it is a good or a bad shot. There are an endless number of sensations that can be described, but basically they fall into two general categories: cutaneous sensation and proprioception.

Touch

Cutaneous sensation allows the perception of touch (pressure, vibration, tickle, texture), temperature (hot/cold), pain (extreme temperatures, tissue damage, mechanical force), and itch via the activation of specific sensory receptors that respond to unique stimulus characteristics. **Touch receptors** can collectively be referred to as *mechanoreceptors*, encompassing Pacinian corpuscles, Meissner corpuscles, Merkel disks, and Ruffini endings (Table 3-1, Figure 3-1); these receptors are also designated by their mode of adaptation (rapid or slow) and their location in the skin (superficial = 1, deep = 2). Slow adapting receptors are activated by a maintained stimulus and continue firing for the duration of the stimulus; conversely, rapidly adapting receptors respond quickly to stimulus change, including the initiation or cessation of a stimulus, but cease activation during a maintained stimulation. Mechanoreceptors project centrally via large diameter, heavily myelinated neurons (A alpha). These receptors collectively allow humans to discriminate a vast array of sensations, including but not limited to: touch perception and localization; two point, texture, weight, and shape discrimination; and object identification. *Texture discrimination* basically involves distinguishing two dimensions along a continuum of rough to smooth and soft to hard.[1] *Stereognosis* refers to the ability to identify an object by touch alone; we all do this when we reach into our pocket and distinguish a quarter from the other coins without looking. *Graphesthesia* is the ability to identify letters or words drawn on the skin, a common game among school-aged children, and *haptic perception* is the ability to distinguish object or surface characteristics, including shape, texture, and weight, through manipulation. This, of course, is an interaction between the motor system and the sensory system, and therefore, can be interrupted by a disturbance of either system.

Temperature, pain, and itch activate free nerve endings, located superficially in the skin with small receptive areas that project centrally via A delta (Aδ) and C fibers that are minimally or non-myelinated, and therefore, slow conducting. Nerve endings that perceive heat and cold are distinct as are those that are activated by extremes of temperature that are perceived as painful (burning or freezing). Nociceptors (pain receptors) not only respond to extremes of temperature but also to other types of tissue damage from mechanical or chemical sources. Many nociceptors respond to only one type of noxious stimulation while others respond to several and are referred to as polymodal nociceptors.[2]

Aδ fibers are associated with higher threshold and single modality nociceptors; conversely, C fibers attach to polymodal nociceptors.[3] Several types of free nerve endings exist that initiate the perception of itch and project via C fibers. Initially, it was thought that the sensation of itch was created only by a histamine

TABLE 3-1	Receptors				
RECEPTOR	**ADAPTATION**	**SURFACE LOCATION**	**AFFERENT**	**CUTANEOUS FUNCTION**	**PROPRIOCEPTIVE FUNCTION**
Meissner corpuscles (RA1)	Rapid	Superficial	A alpha	Motion on the skin	Meissner corpuscles (RA1)
Pacinian corpuscles (RA2)	Rapid	Deep	A alpha	Vibration, texture	Joint perturbations (motion)
Merkel discs (SA1)	Slow	Superficial	A alpha	Pressure, spatial features	
Ruffini endings (SA2)	Slow	Deep	A alpha	Skin stretch	Joint position and rotation
Golgi tendon organ	Rapid	Musculoskeletal junctions	Ib		Muscle tension
Nuclear bags	Rapid or slow	Within spindle in striate muscle	Ia		Muscle length and rate of change
Nuclear chains	Slow	Within spindle in striate muscle	II		Maintained stretch
Free nerve endings	Slow	Superficial	A delta	Pain	
			C	Temperature, itch	

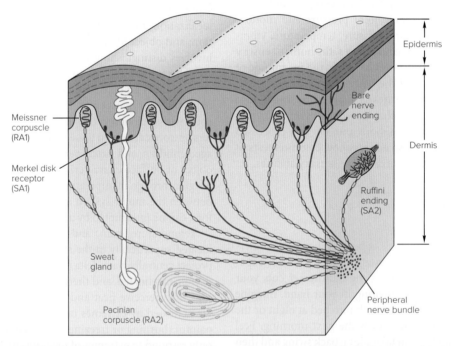

FIGURE 3-1 Illustration of mechanoreceptors. (Reproduced, with permission, from Kandel ER, Schwartz JH, Jessell TM, Siegelbaum SA, Hudspeth AJ. *Principles of Neural Science*, 5th ed. New York, NY: McGraw-Hill; 2013, Fig 23-1, Pg 500.)

reaction, but it has subsequently been noted in the absence of histamine, albeit the precipitating mediator(s) is(are) unclear.

There is another phenomenon associated with pain perception, referred to as hyperalgesia, which likely results from an activation of inflammatory mediators, such as histamine and substance P, and can be localized to the damaged area (primary hyperalgesia) or in adjacent tissues (secondary hyperalgesia).[2] Hyperalgesia, also referred to as allodynia, is exaggerated pain sensitivity such that non-painful stimuli, like light touch, are experienced as pain.

Receptive Fields

A receptive field is the surface area to which a single receptor and its sensory nerve fiber are responsive (Figure 3-2), or in terms of free nerve endings, the area of innervation for a single nerve ending. Each type of mechanoreceptor has a different receptive field with Merkel's disks and Meissner corpuscles having smaller receptive fields than Ruffini endings or Pacinian corpuscles. In turn, receptors are more closely organized in distil body areas (i.e., the hand) than in proximal areas (i.e., the shoulder), and the density of receptors is associated with the tactile sensitivity of the body part. Thus, the hand with its high density of mechanoreceptors is much better at detecting object characteristics than most other areas of the body.

Interestingly, receptors have areas of stronger and lesser sensitivity. For example, Meissner corpuscles have multiple areas of high sensitivity, surrounded by areas of lesser sensitivity, while Pacinian corpuscles are most sensitive in their center with decreasing sensitivity toward their periphery. A given stimulus may activate multiple receptors, especially when applied to the fingertip, and their activation will allow localization of the touch and interpretation of the stimulus characteristics, based on the number and type of receptors that are activated; more intense stimulation may activate a given receptor multiple times, which contributes to the perception of stimulus intensity and duration.

Receptive field 1   Receptive field 2

FIGURE 3-2 Illustration of receptive fields. (Reproduced, with permission, from McKinley M, O'Loughlin VD. *Human Anatomy*, 3 ed. New York, NY: McGraw-Hill; 2012, Fig19.1, pg. 562.)

Proprioception

Proprioception has had many definitions, and there has been considerable confusion in how this term and that of kinesthesia have been used. Most recently proprioception has been used to embody a comprehensive ability to sense: (1) muscle tension, (2) limb or body position and movement, including the velocity and direction of the movement (**kinesthesia**), (3) muscle or movement effort, and (4) balance.[4,5] This chapter will use this comprehensive definition of proprioception and limit the use of kinesthesia to the perception of limb/body position and movement.

Mechanoreceptors, located within joint capsules and ligaments, contribute to proprioception related to joint compression and movement; however, muscle spindles and Ruffini endings are uniquely activated during limb and trunk movement. Muscle spindles within the striate muscle respond to changes in muscle length; similarly, Ruffini endings are activated by skin stretch. In concert, these two receptor types provide a more complete indication of kinesthesia than either alone.[6]

Muscle spindles are unique receptors, located within striate muscle, oriented in parallel to the striate muscle fibers and attached at each end to the adjacent striate muscle fibers; muscle spindles are encapsulated sensory receptors that house two types of tiny muscle fibers (Figure 3-3). To distinguish these tiny spindle muscle fibers from the larger striate muscle fibers, the spindle fibers are referred to as **intrafusal fibers** (within the spindle) and the striate muscle fibers as **extrafusal** fibers (outside of the spindle). Intrafusal fibers have two distinct shapes – one is round in the center like a bag with a handle on each end; the other is long and thin like a chain. Therefore, they are referred to as nuclear bags and nuclear chains. Nuclear bags are larger and the central enlargement, or bag, contains the nuclei of the fiber; the nuclear chains are smaller and narrow with nuclei in a central row in the middle section of the fiber. Each muscle spindle contains one to two nuclear bags and up to 11 nuclear chains. There are two types of nuclear bags (dynamic and static), and it appears that most muscle spindles include one of each.[7]

Muscle spindles project to the spinal cord via two types of afferent fibers (primary and secondary). Each spindle gives rise to a single primary afferent but multiple secondary afferents. **Primary afferents (Ia)** spiral around the central portion of nuclear bags and chains, and their endings that attach to the intrafusal fibers are often referred to as *annulospiral endings*; **secondary afferents** (II) coil around the nuclear chains at each side of the central area with endings that are referred to as *flower spray endings*. The two types of afferents react differently to muscle length, stretch, and maintained tension on the extrafusal fibers. First, stretch of the extrafusal fibers simultaneously stretches the intrafusal fibers, resulting in activation of Ia afferents at a rate comparable to the rate and magnitude of stretch; more specifically, Ia fibers are most responsive at the beginning of a dynamic stretch and decrease their firing rate as the stretch progresses, providing key input toward the perception of movement. It should be noted that for any joint motion, there are muscles that are being elongated (stretched) with heightened spindle activity and those that are shortened with diminished spindle activity; in fact, during muscle shortening, muscles spindles are unloaded and would cease firing unless otherwise activated (see gamma motor innervation). Conversely, group II fibers respond increasingly over the course of a stretch and maximally when the muscle reaches its final tension or length, and thereby, contribute more to the perception of posture than movement.[6]

In the simplest form, the muscle spindle serves a reflex function to prevent excessive stretch to the *homonymous muscle* (muscle in which the Ia fibers originate). Ia afferents project through the dorsal horn of the spinal cord to synapse directly on alpha motor neurons that innervate the homonymous muscle fibers. Once the muscle spindle is activated by stretch, the Ia

A

Flower spray endings

γ-Efferent

Annulospiral endings

Afferents

Nuclear bag

Nuclear chain

INTRAFUSAL FIBERS

C

Muscle fibers

Axon

Tendon

B

Motor

Sensory

Muscle stretch stimulates sensory nerve impulse to travel to the CNS

Muscle spindle

Sensory nerve endings

Motor nerve endings

Muscle

Stretch

FIGURE 3-3 Muscle spindles and Golgi tendon organs. A. Nuclear chains and bags with afferent and efferent innervation. **B.** Muscle spindle illustration within a muscle. (Reproduced, with permission, from Afifi AK, Bergman RA. *Functional Neuroanatomy*. 2nd edition. New York, NY: McGraw-Hill; 2005, Fig 1-13, pg. 17.) **C.** Golgi tendon organ. (Reproduced, with permission, from McKinley M, O'Loughlin VD. *Human Anatomy*, 3 ed. New York, NY: McGraw-Hill; 2012, Fig 16.14, pg. 512.)

fiber's conduction induces alpha motor activation to produce a muscle contraction of the muscle, resulting in shortening of the muscle to prevent excessive stretch. This monosynaptic reflex is easily elicited by tapping a striate muscle tendon (i.e., the patellar tendon of the knee) with subsequent muscle contraction (i.e., quadriceps muscle) and is known as a stretch (tendon, monosynaptic) reflex. Simultaneously, a collateral projection of the Ia fiber also innervates inhibitory interneurons to the antagonistic (heteronymous) muscle's alpha motor neuron to induce relaxation of that muscle to allow the agonist to contract and that heteronymous muscle to elongate.

Secondary afferent (II) fibers synapse within the spinal cord on interneurons that, in turn, project both to the homonymous muscle and heteronymous muscle(s); there is also some evidence that these afferents may impact interneurons at multiple spinal levels. II fibers are smaller and slower conducting than their Ia counterparts. Interestingly, II fibers synapse on both alpha and gamma motor neurons, but, similar to Ia fibers, are primarily excitatory, both to alpha motor neurons and to gamma motor neurons (see subsequent section).

Similar to extrafusal fibers, nuclear bags and chains are innervated by efferent motor neurons, both **beta** and **gamma**, that project from the ventral horn of the spinal cord along with the alpha motor neurons that innervate extrafusal fibers. Beta motoneurons innervate both intrafusal and extrafusal fibers while gamma motoneurons innervate only intrafusal fibers. Intrafusal innervation allows for the responsiveness of the muscle spindle to be up or down regulated under the control of higher motor centers but independent of the muscle length of the homonymous muscle. The structure of intrafusal fibers is unique to their function as stretch receptors; for both bags and chains, the contractile components of the fibers are located at the ends of the fiber. Thus, gamma activations results in contraction of these distil contractile elements with subsequent stretching of the central region where the afferent endings are located. Thus, intrafusal fiber contraction is perceived as extrafusal fiber stretch or lengthening.

Each intrafusal fiber type shortens in response to gamma or beta activation; however, the impact of that shortening creates a slightly different effect. Notably, gamma motor neurons can be divided into two types: dynamic and static. Dynamic gamma motor neurons innervate dynamic nuclear bags; static gamma motor neurons innervate static nuclear bags and/or nuclear chains. Contraction of dynamic nuclear bags in response to gamma activation occurs slowly but increases their overall stiffness such that subsequent extrafusal muscle lengthening rapidly increases the firing of the Ia afferent, and thus, enhances length awareness during motion. When activated by gamma excitation, static nuclear bags rapidly increase the Ia firing rate, facilitating awareness of static muscle length and enhancing force generation within the muscle, especially to maintain posture. Nuclear chain activation, via gamma innervation, is the most rapid of the three intrafusal fiber types and enhances its sensitivity to maintained stretch. See Box 3-1 for a description of the functional application of gamma motor control.

There is another receptor associated with the proprioceptive system called the Golgi tendon organ (GTO); as its name suggests, it is located in the tendon near the junction with the muscle, and each is innervated by a single Ib afferent. As described for other afferents, the Ib has its cell body in the dorsal root with a peripheral projection to the GTO and a central projection into the spinal cord. Unlike the Ia afferent of the muscle spindle, the Ib projects only onto interneurons in the spinal gray rather than directly to alpha motor neurons, creating a polysynaptic reflex loop. These interneurons are inhibitory to the homonymous muscle and excitatory to the heteronymous muscle. As its most simple function, the GTO serves as a protective mechanism to prevent excessive tension generation in the homonymous muscle that could lead to muscle or tendon tearing. When activated, it inhibits the contraction of the homonymous muscle and facilitates the contraction of the

| **BOX 3-1** | **Gamma Motor Control of Muscle Spindles: Why?** |

One key question often asked by the student, struggling to understand muscle spindles and their innervation and function, is why change the sensitivity of the muscle spindle? The following example gives an illustration of how this system is used within complex movement. Visualize, for a moment, a diver on a 10-m platform, preparing to complete a backward 2½ flip. He walks to the end of the platform, turns, and very carefully arranges his feet on the end of the platform, coming to stand precariously on his toes. As he maintains this position, it is critical that he be aware of even the slightest sway of his body so as not to lose his balance. Activation of static nuclear bags will increase his awareness of even minimal muscle length change to assist in balance maintenance as he prepares to dive and enhanced force production as he pushes off of the platform. As he pushes off and leaps up into a pike position (hands on ankles, knees straight), the responsiveness of the spindles needs to be down regulated to avoid a stretch response of the back and hamstring muscles that would pull him out of this position. Yet, toward the end of his second rotation, gamma activation of nuclear chains can enhance his positional awareness in preparation for kicking out of the pike position; similarly, dynamic bags in the hamstrings and back extensors can be activated to facilitate his movement into a fully extended position prior to hitting the water. This integration of gamma and alpha motor activity will be further explored in the chapter on motor control.

heteronymous muscle, which is known as the *autogenic inhibition reflex*. However, the role of the GTO is more complex than this polysynaptic reflex, as it serves as a constant monitor of muscle tension with feedback to higher motor centers. Also, descending corticospinal projections are able to modify the reflexive activity of the GTO at the Ib–interneuronal synapse. See Chapters 2 and 4 for more discussion of how these reflexes are incorporated into function.

● DERMATOMES AND SPINAL NERVE ORGANIZATION

Sensory receptors and their afferents aggregate and enter the spinal cord as spinal nerves with one spinal nerve per segment of the cord (cervical, thoracic, lumbar, sacral) except for the first cervical segment (C1), which does not receive sensory projections. Spinal nerves are organized into the many peripheral nerves, learned in gross anatomy and beyond the scope of this text. A dermatome is the area of the skin innervated by a single spinal nerve (Figure 3-4). Surprisingly, multiple dermatome maps have been developed with varying degrees of commonality. However, recent evidence suggests that the differences in these dermatome maps result from the inherent variability of individual dermatome maps and the significant overlap between adjacent dermatomes, which is greater in the limbs and minimal in the midline of the body.[8]

Anterior view

Posterior view

FIGURE 3-4 Dermatome map. (Reproduced, with permission, from McKinley M, O'Loughlin VD. *Human Anatomy*, 3 ed. New York, NY: McGraw-Hill; 2012, Fig 16.6, pg. 495.)

● CENTRAL PROJECTION SYSTEMS

Receptor activation of a magnitude to initiate transduction (the conversion of a stimulus to an action potential within the sensory neuron) is necessary to begin the central projection of the sensation. Sensory neurons have their cell bodies in the dorsal root ganglia with a long dendritic projection to the periphery, attaching to a mechanoreceptor or ending as a free nerve ending, and an axon or central projection that enters the spinal column through the dorsal root. Within the spinal cord, there are two primary pathways that convey sensation from the periphery to the brain: the dorsal-column-medial lemniscal system and the anterolateral system.

Dorsal-Column-Medial Lemniscal Pathway (DCML)

As sensory neurons, conveying tactile sensation, enter the spinal cord they traverse the dorsal horn and enter the dorsal column in a sequential order from the sacral cord to the cervical cord, beginning medially with the sacral neurons and then filling in toward the lateral margins with fibers from the lumbar, thoracic, and finally cervical regions (Figure 3-5).

From the exterior or cross section, the dorsal column is clearly divided into two columns: the fasciculi gracilis (medially located, conveying lower body neurons) and cuneatus (laterally located, conveying upper body neurons). The primary afferents in this system project all of the way to the medulla where they

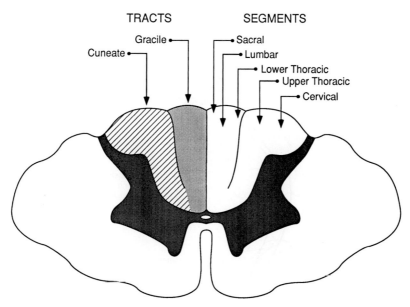

FIGURE 3-5 **Organization of the dorsal column.** (Reproduced, with permission, from Afifi AK, Bergman RA. *Functional Neuroanatomy.* 2nd edition. New York, NY: McGraw-Hill; 2005, Fig 3-8, pg. 53.)

synapse on second-order neurons in their respective nuclei, gracilis and cuneatus, located in the dorsal aspect of the caudal medulla. Here, they synapse on second-order neurons that cross over to the opposite side and then ascend to the thalamus, as the medial lemniscal pathway, where they synapse on third-order neurons in the ventroposteriolateral (VPL) nucleus. These third-order neurons, in turn, project through the posterior limb of the internal capsule, as the thalamic radiations, to the primary sensory cortex (SI), located within the postcentral gyrus (Brodmann's areas 3a, 3b, 1, and 2). The postcentral gyri mirror the primary motor cortices with an inverse body orientation such that the foot is at the top of SI, extending over onto the medial surface of the hemisphere, and the face is located at the bottom of SI (Figure 3-6).

In addition to SI, many other areas are involved in determining the characteristics of sensation: (1) Secondary Somatosensory Cortex (SII) – located above and within the lateral sulcus; (2) Insular Cortex – the cortex deep within the lateral sulcus; (3) Supramarginal gyrus of the temporal lobe; and (4) Posterior Parietal Cortex (Brodmann's areas 5 and 7) – located posterior to SI. There has been much discussion about the projection of sensory information to these higher level processing areas, specifically whether projections are serial, passing through SI to get to other areas, or parallel with third-order sensory neurons projecting directly to SII and the posterior parietal cortex.[9] Of course, some parallel projections could also emanate from the spinothalamic system (see subsequent section). Notably, SI is known to project to each of these sensory areas and interestingly has strong bilateral projections to SI in each hemisphere. We will pick up this discussion in a subsequent section of this chapter.

Anterolateral System (AL)

Just as described in the preceding section for the dorsal column system, nociceptive neurons enter the spinal cord via the dorsal root but differentially enter the posterior aspect of the dorsal horn, forming the Tract of Lissauer, which allows them to ascend or descend up to two spinal segments before synapsing on second-order neurons within the posterior marginalis (Aδ fibers) or nucleus proprious (C fibers) of the dorsal horn within the spinal cord. These second-order neurons then cross to the opposite side of the cord via the anterior commissure and ascend within the anterolateral cord. There are three respective parts to the anterolateral pathway: the spinothalamic tract, the spinoreticular tract, and the spinomesencephalic tract, descriptive of their terminations – the thalamus, reticular formation, and midbrain (Figure 3-6).

The **spinothalamic tract** has, in turn, been identified to have three components: (1) the *neospinothalamic* (ventral spinothalamic) tract, which merges with the medial lemniscal pathway in the brainstem and terminates in the VPL of the thalamus; (2) the *paleospinothalamic* tract (dorsal spinothalamic tract), also called the spinolimbic tract, which is more dorsal and projects to the posterior medial and intralaminar nuclei of the thalamus; and (3) another portion that terminates in the medial central nucleus of the thalamus. Each of these is responsible for different aspects of the pain experience: (1) discrimination of the locus and type of painful stimulus; (2) the motivational component (i.e., the need to change position when you've been sitting or lying too long in one positions); and (3) the affective or emotional response to the stimulus, respectively.[10] It should be noted that spinothalamic fibers also convey a form of crude touch perception, so in the absence of the dorsal column system, some touch information is still conveyed to the cortex via the spinothalamic fibers.

It should be emphasized that the AL ends primarily in the brainstem with only rudimentary projections traversing the brainstem within the spinothalamic projections. The larger **spinoreticular portion** of the AL terminates in two aspects of

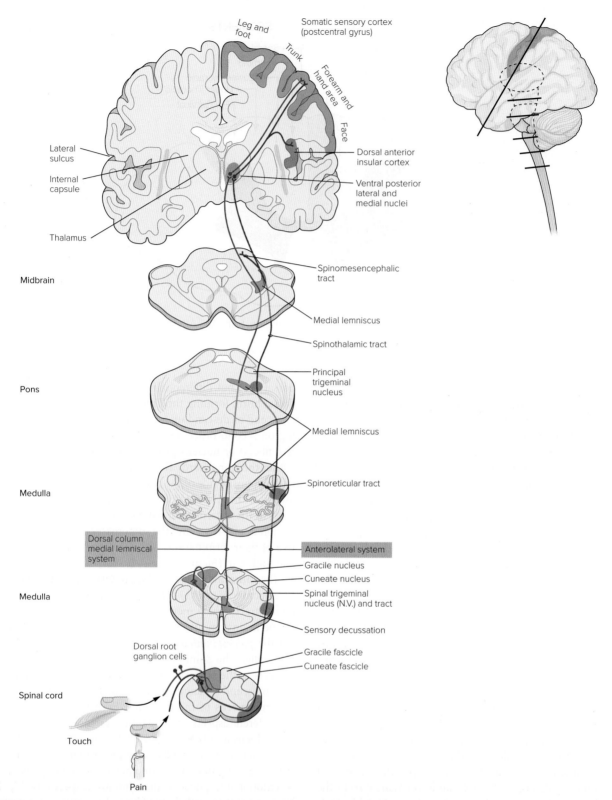

FIGURE 3-6 Ascending somatosensory pathways. (Reproduced, with permission, from Kandel ER, Schwartz JH, Jessell TM, Siegelbaum SA, Hudspeth AJ. *Principles of Neural Science*, 5th ed. New York, NY: McGraw-Hill; 2013, Fig 22-11, Pg 493.)

the reticular formation within the lateral and medial reticular nuclei. The medial nuclei have strong connections to components of the limbic system, and therefore, contribute to the intense emotional responses to persisting pain signals, including depression in chronic pain conditions. The lateral nuclei

also receive input from multiple areas of the motor system, and therefore, may be more involved in the motor response to pain stimuli (i.e., the change in gait pattern to accommodate a painful joint). Interestingly, spinoreticular neurons send collaterals to multiple parts of the brainstem that are associated with pain inhibition (anti-nociception). The **spinomesencephalic** tract also projects to the brainstem, but rather than terminating in the reticular formation, ends in the midbrain, more specifically in the periaqueductal gray (PAG) that surrounds the cerebral aqueduct and the superior colliculus, in the dorsum of the midbrain. Notably, the PAG is an area of anti-nociceptive systems; thus, the spinomesencephalic system along with the collaterals of the spinoreticular pathway work together to activate systems that function to decrease the pain experience. Projections to the superior colliculus are responsible for the reflexive visual orientation to a painful stimulus. See Box 3-2 for a description of pain perception and Box 3-3 for pain modulation.

as the tissue of the cut heals. Without these powerful anti-nociceptive systems, our pain experiences would be much more intense and most likely intolerable; anti-nociceptive activity is noted at every level of the pain projecting pathways to modify our pain experiences. Obviously a paper cut is a minor pain experience; however, this same process occurs in the presence of larger pain situations, and many current treatments for pain are designed to augment the natural endogenous anti-nociception process.

BOX 3-2 What happens when we experience pain?

A simple example of the complexity of the pain experience is a paper cut to your finger. The first thing perceived is a tactile sensation, conveyed by the large A fibers from mechanoreceptors in the fingertip, that your fingertip was "touched" by the paper. This is quickly followed by a perception of acute pain, initiated by Aδ fiber projections from nociceptors (free nerve endings); however, even before your primary sensory cortex has processed where and what has happened, your eyes move to look in the direction of your hand, and you have probably sworn or mumbled a verbal response to the pain that you're now experiencing. The reflexive motions of your hand away from the paper, your eye orientation to look at your hand, and the verbal expletive result from the projections of the spinoreticular and spinomesencephalic tracts as well as reflex units in the spinal cord (look for a detailed explanation in the spinal cord chapter).

However, your pain experience has just begun. Once a painful stimulus is experienced, your body responds in two ways. One, there is a rush of endogenous molecules to the traumatized tissue, including histamine, bradykinin, Substance P, and prostaglandins.[11] These molecules repetitively depolarize nociceptors, activating pain afferent fibers (typically C fibers), and resulting in the ongoing chronic pain perception that will last for several days.

Yet, a second series of events is also in process as collaterals from second-order pain afferents in the brainstem target the sites of powerful endogenous anti-nociceptive (anti-pain) systems, originating in the PAG, reticular formation, and other brainstem nuclei (locus ceruleus, raphe nuclei) (Figure 3-7). These descending pain modulating systems release serotonin, norepinephrine, and other endogenous opiates (opiate-like substances within the body) to decrease the perception of pain. One site of their activity is the synapses in the spinal cord between first- and second-order pain neurons in the anterolateral pathway where they can act as either presynaptic or postsynaptic inhibitors through multiple mechanisms (e.g., neurotransmitter deregulation, postsynaptic hyperpolarization). Similarly, circulating endogenous opiates, such as beta-endorphin, function at the periphery to impede the action of histamine and other nociceptive molecules' depolarization of nociceptors. Thus, this tiny paper cut induces a battle between nociception and anti-nociception that will continue for several days

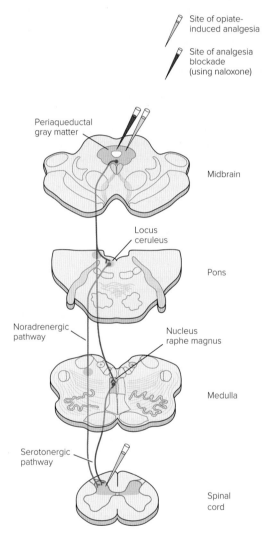

FIGURE 3-7 Descending pain modulating pathways. (Reproduced, with permission, from Kandel ER, Schwartz JH, Jessell TM, Siegelbaum SA, Hudspeth AJ. *Principles of Neural Science*, 5th ed. New York, NY: McGraw-Hill; 2013, Fig 24-15, Pg 548.)

Spinocerebellar Systems

Ia, Ib, and II fibers from muscle spindles and GTOs are not just involved in reflexive mechanisms within the spinal cord; they also contribute to our sense of proprioception through projections to the cerebellum and cortex. Notably, some proprioceptive information is conveyed via mechanoreceptors from the skin and joint capsule, primarily the Ruffini endings, within the

FIGURE 3-8 Schematic of the Gate Theory of Pain. (Reproduced, with permission, from Kandel ER, Schwartz JH, Jessell TM, Siegelbaum SA, Hudspeth AJ. *Principles of Neural Science*, 5th ed. New York, NY: McGraw-Hill; 2013, Fig 24-14, Pg 548.)

DCML system. However, collaterals of the Ia, Ib, and II fibers involved in the spinal reflexes also synapse on second-order neurons within the spinal dorsal gray matter that project rostrally. These second-order neurons convey information to the cerebellum within the spinocerebellar system.

These collaterals of Ia, Ib, and II sensory afferents from the lower extremities and trunk terminate in Clarke's nucleus or column within the lumbar and thoracic dorsal gray matter. Projections from Clarke's nucleus make up both the ventral and dorsal spinocerebellar tracts, which convey information from the lower extremities and trunk to the cerebellum. The dorsal spinocerebellar tract is located in the dorsolateral aspect of the spinal cord, enters the cerebellum via the inferior peduncle, and terminates primarily in the ipsilateral vermis and paravermal cortex but also projects to the deep cerebellar nuclei.[13]

Notably, the dorsal spinocerebellar tract is associated with proprioceptive information from the legs and trunk; however, the ventral spinocerebellar tract, which is also associated with the lower extremities and trunk, appears tightly linked to the descending motor systems, receiving the motor plan during active movement and providing feedback to the cerebellum relative to movement progression. This feedback allows for adaptation of the movement as it is occurring.

Upper extremity proprioception from Ia, Ib, and II fibers is also conveyed centrally, but the systems conveying this information have received little study in humans, in part, because we do not locomote on all fours, and therefore, unconscious proprioception plays a less significant role in arm control. However, proprioception from the arms and upper trunk ascends within the dorsal column and synapses within the external, also called the accessory, cuneate nucleus (ACN) within the medulla adjacent to the cuneate nucleus. From the ACN, it projects to the cerebellum within the inferior cerebellar peduncle, projecting to the interposed nuclei of the cerebellum.

SENSORY PROJECTIONS FROM THE FACE

The preceding discussion of sensory systems has focused on sensation emanating from the extremities and trunk; however, the structures of the face, including the eyes, nose, and ears, and oral cavity also have well-organized sensory projections. Tactile sensitivity from the face and many oral structures (2/3 of the tongue as well as the teeth, cheeks, and gums) is conveyed within the trigeminal nerve (cranial nerve V); the remainder of the tongue is conveyed via the glossopharyngeal nerve (IX). The vagus nerve (X) transmits tactile sensation from the external and internal ear as well as the internal organs (Table 3-2).

Similar to what has been described for sensation from the body, sensation from the face and oral structures involves mechanoreceptors, proprioceptors, and free nerve endings to

TABLE 3-2	Somatosensory Function from the Head and Internal Organs
CRANIAL NERVE	**AREAS OF SOMATOSENSORY FUNCTION**
V	Ophthalmic branch: Cornea, nose, upper eyelid, forehead, anterior scalp Maxillary branch: Lower eyelid, nasal mucosa, upper lip, palate, gums, cheek Mandibular branch: Anterior 2/3 tongue, chin, lower jaw and teeth, 1/3 auricle of ear
IX	Posterior 1/3 of tongue
X	Pharynx, larynx, chest and abdominal organs, external ear

allow detection of cutaneous sensations. In fact, in should be evident that the face, and more specifically the mouth, is capable of the highest level of sensory discrimination.

First-order sensory neurons within the trigeminal nerve have their cell bodies in what is known as the trigeminal ganglion, located within the skull just above the cheekbone (maxilla), with a central projection that terminates in the sensory nuclear complex of cranial nerve V in the pons, medulla, and upper spinal cord. Sensory fibers from both CN IX and X have their cell bodies in the superior and inferior ganglia, located caudal to the trigeminal ganglion, just inside the jugular foramina.

This trigeminal sensory complex is divided into the principal nucleus in the pons and the elongated spinal nucleus in the medulla. Trigeminal sensory fibers enter the brainstem and course upward or downward to these two nuclei within the trigeminal sensory tract, which caudally aligns with the dorsal horn of the spinal cord and is evident in the upper cervical segments (C1–C3). Both nuclei have a somatotropic organization related to the fiber origination from the face; most caudal are the fibers innervating the mandibular area, followed by the maxillary representation and finally the ophthalmic portion

most rostral; however, the most ventral segments of the face (e.g., the nose) are more dorsal and the more dorsal aspects (e.g., the ears) are more ventral within the tract.[14] There is also a separation within the sensory complex of V between large and small diameter neuron projections with large diameter fibers located dorsally and terminating primarily in the principal nucleus and rostral portions of the spinal nucleus while smaller diameter projections course ventrally and terminate in the caudal portion of the spinal nucleus.

Those fibers conveying tactile information merge in the rostral or principal portion of the trigeminal complex, decussate upon exiting within the pons, and join the DCML system on its way to the thalamus where they synapse primarily in the ventroposteriomedial (VPM) nucleus; thereafter, their third-order projections travel with those of the DCML to the sensory cortex within the thalamic radiations (Figure 3-9). Within the primary sensory cortex, there is a large somatotropic representation of the face and oral structures, allowing for the high level of sensory processing of sensation from these areas.

Fibers from cranial nerves IX (glossopharyngeal) and X (vegas) that are conveying pain join with those from the

Cerebral cortex and thalamus

Posterior limb of internal capsule

Primary somatic sensory cortex

Secondary somatic sensory cortex

Ventral posterior medial nucleus

Midbrain

Dorsal trigemino-thalamic tract

Trigeminal lemniscus

Pons

Main trigeminal sensory nucleus

Mechanoreceptive fibers in cranial nerves V, VII, IX, and X

FIGURE 3-9 Trigeminal pathways for somatosensory function. (Reproduced with permission, from Martin JH. *Neuroanatomy Text and Atlas*, 4th ed. New York, NY: McGraw-Hill; 2012, Figure 6-8, pg. 139.)

face (CN V) within the spinal portion of the trigeminal sensory nucleus. Ultimately each crosses to the opposite side within the anterior commissure of the upper cervical segments of the spinal cord and then ascends through the spinal cord and brainstem along with the anterolateral pathway, terminating and sending collaterals to the same areas already discussed for that pathway; however, those aligning with the lateral spinothalamic pathway terminate in VPM along with the facial tactile fibers.

HIGHER LEVEL SENSORY PROCESSING

A growing area of research is aimed at determining how the brain interprets sensation. Our ability to distinguish tactile stimulus characteristics is complex, ranging from the most simple identification of stimulation detection that allows the determination of location, duration, and intensity of the stimulus to the complex determination of multiple object characteristics such as shape, weight, size, texture, and temperature, and the more complex abilities of stereognosis and graphesthesia. Research, using multiple imaging modalities, has allowed us to identify the many areas of the brain involved in these simple and complex sensory perception and discrimination abilities.

As mentioned earlier in the chapter, sensory projecting systems, DCML and AL, have third-order projections that terminate in the primary sensory cortex (SI). Direct thalamic projections have also been found to the secondary sensory cortex (SII), so there is some level of both parallel (at the same time) and sequential (SI first, then SII) sensory processing within these two areas. For the most part, parallel processing is most associated with temperature, pain and vibration perception, and serial processing with most tactile stimuli.[9] SI is uniquely organized into four distinct sensory areas (3a, 3b, 1, and 2), associated with the originating sensory receptor type and resulting in four somatotopic representations of each area of the body.[15] SI is also known to project to the ipsilateral posterior parietal (areas 5 and 7), supramarginal gyrus, intraparietal sulcus, and insular cortex; these latter areas are also known as the lateral somatosensory area. Neurons in SI also project to the contralateral SII and posterior parietal cortex. The insular cortex may also receive some direct sensory projections from dorsal column neurons.

The intricacies in the organization of SI and the connections radiating from its four subareas to SII, the posterior parietal cortex, the lateral sensory area, and the contralateral hemisphere induce activation in an even broader neural network for the determination of object characteristics (Figure 3-10). This network includes dorsal aspects of the prefrontal cortex bilaterally with a dominant level of activity in the right hemisphere.[16,17] There are also connections with speech centers to allow object identification/naming and memory areas within the temporal lobe to maintain tactile memories; the latter is also thought to involve SII. Since active touch to identify object characteristics (haptics) involves active manipulation of the object, activity within the primary motor area (M1) is typically reported with this active exploration. Simple touch perception is associated

FIGURE 3-10 Sensory discrimination: Is associated with functional magnetic resonance activation in a network of SI and lateral somatosensory area, bilateral SII, and dorsal prefrontal cortex bilaterally. (Used with permission of Deborah S. Nichols Larsen, PT, PhD. The Ohio State University.)

with localized activity in SI contralateral to the stimulation, but any type of tactile discrimination, whether for texture, weight, or size, initiates activation in this broader network of SII, the lateral sensory area, and the dorsal prefrontal cortex. Stereognosis, as one of the most complex sensory discrimination abilities, requires activation in memory and speech centers.

Sensory Testing

Common sensory screening techniques are described in Chapter 9 (Evaluation). Logically, sensory screening focuses on touch localization, the discrimination of sharp versus dull stimuli, hot/cold discrimination, and simple proprioception and kinesthesia awareness by having patients identify where a limb or body part is in space or mirroring passive movement of a limb or body part by the examiner with movement of the opposite limb or body part. This method of screening provides insight into potential sensory deficits; however, further testing is warranted if any of these simple screening methods identify deficits. Notably, some sensory deficits are missed when only these screening tests are completed, since there are conditions that disrupt higher level sensory discrimination ability but have little impact on touch localization or proprioception. Table 3-3 highlights a few tests that can be used in the clinic to evaluate sensory skills; these are especially focused on hand and upper extremity function, since most higher level sensory discrimination involves use of the hands. For many of these tests, there are commercial items available for purchase; a few of these that should be used in the clinic are described. However, adequate testing can often be completed with constructed materials or items easily available to the practitioner. Some of these methods are also described in Table 9-4. It is important for the clinician to incorporate these methods into their assessment and progressive evaluation during treatment to determine improvement in dysfunction and improvement in many neurologic conditions. Recently, training paradigms that focus on improving sensation and movement have been described.

TABLE 3-3	Somatosensory Testing Methods	
DOMAIN	**TEST**	**DESCRIPTION**
TOUCH PERCEPTION	Semmes Weinstein Monofilaments™	Monofilaments applied in a descending order until the subject is unable to detect a stimulus; identifies the lightest filament detected.
	WEST (Weinstein enhanced Sensory Test)™	Five monofilaments have been selected from the Semmes Weinstein battery to provide an abbreviated testing procedure; sensitivity is identified as the smallest filament detected.
	Locognosia	The fingertip is divided into specific areas and the individual detects the area of the touch. Stimulus is a monofilament determined to be detectible by the individual.[18]
TWO POINT DISCRIMINATION	Static	Testing is done with a Disk-Criminator™ (or other device) to allow the smallest distance that two points of contact on the skin can be differentiated from a single point. Norms are available.
	Moving	Similar to static testing, a device is used with two points separated by different distances versus a single point. The smallest two point separation that can be distinguished as they are drawn across the hand or other body part is recorded.
SENSORY DISCRIMINATION	Sharp/dull	Frequently uses random application of a pencil eraser and a pin for discrimination of the two sensations. Used frequently with spinal cord injuries to screen the integrity of the two ascending systems.
	Hot/Cold	Multiple testing methods are available for purchase, but testing can include hot/cold water tubs or test tubes, plastic "ice" cubes frozen versus room temperature, or another method.
	Tactile Grating Orientation	Typically uses a set of plastic domes. Each dome has groves/ridges of equal width. The widths vary in decreasing distances. The domes are oriented either parallel or perpendicular to the finger alignment. Response as to orientation is recorded.[19]
	Roughness	There are a variety of commercially available devices to test roughness discrimination, including the domes used for tactile grating orientation. Some involve a continuous progressive grating device engraved with wide to small ridges; testing involves swiping the fingertip across the device and stopping when the ridges can no longer be detected.
	Weight	Can be done with different weights in each hand or comparing weights with the same hand. The heavier the weights, the larger the difference necessary for a detectable difference (e.g., at <10 g, a 1-g difference can be detected; at 100 g, a 7–10 g difference can be detected).
	Stereognosis	A variety of familiar objects can be used that should fit into the hand (e.g., paperclip, coin, marble); verbal influences can be eliminated by providing a picture array of included objects (some non-included objects in the picture array will make the task more challenging). Also, familiar/unfamiliar shapes can be used (circle, oval, square, octagon, or irregular shapes such as a puzzle piece) as well as letters (e.g., plastic or wood children's toys). Commercially available tests can be used.
	Graphesthesia	Letters or numbers can be drawn with the tester's fingertip or utensil (i.e., eraser end of a pencil) on hand or other body part. Verbal response or matching to a visual array can be used.

REFERENCES

1. Libouton X, Barbier O, Plaghki L, Thonnard J. Tactile roughness discrimination threshold is unrelated to tactile spatial acuity. *Behav Brain Res.* 2010;28:473-478.

2. McGlone F, Reilly D. The cutaneous system. *Neurosci Behav Rev.* 2010;34:148-159.

3. Godfrey H. Understanding pain, part 1: physiology of pain. *Brit J Nursing.* 2003;14(16):846-852.

4. Fortier S, Basset FA. The effects of exercise on limb proprioceptive signals. *J Electromyogr Kinesiol.* 2012;22:795-802.

5. Gilman S. Joint position sense and vibration sense: anatomical organization and assessment. *J Neurol Neurosurg Psychiatry.* 2002;73:473-477.

6. Proske U, Ganegia, SC. The kinaesthetic senses. *J Physiol.* 2009;17:4139-4146.

7. Fitz-Ritson D. The anatomy and physiology of the muscle spindle and its role in posture and movement: a review. *J Can Chiropractic Assoc.* 1982;26(4):144-150.

8. Lee MWL, McPhee RW, Stringer MD. An evidence-based approach to human dermatomes. *Clin Anat.* 2008;21:363-373.

9. Knecht S, Kunesch E, Schnitzler A. Parallel and serial processing of haptic information in man: effects of parietal lesions on sensorimotor hand function. *Neuropsychologia*. 1996;34(7):669-687.

10. Almeida TF, Roizenblatt S, Tufik S. Afferent pain pathways: a neuroanatomical review. *Brain Res*. 2004;1000:40-56.

11. Pergolizzi J, Ahlbeck K, Aldington D, Alon E, et al. The development of chronic pain: physiological CHANGE necessitates a multidisciplinary approach to treatment. *Curr Med Res Opin*. 2013;1-9.

12. Melzack R, Wall PD. Pain mechanisms: a new theory. *Science*. 1965;150:971-979.

13. Bosco G, Poppele RE. Proprioception from a spinocerebellar perspective. *Physiol Rev*. 2001;81(2):539-568.

14. DaSilva AFM, Becerra L, Makris N, Strassman AM, et al. Somatotopic activation in the human trigeminal pain pathway. *J Neurosci*. 2002;22(18):8183-8192.

15. Romo R, Lemus L, de Lafuente V. Sense, memory, and decision-making in the somatosensory cortical network. *Curr Opin Neurol*. 2012; 22:914-919.

16. Harada T, Saito DN, Kashikura K, Sato T, et al. Asymmetrical neural substrates of tactile discrimination in humans: a functional magnetic resonance imaging study. *J Neurosci*. 2004;24(34):7524-7530.

17. Borstad A, Schmalbrock P, Choi S, Nichols-Larsen DS. Neural correlates supporting sensory discrimination after left hemispheric stroke. *Brain Res*. 2012;1460:78-87.

18. Jerosch-Herold C, Rosen B, Shepstone L. The reliability and validity of the Locognosia test after injuries to peripheral nerves in hand. *J Bone Joint Surg*. 2006;88-B:1048-1052.

19. Bleyenheuft Y, Thonnard JL. Tactile spatial resolution measured manually: a validation study. *Somatosens Mot Res*. 2007;24(3):111-114.

Review Questions

1. **Your patient is experiencing contralateral loss of pain and ipsilateral loss of touch on their right leg; where would a lesion be to produce these symptoms?**
   A. Spinal cord
   B. Upper medulla
   C. Ventroposterior nucleus of the thalamus
   D. Sensory cortex

2. **Similarly, at what level in the projections of sensation, would you expect a lesion to create contralateral loss of both pain/temperature and touch?**
   A. Above the lower medulla
   B. Below the lower medulla

3. **If there were a condition that resulted in the absence of Ruffini receptors, what types of sensation would be disrupted?**
   A. Tension and touch
   B. Touch and stretch
   C. Pain and touch
   D. Tension and pain

4. **Which is a monosynaptic reflex?**
   A. Ib activation of the heteronymous muscle
   B. Ib activation of the homonymous muscle
   C. Ia activation of the heteronymous muscle
   D. Ia activation of the homonymous muscle

5. **Which commonly used sensory test requires no additional equipment to perform?**
   A. Sharp/dull
   B. Graphesthesia
   C. Stereognosis
   D. Two point discrimination

6. **A stroke disrupting the medial posterior thalamic nucleus would disrupt sensation from which part of the body?**
   A. Arms
   B. Legs
   C. Face
   D. Trunk

7. **Your patient is experiencing hyperalgesia on the left side of her face, occurring when her hair touches it. Damage to what cranial nerve, associated with facial sensation, would it most likely be associated with?**
   A. Cranial nerve V
   B. Cranial nerve VII
   C. Cranial nerve IX
   D. Cranial nerve X

8. **Damage to the most medial part of the dorsal column in the cervical spinal cord would disrupt sensation from which spinal nerve roots?**
   A. Cervical
   B. Thoracic
   C. Lumbar
   D. Sacral

9. **Damage to Clarke's nucleus would disrupt what sensory function emanating from the legs?**
   A. Pain
   B. Proprioception
   C. Touch perception
   D. Stereognosis

10. **Of the components of the anterolateral pathway, which is most associated with the emotional aspects of our pain experience?**
    A. Neospinothalamic tract
    B. Spinomesencephalic tract
    C. Spinoreticular tract
    D. Ventral spinothalamic tract

Answers

1. A	**2.** A	**3.** B
6. C	**7.** A	**8.** D

4. D	**5.** B
9. B	**10.** B

Sensorimotor Systems of the Spinal Cord

D. Michele Basso

4

● INTRODUCTION

This chapter will explore how the spinal cord is organized to produce complex movements. There is an orchestrated, precise balance between the type of afferent information entering the cord and how it is integrated by neurons in the gray matter of the spinal cord to activate muscles. The difference between a simple movement like the patellar tendon reflex and running on a treadmill can be as little as adding a set of interneurons to the monosynaptic circuit. We will consider how the spinal cord is designed to support multi-joint movements that adapt to the changing environment and unexpected perturbations within milliseconds. This chapter will show you that the spinal cord is organized in remarkable ways so that even a few neurons can mediate and sustain intricate, complex movements without input from the brain. Probably the most exciting feature we will consider is that the spinal cord can learn tasks independent of the brain. With this functional capacity existing in the cord, the brain can provide descending input and create even more complex, skilled movements.

Structure and Organization of the Spinal Cord

The human spinal cord extends from the base of the skull to the vertebral level between L1 and L2 (Figure 4-1). It contains four general regions named for the body location in which it resides – cervical, thoracic, lumbar, and sacral. Each region receives afferent information and sends motor signals to nearby muscles – **Cervical** supplies the arms and hands; **Thoracic** supplies the trunk; **Lumbar** supplies the legs and feet; and **Sacral** supplies the bowel, bladder, and genitalia.

The spinal cord is comprised of **gray matter** where neuronal cell bodies reside, surrounded by **white matter** that consists of ascending axons to the brain, descending axons from the brain, and propriospinal axons connecting different regions of the cord (Figure 4-2). **Myelin**, a white protein, wraps each ascending, descending, and propriospinal axon and is critical in facilitating fast signal propagation. It is possible to identify specific regions of the cord from cross sections based on the relationship between the gray matter and the white matter.

In regions that supply many muscles as in the upper and lower extremities, the gray matter will be larger, since more motor neurons will reside there than in areas like the thoracic cord, which primarily supplies intercostal muscles. In addition, the area of white matter will be larger in the cervical region than in the lumbar or sacral region because ascending branches of sensory axons are continually added from the sacral cord to the brain and few descending axons extend all the way to the sacral cord.

The gray matter also has a standard organization throughout the length of the cord. The shape of the gray matter resembles a butterfly and can be divided into three broad regions: the dorsal horn, the ventral horn, and the intermediate or interneuronal region between the two.

The **dorsal horn** consists of several layers of neurons that receive afferent input, described in detail in Chapter 3 – Sensory Pathways and Perception. The **ventral horn** contains alpha motor neuron pools for each of the muscles in the body (Figure 4-2). These pools are generally divided into **medial groups** that supply axial muscles and **lateral groups** that innervate distal muscle groups. The **spinal interneurons** in the **intermediate zone** make up networks for organization of multi-joint muscle synergies within a limb and other typical movement patterns. They connect both sides of the cord and coordinate the action of the axial motor pools to allow for alternating movements of the legs and arms while walking as well as other actions. In contrast, the lateral motor pools have few interneuronal connections with the opposite side of the cord. This allows us to move each hand or foot independent of each other. In the thoracic and upper lumbar regions of the cord, the intermediate gray matter has a prominent lateral horn where neurons of the autonomic nervous system are located. These neurons make up the sympathetic nervous system that controls body responses in emergency situations like dilating the pupils and increasing the heart rate as introduced in Chapter 1.

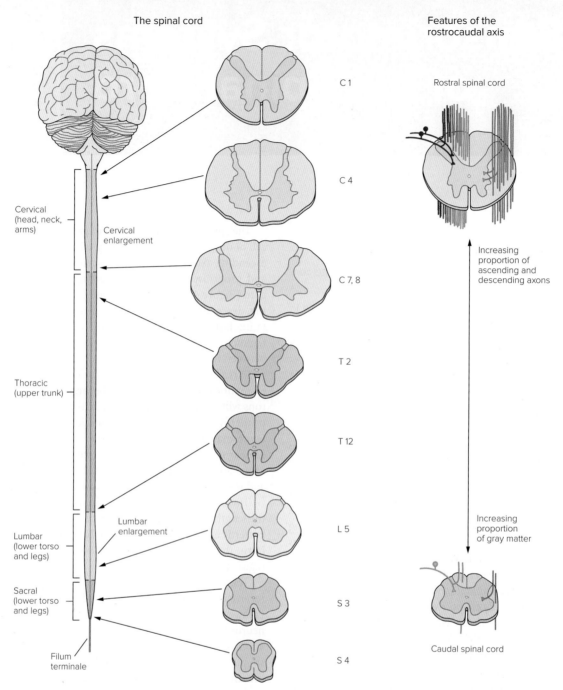

FIGURE 4-1 Internal and external appearance of the spinal cord. (Reproduced with permission from Kandel ER, Schwartz JH, Jessell TM, Siegelbaum SA, Hudspeth AJ. *Principles of Neural Science*, 5th ed. New York, NY: McGraw-Hill; 2013, Figure 16-2, pg 359.)

● BUILDING BLOCKS OF MOVEMENT: MUSCLES AND MOTOR NEURONS

In normal movement, we do not recruit one muscle cell at a time; we recruit an entire **motor unit**, which is defined as one alpha motoneuron and the muscle cells it innervates. In the normal, healthy condition, each time that an alpha motoneuron generates an action potential at the neuromuscular junctions of the innervated muscle, a muscle twitch occurs in every one of its muscle cells. This is the most basic level of movement that can

occur. The job of the nervous system is to organize the multitude of twitches into simple movements like finger tapping as well as the precise movements of ballet or the strength and agility of a running back.

Not all motor units are identical. Several factors differ between motor units, including the number and type of muscle fibers that make up the unit. Some have a relatively small number of muscle fibers in the motor unit, and some have many. Some are comprised of small, **slow twitch** muscle fibers with good endurance that produce low force while some are

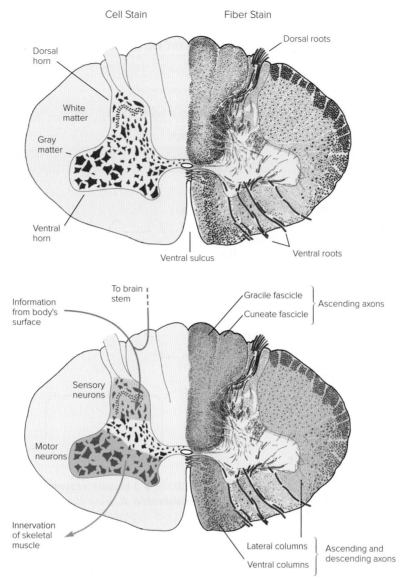

FIGURE 4-2 Organization of the gray and white matter of the spinal cord. (Reproduced with permission from Kandel ER, Schwartz JH, Jessell TM, Siegelbaum SA, Hudspeth AJ. *Principles of Neural Science*, 5th ed. New York, NY: McGraw-Hill; 2013, Figure 16-1, pg 357.)

composed of large, **fast twitch** muscle fibers with high force production capacity but fatigue quickly. And, some are intermediate in these properties. As illustrated in Table 4-1, these properties all go together in certain combinations that provide the nervous system with a menu of choices for the control of movement. For example, whether standing in front of a class or sitting on a stool, we control posture using relatively low force and lasting endurance, recruiting primarily muscle tissue that is highly resistant to fatigue. Smaller motor units with slow twitch muscle fibers are ideally suited to this task. If the person who is standing or sitting reaches for a pen, a greater force impulse will be needed to launch the hand on its trajectory while maintaining a stable posture, but full-blown effort won't be used. Here, a combination of small and intermediate motor units would be recruited to perform these postural and reaching tasks. This reaching task would not require much, if any, recruitment of the largest motor units. However, if we were to throw a ball across the room from our standing or sitting posture, we would

need to recruit additional motor units that produce high force for brief periods. Thus, layered with small, slow motor units for postural control, we would add intermediate motor units to initiate arm trajectory and lastly, our largest, fast twitch-high force motor units would be needed to produce enough arm velocity to propel the ball a long distance.

One of the more convenient tricks of biology for the control of muscle recruitment is described in a phenomenon called the **size principle**, which was extensively studied by E. Henneman.[1] As described above, we would like the first motor units brought into use for the control of low-level effort, where subtle modulation of force is required, to be the smaller motor units with slow twitch muscle fibers. We would not want the largest ones active in this situation because they would make us overshoot the mark. Conversely, if we are in a circumstance where we need maximum muscle force, the slow twitch, smaller motor units are welcome to join in the effort, but we will ultimately need the largest, fast twitch units to get the job done. With few

TABLE 4-1	Classification of Motor Units		
	SLOW	**FAST FATIGABLE**	**FAST FATIGUE RESISTANT**
Fiber type	Type 1; red	Type IIb, IIx; white	Type IIa; red
Motor unit size	Small	Intermediate	Large
Oxidative capacity	High, aerobic	Low, anaerobic	Mix, anaerobic
Force production	Low	High	Intermediate
Contraction time	Long	Rapid	Rapid

exceptions, the nervous system follows this principle of size in recruitment order.

This occurs somewhat automatically because the alpha motoneurons for the smaller, slow twitch motor units are smaller neurons. With a given amount of synaptic drive for excitation, a smaller motoneuron experiences a more substantial voltage change and is, therefore, easier to bring above threshold for an action potential. A larger motoneuron requires a greater amount of synaptic input to become excited. Hence, if the nervous system simply targets small and large motoneurons equally and drives them all without distinction, the natural result is that with low levels of drive to the motoneurons, only the smaller ones will be activated. With a full-blown effort, the small and the large will be activated. Hence, the proper recruitment order comes about naturally, simply based on the sizes of the alpha motoneurons.

Putting the Building Blocks Together

The nervous system activates the different motor units in a selective, organized way to produce finely graded force. For small precise movements like those of the eye and eardrum, small motor units are recruited that have very few muscle fibers. A motor unit in an extraoccular muscle has about 10 fibers. When intermediate control is needed, such as hoisting a hammer, units with more muscle fibers will be recruited. The intrinsic muscles of the hand have a few hundred fibers in each motor unit. When general motor function with a high level of force is required like jumping up to catch a rebound, motor units with a high number of muscle fibers will be activated. In the gastrocnemius, a single motor unit contains about 2000 muscle fibers. We can now see that the muscular system is capable of contracting in a graded fashion to produce forces that match the needs of the task. These gradations are determined by the firing rate of the alpha motor neuron.

The force, speed, and duration of muscle contraction are determined in the spinal cord. The firing rate of the alpha motor neuron modulates muscle force. A slow firing rate of the motor neuron means that the time between one action potential and the next is long enough to allow the motor unit (all muscle cells innervated by a single alpha motor neuron) to fully relax before the next action potential arrives. The long intervals and slow firing rate produce low levels of muscle force that quickly dissipate (Figure 4-3). This type of activity would be a muscle twitch. When the firing rate is increased to an intermediate level, the interval between action potentials shortens and the muscle doesn't fully relax before the second action potential causes a contraction. The contractile force from the second impulse piggybacks on the first, which is known as **summation**, and causes

FIGURE 4-3 Muscle activation and force production relationship. A. Slow firing rate with muscle relaxation between next action potential. **B.** Intermediate firing rate with summation of muscle contraction and greater force. **C.** Fast firing rate with only minimal relaxation and greater force production. **D.** Maximal firing rate and maximal force.

greater force production. In this way, even a slightly faster firing rate can produce substantially higher contraction forces. This type of activity would occur when standing upright to overcome gravity. With a fast firing rate of the motor neuron, the interval between action potentials is very short, so muscle force increases quickly and very little relaxation occurs. Therefore, force levels remain high and each successive action potential produces small fluctuations in force. This is called **unfused tetanus** and occurs during high force activities like weight lifting or a maximal voluntary contraction. There is also an experimental condition that can produce even greater contractile forces; the motor axon is stimulated at a very fast rate, which is higher than the motor neuron can produce on its own. In this condition, there is almost no interval between action potentials and maximum force is immediately generated. Because there is no relaxation, the force is sustained without fluctuation and is called **fused tetanus**.

How much does the firing have to change to produce gradations in muscle force? Even very small changes to the firing rate can modulate muscle force and produce different patterns of movement. Adding an extra action potential or eliminating

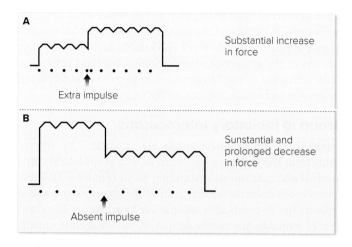

FIGURE 4-4 Gradations in force. Changes in force generation accompany changes in action potential train generation. **A.** An additional impulse creates an increase in force. **B.** An omitted impulse will decrease force.

one from a train of impulses will reset the contractile force. In studies by Burke, adding a single extra impulse to a high firing rate caused the force to summate. This higher level of force was maintained throughout the train of impulses (Figure 4-4A). Likewise, removing a single impulse from a train of action potentials immediately reduces muscle force that is sustained with each subsequent impulse (Figure 4-4B). This means that if the alpha motor neuron simply adds or omits a single action potential from a group of impulses, then a substantial and sustained change in muscle force occurs. The next chapter will consider how features of the muscle and motor neuron recruitment contribute to contractile force determination.

We know that muscle activity is dictated by the firing rate and pattern of the alpha motor neuron, so the next factor to consider is how alpha motor neuron firing is controlled. There are three sources of input that drive motor neuron activity – descending axons from nuclei in the brain, sensory afferents from the periphery, and interneurons within the spinal cord. Descending brain systems will be discussed in the next chapter.

Afferent Drive

Organization of complex movements begins at the level of the spinal cord and builds upon the simplest movement – the muscle spindle stretch reflex. As we have seen in the previous chapter, the stretch reflex is monosynaptic, meaning that the primary sensory afferents from the muscle spindle synapse directly on the motor neuron. A quick stretch of the muscle stimulates the Ia afferent, which elicits firing of the alpha motor neurons that innervate the stretched muscle. The resulting muscle contraction relieves the stretch. This monosynaptic relationship allows for rapid changes in motor neuron firing based on proprioceptive feedback from the periphery. Small stretches of the muscle will change the firing rate, which in turn will produce gradations in force and movement. In this way, proprioceptive input to the cord influences motor neuron activation. It is upon this background that all volitional, purposeful movement is orchestrated.

To engage in purposeful movement, the activation and coordination of many motor neurons and the muscles they innervate

must occur. One process, called **divergence**, creates widely distributed motor neuron ensembles. In divergence, axon collaterals from a single neuron synapse on specific, distributed groups of neurons and, when activated, produce coordinated responses. Divergence occurs in the monosynaptic reflex where the afferent axon sends collateral branches to motor neurons of synergist muscles and to interneurons in the gray matter.[2] The input to the synergistic motor neurons enables a more effective movement. Divergence of afferent drive also occurs within a single muscle that has several divisions like the extensor digitorum (ED) of the hand. By ordering synaptic input to subsets of motor neurons for the ED, extension of one finger is synchronized with the other fingers.[3] Thus, we can begin to see that sending common proprioceptive input to distributed neurons will produce coordinated, synchronized muscle action across multiple joints. Divergence of synaptic input occurs in all neurons in the nervous system.

Spinal Interneurons

Interneurons are located in the gray matter of the spinal cord and receive inputs from peripheral afferents and descending axons from brain nuclei. Interneurons consolidate these multiple signals, compare them, and determine whether the signal is passed onto the motor neuron. Interneurons can be defined by their relationship to the motor neuron, the type of afferent input they receive, and whether they are excitatory or inhibitory. The last interneuron to synapse onto the motor neuron is called the **last order interneuron**, and these have been the most studied type of interneurons in the spinal cord. While many last order interneurons have been identified in mammals (Figure 4-5), three have been characterized in terms of their role in

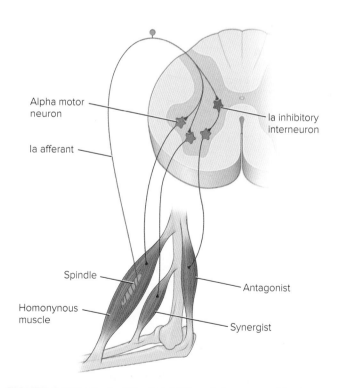

FIGURE 4-5 Diagram of the Ia inhibitory interneuron. The Ia inhibitory interneuron is activated by a collateral of the Ia afferent and serves to inhibit the antagonistic muscle to allow the reflexive contraction of the homonymous muscle and its agonists.

modulating muscle contraction: the 1a inhibitory interneuron, the Renshaw cell, and the 1b inhibitory interneuron.

Ia Inhibitory Interneuron

The Ia inhibitory interneuron plays an important role in the stretch reflex. If we consider a stretch reflex of the biceps tendon, the Ia afferent from the muscle spindle sends axon collaterals not only to the motor neurons of the biceps and the synergistic brachioradialis muscle but also sends a branch to the Ia inhibitory interneuron (Figure 4-5). The Ia inhibitory interneuron synapses on the motor neurons of the antagonist triceps muscle and stops its activity. This is another example of the process of divergence used by the nervous system to produce coordinated, distributed control because at the same time the elbow flexors are contracting, the extensor is relaxed. In this way, there is little opposing force to overcome as the elbow flexes.

The spinal cord interneurons play an important role in goal-directed movements. The Ia inhibitory interneuron receives a convergence of synapses from the primary afferents, corticospinal axons, other descending axons from the brain and brainstem as well as other interneurons (Figure 4-6A). The output of the Ia interneuron is the sum of these excitatory and inhibitory inputs. The higher brain centers control the activity of the opposing muscle at a joint through a single command. A descending signal that stimulates muscle contraction at a joint will also simultaneously relax the opposing muscle.

Renshaw Cells

Renshaw cells are inhibitory and synapse back on alpha and gamma motor neurons of the agonist and synergists, which is called **recurrent inhibition**; they receive input from descending brainstem nuclei and are also stimulated by motor neurons (Figure 4-6B). The Renshaw cell also inhibits Ia inhibitory interneurons to the antagonist, thereby facilitating their activation. Thus, activation of the Renshaw cell controls the excitability of the agonist and antagonist around the joint.

Group Ib Inhibitory Interneurons

Group Ib inhibitory interneurons are innervated by afferent axons from the Golgi tendon organ as well as ipsilateral corticospinal and rubrospinal descending axons (Figure 4-7). These interneurons decrease the firing rate of the homonymous motor neuron. The Ib axons also synapse on Ib excitatory interneurons to stimulate the motor neuron of the antagonist muscle. In this way, while the contracting force of the agonist muscle is controlled or decreased, the opposing resistance is increased. Convergence of input from cutaneous afferents and joint afferents also occurs on Ib inhibitory interneurons to reinforce and integrate multiple inputs.

Importance of Interneurons

Remarkably intricate and orchestrated multi-joint movements emerge by combining excitatory and inhibitory interneurons into circuits within the spinal cord. The spinal cord controls bilateral limb movements without descending brain input by using interneurons to take a single input and convey it throughout a limb and to the opposite limb. This is called divergence.

The flexor withdrawal reflex is a good example of how the spinal cord integrates afferent input through the interneuronal

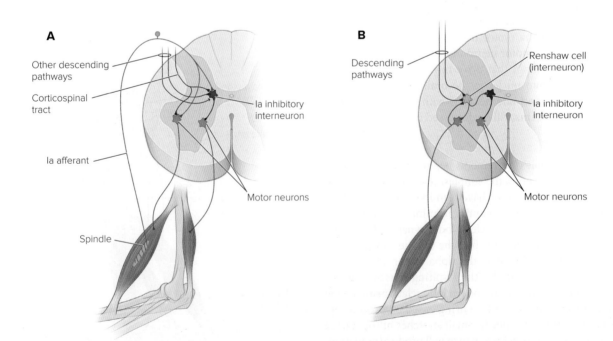

FIGURE 4-6 Illustration of Ia inhibitory neuron and Renshaw cell control. A. Convergence of input from descending pathways and primary afferents converge on the Ia inhibitory interneuron as part of coordinated movement; the sum of these inputs will excite or inhibit the Ia inhibitory interneuron. **B.** Renshaw cells serve to inhibit their agonist and synergists and inhibit the antagonist, which serves to protect the homonymous muscle(s) from excessive exertion or to refine movement; they are activated by motor neurons and descending brainstem pathways.

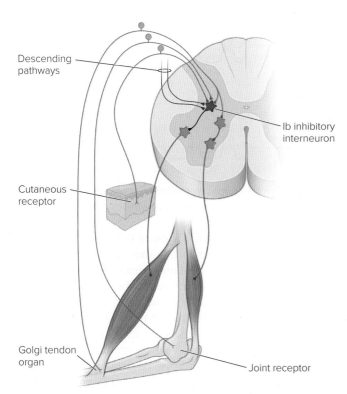

FIGURE 4-7 Ib inhibitory interneurons. The Ib inhibitory interneuron is part of the Golgi tendon organ's homonymous inhibitory circuit, decreasing activation to the homonymous muscle and its synergists while facilitating the antagonist; descending motor systems also can activate the Ib inhibitory interneuron to achieve coordinated muscle activity.

networks to produce coordinated movement across both legs. Figure 4-8 shows the interneuronal pathways activated by a painful stimulus. By stepping on a tack, action potentials in small unmyelinated A-delta fibers from the skin are transmitted to many excitatory and inhibitory interneurons. On the painful leg, the motor neurons that control the flexors receive excitatory input so the leg can be lifted off the tack. However, raising the leg will only happen if the extensor muscles are inhibited. At the same time, the painful input diverges through interneurons that cross the gray matter to the motor neurons of the opposite leg. In this limb, the extensor motor neurons are activated and the flexor motor neurons are inhibited. In this way, the spinal cord insures that while the painful leg is lifted off the tack, the opposite leg is stiffened to support the weight of the person. Otherwise, the person literally wouldn't have a leg to stand on.

These interneuronal networks are not only used to control reflexes but also to coordinate, complex voluntary movements. Depending on the convergence and divergence in the circuit, a single input signal can create a response that outlasts the stimulus (Figure 4-9). This type of processing is called a **reverberating circuit** and is made up of at least three excitatory interneurons. Excitation of the first interneuron diverges and causes excitation of other interneurons that converge back on the original interneuron.

Adding inhibitory interneurons to a reverberating circuit converts afferent activity or tonic, continuous neural drive into alternating activation of flexor and extensor muscle groups

Cutaneous receptor in plantar surface of foot

FIGURE 4-8 Interneuronal network for the spinal flexor withdrawal reflex.

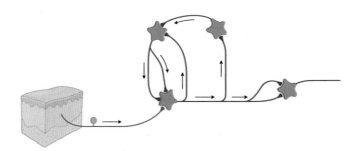

FIGURE 4-9 Illustration of a reverberating excitatory circuit. Initial sensory neuron activation can induce activity in a reverberating circuit that produces ongoing excitation as the circuit feeds back onto the original second-order neuron; this type of activity plays a role in ongoing pain experiences that continue long after the pain stimulus is removed.

(Figure 4-10). This type of organization is thought to be part of the **central pattern generator** (CPG). A CPG produces rhythmic motor patterns without input from the brain or sensory input. Once they receive a "go signal" they become self-stimulating and produce repetitive synchronized activity that continues until a "stop signal" occurs. While there are examples

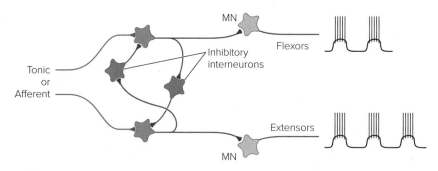

FIGURE 4-10 Inhibitory interneurons within a reverberating circuit. When inhibitory interneurons exist within a reverberating circuit, they induce alternating inhibition within the existing excitation of the circuit, consistent with the repetitive excitation–inhibition of the gait cycle.

of CPGs in various parts of the nervous system, the CPGs in the spinal cord produce locomotion (Figure 4-11; Box 4-1).

The influence of a small portion of descending motor axons from the brain on spinal cord plasticity and learning was recently shown, using a sensitive indicator of learning. In rats with a spinal cord injury in the thoracic region, some descending axons are spared and reach the lumbar enlargement where they change lumbar cord functions. In one group, the lumbar cord had recovered for several weeks in the presence of spared axons. In the other group, recovery occurred in the absence of spared axons. Next, the lumbar cord was isolated from the brain

by complete transection and a learning test was applied to show the capacity of the lumbar cord in these groups (Figure 4-12). In the learning test, the hindlimb is suspended over a saline solution and a contact rod was taped to the paw. When the limb dangles in an extended position, the rod contacts the solution, which completes an electrical circuit and delivers a small electrical stimulation to the leg. If the lumbar cord learns, the leg will be held out of the solution to avoid the stimulation, but if there is no learning, stimulation time will be greater. In this study, the lumbar cord that recovered in the presence of some sparing was able to keep the limb elevated out of the solution longer and

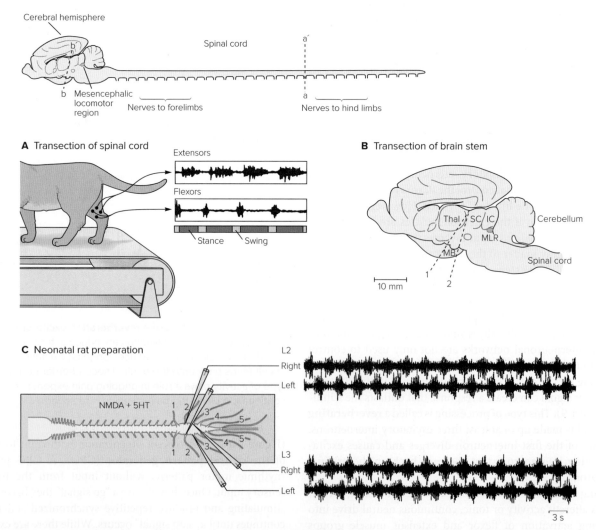

FIGURE 4-11 Evidence of CPG in the spinal cord that produces locomotion. (Adapted with permission from Cazalets J-R, Borde M, Clarc F: Localization and organization of the central pattern generator for hindlimb locomotion in newborn rat, *J Neurosci* 1995 Jul;15(7 Pt 1):4943-4951.)

make fewer mistakes than when no sparing occurred. This study is important because it shows that even small amounts of sparing can greatly change the functional plasticity of neural systems that are likely part of CPGs for walking. It is this plasticity that rehabilitation may be able to capitalize on to improve function.

What are the Clinical Implications of CPGs and Spinal Learning?

Central pattern generators for locomotion have been well-described in a variety of animals but cannot be definitively proven in the human spinal cord because all input from the brain must be eliminated. To assure complete transection of the cord after injury and isolation from brain input, microscopic examination of the injury is required that cannot be performed in people living with spinal cord injury. The best evidence of CPG in the human cord is provided by Blaire Calancie's report from 1994.[7] This study is of a man who experienced a spinal cord injury 17 years earlier that resulted in incomplete paralysis below the injury. He started intensive walking training, and shortly thereafter, found that when he laid supine with his hips fully extended, his legs began moving. The movements were involuntary and moved in

Isolated lumbar cord

CPG interneurons

Computer

FIGURE 4-12 Experimental test of learning and plasticity in the lumbar cord. A mild stimulus over the front of leg activates lumbar interneurons. With good learning and plasticity, the motor neurons are activated and the paw is held out of the water to avoid the stimulus.

an alternating, stepping-like manner. He could not voluntarily suppress these rhythmic movements, and they would continue until he moved out of supine or hip extension. These stepping-like movements emerged during sleeping and awakened him several times a night. Several characteristics of these movements match those produced by CPGs in animal studies, including the fact that rhythmicity occurred without brain input, the stepping movements responded to hip angle, and muscle activation occurred in a strict timing pattern. Availability of human CPGs for locomotion holds promise for improving recovery after CNS injury, since they would remain largely intact after brain or spinal cord injury and be capable of producing coordinated, functional leg movements that respond to changes in the environment.

REFERENCES

1. Henneman E, Somjen G, Carpenter DO. Functional significance of cell size in spinal motoneurons. *J. Neurophysiol.* 1965;28:560-580.

2. Mendell LM, Henneman E. 1971 Terminals of single Ia fibers: location, density, and distribution within a pool of 300 homonymous motoneurons. *J Neurophysiol.* 1971;34(1):171-187.

3. Keen DA, Fuglevand AJ. 2003 Role of intertendinous connections in distribution of force in the human extensor digitorum muscle. *Muscle Nerve.* 2003;28(5):614-622.

4. Stuart DG, Hultborn H. Thomas Graham Brown (1882–1965), Anders Lundberg (1920–) and the neural control of stepping. *Brain Res Rev.* 2008;59:74-95.

5. Zhong H, Roy RR, Nakada KK, Zdunowski S, Khalili N, de Leon RD, Edgerton VR. 2012 Accommodation of the spinal cat to a tripping perturbation. *Front Physiol.* 2012;3:112. doi: 10.3389/fphys.2012.00112.

6. Hodgson JA, Roy RR, de Leon R, Dobkin B, Edgerton VR. Can the mammalian lumbar spinal cord learn a motor task? *Med Sci Sports Exerc.* 1994;26(12):1491-1497.

7. Calancie B, Needham-Shropshire B, Jacobs P, Willer K, Zych G, Green BA. Involuntary stepping after chronic spinal cord injury. Evidence for a central rhythm generator for locomotion in man. *Brain.* 1994;117(Pt 5): 1143-1159.

Review Questions

1. **In an elite weight lifter, name a mechanism to increase force when most or all motor units have been activated.**

   A. Modulate the firing rate through summation

   B. Recruit primarily slow twitch motor units

   C. Use short muscle length

   D. Activate small motor neurons only

2. **Part of any purposeful movement is to adapt to the demands of the environment. How does afferent input from the muscle spindle help to produce purposeful movement?**

   A. Alpha-gamma co-activation helps detect the rate of change in limb position

   B. Afferents converge to activate agonist motor neurons

   C. Afferents diverge to activate inhibitory interneurons to agonist motor neurons

   D. All of the above

3. **In a patient that has sustained a partial spinal cord injury, how would inhibitory interneurons be affected?**

   A. Descending drive to the inhibitory interneurons will increase

   B. Inhibitory interneurons will increase in number

   C. Excitatory interneurons will increase in number

   D. Descending drive to the inhibitory interneurons will decrease

4. **What organizational structures within the spinal cord can produce complex limb movements?**

   A. Central pattern generators

   B. Muscle spindles

   C. Gamma motor neurons

   D. All of the above

5. **How will treadmill training change neural systems in the lumbar cord after spinal cord injury?**

   A. Alternating contraction patterns between muscles of the legs will increase

   B. Neural activation will adapt to afferent input according to the environmental context

   C. Learning and plasticity will occur

   D. All of the above

6. **Increased muscle tone and spasticity typically occurs after spinal cord injury. What spinal cord structures are affected and how?**

   A. Direct damage and loss of alpha motor neurons which innervate the spastic muscle

   B. Muscle atrophy results in loss of motor neurons and their neural input shifts to nearby neurons causing higher firing frequencies

   C. Inhibitory interneurons receive less descending input which lowers their firing rate and allows increased motor neuron firing

   D. None of the above

Answers

1. A   **2.** B   **3.** D   **4.** A   **5.** D

6. C

Motor Control and the Descending Systems

John A. Buford

5

OVERVIEW OF MOTOR CONTROL

The primary difference between animals and plants is the ability to move, and the organ most responsible for this difference is the brain. Some have argued, in fact, that the entire purpose of the nervous system is the control of movement. Perhaps it is no coincidence, then, that the earliest studies of neuroscience began with studies of the control of movement.

To understand the control of movement, one must first have an appreciation for the musculoskeletal system. While that is beyond the scope of this text, a few important principles are worth emphasizing before we explore in any detail what the nervous system does to control movement.

Motor Control Inherent in the Musculoskeletal System

- Many of the characteristics of movements observed are dictated by the biomechanical constraints of the musculoskeletal system, which simplifies the problem of neural control.

- Muscle is the source of power for movement. The nervous system must control the muscles, and therefore, some understanding of muscle physiology is required to understand neural control of movement.

- The nervous system devotes considerable resources to proprioception, the conscious and subconscious sensation of the state of the muscles, and the musculoskeletal system, in order to provide accurate feedback for motor control.

The student of motor control should already possess a basic understanding of the musculoskeletal system and of muscle physiology. Proprioception is covered in Chapter 3 of this book. As we consider the systems for control of movement, we will refer back to and expand upon these concepts.

AN EXAMPLE OF A COMMON MOVEMENT TASK

What is required to sit in a chair and press a specific key on a computer keyboard, and then reach for the computer mouse (Figure 5-1)? First, we need to have the postural control system sufficient to hold our trunk and lower limbs stable in the sitting position. This will require steady, low level activation of trunk and lower limb muscles and the ability to modulate muscle activity as our body sways about in space. We will need the ability to sense body position and a sense of balance to keep upright against gravity. We would also like to be able to do this efficiently, with very little mental or physical effort.

We will simultaneously need to be able to see the keyboard, or perhaps having memorized it, recall the layout from memory as we look at the screen. Either way, we will need to know where the key is that we would like to press. We will need a stable position of our head, from which to direct the gaze of our eyes, as well as a stable position of our shoulders and arms, from which to direct our finger movement. Most likely, in order to simplify the task, we will have our forearms and wrists resting in front of the keyboard so that only a combination of wrist and finger movements is needed to reach the key. Nonetheless, there is subtle modulation of shoulder and arm muscle activity to provide that stability.

As we go to strike the key, we will need to recruit a very specific subset of wrist and finger muscles in a controlled, delicate manner to position the finger over the key and depress it with sufficient but not excessive force. We will pay close attention to the sensory feedback from our fingers, and perhaps use auditory feedback from the key and vision of the character appearing on the screen for confirmation that the key was really pressed. Having accomplished that task and seeing the feedback on the screen, we are now ready to reach for the mouse. We will need to pick up our hand and begin to move it in space toward the mouse. Again, we would like to do this efficiently. Our peripheral vision has already located the mouse, and we do not need to look directly at it to know where to put our hand. Before we finish pressing the key, the brain has already

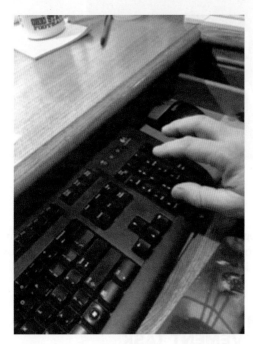

FIGURE 5-1 As a person performs even a seemingly simple task, typing and then reaching for a computer mouse, a complex series of sensory and motor actions is required throughout the central nervous system to control the musculoskeletal system for successful performance. (Used with permission of John A. Buford, PT, PhD).

plotted a trajectory for the hand to reach the mouse, probably in our subconscious, so we have this movement planned and prepared before we make it.

A problem to be solved here is that the inertial mass of our arm, being accelerated toward the mouse, will tend to drive our body toward the opposite direction. This introduces a more dynamic trajectory control problem. Over time, our brain has become familiar enough with the mass properties of our arm that it can predict quite accurately what those inertial consequences will be. Rather than initiating the movement and waiting for the consequences to occur, the brain will actually employ a predictive strategy called feedforward control. We will initiate a slight trunk and shoulder lean toward the mouse immediately prior to reaching. If we execute this feed forward strategy perfectly, this preparatory movement will be just enough to counteract the inertial consequences of the reach so that, to the outside observer, there will appear to be no disturbance of trunk position caused by the reach. This amazing process occurs without our conscious effort and occupies perhaps a tenth of a second, playing out before we even realize that we have begun to reach.

As our hand begins to move toward the mouse, two things are happening at once. First, the hand is being transported along an efficient trajectory, avoiding obstacles on the way to the mouse. For a short movement like this to an object in a known location, we are probably not expecting to make corrections along the way. If it was a living mouse and we were trying to catch it, then that would be a different problem! But with a computer mouse, our plan is likely to succeed without the need to watch the movement and initiate corrections along the way.

The reaching movement occurs with a smooth acceleration profile such that there is very little jerkiness evident in the movement, and the hand comes to rest over the mouse without knocking the mouse out of position in the process. A second aspect of this control process occurs in parallel with the reach. The shape of the hand is being morphed from the shape appropriate for typing into a shape intended to hold the mouse in a gentle grasp, with the index and long fingers free to use the buttons. Having worked with the mouse extensively, we have that shape memorized, and our hand is shaped for the mouse before it gets there. As our hand grasps the mouse, we need sensation to tell us that we have completed the task and to help finish the completion of the grasp with the appropriate positioning and force.

If we break this task down, we will see that we need a number of capabilities to succeed. We need a system for posture and balance that helps us stay upright in a stable position, and we would prefer not to have to give this very much thought or energy. We need the ability to use spatial memory to plan and guide movements in space, or as a novice, the ability to locate a thing in space, usually based on vision, and guide our movement to that spot. We need some knowledge of the way our musculoskeletal system works, how much force our muscles can produce and what the inertial properties of our limbs are, in order to plan and control movements. We need the capacity to do more than one thing at a time to both transport the hand and shape it. And we need sensory feedback to guide movement and to give us knowledge of the outcome of our effort.

As we work through this chapter, we will see how the motor control system is organized in a manner to help us accomplish all of these aspects of the neural control of movement. Before we can integrate our knowledge at that level, however, we will need a foundation. There are certain facts to be learned about the nervous system and its pathways for control of movement. The reader must first understand the muscles and the motoneurons, the means by which the nervous system produces the forces to control movement. This is covered in Chapter 4. From there, we can consider the descending systems for motor control, the pathways from the brain that control the recruitment of motoneurons. Finally, we will consider systems within the brain that organize the control of movement.

● MAJOR DESCENDING SYSTEMS FOR MOTOR CONTROL

There are four major descending systems for motor control: the corticospinal system, the rubrospinal tract, the reticulospinal system, and the vestibulospinal system. Each of these systems has certain preferred functions.

Understanding this organization of the spinal gray helps to understand the functions of the descending systems. For example, the vestibulospinal system is important in postural reactions for standing balance.[1,2] As such, it sends axons to control recruitment of both axial and limb muscles. It should be no surprise, then, to find that vestibulospinal projections can be found in the medial and lateral parts of the ventral horn, as well as in the intermediate zone. Hence, one of the basic anatomical facts we must know about a descending system is where its axons terminate. We will want to know this both in terms of the regions of the gray matter, as described in Chapter 4 and above, and in terms of the segmental levels of the spinal cord contacted. For example, a system that terminates only in cervical levels could not be expected to control the legs.

Another fact about descending systems that we will need to know is where the cells originate. In some cases, this will be a particular nucleus in the brain, and in others, it will be a specific type of neuron. Sometimes, we will know both. In order to appreciate the literature, where these terms may be used interchangeably, we will need to be well versed in the most common ways of speaking about the origins of the descending systems. If a certain part of the brain is lesioned that we know is the location for neurons with axons to a certain descending system, then we will understand why there would be certain deficits in motor control.

We will also want to know the pathways through the nervous system by which the axons of the descending system travel to reach the spinal cord. This will include the names of the major structures through which the axons travel, their general location in that structure, and the location of the axons in the white matter of the spinal cord. Again, this will make it possible to make sense out of the deficits that result from lesions in certain places in the nervous system.

Finally, where possible, we would like to know something about how the axon terminals of any particular descending system ultimately influence the motoneurons. Are there direct connections to the motoneurons themselves, or does a particular descending system only work through the interneuronal networks? Or, is there some combination of both kinds of projection? Does the descending system have a tendency to contact interneurons in the medial gray matter that cross over to the other side, thereby exerting bilateral control, or does the descending system only influence movement on one side at a time? Where possible, integrating an understanding of how a particular descending system ultimately connects to the motoneurons will help explain why that descending system has certain functions.

On the following pages, there are diagrams of the cortical motor areas (Figure 5-2) and the four major descending systems (Figure 5-3), and there are also tables, detailing the origins and destinations of these pathways, along with details of how the system travels through the nervous system. In the text, we will describe one system at a time, integrating this information to paint a functional picture at the end.

DESCENDING SYSTEMS FOR MOTOR CONTROL

Corticospinal Tract

Origins and Inputs

A single neuron in the corticospinal system will have its cell body in the gray matter of the cerebral cortex, and by definition, will produce an axon that ultimately reaches the gray matter

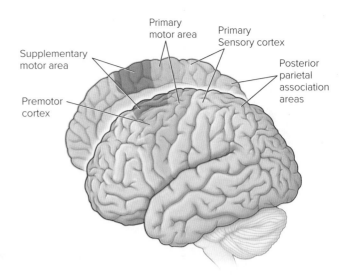

FIGURE 5-2 Cortical motor areas. The lower part of the image represents a lateral view of the left brain. The upper part shows the mesial surface as a reflection. (Modified with permission from Kandel ER, Schwartz JH, Jessell TM, Siegelbaum SA, Hudspeth AJ (Eds). *Principles of Neural Science*, 5th ed. New York, NY: McGraw-Hill; 2013. Figure 37-4A, Pg 840.)

of the spinal cord.[1,2] The type of cell that makes a corticospinal axon is a **pyramidal cell**. The cell body of a pyramidal neuron will be in layer 5 of the cortical gray matter (cortical tissue in this part of the brain has six layers).

About 30–40% of corticospinal neurons have their cell body in the **precentral gyrus**, also known as the primary motor cortex (Brodmann's Area [BA] 4).[2-4] This may be called M1 ("M-one") or simply "the motor cortex." The precentral gyrus is the strip of brain tissue just rostral to the central sulcus. The vast majority of corticomotoneuronal cells in the corticospinal system will emanate from M1, principally from areas devoted to control of the hand and face, and predominately from the part of M1 found buried within the central sulcus.

M1 contains neurons projecting to motor pools for control of virtually any muscle in the body. These are organized in a somatotopic map of the body that is arranged, at the macroscopic level, in a consistent manner among individuals. The foot and leg are most medial, on the mesial surface. The trunk is around the top of the cortex, and then come arm, hand, face, and mouth. A disproportionately large area of cortex in the human and other dexterous primates is devoted to the hand, largely in the part that is enfolded into the central sulcus. Functionally, when MI is activated and these corticospinal cells are creating action potentials, the synaptic strengths of connection to the motor pools is such that movement will invariably occur. Electrical stimulation with a microelectrode placed with its tip in layer 5 of M1 will elicit visible muscle twitches with very low currents, ranging from a few micro amperes up to about 30 microamps.[5] With this method of intracortical microstimulation, a very fine-grained map of the motor cortex outputs can be revealed. Comparable maps on a much grosser scale can also be obtained with noninvasive methods such as transcranial magnetic stimulation.

FIGURE 5-3 Descending systems for motor control. For each system, the path of an axon for a typical neuron is illustrated, along with the pattern of terminations. For the corticospinal system, the lateral corticospinal tract is illustrated in magenta, and the anterior corticospinal tract is blue. From the midbrain, the tectospinal tract is blue, and the rubrospinal tract is magenta. For both the vestibulospinal and reticulospinal systems, the lateral tract is magenta, and the medial tract is blue. In addition to the paths of typical axons, the locations of all fibers in the tract are shown on the spinal cord sections, as is the overall sphere of influence of axon terminals from each tract.

But with only 40% of the corticospinal tract originating from the primary motor cortex, where does the rest of it come from? About 30% of the corticospinal cells originate from areas rostral to M1. In Brodmann's numbering system, most of this broad region is called area 6. In general, this region is active for motor planning in advance of movement, and many of the neurons

in area 6 serve to project to MI to govern movement.[4,6,7] There are also many corticospinal neurons in area 6. Modern neuroscientists have found several subdivisions of area 6, but for this chapter we will consider two.

On the mesial surface of the superior frontal gyrus, there is a region of area 6 called the **supplementary motor area,** abbreviated SMA.[6,8,9] This is also called M2 (M-"two"). This area is sensitive to electrical stimulation, but more current (40–80 microamps) is typically required to evoke movement. The SMA is the second largest contributor to the corticospinal tract, and also contains a somatotopic map. This map is less detailed, however, and it is typical to elicit multi-joint or even bilateral movements from SMA. SMA is most concerned with motor planning and performance for complex, memorized movements such as sequences, and is also critical for bimanual tasks where both hands must be used in conjunction (e.g., buttoning a shirt).[1,9]

The remainder of area 6 is typically called the **premotor cortex** (PM), which is located on the lateral surface of the cortex rostral to M1.[2,4,6,10] This area is concerned with planning for movements like reaching to an object or kicking a ball, where the limb movement must be directed at an external object, especially if the object must be moved in certain directions with respect to the outside world. PM is especially interested in learning arbitrary links between external stimuli and responses, such as learning to respond to traffic lights, turn signals, horns and brake lights to drive a car in city traffic.[11] In the area for hand control, there is a concentration of the ability to imagine moving, based on observation and imitation.[12] As with SMA, much of the output from PM is directed toward MI to coordinate motor outputs there, but some corticospinal neurons emanate directly from PM itself.[2]

With about 70% of the corticospinal tract emanating from these and other frontal lobe areas that have clear relationships to motor control, where does the rest of the corticospinal tract come from? Surprisingly, much of the corticospinal tract comes from the parietal lobe,[1,2] which is typically associated with sensory function, not motor function. Some of these corticospinal projections from sensory areas are thought to help the nervous system focus on aspects of sensory information critical to movement.[13] Further, in order to have control over movement, one must control reflexes. In this regard, it makes sense that the sensory areas of the cerebral cortex contribute to the corticospinal tract. Indeed, in lower animals, the corticospinal tract has no projections directly to motoneurons and has as many terminals in the dorsal horn as in the intermediate zone.[14] In this sense, regulation of reflexes as a prerequisite to voluntary motor control may be the original purpose of the corticospinal tract. Direct voluntary control of motor pools seems to be a more recent development.

In sum, the corticospinal tract originates from a wide region of the parietal and frontal lobes. Most of the projections come from MI and SMA, but the PM and sensory cortical areas also make substantial contributions. The various cortical areas contributing to the corticospinal tract operate in parallel to govern this one descending system just as the four major descending systems work together on a larger scale.

Each of these cortical motor areas that contributes to the corticospinal system receives inputs that are specific to its functions. All receive input to a greater or lesser extent from the basal ganglia and cerebellum via relays in the thalamus. A detailed description of these brain areas is covered later, but a simple characterization is that the basal ganglia are important for selection of movement components and switching from one movement to the next, whereas the cerebellum coordinates

movement and anticipates coordination required for upcoming movements.

Among the cortical motor areas, M1 is principally concerned with real time performance of movement.[15] In other words, if M1 is activated, then there is movement being produced. The major sources of input to M1 are SMA and PM, which relay the movement plans to M1. M1 also receives detailed sensory perceptions from the primary sensory cortex (S1). The premotor cortical areas receive higher order perceptual information that combines things such as whole body image for SMA to govern memorized movements and the perception of the body's position with respect to the outside world for PM to govern targeted limb movements. These integrated perceptions come from the posterior parietal area (PPA; BA 5, 7; Figure 5-2).[12] The prefrontal cortex (PF) is also a strong source of input to SMA and PM. PF is the source of executive functions such as decision making to choose the appropriate action from among many possibilities. In essence, PF chooses what we should do, SMA and PM figure out how, and MI does it.[16-18] These areas can be subdivided further into parts that parcel out certain aspects of the function, but that level of detail is beyond the scope of this chapter.

Destinations

From the primary motor cortex, corticospinal cells often make strong synaptic connections directly to alpha motoneurons for the limb muscles, especially muscles of the hands and feet.[3,7,19-21] This means increased corticospinal activity can reliably and specifically recruit muscles in these body parts, potentially overwhelming competing influences from other descending systems. However, even for the hands, 50% or more of the corticospinal cells will not contact the motoneurons directly. Instead, they will work through interneuronal networks to have their influence, as described in Chapter 4. In other words, the corticospinal cells will synapse on a set of local neurons in the spinal cord and those cells will, in turn, connect to the motoneurons. Corticomotoneuronal cells themselves will also send collateral branches of their axons to interneuronal networks to recruit these in parallel with the motor pool. When the corticospinal projections from areas other than M1 are considered, it becomes even more uncommon for corticospinal cells to synapse directly on alpha motoneurons, and even more likely that this will only occur for control of the hands and feet.[7,8] The point here is that to a great extent, the corticospinal system relies upon well-established networks of neural connections in the spinal cord to produce most movements. Only for the details of the hand and finger movements, and to some extent for limb movements, does the corticospinal system take it upon itself to choose relatively specifically which muscles to recruit for a particular movement.

For control of proximal limb girdle muscles and muscles of the trunk and spinal column, there is very little potential for corticospinal cells to directly control motoneurons. Rather, the corticospinal system works through spinal networks that are responsible for coordination of responses among these axial muscles. Indeed, other descending systems are probably more influential on these girdle and core muscles than the corticospinal tract. Finally, a substantial portion of the corticospinal tract is targeted for the intermediate zone and dorsal horn of the gray matter in the spinal cord. In other words, a large responsibility of the corticospinal tract is to govern the neurons that are involved in reflexes and sensory inputs.

There are actually two main divisions of the corticospinal tract. The **lateral corticospinal tract** is almost completely a contralateral system, with the left brain projecting to the right half of the spinal cord, and the right projecting to the left.[1,2] In total, about 90% of the corticospinal tract decussates and comprises the lateral corticospinal tract, which is located in the white matter of the lateral funiculus in the spinal cord. There are a very small number of corticospinal axons that travel in the ipsilateral lateral funiculus. We have no direct data about what these do, but anatomical studies reveal their presence. The remaining 9–10% stays ipsilateral and descends in the ventral funiculus; this is called the **ventral** (or anterior) **corticospinal tract**. The ventral corticospinal tract is mainly concerned with control of axial muscles and terminates medially in the gray matter of the spinal cord, in Rexed's lamina number VIII, which is where motoneurons and interneurons concerned with trunk and proximal limb girdle muscles are located. The lateral corticospinal tract, in contrast, terminates in the motor pools of the ventral horn, as well as in the intermediate zone and in the dorsal horn. The lateral portions of the ventral horn are where the motoneurons for limb, and especially distal muscles, are located.

Single corticospinal cells in the lateral corticospinal tract will terminate in just a few motor pools spanning just a few spinal segments. This provides a substrate for single corticospinal neurons of the lateral corticospinal tract to recruit just a few muscles at a time. For the ventral corticospinal tract, the terminations in the medial part of the spinal cord often contact interneurons that cross to influence movements on the other side. In other words, the ventral corticospinal tract can influence both sides of the body, but only for the trunk and proximal muscles to which it connects.[8,22]

Functions

From the preceding discussion of the sources and inputs to the corticospinal tracts and their destinations in the spinal cord, we can already glean a good idea of the function of the corticospinal tract. Not surprisingly, the corticospinal tract is critical for **skilled, voluntary movement** throughout the body. This is not to say that voluntary movement cannot occur if the corticospinal tract is damaged, but the movement will not be well controlled. Movements made in the absence of corticospinal function occur in gross, stereotyped synergies reflective of patterns of connections in the brainstem and spinal cord.[2,23] These gross movements are useful in functional tasks such as weight-bearing, but are not specific enough to allow the kinds of arbitrary, learned movements that humans rely upon for things like skilled use of tools or competitive sports. Control of the hand and finger movement is dramatically impaired by damage to the corticospinal tract. Reaching in a variety of directions with reasonably equal accuracy in all directions is also impaired when the corticospinal tract is damaged.

In addition to problems with motor control, there are problems in the regulation of reflexes when the corticospinal tract is damaged, and this should not be surprising given the large number of corticospinal projections to the intermediate zone and dorsal horn of the spinal cord. The most common symptom is spasticity, an inability to govern the stretch reflex.[24,25] Interestingly, the size of the stretch reflex can be learned with practice, and the corticospinal tract is critical for this learning to occur and for its preservation.[26,27] In other words, part of learning a new skill is not just learning how to turn on the proper muscles in the proper sequence, it is also learning how to set up the strengths of the reflexes that will be occurring in parallel with the movement. When the corticospinal tract is damaged, this aspect of motor control is impaired, and patients will have difficulty regulating muscle tone in concert with movement. When we see this, we call it **spasticity**. This emphasizes that regulation of reflexes, and more generally, attention to and regulation of incoming proprioceptive and cutaneous information in concert with movement is also a part of the motor control problem for the nervous system.

Rubrospinal Tract

The rubrospinal tract is greatly overshadowed by the corticospinal tract in the human and does not appear to be as large in relative terms as it is in the cat.[1] However, this is a poor standard by which to judge importance. There is a tract called the raphe spinal system that descends from the brainstem to the dorsal horn. This system is critical for modulation of pain and is much smaller than the rubrospinal tract, but does this make it unimportant? A better question would be, "what is the function of the rubrospinal tract, and is that type of thing critical to human function?"

Origins and Inputs

The rubrospinal tract originates from the **red nucleus**, which is in the midbrain. Like the lateral corticospinal tract, the rubrospinal tract is a crossed system. The neurons that actually contribute to the rubrospinal tract are called **magnocellular neurons** because they are large. There are two principal sources of input to the red nucleus. One is the cortical motor areas in the frontal lobe. The other main source of input to the red nucleus is the cerebellum. The cerebellum uses the rubrospinal tract as one of its outputs for the coordination of movement. Hence, the red nucleus is a center for integrating the motor commands from the motor cortex with coordination from the cerebellum.

Destinations

The rubrospinal tract projects to the lateral motor pools in the anterior horn of the spinal cord, as well as to interneurons projecting to the motor pools. Many of the rubrospinal projections are monosynaptic. In higher primates, including humans, the rubrospinal tract has little to no influence below the cervical spinal cord. Unlike the corticospinal system, rubrospinal connections are not typically sent to motoneurons for distal muscles intrinsic to the hands. Rather, rubrospinal connections are to the **extrinsic muscles** of the hand, wrist, and upper limb (shoulder/elbow).[20] Like corticospinal cells, rubrospinal projections are to selected groups of muscles, but single rubrospinal tract cells are more likely to affect muscles at multiple joints (e.g., shoulder, elbow, and wrist), whereas corticospinal projections are more likely to allow for control of one joint at a time.

Functions

There have been many ideas in the literature about the potential function of the rubrospinal tract. Current evidence is that it is important for rapid, coordinated movement of the entire limb, especially when the reach must be set so the hand can be adapted to the shape of an object.[28,29] Early findings noted that the rubrospinal tract was highly active during the swing phase of walking in the cat. The conclusion was erroneously drawn that rubrospinal tract cells might be important for control of flexors. There seems to have been a desire in the field, in the early studies of motor control, to say that this tract controls flexors, that one controls extensors, etc. These simple ideas have been largely discarded. In the cat, as in the human, the end of swing phase is a time of rapid, accurate limb movement where the positioning for limb placement must be precisely controlled.[30,31] For the upper limb in particular, this is essentially a reaching movement for a quadruped, and there is as much or more extensor activity as flexor activity at this point in the gait cycle. From detailed studies in nonhuman primate, it is clear that rubrospinal tract neurons are quite effective at recruiting extensor muscles around the wrist. Hence, by integrating commands from the cerebellum and MI to affect muscles throughout the limb, it seems likely that the rubrospinal tract is used for rapid correction of limb movements, especially when there is a requirement for both speed and accuracy in the movement. And in particular, the parallel coordination for control of shaping of the hand, during a reaching movement, seems to make rubrospinal cells more active than either task alone.[28,29] With that as the critical function of the rubrospinal tract, even if it is small in the human, it still may be quite important.

Vestibulospinal Tracts

The **vestibular nuclei** in the pons and medulla are centers of integration for inputs from the vestibular system (utricle, saccule, semicircular canals) with the control of eye movements, head and neck movements, and postural reactions for balance. Cortical projections to the vestibular nuclei are sparse and thought to subconsciously inhibit vestibular reflexes that would interfere with voluntary movement; the vestibulospinal tracts are not thought to be under direct conscious control.[32,33] These systems serve in an automatic, regulatory fashion, but that does not mean the vestibulospinal systems are not important for motor learning. Rather, for these systems to make their respective contributions to learning and adaptation, practice is required.

Origins and Inputs

Much of the vestibular system is devoted to internal processing of vestibular information and control and coordination of eye movements, but there are two components that descend to the spinal cord for control of the trunk and limbs. The **medial vestibulospinal tract** is an extension of the head and eye control and coordination system. It originates from the **medial vestibular nucleus**. Inputs to the medial vestibular nucleus arise from all components of the vestibular apparatus, including the semicircular canals, sensing head rotation, as well as the utricle and saccule, sensing linear acceleration of the head in up/down

and anterior/posterior directions (see Chapter 6 for details). The **lateral vestibulospinal tract** originates in the **lateral vestibular nucleus** and receives mainly utricle and saccule inputs, so it senses mainly the linear acceleration components of head movement. The other strong source of input to the vestibular nuclei, in addition to the vestibular apparatus, is the cerebellum. Hence, to the extent the cerebellum is involved in coordination of limb and body movements for postural reactions and adjustments in support of movement, some of that cerebellar influence is exerted through the descending control afforded by the vestibulospinal systems.

Destinations

The medial vestibulospinal system is bilateral. Cells in the medial vestibular nucleus project to the left and right sides of the spinal cord. These projections are limited to the cervical and upper thoracic segments where motor pools to be recruited in support of head movements are located. Medial vestibulospinal projections are concentrated in the medial part of the spinal gray, lamina VIII, where axial muscles are controlled. The lateral vestibulospinal tract projects through the length of the spinal cord and can influence muscles throughout the body. It provides ipsilateral projections, so the left lateral vestibular nucleus projects to the left side of the body. These projections are targeted to facilitate extensor muscles used for postural reactions. Many synapse directly on the motoneurons of the extensor muscles for rapid and secure control of the muscles. Another output of the lateral vestibular nucleus is the reticulospinal system, which, as we will see below, also contributes to postural reactions.

Functions

The medial vestibulospinal tracts govern head and neck movements used to maintain a stable position of gaze, despite fluctuations imposed from the outside. Functionally, this is called the **vestibulo-ocular reflex** (VOR). If something turns your body to the right, your eyes and head will counter-rotate to the left in order to keep your vision on the same object.

The lateral vestibulospinal tracts are used for the control of antigravity muscles required for posture and balance. For example, when something perturbs the body and tends to pitch you forward, you will need to recruit the plantarflexors to restrain that movement. Much of this may be accomplished by the stretch reflex to the extent the ankles themselves sense the change in body position.[34,35] However, when the perturbation is felt by the head, then the lateral vestibulospinal tracts will be driven to recruit extensor muscles in an effort to resist falling.

Reticulospinal Tracts

The reticulospinal tracts are the last of the descending systems we will consider in detail. As with the vestibulospinal tracts, they are divided into two parts, but unlike the vestibulospinal tracts, the reticulospinal tracts are thought to be under some degree of conscious control.[36] In lower animals, the reticulospinal system is the principal descending system for motor control. It has access to a variety of information from the cortex, cerebellum, vestibular systems, and somatosensory systems. And, it has outputs directed toward the limbs and the trunk throughout the body. Hence, the reticulospinal system plays a supporting role, and sometimes a leading role, in control of virtually every functional movement.

Origins and Inputs

The **reticular formation** is a network of neurons located in the core of the brainstem, especially in the pons and medulla. In the caudal part of the pons and rostral medulla, in the vicinity of the vestibular nuclei around the dorsal aspect of the reticular formation, there is an area called **Nucleus Reticularis Pontis Caudalis**. In this region, there are large neurons that produce reticulospinal axons that form one part of the reticulospinal system, the **medial reticulospinal tract**. Moving slightly caudally into the medulla, and also somewhat ventrally toward the medullary pyramids, we find a nucleus called **Nucleus Reticularis Gigantocellularis**. This is also a source of reticulospinal neurons. Some of these contribute to the medial reticulospinal tracts, whereas others descend through the **lateral reticulospinal tracts**.

Destinations

Many texts seem to tell a compellingly simple story about the differences between the functions of the lateral and medial reticulospinal tracts. A careful reading of the original literature, however, reveals no such simple story. It appears to be more based on legend than fact. Modern studies have yet to provide a means to reliably test the differences in function between these two parts of the reticulospinal system. A few findings, however, seem reliable and may reveal some insight, and these are described below.

Neurons of the lateral reticulospinal system tend to have relatively small axons with slower conduction velocities, whereas the medial reticulospinal system is comprised of large axons, often larger and faster than those of the corticospinal system.[1,36] Medial reticulospinal tract axons often travel the length of the spinal cord and deliver collateral branches at multiple levels.[37,38] These single cells may have axons that influence cervical, thoracic, lumbar, and sacral segments of the spinal cord. In many cases, there may be branches on the ipsilateral and contralateral sides of the spinal cord. Lateral reticulospinal tract cells do not seems to have this pattern. Rather, they tend to terminate at only a few levels on the ipsilateral side, and therefore, have a more limited sphere of influence.

For the medial reticulospinal tract, the typical destination is motoneurons and interneurons for motor control in lamina VIII of the spinal gray, where proximal limb muscles and axial muscles are controlled. There are also interneurons called commissural interneurons that coordinate responses between the left and right sides of the spinal cord. For example, in the flexor withdrawal and crossed extension response (described in Chapter 4), stepping on a nail with your right foot causes right leg flexion and left leg extension. The left leg response is mediated through these commissural interneurons. The reticulospinal tract uses commissural interneurons as well to produce bilateral influences.[39] For the medial reticulospinal tract, there are also some fibers that produce terminals in both sides of the spinal cord, so responses are promoted on both sides simultaneously in response to the activity of single neurons. The medial reticulospinal neurons are rapidly conducting, so that responses may occur almost simultaneously in the arms and legs.

The lateral reticulospinal tract tends to have more limited influences at a smaller number of spinal segments. Lesioning of the spinal cord laterally, where this tract descends, is particularly detrimental to the brain's ability to activate the spinal central pattern generator for locomotion.[40]

Based on physiological data and anatomical connections, a reasonable hypothesis is that the **lateral reticulospinal tracts** may be more the route for activation of **central pattern generation circuits** (defined later) in control of locomotion, and the **medial reticulospinal tracts** are more for **rapid postural reactions** and cortico-reticular pathways for **gross limb movements**.

Functions

As those involved in neurological rehabilitation well know, a critical part of distal mobility is proximal stability. Hence, while the person who is making a reaching movement is thinking about what to do with the hand, there are postural responses and coordination of shoulder girdle and arm movements that must occur for the reach to succeed. The person may be subtly aware that these components of movement are occurring but does not usually think about them overtly. But when a clinician sees a person moving, we often pay more attention to these proximal bases of the movement than to exactly what is going on with the hand because we know that problems with proximal stability are going to lead to problems with distal control. These proximal adjustments that occur in conjunction with skilled movement are largely the domain of the reticulospinal system.

There are projections from the cortical motor areas to reticulospinal neurons in the brainstem, especially from PM and SMA.[36] There are also projections from the cerebellum to the reticulospinal neurons. Thus, as we begin to plan movement and make the early parts of movement, we are typically making postural adjustments that we have learned through practice must precede and accompany our limb movement. Otherwise, the limb movement will destabilize the trunk, and our limb will not go where we expect. Reticulospinal neurons are activated in the early stages of movement, even when the movement is just being planned, presumably to help setup the right state in the postural control system and the proximal limb to support the distal movement that is about to occur. Reticulospinal outputs can coordinate trunk and limb movements bilaterally. The typical output of the reticulospinal system to the upper limb is a reciprocal action that resembles the asymmetric tonic neck reflex: ipsilateral limb flexion and contralateral limb extension. This typical reticulospinal output pattern is an obvious component of the basic alternating limb movements that have their roots in locomotion. In fact, the neural systems that initiate and regulate locomotion depend heavily on the reticulospinal tracts to do so.

● FUNCTIONAL SCHEME FOR UNDERSTANDING THE TRACTS

One useful way for dividing the descending systems is into the **lateral systems**, including the lateral corticospinal and rubrospinal systems, and the **ventromedial systems**, including the ventral corticospinal, vestibulospinal, and reticulospinal systems.[1] The following sections integrate the details for the descending systems into this functional scheme for understanding.

Lateral Systems: Corticospinal and Rubrospinal

Lateral Systems Govern Voluntary Movements and Fine Motor Control

Working together, the lateral systems are most responsible for controlling the distal components of limb movements, especially the parts we think about and try to control voluntarily. The extreme example of this is using the hands to manipulate small objects. Yet, whenever we make a discrete movement such as reaching out for an object or placing our foot in a particular spot such as a rung on a ladder, we are depending on the corticospinal system.

Lateral Systems Are Especially Important for Limb Movement

As indicated by the location of projections to the spinal cord in the lateral parts of the spinal gray, the lateral systems are especially important for limb movement. For the corticospinal system, this is evident in the homunculus by the amount of cortex devoted to the limbs, especially the hands and feet, and also the face. For the rubrospinal tract, it is mainly concerned with reaching movements, especially rapid movements to position the limb.

Lateral Systems Are Focused on Distal Muscles and Parametric Motor Control at the Interface with the Environment

The corticospinal system, in particular, controls our ability to produce finely graded amounts of force in specific directions for specific periods of time. To accomplish this, the lateral systems employ the immense sensory systems devoted to conscious perception of the hands and feet. Consider this: take a small sewing needle and try to thread it with poor lighting. You probably will not succeed. Now, add bright light, stick the needle in a pin cushion, and use a magnifying glass. You will find yourself able to thread the needle straight through the middle of the hole. Why should it be possible for us to visually control our fingers with many times the accuracy than we could ever expect to have in a natural environment? Normally, we use the immensely accurate sensory perceptions from our fingers to control precision grip of small objects. When the nervous system is provided visual input at a level of accuracy to match, it has more than enough precision in motor control and proprioceptive acuity to capitalize on the augmented visual feedback. All of this interaction is occurring in the cerebral cortex. Without the corticospinal tract, a magnifying glass would mainly make it easier to see how badly you were missing the hole with the thread.

Ventromedial Systems: Vestibulospinal and Reticulospinal

The ventromedial system includes the reticulospinal and vestibulospinal tracts, as well as the ventral corticospinal tract. The ventromedial systems operate in parallel with the lateral systems, and to a great extent are governed by different subsystems in the brain. While lateral systems are mainly driven by the cortex with modulation by subcortical systems, the ventromedial systems are in some cases completely dependent on subcortical centers such as the cerebellum and vestibular system. Even for the reticulospinal tract, which does receive cortical control, the cerebellar inputs are highly influential. Hence, a large proportion of the ventromedial system is not directly accessible to our imagination. We will tend to do things in the way we have practiced, not the way we intend, for movements where the ventromedial systems are a strong component of control.

Ventromedial Systems Govern Whole Body Postural Reactions, Trunk Control

When the surface under your body moves, such as an elevator or a moving walkway, you need a whole body reaction to maintain your balance as you reach for the elevator button or struggle to control your luggage. Likewise, when your body is perturbed from above, like having a patient slip while you hold her gait belt, you also need a whole body reaction to remain stable. These kinds of movements are the domain of the ventromedial systems. Of course, to do this, these systems connect preferentially to trunk and proximal limb muscles and have relatively weak influence in the hands or feet. Further, it makes little sense to move one side of your trunk at a time, and it may rarely be useful to react with only one limb. Hence, single neurons from the ventromedial systems tend to have bilateral influences, and may even affect the upper and lower limbs simultaneously.

Ventromedial Systems Produce Gross Limb Movements in Synergy

The ventromedial systems can move the limbs, to some extent under voluntary control through cortical projections to the reticulospinal system. However, the limb movements produced are stereotyped into synergies, organized through the interneuronal networks in the spinal cord. During walking, there are also basic limb synergies that dominate the motor pattern. These gross limb movements show the prevalent outputs of the ventromedial systems. The lateral systems depend on these basic limb movement synergies as a starting point upon which to superimpose control for specific skills.

Ventromedial Systems May Provide Most of the Power for Functional Tasks, Especially Trunk Stability Required for Limb Movement

When it comes to control of the trunk, one need only look at the homunculus of the cerebral cortex to realize that something else is in charge of trunk movement. Many functional tasks, such as getting in and out of bed or walking, require substantial trunk control. Neurologic rehabilitation is often focused on trunk control for these tasks, and our clients often have trouble controlling their trunk in the ways we ask. When we stop to realize the trunk control is largely automatic and under the control of the ventromedial systems, not the lateral systems, this should come as no surprise. This means we cannot expect to make much progress in these tasks by talking to the patient. We need to create situations where they can practice the skill in a way that demands and promotes the components they lack, and then, keep them working on it to develop the skill. When a limb movement must be made, the ventromedial systems may be engaged right away by the SMA and PM projections to reticulospinal systems and by cerebellar coordination produced in anticipation of the movement. These components of movement for stability of the trunk will actually precede the movement of the limb.

Elements of Control for Reaching

Control of reaching provides an example that contrasts the roles of the lateral and ventromedial systems. Here, we are considering a movement largely driven by the lateral systems, where support from the ventromedial systems is crucial for success.

Endpoint Accuracy – Lateral Systems

Generally when reaching, we look at an object and reach out to grasp it in some way. The endpoint accuracy of our movement is the domain of the lateral systems. Without the lateral systems functioning properly, our movement will tend to go the wrong distance and to the wrong location, though we may still grossly extend the limb in an effort to make the reach. Our PM will use perception of the object to recruit the motor cortex to produce the proper limb movements to make the reach and shape the hand as needed to conform to the object to be reached. With coordinated control from the cerebellum and motor cortex, rubrospinal systems will participate and help coordinate the actions and adjust to errors made along the way.

Dynamic Postural Control – Ventromedial Systems

As the PM is preparing in advance of the reach, part of its responsibility is to engage preparatory actions in the trunk and proximal limb. Not surprisingly, the PM is a strong source of control over the reticulospinal system, which has access to these parts of the body. By pre-engaging well-established trunk movement and gross limb movements in synergy, the problem faced by the cerebral cortex to govern movement through the lateral systems is simplified. In engineering terms, this is called constraining the **degrees of freedom**. With an automated system, such as the ventromedial system, taking care of details such as setting up the posture and recruiting limb extensors in a coordinated synergy, the lateral systems can focus on details of the distil limb, such as putting a key in a lock. Without the ventromedial systems providing their influence, the arm would tend to hang limp at the side, with the hand moving well, but not enough power or proximal stability to support extending the limb in space.

Elements of Control for Gait

For gait, the situation is almost the opposite. Gait is a gross motor behavior relying heavily on trunk control and movement of all four limbs in a stereotyped pattern. The ventromedial systems are really the principal systems governing the behavior, and the lateral systems play a supporting role.

Central Pattern Generation – Ventromedial Systems

At the heart of neural control for locomotion is a set of neural circuits known as a **central pattern generator**. The existence of a central pattern generator for locomotion has been confirmed for every animal in which it has been studied. In humans with spinal cord injuries that are apparently motor complete, treadmill training with a body-weight supported harness system can lead to reemergence of locomotor EMG patterns, and in some cases, a return to independent locomotion with assistive devices even in patients who are years out after their injury. When various aspects of the neuromotor control patterns in these patients are probed, certain features of the responses mimic what has been observed in animal models with a complete spinal cord transection. Tonic stimulation of the lumbar spinal cord in a spinal cord injured adult can lead to alternating left and right kicking movements.[41,42] These findings make it hard to argue that there is not a central pattern generator for locomotion in the human.

Interestingly, in the animal models, the evidence is clear that the locomotion-initiating systems in the brainstem rely upon the reticulospinal tracts as the principal route for initiation and regulation of locomotion. It seems clear that the reticulospinal systems are part of the normal route for activation of the central pattern generators in the spinal cord. If this is true, then, it would be unnatural to ask a person to try to voluntarily use a little more dorsiflexor effort during swing. Their normal means of walking is not to have their corticospinal tract control that muscle in swing. The recruitment of the proper muscles in the proper sequence is built into the brainstem and spinal cord, and the ventromedial systems utilize that for control. To increase a certain element of the locomotor pattern, the client should practice with a task that demands the missing component, such as walking up a ramp.

The Obstacle Course – Lateral Systems

When walking must occur on unusual surfaces, such as an obstacle course, then the lateral systems are required to translate the visual perception of the safe places to step into accurate placement of the foot.[30] In this situation, the central pattern generator continues to operate, but the lateral systems make specific adjustments as required. When running or walking, the adjustments we can make voluntarily, in deviation from the typical pattern, are limited. The ventromedial systems and central pattern generators have largely taken over the circuits in the spinal cord, and the lateral systems can add or subtract from what is already going on but will have a hard time completely changing the motor pattern.

● FUNCTIONS OF THE BASAL GANGLIA AND CEREBELLUM IN MOTOR CONTROL

The basal ganglia and the cerebellum play key roles in motor control. The **basal ganglia** are a set of large nuclei within the cerebral cortex. In general, they provide a set of pathways for information, originating in the cerebral cortex, to be processed and relayed through the thalamus back up to the cerebral cortex. There are many theories of basal ganglia function. Two, which we will consider here, are that this system helps select certain actions, to the exclusion of others, and helps regulate the effort for movement. The **cerebellum** is a structure attached to the dorsal aspect of the brainstem. This complex structure receives sensory inputs from the spinal cord and information about the movements, being planned and performed from the cortex, and it is able to influence and adjust planning and performance of movement to provide for better coordination and control.

Basal Ganglia

For the basal ganglia, there are two pathways, the direct and the indirect (Figure 5-4). For the **direct pathway**, cortical neurons send information through the basal ganglia, and the net result is increased facilitation sent back to the cortex. For the **indirect pathway**, the net result is decreased cortical excitation. At the simplest level, we can understand this as a way to promote activity in certain cortical neurons while suppressing activity in others. Hence, this system can help select certain actions to the exclusion of others.[43,44] At the same time, the relative strength with which one activity is promoted and competing activities are suppressed can result in larger or smaller efforts being required.

Consider our example of typing and using the mouse. The most natural way to use the hand is either to extend all the fingers or to flex them all. Selecting one finger to the exclusion of others requires more control. As we move to strike one key to the exclusion of others, circuits in the direct pathway would be promoting movement of one finger while activation of nearby circuits through the indirect pathway would be suppressing

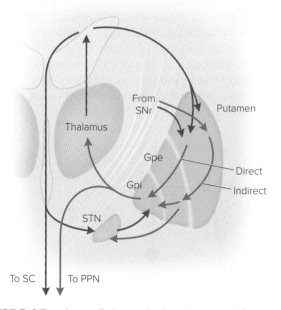

FIGURE 5-4 Basal ganglia loops. In the diagram, pink arrows show excitatory effects, blue arrows inhibitory. Abbreviations: GPi, globus pallidus internal segment; GPe, glocus pallidus external segment; SNr, substantia nigra pars reticulate; STN, subthalamic nucleus; SC, spinal cord; PPN, pedunculopontine nucleus. (Modified with permission from Kandel ER, Schwartz JH, Jessell TM, Siegelbaum SA, Hudspeth AJ (Eds). *Principles of Neural Science*, 5th ed. New York, NY: McGraw-Hill; 2013. Figure 43-2, Pg 984.)

similar movements in other fingers. If we move our example to the difference between typing and reaching for the mouse, then in the motor planning areas, to move the hand, without also reaching, requires a selection, promoting the plan to move the hand while suppressing nearby plans to move the arm. But then to reach, the active area would need to be switched. Hence, not only can the basal ganglia help us choose to move one body part and not another, it can help us choose on action and not another, and then, to switch to the reverse actions.

Dopamine is a neuromodulator that is critical to normal function of the basal ganglia. Dopamine regulates the transmission of information through the direct and indirect loops. Normally, dopamine makes it easier for information to pass through the direct loop but more difficult for it to pass through the indirect loop. In a normal nervous system, the precise location of dopamine release is regulated in concert with the movement such that only certain parts of the direct pathway and certain parts of the indirect pathway are affected, so we can choose what to promote and what to suppress and how strongly to do so.

The cells that make dopamine are in the substantia nigra, pars compacta. The axons of these neurons terminate in the caudate and putamen, the nuclei in the basal ganglia where the cortical information is first delivered. In parkinsonism, these dopamine-producing neurons begin to be lost, and the overall number of these cells is reduced. At first, the nervous system can compensate for this by having the remaining dopamine-producing cells grow new axon collaterals and take over slightly larger regions of responsibility in the caudate and putamen. Eventually, however, there are simply not enough dopamine-producing cells for sufficient dopamine release. The result of this is a relative imbalance between promotion of the direct pathway and suppression of the indirect. As it so happens, the imbalance favors the lack of suppression of the indirect pathway, and the result is a stiff state known as rigidity, with difficulty relaxing and activating the muscles to produce one movement to the exclusion of others. When the patient attempts to move, not only are the agonists recruited, the antagonists are, as well.

Another consequence of basal ganglia dysfunction is slow movement (bradykinesia) and reduced movement amplitude (hypokinesia). In part, this may be a consequence of the excessive co-contraction and rigidity. But another factor seems to be an altered perception of movement velocity and amplitude. The person with parkinsonism thinks he is moving faster and farther than he really is.[45] Basal ganglia circuits are also connected to frontal and parietal lobe areas related to regulation and perception of sensation, so it is not unexpected that there would be some alterations in this system, as well. As described in Chapter 14's discussion of Parkinson Disease, a deliberate and practiced attempt to make big movements can result in some improvement.

Cerebellum

The cerebellum is a structure attached to the back of the brainstem. Its first recognized role was in balance and motor coordination, but it is now accepted that some functions associated with motor planning, which might be considered cognitive, also engage the cerebellum.[46] The cerebellum has three main functional divisions. The **vestibulocerebellum** receives information from the vestibular nuclei about balance and eye/head movements and helps regulate these. The **spinocerebellum** receives sensory and proprioceptive inputs from the spinal cord and influences the activity of the descending systems through the reticulospinal system, rubrospinal system, and via the motor cortex, the corticospinal system. The **cerebrocerebellum** receives inputs from the cerebral cortex and projects back up to the cerebral cortex in order to help maintain coordinated neural activity in support of movement and motor planning.

At its core, the cerebellum helps improve motor control in two ways, adjustment and coordination. **Adjustment** is the ability to do slightly more or less. For example, in trying to thread a needle, you will watch the thread as you move it toward the needle's eye. If you are slightly left of the target, you will adjust to move slightly right. **Coordination** is the ability to link together control of two or more actions. If a glass is tipping over and you reach out to grab it, you will not only need to move your arm rapidly to the proper location, you will need your trunk to support the reaching action and your hand to open in preparation. There are two distinct features of the circuits through the cerebellum that support adjustment and coordination. The same circuits are used in each functional division of the cerebellum.

The first circuit is shown in Figure 5-5. The inputs to the cerebellum come in via axons that are called **mossy fibers**. These come from one of the three places mentioned above, the vestibular nuclei, spinal cord, or brainstem. In the case of the vestibular nuclei, the mossy fibers come directly from vestibular nucleus neurons. For the spinal cord and cerebrum there will be at least one synapse between the origin of the information (a primary sensory neuron or a cortical neuron) and the mossy fiber. For the spinocerebellum, the mossy fiber will come from a cell in **Clarke's column** of the lumbar spinal cord or from the **accessory cuneate nucleus** for upper thoracic and cervical segments. For information coming from the cerebrum, the synapse will be in the pontine nuclei.

Once the mossy fiber carries its information into the cerebellum, it will make excitatory synapses in two places. One branch will go to a neuron in a **deep cerebellar nucleus** (DCN), and the other will synapse in the cerebellar cortex on a type of cell called a **granule cell**. The cell in the DCN will convey the output of the cerebellum, so for this part of the circuit, a higher level of activity coming in on the mossy fiber will tend to lead to a higher level of activity going out. At the same time, however, the activity from the mossy fiber is driving the granule cell. The granule cell will, in turn, synapse on a type of cell in the cerebellar cortex called the **Purkinje cell**. The Purkinje cells make inhibitory synapses on the neurons in the DCN, so through this side of the circuit, increased activity on the mossy fiber coming in will lead to less output from the DCN. The ultimate effect is a contest. Through a process described below, the relative strengths of the excitatory and inhibitory drive to the DCN cells is adjusted with practice so that the proper amount of DCN output is produced. For DCN output cells with influence over the position of the fingers, decreased activity might move the thread slightly left, and increased activity might move it slightly right. Hence, this circuit is well suited for adjustments in motor control.

The feature of cerebellar circuitry that supports coordination of actions across joints is the way in which the granule cells themselves connect to the Purkinje cells. When the granule cell's axon reaches the upper layers of the cerebellar cortex, it splits into two branches, each of which runs parallel to the folia of the cerebellar cortex. These axons are thus aptly named **parallel fibers**. The parallel fibers are what synapse on the Purkinje cells. Each parallel fiber spans relatively far, as much as one-third the width of the cerebellum. Across this much span, there is the possibility that a single parallel fiber in the spinocerebellum could contact various Purkinje cells to influence motor outputs for the legs, trunk, and arms. As such, parallel fibers provide the substrate for coordination of activity across these body parts. In the vestibulocerebellum, the parallel fibers could link balance and postural reactions to movements of the eyes and the head. And in the cerebrocerebellum, they could link past experience with future expectations to provide for anticipatory motor control.

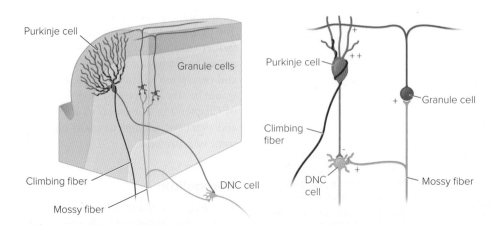

FIGURE 5-5 Cerebellar circuits. On the left, an anatomical cross section of the cerebellar cortex is illustrated, and on the right, a schematic diagram of the circuit is shown. For simplicity, this diagram shows only a part of the cerebellar circuit.

The last aspect of cerebellar function that we will consider is the basis for motor learning provided by the climbing fibers. A **climbing fiber** is a special type of axon that climbs up and around the soma and proximal dendrites of each Purkinje cell. There is only one climbing fiber per Purkinje cell. The **inferior olivary nucleus** in the medulla is where we find the cell bodies of the neurons that produce the climbing fibers. As noted earlier, for adjustments to occur, the relative strengths of the Purkinje cell and mossy fiber influences on the DCN cell must be adjustable. There are two ways in which this occurs. First, there is a principle of operation in the nervous system called **long-term potentiation**. A simple catch phrase used to describe this is that "neurons that fire together wire together." What this mean is that if a Purkinje cell tends to make an action potential every time a particular parallel fiber synapse fires to excite it, that synapse will strengthen over time. At first glance, this might seem inevitable, but there are millions of parallel fibers for each Purkinje cell. One parallel fiber firing alone, therefore, is not sufficient to make the Purkinje cell fire. But if the whole set of parallel fibers influence is such that the Purkinje cell fires, then those parallel fibers that are active when the Purkinje cell does make an action potential will tend to see their synaptic influence increase over time. Hence, there is a natural way for synapses between parallel fibers and Purkinje cells that are involved in similar actions to strengthen their connections with each other.

However, what if the action made was a mistake? This is where the climbing fibers come in. Projections to the inferior olivary nucleus will produce action potentials in climbing fibers going to Purkinje cells that were active in association with the mistake. When the climbing fiber makes an action potential, its influence upon the Purkinje cell is profound. The electrical potential created by the climbing fiber is so strong that it creates a special kind of action potential in the Purkinje cell called a **complex spike**. After a complex spike occurs, any parallel fiber synapses that were recently active in that Purkinje cell get weaker, and this is called **long-term depression**. Presumably, these were parallel fiber inputs to the Purkinje cell that were associated with the mistake, so in a way of thinking, they get the blame.

Thus, parallel fiber to Purkinje cell synapses that are not associated with errors will naturally tend to get stronger via long-term potentiation, and those that are associated with errors are made weaker through long-term depression. This allows the adjustment of Purkinje cell influence on the DCN cell. And just as this can occur in any given Purkinje cell to make adjustments in the control of a single aspect of the motor control problem, it can occur in a whole set of parallel fiber to Purkinje cell connections all at once as a means to adjust the coordination of activity among the Purkinje cells, and hence, coordination among multiple aspects of the motor control task.

• PUTTING IT ALL TOGETHER

We now return to the example of the person typing and reaching for the mouse. At this point, we can attach specific tracts and their functions to the example. As the person is typing, there will be tonic activity in the ventromedial systems, including the reticulospinal and vestibulospinal systems, to maintain a stable sitting posture. The primary motor cortex and supplementary motor areas will be active on both sides to select the appropriate sequencing of finger movements to type the text. There will be engagement of the basal ganglia circuits to select the sequence of keystrokes for typing and to select the particular muscles to recruit and relax to perform the actual wrist and finger movements. While the typist will be somewhat unaware of this, there will also be subtle modulation of shoulder and upper trunk activity so that the small shifts in hand and forearm position are made from a stable base. Cerebellar activity will be constantly coordinating these actions, maintaining appropriate forces of the keystrokes and locations of the keys as time passes.

When it is time to reach for the mouse, cortical sensory areas will have a memory of the mouse's location and weight and size and will transfer this memory to the frontal lobe, which will engage motor memory of the action to grasp the mouse through basal ganglia (selection and initiation) and cerebellar (anticipation, coordination, and adjustment) circuits as soon as the desire to use the mouse enters the author's mind. The trajectory to the mouse will be planned, and before the hands are raised from the keyboard, neural activity in the PM and supplementary motor areas will begin to create a subtle postural shift of the shoulders and upper trunk to prepare for the expected inertial consequence of moving the arm. These outputs will be conveyed to some extent through the corticospinal system, which does originate, in part, from these premotor areas. In addition, corticoreticular projections will engage the reticulospinal system to provide the dynamic, anticipatory postural adjustment prior to the reach.

As the reach for the mouse occurs, the author will most likely maintain a visual gaze toward the computer monitor. To the extent that the anticipatory postural adjustment, prior to reaching, along with the arm movement itself, during the reach, result in subtle head movements in reaction, the VOR will operate through the medial vestibulospinal tracts to help keep the eyes pointed to the correct location.

As the reach occurs, the lateral corticospinal tract will be heavily engaged to move the arm in the proper direction and the hand and fingers into a position to grasp the mouse. The rubrospinal tract will also help with this rapid, coordinated reaching action to help shape the hand for grasping the mouse. Cerebellar circuits will help coordinate the forces and torques throughout the upper limb for a smooth movement, making adjustments along the way. As the mouse is grasped, sensory systems will be attuned to the shape and texture of the mouse, helping guide the motor actions required for final placement of the hand around the mouse to use it properly. This seemingly simple action requires cooperation throughout the motor system.

REFERENCES

1. Kuypers HG. Anatomy of descending pathways. *Handbook of Physiology. Sect. I. The Nervous System. Vol. II. Motor Control, pt 1*. Bethesda, MD: The American Physiological Society; 1981: 597–666.

2. Lemon RN. Descending pathways in motor control. *Ann. Rev Neurosci.* 2008;31(1):195-218.

3. Bortoff GA, Strick PL. Corticospinal terminations in two new-world primates: further evidence that corticomotoneuronal connections provide part of the neural substrate for manual dexterity. *J Neurosci.* 1993;13:5105-5118.

4. Dum RP, Strick PL. Motor areas in the frontal lobe of the primate. *Physiol Behav.* 2002;77(4-5):677-682.

5. Strick PL. Stimulating research on motor cortex. *Nat Neurosci.* 2002;5(8):714-715.

6. Freund HJ. Premotor areas in man. In: Evarts EE, Wise SP, Bousfield D, eds. *The Motor System in Neurobiology.* New York, NY: Elsevier; 1985: 332-335.

7. Maier MA, Armand J, Kirkwood PA, Yang HW, Davis JN, Lemon RN. Differences in the corticospinal projection from primary motor cortex and supplementary motor area to macaque upper limb motoneurons: an anatomical and electrophysiological study. *Cereb Cortex.* 2002;12(3):281-296.

8. Dum RP, Strick PL. Spinal cord terminations of the medial wall motor areas in macaque monkeys. *J Neurosci.* 1996;16(20):6513-6525.

9. Roland PE, Larsen B, Lassen NA, Skinhoj E. Supplementary motor area and other cortical areas in organization of voluntary movements in man. *J Neurophysiol.* 1980;43(1):118-136.

10. Cheney PD, Hill-Karrer J, Belhaj-Saif A, McKiernan BJ, Park MC, Marcario JK. Cortical motor areas and their properties: implications for neuroprosthetics. *Prog Brain Res.* 2000;128:135-160.

11. Wise SP, di Pellegrino G, Boussaoud D. Primate premotor cortex: dissociation of visuomotor from sensory signals. *J Neurophysiol.* 1992;68(3): 969-972.

12. Halsband U, Lange RK. Motor learning in man: a review of functional and clinical studies. *J Physiol Paris.* 2006;99(4-6):414-424.

13. Vaseghi B, Zoghi M, Jaberzadeh S. Does anodal transcranial direct current stimulation modulate sensory perception and pain? A meta-analysis study. *Clin Neurophysiol.* 2014;125(9):1847-1858.

14. Courtine G, Bunge MB, Fawcett JW, et al. Can experiments in nonhuman primates expedite the translation of treatments for spinal cord injury in humans? *Nat Med.* 2007;13(5):561-566.

15. Schwartz AB. Useful signals from motor cortex. *J Physiol.* 2007;579(Pt 3): 581-601.

16. Seidler RD, Bo J, Anguera JA. Neurocognitive contributions to motor skill learning: the role of working memory. *J Mot Behav.* 2012;44(6):445-453.

17. Petrides M. Lateral prefrontal cortex: architectonic and functional organization. *Philos Trans R Soc Lond B Biol Sci.* 2005;360(1456):781-795.

18. Goldman-Rakic PS. Motor control function of the prefrontal cortex. *Ciba Found Symp.* 1987;132:187-200.

19. Buys EJ, Lemon RN, Mantel GW, Muir RB. Selective facilitation of different hand muscles by single corticospinal neurons in the conscious monkey. *J Physiol.* 1986;381:529-549.

20. Fetz EE, Cheney PD, Mewes K, Palmer S. Control of forelimb muscle activity by populations of corticomotoneuronal and rubromotoneuronal cells. *Prog Brain Res.* 1989;80:437-449.

21. McKiernan BJ, Marcario JK, Karrer JH, Cheney PD. Corticomotoneuronal postspike effects in shoulder, elbow, wrist, digit, and intrinsic hand muscles during a reach and prehension task. *J Neurophysiol.* 1998;80(4):1961-1980.

22. Jankowska E, Edgley SA. How can corticospinal tract neurons contribute to ipsilateral movements? A question with implications for recovery of motor functions. *Neuroscientist.* 2006;12(1):67-79.

23. Denny-Brown D. *The cerebral control of movement.* Springfield, IL: Charles C Thomas; 1966.

24. Bourbonnais D, Vanden Noven S, Pelletier R. Incoordination in patients with hemiparesis. *Can J Public Health.* 1992;83(Suppl 2):S58-S63.

25. Porter B. A review of intrathecal baclofen in the management of spasticity. *Br J Nurs.* 1997;6(5):253-260, 262.

26. Thompson AK, Wolpaw JR. Operant conditioning of spinal reflexes: from basic science to clinical therapy. *Front Integr Neurosci.* 2014;8:25.

27. Chen XY, Chen Y, Wang Y, et al. Reflex conditioning: a new strategy for improving motor function after spinal cord injury. *Ann N Y Acad Sci.* 2010;1198(Suppl 1):E12-E21.

28. Van Kan PL, McCurdy ML. Role of primate magnocellular red nucleus neurons in controlling hand preshaping during reaching to grasp. *J Neurophysiol.* 2001;85(4):1461-1478.

29. Van Kan PL, McCurdy ML. Discharge of primate magnocellular red nucleus neurons during reaching to grasp in different spatial locations. *Exp Brain Res.* 2002;142(1):151-157.

30. Drew T, Andujar JE, Lajoie K, Yakovenko S. Cortical mechanisms involved in visuomotor coordination during precision walking. *Brain Res Rev.* 2008;57(1):199-211.

31. Rho MJ, Lavoie S, Drew T. Effects of red nucleus microstimulation on the locomotor pattern and timing in the intact cat: a comparison with the motor cortex. *J Neurophysiol.* 1999;81(5):2297-2315.

32. Fukushima K. Corticovestibular interactions: anatomy, electrophysiology, and functional considerations. *Exp Brain Res.* 1997;117(1):1-16.

33. Sugiuchi Y, Izawa Y, Ebata S, Shinoda Y. Vestibular cortical area in the periarcuate cortex: its afferent and efferent projections. *Ann N Y Acad Sci.* 2005;1039:111-123.

34. Horak FB. Postural compensation for vestibular loss. *Ann N Y Acad Sci.* 2009;1164:76-81.

35. Horak FB, Henry SM, Shumway-Cook A. Postural perturbations: new insights for treatment of balance disorders. *Phys Ther.* 1997;77(5):517-533.

36. Buford JA. Reticulospinal system. In: Squire L, ed. *The New Encyclopedia of Neuroscience.* Elsevier; 2008. Available at http://store.elsevier.com/product.jsp?isbn=9780080446172.

37. Matsuyama K, Takakusaki K, Nakajima K, Mori S. Multi-segmental innervation of single pontine reticulospinal axons in the cervico-thoracic region of the cat: anterograde PHA-L tracing study. *J Comp Neurol.* 1997;377(2):234-250.

38. Matsuyama K, Mori F, Kuze B, Mori S. Morphology of single pontine reticulospinal axons in the lumbar enlargement of the cat: a study using the anterograde tracer PHA-L. *J Comp Neurol.* 1999;410(3):413-430.

39. Jankowska E. Spinal interneuronal networks in the cat: elementary components. *Brain Res Rev.* 2007;57:46-55.

40. Steeves JD, Jordan LM. Localization of a descending pathway in the spinal cord which is necessary for controlled treadmill locomotion. *Neurosci Lett.* 1980;20(3):283-288.

41. Angeli CA, Edgerton VR, Gerasimenko YP, Harkema SJ. Altering spinal cord excitability enables voluntary movements after chronic complete paralysis in humans. *Brain.* 2014;137(Pt 5):1394-1409.

42. Edgerton VR, Roy RR. A new age for rehabilitation. *Eur J Phys Rehabil Med.* 2012;48(1):99-109.

43. Mink JW. The basal ganglia: focused selection and inhibition of competing motor programs. *Prog Neurobiol.* 1996;50(4):381-425.

44. Mink JW. The basal ganglia and involuntary movements: impaired inhibition of competing motor patterns. *Arch Neurol.* 2003;60(10):1365-1368.

45. Konczak J, Corcos DM, Horak F, et al. Proprioception and motor control in Parkinson's disease. *J Mot Behav.* 2009;41(6):543-552.

46. Bostan AC, Dum RP, Strick PL. Cerebellar networks with the cerebral cortex and basal ganglia. *Trends Cogn Sci.* 2013;17(5):241-254.

Review Questions

1. **What is the best example of feed-forward control?**
   A. A stretch reflex resisting forward sway when a person is pushed from behind
   B. Looking at a mouse before reaching for it
   C. Leaning forward before reaching forward
   D. Moving one finger while holding the wrist stable

2. **Which of the cortical motor areas is most likely to produce a corticospinal cell that synapses directly on an alpha motoneuron?**
   A. Primary motor cortex
   B. Supplementary motor area
   C. Premotor cortex
   D. All are equal in this regard

3. **Which body area has a disproportionately small representation in the primary motor cortex?**
   A. Face (mouth)
   B. Arm and hands
   C. Trunk
   D. Legs and feet

4. **In which part of the spinal cord would we expect to find a complete absence of the ventral (anterior) corticospinal tract?**
   A. Upper cervical
   B. Cervical enlargement
   C. Thoracic
   D. Lumbosacral enlargement

5. **Which of the descending systems listed here has bilateral influence?**
   A. Rubrospinal
   B. Lateral reticulospinal
   C. Medial reticulospinal
   D. Lateral vestibulospinal

6. **A patient in a neurologic clinic has trouble moving the right side of her body, reaches with her right arm in a very limited way, and does not seem able to use her right hand. She can sit and can walk with a cane, but there is** also some difficulty in the right leg. She is speaking and her eye movements and facial function seem fairly normal. Where would you most expect the lesion in this person's nervous system to be found?
   A. Left cervical spinal cord
   B. Left motor cortex
   C. Left brainstem
   D. Left cerebellum

7. **What additional motor deficit would you expect to discover upon testing this individual?**
   A. Marked weakness in the left hand
   B. Spasticity (difficulty regulating reflexes) in the right arm and/or leg
   C. Inability to swallow
   D. Ataxia (discoordinated, flailing movements) on the left side

8. **In the basal ganglia, which pathway includes the subthalamic nucleus?**
   A. The direct pathway
   B. The indirect pathway
   C. The thalamocortical pathway
   D. The substantia nigra pathway

9. **What happens when a climbing fiber sets off a complex spike in a Purkinje cell?**
   A. Synapses of mossy fibers on DCN cells get stronger if they were silent
   B. Synapses of parallel fibers on the Purkinje cell get weaker if they were active
   C. Synapses of the Purkinje cell on the DCN cell get stronger
   D. Synapses of the granule cell on the climbing fiber get weaker

10. **The ventromedial systems for motor control serve what general function?**
    A. Control of the adductor and extensor muscles
    B. Control of the postural and proximal limb muscles
    C. Control of the distal hand and foot muscles
    D. Control of the abdominal and low back muscles

Answers

| 1. C | 2. A | 3. C | 4. D | 5. C |
| 6. B | 7. B | 8. B | 9. B | 10. B |

The Special Senses

Deborah S. Nichols-Larsen and Anne D. Kloos

6

OBJECTIVES

1) Review the neuroanatomical basis of vision, hearing, smell, taste, and vestibular system function

2) Develop a foundation for the discussion of sensory dysfunction associated with neurologic conditions

3) Examine common testing methods to identify sensory system integrity

In this chapter, we will review the organization and function of the special senses, focusing on vision, vestibular, hearing, taste, and proprioception. These special senses, like somatosensation, each have specific receptors that translate external stimuli to neural coding, neural projections that convey these neural impulses centrally, and brain networks that decode the sensation. This review should help the reader with later chapters, when these systems are disrupted by neurologic injury or disease.

● VISION

The Eye

The visual system, of course, starts with the eye. The eye is uniquely shaped to allow perception of our environment; its rounded shape allows the projection of almost 180 degrees of horizontal vision without head or eye movement and nearly 130 degrees of vertical vision. The eye is protected from the environment by a tough external membrane, the **sclera**, which is opaque (white); interestingly, the sclera is continuous with the dura mater (the protective covering of the brain). The **cornea** makes up the most central portion of the sclera, over the iris, and refracts light toward the lens as it enters the pupil. The eye and, more specifically, the retina are nourished by the underlying choroid, which is a highly vascular tissue that provides critical nutrients to maintain eye health. Light is projected by the cornea, through the **pupil** (the central opening of the eye) onto the **lens**, which in turn, focuses it onto the retina (Figure 6-1). The pupil is surrounded by the iris that is comprised of muscles that control the pupils' size: the sphincter pupillae muscle constricts the pupil in bright light, and the dilator pupillae muscle dilates the pupil when light is low. Although the pupil determines the amount of light that enters the eye, it does not play a critical role in focusing the light. This is done by the cornea and the lens. The **lens** sits behind the pupil and is controlled by the ciliary muscles. Both the muscles of the iris and those for the pupil are controlled by the autonomic nervous system via CN III: sympathetic activity dilates the pupil; parasympathetic activity constricts the pupil and contracts the ciliary muscle for lens control (see Box 6-1). Although the greatest amount of light refraction occurs at the cornea, the lens is critical for finely focusing light on the fovea. In the center of the eye, between the lens and retina, there's a gelatinous substance, known as the **vitreous humor** that serves to maintain the shape of the eye. The retina is a layered structure at the rear of the eye that contains the photosensitive receptors of the eye and the transmission neurons of optic projections.

Visual Field(s)

The shape of the eye along with the unique characteristics of the cornea and lens allows for projection of our visual environment with duplication of the central portion of our visual field onto the retinas of both eyes; this explains our enhanced central vision, compared to our peripheral vision, and allows some visual preservation with certain neural injuries. The view of our environment that is visible without eye movement is referred to as our *visual field* (Figure 6-2). Information from the right visual field is conveyed to the nasal retina of the right eye and the temporal retina of the left eye and vice versa for the left visual field; there is a portion of the extreme peripheral visual field that is only projected to the ipsilateral eye because the nose blocks its projection to the opposite eye; this information is projected to the most nasal portion of the ipsilateral eye. For the most part, however, our visual field is binocular.

Visual Receptors

The eye possesses a unique filtering system and sensory receptors that encode light into neural signals. As light enters the eye through the pupil, the lens focuses the incoming image centrally, aiming for the tightest cluster of receptors, located in the central portion of the retina, known as the **fovea**, which is the central area of the **macula**, a lightly colored area in the central retina that is dense with receptors and ganglion cells. The receptors of the eye are **rod and cone cells**; both are photosensitive due to special pigments within them. The fovea contains only cones, which are color receptors that are less sensitive to light but provide better visual acuity. There are three types of cones, responding to different portions of the light spectrum: red – longest rays of the spectrum, L cones; green – middle portion

FIGURE 6-1 Anatomy of the eye. (Reproduced with permission from McKinley M, O'Laughlin VD. *Human Anatomy* 3rd Ed, New York, NY: McGraw-Hill; 2012, Fig. 19.12B, P. 576.)

BOX 6-1 Pupil and Lens Control

Pupillary reflexes:

Constriction: When a strong light hits the retina, it induces constriction of the pupil through a reflexive response. This reflex is mediated by sequential projections from the retina to the midbrain's pretectal nucleus, to the Edinger–Westphal nuclei (also in the midbrain), to the ciliary ganglion and ultimately to the ciliary muscles that constrict the pupil via parasympathetic fibers in CN III. Each Edinger–Westphal muscle connects to its counterpart on the opposite side such that pupillary constriction occurs bilaterally and symmetrically.

Dilation: Dilation can be achieved by inhibition of the reflexive loop that produces constriction or activation of the iris dilator muscle via the sympathetic nervous system component of the ciliary ganglion.

Accommodation:

Changing of the shape of the lens within the eye allows us to orient to objects near to us as well as those far away. To allow us to focus on objects in the distance, the lens becomes elongated, associated with ciliary muscle relaxation, while focus on near objects is achieved by a thickening of the lens via ciliary muscle contraction; both of these changes serve to focus the image on the retina. The ciliary muscles of the lens create this change in lens shape through the same series of projections that control the pupillary reflexes; in fact, accommodation for near vision is also associated with pupil constriction and eye convergence (slight adduction), requiring integration via these brainstem nuclei.

Myopia (nearsightedness): Light is focused short of the retina, making distance vision poor, associated with poor elongation of the lens or an eye that is too long.

Hyperopia (farsightedness): Poor near vision caused by poor accommodation (inability of the lens to achieve a sufficiently round shape) or an eye that is too short.

Presbyopia: Age-induced change in the ability to accommodate, resulting in poorer near vision.

---

of the spectrum, M cones; blue – shortest rays of the spectrum, S cones. However, since cones are less light sensitive, they are inactive in dim light, rendering us "color blind" in low levels of light. Conversely, rods are highly light sensitive, capable of being activated by a single photon of light, and responsible for our vision at night and in poorly lit environments. However,

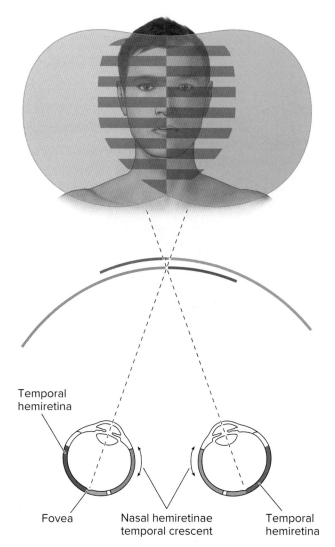

Temporal
hemiretina

Fovea   Nasal hemiretinae   Temporal
        temporal crescent   hemiretina

FIGURE 6-2 Schematic of visual field projections. Projections to the retina: The central striped area illustrates the overlapping binocular visual field, conveyed to the temporal retina of each eye. The solid colored fields are unique to each eye. The right monocular visual field (green) is transmitted to the right nasal retina while the left (blue) is transmitted to the left nasal retina. This allows the projections from the right field to come together as the nasal fibers cross at the optic chiasm. (Reproduced with permission from Martin JH. *Neuroanatomy Text and Atlas*, Ed 4. New York, NY: McGraw-Hill; 2012, Fig 7-5, pg. 161.)

they quickly become saturated, and therefore inactive, in bright light. Notably, cones are clustered tightly in the fovea and then progressively decrease toward the periphery of the retina; conversely, rods are absent in the fovea, more dense in the area surrounding it, and also become progressively less dense toward the periphery.

The Retina

Although rods and cones are the photosensitive receptors for vision, they are uniquely located in the layer of the retina furthest from the pupil where light enters the eye (Figure 6-3).

Thus, light must travel through multiple cellular layers of the retina before reaching these critical receptors; interestingly, the pigment epithelium also absorbs light to prevent it from "bouncing back" through the eye. The middle cellular layer of the retina houses the interneuronal complex that transmits signals from the receptors to the ganglion cells. This interneuronal complex is comprised of three types of interneurons: bipolar, horizontal, and amacrine cells. **Bipolar cells** are the primary transmission interneurons, connecting the receptors to the ganglion cells that make up the optic nerve; the **horizontal** and **amacrine** cellular networks function as modulators of neural transmission by increasing or decreasing the effectiveness of bipolar cell activation of ganglion cells, and thereby, adjusting spatial sensitivity and acuity. Ganglion cells are more superficial in the retina, closest to the incoming light; their axons come together in the optic disc, also known as the **blind spot** of the eye, as they exit the eye to convey visual information centrally as the optic nerve (CN II).

Optic Projections and Visual Processing

As mentioned, the visual environment is projected such that each eye receives information from the right and left environment: ipsilateral peripheral vision to the nasal retina and contralateral central vision to the temporal retina. As the ganglion cell axons merge into the optic nerve, those from the nasal retina are more medial and those from the temporal retina more lateral. Just above the pituitary gland, the two optic nerves come together in the **optic chiasm**; it is here that the central fibers cross and merge with the temporal fibers of the contralateral eye. This crossing brings all of the fibers for a **hemifield** (1/2 of the entire visual field) into the contralateral **optic tract** that projects to the **lateral geniculate** of the thalamus; a small number of fibers bypass the lateral geniculate and project to the **superior colliculus**, which is involved in the assessment of object versus self-movement and visual reflexes. Visual neurons from the lateral geniculate project as the **optic radiations** to the primary visual cortex in the occipital lobe (Brodmann's area 17; striate cortex); the optic radiations split as they leave the lateral geniculate, to accommodate the lateral ventricles, with the upper visual field fibers (lower retinal fibers) traversing laterally within the temporal lobe as **Meyer's loop** and the lower visual field fibers (upper retinal fibers) coursing superiorly through the parietal lobe to the striate (calcarine) cortex of the occipital lobe, which is the primary visual cortex (Brodmann's area 17) (Figure 6-4). It is referred to as the calcarine cortex because it straddles the calcarine sulcus on the medial surface of the hemisphere as well as the striate cortex because of its layered or striped appearance. Terminations of the optic radiations place the information from the fovea more posteriorly and that from the periphery more anteriorly with the upper visual field in the lower striate cortex and the lower visual field in the upper striate cortex; thus, the visual image is upside down in the primary visual cortex. Visual processing begins in the striate cortex but relies heavily on the surrounding occipital lobe, or non-striate cortex (areas 18 and 19). The cortical processing of visual stimuli occurs through interconnections within these three occipital areas to separately decode for color, shape, and location/movement.

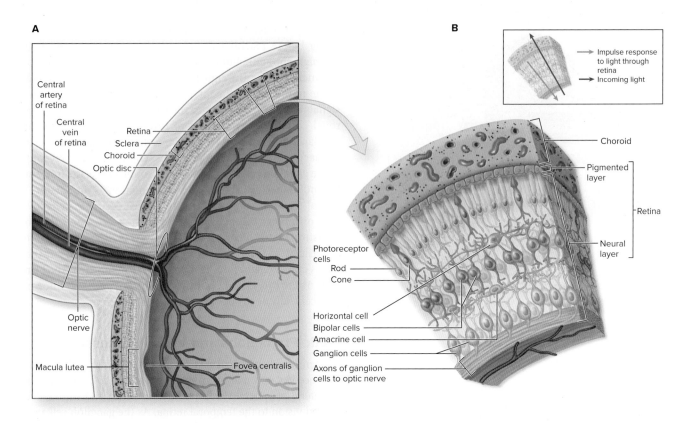

FIGURE 6-3 Diagram of eye and retina. Light enters the front of the eye and passes through the lens, vitreous humor to the retina, where it passes first through the interneural complex of ganglion, bipolar, and horizontal cells before hitting the photosensitive rods and cones. Transduction retraces this pathway with sequential activation of the bipolar cells and then the ganglion cells that form the optic nerve. Horizontal and amacrine cells modulate the cellular activity between the bipolar and ganglion cells. (Reproduced with permission from McKinley M, O'Laughlin VD. *Human Anatomy.* 3rd ed. McGraw Hill, Inc., 2012; Figure 19.14, p. 578.)

Additional connections between the two hemispheres allow for a complete reproduction of the visual environment to occur. More sophisticated analysis of object recognition and localization relies on two separate networks between the occipital lobe and the temporal and parietal lobes, respectively (Figure 6-5).

One method of testing for visual system integrity is through the **visual evoked potential** (VEP). The VEP measures the time it takes a presented stimulus to move through the visual system to the occipital cortex, using electroencephalographic (EEG) measurement. The typical stimulus is a checkerboard pattern, introduced in an alternating fashion to each eye, or a flashing light, used mostly in children. The N100 wave is a spike that can be seen when the visual signal reaches the occipital cortex, named for the characteristic 100 seconds this transmission takes in most people. A delay in the N100 is indicative of disruption in the visual projections, associated with multiple sclerosis, optic neuritis or other conditions that impede neuronal transmission.[1]

Eye Movement and Visual Pursuit

The eye has a dynamic group of six muscles, innervated by three cranial nerves (III, IV, and VI) that allow its unique and complex movement abilities: superior rectus, inferior rectus, medial rectus, and inferior oblique, innervated by CN III; superior oblique (CN IV); and lateral rectus (CN VI). The medial and lateral recti produce medial (adduction) and lateral (abduction)

horizontal movements, consistent with their names. Similarly, the superior and inferior recti pull the eye upward (elevation) and downward (depression), respectively, but due to their off-center insertions on the eye, also pull the eyes inward, so with superior rectus contraction the eye moves up and in, and conversely, the inferior rectus contraction pulls the eye down and in to look at the tip of the nose. Both of the oblique muscles attach to the eye on the posterolateral surface and have actions in opposition of their name but consistent with their attachment on the eye. The superior oblique attaches on the superior aspect of the eye and orients the eye downward and laterally (lower corner of the room) by pulling the back of the eye up and in, while the inferior oblique attaches on the inferior aspect and orients the eye upward and laterally (to look at the upper corner of the room) by pulling the back of the eye down and medially.

Although these extraocular muscles can be controlled individually or in combination through upper motor neuron activation of their respective cranial nuclei and nerves, eye control is also maintained through a series of brainstem networks, and as you have likely experienced, moving just one eye is very difficult as they are controlled in tandem through these networks. First, the paramedian pontine reticular formation controls lateral eye coordination, referred to as **horizontal saccades**, through its projections to the abducens nucleus; neurons within this nucleus directly produce lateral rectus contractions of the

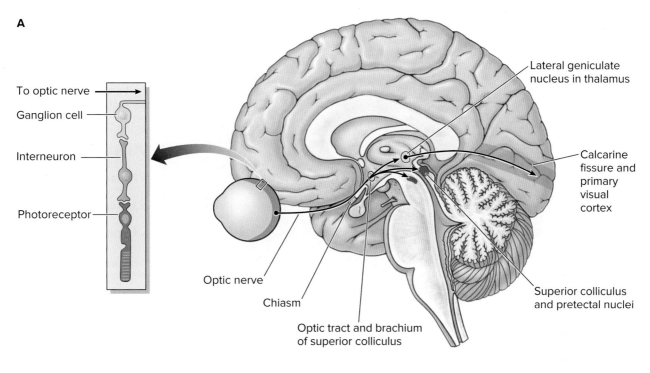

A

To optic nerve

Ganglion cell

Interneuron

Photoreceptor

Lateral geniculate nucleus in thalamus

Calcarine fissure and primary visual cortex

Optic nerve

Chiasm

Optic tract and brachium of superior colliculus

Superior colliculus and pretectal nuclei

B

Frontal pole

Optic nerve

Optic chiasm

Optic tract

Optic radiation

Primary visual cortex

Lateral geniculate nucleus

Occipital pole

C

Pretectal nuclei

Brachium of superior colliculus

Superior colliculus

FIGURE 6-4 Visual projections from the retina to the visual cortex. (Reproduced with permission from Martin JH. *Neuroanatomy Text and Atlas*, Ed 4. New York, NY: McGraw-Hill; 2012, Fig 7-2, pg. 158.)

ipsilateral eye and indirectly produce medial rectus contractions of the contralateral eye via the oculomotor nucleus. A group of neurons within the abducens nucleus, known as internuclear neurons, decussate and project to the contralateral oculomotor nucleus, thus activating the medial rectus of the opposite eye. Thus, abduction of the ipsilateral eye and adduction of the contralateral eye can be produced in unison to achieve smooth horizontal motion of the eye. Horizontal saccades can be initiated via projections from the frontal eye fields within the frontal lobe to the superior colliculi in the midbrain but are also controlled by projections from the medial vestibular nuclei in the adjacent brainstem and ultimately their cerebellar connections to maintain vision when the head is turned (see vestibular section of this chapter).

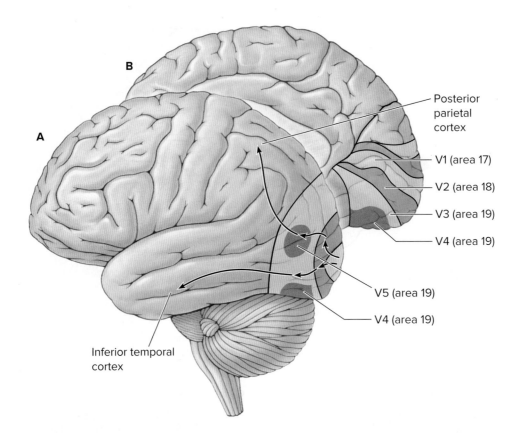

FIGURE 6-5 Areas involved in visual image processing. V1, primary visual cortex (area 17); V2, secondary visual cortex (area 18); V3, V4, V5, distinct regions of area 19. V2–V5 are referred to as the extrastriate cortex as well as visual association cortex. Areas 18 and 19 surround area 17 in a circular fashion. These areas are highly interconnected with many subdivisions, allowing for the complex interpretation of object shape, color, orientation, and movement. Ventral projections to the temporal lobe are associated with object recognition. Dorsal projections to the posterior parietal cortex are associated with object location. (Reproduced with permission from Martin JH. *Neuroanatomy Text and Atlas*, Ed 4. New York, NY: McGraw-Hill; 2012, Fig 7-15, pg. 171.)

Similarly, smooth **vertical saccades** (upward–downward motions) of both eyes are achieved by a network that includes the mesencephalic reticular formation (MRF), the medial longitudinal fasciculi, and the oculomotor nuclei bilaterally. The mesencephalic reticular formations of each side of the brainstem interconnect via projections through the posterior commissure in the midbrain, allowing bilateral control of vertical saccades. The medial longitudinal fasciculus runs between the MRF and the ipsilateral oculomotor nucleus on each side of the brainstem, which innervates both the superior and inferior recti. Thus, simultaneous activation of the respective oculomotor neurons will generate smooth up and down movements. Vertical saccades are also controlled by the frontal eye field via the superior colliculus as well as through inputs from the cerebellum and vestibular nuclei.

This link between eye movement and the vestibular system serves to facilitate eye orientation with head movement via a reflexive response known as the optokinetic reflexes (see vestibular section of this chapter).

Visual Testing

Evaluation of visual function and system integrity is highly complex; here we will discuss briefly some of the measures currently used to examine visual acuity, which should look at each eye and both eyes together, color vision, the ophthalmoscopic assessment of the inner eye, visual field analysis, ocular motility, and pupil responsiveness. Almost everyone has experienced a **high-contrast visual acuity** examination, using a Snellen Chart (lines of letters and numbers of progressively diminishing size) with each line marked by an acuity level. Normal vision is 20/20 or the ability to read at 20 feet what is considered "typical." If you have a visual acuity deficit, this is represented by an increase in the denominator of this fraction (e.g., 20/40), indicating that you see at 20 feet what others see clearly at 40 feet; over correction or enhanced vision is similarly represented by a smaller denominator (e.g., 20/10), indicating that you see at 20 feet what others must be at 10 feet to see. Visual acuity can also be examined at bedside, using a Rosenbaum visual acuity card held 14 inches from the face with a similar acuity outcome measure to a Snellen chart. Visual acuity testing is also the best way to confirm CN II function.[2]

Color perception is trichromatic (red, green, blue) and achieved by the sensitivity of different cone subtypes to specific light spectra; color "blindness" results from a change in the prevalence or functioning of a cone subtype. For many of those affected, the deficit is incomplete with three cone subtypes present but one is impaired, resulting in what is known as an **anomalous trichromatic** deficit; in others, there's an absence of one cone subtype, which is referred to as **dichromatic vision**. For these individuals, they perceive the two remaining color spectra but see the missing spectra as gray or black. Although true color blindness is rare, partial deficits are present in up to 10% of the male population; females rarely experience this deficit because red and green deficits are primarily genetically acquired via X-linked inheritance so that females are carriers but males are affected. Blue color blindness is associated with chromosome 7 mutation, so may be found in both men and women but is much rarer than red or green deficits. Testing for color vision is typically done with Ishihara plates, which are spheres with a background of multicolored dots with an embedded number or letter, also constructed of multicolored dots. The plates are designed to distinguish the different color deficits, listed in Table 6-1 so that the background would be shades of one hue (e.g., green) and the embedded figure would be shades of another (e.g., red) to identify those with an anomalous trichromatic deficit or dichromatic deficit (e.g., protanomaly).[3]

The **ophthalmoscope assessment** of the inner eye allows magnified scrutiny of the external (cornea) and internal eye (lens, vitreous humor, retina), with close attention paid to the **fundus** of the eye, which includes the fovea, macula, optic disk, retina and retinal blood vessels, and is a critical part of evaluation of eye integrity.

To assess **visual fields**, it is best to have the individual look straight ahead; the examiner can then introduce their finger into the peripheral vision from the left and right above and below eye level (upper and lower visual fields), thus, checking peripheral vision by quadrant. It is important that no eye movement be allowed so that "true" peripheral vision is tested.

Optic muscle function should first be evaluated by assessing the resting position of the eye when the individual is looking straight ahead. Second, having the individual track your finger as it moves in all directions will identify disparities between the two eyes indicative of cranial nerve dysfunction and subsequent muscle dysfunction, since these are typically unilateral. Table 6-2 provides details on loss of function with cranial nerve damage.

TABLE 6-1 Color Vision Deficits

TERM		CONES/WAVELENGTH DISRUPTED	COLOR VISUAL DEFICIT
Protanomaly		L Cones – long wavelength	Red
Deuteranomaly		M Cones – middle wavelength	Green
Tritanomaly		S Cones – short wavelength	Blue
Achromatopsia	Rod monochromatism	Loss of all cone function	Photophobia Nystagmus Poor acuity No color vision
	Cone monochromatism	Blue cone function without red or green function but very few blue cones	

TABLE 6-2 Ocular Cranial Nerve Function and Dysfunction

CRANIAL NERVE	FUNCTION	DYSFUNCTION
III	Medial, inferior and superior recti, and inferior oblique; pupil constriction; eyelid lifting (opening); accommodation	Pupil dilation; at rest, pull of superior oblique and lateral rectus is unopposed, so eye looks down and outward. Can't look directly downward due to absence of inferior rectus (eye deviates outward due to pull of superior oblique), medially or upward. Pupil is dilated; eyelid droops; and vision is blurry (lack of accommodation)
IV	Superior oblique	At rest, eye is elevated. When eye is adducted, elevation increases. When eye is abducted, elevation decreases
VI	Lateral rectus	Unable to abduct eye

Pupillary responsiveness should be evaluated in a semi-darkened room with the person looking to an object straight ahead on the wall; this will produce pupil dilation. Then, introduce a pen light from below and watch for the response; both pupils should constrict equally. It is not unusual for people to have a slight difference in the size of their pupils, but the degree of the response should be the same.[2]

OLFACTION: THE SENSE OF SMELL

Our sense of smell, or olfaction, is phylogenetically the oldest sensory system, and in nonhumans plays a critical role in survival, enabling the identification and location of food. Thus, in most animals, the olfactory system is much larger, respectively, than in humans, who rarely rely on their nose to find their food except perhaps when they are awakened by the smell of fresh coffee brewing or bacon frying.

Olfactory Receptors

Olfaction originates in the **bipolar cells** of the nasal epithelium. These cells project multiple **cilia** (hair like projections) into the mucosa that covers the epithelial layer. Only airborne chemicals, known as **odorants**, that are soluble in the mucosa can activate the olfactory neurons and be perceived, yet the wide degree of odors perceived and the sensitivity of the olfactory system to minor variations of odor is quite impressive. The mucosa, itself, facilitates the transportation of these soluble chemicals toward the epithelial layer. Odorants enter the nose through breathing or sniffing as well as through the nasopharyngeal corridor during eating. The axons of the olfactory bipolar cells bundle together into axons that pass through the bony cribriform plate at the top of the nasal passage; these bundled axons, though not tightly organized, make up the **Olfactory Nerve** (CN I), synapsing on second-order neurons, called **mitral cells**, in the olfactory bulb. The connection between the mitral cells and bipolar axons is quite complex with multiple bipolar axons synapsing on each mitral cell, serving to magnify the olfactory signal. The mitral cell axons merge to form the olfactory tract as it exits the olfactory bulb and projects directly to cortical processing centers. See Figure 6-6 for the olfactory projections. Notably, the sense of smell is the only sense that does not project initially to the thalamus before proceeding to the cortex; however, there are projections from the olfactory cortical areas to the thalamus.

Cortical Processing of Olfaction

The areas of the cortex that receive direct olfactory projections are collectively called the olfactory cortex and are located together in the dorsal aspect of the brain: the anterior olfactory nucleus, the olfactory tubercle, the amygdala, the piriform cortex, and the rostral entorhinal cortex (Figure 6-7). The connections with the amygdala and olfactory tubercle are likely related to the strong emotional responses generated by many smells, while the piriform cortex is thought to be the source of odor identification and the entorhinal cortex the source of memories, associated with specific smells. The

Olfactory receptor cells

FIGURE 6-6 Olfactory receptors and projections. Bipolar cells within the nasal epithelium project through the cribriform plate to the olfactory tubercle, activating mitral cells that project as the olfactory tract to the olfactory cortex in structures on the dorsum of the brain. (Reproduced with permission from McKinley M, O'Laughlin VD. *Human Anatomy* 3rd Ed, New York, NY: McGraw-Hill; 2012, Fig. 19.9A, P. 572.)

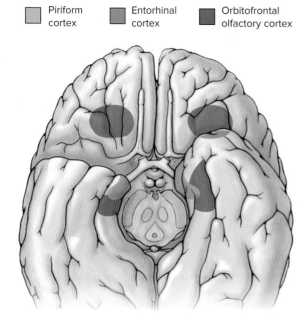

Piriform cortex ▪ Entorhinal cortex ▪ Orbitofrontal olfactory cortex

FIGURE 6-7 Olfactory cortex. (Reproduced with permission from Martin JH. *Neuroanatomy Text and Atlas*, Ed 4. New York, NY: McGraw-Hill; 2012, Fig 9-11, pg. 215.)

anterior olfactory nucleus not only receives projections from the olfactory tract but also projects multiple projections back to the olfactory bulbs bilaterally, and thereby, may serve most to modulate our olfactory experience, either enhancing or diminishing it.

The olfactory tubercle, piriform and entorhinal cortices serve as primary cortical areas for olfaction along with the amygdala, which is deep within temporal lobe, and the anterior olfactory nucleus, which is located along the olfactory tract. The orbitofrontal olfactory cortex receives secondary and tertiary projections from the other olfactory cortices and the thalamus, respectively; it is thought that this area is critical in olfactory discrimination and identification.

Olfactory Testing

Testing olfactory function is relatively simple: choose common liquids with distinct and familiar odors (e.g., vanilla, peppermint extract, or diluted ammonia); wet a cotton swab with the liquid and bring it to a distance of about 1 inch from each nostril. The other nostril should be pushed close with the tester's finger. Using several different odors will yield a more reliable measure.

● GUSTATION: THE SENSE OF TASTE

Similar to olfaction, our perception of taste is based on the transduction of chemicals (**tastants**) within food to neural signals and starts with the taste (gustatory) receptors that are arranged within taste buds. Taste buds are located on the tongue, pharynx, soft palate, epiglottis, and larynx; the taste

buds on the tongue are located within papillae while those on the other surfaces are embedded in the epithelium. Although there are taste buds on the anterior 2/3 of the tongue, they have fewer receptors and play a lesser role in taste differentiation; the lateral edges and posterior 1/3 of the tongue have the largest number of taste receptors, and thereby, play a more critical role in taste along with the other areas in the back of the oral cavity (soft palate, epiglottis, larynx, pharynx). See Box 6-2 for the relationship between taste and smell.

Taste Receptors

There are five identified taste qualities perceived by specific taste receptors: salty – responding to potassium, sodium, or other ionized metals; sweet – responding to sugars; sour – responding to acid released hydrogen ions; bitter – responding to toxins or alkaloids; and umami, which is a Japanese word that translates as a pleasant or savory taste, typically associated with meats and cheeses due to their amino acid content. Some taste receptors respond to only one quality while others respond to several. Unlike other sensory cells, taste receptors die after about 10 days and are replaced with new cells; this most likely assures ongoing responsiveness to tastants.

Why is taste so important? It allows us to identify potential poisons or impurities in our food.

Central Processing of Taste

Taste is projected centrally via three cranial nerves: VII (anterior 2/3 of the tongue), IX (posterior 1/3 of tongue, pharynx), and X (epiglottis, larynx). Figure 6-8 illustrates these projections. Analogous to the primary sensory receptors, these are pseudounipolar neurons with cell bodies in peripheral ganglia encased within the skull; their central projections all terminate in the solitary nucleus of the medulla. Second-order neurons project from the solitary nucleus to the ventral posterior medial nucleus of the thalamus along with somatosensory information from the face. Tertiary projections convey information from the thalamus to the gustatory cortex within the insula and adjacent operculum.

Taste Testing

Similar to the testing of smell, taste can easily be tested by wetting a cotton swab with water flavored with sugar, salt, or lemon juice. Due to the complexity of the innervation for

A

Facial nerve motor root (VII)
Intermediate (VII)
Geniculate ganglion
Glossopharyngeal (IX)
Inferior ganglia
Vagus (X)

Olfactory epithelium
Palate
Tongue
1/3
2/3
Epiglottis

B

Ventral posterior medial nucleus (parvocellular division)
Central tegmental tract
Facial, glossopharyngeal, and vagus nerves
Rostral solitary nucleus
Caudal solitary nucleus

FIGURE 6-8 Cranial nerve projections of taste. A. The three cranial nerves (VII, IX, and X) innervate the oral cavity through long dendritic projections from the cells within the peripheral ganglia (inferior, geniculate) with axonal projections to the solitary nucleus. **B.** Gustatory projections from the solitary nucleus project to the ventral posterior medial nucleus of the thalamus. (Reproduced with permission from Martin JH. *Neuroanatomy Text and Atlas*, Ed 4. New York, NY: McGraw-Hill; 2012, Fig 9-4 and 9-5, pg. 206 and 207.)

taste, testing should include the anterior 2/3 of the tongue (CN VII) as well as the posterior 1/3 of the tongue (CN IX); although taste also originates from receptors in the epiglottis and throat, testing here is most likely to cause gagging, and therefore, is not done.

● HEARING: THE AUDITORY SYSTEM

The Ear's Organization and Auditory Apparatus

The ear is the location for two sensory functions: hearing and vestibular. This section will address the sense of hearing. The external ear (**auricle**) and the **external acoustic meatus** (ear canal) are uniquely funnel-shaped, directing sound inward and toward the **tympanic membrane** (eardrum). Sound waves press upon the tympanic membrane, and this pressure-release phenomenon creates a chain reaction vibration within the middle ear's three ossicles (tiny bones): stapes, incus, and malleus. The vibrating of these tiny auditory ossicles amplifies the sound wave and causes the stapes (the third bone in the chain) to push in and out of the **oval window**, which is the membranous covering for the inner ear. The middle ear is also connected to the nasopharynx via the **Eustachian tube**, which allows the relief of pressure that can develop in the ear (e.g., changes in external pressure while flying) as well as a means of clearing mucus from the middle ear.

The inner ear is comprised of the cochlea and vestibular apparatus or labyrinths that are part of what is referred to as the **bony labyrinth**, a part of the temporal bone that is pitted with cavities and tunnels, lined with a **membranous labyrinth**. The space between the bony and membranous labyrinths is fluid-filled with a substance known as **perilymph** that serves as a protective cushion for the membranous labyrinth. The membranous labyrinth is also filled with fluid, called **endolymph**. The **cochlea** is coiled like a snail with the **cochlear duct** (scalia media) in its center, enclosed by the vestibular membrane above and basilar membrane below. These two membranes also partition the cochlea into two additional chambers, the **vestibular duct** and **tympanic duct** that are connected by a tiny opening. The cochlear duct has an area of thick epithelium, called the **spiral organ** or **organ of Corti** that is embedded with **hair cells**, which are the sensory receptors for sound. The hair cells lie in a supporting matrix of cells just above the basilar membrane but project tiny extensions (stereocilia) upward into a gelatinous mass, known as the **tectorial membrane**. When the oval window is struck by the stapes, vibrations are transmitted into the vestibular duct and successively to the tympanic duct via movement of the endolymph, which, in turn, generates movement of the basilar membrane and the hair cells resting above it. However, the stereocilia are more rigid within the tectorial membrane, causing a shearing force between them and their respective hair cell; this shearing activates the hair cell and induces transduction of the vibration to a neural impulse. There are two types of hairs cells, identified by their location as inner and outer hair cells. The **inner cells** are fewer but receive extensive innervation from CN VIII

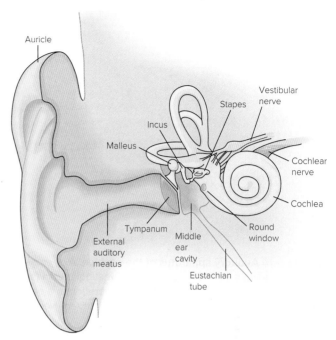

FIGURE 6-9 The three components of the ear. The ear has three functional components: (1) the external ear (auricle, external acoustic meatus, and tympanic membrane) that funnels sound to the interior of the ear; (2) the middle ear (auditory ossicles — malleus, incus, and stapes) that transmits vibration to the ear drum; and (3) the inner ear (cochlea) that allows the transduction of sound to neural signals. (Reproduced with permission from Kandel ER, Schwartz JH, Jessell TM, Siegelbaum SA, Hudspeth AJ. *Principles of neural Science*, 5th Ed., New York, NY: McGraw-Hill; 2013, Fig 30-1, Pg 655.)

fibers; these cells are principally responsible for the transduction of auditory information. **Outer hair cells** outnumber inner cells 3:1 but appear to have more of an efferent function, modulating the activity of inner cells, and thereby, enhancing the amplification of the auditory signal. The vibration dissipates as it passes through the tympanic duct and, then, dissipates through the **round window**, back into the middle ear cavity. See Figure 6-9 for the components of the ear and 6-10 for the auditory apparatus.

Central Processing of Hearing

Similar to other cranial nerves, the neurons that make up the cochlear portion of CN VIII have their cell bodies in peripheral ganglia, the **spiral ganglia**, with long central axons that terminate in the ventral and dorsal **cochlear nuclei** of the rostral medulla. CN VIII neurons convey information from specific areas of the cochlea, associated with sound frequencies, with those transmitting low frequencies originating from the apical portion of the cochlea (narrow tip) and those transmitting higher frequencies originating from the basal cochlea (area closest to the middle ear). Similarly, these projections terminate within the cochlear nuclei such that the ventral portion receives the apical projections and the dorsal portion receives basal projections. This organization is referred

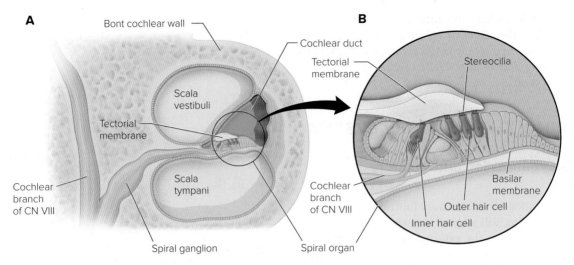

FIGURE 6-10 Auditory apparatus of the cochlea. A. A cross section and close up view of the cochlea with the membranous labyrinth dividing it into the cochlear duct, vestibular duct (scala vestibuli), and tympanic duct (scala tympani). **B.** The spiral organ houses the hair cells that transduce sound vibration to a neural signal within cranial nerve VIII. (Reproduced with permission from McKinley M, O'Laughlin VD. *Human Anatomy.* 3rd ed. New York, NY: McGraw-Hill; 2012, Figure 19.27, p. 595.)

to as tonatopic, meaning it is organized by the tone of the sounds. Second-order projections from the cochlear nuclei project bilaterally to the **superior olivary nuclear complex** and the contralateral inferior colliculus. Tertiary projections from these two areas project within the lateral lemniscus to **the lateral geniculate nucleus** of the thalamus with a fourth level projection to the auditory cortex, located in Herschl's gyrus within the lateral sulcus, which is part of the temporal lobe. Surrounding Herschl's gyrus in a circular fashion are the secondary and higher-order auditory processing areas. From these initial auditory processing cortices, auditory information is projected to numerous areas of the brain, including the posterior parietal cortex, where it is integrated with somatosensory and visual information, and the language centers in the temporal and frontal lobes. See Figure 6-11 for central auditory projections.

Sound Localization

The localization of sound is complex, since most sounds are transmitted to both ears. However, sound to the right of midline will reach the right ear before it hits the left ear, and vice versa, resulting in an interaural time difference. The more lateral a sound, the greater the interaural difference. For higher frequencies, location is primarily determined by what is referred to as an interaural intensity difference with a stronger signal received by the closest ear. Either way, we can determine the horizontal location of sound, based on the difference in interaural activation.

Auditory Testing

The complexity of the hearing apparatus requires complex testing to assure adequate analysis of the different parts of the system. The first step in an auditory assessment is typically **behavioral audiometry**, also known as air conduction testing or pure tone audiometry; this is the presentation of sounds via earphones or headphones, at a range of frequencies (0.25–8 Hz), to each ear in a random order; patients are instructed to raise their hand on the side that the sound is heard. **Speech audiometry** may be done to further clarify a hearing deficit, identified through behavioral audiometry, and includes two components: (1) **speech recognition** – the ability to repeat word phrases heard through the audiometry headphones at different decibel levels; and (2) **word recognition** – the ability to hear single words in a quiet environment. Also, if behavioral audiometry is abnormal, a second measure, known as **bone conduction**, may be completed. With bone conduction, vibration is introduced to the forehead or mastoid via a tuning fork or audiometer to activate the cochlea while bypassing the external and middle ear. An audiograph is developed that illustrates the perceived frequencies from both tests in comparison to normal levels. A hearing loss characterized by an abnormal pure tone audiometry but normal bone conduction is referred to as a **conductive loss**, associated with abnormalities of the middle ear. When the two tests yield similar results, it is most likely that there is a **sensorineural hearing loss**, involving the cochlea or other neural projections; however, some hearing deficits result from a combined loss (both conductive and sensorineural). Further clarification of a sensorineural hearing loss may be provided by the auditory brainstem evoked potential, also known as the **auditory brainstem response** (ABR). Similar to the VEP, the ABR tracks the neural conduction of sound from its presentation to sequential neural structures: CN VIII, cochlear nucleus in the medulla, superior olivary complex, and inferior colliculi in the midbrain; each of these

1. Movement of basilar membrane produces a nerve impulse that travels in cochlear nerve axons.

2. Sensory axons terminate in the cochlear nucleus in the brainstem.

3. Some axons from the neurons in the cochlear nucleus project to the inferior colliculi, and others project to the superior olivary nucleus.

4. Axons from the inferior colliculus project to the medial geniculate nucleus of the thalamus.

5. Thalamic neurons project to the primary auditory cortex, where the impulse is perceived as sound.

FIGURE 6-11 **Auditory projections.** (Reproduced with permission from McKinley M, O'Laughlin VD. *Human Anatomy* 3rd Ed, New York, NY: McGraw-Hill; 2012, Fig. 19.30, P. 598.)

structures is associated with a specific wave change with a predictable time delay.[4]

HEAD POSITION AND MOVEMENT: THE VESTIBULAR SYSTEM

The purpose of the vestibular system is to detect the position and motion of your head in space. It does this by measuring **linear** and **angular acceleration** of the head through five receptor organs in the portion of the inner ear called the **vestibular labyrinth**. Information conveyed by the vestibular system helps us to maintain balance through its roles in our subjective perceptions of movement and spatial orientation, in postural reflexes that allow us to adjust muscle activity and body position to stay upright, and in control of reflex eye movements that stabilize the eyes in space during head movements.

The Vestibular Labyrinths

The vestibular labyrinths are mirror-symmetric structures on both sides of the head that are composed of three **semicircular canals** (SCCs) and two **otolithic organs**, the **utricle** and **saccule** (Figure 6-12). The vestibular portion of the **bony labyrinth** consists of a central area called the **vestibule** and the three SCCs that are attached to the vestibule. Suspended within each SCC is a semicircular duct that corresponds to the **membranous**

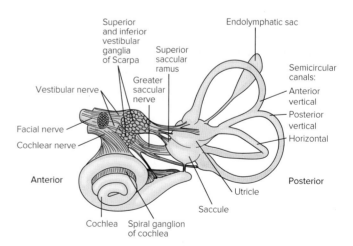

FIGURE 6-12 **Vestibular labyrinths: This schematic illustrates the relationship of the cochlea and the components of the vestibular labyrinth: the vestibule with its saccule and utricle and the three semicircular canals.** (Reproduced with permission from Kandel ER, Schwartz JH, Jessell TM, Siegelbaum SA, Hudspeth AJ. *Principles of Neural Science*, 4th Ed., New York, NY: McGraw-Hill; 2000; Figure 40-1, Pg. 802.)

labyrinth. The two otolithic organs, the **utricle** and **saccule**, are each a dilation of the membranous labyrinth within the vestibule. As in the cochlea, the space between the bony and membranous labyrinths is fluid-filled with **perilymph** while the membranous labyrinth is filled with **endolymph**.

The sensory cells in each organ are specialized epithelial cells called **hair cells** which transduce mechanical signals into neural signals. Similar to the hair cells in the cochlea for hearing, each hair cell in the vestibular labyrinth has a graduated array of **stereocilia**, protruding into the endolymph-filled space within the membranous labyrinth. At one end of the stereocilia is a particularly long process called the **kinocilium**. When a hair cell is in a resting state (i.e., no deflection of sterocilia) there is generally some amount of tonic firing, recorded from the connecting vestibular nerves. Displacement of the sterocilia toward the kinocilium elicits a depolarization (i.e., excitation) of the hair cell membrane and leads to greater release of an excitatory neurotransmitter onto the vestibular nerve endings, which in turn, increase their firing frequencies. In contrast, deflection of stereocilia away from the kinocilium causes hyperpolarization (i.e., inhibition) and leads to a reduction in neurotransmitter release, thereby decreasing vestibular nerve firing rate (see Figure 6-13).

Semicircular Canals Detect Angular Acceleration

Angular accelerations caused by rotations of the head, such as when you turn or tilt your head, rotate your body, or make turns during walking, are measured by the SCCs. The three SCCs – horizontal, anterior, and posterior – are oriented almost precisely perpendicular to each other (analogous to the spatial relationship between two walls and the floor of a rectangular room), so that each canal detects motion in a single plane (Figure 6-14). The horizontal canal as its name implies is roughly horizontal (although it's actually tilted backwards about 30 degrees) when the head is in its typical, upright position. This canal is, therefore, sensitive to head rotations about a vertical axis. Each anterior and posterior canal is roughly vertical. However, the anterior and posterior canals are oriented at 45-degree angles from the sagittal plane in opposite directions from each other.

The anterior canal of one side is, therefore, parallel to the posterior canal of the other side, so movements that affect one will affect the other. Thus, the two horizontal canals lie in the same plane and function together, while the anterior canal of one side functions as a pair with the contralateral posterior canal.

Each SCC is a continuous endolymph-filled hoop that connects with the utricle. In one end of each semicircular duct is a swelling called the **ampulla**. Within each ampulla is a **crista**, a saddle-shaped ridge of tissue that contains the sensory hair cells. The hair cells are arranged as a single tuft that projects up into the **cupula**, a gelatinous mass that stretches from the crista to the roof of the ampulla (Figure 6-15). Rotation of a SCC around an axis perpendicular to it (like a wheel on an axis) is the best way to deflect a cupula. Consider the example of an ice skater who performs a basic upright spin. At the beginning of such a spin, the horizontal SCCs will rotate around their vertical axes. However, movement of the endolymph inside the canals lags behind because of inertia, which causes it to slosh against the cupula and deflect the hair cells to stimulate them. With continued rotations, the endolymph will eventually "catch up" so that the cupula is no longer deflected and stimulation of hair cells ceases. When the rotation stops, the endolymph sloshes up against a suddenly still cupula (again because of inertia), and the cupula bulges in the opposite direction and the person experiences a feeling that he or she is turning in the other direction. Thus, each SCC responds best to changes in the speed of rotation in a particular plane (i.e., angular acceleration), making them particularly sensitive to higher-frequency motion, such as head movements that occur during walking. The SCCs are normally insensitive to linear accelerations or gravitational forces because the densities of the cupula and endolymph are equal. Since all of the hair cells of a given crista are aligned so that their kinocilia are facing in the same direction, angular acceleration in one direction causes the vestibular afferents that innervate the crista to increase their firing rates, while acceleration in the opposite direction causes them to decrease their firing rates. Because the three SCCs are oriented in roughly orthogonal planes (Figure 6-14), and most head movements have a rotational component, movements in any direction can be detected.

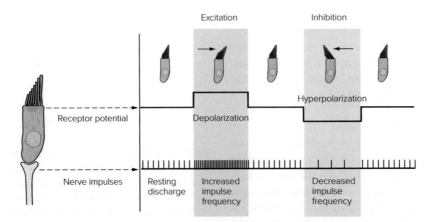

FIGURE 6-13 Hair cells of the vestibular labyrinth. In the resting state, the stereocilia are upright, with depolarization they bend in the direction of the kinocilium and with hyperpolarization they bend away from the kinocilium. (Adapted with permission from Flock A. 1965. Transducing mechanisms in the lateral line canal organ receptors. *Cold Spring Harbor Symp Quant Biol* 30:133-145.)

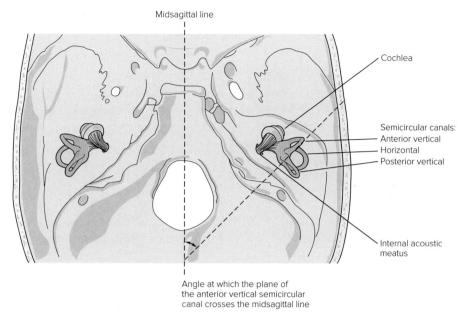

FIGURE 6-14 Alignment of the anterior semicircular canal. With the head upright, the anterior vertical canal is at a 45-degree angle from the sagittal plane as is the posterior vertical canal (angle not drawn). (Reproduced with permission from Kandel ER, Schwartz JH, Jessell TM, Siegelbaum SA, Hudspeth AJ. *Principles of neural Science*, 5th Ed., New York, NY: McGraw-Hill; 2013; Figure 40-4, pg. 921.)

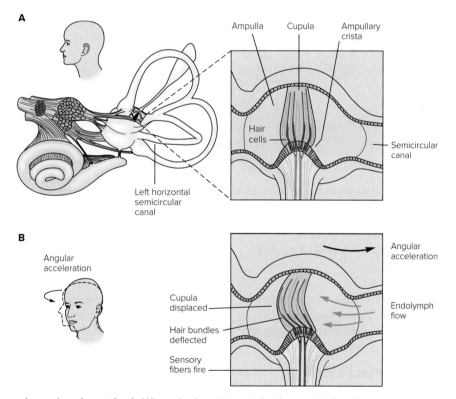

FIGURE 6-15 Ampulla and cupula schematic. A. When the head is upright, the cupula (a gelatinous mass) and its hair cells are stationary within the ampulla (swelling within the canals). **B.** As the head moves, the ampulla and its hair cells are moved by the motion of the endolymph. (Reproduced with permission from Kandel ER, Schwartz JH, Jessell TM, Siegelbaum SA, Hudspeth AJ. *Principles of Neural Science.* 5th ed. McGraw Hill, Inc.; 2013, Figure 40-3A and B, p. 920.)

Since most people don't typically experience maintained rotations (except at amusement parks), the fact that the SCC cannot detect maintained rotation is not a great disadvantage.

Each coplanar pair of canals (i.e., right and left horizontal, left anterior and right posterior, and left posterior and right anterior) on either side of the head will generally be operating in a push–pull rhythm; when one is excited, the other is inhibited. This occurs because head motion within their shared plane causes the endolymph of the pair to be displaced in opposite directions with respect to their ampullae, resulting in increased

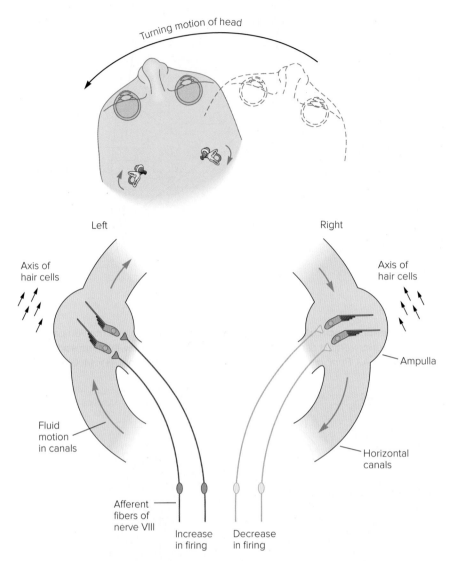

FIGURE 6-16 Complimentary function between the pairs of semicircular canals. This schematic illustrates the push–pull relationship of the complimentary SCC pairings. With a slight head turn to the left, the left hair cells are excited, moving toward the kinocilium while the hair cells in the right canal are inhibited (moving away from the kinocilium) in association with the movement of the endolymph. (Reproduced with permission from Kandel ER, Schwartz JH, Jessell TM, Siegelbaum SA, Hudspeth AJ. *Principles of Neural Science*, 5th Ed., New York, NY: McGraw-Hill; 2013; Figure 40-9, pg. 925.)

firing in one vestibular nerve and decreased firing in the other (Figure 6-16). Disruption of this relationship between sides, as in vestibular neuritis, will cause a person to feel debilitating vertigo and nausea.

The Utricle and Saccule Detect Linear Acceleration and Static Head Position

Linear accelerations, such as when a person steps onto a moving sidewalk or when you lean to one side, and static head positions are detected by the utricle and the saccule. Each organ has a sheet of hair cells located in a portion of its wall called the **macula**. Macular hair cells are also embedded in a gelatinous mass similar in composition to the cupula. However, the gelatinous substance also contains clumps of small crystals of calcium carbonate, called **otoconia** or **otoliths**, and thus, is called an **otolithic membrane**, from which the otolithic organs get their name. The otoconia make the otolithic membrane denser than

endolymph, thereby, making the otolithic organs sensitive to gravity and linear accelerations such as experienced in elevators and automobiles. When the head changes position or begins a movement, the weight of the membrane bends the stereocilia of the macular hair cells (Figure 6-17). This stimulates the hair cells, which then signal the new head position. The orientation of the utricular macula is roughly horizontal (near the plane of the horizontal SCCs), while that of the saccular macula is roughly vertical when the head is in its typical upright position. Thus, in the upright position, the utricle is particularly sensitive to any accelerations in the horizontal plane (i.e., side-to-side and anterior–posterior motions) and the saccule particularly senses any accelerations along a sagittal plane (i.e., up and down motions) as well as anterior–posterior motions. As in the SCCs there is push–pull processing of the otolithic organs between the two sides of the head. In addition, the hair cells within each otolithic macula are oriented with their kinocilia in different directions

Head tilting downward

Stereocilia of hair cells bend

Otolithic membrane sags

Gravitational force

FIGURE 6-17 Movement of the stereocilia within the otolith. (Reproduced with permission from McKinley M & O'Loughlin VD. *Human Anatomy* 3rd Edition. New York, NY: McGraw-Hill; 2012. Figure 19.24 Right Side, pg 592.)

along a curving zone called the **striola**, so that head movement causes excitation of a group of hair cells from one portion of the macula while those in another portion of the same macula are inhibited. This extra redundancy probably explains why the otolithic organs are less impacted by unilateral vestibular lesions than the SCCs. The otoliths are most sensitive to lower-frequency motion, such as motion that occurs while standing in place, and thus, they are particularly important for postural control.

As the head tilts, the otolithic membrane sags, bending the stereocilia of the hair cells and generating activation of these receptors.

Although the actions of the vestibular labyrinths have been discussed separately, most human movements produce complex patterns of excitation and inhibition in several receptor organs on both sides of the body (see Box 6-3 for an example).

Vestibular Pathways

Vestibular primary afferents have cell bodies in the vestibular ganglion (also called Scarpa's ganglion), which lies in a swelling of the nerve within the internal auditory canal (Figure 6-15). Their central processes travel within the eighth cranial nerve and enter the brainstem at the pontomedullary junction. The main targets of the vestibular primary afferents are the cerebellum and the vestibular nuclei. Vestibular afferents to the cerebellum enter through the inferior cerebellar peduncle and terminate in the flocculonodular lobe (or vestibulocerebellum) and other parts of the cerebellar vermis (i.e., middle part of the

| BOX 6-3 | What would be the pattern of stimulation of the vestibular labyrinths when a person arises from the driver's seat of an automobile? |

As a person begins to swivel toward the door, both horizontal SCCs are strongly stimulated. Simultaneous lateral movement out of the car's door stimulates hair cells in both utricles in a pattern that changes as the head turns in respect to the direction of bodily movement. Vertical acceleration to arise to the standing position stimulates certain hair cells in the saccules, while oppositely oriented saccular hair cells are inhibited. As the movement is completed, linear and angular accelerations in the opposite direction to the initial movement stimulate other hair cells in the utricles and SCCs.

cerebellum). The primary roles of the cerebellum, related to the vestibular system, are to monitor vestibular performance and make adaptive adjustments to central vestibular processing as needed. More specifically, the cerebellar flocculus adjusts and maintains the gain (ratio of head to compensatory eye movement) of the vestibulo-ocular reflex (VOR), the cerebellar nodulus regulates the duration of VOR responses and processing of otolith input, and the anterior–superior portion of the vermis of the cerebellum regulates the vestibulospinal reflex (VSR) to maintain postural and gait stability.[5]

Most primary vestibular afferents project to the vestibular nuclear complex, a large structure containing four main nuclei (superior, medial, lateral, and descending) located within the pons and medulla. The vestibular nuclei integrate inputs from the primary vestibular afferents with those from the visual system, spinal cord, and cerebellum and project to several central targets: the oculomotor nuclei (i.e., cranial nerves III, IV, and VI), the spinal cord (via the lateral and medial vestibulospinal tracts), parts of the cerebellum (i.e., same areas as do primary vestibular afferents), the parietal cortex (via the thalamus), and the contralateral vestibular nuclear complex.

The major vestibular nuclei subserve different functions (Figure 6-18). The superior and medial nuclei receive inputs primarily from the SCCs and send ascending projections via the **medial longitudinal fasciculus** (MLF) to the oculomotor nuclei (i.e., cranial nerves III, IV, VI) that are responsible for mediating the VOR. In addition the medial nucleus sends descending projections via the **medial vestibulospinal tract** that travel within the MLF to cervical areas of the spinal cord. These projections function to stabilize the head position, during activities like walking, and to coordinate head with eye movements. The lateral nucleus (Deiter's nucleus) receives inputs from the SCCs and the otolithic organs and projects via the **lateral vestibulospinal tract** to the motor neurons for antigravity muscles at all areas of the spinal cord (Table 6-3). This tract, along with the medial vestibulospinal tract, is responsible for mediating the vestibulospinal reflexes that compensate for tilts and movements of the body. The inferior nucleus receives predominantly input from the otolithic organs and projects to the cerebellum, reticular formation, spinal cord, and contralateral vestibular nuclei. This nucleus primarily functions to integrate vestibular and central motor system activity for postural control.

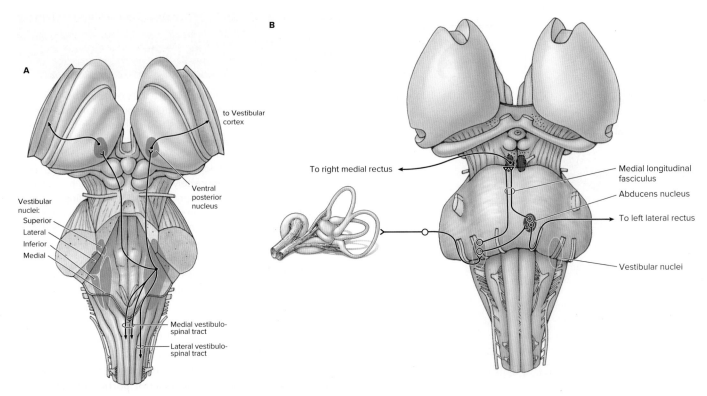

FIGURE 6-18 A and B. The vestibular nuclei. The four vestibular nuclei can be visualized in this diagram along with their projections to the thalamus and spinal cord. (Reproduced with permission from Martin JH. *Neuroanatomy Text and Atlas*, 4th Ed. New York, NY: McGraw-Hill; 2012. Figure 12-2 (A) and 12-6 (B) pgs 280 and 285, respectively.)

TABLE 6-3	Vestibular Nuclei Function and Efferents	
NUCLEUS	**EFFERENTS**	**FUNCTIONS**
Superior	Axons ascend in ipsilateral MLF to nuclei of extraocular muscles (CN III, IV, VI) and bilateral thalamus	Mediates vestibulo-ocular reflex (VOR)
Lateral	Axons descend in lateral vestibulospinal tract to anterior horns cells throughout cord	Mediates vestibulospinal reflex (VSR)
Medial	Axons ascend in contralateral MLF to nuclei of extraocular muscles and descend in medial vestibulospinal tract to cervical area of cord	Mediates VOR and VSR reflexes, coordinates eye and head movements that occur together
Inferior (Spinal)	Axons project to reticular formation, cerebellum, and contralateral medial lateral and inferior vestibular nuclei	Mediates postural adjustments via reticular formation; allows sharing of information between vestibular nuclei bilaterally

Vestibulo-Ocular Reflex

The vestibulo-ocular reflex (VOR) is the means by which a person's gaze can stay fixed on a target even though his or her head is moving or is being moved. To illustrate how the eyes are kept still by the VOR, shake your head side to side quickly while you read this paragraph. The VOR allows you to continue reading even with head movement. However, if you move this book at the same speed and try to read it, you will have difficulty because visual processing takes longer and is less efficient than vestibular processing for image stabilization. The neural pathways of the reflex are shown in Figure 6-18. The direction of the three planes of the SCCs are matched closely by the directions of motion of the three pairs of muscles that

control eye movements (medial/lateral recti; superior/inferior recti; inferior/superior obliques), so that a single canal interacts with a single muscle pair. Each horizontal canal controls motoneurons that innervate the ipsilateral medial rectus (via ipsilateral CN III) and contralateral lateral rectus muscles (via contralateral CN VI). At the same time, they inhibit the antagonist eye muscles (Figure 6-19). Anterior canals control motoneurons to ipsilateral superior rectus and contralateral inferior oblique muscles (via contralateral CN III), while posterior canals control motoneurons to ipsilateral superior oblique (via contralateral CN IV) and contralateral inferior rectus muscles (via contralateral CN III). Thus, downward rotation of the head stimulates the anterior canals and causes compensatory

A

Right

Left

Direction of
head rotation

Direction of
eye movement

Target

B

FIGURE 6-19 VOR and its neural connections. A. Head rotation to the right excites hair cells in the right horizontal SCC and signals are sent via the right vestibular nerve to the right medial and lateral vestibular nuclei. Neurons from these nuclei in turn stimulate neurons in the right oculomotor nucleus to excite the right medial rectus muscle and simultaneously stimulate neurons in the left abducens nucleus to excite the left lateral rectus muscle, thereby, evoking conjugate eye movements to the left. At the same time, neurons that excite the right lateral rectus and left medial rectus muscles are inhibited. **B.** Neural pathway projections active during the VOR described above. (Reproduced with permission from Martin JH: *Neuroanatomy Text and Atlas*, 4th Ed. New York, NY: McGraw-Hill; 2012. Figure 12-6A, P. 285.)

upward eye movement, while upward head rotation stimulates the posterior canals and the eyes move downward. There are also VOR reflexes that involve the otolithic organs to compensate for linear and head tilt away from the vertical movements. The "gain" of the rotational VOR is defined as the change in the eye angle divided by the change in the head angle, during the head turn, and is normally 1.0. There are some situations where a VOR is not a good thing, such as when we want to direct our gaze in the same direction that our head is turning. In that case, the VOR is suppressed by the central nervous system, which is referred to as **VOR cancellation**. Two mechanisms that have been proposed to explain this cancellation are a reduction of the VOR gain by the flocculus of the cerebellum or activation of smooth pursuit eye movements in the opposite direction.[6] Individuals who lose this reflex experience **oscillopsia**, in which the visual world is unstable and objects appear blurry. In comatose individuals, the VOR can be used to test the integrity of brainstem eye movement pathways. The **oculocephalic reflex**, a form of the VOR, is tested by holding the person's eyes open and rotating the head quickly from side to side or up and down. The reflex is present if the eyes move in the opposite direction of the head movements, and it is often referred to as **doll's eyes**. Doll's eyes are typically not present in conscious individuals because they will usually suppress the reflex. Thus, the absence of doll's eyes suggests brainstem dysfunction in the comatose person but can be normal in the conscious individual. The afferent limb of the oculocephalic reflex probably also includes proprioceptors of the neck because some reflex movement can be elicited in individuals with nonfunctioning labyrinths.[7]

Vestibulospinal Reflex

The vestibulospinal reflex (VSR) functions to help us maintain our balance. For example, consider the situation where a person is walking and slips on an icy sidewalk. The person's feet fly to the right and his or her upper body and head fly to the left (left ear down). The head movement to the left will stimulate the vestibular labyrinths on the left side and increase the firing rate of the left vestibular nerve, which in turn will increase activity in the left vestibular nuclei. Activation of neurons in the lateral and medial vestibular nuclei that project to the spinal cord (via the lateral and medial vestibulospinal tracts respectively) will excite motoneurons to extensor muscles and inhibit motoneurons to the flexor muscles in the left arm and leg in order to right the person and prevent the person from falling.

Nystagmus

With sustained head rotations that are too large to be compensated for by the vestibulo-ocular reflex, the VOR is periodically interrupted by rapid eye movements in the opposite direction. The back-and-forth eye movements, with a slow phase in one direction and a fast phase in the other, are called **nystagmus**. The eye movements of nystagmus can be in any direction (i.e., horizontal, vertical, or torsional). Eye movements of nystagmus may be faster in one direction, or the movements in both directions may be the same. Certain types of nystagmus are a normal physiological response to vestibular or visual system stimulation, but other types of nystagmus are due to neuropathology.

There are three main ways to cause nystagmus physiologically. Sustained head rotation is one example. Consider again the ice skater who performs a basic upright spin. As the skater begins to rotate to the left, the VOR, as explained previously, will cause compensatory deviation of the eyes to the right. As rotation to the left continues, one would think that the skater's eyes would move to the edge of the orbit and stay there. However, this doesn't happen because the eyes make a very rapid or **saccadic** resetting movement to the left back across the center of the gaze. The nystagmus is named for the direction of rapid movement (i.e., in this case, the eyes move slowly to the right and rapidly back to the left, so it would be called **nystagmus to the left** or **left-beating nystagmus**). During the period of sustained rotation, when the cupula "catches up" and is not deflected, the eye movement response depends on the light condition. In the dark or with the person's eyes closed, nystagmus would cease; with visual input, for reasons explained below, left-beating nystagmus might continue throughout the rotation. When the rotation is suddenly stopped, movement of the cupula in the opposite direction tricks the brainstem into thinking that the direction of head rotation has reversed (to the right), which causes a brief period of right-beating **postrotatory nystagmus**. Another consequence of rotation in the postrotatory period is **past pointing**. If a person is asked to point at a target immediately upon being stopped from a sustained rotation with eyes closed, the person will consistently point inaccurately with the deviation always in the direction of the previous rotation. The person will also tend to fall in the direction of the previous rotation when walking. Thus, if the rotation was to the left, the person will past point to the left of the target and tend to fall to the left when walking. The postrotatory past pointing and falling is due to an imbalance of the lateral vestibulospinal tracts.

A second way to cause physiological nystagmus is with a moving visual stimuli. Consider the situation of a person sitting in a rapidly moving bus who is watching regularly spaced telephone poles fly by. The person's eyes will slowly follow a particular pole toward the rear of the bus and then rapidly flick back toward the front of the bus to find a new pole to fixate on. If the individual is seated on the right side of the bus, looking out the window, the movement of the series of telephone poles to the right across the person's visual field would cause slow pursuit tracking eye movements to the right followed by fast saccadic "reset" movements to the left or nystagmus to the left. Because it is induced by moving visual stimuli, it is called **optokinetic nystagmus** (OKN) and the reflex that causes OKN is called the **optokinetic reflex**. In the clinic, a rotating striped drum or moving piece of striped cloth is typically used to test the reflex. OKN is the reason for the continued nystagmus, during sustained rotations in a lighted room.

A third way to cause physiological nystagmus is by means of the **caloric test**. For this test, a person's head is tilted backward by about 60 degrees to bring the horizontal SCCs into a vertical position. Cold or warm water or air is then introduced into the person's ear. The temperature difference between the body and the injected water or air creates a convective current in the endolymph of the nearby horizontal SCC. Hot and cold water produce currents in opposite directions, and therefore, a horizontal nystagmus in opposite directions. If the water is warm (44°C or above), endolymph in the ipsilateral horizontal SCC

rises, causing an increased rate of firing in the vestibular afferent nerve. This situation mimics a head turn to the ipsilateral side, creating horizontal nystagmus to the ipsilateral ear. For example, irrigation of the left ear with warm water will cause the endolymph in the left horizontal SCC to move in the direction that causes an increased rate of firing in the left vestibular nerve, mimicking a left head turn. This, in turn, will cause conjugate eye movements to the right via the VOR followed by fast saccadic movements to the left or left-beating nystagmus. If the water is cold (3°C or below), the endolymph falls within the SCC, decreasing the rate of vestibular afferent firing. The eyes then deviate toward the ipsilateral ear, with horizontal nystagmus induced to the contralateral ear. One mnemonic used to remember the fast direction of nystagmus with caloric testing is *COWS*. With *C*old water irrigation, the fast phase of nystagmus is to the *O*pposite side from the filled ear; with *W*arm water irrigation the fast phase of nystagmus is to the *S*ame side as the filled ear.

Nystagmus can be caused by pathology to a variety of nervous system structures including the labyrinths, vestibular nerves, vestibular nuclei, oculomotor nerves, and the cerebellum. Peripheral vestibular disorders involve the vestibular nerve and all distal structures. Patients with a unilateral peripheral disorder typically demonstrate horizontal nystagmus to the contralateral side which suppresses with visual fixation. Unlike peripheral lesions, nystagmus of central pathology usually changes direction with gaze, is unaffected by fixation, and may be purely vertical or torsional.

Balance Control

The ability to balance or maintain vertical orientation of the body requires perception and action. Perception is the integration of sensory information to assess the position and motion of the body in space, involving sensory and higher-level cognitive processes. Action is the ability to generate forces for controlling body position, involving motor systems. The main sensory inputs that the central nervous system uses for determining the body's position and movement in space are visual, somatosensory, and vestibular. The visual system provides information about body movement with respect to surrounding objects and helps us determine what is upright. The vestibular system provides information about head position with respect to gravity and inertial forces and about head movement. The somatosensory system (i.e., proprioception, touch) provides information about the body with reference to supporting surfaces (i.e., weight-bearing) and the relative positions of body parts. Auditory inputs assist with maintenance of upright posture by alerting us to objects in the environment (i.e., cars, buses) that might destabilize us.

REFERENCES

1. San T, Kvaloy MB, Hovdat T. Evoked potential tests in clinical diagnosis. *Tidsskr Nor Legeforen.* 2013;133(9):960-965.

2. Corbet JJ. The bedside and office neuro-ophthalmology examination. *Semin Neurol.* 2003;22(1):63-76.

3. Melamud A, Hagstrom S, Traboulsi EI. Color vision testing. *Ophthalmic Genet.* 2004;25(3):159-187.

4. Baiduc RR, Poling GL, Hong O, Dhar S. Clinical measures of auditory function: the cochlea and beyond. *Dis Mon*. 2013;59(4):147-156.

5. Hain TC, Helminski JO. Anatomy and physiology of the normal vestibular system. In: Herdman SJ, ed. *Vestibular Rehabilitation*. 3rd ed. Philadelphia, PA: FA Davis Co; 2007.

6. Gordon CR, Caspi A, Levite R, Zivotofsky AZ. Mechanisms of vestibulo-ocular reflex (VOR) cancellation in spinocerebellar ataxia type 3 (SCA-3) and episodic ataxia type 2 (EA-2). *Prog Brain Res*. 2008;171:519-525.

7. Singh HH. The comatose patient (chapter 13). In: *Clinical Examination: A Practical Guide to Medicine*. New Delhi, India: Jaypee Brothers Medical Publishers; 2011.

Review Questions

1. **Which two structures are responsible for focusing light onto the retina of the eye?**
   A. Iris and pupil
   B. Pupil and cornea
   C. Cornea and lens
   D. Lens and vitreous humor

2. **Which of the following correctly describes the projection of the right visual field onto the retina of the eye?**
   A. The right monocular visual field projects to the temporal retina of the left eye
   B. The right monocular visual field projects to the nasal retina of the left eye
   C. The right monocular visual field projects to the temporal retina of the right eye
   D. The right monocular visual field projects to the nasal retina of the right eye

3. **Meyer's loop contains what aspect of the visual field?**
   A. The ipsilateral upper visual field (lower retinal fibers)
   B. The contralateral upper visual field (lower retinal fibers)
   C. The ipsilateral lower visual field (upper retinal fibers)
   D. The contralateral lower visual field (upper retinal fibers)

4. **The lateral rectus muscle of the eye is innervated by what cranial nerve?**
   A. CN II
   B. CN III
   C. CN IV
   D. CN VI

5. **Which sense discussed in this chapter projects directly to the cortex without going through the thalamus?**
   A. Hearing
   B. Olfaction
   C. Taste
   D. Vestibular
   E. Vision

6. **The strong emotional response that we have to many smells is most likely associated with what part of the olfactory cortex?**
   A. Amygdala
   B. Entorhinal cortex
   C. Olfactory tubercle
   D. Piriform cortex

7. **Which of the cells listed below is the receptor cell for the sense that it is paired with?**
   A. Bipolar cells – vision
   B. Hair cells – hearing
   C. Mitral cells – olfaction
   D. Papillae – taste

8. **The gustatory cortex (taste) is located where?**
   A. Dorsal temporal cortex
   B. Insular cortex
   C. Anterior frontal lobe
   D. Posterior occipital lobe
   E. Ventral parietal lobe

9. **Taste receptors are more dense on what aspect of the oral structures?**
   A. Tip of the tongue
   B. Anterior 2/3 of tongue
   C. Posterior 1/3 of tongue
   D. Inner cheeks
   E. Inner gums

10. **What nucleus in the brainstem receives all gustatory projections?**
    A. Abducens
    B. Cochlear
    C. Solitary
    D. Superior colliculus

11. **The middle ear cavity contains which of the following structures?**
    A. Bony labyrinth
    B. Incus, malleus, and stapes

C. Eustachian tube

D. Tympanum

12. **The thick epithelium that holds the auditory receptors is called what?**

   A. Bony labyrinth

   B. Cochlear duct

   C. Endolymph

   D. Spiral organ

13. **The otolithic organs (utricle and saccule):**

   A. Are part of the central vestibular system

   B. Detect rotational movement and velocity of the head

C. Detect linear acceleration and static position of the head

D. Mediate the vestibulo-ocular reflex

14. **In a healthy individual, rotation of the head to the right produces which of the following in the hair cells in the horizontal semicircular canals (SCCs):**

   A. Hyperpolarization of hair cells in the right SC; depolarization of hair cells in the left SC

   B. Depolarization of hair cells in the right SC; hyperpolarization of hair cells in the left SC

   C. No change in the activity of the hair cells on either side

   D. Depolarization of the hair cells on both sides

Answers

1. C	2. D	3. B	4. D	5. B
6. A	7. B	8. B	9. C	10. C
11. B	12. D	13. C	14. B	

Cognition, Emotion, and Language

Deborah S. Nichols-Larsen

7

1) Differentiate the abilities that comprise cognition, including executive function and memory, and the neural networks that support them

2) Distinguish the neural networks responsible for language production and language comprehension

3) Discern feelings from emotions and the neural networks that support these concepts

This chapter focuses on the most complex of abilities (cognition, emotion, and language), and in many ways, the areas of functioning that most differentiate humans from other animals, or at least we like to think so. Although these functions are highly interrelated, we will talk about each and the neural networks that support them individually.

• COGNITION

Cognition is an expansive term used to describe our ability to perceive the world around us, interact with it, remember our past experiences in it, and imagine potential experiences with it; the concepts of thinking, memory, imagery, problem-solving, and decision-making are all included within the term cognition. Obviously, these skills are extensive and span multiple neural networks. Within this chapter, we will discuss some of the components of cognition and the neural networks that are involved in cognitive processes, specifically executive function and memory. Our ability to understand and produce language is critically tied to our cognitive abilities and vice versa. In addition, our emotional state plays a significant part in cognition; thus, this chapter will also explore the neural control of language and emotion.

Executive Function

Executive function (EF) is a term that refers to a spectrum of abilities, including attention, working memory, inhibition, task switching, abstract thought and behavioral regulation as well as decision-making, sequence planning, and initiation. First, we will explore these skills under the executive function umbrella, and then, we'll look at the areas of the brain that give rise to these abilities.

Attention is the ability to focus your awareness on visual, auditory, tactile, or other sensory stimuli (**sustained attention**) but also involves the ability to prioritize your attention on one among competing stimuli as well as to switch your attention from one stimulus to another (see Box 7-1).

Task switching, just as it sounds, is the ability to focus on one task, and then, immediately switch to another task. There is some natural overlap between this skill and that of attention, as it requires us to switch our attention to different cues to complete each task. For example, if I asked you to sort playing cards by suit and then by number, you would first pay attention to the suit designation without need to look at the number, and then, you would focus on the number while disregarding the suit. **Perseveration** occurs when we fail to switch our attention to the appropriate cue and continue to sort by suit instead of by number. The more similar the task, the more likely we are to make perseverative errors.

Working memory refers to the ability to retain or manipulate information cognitively for immediate use; the most common example used to illustrate this is retaining a phone number for the brief amount of time needed to punch it into your cell phone, after your friend gives it to you. How many times have you been distracted in this process and forgotten the number, requiring you to ask your friend to repeat it. Thus, working memory is of short duration, for small amounts of information, and does not indicate that learning has taken place; also, any

---

BOX 7-1 | Types of Attention

As you read this paragraph, let's propose that you are also listening to the radio (a cognitive-cognitive dual task); this requires **divided attention** between the two activities, yet, to fully understand the words on the page, you will need to focus more of your attention on the printed word than on the music (**prioritization of attention**). However, if your favorite song comes on the radio, you are able to switch your attention quickly to listen to the song and then switch back to prioritizing reading again, once the song is done (**shifting attention**). This ability to divide, prioritize, and switch your attention from one stimulus to another is critical for functioning in our complex environment and often disrupted in many neurologic conditions. However, as the many instances of accidents when driving or walking while texting or talking on the phone indicate, there are limitations in our ability to divide our attention, and at times, we prioritize the wrong task (e.g., texting when we need to focus on driving).

disruption will typically impede our ability to retain information within the working memory circuits.

Inhibition is a complex ability that involves delaying our verbal or physical response to a stimulus, or in many instances, simply waiting; interestingly, we are constantly in a state of cognitive inhibition. How many times do you think of something but know not to say it, or similarly, how many times you find yourself doing something (e.g., tapping your pencil), when you are really focused on something else. The first is an example of inhibition; the second, an example of failure of inhibition or **disinhibition**. Thus, inhibition is a willful blockade of attention, movement, verbalization, or other behavior, while disinhibition is a failure of inhibition. Disinhibition is also apparent in young children, who are likely to say whatever they are thinking or to reach out and touch things, even after being told "no," because they haven't yet learned to inhibit their behavior. Inhibition is tightly linked to **behavioral or self-regulation**, which refers to our ability to learn the rules of behavior in society and respond accordingly, even in novel situations. For example, we learn to take turns in conversations – listening and then talking; we learn to be quiet in libraries and cheer at sporting events; we learn to sit quietly in school and run freely at recess. And perhaps most importantly, we learn to observe others' behavior in new situations and regulate our own in accordance to their example. Finally, **abstract thought** is the highest of human abilities; it refers to our ability to combine information in novel ways so as to generalize to new situations, to use logic or deductive reasoning to solve problems, or to be adaptable in one's thinking such that new information can be used to form new opinions. All of these abilities, along with memory, contribute to the capacity for **decision-making**, based on relevant information, past experience, environmental factors, and our current emotional state; decision-making requires the comparison of current factors with past experience to make a choice between multiple potential solutions.

The Neural Networks Supporting Executive Function

With the vastness of capabilities subsumed in the term EF, it should not be surprising that multiple brain regions contribute to these high-level skills. However, the frontal lobe has three areas that play critical roles in these functions: the dorsolateral prefrontal cortex, the orbitofrontal or ventromedial prefrontal cortex, and the anterior cingulate cortex[1] (Figures 7-1 and 7-2). Each of these areas is linked to multiple other areas that appear to contribute to our EF abilities.

Dorsolateral Prefrontal Cortex (DLPFC)

As indicated by its label, the DLPFC is located just in front of the premotor cortex on the dorsolateral aspect of the frontal lobe. It has projections to and from the temporal and parietal lobes, the basal ganglia (globus pallidus and substantia nigra), and hypothalamus. The temporal lobe is our emotional center, and the DLPFC has connections to temporal structures, including the nucleus accumbens, the hippocampus, the amygdala, and the entorhinal cortex, all of which are implicated in emotion. The DLPFC is critical in working memory as well as memory retrieval from the temporal and posterior association cortices

FIGURE 7-1 Frontal areas associated with executive function.

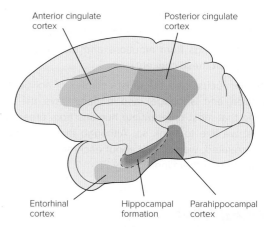

FIGURE 7-2 Anterior cingulate (ACC) and its connections with the limbic system. The ACC, as depicted here, is the anterior portion of the cingulate gyrus within the frontal lobe on the medial surface of the hemisphere. Its interconnections with the medial temporal lobe structures of the limbic system contributes to our awareness of emotion. (Reproduced with permission from Kandel ER, Schwartz JH, Jessell TM, Siegelbaum SA, Hudspeth AJ. *Principles of Neural Science*, 5th Ed. New York, NY: McGraw-Hill; 2013. Figure 19-5, Pg 409.)

for use in problem-solving activities. Damage to the DLPFC is associated with perseveration, lack of attention, difficulty following instructions or maintaining the goal of a task in mind, poor planning or strategy development, impaired decision-making, especially related to moral dilemmas, and changes in personality. Along with these, there is an obvious loss of inhibition. This myriad of deficits has been referred to as **frontal dysexecutive syndrome**.[1]

Orbitofrontal Cortex (OFC)

The OFC encompasses Brodmann's areas 11–14 and 47 and can be visualized as the most ventral part of the frontal lobes; in association with the anterior cingulate cortex and frontal polar cortex, it is referred to as the **orbitofrontal ventromedial cortex (OFVMC)** or **ventromedial prefrontal cortex (VMPC)**. The OFC is an area of integration for sensory processing of visual, auditory, and somatosensory stimuli, receiving information from the inferior temporal lobe, secondary and tertiary auditory cortex, and the parietal lobe's secondary somatosensory area; each conveying their respective information. The VMPC is also interconnected with the DLPFC; areas of memory in the insular cortex, temporal lobe, and hippocampus; as well as areas associated with emotion and homeostasis in the amygdala and hypothalamus. Ultimately, this area is associated with determining the motivational aspects of decision-making, whether for reward or to avoid punishment. Damage to this region impairs social awareness, reflected as the inability to interpret other people's emotions and to demonstrate appropriate behavior in social situations. This also manifests as impulsive behavior and risk-taking due to the inability to see the potential consequences of actions.[1]

Anterior Cingulate Cortex (ACC)

Located on the medial surface of the frontal lobe, the ACC is an area of convergence for projections from the other two critical areas, the DLPFC and OFVMC, but also has reciprocal connections to these areas. It appears to contribute to our ability to shift our attention from one task feature to another and also has been associated with our awareness of emotion, resulting from its strong connections to the limbic system, including the amygdala, hippocampus, entorhinal cortex, and parahippocampal cortex[2] (see Figure 7-2). It works with the DLPFC and OFVMC for executive function but seems particularly essential for decisions where the outcome is ambiguous or incongruent (e.g., reading the word RED when printed in blue as in the Stroop test). Damage to this area exacerbates the poor social awareness, demonstrated with OFVMC damage, and results in a condition, referred to as **alexithymia**, which is the inability to describe one's emotions.[3]

Other Networks Involved in EF

It is too simplistic to think that the three areas discussed in the previous sections act exclusively to mediate executive function. First, as mentioned, these three areas are interconnected with multiple other regions of the cerebral cortex, basal ganglia, and limbic system. For example, the **posterior parietal cortex**, with its links to the DLPFC, contributes to working memory, and more specifically is thought to be active when we compare, evaluate, or manipulate information held in working memory (e.g., picking out a picture of an object recently held in the hand). An adjacent area within the intraparietal sulcus has been linked to our ability to orient to objects and space, including our ability to mentally realign objects to their appropriate orientation, if they are presented upside down or sideways. The basal ganglia also plays a role in working memory and our ability to benefit from errors while learning a task as well as shifting from one strategy to another, as in the card sorting task described earlier.[2] Such learning contributes to the development of behavioral habits.

Memory

The concepts of learning and memory are linked; historically, learning has been defined as a permanent change in behavior that results from experience or practice with memory being the method by which learning is stored. Even memory is not a simple concept because we have different types of learning and thereby memory. Do you know how to ride a bicycle? Most of us do, but if asked to describe how it is done, we would all struggle a bit with verbalizing the combination of movements and awareness necessary to successfully ride a bike. Such a skill is typically learned by practice through what is referred to as **procedural learning** and stored as a **nondeclarative** or **implicit** memory. On the other hand, when we learn facts or remember events from our childhood, it is much easier to verbalize them; this type of learning and memory is referred to as **declarative** or **explicit**. The neural structures and networks supporting these two types of memory are different. It should be noted, that memories are not stored in a single region; rather, memory seems to be a distributed function with many brain regions involved. Memory duration also differentiates memory characteristics, and neural networks that support working (short-term) memory are different from those supporting long-term memory. We have already discussed the network associated with working memory, so in this section we will focus on long-term memory and the networks that support procedural versus declarative memory.

Declarative (Explicit) Memory

Declarative memory includes retention of our personal experiences (**episodic memory**) as well as retention of facts and concepts (**semantic memory**). Further, declarative memory involves at least three separate processes. The initial phase is known as **encoding**, referring to the neural process of translating what is to be remembered to activity in neural circuits that link new experiences/information to prior related memories. Second, permanent changes in synaptic activity occur as the "new memory" is **consolidated** into a more stable memory within widespread neural areas with similar memories aligned in given brain networks.[4] Ultimately, our ability to recall our memories in the future is based on the process of **retrieval**. These sequential stages of memory (encoding, consolidation, and retrieval) help to explain why some events or facts are well remembered and others not. If we lack related memories with which to link new information, we are likely to lay down a weak memory or one that is difficult to retrieve. Further, if the process of consolidation is disrupted, as often happens with a brain injury, a stable memory may fail to form, resulting in the common inability to remember the accident that produced the brain injury as well as events leading up to the accident. Lastly, our ability to retrieve a memory is reliant on appropriate cues that direct our recall; if there aren't appropriate cues, we are unlikely to retrieve the memory. Interestingly, perceived or imagined events can disrupt the consolidation of memories, leading to a "false" memory; similarly, competing information/events can disrupt the encoding or consolidation of memories. Sleep can facilitate memory consolidation but has also been found to distort memories as perceived attributes may be added to the "true" memory.[5]

Structures in the medial temporal lobe are critical for declarative memory; these include the hippocampal formation (hippocampus, dentate gyrus, and subiculum) as well as the lateral entorhinal, perirhinal, medial entorhinal, and parahippocampal cortices (Figure 7-3). These medial temporal lobe structures

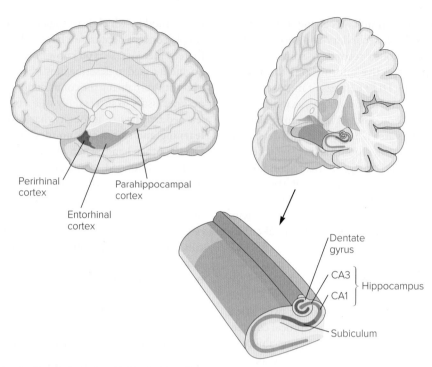

FIGURE 7-3 Medial temporal lobe structures Associated with memory. Within the medial temporal lobe, the hippocampal formation, and the surrounding cortex – rhinal (perirhinal, entorhinal) and parahippocampal – are critical for the encoding of memories. The hippocampal formation consists of the dentate gyrus, subiculum, and hippocampus, which has two layers of pyramidal neurons (CA1 and CA3). These pyramidal neurons are activated by projections from the entorhinal cortex and subsequently activate projection fibers that exit through the subiculum to the prefrontal cortex. (Reproduced with permission from Kandel ER, Schwartz JH, Jessell TM, Siegelbaum SA, Hudspeth AJ. *Principles of Neural Science*, 5th Ed. New York, NY: McGraw-Hill; 2013. Figure 65-2 PartA, Pg 1444.)

have reciprocal connections with the association cortices that are areas of convergence for sensory, motor, emotion, and cognitive brain regions. Notably, these temporal lobe areas appear to be differentially responsible for separate aspects of a given experience with the entorhinal and perirhinal cortices active in response to "what" was experienced and the medial entorhinal and parahippocampal cortices active with regard to the spatiotemporal context or the "where/when" of the experience.[4] Each of these areas has reciprocal connections with the hippocampus, which in turn, is reciprocally connected to the prefrontal cortex via the subiculum. The prefrontal cortex appears instrumental in both memory consolidation and retrieval, likely playing a role in organizing similar memories and their respective/distinctive features and helping us to discern critical cues to achieve memory retrieval. However, the locus of memories seems well distributed throughout many cortical areas, protecting us from losing all of our memories with any focal injury. Yet, damage to the medial temporal lobe will disrupt memory encoding (**anterograde amnesia**) and may disrupt access to some recent memories as the hippocampus continues to play a role in memory retrieval for some time after the memory origin. Over time, as memories are consolidated, they become "cortical," losing some of the contextual details of the original experience and becoming less reliant on the hippocampus for retrieval. However, memories that retain a strong emotional context for us may always rely on the hippocampus for retrieval.[6]

Other areas linked to declarative memory functions are the anterior and mediodorsal nuclei of the thalamus and the mammillary bodies. The mammillary bodies are part of the diencephalon and seem to serve a relay function between the hippocampus and the anterior thalamus, which in turn, projects to the cingulate cortex, another area implicated in memory recall. The mediodorsal nuclei have reciprocal projections to both the prefrontal cortex and the medial temporal lobe structures; this network is active in distinguishing novel from familiar events or objects.[7] One can also make a distinction between recollection of an event and the determination of something as familiar; in recollecting an event, all of the characteristics of the event would be remembered. However, there is a lack of detail associated with the determination of something as familiar versus novel. We have all experienced this phenomenon while at a party where we are meeting new people; we often recognize someone later in the evening that we met earlier without remembering the details of the introduction (name, relationship to the host, etc.). Anatomically, the hippocampus is routinely active in recollection but not in determining familiarity, which is associated more with activity in the rhinal cortex.

Nondeclarative (Implicit) Memory

Nondeclarative or implicit learning and memory refers to our ability to learn without conscious awareness of that learning. Although much of implicit learning is related to the learning of movements or procedures, and often referred to as **procedural learning**, we are also capable of learning other types of information in this manner, including habits, classical conditioning responses, mirror reading, distinguishing familiar from novel stimuli, and many others. For example, when presented with a hidden repeating sequence of letters within a long series of letters, most people will not be able to verbalize the sequence but will react to it as familiar when presented with it later (Box 7-2). While explicit memories have been well documented to incorporate the medial temporal lobe structures, thalamus, and prefrontal and cingulate cortices, implicit learning is thought to be possible in multiple brain systems through changes in synaptic activity within neuronal networks (Figure 7-4).

These synaptic changes can largely be defined by two mechanisms: long-term potentiation and long-term depression, as initially discussed in Chapter 5. **Long-term potentiation (LTP)** results from an increased level of activity within a synapse in response to a given stimulus. Conversely, **long-term depression (LTD)** is associated with a decreased level of responsiveness within a synapse.[8] Both are long-lasting and occur in response to repeated exposure to specific stimuli. [**It should be noted that explicit memory consolidation also involves**

these mechanisms.] Thus, groups of neurons that are activated or inhibited in the presence of a given sensory or motor experience will begin to fire as a group with subsequent exposure to the same or very similar experiences. Based on this premise, implicit learning can involve almost any area of the brain. For **sensorimotor skills**, the cerebellum, basal ganglia, and the premotor and motor cortices are active during learning and remembering of these skills. The striatum of the basal ganglia is active when **habits** are learned, such as our method of combing our hair or brushing our teeth. Both the visual and auditory sensory cortices have been found to develop specific neuronal responses, known as **priming**, to repeated exposure to a given salient stimulus; priming results in less neural activity to a repetition of the stimulus that is characterized by fewer neurons firing for a shorter length of time, but the onset of the activity is quicker than for novel stimuli. These changes are thought to represent efficiency within the sensory system. Similar priming effects are also though to mediate other types of implicit learning like the response to the hidden sequence of letters within the implicit learning paradigm, described in Box 7-2.[9] Similarly, repeated exposure to sensory stimuli can result in decreased responsiveness (**habituation**) or increased responsiveness (**sensitization**); these terms have been generated from animal experiments where animals are presented with threatening or nonthreatening stimuli. Over time, they ignore the nonthreatening stimuli (habituation) but show heightened responses to the threatening stimuli (sensitivity).[10] An example for humans may be a young child's initial fear response to fireworks on the 4th of July that over time becomes an enjoyable experience with limited response to each "pop" (habituation). Conversely, a bumble bee may be just another pretty insect to a young child, but once stung, sighting a bee may elicit a strong fear response (**sensitivity**). This type of classical or operant conditioning, where a neutral stimulus is associated with a reward or punishment, is

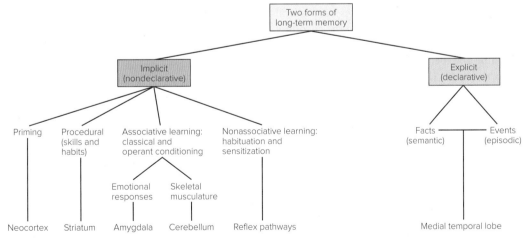

FIGURE 7-4 Schematic of implicit and explicit memory systems. Long-term memory can be divided into explicit (semantic – facts; episodic – events) and implicit (procedural) memories. Explicit memories are encoded by the medial temporal lobe structures and their connections to the anterior cingulate and prefrontal cortices. Implicit memories are generated within an array of networks, including the sensory cortices (priming), striatum of the basal ganglia and cerebellum (motor skills, habits), the cerebellum and amygdala (classical and operant conditioning), and reflex networks of the brainstem. (Reproduced with permission from Kandel ER, Schwartz JH, Jessell TM, Siegelbaum SA, Hudspeth AJ. *Principles of Neural Science*, 5th Ed. New York, NY: McGraw-Hill; 2013. Figure 66-1 Top Section, Pg 1462.)

linked to activity in both the cerebellum (motor response) and the amygdala (emotional response). As a reminder, classical conditioning involves the presentation of a neutral stimulus followed by the presentation of another stimulus (positive or negative), where the response to the second stimulus becomes tied to the first. Similarly, operant conditioning is behavior that is developed as a result of the consequence of that behavior. So, a young child may initially grab a bee, but after being stung, may cry at the sight of a bee (operant conditioning). The pretty firework, followed by the loud sound, may generate a fear response to the sight of the firework (classical conditioning).

Emotion

Emotions are complex learned responses elicited by sensory stimuli that produce physiologic changes (heart and respiration rate, sweating, etc.), motor responses (muscle tensing, facial expression, movement), and motivate us to action (attraction, avoidance).[11] The culmination of these induced changes are interpreted cognitively, resulting in what humans call feelings, ranging from happiness to sadness, hope to fear, attraction to disgust, and gratitude to anger.

The neural center for emotional control is the limbic system, which includes the hippocampus, amygdala, striatum, fornix, hypothalamus, mammillary bodies, anterior thalamic nuclei, areas of the cingulate gyrus, and the insular cortex.[12] Fibers from the hippocampus project through the fornix to the mammillary bodies, thalamus, and hypothalamus and ultimately to the cingulate cortex, which connects to the prefrontal cortex; however, this circuit primarily supports memory function rather than emotions but may connect emotion to our memories (Figure 7-5). Thus, although the limbic system is often solely referred to as our emotional system, it is important to remember its critical role in memory.

A second network links the amygdala to the insular and orbitofrontal cortices via the uncinated fasciculus (a fiber bundle running from the temporal lobe to the frontal lobe). This network (temporo-amygdala-orbitofrontal) integrates our visceral sensations with our cognitive activities, including the encoding of memories, thus, accounting for the impact of reward and punishment on learning and memory and contributing to emotions, especially fear and anger (Figure 7-5). More recently, the dorsomedial default-mode network, which includes the anterior cingulate and medial prefrontal cortex, has been identified. This network, as its name implies, is active in the absence of a goal-directed activity and seems to be responsible for internalized activities such as daydreaming or introspection, which may contribute to the monitoring of our emotional state (Figure 7-5).

The **amygdala** is another medial temporal lobe structure that is adjacent to the hippocampus and the other structures associated with memory. The amygdala has reciprocal connections to the medial prefrontal and orbitofrontal cortices and also projects to the hypothalamus and brainstem nuclei that contribute to the control of respiration, heart rate, postural muscle control, and other autonomic responses (e.g., sweating, chills). The amygdala is core to our fear responses and to the heightened vigilance that we display in fearful situations; for example, when you are walking down a dark alley or street by yourself, your heart rate increases, you may have goose bumps, and are likely to react in an exaggerated way to any noise. This vigilance and hyper-responsiveness is triggered by activity in the amygdala through its connections to the hypothalamus and its related brainstem nuclei. Notably, the afferent connections from the medial prefrontal cortex to the amygdala are critical for suppression of these natural fear and avoidance responses, suggesting that stimuli are analyzed by the frontal cortex with subsequent inhibition of amygdala activity.[13] The amygdala also appears to contribute to the analysis of social situations as well as encoding the emotional components of memory via its connections with the hippocampus, which may explain why some of our strongest memories are associated with fearful experiences.

Similar to the amygdala's connection to fear responsiveness, other areas of the limbic system seem to be linked to specific emotions. The **ACC** is most active when people describe sadness and has been found to be less active in those diagnosed with depression, increasing its level of activity in the presence of antidepressant medications.[14] In addition, the ACC seems to be involved in our conscious awareness of our emotions.[15] Conversely, the **basal ganglia** is linked to happiness or positively motivating activities but is also tied to our disgust response.[14] This activity in the basal ganglia may be related to the potential motor response to situations/things that elicit happiness (movement toward) or avoidance of those that elicit disgust (movement away). The basal ganglia exert their role in emotion through projections from the dorsal caudate to the amygdala, insular cortex, and prefrontal cortex. Interestingly, this connection between the dorsal caudate and the limbic areas has been found to have exaggerated activity in response to pictures of food in morbidly obese individuals,[16] supporting its role in motivation. Disorders of the basal ganglia, such as Parkinson's disease, are often associated with emotional changes, further illustrating its contributory role in emotion.

Finally, the **medial prefrontal cortex** appears to have a significant role in emotional processing that may comprise the analysis of contextual cues to determine the appropriate emotion, including the comparison of the current situation to our memories of similar situations, as well as self-assessment of our current emotional state. Its interconnections with the hippocampus likely facilitate this comparison. The **insular cortex** is an area of convergence for visceral sensations (e.g., heart and respiration rate, sweeting), which contribute to our interpretation of our emotional response. Further, this area of the brain seems to play a critical role in our interpretation of reward and punishment and interestingly appears to also contribute to the development of addiction.[14]

Language

Of all of the higher level skills that differentiate humans from other animals, none is as obvious as language. Our understanding of the neural substrates that support our language abilities continues to evolve as our ability to image and use electrical stimulation to evaluate this system expands. Our language skills and the systems that support them are typically divided into reception (our ability to recognize and understand language) and production (our ability to produce speech).

FIGURE 7-5 A and B. Circuits of the limbic system. These two figures schematically illustrate the two circuits of the limbic system: **A** illustrates the temporo-amygdala-orbitofrontal network that supports emotions (especially fear) and impacts learning related to reward and punishment. **B** – illustrates the hippocampal formation's connections to the mammillary bodies and areas of the cingulate and insular cortex; this network subserves memory and emotion. (Reproduced with permission from Martin JH. *Neuroanatomy Text and Atlas*, 4th Ed. New York, NY: McGraw-Hill; 2012. Figure 16-6A&B, Pg 393.)

A few common terms, associated with language, will be important for our discussion of the neural systems supporting our language abilities. **Phonology** or **phonetics** refers to the way sounds are put together to form words while **syntax**, also known as grammar, is the way words are organized within a phrase or sentence. **Semantics** refers to the meaning of words or sounds, such as "un" referring to "not."

In the 1800s two centers were identified that seemed to support these two functions, based on the presentation of patients that had damage to one or the other area. Broca's area, named for Paul Broca, is located in the frontal lobe, just anterior to the primary motor area on the lateral surface of the hemisphere, and was linked to language production; damage to this area was reported to result in difficulty with word selection and, thereby, limited speech output but good speech understanding (**nonfluent aphasia**). Wernicke's area, named for Carl Wernicke, is located in the posterior aspect of the temporal lobe and associated with language reception; damage to this area resulted in loss of speech understanding with fluid but nonresponsive speech production thought to be the result of limited comprehension of what others say as well as the inability to monitor self-generated speech (**fluent aphasia**). These two areas were found to interconnect via the arcuate fasciculus and damage to these fibers resulted in **conductive aphasia**, associated with disordered ordering of syllables (phonology). Further, the left hemisphere was found to be dominant for language in most individuals, but with a small percentage of left-handed individuals showing right dominance. However, several hundred years of research, since these early descriptions, has determined them to be a simplistic view of human language systems, so our complex language abilities are now believed to be supported by a more expansive neural network that spans the temporal, parietal, and frontal lobes.[17] However, many clinicians still rely on these original definitions of **aphasia** (disrupted speech).

The neural networks, supporting language perception and production, involve two projection streams and their respective connections. Although speech sounds are processed initially by the same neurologic substrates as any other sounds, as described in Chapter 6, the superior temporal gyrus (STG) is active bilaterally when speech is heard and appears to be the first processing area of our language system, likely playing a role in distinguishing verbal from nonverbal stimuli. In fact, damage to the STG bilaterally results in a severe phenomenon, known as **word deafness**, which literally is the inability to distinguish speech from other sounds. Fortunately, this is an extremely rare disorder.

Subsequent to activity in the STG, verbal processing appears to use two projection streams that are lateralized primarily to the left hemisphere in most individuals (a small percent of left-handed individuals do have their language centers on the right). A **dorsal stream** projects from Wernicke's area to the parietal lobe within the Sylvian fissure and then to Broca's area in the frontal lobe (inferior frontal gyrus, Brodmann's areas 44 and 45) via the arcuate fasciculus and superior longitudinal fasciculus; this stream is critical for transforming what we want to say into appropriately articulated sentences (syntax). Therefore, the historic non-fluent aphasia is a disruption of the dorsal stream, resulting in disordered syntax. Interestingly, the basal ganglia and cerebellum play a role in the fluidity of our speech, contributing to the rate at which we say words as well as the word spacing.[18] The **ventral stream** connects the superior temporal sulcus, middle temporal gyrus, and inferior temporal gyrus as well as the visual cortex to the DLPFC, frontal operculum, and areas 45 (part of Broca's area) and 47 via the uncinate fasciculus and inferior fronto-occipital fasciculus. The temporal lobe regions are tightly linked to semantic memory areas and visual areas in the frontal, parietal, and occipital lobes. This ventral stream principally supports the conversion of what is heard and seen to its meaning for both understanding what is

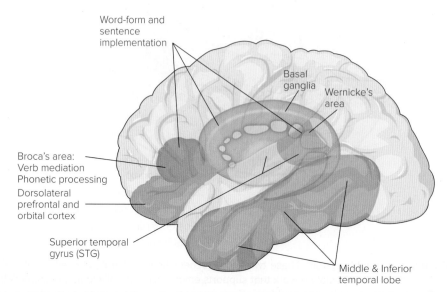

FIGURE 7-6 Language centers. The historic Broca's and Wernicke's areas are depicted in association with the surrounding areas that contribute to language skills (dorsolateral and orbitofrontal cortex, middle and inferior temporal lobes, basal ganglia). (Reproduced with permission from Kandel ER, Schwartz JH, Jessell TM, Siegelbaum SA, Hudspeth AJ. *Principles of Neural Science*, 5th Ed. New York, NY: McGraw-Hill; 2013. Figure 60-5, Pg 1364.)

said (semantics) and planning what one wants to say, including naming visually presented objects. Thus, the fluent aphasia, previously associated with Wernicke's area, results from disruption to the ventral stream with subsequent disordered semantics. Both streams are bidirectional, allowing for the integration of speech production with speech perception. Obviously, damage to many areas, surrounding the historic Broca's and Wernicke's areas will result in disruption of language abilities (Figure 7-6). However, this expanded network also explains the preservation of many language skills after brain damage as well as the more variable presentations of some survivors of stroke, brain injury, or other disorders.[19]

The historic view of **conduction aphasia** is that it is caused by damage to the arcuate fasciculus, which, in effect, disrupted the connection between speech perception centers in the temporal lobe and speech production centers in the frontal lobe. This resulted in disruption in speech production that included difficulties in repeating what someone else has said, disordered phonology (syllable ordering within a word or word order within a sentence), and problems with naming of objects. More recent evidence suggests that conduction aphasia is more likely the result of damage to the superior temporal sulcus and subsequently the temporal–parietal lobe interconnections rather than the arcuate fasciculus.[18]

● SUMMARY

The higher level functions discussed in this chapter – executive function, memory, emotion, and language – demonstrate the complexity of the human brain. They also illustrate the multiple interconnections between these functions and the neural systems that support them, which is the reason that they were presented in a single chapter. In the presence of neurologic injury or disease, these higher level functions are often disrupted in combination with highly variable presentations, since brain damage is rarely the same between individuals with similar conditions. In the disease-focused chapters of this text, the impact of brain damage on higher level functions will be discussed.

REFERENCES

1. Rosenbloom MH, Schmahmann JD, Price BH. The functional neuroanatomy of decision-making. *J Neuropscyh Clin Neurosci*. 2012;24(3):266-277.

2. Leh SE, Petrides M, Strafelia AP. The neural circuitry of executive functions in healthy subjects and Parkinson's disease. *Neuropsychopharmacology*. 2010;35:70-85.

3. Meriau K, Wartenburger I, Kazzer P, et al. A neural network reflecting individual differences in cognitive processing of emotions during perceptual decision making. *Neuroimage*. 2006;33(3):1016-1027.

4. Preston AR, Eichenbaum H. Interplay of hippocampus and prefrontal cortex in memory. *Current Biol*. 2013;23:R764-R773.

5. Staube B. An overview of the neuro-cognitive processes involved in the encoding, consolidation and retrieval of true and false memories. *Behav Brain Funct*. 2012;8:35-45.

6. Winocur G, Moscovitch M, Bontempi B. Memory formation and long-term retention in humans and animals: convergence towards a transformation account of hippocampal-neocortical interactions. *Neuropsychologia*. 2010;48:2339-2356.

7. Metzger CD, van der Werl YD, Walter M. Functional mapping of thalamic nuclei and their integration into cortico-striatal-thalamo-cortical loops via ultra-high resolution imaging – from animal anatomy to in vivo imaging in humans. *Front Neurosci*. 2013;7:1-14.

8. Gold MG. A frontier in the understanding of synaptic plasticity: solving the structure of the postsynaptic density. *Bioessays*. 34:599-608.

9. Reber PJ. The neural basis of implicit learning and memory: a review of neuropsychological and neuroimaging research. *Neuropsychologia*. 2013;51:2026-2042.

10. Cellular mechanisms of implicit memory storage and the biological basis of individuality. In: Kandel ER, Shwartz JH, Jessel TM, Siegelbaum SA, and Hudspeth AJ, eds. *Principles of Neural Science*. 5th ed. Chapter 66. Chicago, IL: McGraw Hill; 2013:1461–4185.

11. Brosch T, Scherer KR, Grandjean D, Sander D. The impact of emotion on perception, attention, memory, and decision-making. *Eur J Med Sci.; Swiss Med Wkly*. 2013;143:w13786.

12. Catani M, Dell'Acqua F, deSchotten MT. A revised limbic system model for memory, emotion and behavior. *Neurosci Biobehav Rev*. 2013;37:1724-1737.

13. Kim MJ, Loucks RA, Palmer AL, Brown AC, Solomon KM, Marchante AN, Whalen PJ. The structural and functional connectivity of the amygdala: from normal emotion to pathological anxiety. *Behav Brain Res*. 2011;223(2):403-410.

14. Phan KL, Wager T, Taylor SF, Liberzon I. Functional neuroanatomy of emotion: a meta-analysis of emotion activation studies in PET and fMRI. *Neuroimage*. 2002;16:33-348.

15. Dalgleish T. The emotional brain. *Perspectives*. 2004;5:582-589.

16. Nummenmaa L, Hirvonen J, Hannukainen JC, Immonen H, Lindroos MM, Salminen P, Nuutila P. Dorsal striatum and its limbic connectivity mediate abnormal anticipatory reward processing in obesity. *PLoS One*. 2012;7(2):e31089.

17. Dick F, Bates E, Wulfeck B, Utman JA, Dronkers N, Gernsbacher MA. Language deficits, localization and grammar: evidence for a distributive model of language breakdown in aphasic patients and neurologically intact individuals. *Psychol Rev*. 2001;108(4):759-788.

18. Reilly KJ, Spencer KA. Speech serial control in healthy speakers and speakers with hypokinetic or ataxic dysarthria: effects of sequence length and practice. *Front Hum Neurosci*. 2013;7(article 665):1-17.

19. Hickok G, Poeppel D. Dorsal and ventral streams: a framework for understanding aspects of functional anatomy of language. *Cognition*. 2004;92:67-99.

Review Questions

1. **Failure to switch attention from one cue to another in a task switching paradigm is known as:**

   A. Disinhibition

   B. Dysregulation

   C. Perseveration

   D. Prioritization

2. **Frontal dysexecutive syndrome is associated with damage to:**

   A. Anterior cingulate cortex

   B. Dorsolateral prefrontal cortex

   C. Orbitofrontal cortex

   D. Premotor cortex

3. **What brain region is critical to working memory?**
   A. Anterior cingulate
   B. Dorsolateral prefrontal cortex
   C. Orbitofrontal cortex
   D. Ventromedial cortex

4. **Our ability to remember a skill, like how to hit a baseball, is referred to as:**
   A. Declarative memory
   B. Episodic memory
   C. Implicit memory
   D. Semantic memory

5. **Permanent changes in synaptic activity, in association with memory creation, are associated with what process?**
   A. Consolidation
   B. Encoding
   C. Retrieval
   D. Priming

6. **Anterograde amnesia is associated with damage to what anatomical area?**
   A. Amygdala
   B. Hippocampus
   C. Prefrontal cortex
   D. Thalamus

7. **Increased responsiveness of a synapse to a given stimulus, associated with memory, is known as:**
   A. Long-term depression
   B. Long-term excitation
   C. Long-term potentiation
   D. Priming

8. **The amygdala is most strongly linked to what emotion?**
   A. Disgust
   B. Fear
   C. Happiness
   D. Sadness

9. **Monitoring of our internal emotional state is likely related to what emotional network?**
   A. Caudate–amygdala–prefrontal cortex network
   B. Hippocampal-mammillary body–hypothalamus–cingulate network
   C. Resting state network
   D. Temporo-amygdala–orbitofrontal network

10. **What area of convergence for visceral sensation is active in our interpretation of reward and punishment?**
    A. Anterior cingulate
    B. Basal ganglia
    C. Insular cortex
    D. Medial prefrontal cortex

11. **In language, the way sounds are organized into words is known as what?**
    A. Grammar
    B. Phonetics
    C. Semantics
    D. Syntax

12. **Which language network supports syntax?**
    A. Dorsal stream
    B. Fronto-occipital stream
    C. Uncinate stream
    D. Ventral stream

13. **Fluent aphasia is characterized by disruption of what language skill?**
    A. Phonetics
    B. Repetition
    C. Semantics
    D. Syntax

14. **Damage to the superior temporal sulcus is associated with what type of aphasia**
    A. Conductive aphasia
    B. Fluent aphasia
    C. Non-fluent aphasia
    D. Receptive aphasia

15. **Which area of the brain has been found to be associated with learning, emotion, language, and working memory?**
    A. Amygdala
    B. Basal ganglia
    C. Hippocampus
    D. Parietal cortex

Answers

1. C	2. B	3. B	4. C	5. A
6. B	7. C	8. B	9. C	10. C
11. B	12. A	13. D	14. B	15. B

Neuroplasticity

8

Deborah S. Nichols-Larsen
and D. Michele Basso

● DEVELOPMENTAL NEUROGENESIS

As described in Chapter 18 (Neural Tube Disorders), the nervous system arises from neural crest cells within the ectodermal layer of the developing embryo. Cell proliferation transforms the neural plate into the neural tube that is initially differentiated into three vesicles from rostral to caudal: prosencephalon, mesencephalon, and rhombencephalon. Further cell proliferation results in a five-vesicle structure: telencephalon (cerebral hemispheres), diencephalon (retina, hypothalamus, thalamus, epithalamus, and subthalamus), mesencephalon (midbrain), metencephalon (pons, cerebellum), and myelencephalon (medulla), which is contiguous with the remainder of the neural tube that forms the spinal cord. The lumen of the neural tube develops into the ventricular system and central spinal canal.

Initially, the tissue of the neural tube expands into three layers (see Figure 8-1): ependymal layer, mantel layer, and marginal layer. The **ependymal layer** provides the border for the developing ventricular system and is cell rich with rapidly dividing cells. The **mantel layer** will become the gray matter (cortex and deep nuclei), and the **marginal layer** will be filled with axons (white matter). Within weeks, there will be five identifiable layers: (1) **ventricular zone** – area of rapid cell proliferation; (2) **subventricular zone** – second area of cell proliferation; (3) **intermediate zone** – developing white matter; (4) **subplate** – early neurons and glial cells that facilitate connections between

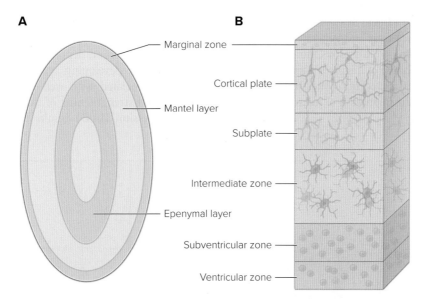

A **B**

- Marginal zone
- Cortical plate
- Mantel layer
- Subplate
- Intermediate zone
- Epenymal layer
- Subventricular zone
- Ventricular zone

FIGURE 8-1 Cell proliferation in the developing CNS. A. Three layered neural tube with cell proliferation in the ependymal layer and cell poor mantel and marginal layers. **B.** Five layers of developing brain: ventricular and subventricular zones are areas of cell proliferation filled with neural stem cells; intermediate zone will be filled with glial cells and become the white matter; the subplate will house early neurons that will connect the cortex to the thalamus; the cortical plate will become the cortex ; the marginal zone is cell poor but will contain axons and a few neurons. (Used with permission of Deborah S. Nichols Larsen, PT, PhD. The Ohio State University.)

the cortex and thalamus;[1] (5) **cortical plate** – developing cortex; and (6) **marginal zone** – cell poor with surface neurons and horizontal fibers.[2]

Cell Proliferation

Neurogenesis refers to the development of neurons, while **gliogenesis** is the development of glial cells; these are interrelated processes. **Neural stem cells** (**NSCs**) are progenitor cells for both neurons and glia that can be found initially in the ventricular zone and, then, also in the subventricular zone, where they undergo rapid cell divisions. While NSCs appear undifferentiated, they actually differ in their mitotic activity, cellular and molecular characteristics, transcription factor expression, and the types of cells that they produce.[3,4] One of the first cells to develop from the NSCs of the ependymal layer is the **radial glial cell** (**RGC**). RGCs extend a projection to the ependymal lining of the ventricle and another to the pial lining, which covers the outside of the developing neural tube.

These cells replicate, initially forming neurons but ultimately forming glia – astrocytes and ependymal cells along with oligodendrocyte progenitor cells that proliferate to produce these crucial glia.[5] In addition, the RGCs form a matrix that helps to guide the neurons to their ultimate settling point in the cortical plate[6] (see Figure 8-2). While RGCs are the first progenitor cells to develop, eventually there are multiple progenitor cells, derived from ependymal cells, referred to as short neural precursors, intermediate progenitor cells, and basal radial glial cells.[3] As a group, these neural stem cells populate the neurons of the mature brain. Cell proliferation is stimulated and controlled by signaling **morphogens**; these are found within the cerebrospinal fluid and enter the ventricular and subventricular zones via the primary cilium (projection adhered to the ventricular lining). Morphogens include sonic hedgehog (SHH), growth factors (fibroblast and insulin), and bone morphogenic proteins (BMPs).[7] Within the VC and SVC, progenitor cells distribute themselves in distinct areas and generate unique neural cell types. Again, signaling from various morphogens and microRNAs trigger the migration of the progenitor cells to specific regions of the subcortical and cortical plates and apparently play a role in the ultimate differentiation of neuronal cell type (e.g., excitatory or inhibitory).[8]

Developmental Neuroplasticity: Connectivity and Pruning

Following cell migration, networks of neurons develop that tie critical areas of the brain together through axonal growth to specific synaptic targets (e.g., corticocortical, thalamocortical). This process begins early in the second trimester of gestation. Axonal growth and the sprouting of terminal axon boutons are guided by neurotrophic and morphogenic factors, secreted by glial cells. For example, oligodendrocytes are known to secrete nerve growth factor and brain-derived neurotrophic factor (BDNF) that contribute to axonal outgrowth. Cell adhesion molecules on the surface of target neurons also appear to guide synapse formation.[9] Eventually, however, it is activity within the neural circuits that fine tunes ultimate synaptic connectivity; this second stage of axonal growth seems to be facilitated by neurotrophic factors (e.g., BDNF).[10] Initially, there is an overproduction of axon collaterals, and synaptic contacts, followed by remodeling that eliminates poorly connected axons, excessive synapses, and ultimately neuron overpopulation. The elimination of unnecessary axon collaterals is known as **pruning**, and the destruction of neurons is referred to as **programmed cell death**.[11] One determinant of axonal pruning is the need for each axonal collateral to establish effective synapses with postsynaptic neurons; poorly connected axons are eliminated. This involves reabsorption of the axon fragment back into the proximal axon or disconnection of the distil axon component as a fragment that is then, phagocytized by surrounding microglia. Figure 8-3 illustrates these changes.

Similarly, dendrites that do not establish connections are eliminated. Ultimately, neurons that are poorly connected or remain inactive go through programmed cell death so that effective neural networks remain. This process extends into the first 6 months of neonatal life.[9] In addition, myelination of developing neurons continues well into the second year of life, associated with developmental maturation. The efficacy of synapses, within the developing nervous system, is honed by long-term potentiation and depression (as described in Chapter 7). In the case of developing synapses, **long-term potentiation** (**LTP**) is associated with well-established connections, axon survival, and strengthening of the network. Conversely, **long-term depression** (**LTD**) results from poor connectivity and

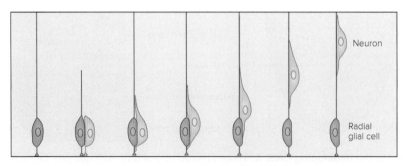

Neuron

Radial glial cell

Radial glial cell division generates neurons

Neuronal migration on radial glial cells

FIGURE 8-2 Neuronal migration along radial glial cells. Radial glial cells produce neurons and then guide them along their apical projection to the cortical plate. (Adapted with permission from Kandel ER, Schwartz JH, Jessell TM, Siegelbaum SA, Hudspeth AJ. *Principles of Neural Science*, 5th ED, New York, NY: McGraw-Hill; 2013. Figure 53-2, p. 1190.)

FIGURE 8-3 **Synaptogenesis, pruning, and sprouting – mechanisms of neural development and injury repair. A.** An axon passing by a cell can develop a new branch called a filopodium, which begins to form a synapse, and eventually becomes functional. The postsynaptic member begins to develop a synaptic spine. **B.** When a synapse strengthens over time, the presynaptic and postsynaptic elements can enlarge, and eventually, a second synapse can develop. **C.** As neurons develop, they initially lack synaptic spines. In the middle phase of development, they have an overabundance. As the connections mature, there is pruning, and some spines are eliminated. **D.** A dendritic spine can become stronger or weaker over time as the plasticity develops. **E.** In a circuit with alternative pathways, if one route is lesioned, the other can become stronger and replace the lost function. (A: Reproduced with permission from Kandel ER, Schwartz JH, Jessell TM, Siegelbaum SA, Hudspeth AJ. *Principles of Neural Science*, 5th ED, New York, NY: McGraw-Hill; 2013. Figure 55-14A, Pg 1250.) (C: Reproduced with permission from Kandel ER, Schwartz JH, Jessell TM, Siegelbaum SA, Hudspeth AJ. *Principles of Neural Science*, 5th ED, New York, NY: McGraw-Hill; 2013. Figure 54-3, Pg 1213.) (Parts B, D, and E: Used with permission of John A. Buford, PT, PhD.)

induces axonal pruning and potentially cell death. Network remodeling occurs as a result of experience within critical periods; hence, inactivity, during a critical period, can result in loss of essential neurons. Importantly, critical periods are associated with a greater capacity for plasticity than at other times of development and are associated with increased GABA inhibition. BDNF is thought to play an important role in these critical periods through the stimulation of GABA neuron maturation. Other molecular changes, then, apparently impose a blockade to the critical period potentiation. Notably, premature birth or developmental trauma may block neural network formation within critical periods.[9]

ADULT NEUROGENESIS

Interestingly, gliogenesis continues throughout the brain and spinal cord into adult life, while neurogenesis is largely confined to embryonic and early postnatal development. However, adult neurogenesis does exist in discrete areas of the nervous system, referred to as neurogenic niches; in humans, these appear localized in the subgranular and subventricular zones adjacent to the hippocampus, supporting new neurons for the dentate gyrus of the hippocampus and the olfactory bulb. Neurogenesis has also been described in the motor cortex in primates and the progenitor cells are thought to come from the subventricular zone.[12] It is important to note that progenitor cells in the embryonic period can produce both neurons and glial cells; thus, limitations in neurogenesis in adulthood likely stem from changes in the microenvironment necessary for the generation of neurons, including the absence of appropriate growth factors and the presence of cytokines, chemokines, and other signaling molecules that block the production of neurons.[4,13] Further, neurogenesis is slower in the mature brain, and axonal projections typically target active synapses to insure viability; therefore, synaptogenesis in pathways damaged by disease is unlikely. However, synaptogenesis of bystander pathways, that is, pathways not directly damaged by trauma or disease, has been widely reported in animal studies.[14] There is also some indication that an enriched environment, exercise, and diet facilitate neurogenesis in adults, which, in turn, can be disrupted by aging and stress[13] as well as pathologic conditions such as seizures.[4] Aging appears to induce a state of quiescence (inactivity) in stem cells as well as a moderate inflammation, resulting in limited cell proliferation.[4]

LEARNING-ASSOCIATED NEUROPLASTICITY

Similar to the earlier discussion of developmental plasticity, a significant body of evidence has emerged to support that the brain continues to be highly malleable throughout our lives, adapting and reorganizing in response to the level of activity it experiences. In Chapter 7, we discussed this in terms of memory; however, any skill acquisition is associated with neuroplastic changes within those neural networks activated during practice. For example, the motor area of the hand, in the primary motor cortex (precentral gyrus, M1), expands in response to specific training paradigms; this expansion is associated with: (1) **synaptogenesis** evident through new dendritic spines and more synapses per neuron; (2) **microstructural changes** in white matter with greater myelin density; and (3) alterations in specific **gene expression** that seem to align with the changes in synapses and white matter. Of interest, tegmental dopamine projections to M1 seem to play a critical role in these mechanisms of learning-induced plasticity, and there is some speculation that naturally occurring differences in the density of these dopamine projections may underlie individual differences in motor ability.[10,15]

LTP, as previously discussed, occurs in the presence of heightened neuronal activity, associated with skill acquisition. Modulation of synaptic activity is mediated by multiple factors, including interleukin-1β (IL-1β) and tumor necrosis factor (TNFα). One method for synaptic modulation, known as synaptic scaling, is induced by TNFα and associated with an increase in the density of receptors at the synapse, specifically glutamate receptors [N-methyl-D-asparate (NMDA)].[16] Other mechanisms of LTP include: (1) increased calcium permeability; (2) dendritic spine enlargement; (3) increased protein synthesis; and (4) enhanced actin polymerization.[17] Calcium influx appears to trigger several different enzymatic cascades that enhance existing receptor function but also stimulate new receptor generation in postsynaptic neurons. Interestingly, different cascades respond to different stimulus characteristics (e.g., intensity versus frequency), suggesting that LTP likely involves different mechanisms at different synapses.[17] Actin polymerization is thought to be involved in early stage LTP, providing reorganization of the cytoskeletal structure of active synapses, specifically to facilitate dendritic spine formation. Changes in actin are followed by the appearance of membrane attachment proteins that further consolidate LTP changes at the synapse.[18]

BDNF also appears to contribute to motor map reorganization and synaptogenesis, associated with motor learning, through stimulating protein synthesis to support synapse formation.[19] Neural reorganization increases the metabolic demands of the tissue and triggers the expansion of the capillary bed, known as **angiogenesis**. This involves either: (1) the splitting of capillaries into two branches by a process called intussusception, or (2) the projection of new vascular "sprouts" that connect to a second capillary. This results in increased vascular density and the ability to meet the oxygen and nutritional demand of the new synapses.[20] Angiogenesis is mediated by endothelial progenitor cells that migrate to areas of need and secrete VEGF and cytokines necessary for angiogenesis.[21]

As discussed with developmental neuroplasticity, a second mechanism of plasticity with learning is LTD. In this case, synapses with limited activity levels can be eliminated; this may contribute to forgetting but is also a mechanism for honing neural pathways that are critical to function by eliminating those that are not as critical. This, in effect, is a method for achieving synaptic efficiency. Surprisingly, LTD is also characterized by an increase in calcium influx; however, in this instance, the increase is slow and prolonged. These two neural processes (LTP and LTD) occur simultaneously at adjacent synapses of the same neuron to maximize synaptic efficiency. LTD at some synapses can induce **microglial synaptic pruning**; this involves phagocytosis of the synaptic components in both the pre and postsynaptic neurons of inactive synapses by resident microglia.[16]

● NEURAL RESPONSE TO INJURY

Focal Degeneration

Neural injury typically involves both focal damage (at the site of the injury) and secondary remote damage downstream from the initial injury. With **focal damage** there is disruption of cellular function within the soma (cell body) of neurons at the immediate site of injury, leading to cell death. Additionally, neurons that experience axon disruption (axotomy) will undergo either retrograde or anterograde degeneration or both. **Anterograde degeneration**, also known as **Wallerian** or **orthograde** degeneration, occurs in the distal segment or fragment that has been separated from the proximal component; since axonal transport is lost, this segment rapidly undergoes degeneration and is phagocytized by the circulating microglia. The proximal component may also undergo a series of intracellular changes that ultimately lead to degeneration of the axon (dying back), known as **retrograde degeneration**; this is dependent on the location of the injury and whether some axonal projections maintain functional synapses. If some projections remain, the axon may survive. However, completely axotomized neurons, in which no collaterals remain, undergo pronounced changes including swelling, chromatolysis, damage to cellular components, impaired protein synthesis among other mechanisms that disrupt endoplasmic reticulum function and cytoskeleton integrity, ultimately resulting in cellular shrinkage and cell death.[22] This loss of axons results in synaptic stripping on the somas and dendrites of postsynaptic neurons, to which the axotomized neurons project.[23]

Remote Neurodegeneration

Secondary retrograde and anterograde degeneration can result from loss of connectivity with neurons lost at the site of the focal injury. Those neurons that project onto the lost neurons have lost their functional connections; thus, they may undergo **retrograde transneuronal degeneration**. Similarly, those neurons that typically receive axonal connections from the lost neurons have lost at least a portion of their activation source, and thus, may undergo **anterograde transneuronal degeneration**.[22] This secondary neurodegeneration (e.g., retrograde and anterograde transneuronal degeneration) is common after neural injury, leading to loss of neurons in the area surrounding the focal injury and at sites distal to but functionally related to the injured area. While several factors impact the degree of remote cell death, including magnitude of the original injury, patient age, and connectivity characteristics of the damaged neuronal networks, several mechanisms contribute to cell survival or death.[22] In the subsequent sections, we will discuss the mechanisms of secondary cell damage.

Inflammation

Inflammation at the site of injury and in areas well away from the primary injury is mediated by both microglia and astrocytes that secrete pro-inflammatory chemokines and cytokines. The astrocytes function to reestablish the blood–brain barrier, stimulate glutamate reabsorption, and limit the spread of damage. In contrast, microglia produce inflammatory mediators, including free radicals, glutamate, TNF-α, IL-1β, nitric oxide along with pro-inflammatory chemokines and cytokines, that function to prolong the inflammatory period and exacerbate neural damage at the site of injury. While most people consider that inflammation spreads slowly to remote regions over the course of 2–3 weeks, recent findings in the spinal cord showed profound microglial activation and inflammation within 24 hours of an injury at least 10 segments away.[24] In these remote regions, changes in structural neural plasticity and dendritic spines can be seen within 7 days. Some have noted that the behavior of these glial cells is reversed, at these distal sites, with astrocytes triggering greater degeneration through mechanisms attributed to microglia at the site of the injury, and microglia functioning to minimize remote damage;[22] however, this may vary by site, as it is not seen in the spinal cord.

Excitotoxicity

Excessive release of glutamate, dopamine, and norepinephrine occurs as a result of CNS trauma or ischemia, as experienced with head injury, prolonged seizures (e.g., status epilepticus – see Chapter 19), or stroke. Reduced glial function may limit the scavenging of glutamate, also increasing its extracellular concentration. Excessive glutamate results in an influx of Na^+ and Ca^{++} into the cell with subsequent cellular edema and contraction of the extracellular space. Similarly, glutamate also stimulates reactive oxygen species production (see later section on oxidative stress).[25] Likewise, there is often an exaggerated release of dopamine and norepinephrine with a buildup of their toxic by-products. Together, these factors create a toxic environment and ultimately contribute to neuronal death.[25]

Apoptosis

Programmed cell death not only occurs as a process in neural development, but it is also found in response to neural injury and is known as apoptosis. There are two pathways that induce apoptosis. The first is known as the **external pathway** and involves surface receptors, known as death receptors that trigger a cascade of caspase activity.[22] **Caspases** are endoprotease enzymes that exist in an inactive form until neural damage transforms them into active molecules. The first caspases to be activated are known as initiators (caspases 8 and 9); these, in turn, activate executioner caspases (3, 6, and 7), which disrupt cellular structural proteins and other cellular components, leading to cell death.[26] The second pathway also involves caspase activity, targeting the cell's mitochondria. Multiple factors can trigger this **internal pathway**, including loss of specific growth factors, cell membrane disruption, hypoxia, and certain hormones. This pathway is the one active in developmental programmed cell death.

Autophagy

Autophagy is a natural process to eliminate damaged proteins or organelles within the cell body to promote optimal cell functioning; mitochondria and the endoplasmic reticulum play a critical role in the regulation of autophagy. While autophagy, after focal injury, may initially be triggered to eliminate damaged organelles in injured neurons to promote homeostasis, it may actually determine cell survival and ultimately become a secondary pathway for cell death. Of interest, autophagy has been identified in remote neurons; however, the triggers for this occurrence remain elusive. Autophagy and apoptosis may share common mechanisms and have been found to occur simultaneously; however, there is some suggestion that apoptosis occurs when autophagy is ineffective in achieving homeostasis.[22] Of note, autophagy has also been linked to multiple neurodegenerative disorders and cancers (e.g., Amyotrophic Lateral Sclerosis).[27]

Oxidative and Nitrosative Stress

Following neural injury, there is a proliferation of reactive oxygen species (ROS) and reactive nitrogen species (RNS), both of which are detrimental to neurons. ROS are produced by mitochondria, and when mitochondria are damaged, there is excessive accumulation of ROS, which attack the cell membrane and degrade other key cellular components (e.g., proteins). Similarly, nitric oxide, an RNS, is toxic to neurons, leading to cell death by damaging key proteins and lipids.[22]

The mechanisms, discussed here, all contribute to secondary cell death after initial CNS injury; current treatment methods, both medical and rehabilitative, are focused on blocking this secondary cell loss to improve outcomes. Some of these methods will be discussed in the second half of this book, along with the disease processes; however, in the next section, we will review the general processes for neural plasticity associated with CNS injury or disease.

● NEUROPLASTICITY AFTER CNS INJURY

Plasticity Promoters

Neural changes, post-injury or during neurologic disease, target the salvaging and strengthening of survivor neurons and their synapses and facilitation of new axonal–dendritic connections. For example, after a spinal cord injury, astrocytes rush to the lesion, restoring blood flow, blocking the activity of peripheral leukocytes and promoting revascularization.[23] Alternatively, after many types of neural injury, microglia stimulate the retraction of excitatory axonal boutons to protect surviving neurons from excessive excitation, known as **excitatory stripping**. There are several endogenous plasticity promotors, specifically **neurotrophins** (BDNF, NT-3) that may facilitate plasticity post-injury. These seem to promote cell survival, strengthen synaptic connections, and promote axonal growth and sprouting, yet following spinal cord injury, they are downregulated. Thus, research is targeting the application of these neurotrophins in the spinal cord to promote recovery, which in animal models of SCI has improved axonal regrowth around the lesion, prevented

synaptic stripping, and protected against excitotoxicity by promoting inhibitory synapse connections.[23] Importantly, BDNF and NT-3 are regulated by exercise within the spinal cord and muscle.[28] After SCI in rodents, treadmill training increased BDNF and was associated with resolution of neuropathic pain.[28] Interestingly, static standing exercise or rhythmic non-weight-bearing swimming exercise did not produce the neurotrophin or sensory effects and neuropathic pain remained.[28]

Spontaneous Recovery

Early spontaneous recover is likely dependent on recovered activity of surviving neurons in the penumbra (area surrounding the lesion). Immediately following injury, a period of neural "shock" exists, known as diaschisis, whereby neurons in the penumbra and areas, connecting to the lesioned area, demonstrate limited activity. This resolves over a matter of weeks. During this time period, studies have demonstrated neurite outgrowth, local sprouting, synaptogenesis, and angiogenesis.[10] Sprouting is a mechanism by which axons grow additional distal projections to fill vacated receptor sites. In animal models, improved motor performance has also demonstrated a reliance on compensation and expansion of motor maps, corresponding to the compensating muscle groups (e.g., trunk muscles compensating for shoulder muscles).[10] Additionally, there is a bilateral change in NMDA and GABA receptors, with upregulation of the former and downregulation of the latter, and sprouting of neurons that project to the peri-infarct area, including transcallosal projections from the non-lesioned hemisphere. Notably, interhemispheric connections likely play a greater role in recovery from larger lesions than smaller lesions.[10] In the motor cortex, there are also increased projections to the peri-infarct area from the surrounding motor areas (e.g., premotor).

Experience-dependent Plasticity

Earlier in this chapter, we discussed the role of experience in the development of neural connections. Following neural injury, the nervous system demonstrates a remarkable capacity to repair and remodel itself. More important to the rehabilitation community, evidence over the last few decades has shown that this repair and remodeling responds to the experience of the patient following injury, and therefore, is influenced by the therapy (or lack thereof) provided. Thus, experience-dependent plasticity is a critical process in the recovery of all patients with neurologic injuries/diseases. However, it should be noted that this plasticity can be adaptive or maladaptive, promoting recovery of lost function or preventing that recovery.

Maladaptive Plasticity

Perhaps the best example of maladaptive plasticity is the phenomenon that is known as **learned nonuse**. Briefly, this is a process, whereby patients post-stroke experience negative feedback, when initially trying to use the paretic arm (e.g., limited success, pain); this feedback discourages subsequent use of the arm even as spontaneous recovery is occurring. Thus, patients fail to use retained function. Further, they are positively rewarded for developing compensatory strategies (e.g., trunk motion to achieve shoulder abduction) or using the non-paretic limb to achieve function, resulting in limited use of the paretic limb, despite greater movement ability than demonstrated. Interestingly, compensatory use of the non-paretic limb may disrupt plasticity in the peri-infarct area by targeting synaptogenesis within the contralesional hemisphere.[10] These findings are critical for rehabilitationists, since they suggest that early treatment, which can be aimed at compensation due to minimal motor ability in the paretic limbs, may, in fact, stimulate expansion of motor maps in the contralesional hemisphere rather than promoting plasticity changes in the lesioned hemisphere. There is some suggestion that excessive activity in the contralesional hemisphere, measured by functional magnetic resonance imaging (fMRI), is maladaptive rather than adaptive, especially in the acute stage post-injury, where it has been linked to poorer recovery; however, many stroke survivors with good recovery demonstrate some contralesional control of the ipsilateral extremities.[25] Another example of maladaptive plasticity, is the emergence of allodynia, following spinal cord injury, which seems to emerge from neural remodeling within the pain centers, responding to non-noxious inputs post-injury.[23] In addition, new evidence is emerging that spasticity may result from maladaptive plasticity within the gray matter of the spinal cord.[29] An increased density of dendrites combined with neuronal atrophy lead to heightened excitability of neurons that produces hyperreflexia.[29]

Adaptive Plasticity

Constraint-induced movement therapy (CIMT), which will be discussed in more detail in Chapter 10 (Stroke), is partially effective in reducing learned-nonuse, as described in the preceding section, and to expand the motor map of the paretic hand, as measured by TMS,[30] as well as shift the locus of control of the hand back to the ipsilesional motor cortex as shown on fMRI.[31] These findings illustrate the importance of focused training to promote plasticity in better recovery post-injury (see Figure 8-4).

Kleim reviewed multiple factors that seem critical to inducing adaptive plasticity in the injured CNS[32] (see Box 8-1).

FIGURE 8-4 Imaging documentation of neural remodeling. A. Initial motor map of the paretic hand post-stroke before treatment; (**B**) post-training motor map illustrating expansion of the ipsilesional (right) motor cortex; (**C**) diffusion tensor imaging illustrates integrity of fibers within the internal capsule, associated with improved function, which could be the product of greater neuronal survival, enhanced sprouting, or a combination of the two; and (**D**) demonstrates localized activity in the sensory discrimination network (ipsilesional primary sensory cortex, contralesional secondary sensory cortex, and right superior frontal cortex) of a left stroke survivor with full recovery of sensory ability (imaging view – right is anatomical left). (C and D: Used with permission of Deborah S. Nichols Larsen, PT, PhD. The Ohio State University.)

BOX 8-1	Critical Factors for Adaptive Neural Plasticity[32]

- Activity must target neural networks, in which plasticity is desired.
- Activity can prevent secondary damage.
- Activity must target specific movements and skills that are salient to the patient to induce change in desired neural networks; saliency may activate critical emotional networks to facilitate plasticity.
- Neural plasticity requires repetition at an intensity that challenges the nervous system.
- The timing of activity is critical: (1) too much too early can exacerbate the lesion; (2) some early level of activity may be neuroprotective; (3) there may be a critical period or periods when plasticity is more likely; and (4) the window for plasticity is restricted and doesn't continue indefinitely.
- Older brains do not have the same capacity for remodeling that is available to younger brains.
- Plasticity in one neural network may facilitate (transference) or inhibit (interference) plasticity in other networks.

Thus, as rehabilitation practitioners, physical, occupational, and speech therapists play a critical role in neural recovery through the implementation of targeted treatment programs. Most notable, there is potentially a critical period post-injury, where the nervous system is maximally able to remodel itself, when protein and growth hormone upregulation peaks to promote neural regrowth and axonal sprouting. Thus, it is critical for us to identify that time period and provide therapy directed at promoting adaptive plasticity.[10] While specificity of training appears to be critical for new skill acquisition, there is evidence that aerobic activity (e.g., treadmill training or cycling) can raise BDNF, protein, and microRNA levels that support neuroplasticity mechanisms. Thus, this may also be an essential component of a rehabilitation program.[23]

REFERENCES

1. Hoerder-Suabedissen A, Molnar Z. Development, evolution and pathology of neocortical subplate neurons. *Nat Rev Neurosci.* 2015;16:133-146.
2. Kandel ER, Schwartz JH, Jessell TM, Siegelbaum SA, Hudspeth AJ. Chapter 53: Differentiation and survival of nerve cells. In: *Principles of Neural Science.* New York, NY: McGraw Hill; 2013:1187-1208.
3. Laguesse S, Peyre E, Nguyen L. Progenitor genealogy in the developing cerebral cortex. *Cell Tissue Res.* 2015;359:17-32.
4. Urban N, Guillemot F. Neurogenesis in the embryonic and adult brain: same regulators, different roles. *Front Cell Neurosci.* 2014;9(article 396):1-19.
5. Dimou L, Gotz M. Glial cells as progenitors and stem cells: new roles in the healthy and diseased brain. *Physiol Rev.* 2014;94:709-737.
6. Tan X, Shhi SH. Neocortical neurogenesis and neuronal migration. *Wiley Interdiscip Rev Dev Biol.* 2013;2(4):443-459.
7. Taverna E, Götz M, Huttner WB. The cell biology of neurogenesis: toward an understanding of the development and evolution of the neocortex. *Annu Rev Cell Dev Biol.* 2014;30:465-502.
8. Stappert L, Roese-Koerner B, Brüstle O. The role of microRNAs in human stem cells, neuronal differentiation and subtype specification. *Cell Tissue Res.* 2015;359:47-64.
9. Kiss JZ, Vasung L, Petrenko V. Process of cortical network formation and impact of early brain damage. *Curr Opin Neurol.* 2014;27:133-141.
10. Nudo RJ. Recovery after brain injury: mechanisms and principles. *Front Human Neurosci.* 2013;7(article 887):1-14.
11. Shuldiner O, Yaron A. Mechanisms of developmental neurite pruning. *Cell Mol Life Sci.* 2015;72:101-119.
12. Gould E, Reeves AJ, Graziano MSA, Gross CG. Neurogenesis in the neocortex of adult primates. *Science.* 1999;286(5439):548-552.
13. Aimone JB, Li Y, Lee SW, Clemenson GD, Deng W, Gage FH. Regulation and function of adult neurogenesis: from genes to cognition. *Physiol Rev.* 2014;94:991-1028.
14. Cotman CW. Axon sprouting and reactive synaptogenesis. In: Siegel GJ, Agranoff BW, Albers RW, et al., eds. *Basic Neurochemistry: Molecular, Cellular and Medical Aspects.* 6th ed. Philadelphia, PA: Lippincott-Raven; 1999. Available at: http://www.ncbi.nlm.nih.gov/books/NBK28183/
15. Heijtz RD, Forssberg H. Translational studies exploring neuroplasticity associated with motor skill learning and the regulatory role of the dopamine system. *Dev Med Child Neurol.* 2015;57(suppl 2):10-14.
16. Delpech JC, Madore C, Nadjar A, Joffre C, Wohleb ES, Layé S. Microglia in neuronal plasticity: influence of stress. *Neuropharmacology.* 2015. Available at: http://dx.doi.org/10.1016/j.neuropharm.2014.12.034.
17. Baudry M, Zhu G, Liu Y, Wang Y, Briz V, Bi X. Multiple cellular cascades participate in long-term potentiation and in hippocampus-dependent learning. *Brain Res.* 2014. Available at: http://dx.doi.org/10.1016/j.brainres.2014.11.033.
18. Kramár EA, Lin B, Rex CS, Gall CM, Lynch G. Integrin-driven actin polymerization consolidates long-term potentiation. *PNAS.* 2006;103(14):5579-5584.
19. Adkins DL, Boychuk J, Remple MS, Kleim JA. Motor training induces experience-specific patterns of plasticity across motor cortex and spinal cord. *J Appl Physiol.* 2006;101:1776-1782.
20. Thomas AG, Dennis A, Bandettini PA, Johansen-Berg H. The effects of aerobic activity on brain structure. *Front Psychol.* 2012;3(article 86):1-9.
21. Ma F, Morancho A, Montaner J, Rosell A. Endothelial progenitor cells and revascularization following stroke. *Brain Res.* 2015. Available at: http://dx.doi.org/10.1016/j.brainres.2015.02.010.
22. Viscomi MT, Molinari M. Remote neurodegeneration: multiple actors for one play. *Mol Neurobiol.* 2014;50:368-389.
23. Spejo AB, Oliveira ALR. Synaptic rearrangement following axonal injury: old and new players. *Neuropharmacology.* 2014. Available at: http://dx.doi.org/10.1016/j.neuropharm.2014.11.002.
24. Hansen CN, Fisher L, Deibert RJ, Jakeman LB, Zhang H, Noble-Haeusslein L, White S, Basso DM. Elevated MMP-9 in the lumbar cord early after thoracic spinal cord injury impedes motor relearning in mice. *J Neurosci.* 2013;33(32):13101-13111.
25. Brassai A, Suvanjeiev RG, Bán EG, Lakatos M. Role of synaptic and non-synaptic glutamate receptors in ischaemia induced neurotoxicity. *Brain Res Bull.* 2015;112:1-6.
26. McIlwain DR, Berger T, Mak TW. Caspase functions in cell death and disease. *Cold Spring Harb Perspect Biol.* 2013;5:a008656.1-28.
27. Ghavami S, Shojaei S, Yeganeh B, et al. Autophagy and apoptosis dysfunction in neurogenerative disorders. *Prog Neurobiol.* 2014;112:24-49.
28. Hutchinson KJ, Gomez-Pinilla F, Crowe MJ, Ying Z, Basso DM. Three exercise paradigms differentially improve sensory recovery after spinal cord contusion in rats. *Brain.* 2004;127:1403-1414.
29. Hansen CN, Faw TD, Kerr S, et al. Sparing of descending systems modulates pre-motor interneuron plasticity in the lumbar cord after thoracic spinal cord injury. *Exp Neurol.* 2015; (In Review).
30. Sawaki L, Butler AJ, Leng X, et al. Constraint-induced movement therapy results in increased motor map in subjects 3 to 9 months after stroke. *Neurorehabil Neural Repair.* 2008;22(5):505-513.
31. Liepert J, Hamzei F, Weiller C. Lesion-induced and training-induced brain reorganization. *Restor Neurol Neurosci.* 2004;22(3-5):269-277.
32. Kleim JA, Jones TA. Principles of experience-dependent neural plasticity: implications for rehabilitation after brain damage. *J Speech Lang Hear Res.* 2008;51:S225-S239.

Review Questions

1. Cell proliferation in the developing nervous system begins in which area?
   A. Cortical plate
   B. Intermediate zone
   C. Subplate
   D. Ventricular zone

2. Which progenitor cells help to guide developing neurons to the cortical plate?
   A. Ependymal cells
   B. Intermediate progenitor cells
   C. Radial glial cells
   D. Short neural precursors

3. The overproduction of axonal projections is balanced by what process that eliminates some of these projections?
   A. Apoptosis
   B. Cell migration
   C. Pruning
   D. Programmed cell death

4. Adult neurogenesis differs from that in the developmental period by which of the following?
   A. It occurs only in the cortical plate of the mature brain
   B. It occurs only in neurogenic niches in the mature brain
   C. It occurs faster in the mature brain than the immature brain
   D. It occurs more easily than gliogenesis in the mature brain

5. Long-term potentiation is associated with which mechanism?
   A. Decreased calcium permeability
   B. Enlargement of dendritic spines
   C. Decreased protein synthesis
   D. Diminished actin polymerization

6. Angiogenesis involves the creation of new blood vessels in the mature brain.
   A. True
   B. False

7. Microglial synaptic pruning is associated with
   A. LTD
   B. LTP
   C. synaptic scaling
   D. enhanced actin polymerization

8. Dying back of the proximal segment of the axon is known as:
   A. Anterograde degeneration
   B. Orthograde degeneration
   C. Retrograde degeneration
   D. Wallerian degeneration

9. The loss of neurons that normally synapse on neurons in the lesioned area is referred to as:
   A. Anterograde transneural degeneration
   B. Retrograde transneural degeneration
   C. Apoptosis
   D. Necrosis

10. The primary cause of excitotoxicity post-CNS injury is:
    A. Dopamine
    B. GABA
    C. Glutamate
    D. Norepinephrine

11. The internal pathway of apoptosis targets which organelle?
    A. Endoplasmic reticulum
    B. Golgi apparatus
    C. Mitochondria
    D. Ribosomes

12. Which of the following mechanisms is unlikely during spontaneous recovery from a small ischemic lesion?
    A. Angiogenesis
    B. Interhemispheric connections
    C. Sprouting
    D. Synaptogenesis

13. Teaching a patient to get out of bed by lifting the paretic leg with the non-paretic leg is likely to lead to:
    A. Adaptive plasticity
    B. Maladaptive plasticity
    C. Synaptogenesis
    D. Apoptosis

14. To treat a patient, based on the critical factors for adaptive neural plasticity, it would be best to:
    A. Isolate joint activities to improve kinematics during gait
    B. Walk at the peak speed that the patient can tolerate
    C. Use an AFO to control ankle dorsiflexion
    D. Wait to ambulate until the patient can stand independently

Answers

1. D	2. C	3. C	4. B	5. B
6. B	7. A	8. C	9. A	10. C
11. C	12. B	13. B	14. B	

NEUROLOGIC CONDITIONS – NEUROPATHOLOGY AND PHYSICAL THERAPY MANAGEMENT

Neurologic Exam

Deborah A. Kegelmeyer,
Jill C. Heathcock
and Deborah S. Nichols-Larsen

9

OBJECTIVES

1) Understand the parts of the neurologic examination and how they are performed

2) Determine when the systems review indicates the need for further evaluation and which evaluative methods to utilize

3) Choose appropriate outcome measures based on both the individual characteristics of the client as well as the measurement characteristics of the tool

4) Determine how to adapt and modify the neurologic examination based on the individual characteristics of the client

● OVERVIEW OF THE NEUROLOGIC EVALUATION AS A PROCESS

An examination of the neurologic system is an essential component of a comprehensive physical examination for every client that a physical therapist sees. The examination may be limited to a screening as described under the System Review section, or in those clients who have sustained damage to any aspect of the neurologic system, it should be a comprehensive and systematic examination that surveys the functioning of nerves delivering sensory information to the brain and those carrying motor commands to muscles and organs (peripheral nervous system) as well as neural networks that support high level multisystem processing and coordination of sensorimotor function (central nervous system). A careful neurological examination can help to determine impairments and their possible cause(s), functional loss, and focus of treatment.

The examination begins with a history that helps the clinician to localize the problem. For example, symptoms that occur unexpectedly might suggest a blood vessel or seizure problem. Those that are not as sudden might suggest a possible tumor. Symptoms that have a variable course with recurrences and remissions but worsen over time suggest a disease that destroys nerve cells. Others that are chronic and progressive indicate a degenerative disorder. In cases of trauma, symptoms may be evident upon inspection, and causes may be explained by third-party witnesses. The history assists the clinician to diagnose conditions and better focus their examination.

The examination is an ongoing process and continues throughout the course of treatment. While this chapter will attempt to lay out the path of the evaluation in a more

step-by-step manner, it is actually more of a cyclical process. As the clinician generates hypotheses, based on the examination, they then design the intervention to address these hypotheses. After trying the intervention and observing the response, the original hypothesis is modified, and the impact on activity limitations is reassessed. Thus, the examination informs the intervention, which in turn, informs the examination (Figure 9-1).

● COMPONENTS OF THE ADULT NEUROLOGIC EVALUATION

CASE A , PART I

Trisha is a 50-year-old female who is complaining of increasing weakness in her legs along with problems with falling and tingling in all of her limbs. She reports a history that includes multiple ear and sinus infections, hypertension, two pregnancies with natural birth (children are 15 and 17), and diabetes of 15 years' duration. She is managing her diabetes with diet and her most recent A1C was 12. She lives in a two-story home with her husband, children, and dog and enjoys knitting and hiking.

History

A careful history will allow you to prioritize the examination. A well-done history should be brief yet comprehensive and result in the generation of several hypotheses as to why the

FIGURE 9-1 Diagram of the relationship between evaluation and treatment.

client is experiencing the symptoms and limitations that have brought her to the clinic. The role of the clinician is to be open and receptive to receiving information and to put the client at ease so that she is comfortable providing an adequate history. Secondarily, the clinician must be skilled at guiding the process so that it remains focused, does not stray off course nor take up unnecessary time from that allotted for the examination.

A history starts with baseline data such as name and age and then moves on to the past and current medical history. It is important to gather this information from both the client and the medical record, if available (Box 9-1). The medical record provides an objective report of the condition(s) other professionals have identified, while the client's report provides insight into her understanding of her health status. In addition, the client may provide information that has been left out of the medical record that is pertinent to her present health status. Identification of medications and supplements that have been prescribed, as well as what is actually being taken, is critical as medication side effects are common and should be ruled out before moving onto other potential causes of the present change in health status. This initial history is essential as it provides the therapist with an indication of any precautions or limitations that may impact elements of the neuromuscular examination, such as weight-bearing limitations or cardiac precautions.

Finally, and most importantly, the therapist needs to find out what the client hopes to achieve through their therapy. If their goals seem low, then, the therapist should encourage them to be optimistic and not aim too low, based on their present status. The therapist must also be realistic and consider the client's status, prior to this current situation, and set goals with the client that are appropriate and individualized to her unique needs. At times, clients have difficulty identifying what activities they are or will have difficulty participating in, and therefore, would like to work on in therapy. There are tools that can help both the therapist and client get a better grasp on this if the client is having difficulty such as the OPTIMAL scale (APTA)[1] and the Physical Self Maintenance scale,[2] which can be utilized to determine activity level limitations and assist in goal setting.

BOX 9-1 | Home Assessment

Note:
An area of the history that is often neglected is the assessment of home status. The type of living environment and support system available will play a large role in discharge planning and goal setting. Therefore at a minimum the following questions should be addressed:

- Does the client live alone or with a spouse or companion? If alone, do they have assistance from neighbors or family?
- What architectural barriers exist at home? Stairs inside or outside the home? Bathroom location, shower set up (grab bars, in a tub, seat or not), etc.?
- What equipment does the client have?
- What is the client's occupation? What is their role in the home?
- What is their community or leisure integration like?

CASE A, PART II

Trisha has revealed in her history that she has diabetes. Based on her A1C is her diabetes well managed?

No – normal A1C is between 4.5% and 6%; for diabetics, the goal is to keep A1C below 7%. Given that Trisha's diabetes is not well managed, we might suspect that she has peripheral neuropathy, leading to weakness and tingling. We cannot rule out an upper motor neuron lesion, however, as cardio-vascular disease and stroke are often secondary complications of poorly managed endocrine disease. We know that her functional goals will likely include fine motor skills, since she enjoys knitting, and we know that she needs adequate lower extremity strength and power to ascend stairs in her home. With her history, we know that a careful systems review will be necessary as endocrine disorders can impact every system in the body.

Systems Review

A neurological screening is an essential component of every comprehensive physical examination. In cases of neurological trauma, disease, or psychological disorders, patients are usually given a very in-depth neurological examination. The examination is best performed in a systematic manner, which means that there is a recommended order for procedures.

Elements of the Systems Review (Screening)

The systems review is a general review of each of the body systems and is a guide for what areas should be investigated more thoroughly, dictate referral to another medical professional, or may impact the PT plan of care, as indicated by an impaired item. Each item on the systems review is marked as impaired or not impaired, meaning within normal limits. On documentation templates, either paper-based or as part of an electronic medical record, there is typically a small space available for brief comments under each system. At a minimum, the system's review should include a brief assessment of all of the following:

- Mental status: Are they alert? Are they alert to: Person? Place? Time? Situation? Do they remember recent events? Are they able to do simple problem solving, such as figuring out how to lock a wheelchair?
- Cranial nerves should be screened by observing eye and facial movements.
- Sensory: Screen for adequate vision and hearing to participate in therapeutic activities. Also screen the ability to sense light touch and location of limbs.
- Integumentary: Examine for the presence of incisions, wounds, burns, inflammation;
  Note: Screening of the integumentary system is especially critical when diseases of the endocrine system are diagnosed or suspected because of their impact on the skin; similarly, pulmonary dysfunction may also affect the integumentary system (e.g., bluish nail beds).

BOX 9-2   Upper Motor Neuron Screening Tests

Babinski (plantar reflex) – Stroke bottom of foot from heel to toes, using your thumb or the end of a reflex hammer, this should elicit flexion of the big toe and perhaps the other toes (negative sign); in very young infants (<24 months) and those with upper motor neuron injuries (stroke, brain injury, etc.), the big toe will extend and the other toes will splay out (positive sign).

Hoffman test/reflex – Flick the fingernail of the middle finger by squeezing the tip of the finger between your thumb and index finger and then rapidly releasing their finger in a flicking motion; watch for flexion of the thumb or index finger. This should be done on both sides. If flexion occurs, this is a positive Hoffman sign and can be an indication of upper motor neuron disease. However, some people without neurologic injury will have a positive Hoffman sign, so the tester should look for asymmetry in this reflex or the emergence of it after a neurologic injury, when it suggests corticospinal disruption.

- Cardiopulmonary: Vitals – heart rate, blood pressure, respiration rate.
- Musculoskeletal: Rule out contraindications for further evaluation and treatment. Is the patient capable of doing examination activities? (Gross screen of strength and range of motion - ROM)
- Neuromuscular: Screen for muscle tone, strength, and functional movement/coordination by observing mobility as the patient enters the evaluation area (e.g., gait and transfers) and performs gross movements; screen for coordination, using the finger to nose test or heel to shin test. Deep Tendon Reflexes (DTRs) should be checked along with screening for the presence of clonus at the wrist and ankle and upper motor neuron signs, using the Babinski and Hoffman tests (see Box 9-2).
- Genito-urinary systems: Ask about continence, urgency of voiding, any recent changes? Age-related changes? Also inquire about a history of bladder or urinary tract infections, which can be signs of incomplete voiding.
- Gastrointestinal, hepatic, and biliary: Ask about regularity, frequency, nausea, recent changes? Positional issues such as heartburn on going into supine?

In individuals who have a known neurologic disorder or, are found to have deficits in the neuromuscular system during the systems review,, the clinician should progress to the neurologic examination, targeting those areas of concern from the screening.

● NEUROLOGICAL EXAMINATION: BODY STRUCTURE AND FUNCTION

The neurologic examination should be performed on any individual suspected of having any neurologic disorder or psychological diseases. This examination is performed in a systematic and comprehensive manner and consists of several thorough and in-depth assessments of mental status, cranial nerves, motor examination, reflexes, sensory examination, and posture and mobility analysis.

Mental Status Examination

The first item to be examined is always mental status. It is not possible to conduct the rest of the examination without first determining how the individual is interacting with the environment and whether or not he/she is able to follow directions partially or completely. There are two types of mental status examination: informal and formal. The **informal mental status exam** is usually done while clinicians are obtaining historical information from a patient when a neurological problem is suspected. For the informal assessment, the client is commonly asked: his/her name (person); the location of the testing (place); the day of the week and date (time); and why she is there (situation). This is typically documented as Alert and Oriented $\times$ 1, 2, 3, or 4 (A & O $\times$ #). The numbers 1–4 stand for person, place, time, and situation. If it is documented that a patient is O $\times$ 2, then, the area(s) of disorientation are indicated (e.g., "not oriented to place or time"), or conversely, if O $\times$ 1, the area of orientation is stated (e.g., "oriented to person"). This is a very basic assessment of mental status and does not give an indication of ability to follow directions or problem solve. Therefore, mental status should be assessed in more detail in individuals suspected of a neurologic disorder, even when orientation $\times$ 4 is present. This should include:

- **Retentive memory capability and immediate recall** – assessed by determining the number of digits that can be repeated in sequence from a string recited by the examiner;
- **Recent memory** – typically examined by testing recall of a series of three to five objects immediately, then after 5 and 15 minutes with intervening activities (e.g., other parts of this exam);
- **Remote memory** – assessed by asking the patient to review in a chronological fashion, his or her illness or personal life events that the patient feels comfortable talking about (e.g., dates of birth of children and where they currently live);
- **General knowledge** – assessed by asking the patient to recall common historical or current events;
- **Higher functioning** (referring to brain processing capabilities) – assessed by spontaneous speech and repetition, reading, naming, writing, and comprehension of written and oral information;
- The patient may be asked to perform further tasks such as identification of fingers, whistling, saluting, brushing teeth motions, combing hair, drawing, and tracing figures. These procedures will assess the intactness of what is called dominant (left-sided brain) functioning or **higher cortical function**, referring to the portion of the brain that regulates these activities.

Other areas for assessment of mental function are delineated in Table 9-1 with their potential for providing information about mental function and potential areas that may be involved when dysfunction is seen. Box 9-3 describes two easy measures to objectively assess mental function.

TABLE 9-1	Mental Function Assessment for the PT	
AREA TO BE EXAMINED	**WHAT TO LOOK FOR**	**INSIGHT**
Appearance	Clothes, posture, grooming, alertness	Ability to take care of themselves; mood/affect
Behavior	Impulse control, fidgeting, overall movements	
Speech	Volume/Rate	Mood (e.g., loud and fast speech-related to mania; soft and slow – related to depression)
	Coherence	Indication of higher level processing
Mood/Affect	Flat – minimal or absent affective response to situation	Signs of mental illness or cortical disease
	Labile – shifting emotional outbursts (e.g., crying/laughing)	
	Blunted – some emotional response but less than would be expected for the situation	
	Constructed/Inappropriate – responses that are inconsistent with the situation (e.g., laughing at a sad situation)	
Thought processing	Word usage	Language issues (agnosia, expressive aphasia)
	Thought stream	Slow versus overabundant gives an indication of mood and cognition
	Continuity – coherence of thought and idea association	Ability to follow the discussion and respond accordingly – Higher level cognition or receptive language problems
	Content – complete/incomplete responses	Higher level cognition/language issues, delusions suggest mental disorders
Perception	Screening of vision, hearing, touch, taste, and smell	General system integrity/dysfunction; potential medication side effects
Attention/Concentration	Ability to stay focused on a task	Frontal lobe dysfunction; anxiety
Memory	Long-term and current episodic memory (client's history and current events); immediate memory (naming 3 objects immediately and then in 5 and 15 minutes)	Temporal and frontal lobe function/dysfunction
Judgment	Decision-making in complex situations (safe versus unsafe)	Executive function (frontal lobe function)
Intelligence	Requires specific testing but a general sense can be obtained by responses to questions, general language used, etc.	Overall ability to participate in treatment/cortical deficits
Insight	Understanding of the current illness and potential limitations	Executive function

Communication

While physical therapists are not the primary practitioner to evaluate communication disorders, it is important that we have an understanding of the presentation and consequences of these disorders in our patients. First, it is important to assess hearing ability very early in the examination and to adjust your communication appropriately, if the individual has hearing deficits. This can easily be done, while taking the history, by noting the patient's ability to hear questions and respond to what was asked. At a minimum, physical therapists should report the patient's comprehension and ability to express himself verbally or nonverbally. Assessment should answer the following questions (specific descriptions of these disorders are discussed in Chapter 10 relative to Stroke):

- Can the client speak? Does he have word finding problems consistent with **Expressive Aphasia** or trouble enunciating consistent with **dysarthria**?
- Note voice quality, is volume adequate?
- Does the individual understand language or show signs of **receptive aphasia**?

Mental Status Evaluation Tools for Use in Physical Therapy Assessment

The **Folstein Mini Mental Status Exam**[3] is the most common screening tool for cognitive issues, but clinics must obtain permission to use it. Other common, easy to use cognitive screening tools are the **Quick Mild Cognitive Impairment Screen** (**Qmci**)[4] and the **Montreal Cognitive Assessment** (**MoCA**).[5] It is important to remember that these tools do not fully assess all domains of cognition and mental function but are appropriate screening tools (not to be used for diagnostic purposes). Clients, who have deficits when screened, should be referred to a neurologist or cognitive psychologist for a diagnostic work-up. In addition, therapists should be aware that there are transient conditions that can lead to lower scores on these screening tools, including the use of some medications, post-anesthesia and delirium (a transient condition brought on by an acute change in status – urinary tract infection, pneumonia, etc., most commonly in elderly people).

Motor Examination

The motor examination assesses the individual's muscle strength, tone, and shape; passive versus active range of motion; and sustained postures versus functional movement. Findings will give an indication of whether the presenting disorder is muscular, neural (lower motor neuron, upper motor neuron), perceptual, or associated with the motor control system. It is important to look for abnormal movements (tics, myoclonus) as well as to observe the patient in multiple positions and activities.

Muscles could be hypertrophied, due to overuse or some neurologic disorders, or atrophied, secondary to weakness, inactivity, or tissue destruction; asymmetry in muscle size suggests a unilateral problem (e.g., neuropathy, stroke), while bilateral changes are associated with a more systemic disorder (e.g., Multiple Sclerosis, Parkinson's). It is important to look for twitching or abnormal movements, which are best observed while the individual is at rest, yet are characteristic of specific conditions (e.g., Amyotrophic Lateral Sclerosis). Additionally, muscle activity can be abnormal during maintained postures in neurological disorders such as Parkinson's disease. Muscle tone is usually tested by performing passive motion of a relaxed limb first at a slow speed and then at a faster speed to determine the impact of speed of movement on tone. Decreases or increases in muscle tone can help the examiner localize the problem.

Strength (Force Production)

The examination of strength in individuals with neurologic disorders can be challenging as they often have impaired trunk control that can negatively impact their ability to stabilize themselves, while undergoing a manual muscle test. Therapists should be sure to set up the test so that sufficient support is provided to stabilize the trunk for the client during strength testing. Individuals who have significant motor impairments will attempt to substitute motions during strength testing (e.g., trunk extension to assist shoulder flexion). It is especially important to be cognizant of this in individuals with neurologic disorders

and to take steps to prevent substitution. Notably, **the manual muscle test** can be invalidated by the presence of limited ROM, synergies, or disturbances of tone; when these are present, a functional test of strength should be used and any modifications to the test should be noted. Strength is first assessed by asking the client to move the limb through the range of motion against gravity (fair grade), and then, by determining the amount of resistance, against which the individual can maintain a mid-range position. If the individual is not able to move the limb against gravity, they should be placed in a position that allows movement through the range of motion with gravity eliminated (e.g., side-lying).

When testing strength, document the following:

- What range did the individual move through?
- Was gravity eliminated or not?
- Did synergy (see description later in this chapter) influence the movement? If so, how?

The manual muscle test does not test the individual's ability to perform functional activities, and for strength grades above fair (3/5), it only examines the ability to produce an isometric contraction at one point in the range of motion. Therefore, the manual muscle test does not fully inform us about the force production capabilities of the individual within functional activities. Individuals with upper motor neuron disorders often have difficulty developing consistent force over time such that force production may vary throughout the range of motion. Methods for examining isotonic strength are standard manual muscle testing (Daniels and Worthingham method[6]), use of equipment such as a dynamometer, and functional muscle testing. Power is an important aspect of strength that relates to the ability to maintain force and speed to move a limb or an object (resistance), which is difficult to assess unless the clinician has access to isokinetic equipment.

Functional Muscle Testing involves evaluating the muscle's performance as the client performs activities or maintains postures consistent with normal daily conditions. The therapist then documents by describing the range of motion that key joints moved through, in what position the activity was performed, and what was the relation of the limb to gravity. Some examples of things to consider when functionally testing the upper extremity are:

- Does the individual use both arms equally? If not, does the individual use the weaker/paretic arm at all or for what tasks? For support? For reaching?
- Does the individual have functional grasp bilaterally? If not, what was observed (e.g., fisting during the attempt to grasp)?
- Can the individual manipulate objects?
- Does the individual have fine motor coordination in their fingers (e.g., can they touch the fingertips of the thumb to each)?

Tone

Abnormal tone is a common finding in individuals with neurologic disorders. It can be hypertonic or hypotonic. Tone is assessed by performing passive range of motion, in which the limb is moved through the range of motion in a slow manner, while noting the resistance to the motion. If this is not painful, the limb is then moved through the range of motion more rapidly. An increase in tone, **hypertonicity**, is present when the examiner notes an increased resistance to passive movement. There are two types of hypertonicity: spasticity and rigidity. **Spasticity** is characterized by increased resistance to passive movement, as the velocity of the movement is increased (velocity dependent), and hyperreflexia (exaggerated monosynaptic reflexes). The most common method for objectively documenting hypertonicity is the Ashworth Scale[7] (Box 9-4). While there are some issues with inter and intra-rater reliability for the Ashworth Scale, this remains the only clinically accessible means of objectively measuring tone at this time. **Rigidity** is increased resistance throughout the range of motion that is independent of the velocity of the movement; reflexes are typically normal with rigidity. The causes of spasticity and rigidity are different and will be discussed with the conditions that are associated with them (e.g., stroke, Parkinson's disease). A limb that feels heavy or "floppy" is **hypotonic**, demonstrating limited resistance to passive movement and poor ability to sustain power or maintain a given posture. Because hypotonia can be caused by both central and peripheral nervous system disorders, reflexes can be decreased (hyporeflexia), normal, or exaggerated (hyperreflexia), depending on the cause of the hypotonia. Since tone can fluctuate over the course of the day and due to other factors, such as level of stimulation and room temperature, the assessment should always be performed at the same time of day, in the same room, and, if possible, by the same person. The examiner needs to be aware of things that can influence tone such as:

- Infections or fevers
- Stress and anxiety
- Volitional effort and movement
- Medications
- General health
- Environmental temperature
- State of central nervous system arousal or alertness
- Position interaction of tonic reflexes (see pediatric evaluation later in this chapter)

Additionally, the examiner should observe how the individual "holds" herself. An arm that is held in an antigravity position may indicate the presence of hypertonicity. Movement can also be impacted by tone, and the examiner should observe movements for signs of high tone, such as moving through a more limited range of motion than is typical for the activity.

Synergistic Movement Patterns (Synergies)

It is common for individuals, who have had an upper motor neuron lesion, to exhibit movements that are highly influenced by or bound in synergistic movement patterns, which refers to multijoint movements that occur simultaneously when trying to move an isolated joint (e.g., finger, wrist, elbow, and shoulder flexion when bringing the hand to the mouth to stifle a yawn). In Chapter 10, a description of synergy patterns seen after stroke is provided. To examine for the presence of synergy patterns, the examiner should watch the client while they perform active range of motion as well as functional movements (e.g., grasping, walking). If the client is able to achieve movement only through one rigid movement pattern, then, they are said to be bound in synergy. When synergistic movement patterns are noted, the examiner should ask

BOX 9-4	**Modified Ashworth Scale[7]**

0	No increase in muscle tone
1	Slight increase in muscle tone, manifested by a catch or by minimal resistance at the end of the range of motion (ROM) when the affected part(s) is moved in flexion or extension
1+	Slight increase in muscle tone, manifested by a catch, followed by minimal resistance throughout the remainder (less than half) of the ROM
2	More marked increase in muscle tone through most of the ROM, but affected part(s) easily moved
3	Considerable increase in muscle tone, passive movement difficult
4	Affected part(s) rigid in flexion or extension
9	Unable to test

Adapted with permission of Pandyan AD1, Johnson GR, Price CI, Curless RH, Barnes MP, Rodgers H. A review of the properties and limitations of the Ashworth and modified Ashworth Scales as measures of spasticity. *Clin Rehabil*. 1999 May;13(5):373–383

the client to move out of these patterns such as asking them to flex the shoulder while extending the wrist and elbow, and observe whether or not the client can perform movements out of the synergy pattern. The Fugl-Meyer[8] is the most common assessment tool for objectively examining synergistic movement patterns.

Reflexes

The patient's DTRs are tested by using a reflex hammer. The clinician will tap the rubber triangular shaped end over key tendon insertions, in the arms (biceps, triceps, brachioradialis), knees (quadriceps, hamstrings), and heals (Achilles). If there is a difference in response from the left to the right, there may be an underlying problem that merits further evaluation. A difference in reflexes between the arms and legs usually indicates a lesion involving the spinal cord. Depressed reflexes in only one limb, while the other limbs demonstrate a normal response usually indicates a peripheral nerve lesion. Hyperactive reflexes indicate a lesion in the central nervous system. DTRs are reported on a numerical scale (Table 9-2), and at a minimum, the biceps, triceps, quadriceps, and Achilles reflexes should be tested. In addition, the examination should include the Hoffman and Babinski reflex testing, for an upper motor neuron lesion, and examination for clonus at the wrist and ankle. In general, the presence of clonus is indicative of an upper motor neuron lesion; although, there are rare muscle disorders that can also lead to clonus.

Cranial Nerves (CN)

Cranial nerves are specialized nerves that originate in the brainstem and innervate the muscles of the face and eyes, sensory receptors throughout the cranium and internal organs, and support the special senses (vision, hearing, smell, taste, vestibular function). Physical therapist should always grossly screen these nerves by observing facial and eye movement as well as eye reflexes (response to light or turning of the head). Table 9-3 provides general screening methods for the CN.

TABLE 9-2	Deep Tendon Reflex Grades	
REFLEX GRADE	**EVALUATION**	**RESPONSE CHARACTERISTICS**
0	Absent	No visible or palpable muscle contraction
1+	Hyporeflexia	Slight or sluggish muscle contraction with little or no joint movement. Reinforcement may be required to elicit a reflex response.
2+	Normal	Slight muscle contraction with slight joint movement
3+	Hyperreflexia	Clearly visible, brisk muscle contraction with moderate joint movement
4+	Abnormal	Strong muscle contraction with one to three beats of clonus. Reflex spread to contralateral side may be noted.
5+	Abnormal	Strong muscle contraction with sustained clonus. Reflex spread to contralateral side may be noted.

TABLE 9-3	Cranial Nerve Function and Screening Methods		
CRANIAL NERVE	**NAME**	**FUNCTION**	**SCREENING**
I	Olfactory	Smell	Have patient identify familiar smells (vanilla); there are vials that can be purchased or therapists can make their own.
II	Optic	Vision	Reading close and distant items
III	Oculomotor	Eye movement, pupillary reflexes	Eye tracking in all directions, pupillary response to light; at rest, eye will be slightly depressed and rotated toward the nose, when damaged.
IV	Trochlear	Superior oblique eye muscle innervation	Observe eye position at rest; will be elevated if there's a problem.
V	Trigeminal	Muscles of mastication and sensation of the face	Observe jaw motion (resistance to motion, opening, side-to-side mobility), temporalis muscles can be palpated.
VI	Abducens	Lateral rectus of the eye innervation	Look at eye movement; if damaged, there will be an inability to look outward (abduct the eye)
VII	Facial	Muscles of facial expression, taste for the anterior 2/3 tongue	Look for facial asymmetries, observe motions (raising eyebrows, wrinkling forehead, closing eyes, frowning/smiling, lip pursing, etc.). Taste with common liquids (lemon juice, honey) can also be tested.
VIII	Vestibulocochlear	Hearing and Vestibular	Can use the "rub test" – rub thumb and forefinger together next to the ear. Ask the patient to point to which ear they hear it in. Check both. Look for differences. You can use a tuning fork, which tests for air conduction and structural problems that can occur inside the ear – strike tuning fork on your hand and place behind the ear on the bony surface. Observe balance.
IX	Glossopharyngeal	Sensation and taste for posterior tongue and pharynx	Ask about swallowing, which may be impaired, have them say "ahh" and watch for palatal-uvula movement; unilateral nerve damage can yield asymmetric motion; absent gag reflex is also a sign of damage (stimulate with tongue depressor)
X	Vagus	Innervates epiglottis and larynx, parasympathetic innervation of internal organs	Voice hoarseness with increased heart and respiration rate are signs of CN X damage.
XI	Accessory	Trapezius and sternocleido-mastoid muscle innervation	Observe ability to shrug shoulders and turn head to both sides.
XII	Hypoglossal	Tongue muscles	Observe tongue protrusion and mobility; unilateral lesions will result in lateral movement when protruding tongue.

Sensory Examination

Although a very essential component of the neurologic examination, the sensory examination is the least exacting since it requires patient concentration and cooperation. Five primary sensory categories are assessed: vibration (using a tuning fork), joint position and awareness (examiner moves the limb side-to-side and in a downward position), light touch, pinprick, and temperature. Individuals who have sensory abnormalities may have a lesion at any level of the sensory pathways (see Chapter 3). Spinal cord lesions or disease can possibly be detected by pinprick and temperature assessment. Sensation must always be screened; depending on the individual's problem and reason for therapy, you may or may not do a more detailed exam of any or all of the sensory modalities. For instance, in SCI during the acute stage, sensation by dermatome is assessed to both touch and pain to determine initial lesion level and subsequent recovery.

Tests of Proprioception

Movement Sense – Kinesthesia – The examiner has the client close their eyes and then moves the extremity through a small ROM, the client is asked to indicate verbally the direction of movement while the extremity is in motion. Prior to performing the test, the examiner and client should discuss the terminology that will be used to describe the direction of the motion so that it is clear that any discrepancies are due to actual deficits and not due to miscommunication. Simple terms such as "up," "down", "out" and "in" should be used. The most accurate areas to perform this test are on the hallux, wrist, and fingers. The examiner should use a light touch and grasp the limb at a joint space on the medial and lateral aspects of the joint, in order to minimize cutaneous input. There are also more objective tests, such as the Brief Kinesthesia Test,[9] that will provide measurable errors, if a problem is indicated.

Position Sense – The extremity is placed in a position and the individual is then told to verbally report the position. Another method is to have the client place her opposite extremity (e.g., right) in the same position as the examiner has positioned the tested extremity. This method can only be used in individuals who have full antigravity active movement in the opposite extremity.

Vibration Testing is the most reliable and valid way to test dorsal column–medial lemniscal system integrity. Since this tract carries sensory information, including position sense and kinesthesia, vibration testing can be a highly reliable and valid way to test for deficits in these sensory modalities. Use a 250 mHz tuning fork; strike the fork against the palm of your hand or a solid surface and place it on a bony prominence (e.g., lateral malleolus) and ask the patient "what do you feel."

Cutaneous Sensation is commonly tested by: (1) monofilament testing for sensory threshold; (2) pinprick for pain; and (3) water vials for hot and cold modalities. The examiner should screen for the ability to sense touch as well as to locate the touch. For a screening exam, a light touch is often applied across the surface of both upper/lower limbs, and the individual is asked if she "can feel it" and "does it feel the same." Then, the patient should be asked to close their eyes and identify the location of randomly applied touch along each extremity. If deficits are found, a more thorough sensory exam, including pinprick and temperature, should be conducted. Temperature is typically examined using a vial with cold water and a vial with hot water that are randomly touched to the skin, while asking the client to identify the temperature. Additional tests can be performed, including identification of common objects or shapes (Stereognosis) via manipulation of the object in the hand. See Table 9-4 for a listing of some common sensory disorders and methods for testing for each of them.

CASE A, PART III

Her verbal history indicates that Trisha is experiencing paresthesias, dysesthesia, and pain in both feet and lower legs of 2 years' duration that has worsened lately, especially at night; she has similar but much milder symptoms recently starting in her hands. Light touch, measured by monofilaments on both feet is diminished (>2 SD above normal thresholds for the testing kit used), lower leg (1 SD above normal) and thumb and index fingers (1 SD above normal thresholds) consistent with carpel tunnel; all other areas are normal. Muscle strength is 3/5 in the anterior tibialis but still 5/5 in other muscles, her anterior tibialis reflex is 1+ but all others are 2+ (normal). These are typical symptoms for the most common form of diabetic neuropathy – symmetrical sensorimotor polyneuropathy (See Chapter 15).

Coordination and Balance

Coordination is the ability to execute smooth, accurate, controlled movements. It is characterized by appropriate speed, distance, direction, rhythm, muscle tension, and synergistic movements accomplished via orchestrated reversals of opposing muscle group activations. For well-coordinated movements, the individual must be able to achieve proximal fixation that allows for distal motion or maintenance of a posture. Coordination can be divided into nonequilibrium (does not require upright balance) and equilibrium (requires upright balance). Generally, nonequilibrium tests are completed first, followed by the equilibrium tests. Attention should be given to carefully guarding the patient during testing; use of a safety belt may be warranted. During the testing activities, the following questions can be used to help direct the therapist's observations and the results documented.

1. Are the movements direct, precise, and easily reversed?

2. Do the movements occur within a reasonable or normal amount of time?

TABLE 9-4 | **Common Sensory Impairments and Assessment Methods**

NAME OF SENSORY IMPAIRMENT	DEFINITION OF SENSORY IMPAIRMENT	ASSESSMENT
Abarognosis	The inability to recognize weight	Hold objects of varying weights in each hand and state which is heavier (or the same)
Allodynia	Pain is caused by non-painful stimuli such as light touch	Uncovered in the sensory exam when light touch or other non-painful stimuli elicit pain
Analgesia	A complete loss of pain sensitivity	Lack of pinprick sensation along with findings from the history
Astereognosis	The inability to use touch to recognize the shape or form of an object	Have identify shapes of objects while eyes are closed. Use common shapes like square and ball
Atopognosia	The inability to localize a sensation	During light touch testing ask to localize the touch with eyes closed
Dysesthesia	Abnormal touch sensation that may be experienced as unpleasant or painful	Typically determined during cutaneous testing (touch localization)
Hyperalgesia	Increased sensitivity to pain	Senses pinprick as being more painful than is typical and discovered through the history
Hyperesthesia	Increased sensitivity to sensory stimuli	Noted throughout the exam as an increased sensitivity to stimuli as compared to normal
Hypoalgesia	Decreased response to pain	Identified with the pinprick testing
Paresthesia	Abnormal sensation such as prickly or burning feeling that has no apparent cause	Noted during the history or when asked if they have any burning or prickling sensations

3. Does increased speed of performance affect quality of the motor activity?

4. Can continuous and appropriate motor adjustments be made if speed and direction are changed?

5. Can a position or posture of the body or specific extremity be maintained without swaying, oscillations, or extraneous movements?

6. Are placing movements of both upper and lower extremities exact?

7. Does occluding vision alter the quality of motor activity?

8. Are the problems greater with movement proximally or distally? On one side of the body versus the other?

9. Does the patient fatigue rapidly? Is there a consistency of motor response over time?

Nonequilibrium testing involves repetitive motions as described in Box 9-5. Equilibrium testing begins with observing the ability to perform quiet stance and then progresses to more difficult standing balance tasks, as described in Box 9-6. Table 9-5 outlines common movement and coordination abnormalities and their assessment methods.

BOX 9-5 | **Nonequilibrium Coordination Tests**

Most of these tests should be performed first with eyes open and then with eyes closed to examine the influence of vision on the individual's coordination. After doing each test at a comfortable pace, instruct the client to move faster and examine the influence of speed on coordination:

1. *Finger to nose:* With shoulder in a flexed position, bring the finger to the tip of the nose and back out to the examiner's hand or just straight out in front, repeating several times.

2. *Finger to therapist's finger:* Therapist sits in front of the client and has them alternately touch the therapist's fingertip. The therapist places their fingertip at nose height, arm's length away from the client. The movement is alternated. The therapist can also try moving their own finger so that the client has to make contact with the finger in different locations and can also move their finger, while the client is reaching, to observe how easily and smoothly he can change the trajectory of this movement in response to a moving target.

3. *Opposition of fingers:* The thumb is touched to the tip of each finger on the same hand, moving in

order from the index finger to the pinky and back down to the index finger. Be sure that the client is instructed to fully abduct the thumb after each digit is touched.

4. *Grasp:* The hand is opened and closed with gradually increasing speed. Encourage the client to fully open the hand with each repetition. Failure to fully open the hand or progressive shrinking of movement may be indicative of basal ganglia disorder.

5. *Alternating pronation and supination:* The client is asked to alternately pronate and supinate with the arms held at the sides and elbows flexed (hands can be placed on legs while seated so that palms and back of hands alternately touch the thighs).

6. *Tapping (hand and/or foot):* The arm is placed on a table or on the client's leg and they are instructed to tap the hand on the table or on his knee. For the foot, the client is seated with the knee flexed and foot flat on the floor; then, ask him to tap his toe on the ground.

7. *Rebound test:* The client is positioned with the elbow in 90 degrees of flexion and the therapist applies resistance to elbow flexion. The client is instructed to maintain the flexed posture. The therapist then suddenly releases their resistance and observes the response; since the elbow flexors are active, the arm will begin to flex, when the resistance is released. A normal response involves the opposing muscle group (triceps) rapidly checking the flexion movement with little motion occurring. Abnormal tests involve a large flexion of the elbow or a loss of trunk control in response to the sudden change in resistance.

8. *Heel on shin:* In supine or sitting, the client is asked to slide the heel up the shin from the ankle to the knee and back down again. Any movement off of the shin is considered a coordination deficit.

9. *Toe to examiner's finger:* Examiner holds their finger out and the client is asked to point to it with their great toe. This motion can be alternated

10. *Drawing a circle:* The client is asked to draw a circle on the floor with the big toe. A figure of eight can also be used. In supine, they can be asked to draw the figure in the air. This test can also be done with the upper extremity, using the finger to draw an imaginary circle in the air.

BOX 9-6   Equilibrium Coordination Tests

Tests are listed from least to most difficult

1. Standing in normal, comfortable posture
2. Standing, feet together (narrow base of support)
3. Standing, with one foot directly in front of the other in tandem position (toe of one foot touching heel of other foot)
4. Standing on one foot
5. Arm position may be altered in each of the above postures (i.e., arms at side, over head, hands on waist, and so forth)
6. Displace balance unexpectedly (while carefully guarding the patient, wearing gait belt)
7. Standing, alternate between forward trunk flexion and return to neutral
8. Standing, laterally flex trunk to each side
9. Standing; eyes open to eyes closed; ability to maintain an upright posture without visual input is referred to as a **positive Romberg sign**
10. Standing in tandem position eyes open to eyes closed – **Sharpened Romberg**
11. Walking, placing the heel of one foot directly in front of the toe of the opposite foot (tandem walking)
12. Walking along a straight line drawn or taped to the floor, or place feet on floor markers while walking
13. Walk sideways, backward, or cross stepping
14. March in place
15. Alter speed of ambulatory activities; observe patient walking at normal speed, as fast as possible and as slow as possible
16. Stop and start abruptly while walking
17. Walk and pivot (turn 90, 180, or 360 degrees)
18. Walk in a circle, alternate directions
19. Walk on heels and then on toes
20. Walk with horizontal and vertical head turns
21. Step over or around obstacles
22. Stair climbing with and without using handrail; one step at a time versus step over step
23. Agility activities (coordinated movement with upright balance); jumping jacks, alternate flexing and extending the knees while sitting on a Swiss ball

---

Balance

Balance is a complex concept that is tied to limb and body movements. Clinicians typically examine static and dynamic balance within functional activities such as seated reaching, transfers, and walking. The examination of balance is commonly done through the use of outcome measures such as the Berg Balance Scale (BBS),[10] the Sensory Organization Test (SOT),[11] the Functional Reach Test,[12] and the Romberg test.[13] Each of these tests incorporates standing, assessment of limits of stability, and transfers from sitting to standing. Gait activities, which are a form of dynamic balance, can also give an indication of balance function. These include the Timed Up and Go test (TUG), the Tinetti Mobility Test (TMT), the Dynamic Gait Index (DGI), and the BEST test or mini-BEST test.[14] Clinicians have many outcome measures to choose from and should base their choice on not only the reliability and validity of the measure but also on the goals of the client with whom they are working.

TABLE 9-5	Movement and Coordination Impairments with Assessments Methods	
IMPAIRMENT	**DEFINITION**	**SAMPLE TEST**
Dysdiadochokinesia	Impaired alternating movements	Finger to nose Alternate nose to finger Pronation/Supination Knee flexion/Extension Walking, alter speed or direction
Dysmetria	Uncoordinated movement, characterized by over or under shooting intended position	Pointing to a target Drawing a circle or figure eight Heel on shin Placing feet on floor markers while walking
Dyssynergia	Movement decomposition and loss of coordination	Finger to nose Finger to therapist's finger Alternate heel to knee Toe to examiner's finger
Hypotonia	Diminished muscle tone	Passive movement Deep Tendon Reflexes
Tremor (resting)	Oscillating movements at rest	Observation of patient at rest Observation during functional activities (tremor will diminish or disappear with movement)
Tremor (intentional)	Oscillating movements with movement	Observation during functional activities Alternate nose to finger Finger to finger Finger to therapist's finger Toe to examiner's finger
Termor (postural)	Oscillating trunk movements	Observation of steadiness of normal standing posture
Asthenia	Diminished strength	Fixation or position holding (UE and LE) Application of manual resistance to assess muscle strength
Rigidity	Hypertonia with normal reflexes	Passive movement Observation during functional activities Observation of resting posture(s)
Bradykinesia	Slowness of movement and loss of associated movements (e.g., arm swing)	Walking, observation of arm swing and trunk motions Walking, alter speed and direction Request that a movement or gait activity be stopped abruptly Observation of functional activities; timed tests
Disturbances of posture	Inability to maintain a given position, react to displacement, or adjust one's posture to changing expectations	Fixation or position holding (UE and LE) Displace balance unexpectedly in sitting or standing Standing – alter base of support (e.g., one foot directly in front of the other; standing on one foot)
Disturbance of gait	Any change in the ability to walk under varying conditions	Walk along a straight line Walk sideways, backward March in place Alter speed and direction of ambulatory activities Walk in a circle

CASE A, PART IV

Trisha has reported a history of falls. Based on this, an examination of balance should be included in her assessment. Assessments at the body structure and function level might include the SOT and Romberg tests. These will help elucidate whether or not the balance problem is related to the vestibular or somatosensory systems. Examination of coordination and equilibrium would likely yield positive findings, if the lesion is in the cerebellum. In addition, the clinician may wish to choose one or two outcome measures to better measure baseline and document progress. The BBS, TUG, TMT, DGI, and BEST all give valid and reliable data, regarding functional balance status, and inform the clinician about fall risk. Given that Trisha has already had one or more falls, it is already known that she is a fall risk, but measuring improvement with tools such as these would still be important. Choice of the tool to use should be based on the underlying cause of Trisha's balance problems, as some tools work well in the aged while others may be more appropriate for individuals with a neurologic disorder. In addition, age, level of function, and situation(s), in which falls typically occur, are all factors to consider in choosing the right outcome measure to be used with Trisha.

In the SOT, she is unstable in both conditions where her eyes are closed (Conditions 2 and 5), falling within the first few seconds; she was able to assume a Romberg position but fell when attempting to maintain it with her eyes closed. Both of these findings indicate a strong reliance on vision and a strong likelihood of proprioceptive loss. Her

Berg score was a 50/56 with deductions for standing with feet together and eyes closed (could only hold for 3 seconds before falling), turning 360 degrees in each direction, which was very slow, and placing alternating feet on a low stool (only able to complete four steps in 2 seconds). When reviewing her falls, each has taken place in dim light with tripping over a change in surface height or a throw rug in the house.

NEUROLOGICAL EXAMINATION: ACTIVITY AND PARTICIPATION

Transfers

The examination of transfers includes an assessment of the individual's ability to make position changes in the bed, go from a seated position to standing, go from standing to sitting, and transfer to and from surfaces that are of differing heights and softness. The level of assistance should be described, including any relevant details such as how the assistance is best provided (i.e., guard left knee from buckling during stance phase). Refer to Table 9-6 for descriptions of assistance levels. Bed mobility, including rolling side to side and the ability to go from seated to supine and supine to sitting should be described. Movements should be attempted with and without assistive devices, if possible. Additional details that should be documented include:

- Movement strategy description
- Whether all extremities are used equally (e.g., one arm more than the other?)

TABLE 9-6	Terminology for Levels of Assistance
Independence	Completes the activity with no assistance and is safe while doing it.
Modified independence	Completes the activity with no assistance and is safe but requires the use of an assistive device or orthosis.
Supervision	Completes the activity with no assistance but is not safe <50% of the time. The level of safety risk is minimal. Assistance provided is that of the therapist being in close proximity, in order to assist if needed, but not touching the client.
Contact guard assist (CGA)	Completes the activity with no assistance but there are consistent safety concerns or periodic losses of balance requiring light assistance to regain balance.
Minimal assistance (Min)	Assistance is required but no more than 25% of the work is done by the person helping, during times of assistance.
Moderate assistance (Mod)	Assistance is required but no more than 75% of the work is done by the person helping, during times of assistance.
Maximal assistance (Max)	The majority of the work is done by the person helping (>75%).
Total assist	The patient does not do anything and all work is done by the person(s) helping.

Additional items to document:
Number of helpers should be included. Typically this is documented as +1 Min assist meaning only one person helped. +2 Mod assist would mean that two people helped.
Any assistive device that is used should also be documented. Ie: +1 Min assist with walker.

- Presence of involuntary or uncontrollable movements
- Level of independence or assistance required (how much, what type, assistive device). Are any assistive devices typically used?
- Description of the quality of movement and environment/situation, whether skilled and efficient, or if not, the measurements of the movement for documenting progress.

Sample Movement Description: Sit to stand from firm seat with armrests required vigorous rocking, six to seven times, followed by pushing off with (R) UE and LE. (L) UE and LE were not incorporated.

Walking (Gait)

Normal walking is a complex process and requires the use of many elements such as power, coordination, sensation, and balance working together in a coordinated fashion. The examination of gait can assist in detecting a variety of disease states. A slow velocity gait with short stride length and decreased arm swing could indicate Parkinson's disease, while a wide-based gait with ataxic movement may be indicative of disorders involving the cerebellum. The gait pattern should be carefully observed and documented by gait phase: initial contact, stance (early, mid, and late), push off, and swing. It is essential in the neurologic patient that we determine in which phase(s) of gait the primary problem is occurring so that we can better direct our treatment. Some areas to document under gait analysis include:

- Can the individual ambulate independently? With or without assistive devices? What level of assistance is required from the therapist?
- What gait pattern is used? Be sure to describe what happens at each phase of gait. Describe both lower extremities. Be thorough and clear with this description and make sure that the descriptive terms are measurable.
- Can the individual turn and maneuver around objects? Do they choose a specific direction to turn (e.g., always to the right)?
- Can he walk backwards and sideways, in both directions? Describe the pattern used.
- Can he walk on uneven surfaces like grass, thick carpet, or go from linoleum floor to a carpeted floor? Do he change speed when approaching a different surface?
- With any of the above, is there a loss of balance? Is it consistently in a certain direction? Do the client self-correct or need assistance to prevent a fall?

The use of orthotic and assistive devices needs to be assessed and documented. Consider:

- What assistive devices and/or orthosis is the client presently using and when are they used?
- Observe gait with and without the use of the orthosis. Does the orthosis improve the client's gait pattern?
- Can the client walk without it?
- Is the client using any assistive devices for the upper extremity? If so, what and when? Are the devices effective?

- Are any orthosis and assistive devices in good working order? Would adjustments improve their performance?

Many researchers are now recommending that gait speed become the sixth vital sign.[15] Gait speed has been shown to correlate with measures of health, and therefore, can be a valuable tool for measuring activity status. Studies have shown that a gait speed of .8 m/s is necessary to be a community ambulator while gait speeds less than .4 m/s put individuals at highest risk for negative health outcomes. Fortunately, there are many easy to use outcome measures that examine gait. Some of these tools focus on endurance (6-minute walk test), yet many examine both gait and balance (DGI, TMT, Rivermead mobility test[16]) while others examine both gait and transfers (timed up and go).

Assessment of stair climbing is performed by asking the individual to climb up and down stairs. Optimal stair climbing is the ability to independently ascend and descend in a foot over foot manner without the use of a handrail, and therefore, determining whether or not the individual can do this or how they deviate from this is the goal of the assessment. If the individual cannot climb foot over foot, then, assess the ability to utilize a step-to pattern, and note which extremity is used to step up. Optimally, the individual should be encouraged to try to ascend/descend the stairs without using the handrail, if this is not possible, note which handrail is used or that both handrails are needed. For individuals who use an assistive device, note whether or not they are able to use the assistive device on the stairs. Speed of climbing may also be measured as a means of tracking progress.

For individuals who will need to use a wheelchair for mobility, the ability to propel the chair is assessed. Some individuals find propelling the chair with their feet easier than using their arms; this is common in individuals with Huntington's disease. Other individuals may not be able to propel a standard wheelchair due to hand weakness or coordination problems. Modifications to the wheel or drive mechanism may be necessary for these individuals (this will be discussed related to appropriate disorders in later chapters). Still, other individuals are unable to self-propel due to significant deficits in the upper extremities or cognitive limitations and will, therefore, require an electric wheelchair. Once a means of propulsion has been determined, examine the ability to propel on different surfaces, such as linoleum or carpet and ramps, and to change direction.

CASE A, PART V

Case Report: Trisha remains independent in her walking with only a slight increase in knee flexion, associated with a mild foot drop bilaterally; this likely contributes to her falling in low light situations when encountering a change in surface height (tile floor to carpet) or obstacle (throw rug). On the TUG, her time was 15 seconds or "mostly independent"; there was obvious slowing when she was turning around to walk back to the chair.

● EVALUATION

This is your thought process and should discuss how you have confirmed or refuted your hypotheses regarding the cause of the movement disorders that you as a physical therapist are going to address in treatment. This may include:

- Synthesis of all data and findings gathered from the examination, highlighting pertinent factors
- Various forms of documentation such as a problem list, statement of general assessment with key factors influencing status

---

CASE A, PART VI

Case Report: *What do you think that Tricia's diagnosis should be?* Trisha's symptoms are consistent with bilateral symmetrical peripheral neuropathy secondary to diabetes.

Diagnosis

The diagnosis should describe how the identified limitations in body structure/function (impairment) and activity (functional limitation) restrict the client's desired participation role(s) and whether or not physical therapy can have a beneficial effect. Historically, the pattern from the Guide to Physical Therapy Practice[17] would be given within the diagnosis along with the relevant International Classification for Disease 10 Code (ICD 10); most recently, the Guide (Edition 3.0) has moved away from these pattern designations, as more clinical practice guidelines are created, but some clinics may still use this method of documentation.

CASE A, PART VII

Case Report: *What ICD -10 code and G code would you give Trisha?* Trisha's diagnosis is consistent with an ICD 10 Code of E11.42. The G Code would be OG8978 Mobility: walking & moving around functional limitation at least 1 percent but less than 20 percent impaired, limited or restricted.

Prognosis (Goals and Outcomes)

It is very important to consider and state the long-term functional prognosis as well as identifying the short- and long-term goals for this episode of care (level of care). By focusing on the long-term functional prognosis, it assists the therapist in prioritizing and considering things such as impact on neuroplasticity and negative consequences of compensation techniques on long-term functional prognosis. The prognosis statement should address the following:

1. What is the potential for function or participation for the long term?
2. What specific motor functions should the patient be prepared for at this time (this level of care)?

3. Identify the positive factors that will contribute to the achievement of the goals.
4. Identify the attributes that might prevent or delay the acquisition of the goals.
5. Identify the likely time frame for achieving the long-term goals (include this in the prognosis).

Do NOT say "Good potential for rehab." This is a meaningless statement. Say something like "Trisha has good potential to learn knitting within 2 months because she is highly motivated and retains full strength in (B) hands. Her skill acquisition will be slowed by her sensory loss in (B) hands." Goal setting will be discussed more in the following chapters, in association with the different clinical case studies.

Short-Term and Long-Term Goals

Be sure that the goals are **measurable** and **functional**. Body structure/function (impairment) related goals are acceptable as short-term goals. If underlying impairments are not addressed, the client will not reach her full rehabilitation potential, and therefore, these elements are important to consider in setting goals and designing a treatment plan. Be sure that the long-term goals come from the activity problem list and/or the recorded participation restriction on the examination notes.

● COMPONENTS OF THE PEDIATRIC EVALUATION

Although the evaluation of children with developmental disorders is similar to that for adults, it is complicated by the interplay between the developmental processes of neurologic maturation, engagement with the environment, and neuroplasticity precipitated by an insult to the developing nervous system. As physical therapists, we are charged with not only identifying impairments (ROM, abnormal tone, etc.) but also the relative impact of these impairments on the typical acquisition of developmental milestones. Thus, the pediatric physical therapist must not only be an expert on gross motor development but also have an understanding of psychological, social, language, and fine motor development as these are tightly entwined as the child matures.

CASE B, PART I

Haeley is a 2-year-old Caucasian female born full-term at 38 weeks. She has a history of altered motor and cognitive skills, after a possible incidence of shaken baby syndrome 6 months ago. Besides the recent "incident," she has an unremarkable medical history. Haeley lives in a two-story house with two steps to the front door. Haeley's father is an elementary school teacher, and her mother is a chiropractor. Haeley attended a day-care program until the "incident" but is currently being cared for by a babysitter in the home.

History

The evaluation of the pediatric client includes unique aspects because young infants and most children are not able to answer questions about their medical history or their reasons for coming into the clinic. To begin, the role of the clinician is to be receptive to the expertise of the parent in order to obtain a meaningful and adequate history. Allowing the parents a few minutes to talk candidly about their concerns, may give you unique insight into the medical and functional needs of the child. A pediatric history starts with baseline data such as date of birth and due date plus the current concerns of the parents and child. It is useful to include the child in this line of questioning, if they are able to respond. Some questions that could be asked in addition to the parents' concerns are: What would you like your child to be able to do? And, what is the latest thing your child has learned to do?

The medical history may be available in the medical records of the child, but in some clinical or educational settings, this information must be acquired from the parent, but the referring physician may be contacted to confirm the parent's report or obtain missing information. A clear understanding from the parent and physician regarding any precautions or contraindications to handling or positioning is necessary so the clinician is aware of potential limitations in positioning, during the physical examination. Handling precautions could include things like restricted lower extremity weight-bearing because of a possible hip dislocation or avoidance of pulling to sit (a common physical test to evaluate head and trunk control) after cardiac surgery.

In addition to medical history, **demographics**, including information about the child that is not medical, such as: contact information, the best way to communicate with the family about appointment times, race, religion, occupation of the parents, and any general family information pertinent to the child or potential treatment implementation (e.g., number of siblings in the home). **Medical history** includes current and previous medical diagnosis and concerns, clinical tests that have been completed and their understanding of them (e.g., genetic, imaging, laboratory), medication(s) with dosage and adherence, previous and current diseases, illnesses, and surgical procedures. **Developmental history** includes pre and postnatal information such as gestational age at birth, pregnancy, or postdelivery complications that could affect the child (e.g., a fall during pregnancy, feeding issues); timeline for developmental milestones that have been achieved; growth history (e.g., small for age); adaptive or other equipment used by the child; and previous developmental evaluations. **Family history** includes a general overview of family medical issues, including developmental problems in other family members, especially siblings of the child (e.g., motor, learning, or cognitive impairments). Questions related to the **living environment** and the **support system** available will play a large role in goal setting, prescribing therapeutic exercises for developmental improvement, and designing a meaningful home exercise program (see Box 9-7).

The last question on the list in Box 9-7 (What are the daily activities of the family in the home and in the community?)

leads nicely into the next section of the history – **Programs or related therapy services**. If the child is in a day-care program or school, further information about related therapy services available in either setting, including PT, OT, SP, adaptive physical education, dance, etc., will be helpful. If these programs exist in a currently utilized program, the PT can advocate for related therapy services, if needed. If the child is receiving supportive services, details about the setting, type, frequency, and goals of the treatments are necessary.

BOX 9-7 **Necessary questions to evaluate the living environment and support system should include:**

- In what type of household does the child and family reside – two-story house, a walk-up apartment, etc.? *In some cases, an evaluation of the home might be done to determine assistive technology needs (e.g., before the child receives a wheelchair or for an assessment of where to place a ramp).*
- What is the entry way into the home, does it have stairs or an elevator, and how does the child get in and out – carried, wheeled, ambulates?
- Who lives in the household with the child, including the number of adults and ages of other children?
- Where does the family eat meals (at a table, kitchen counter, etc.)? Does the child sit with the family? How and what does the child eat?
- Where is the child's bedroom and bathroom?
- What adaptive equipment does the child have (e.g., adaptive toilet seat, stander, tub chair)?
- For older children, does the child participate in home chores, like setting the table?
- How is the child transported within the community – car, van, bus; include assessment of car seat or wheelchair, if used?
- What kinds of toys or play equipment, outside of specific adaptive therapy equipment are available?
- What is the support system for the caregivers?
- What types of play activities/toys does the child like?
- What are the daily activities of the family in the home and in the community? Does the child attend day care or school? Does the (older) child have a job? *Asking the caregiver/parent to describe a typical day may be the easiest way to obtain this information.*

CASE B, PART II

Haeley is an only child, conceived after multiple fertility treatments. Mother reports her pregnancy was uncomplicated and delivery lasted 18 hours, aided by an epidural. Her parents also report an uncomplicated medical history, confirmed by the pediatrician's report. Prior to the "incident," she was at the 40th percentile for height, weight, and head circumference. She is currently having eating difficulties so has dropped to the 20th percentile for weight in just the last 4 months. Parents report that she rolled over by 6 months, sat independently at 8 months, walked at 11 months, and was saying multiple words (mama, dada, hi, bye, up, "ba" for bottle, dog, and cat) by 18 months when the incident occurred. They describe that they picked their daughter up from day care and she was unusually sleepy. After inquiring of the day-care provider (a mother of grown children, providing care in her home), she indicated that Haeley might have fallen as they found her on the floor behind a couch during "free play" time, acting sleepy. They were apologetic but did not seem overly concerned. The parents immediately took her to the Emergency Room, where she was found to have retinal hemorrhaging and a mild frontal subdural hematoma and associated mild cerebral edema on magnetic resonance imaging (MRI). She remained hospitalized for 4 days, when the subdural hematoma had resolved. The police investigation did not find sufficient evidence to charge anyone with shaking Haeley, but shaken baby syndrome is suspected; as SBS is difficult to diagnose, they could not rule out that Haeley had fallen (although there was no "bump" evident on her head). On discharge, Haeley was still able to walk, although seemed a little "wobbly" at first; since that time, she seems not to be progressing as she should with little change in motor skills. She is still crawling up and down stairs, does not catch or kick a ball, and is not using a fork or spoon to feed herself (she does feed herself finger foods as she did before the incident). She has acquired a few more words but is not putting two words together yet. Her parents state they can see that she is not progressing the same as others in their "play group." Their goals are for her to get "back on track" with her developmental progression.

Functional Status describes the current functional activities that the child can perform. It is helpful to ask about functional status in a variety of conditions such as at school, in the home, on the playground. Qualify these activities with the type of assistive device that is used. In addition, questions about learning style can be included (Box 9-8) to determine how best to present.

The PEDI[18] and PEDI-CAT[19] are survey-based tools that may be beneficial in assisting caregivers and families in identifying their child's current level of function and help identify areas of need. One advantage to these tools is the wide age range they encompass (PEDI: 6 months–7 years; PEDI-CAT: birth–20 years), so they can be used with a variety of pediatric clients. Either tool can also be used for examination of self-care and home management.

Systems Review

The systems review, for the child, contains many of the elements of the adult exam and some novel elements, specific to children.

> **BOX 9-8** **Questions about Learning can be included in the history interview with the child and caregiver, and modified, if needed, after interacting one-on-one with the child. Important questions to ask are:**
>
> - Does the child learn best with vision, pictures, hearing, or demonstration?
> - Can the child read? Can the child understand what is read to them?
> - Are there any language needs, including the need for an interpreter, if English is not the child's primary language?
>
> **The same questions are repeated about how the adult caregiver learns. During the examination note how the child is attentive, response, cooperative, and what mode of communication is most effective.**

Here, we will focus on the elements that might be different from the adult exam or specific to children:

- Integumentary System review: Although the integumentary review for children mirrors that for adults, the skin areas around braces and weight-bearing surfaces, especially in children with limited movement, should be carefully evaluated. If skin issues are identified, careful review of any adaptive equipment must be completed to determine points of potential pressure.
- Musculoskeletal systems review: Gross ROM, Strength, and Symmetry in sitting and standing are screened and assessed during functional activities, since infants and young children don't typically understand or comply with standard adult-like testing methods. Presence of symmetry or asymmetry should be noted and further examined in the musculoskeletal assessment, as described in the next section.
- Cardiovascular/Pulmonary system review: No specific differences from adults.
- Gait, primary form of locomotion, balance, transitions, coordinated movements, proprioception, motor control, and motor learning are part of the Neuromuscular Systems review. Remember during this level of the review the indication for each item is impaired or not impaired.
- Other systems review: Standard testing for vision, hearing, and the other special senses is not feasible in infants and young children, but tracking visually (following an object with the eyes laterally and vertically) and to sound (turning in the direction of a sound out of the visual field) can be screened even in young infants, using common toys; also, very young infants will blink to a light focused on the eyes. Taste is typically not tested in young children, but the other CNs may be screened by observing eating and facial expressions as well as shoulder movements.

CASE B, PART III

The system review of Haeley is negative for any disturbances of the integumentary, cardiovascular/pulmonary, or other systems. Observation indicates a need for a comprehensive musculoskeletal and neuromuscular examination, as her movements are slow, she walks on her toes with hands at mid-guard position, and she requires an external support to pull to stand.

Examination

Similar to the methods for screening, examination of strength and ROM occurs through structured observation of functional motor skills and some passive handling/positioning. For example, kicking a ball in sitting can assess antigravity quadriceps strength, while squatting to the ground and returning to standing is an indication of good quadriceps strength. If she can also lift an object, during squat to stand, (e.g., a large ball), normal strength is likely. Prone extension over a ball is a nice way to examine antigravity shoulder, back and hip strength; the length of time the position can be held can suggest good or normal strength. Many of these skills are included in standardized tests with increasing time for maintaining the position as an indicator of developmental age. In Box 9-9, standard questions that

BOX 9-9 Questions to be answered while observing a pediatric client:

(*A similar framework is used in the Alberta Infant Motor Scale (AIMS),*[20] *a common scale of infant development.*)
* What is the weight-bearing position?
* What are the antigravity movements, required by the position?
* Is the position/movement symmetrical or asymmetrical?
* What is the midline behavior while in the position?

The answers to these questions give information about strength, ROM, balance, and coordination.

In addition, the following overall questions should be addressed:
* What are the abilities of the child?
* What are the strengths of the child's functional movements?
* What is the quality of the movement?
* Can the child sustain the position?
* Can the child sustain a position and stabilize in order to play or perform ADLs with the arms and hands?
* Is there sufficient variability in the number of postures and positions, or does the child adopt only one position, putting them at risk for a secondary impairment or overuse injury?
* What positions and activities cannot be performed?
* Is the alignment, posture, or movement typical or atypical
* What type of assistance is required to assume a position or perform a skill or task?

the therapist should consider in each position, in which the child is observed, are delineated.

Muscle Tone: Muscle tone is objectively measured with the modified Ashworth, as described for the adult assessment, despite limited evidence of validity or interrater reliability. Commonly, pediatric assessments only describe tone as normal, hypotonic (low tone, floppy), hypertonic (high tone), or mixed (combinations of normal, high, and low tone), which is common in some developmental disorders. Tone should be assessed in all position; at rest; and during passive, active, and challenging (stressful) movements. Tone can impede acquisition of motor milestones, limit function, and interfere with the assessment of strength and muscle power.

CASE B, PART IV

Upper extremity tone is normal, but Haeley demonstrates mild hypertonia in her gastrocs and hip adductors (Ashworth = 1, DTR = 3+).

Range of Motion: Passive and active ROM is assessed while playing with the child or through the observation of functional movements; if there are any contractures or orthopedic deformities, goniometric measurements should be attempted, with help from the caregiver/parent to distract the child.

CASE B, PART V

Haeley has full ROM in her UE, but active dorsiflexion is to neutral when her leg is straight (observed when asking her to touch the examiner's fingers with her toes, while her legs were straight; if external support was not provided, she would flex her knee, when dorsiflexing). She prefers w-sitting to tailor-sitting, assuming this position frequently, consistent with adductor tightness. Abduction with knees flexed is approximately 60 degrees, but should be near 90 degrees.

Strength: Observation of movement against gravity and with resistance in functional activities or during activities that use muscle power is the primary method for assessing strength and power for infants and young children; by the age of 8–10, children can typically understand standard strength testing methods. There is good reliability for using handheld dynamometers for strength assessments in older children, if desired, and dynamometers are frequently available in a pediatric clinical setting. The Biodex offers options for measuring more advanced examination and outcome values of isometric, isokinetic strength especially in the lower extremity but are not common in pediatric clinics.

Case Study

Haeley demonstrates antigravity muscle strength in all major muscle groups. However, she still pulls to stand, requiring an external support, and is not squatting to the ground and returning without an external support, suggesting some LE muscle weakness (Fair+/Good−). She could walk on her hands in a wheelbarrow position, which is indicative of good UE muscle strength.

Anthropometrics: Body weight, length/height, and head circumference are commonly measured good indicators of growth, and important for monitoring growth and development of the body due to nutritional concerns. Head circumference is also an indirect measure of brain growth and can indicate microcephaly and associated lack of brain growth within an expected trajectory. Head circumference may also be needed to monitor hydrocephalus and shunt function (see Chapter 18). Other less routine anthropometrics include limb lengths and circumference, which are used to evaluate asymmetrical growth, secondary joint dislocations, and to fit assistive devices and braces.

CASE B, PART VI

Anthropometrics are unremarkable except for the recent drop in weight.

Sensory Integrity: Many aspects of sensory function are observed simultaneously with motor function and during play. Response to touch can be determined by looking for a withdrawal of the trunk, limb, or digit to a light tickle or pinch but formal sensory testing can't typically be done until the child is 6–8 years of age. Proprioception can be grossly assessed by moving the limb into an awkward position and watching to see if the child moves it (e.g., place the arm under the child). Balance is typically assessed by observation of the child's ability to assume, maintain, and move within a given posture (sitting, standing, supine, prone) during play. Further, there are many reflexes that are present in the infant that come under higher nervous system control with maturation (primitive reflexes) and others that emerge as the child matures (protective, equilibrium, and righting reactions). While **primitive reflexes** (the historical name) are less obvious in the older infant/child/adult, they are often integral parts of coordinated movement patterns or become obvious when we are under stress. For example, while the crossed extensor reflex can't be elicited via the typical testing method after the second month of life, it is often apparent in our response to stubbing our toe or stepping on something. The first response to hitting your toe is to rapidly flex the injured leg with strong extension of the other (stance) leg to maintain an upright posture (often with some hopping and yelling) indicative of a crossed extensor pattern. Figure 9-2 illustrates some of these primitive reflexes while Table 9-7 provides a description of

how they are tested and displayed. Thus, primitive reflexes don't truly disappear; they just become part of our motor program repertoire, and their integration is a sign of nervous system maturation. However, failure to integrate these reflexes at the appropriate age is often a sign of central nervous system dysfunction; similarly, reemergence of these reflexes to their initial stimulus often occurs with nervous system damage. **Righting**, **protective**, and **equilibrium reactions** are mature responses that develop over the first 2 years of life that maintain our body alignment and balance (Figure 9-3 illustrates some of the earliest righting reactions and Table 9-7 describes the testing method and description of the response.)

CASE B, PART VII

Haeley has a mild Babinski in both feet but otherwise demonstrates integration of all primitive reflexes; a Babinski at this age is indicative of a brain injury. She demonstrates normal protective and equilibrium reactions in sitting and quadruped; however, her equilibrium reactions in standing are delayed and not effective to a moderate disturbance (Haeley will fall or reach for a support).

Developmental Assessment and the Examination of Movement

Pediatric evaluation for infants, toddlers, and children with apparent neurological dysfunction include a thorough examination, requiring observation and interaction with the child, usually in the context of play, in four body positions: supine, sitting, prone, and standing. In many settings, standardized assessment tools such as the Bayley Scales of Infant Development[21] (birth–42 months), the Peabody Developmental Motor Scales (birth–72 months),[22] or the AIMS (birth–18 months)[20] are used in conjunction with observation skills of the physical therapist to obtain a comprehensive evaluation. It should be noted that an adjustment is made for any child born prematurely up to age 24 months (Box 9-10). The Gross Motor Function Measure (GMFM)[23] is a common tool used to measure motor function and change in motor function in infants and children with cerebral palsy and has high psychometric properties; in addition, the GMFM-88[23] is validated in other populations, including Down syndrome. There are five domains on the GMFM: lying and rolling; sitting; crawling and kneeling; standing; and walking, running, jumping. Motor function for pediatric patients with neurological disabilities should be measured in all positions and in a functional context similar to those described and measured by the GMFM. When using a specific assessment tool, incorporate appropriate additional items that you would like to observe, while the child is in a given position (e.g., head movement, reaching, etc., while in prone), so that you are not requiring too many forced changes between positions. The more naturalistic the play and observation, the more accurate the examination will be, and the child will demonstrate better compliance. Older children or children with advanced motor skills need not be tested in every position. For all positions, the

FIGURE 9-2 Primitive reflexes in infants. A. Palmar grasp. **B.** Plantar grasp. **C.** Symmetrical tonic neck in prone – flexion of neck is associated with UE flexion and LE extension. **D.** Asymmetrical tonic neck – head turn to side elicits extension (less flexion) of face side extremities and more flexion of skull side extremities. **E.** Moro – quick drop of head backward elicits abduction of arms (shown), followed by adduction as though reaching toward the holder. **F.** Babinski – splaying of toes and hallux extension to stroking the bottom of the foot.

TABLE 9-7   Primitive Reflexes and Righting, Protective, and Equilibrium Reactions

REFLEX	DESCRIPTION	AGE SEEN
Asymmetric Tonic Neck Reflex (ATNR)	Lateral head turning leads to flexion (less extension) of the extremities on the skull side and extension on the face side	0–3 months
Symmetric Tonic Neck Reflex	Neck flexion leads to UE flexion and LE extension; neck extension leads to UE extension and LE flexion	0–4 months
Moro	Quickly moving the child from an upright sitting position backward toward the support surface, elicits abduction of the arms (away from midline), followed by adduction of the arms (toward midline) and trunk flexion	0–6 months
Rooting	Stroking the cheek elicits head turning, as if to find a nipple	0–4 months
Galant (truncal incurvation)	Stroking the lateral part of the trunk produces trunk flexing away from the stimulus (e.g., right stroke – convexity of trunk incurvation to the right)	0–4 months
Palmar grasp	Applying pressure to the palm of the hand elicits grasping (baby will hold the tester's finger)	0–6 months
Plantar grasp	Pressure on the ball of the foot will elicit toe flexion as if to grasp with the toes	0–15 months
Stepping	Placing an infant in a standing position and leaning them forward, will elicit stepping	0–2 months
Positive support (primitive standing)	Placing an infant in a standing position results in leg and trunk extension	0–2 months
Flexor withdrawal reflex	A tap to the heel or pulling of the great toe results in leg flexion away from the stimulus	0–2 months
Extensor thrust	Pushing on the foot elicits strong extension of the leg	0–2 months
Crossed extensor reflex	Passive flexion of one leg is associated with extension of the other leg	0–6 weeks
Righting reactions	Orient head to the body	
Rotational Righting	Turning a segment of the body (e.g., head) elicits rotation of the rest of the body in a "log roll" fashion	Present up to 6–12 months
Body on head	Touching the body to a support services elicits lifting of the head	
	Prone	Emerges 1.5–4 months
	Supine	Emerges 4–6 months
Vertical Righting		
Labyrinthine righting reaction	Hold the child upright and tilt laterally with vision occluded (blindfold), head will be maintained upright or return to upright	Emerges 3–6 months
Optical Righting	Tested same as LRR but with vision; head is maintained upright	Emerges 2.5–6 months
Prone Vertical Righting (Landau)	Hold child in a supported prone position (arms under stomach and hips)	
	Partial – head up to 45 degrees	Emerges 2.5–4 months
	Mature – head up to 90 degrees	Emerges by10 months
Protective Responses		
Prone (parachute)	Support the child under the trunk in prone and quickly but carefully tip them forward toward a mat; the child should extend their hands	Emerges 6–7 months

(Continued)

TABLE 9-7	Primitive Reflexes and Righting, Protective, and Equilibrium Reactions (*Continued*)	
REFLEX	**DESCRIPTION**	**AGE SEEN**
Sitting	While the child is sitting, gently push them in a given direction (can be done on an equilibrium board by tipping the board)	
Forward		Emerges 6–11 months
Lateral (to the side)		Emerges 6–11 months
Backward		Emerges 9–12 months
Tilting/Equilibrium reactions	Typically tested with the child on an equilibrium board (tilting reaction) or by gently pushing the child to destabilize in a given direction (equilibrium):	
Prone	With the child prone, tip board to one side, trunk should curve away from the tip with arm reach toward the top of the board	Emerge 5–9 months
Supine	Tip board with child supine, trunk incurvation away from tip with arm reach toward top of board	Emerges 7–11 months
Sitting	In sitting, the child can be tipped forward/backward and to the side or while sitting on the floor, gently pushed in each direction	Emerge 7–8 months
Quadruped	While child is in quadruped, disturb balance to the side, will curve trunk to opposite side to return to stability	Emerges 8–12 months
Standing	With child in standing, disturb balance in any direction; extreme disturbance may elicit a step	Emerge 12–21 months

child should be observed for symmetry of movement to discern unilateral or asymmetrical abilities/deficits (see Box 9-9). To elicit movements, the therapist will need to make each activity fun, using toys, pictures, family members, or other types of stimulation to entice the child to look, reach, and move.

Table 9-8 describes movements and skills that should be evaluated in each position (supine, side-lying, prone, sitting, quadruped, and standing).

Mobility

In Table 9-8, posture, mobility, and function in supine to standing are discussed in association with the structured observation of the young child to limit the need for many position changes. In the mobile child, the therapist must use their observation skills and creativity to assess the quick transitions and gait of the child (See Box 9-11 for suggestions in movement observation). **Transitions** refer to the movements that children (and adults) use to go (transition) from one position to another. Some transitions elicit new postures for the child that they may maintain during play (e.g., ½ kneeling). The initial transition for typically developing children is rolling, frequently from prone to supine and then supine to prone, occurring between 4 and 6 months. However, since most children are now placed in supine for sleeping, and therefore, may spend limited time in prone, many are rolling supine to prone first. Yet, the timeframe for rolling, 4–6 months, remains the same. Table 9-9 lists common transitions and the ages that most children use them consistently (*notably, child development is highly variable; some children will do things early and others late, but consistently late development is cause for concern*).

Primary form of mobility – There are several forms of independent mobility that allow infants and children to explore their environment. Rolling, belly/commando crawling, creeping in quadruped, bottom scooting, cruising on furniture, and walking are all meaningful ways of mobility and exploration. Assessment of these skills includes observation of the posture, weight-bearing positions of the limbs, movement pattern, symmetry of the movement, and ability to use the position for play. It is helpful to consider why the child is using a certain form of mobility as their primary form (e.g., scooting in sitting rather than creeping due to hemiparesis). When the child is moving, it is critical to observe whether the movements are performed selectively or as a mass movement (e.g., segmental versus log rolling). Is the child purposefully initiating movements, or are they not purposeful? The timing and sequencing of movements should also be considered. It is important to consider if the form of mobility can be used to maneuver around the child's environment, on uneven surfaces or hills, or contributes to functional play and development of new skills.

Walking (gait) is the motor milestone that defines the transition from infancy to toddlerhood; however, it is a skill that is achieved gradually. The average age for taking a few independent steps is 12 months. However, the infant achieves this early stepping ability after spending considerable time in standing. Initial movement in standing begins with bouncing and weight shift, first while supported (4–6 months) and then while holding onto a support (7–9 months); then, cruising around furniture is initiated with side-stepping (8–10 months), progressing to forward stepping with one hand on the support (9–12 months), and at

FIGURE 9-3 Postural reactions. A. Landau – prone support with head to 60 degrees (immature). **B.** Body on body reaction – log roll in association with rotation of the hip. **C.** Optical righting – head up to vertical when body is tipped laterally (labyrinthine can be tested with similar motion when eyes are covered). **D.** Parachute response – forward movement toward mat elicits arm extension in protective manner.

the same time, the child is likely beginning to walk with first both hands held and then, one hand (11–12 months). Finally, the first independent steps are achieved with hands in a high guard position. *Generally, if a child is 18 months or older without taking any steps, he/she is considered delayed in walking.* The primary stepping patterns of alternating, step-to, and side-stepping can be observed in a variety of contexts. Young children take shorter steps, have a wide base of support, keep their arms in a high guard position, and fall a lot. Over the second year of life, gait matures toward an adult-like pattern as different gait parameters, such as toe off, heal strike, and arm swing emerge and gait speed increases. Observation of weight acceptance can be helpful to assess the walking pattern, impairments, and identify asymmetries, as many children will fail to develop a heel-strike and will initiate contact with their toes.

Notably, children with more distal neurological impairment may use a hip strategy primarily for stepping, while those with less impairment may be able to use both a hip and ankle strategy. A complete gait assessment should evaluate heel strike, stance time, weight shifts, knee and hip positioning during swing, forefoot placement and position (pronation/supination), tibial torsions, genu varus/valgus, femoral anteversion/retroversion, pelvic tilt (anterior/posterior) or obliquities, scapular protraction/retraction, and positioning of arms. Further, gait observation should include assessment of postural control, balance, and the ability to use gait for play.

Fine motor skills – Toy manipulation with the hands should be examined in each position mentioned above; this observation should include: unilateral and bilateral reaching in a variety of directions, bringing the hands to middle, crossing midline, and

	YEAR	MONTH	DAYS
Due date	2012	4(3)	15 (45)
Date of birth	2012	2	23
Prematurity correction		1	22
Date of testing	2013 (2)	1(13)	30
Date of birth	2012	2	23
Uncorrected age	0	10	7(37)
Correction		1	22
Corrected age		9	15

Almost every mother will remember her due date and the date of birth of the child. Subtracting the date of birth from the due date will give the prematurity adjustment (in red). An uncorrected age at testing is determined by subtracting the date of birth from the date of testing (this age would be used for any child that is over 2 or not born prematurely). The corrected age is then computed by subtracting the prematurity adjustment from the uncorrected age at testing.

Note, in this instance the due date was the 15th of April with a birthdate of February 23rd, to subtract the 23 from the 15 of the due date, one must add a month (30 days) to make this 45 and then subtract a month to make the 4 a 3. Similarly, a year (12 months) must be added to the months to subtract 2 from 1, when determining the uncorrected age, which subtracts 1 year from the 2013, making it 2012.

manipulating and transferring objects. Grasping skills using a raking, thumb-to-forefinger, and pincer grasp (thumb pad to index finger pad) can easily be evaluated using a small toy or piece of food and are typically evaluated in sitting (with or without support); Table 9-10 identifies key fine motor skills over the first 24 months. It should be noted that hand preference typically isn't consistent until age 5, but most children begin to show some preference by age 3 or so. Fine motor assessment is typically done by an occupational therapist, but it is important for pediatric physical therapists to have some knowledge of fine motor skill development, for which most motor assessments include a fine motor or visuomotor assessment (e.g., the PDMS and Bayley). Examining fine motor skills for the older child with neurological disorders can follow the section in the adult examination (Box 9-5) for coordination. Self-care activities that involve arm and hand control like brushing teeth, eating, or object manipulation can be tested or mimed in the clinical assessment or addressed in the history.

Advanced motor skills – An identical framework of weight-bearing position, antigravity movements, symmetry or asymmetry, and midline positions can be used for advanced motor skills. For some children with neurological impairments, like hemiplegic CP, advanced motors kills may be the only type of motor skills that are delayed or impaired. These tests of motor function should be adapted to the abilities of the child, but include play skills, such as throwing and kicking a ball, advanced mobility, such as running, hopping and skipping, and playground skills such as climbing a ladder. Table 9-11 identifies common ages for the acquisition of some of these milestones.

Adaptive Equipment

Many children with developmental disorders will have been prescribed adaptive equipment. Any subsequent evaluation should

TABLE 9-8	**Observations by Position**
POSITION	**OBSERVATIONS/SKILL TESTING**
Supine	Weight-bearing on the head, back, pelvis, posterior legs, and feet
	Spontaneous movements of arms and legs (frequency, vigor, pattern of leg kicks [unilateral, parallel, alternating])
	Ability to assume and maintain the head in midline (the position of the nose between the nipple line is a good reference for a midline head position) and tuck the chin (neck flexor control)
	Arm movement – length of movement (short or long), antigravity ability, ability to bring arms to midline (on belly or chest), extend to reach a toy, to mouth (self-soothing or toy-mouthing)
	Hand position – open or closed
	Visual tracking of a toy (cephalic, caudal, circular directions) – observe eye and head movements
	Orientation and tracking to sound (mother's voice, toy)
	Passive ROM – determine limitations, feel for tone restrictions (e.g., spasticity), screen for hip dysplasia (see Chapter 18)
	Antigravity movement of legs and pelvis (e.g., bridging) as an indication of abdominal and leg muscle strength
	Pull to sit – observe head position, arm pull and leg movement (see Figure 9-4 and Box 9-11 for descriptions)

(Continued)

TABLE 9-8	Observations by Position (*Continued*)
POSITION	**OBSERVATIONS/SKILL TESTING**
	Rolling to prone – a toy can be used to stimulate this, if not done spontaneously; move a toy laterally in the child's line of vision and encourage reaching; assistance can be provided at the shoulder, hip, or leg, if the child needs assistance. If the child rolls on her own, look at the type of roll (log rolling, segmental – note which body part leads the roll)
Prone	Weight-bearing can be on the head, chest, belly, or hands and knees (in quadruped)
	Antigravity head control – sufficient to turn head and clear airway; distance lifted in degrees (e.g., 45 or 90 degrees for 10 seconds)
	Ability to lift in midline with nose between the nipple lines (harder than asymmetrical lifting with head turned slightly to side)
	Ability to turn the head to track a toy or sound
	Upper extremity weight-bearing – on elbows or hands; elbows flexed or extended; chest on or off the ground; ability to shift weight to reach (controlled or unsteady)
	Rolling to side-lying and supine – initially initiated with the head in a log roll (hip and legs in line) fashion; later led by the shoulders or legs in a segmental fashion (hip or shoulder ahead of the other)
	Movement in prone: • Pivot prone – ability to turn in a whole or partial circle • Commando crawling – ability to move forward, using arms and/or legs, often initially with bilateral motion and later alternating reciprocal motion
Side-lying	Note weight-bearing on the lateral trunk, head, legs, and arm. (*The child can be placed in side-lying, roll into side-lying on their own, or go through side-lying when transition to another position.*)
	Midline and functional play of the arms should be noted, and the position of the legs
	Antigravity movements of lateral head flexion, trunk flexion and rotation
	Upper extremity weight-bearing – ability to prop on elbow
Sitting	Note whether weight-bearing is on the bottom, legs, and/or hands
	Trunk control (antigravity movement with the trunk), needed assistance or support to assume/maintain a sitting position. How the child supports himself – on elbows, hands with elbows flexed or extended, or without arm support, using trunk muscles (*note position of arms, if sitting without arm support – high with shoulder retraction, called a* **high-guard** *position, at the sides [ready to stop a fall] or free to reach and play*)
	Position of the pelvis – anterior tilt/posterior tilt; relation to trunk
	Position of the legs and width of the base of support • Ring-sitting: legs are flexed with feet together, forming a circle or ring • ½ Ring – sitting: one leg straight, the other flexed with foot toward midline • Tailor-sitting: knees bent and hips externally rotated with one leg in front of the other and feet near the opposite knee • W-sitting: legs are internally rotated with heels wide and the bottom between the heels
	Ability to assume and maintain
	Ask the caregiver/parent, whether he can leave the child in sitting when they leave the room; this is a good indication of the child's stability in sitting.
	Ability to weight shift (rotational or planer movements), reach to the side with trunk rotation or above the shoulder for a toy
	Ability to reach for and play with toys, switch objects from hand to hand, and bring hands or toys to midline
	Head righting, protective responses, and equilibrium reactions – elicited by tipping the child, a gentle to firm push, or reaching outside of the base of support, developed over first year of life • Head righting – ability to maintain or return the head to upright when the trunk moves • Protective responses – arm extension to stop a fall • Equilibrium responses – trunk movement to avoid loss of balance

(Continued)

TABLE 9-8	Observations by Position (*Continued*)
POSITION	**OBSERVATIONS/SKILL TESTING**
Quadruped	Weight-bearing is on the hands, knees, and occasionally feet (or foot). *The belly and chest are not on the ground, indicating antigravity movement of the trunk and abdominal control.* Movement in quadruped is observed by noting the coordination and pattern of the arms and legs, such as reciprocal movements, and measuring how far the child can move, if they can perform upper extremity object manipulation, and how they achieve functional play in this position. Weight shits might be cephalic or caudal resulting in rocking in this position, and lateral as infants reach for toys and move forward to creep. Position of the pelvis (e.g., increased lumbar lordosis – indicates decreased abdominal control) Position of the hip relative to the knee and shoulder relative to the elbow Ability to maintain (how long) Ability to shift weight (laterally, cephalic–caudal), rock, reach for toys, functional play Ability to assume the position from prone and sitting and resume prone or sitting Movement – creeping • Reciprocal – alternating opposite arms and legs • Symmetrical (bunny hop) – moving both arms and then both legs
Standing	Weight-bearing position on the feet. (*In older children, a weight-bearing position on the toes can indicate some spasticity in the gastrocnemius, or dorsiflexion ROM deficits.*) Independent or assisted: note how much weight (if any) is taken through the legs, and whether support is needed to assume/maintain (how much) Trunk control – upright or bending forward with UE support (elbows, hands) or resting chest against a support Alignment of the head, shoulders, and hips Ability to weight shift from one foot to the other, lift a foot off the ground Position of the arms, in independent standing: • High guard: hands above shoulders • Mid guard: arms out to the side • Low guard: arms down by their sides Functional activities – maintain for play, reaching in all directions, including to the ground and returning to upright

TABLE 9-9	Transitional Movements	
TRANSITIONAL MOVEMENT	**DESCRIPTION**	**AVERAGE AGE OF CONSISTENT USE**
Sit to prone	Initial – fold forward over their legs, sliding their legs into extension; mature – rotation to the side to place hands on the floor and extend legs	6–9 months
Prone to sit	Initial – push upward into quadruped and then backward into sitting with limited trunk rotation and hip flexion and external rotation Mature – may assume side-lying and push-up or assume quadruped and rotate through the trunk and hips to sit	8–11 months
Sit to quadruped	Similar to sit to prone, initial sit to quadruped transitions are completed with limited trunk rotation but rotation and flexibility in patterns used increases with maturity	9–11 months
Pull to stand	Infants typically assume a kneeling position in front of a support and use both hands to pull to standing, moving both legs into extension simultaneously	9–12 months
Pull to stand with ½ kneeling	Pull to kneeling and then assume ½ kneeling (one knee up with foot flat on the floor) and then pull to stand; this requires less arm pull and more active knee extension in the forward leg	11–13 months

(Continued)

TABLE 9-9	Transitional Movements (*Continued*)	
TRANSITIONAL MOVEMENT	**DESCRIPTION**	**AVERAGE AGE OF CONSISTENT USE**
Standing to sitting (controlled)	Lowers himself to the floor with graduate knee flexion and arm support	11–13 months
Floor to standing without pull	Assumes weight-bearing on feet and hands, shifts weight backward and rises	15–18 months
Squat and return to standing	Flexes at hip and knees into squat and uses leg extension to return, initially with trunk extension	15–18 months

FIGURE 9-4 Development of pull to sit. A. Neonate – pulled to sit with some head lag and no arm pull. **B.** Infant – holds head in line with shoulders, beginning arm pull and LE flexion. **C.** Six-month-old – head ahead of shoulders with strong arm pull and LE flexion.

BOX 9-11	Targeting Quality and Maturity of Movement

During any assessment, the examiner should consider the quality of motor function and movement, including the:
- Maturity of the movement
- Speed of the movement
- Influence of abnormal (primitive) reflexes on the movement
- Coupling and decoupling of the joints during a movement

Other questions to be answered during observation of movement in the child are:
- Can the child play or accomplish a task during a dynamic activity?
- Are there any missing or abnormal components of the movement?
- Is each joint moving through the available ROM needed for the activity?

BOX 9-12	Pull to Sit

Observing the child's response to being pulled to a sitting position, with the examiner pulling at the hands, elbows, or shoulders, can tell the examiner many things about the child's strength and maturity at the neck, shoulders, and legs.

1. Head lag – head remains behind shoulders (ears posterior to shoulders) – normal in young children; abnormal after 4–6 months; persistence is often seen in children with hypotonia

2. Concentric neck flexion – initially keeps head in line with shoulders at approximately 4 months, but eventually the head will lead the shoulders, usually by 6 months

3. Arm pull and leg movement accompany the pull to sit by 6 months to assist in moving toward sitting

4. Lowering the child from sitting to supine, again by holding the hands, arms, or trunk can give additional information about muscle activity and enable the therapist to determine at what point in the movement the child loses control for the child with hypotonia or immature head control

TABLE 9-10	Fine Motor Skills in the First 24 Months	
AGE (MONTHS)	**FINE MOTOR SKILL**	**DESCRIPTION**
0–2	Hand fisting	Hands are closed most of the time
	Palmar grasp	Grasp of any object placed in hand, typically holds for <10 seconds
2–4	Hand opening at rest	Increasing time spent with hand open and not fisted (or loosely fisted)
	Shakes rattle	Will shake rattle when held in hand for <20 seconds
4–6	Plays with hands	Brings hands together and to mouth
	Grasps objects	Will reach for and grasp objects within arm's reach in supine, prone, and supported sitting (whole hand grasp)
	Brings toys together	Will bang blocks or other items within each hand together, briefly
6–8	Grasps block	Uses thumb, index, and middle finger (3 jaw chuck grasp)
	Brings toys to mouth	Toys are typically brought to mouth to chew or "experience"
		Begins transferring items from one hand to the other
8–10	Grasps smaller objects	Will grasp small items (e.g., cereal) with a raking motion of all fingers (thumb will move from middle to lateral over this 2-month period)
	Removes pegs	Will remove peg from pegboard and explore opening with isolated finger
	Claps	Begins clapping hands together in imitation
10–12	Pincer grasp	Will grasp a small item (e.g., cereal) with pad of thumb and index finger
	Places objects	Will place block or other small objects in a container
12–14	Places pegs	Places up to 3 pegs in pegboard
	Puzzles	Begins placing simple shapes in a puzzle (circle, square)
	Feeding	Feeds finger foods to self
14–16	Scribbling	Begins scribbling with crayon, no hand preference; holds crayon with thumb and first finger
	Stacks blocks	Can stack 2–3 blocks
	Utensils for eating	Begins to play with utensil but still primarily uses fingers
16–24	Turns book pages	Can turn pages in books (may tear paper page)
	Vertical drawing	Can draw or imitate drawing a vertical line (still no hand preference)
	Utensil	Improved feeding with fork and spoon – scoops and stabs food

include a check of this equipment, including mobility devices, orthoses, and protective devices, as growth can be a critical factor in their fit and usability. Thus, the fit of equipment and appropriateness (rationale for use, and age-appropriateness) should be assessed, including whether the equipment will grow with the child and is durable given the activity level of the child. Finally, the PT must determine the need for additional equipment. This will be discussed further in the chapters on Neural Tube Disorders (Chapter 18), Cerebral Palsy (Chapter 19), and Developmental Disabilities (Chapter 20).

CASE B, PART VIII

Haeley was evaluated using the Peabody Developmental Motor Scales; her age at the time of testing was 2 years, 3 months (27 months). She received a score of "0" for walking (due to her wide-base), walking up stairs, walking fast, and walking backward. She was able to throw a tennis ball with shoulder extension but not overhand or underhand; she was not able to kick or catch a ball. Her ceiling for her gross motor scale was 15–16 months. She was able to place two shapes in a shape board (not the triangle) and stack six cubes but couldn't remove the top from a bottle, make a vertical mark with a crayon, or snip with scissors, giving her a ceiling of 22 months on the fine motor scale. Thus, she's showing a moderate gross motor delay and a mild fine motor delay. She should be referred for a speech and occupational therapy evaluation, since she is presenting with global delays (see Chapter 20).

TABLE 9-11   **Advanced Motor Skills**

SKILL	DESCRIPTION	AGE (IN MONTHS)
Stair mobility/Climbing		
Creeps up and down stairs	Typically goes up first; alternates hands and knees	12–15
Walks up stairs	Holds rail, brings both feet to each stair (step-to pattern)	15–16
Walks down stairs	With rail or hand held, step-to pattern	16–18
Walks up and down stairs	Alternating pattern (one step/tread) with rail	26–28
Walks up and down with toy	Alternating pattern, no rail, able to carry toy	34–36
Ladder climbing	Climbs 2–3 stairs of toy slide	12–16
Small ladder	Climbs vertical slide, step-to pattern	40–48
Vertical ladder	Climbs vertical ladder, alternating pattern	60–72
Jumping/Hopping	Begins jumping up from ground or down from stair	22–24
	Jumps forward up to 24 inches	30–32
	Jumps 2 inch hurdle	32–34
	Begins hopping	46–48
Advanced walking skills	Walks backward	24–26
	Walks straight line one foot in front of other (not heel to toe)	26–30
	Walks on tiptoes	28–30
Advanced movement		
Galloping	Forward movement with one foot ahead of the other at a fast pace	48–52
Skipping	Alternating feet with hop on each foot	57–64
Ball skills		
Catches large ball	2 handed with arms straight out in front of body	26–34
	2 handed with hands on sides of ball and elbows flexed	40–42
Catches small ball	2 handed catch with hands together	50–52
Kicks ball	Kicks stationary ball (increasing distance)	15–24
	Kicks rolling ball	36–40
Throws ball	Flings ball without directional intent	12–14
	Throws underhand	24–30
	Throws overhand	38–40

REFERENCES

1. Outpatient Physical Therapy Improvement in Movement Assessment Log (OPTIMAL). Available at: http://apta.org/optimal/. Accessed October 20, 2014.

2. Physical Self-Maintenance Scale. Available at: http://aging.ufl.edu/files/2012/05/ADLTable.pdf. Accessed October 20, 2014.

3. Folstein MJ, Folstein SE, McHugh PR. Mini-mental state: a practical method for grading the cognitive state of patients for the clinician. *J Psychiatr Res.* 1975;12(3):189-198.

4. O'Caoimh RO, Gao Y, Gallagher PF, Eustace J, McGlade C, Molloy DW. Which part of the Quick mild cognitive impairment screen (Qmci) discriminates between normal cognition, mild cognitive impairment and dementia? *Age Ageing.* 2013;42:324-330.

5. Nasreddine ZS, Phillips NA, Bedirian V et al. The Montreal Cognitive Assessment, MoCA: a brief screening tool for mild cognitive impairment. *J Geriatr Soc.* 2005;53:695-699.

6. Hislop H, Avers D, Brown M. *Daniels and Worthingham's Muscle Testing.* 9th ed. Philadelphia: Elsevier/Saunders; 2013. ISBN: 9781455706150.

7. Pandyan AD1, Johnson GR, Price CI, Curless RH, Barnes MP, Rodgers H. A review of the properties and limitations of the Ashworth and modified Ashworth Scales as measures of spasticity. *Clin Rehabil.* 1999;13(5):373-83.

8. Fugl-Meyer AR, Jääskö L, Leyman I, Olsson S, Steglind S. The post-stroke hemiplegic patient: a method for evaluation of physical performance. *Scand J Rehabil Med.* 1975;7(1):13-31.

9. Dunn W, Griffith J, Morrison MT, Tanquary J, Sabata D, Victorson D, Carey LM, Gershon RC. Somatosensation assessment using the NIH Toolbox. *Neurology.* 2013;80(11 suppl 3):S41-S44.

10. Berg K, Wood-Dauphinee S, Williams JI. The balance scale: reliability assessment with elderly residents and patients with an acute stroke. *Scand J Rehabil Med.* 1995;27(1):27-36.

11. Cohen H, Blatchly CA, Gombash LL. A study of the clinical test of sensory interaction and balance. *Phys Ther.* 1993;73(6):346-351; discussion 351–344.

12. Duncan PW, Weiner DK, Chandler J, Studenski S. Functional reach: a new clinical measure of balance. *J Gerontol.* 1990;45(6): M192-M197.

13. Black FO, Wall C III, Rockette HE Jr., Kitch R. Normal subject postural sway during the Romberg test. *Am J Otolaryngol.* 1982;3(5):309-318.

14. Langley FA, Mackintosh SF. Timed Up and Go test (TUG), the Tinetti Mobility Test (TMT), the Dynamic Gait Index (DGI) and the BEST test or mini-BEST test. *J Allied Health Sci Pract.* 2007;5(4):1-11.

15. Fritz S1, Lusardi M. White paper: "walking speed: the sixth vital sign". *J Geriatr Phys Ther.* 2009;32(2):46-49.

16. Collen FM, Wade DT, Robb GF, Bradshaw CM. The Rivermead Mobility Index: a further development of the Rivermead Motor Assessment. *Int Disabil Stud.* 1991;13(2):50-54.

17. Guide to Physical Therapy Practice, Edition 3.0. Available at: http://guideto-practice.apta.org.

18. Haley, SM, Coster WJ, Ludlow LH, et al. *Pediatric Evaluation of Disability Inventory: Development, Standardization and Administration Manual.* Boston, MA: Trustees of Boston University; 1992.

19. Haley SM, Coster WJ. *PEDI-CAT: Development, Standardization and Administration Manual.* Boston, MA: CRE-Care, LLC; 2010.

20. Piper MC, Pinnell LE, Darrah J, et al. Construction and validation of the Alberta Infant Motor Scale. *Can J Public Health.* 1992;83:S46-S50.

21. Bayley N. *Bayley Scales of Infant and Toddler Development.* San Antonio, TX: The Psychological Corporation; 2006.

22. Folio MR, Fewell RR. *Peabody Developmental Motor Scales: Examiner's Manual.* Austin TX: Pro-ed; 2000.

23. Russell DJ, Rosenbaum PL, Avery LM, Hamilton ML. *CanChild Centre of Childhood Disability Research. Gross Motor Function Measures (GMFM-66 and GMFM-88) User's Manual.* Hamilton Ontario: Mac Keith Press; 2002.

Review Questions Evaluation Chapter (Adult)

1. A trial of intervention is a part of the adult neurologic evaluation process (True or False)

A. True

B. False

2. If the client is not able to identify which activities they are having trouble with the therapist can facilitate the process by:

A. Determining best activities to focus on from their examination

B. Utilizing an assessment tool to assist the client in identifying activities of interest

C. Focusing on activities of daily living basic to all clients such as sit to stand from a couch

D. Focusing on impairments that have been identified in the examination

3. Which of the following would be included in a review of systems?

A. Detailed examination of range of motion

B. Mental status assessment such as the mini-mental status exam

C. Reflex testing for UMN lesion including the Babinski and the Hoffman

D. Assess blood pressure during position changes from supine to sit to stand

4. Which of the following is a method for examining remote memory?

A. Name three objects and have the client repeat them back to you

B. Name three objects and ask the client to repeat them back to you 5 minutes later

C. Ask the client to recall common historical events

D. Ask for a chronological recall of the client's current illness

5. Mrs. Smith is 4 weeks s/p CVA. On initial examination 1 week prior, her Ashworth scores in her right arm were 2 throughout. On this day Mrs. Smith is tired and Ashworth scores in the right arm are 3–4. One possible cause of this increase in tone would be:

A. Response to resistance exercise you performed the day before

B. She has a urinary tract infection

C. She has contractures in her arm

D. Tone is increased when someone is sleeping or tired

6. Your client exhibits upward rotation of the eye and is complaining of double vision. Which cranial nerve is implicated?

A. CN III: Oculomotor

B. CN IV: Trochlear

C. CN V: Trigeminal

D. CN VI: Abducens

7. The most reliable way to evaluate position sense and kinesthesia is to:

A. Use a 250 mHz tuning fork on the bony prominence

B. Have the client perform finger to nose testing

C. Have the client perform alternating supination and pronation

D. Move the limb up or down and ask the client what direction it moved

8. When performing finger to examiner's finger testing, your client exhibits jerky movements and his finger goes past the examiner's finger and sometimes stops short of the examiner's finger. This type of movement would be called:

A. Dysdiadochokinesia

B. Dysmetria

C. Tremor

D. Asthenia

9. Mrs. Smith is unable to advance her right leg without some assistance to clear her foot. The therapist provides physical assistance for mid-swing to terminal swing to help the foot clear the floor. Mrs. Smith is able to balance herself, manage stance and her quad cane without assistance. Her assistance level should be documented as:

A. Modified independence

B. Contact guard assist

C. Minimal assistance

D. Moderate assistance

10. The sixth vital sign is:

A. Temperature

B. Level of assistance

C. Gait speed

D. Capillary refill time

11. In examining an infant, you notice his right arm and leg flex when he looks to the left; what reflex would this be:

A. ATNR

B. Moro

C. Galant

D. STNR

12. What are components of motor skill evaluation that are also used on clinical assessment tools like the AIMS?

A. Weight-bearing, posture, head control

B. Head control, reaching ability, locomotion

C. Antigravity movements, posture, weight-bearing

D. Arm support, lower extremity position, trunk control

13. The average age of independent walking (three steps) in typically developing children is

A. 6 months

B. 12 months

C. 18 months

D. 24 months

14. For most children, the first form of independent mobility is?

A. Belly crawling

B. Rolling

C. Scooting

D. Walking

15. For an integumentary systems review in pediatrics it is important to check

A. Integumentary checks are not performed in infants

B. The skin areas around braces and weight-bearing surfaces

C. Tissue damage related to falling

D. Pressure from spending too much time in one position

16. In typical development, the transition of infant to toddler is around what milestone?

A. Skipping

B. Crawling

C. Creeping

D. Walking

17. The PT systems review part of the examination includes reviewing

A. Observation of motor milestones

B. Use of the GMFM

C. Cardio/Pulmonary function and special senses systems

D. Getting a through history from the parent

18. How is strength measured in a toddler?

A. Manual muscle testing

B. Biodex

C. Passive movement to feel for resistance

D. Observations of movement against gravity

19. What is head lag?

A. The head remains behind the shoulders in a pull to sit task

B. The inability to maintain the head in midline in supine lying

C. A roll that is initiated by the arm and not the head

D. Optical righting without labyrinthine righting

20. A 40-month old child should be able to do which of the following?

A. Hop on one foot

B. Skip

C. Kick a ball

D. Gallop

Answers

1. A	2. B	3. C	4. D	5. B
6. B	7. A	8. B	9. C	10. C
11. A	12. C	13. B	14. B	15. B
16. D	17. C	18. D	19. A	20. C

Stroke

Deborah S. Nichols-Larsen
and Deborah A. Kegelmeyer

10

OBJECTIVES

1) Understand the pathophysiology of stroke
2) Relate the common risk factors for stroke to the cardiovascular changes created
3) Identify the typical symptoms of common stroke syndromes and the associated areas of brain damage
4) Identify assessment tools for use in individuals post-stroke across all settings
5) Identify and choose optimal treatment interventions for individuals post-stroke

PATHOPHYSIOLOGY

What Is a stroke?

Stroke, or cerebrovascular accident, is the leading cause of adult disability with an estimated 15 million people around the world experiencing a stroke each year.[1] In the United States, it is estimated that more than 7 million people are living with disability post-stroke. A stroke occurs when there is interruption of blood flow within brain blood vessels; this can result from either blockage of the vessel (ischemia) or rupture of the vessel (hemorrhage). Ischemic strokes are about seven times more common than hemorrhagic strokes, accounting for 87% of strokes[2]; conversely, hemorrhagic strokes typically produce much greater consequences than ischemic strokes and are more likely to result in death.

Ischemia can result from either an **embolism**, which is a clot that forms elsewhere, often in the heart, and then travels to the brain and lodges in one of the cerebral vessels, or a **thrombus**, which is a blockage of an artery that develops from a build-up of plaques, typically made up of fatty cells and cholesterol, within the wall of the vessel that eventually slows blood flow substantially or blocks it all together (Figure 10-1A). Ischemic stroke in a large blood vessel of the brain is referred to as a **thrombotic stroke** with neural consequences that relate to the vessel injured and the duration of the ischemia. Ischemic stroke in small vessels, referred to as **lacunar stroke**, may go undiagnosed until many such strokes have occurred and larger areas of damage, from these multiple strokes, have developed. **Transient ischemic attacks (TIAs)** are the result of brief blockages with associated stroke symptoms that resolve quickly (<24 hours) and are not associated with permanent consequences. However, TIAs are a sign of circulation disruption and the potential for subsequent stroke.

Hemorrhagic strokes occur in cases of poorly controlled and typically long-term hypertension, resulting in leakage or bursting of a small- or medium-sized vessel. Alternatively, they are the result of a weakening in the vascular wall, associated with an aneurysm or other vascular anomaly. Hemorrhage within the cerebral vessels is referred to as an **intracerebral hemorrhage**; if it occurs in a surface vessel within the pial lining of the brain, it is called a **subarachnoid hemorrhage** because the blood flows into the subarachnoid space (Figure 10-2).

RISK FACTORS

Why do Strokes Occur?

Risk factors for stroke include obesity, high cholesterol, heart disease (hypertension, atrial fibrillation, and congenital heart anomalies), atherosclerosis, diabetes, and substance abuse (smoking, alcohol, drugs, especially cocaine). Many of these risk factors are also associated with a sedentary lifestyle and are considered controllable, either by lifestyle change, medication, or both.

FIGURE 10-1 Ischemic stroke pathology. A. Right – Schematic of embolus from heart that enters cerebral circulation and is caught in the atherosclerotic cerebral artery. Left – Stenosis of the carotid artery can result in diminished cerebral blood flow and ischemia within the penetrating arteries of the cerebral hemispheres. **B.** Illustrates the division of the common carotid into the internal and external carotids. **C.** A CT image of the carotid arteries as they enter the cranium. (Adapted with permission from Hauser SL (ED) *Harrison's Neurology in Clinical Medicine* 3rd Ed, New York, NY: McGraw-Hill; 2013, Fig 27-3, pg. 262.)

FIGURE 10-2 Illustration of cerebral artery within subarachnoid space. As illustrated, cerebral arteries lie within the subarachnoid space; thus, hemorrhage of one of the major vessels will result in bleeding into the space, referred to as a subarachnoid hemorrhage. (Adapted with permission from Parent A. *Carpenter's Human Neuroanatomy*, 9th ed. Williams & Wilkins; 1996.)

Additionally, stroke is greater with advancing age, in certain racial/ethnic groups, and in people with a family history of cardiovascular disease or stroke. See Table 10-1 for a discussion of risk factors and their relationship with stroke. However, it should be noted that strokes can occur in those without known risk factors and are referred to as idiopathic (without known cause).

● CEREBRAL CIRCULATION

Why Are the Results of Strokes so Variable?

The brain is perfused by a complex system of arteries and their tributaries, originating from two ascending systems. The first is the **carotid artery system**, originating from the common carotid bilaterally, which bifurcates into the internal and external carotid arteries on each side (Figure 10-1B and C). The smaller external carotids are responsible for perfusion of the muscles and other tissues of the face. However, the large internal carotids enter the cranium through the carotid canal bilaterally and then split on each side into: a larger middle cerebral artery, the smaller anterior cerebral artery, and the even smaller posterior communicating artery. The **anterior cerebral arteries** supply the medial surfaces of the cerebral hemispheres, including the anterior portion of the corpus callosum, and the superior aspect of the lateral surface of the frontal and parietal lobes. The **middle cerebral arteries** supply most of the lateral surface of the frontal, parietal, and temporal lobes, including penetrating arterial branches to the basal ganglia, internal capsule, and insular cortex. The **anterior communicating artery** connects the two anterior cerebral arteries and forms the anterior portion of the **Circle of Willis**. The **posterior communicating arteries** project back to the posterior cerebral arteries, completing the Circle of Willis (Figure 10-3).

The second ascending arterial system is the vertebral artery system. The **vertebral arteries** are bilateral branches of the subclavian arteries and enter the skull via the foramen magnum. At the level of the medulla, the two arteries merge to form the large basilar artery. The **basilar artery** supplies most of the medulla and then gives rise to two cerebellar arteries (**anterior inferior cerebellar** and **superior cerebellar**) that supply the cerebellum and components of the brainstem, a series of **pontine arteries** to perfuse the posterior pons and midbrain, the **superior cerebellar artery**, and finally the **posterior cerebral artery** (Figure 10-3B).

The **posterior cerebral artery** provides the blood supply for the occipital lobe and the inferior and partial medial surface of

TABLE 10-1 Stroke Risk Factors and their Cardiovascular Consequences

RISK FACTOR	EXPLANATION OF RELATIONSHIP WITH STROKE[*,**,***,****]
Age	With increasing age, the frequency and severity of many other risk factors increases and multiple comorbidities are common, thus increasing the risk for stroke.
Gender	Men are more likely to have strokes at younger ages, but more women than men have strokes annually (NSA), perhaps due to the greater number of women living longer.
Race	Stroke is more common in African, Asian, and Hispanic Americans than in Caucasians. This partially reflects disparities in health care and the delay in diagnosis and treatment of risk factors in these racial groups. It may also relate to differences in diet or access to health literature.
Hypertension	Uncontrolled hypertension stresses blood vessels, decreasing their pliability and causing thickening of the arterial walls, which in turn, makes them susceptible to clot formation and hemorrhage.
High cholesterol	Cholesterol is an essential lipid for cell maintenance; cholesterol, specifically low density lipoproteins (LDL), contributes to plaque formation in vessel walls.
Obesity	Stresses the cardiovascular system and is often associated with hypertension, high cholesterol, and diabetes (metabolic syndrome)
Atrial fibrillation	AF is associated with a high incidence of embolism formation and subsequent embolic stroke.
Congenital heart anomaly	A high incidence of stroke has been associated with a patent foramen ovale (PFO), which is the persistence of the fetal connection between the right and left atria that typically closes at birth. PFO is associated with embolitic stroke.
Atherosclerosis	Plaque buildup in blood vessels (atherosclerosis) throughout the body is associated with both embolitic and thrombotic stroke.
Diabetes	Vascular changes are common in type 2 diabetes, increasing the stiffness of the vascular wall and resulting in decreased capacity for vasodilation.
Alcohol abuse	Excessive alcohol consumption is associated with increased clotting and thereby stroke.
Smoking	Smoking increases the likelihood of blood clots and contributes to the development of atherosclerosis.
Drug abuse	Many drugs (cocaine, LSD, amphetamines, heroin, opiates, Ecstasy, PCP) are associated with risk of stroke, often associated with induced hypertension, vasospasm with/without tachycardia. Heroin/opiates/LSD are more likely to induce stroke by cardioembolism

*Ihle-Hansen H, Thommassen B, Wyllar TB, Engedal K, Fure B. Risk factors for and incidence of subtypes of ischemic stroke. *Funct Neurol.* 2012;27(1):35-40.
**Roda L, McCrindle BW, Manlhiot C, Macgregor DL, Askalan R, Moharir M, deVeber G. Stroke recurrence in children with congenital heart disease. *Ann Neurol.* 2012;72:103-111.
***Esse K, Fossati-Bellani M, Traylor A, Martin-Schild S. Epidemic of illicit drug use, mechanisms of action/addition and stroke as a health hazard. *Brain Behav.* 2011;1(1):44-54.
****Parry CD, Patra J, Rehm J. Alcohol consumption and non-communicable diseases: epidemiology and policy implications. *Addiction.* 2011;106:1718-1724.

the temporal lobe, including part of the insular cortex and hippocampus; it also supplies the thalamus and ventral surface of the midbrain, including the cerebral peduncles. The **anterior inferior cerebellar artery** (AICA), as the name implies, provides circulation to the anterior and inferior cerebellum as well as the flocculus; it also gives off a branch that supplies the internal ear (labyrinthine artery). Other branches supply the inferolateral pons and middle cerebellar peduncle. It anastomoses with the posterior inferior cerebellar artery such that the actual area supplied by these two arteries is highly variable between individuals. However, the **posterior inferior cerebellar artery** (PICA) typically supplies the posteroinferior cerebellum, including the vermis, and the inferior portion of the medulla. Strokes affecting the AICA or PICA are less common, in part, because of their anastomoses and thereby, overlapping circulation. Finally, the **superior cerebellar artery** supplies the upper (superior) half of the cerebellum and components of the midbrain. It also anastomoses with the AICA and PICA, and strokes are rare within this artery. Symptoms can be either cerebellar only or combined with midbrain dysfunction, depending on whether the terminal portion of the artery or its brainstem projections near its origin are the site of infarction.

Stroke Consequences: How do the Symptoms of Stroke Relate to Circulation Compromise?

Stroke, within a given artery, presents with symptoms indicative of the brain regions supplied by that artery and their respective functions (Figure 10-4). Variability in symptomology relates to the site of artery occlusion or hemorrhage – the main artery or its branches – and the relative length of time of the occlusion or severity of the hemorrhage. Table 10-2 outlines specific stroke symptoms associated with the primary vasculature and

A

B

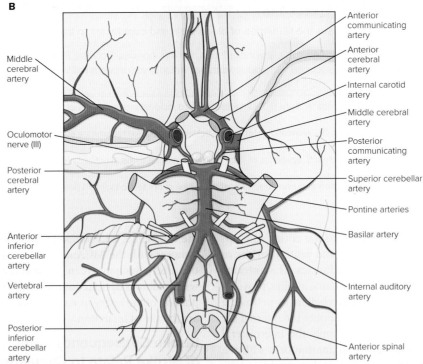

FIGURE 10-3 Schematic of the major blood vessels of the brain and the Circle of Willis. A. The brain is supplied by two networks, arising from the aorta: the internal carotid network, branching into the anterior and middle cerebral arteries that supply the anterior 2/3 of the cerebral hemispheres and the vertebral artery system that supplies the posterior 1/3 and the brainstem and cerebellum. **B.** The Circle of Willis is comprised of the anterior cerebral arteries, the anterior communicating arteries, and the internal carotid arteries (components of the carotid artery system), as well as the posterior communicating arteries and the posterior cerebral arteries (components of the vertebral artery system). The vertebral artery distribution illustrated on the dorsal surface of the brainstem, supplies the brainstem and cerebellum as well as the posterior cerebrum. (Reproduced with permission from Kandel ER, Schwartz JH, Jessell TM, Siegelbaum SA, Hudspeth AJ. *Principles of Neural Science*, 5th ED, New York, NY: McGraw-Hill; 2013. Figure C-1, p. 1551.)

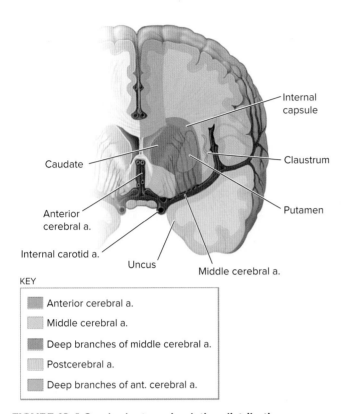

FIGURE 10-4 Cerebral artery circulation distribution.
(Reproduced with permission from from Hauser SL (ED) *Harrison's Neurology in Clinical Medicine* 3rd Ed, New York, NY: McGraw-Hill; 2013. Figure 27-6, p 274.)

common areas of damage. Figure 10-5 illustrates the complexity of impairments with disruption of brainstem circulation. It should be noted that patients will present with some or all of these symptoms, varying in severity, but can also present with a combination of symptoms from the different syndromes due to variability in individual circulation patterns.

Based on the stroke syndromes, what stroke syndrome has Mr. Brown experienced?

MCA

What cortical areas are most likely affected to create Mr. Brown's symptoms?

Primary motor (hemiparesis), primary sensory (sensory loss), Broca's area (expressive aphasia), optic radiations (upper and lower – homonymous hemianopia).

● MIDDLE CEREBRAL ARTERY (MCA) INFARCTION AS AN EXAMPLE OF STROKE

MCA strokes are the most common of the stroke syndromes, accounting for 51% of known stroke occurrences,[3] and their presentation is a good starting point for a discussion of stroke consequences, treatment, and outcomes. Onset of an MCA stroke is often associated with slurring of speech; tingling or numbness of the face, arm, and/or leg; loss of movement in corresponding body parts, or a combination of any of these. Consciousness is

typically maintained; however, when consciousness is lost, it is usually associated with a seizure or significant cerebral edema.

Motor Dysfunction

The motor consequences of an MCA stroke vary but can include early **flaccidity** (complete loss of movement and muscle tone) in the limbs contralateral to the lesion; this is referred to as **hemiparesis** (decreased movement) or sometimes **hemiplegia** (absence of movement). Corticospinal and corticobulbar projections are typically damaged with an MCA stroke, and often other stroke syndromes, either at the site of origin (the cortex) or as they pass through the internal capsule. Loss of corticospinal fibers, originating from the primary motor cortex, disrupts isolated muscle control in limb muscles. Loss of corticospinal fibers, originating in the premotor cortex, as well as corticobulbar fibers that project to brainstem nuclei, results in disruption of postural control, primarily within trunk and proximal muscles. Some patients will have diminished movement and muscle tone early but not flaccidity. It is rare for the limbs to remain flaccid, so the use of the term hemiplegia is an inaccurate representation of the movement abilities of most people post-stroke even though it is often used.

Motor recovery is complex and may be characterized by either return of isolated muscle control (partial or complete) or synergistic motor control. **Synergistic motor control** refers to activation of flexors or extensors in combination or synergy. For example, flexion of the shoulder is associated with elbow and wrist flexion and hand closing; conversely, extension of the shoulder is accompanied by elbow and wrist extension with hand opening. Similar flexion and extension patterns may be seen in the leg. This type of movement is associated with brainstem level motor control. **Isolated muscle control** is the ability to activate individual muscles to produce isolated movements in any combination (i.e., wrist flexion with finger extension) that is characteristic of typical motor control and is associated with motor cortex control. Although some patients will progress from synergistic movement to isolated motor control, others will develop synergistic movements and fail to develop isolated movements. Despite regaining isolated muscle control, some stroke survivors will not have the variety of movement, dexterity, or force generation that they had pre-stroke even after years of treatment and recovery. Damage to the prefrontal cortex, including the premotor and/or supplementary motor cortices, results frequently in disturbed motor planning abilities, referred to as **apraxia**. Patients with apraxia may be able to perform a given motion but may have difficulty incorporating that motion into a complex movement; as a consequence, their movements look clumsy, and they will often have trouble achieving the goal of the movement.

Since motor planning is a bilateral activity, apraxia may be noted bilaterally post-stroke. So, although post-stroke motor impairment has historically been referred to as hemiparesis, it is not uncommon to see subtle changes in motor control in the ipsilesional extremities that may not be apparent to the stroke survivor, or the novice clinician, but may impact recovery. Specific deficits have been noted in inter-digit coordination (finger tapping) and hand dexterity that can impact many functional skills. These deficits may relate to loss of ipsilateral

TABLE 10-2 Stroke Syndromes and Associated Symptoms

ARTERY	AREAS OF DAMAGE	COMMON SYMPTOMS
Anterior cerebral A*	Frontal lobe	
	Medial surface	Apathy/lack of spontaneity
	Anterior and superior aspect of primary motor area	Contralateral motor dysfunction of the lower leg and foot
		Bladder incontinence
	Anterior and superior aspect of premotor cortex	Gait apraxia
	Parietal lobe	
	Medial surface	Contralateral sensory dysfunction of leg and foot
	Superior aspect of lateral surface	
Middle cerebral B****	Lateral surface of frontal lobe	
	Primary motor area	Contralateral hemiparesis (UE>LE)
	Premotor area	Apraxia
	Broca's area	Expressive aphasia (left)**
	Lateral surface of parietal lobe	Contralateral hemisensory loss
	Parietal lobe projections to frontal lobe and contralesional parietal lobe	Contralateral neglect syndrome (right)
		Bilateral sensory discrimination loss
	Internal capsule (posterior limb)	Contralateral hemiparesis and hemisensory loss
	Optic radiations	
	Superior (parietal lobe)	Inferior quadrantanopia
	Inferior (temporal lobe, "Meyer's loop")	Superior quadrantanopia
	Both	Homonymous hemianopia
	Temporal lobe (Wernicke's area)	Receptive aphasia (left)**
Carotid artery	Distribution of both anterior and middle cerebral arteries	Combination of anterior and middle cerebral artery symptoms

Anterior cerebral artery infarct — Superior frontal gyrus, Cingulate gyrus, Corpus callosum, Insular cortex, Putamen, Globus pallidus, Thalamus, Third ventricle

Middle cerebral artery infarct — Cingulate gyrus, Caudate nucleus, head, Internal capsule, anterior limb, External capsule, Putamen, Insular cortex, Claustrum, Globus pallidus, Anterior commissure, Optic tract

Artery	Structure	Symptoms
Posterior Cerebral	Occipital lobe	Contralateral hemianopia or quadrantanopia
		Cortical blindness (bilateral)
		Visual agnosia, agraphia (dominant)
		Prosopagnosia – loss of facial recognition
	Thalamus	Contralateral hemisensory loss
	Hippocampus (temporal lobe)	Memory loss (dominant hemisphere)
	Cerebral peduncle/midbrain	
	Lateral geniculate	Hemianopia/quadrantanopia
		Ophthalmoplegia:
	Cranial nerve III	Ipsilateral gaze deviation – down and out (unopposed pull of superior oblique and lateral rectus)
		Double vision, lack of accommodation
Basilar	Medulla	Death is common due to loss of medullary centers associated with respiration control
	Reticular activating system	Loss of consciousness, coma
	Cranial nerve disruption	
	Cr N IX and XII	Tongue paresis, loss of taste, swallowing deficits (dysphagia)Vocal loss (dysphonia)
		Ipsilateral/bilateral
	Pons	
	Cr N III	Dilated pupil(s) – ipsilateral/bilateral
	Cr N V and VII	Facial muscle paresis and sensory loss (dysarthria) – ipsilateral/bilateral
	Cr N VI	Horizontal gaze paresis – bilateral eye turns in – ipsilateral
	Descending motor fibers	Contralateral hemiparesis or quadreparesis (pure motor stroke)
	Ascending sensory fibers	Contralateral hemisensory loss
	Cerebellum	Ipsilateral/bilateral ataxia, vertigo, nystagmus (ipsilateral/bilateral)
	Distribution of posterior cerebral artery	Same symptoms as above

(Continued)

TABLE 10-2 Stroke Syndromes and Associated Symptoms (*Continued*)

ARTERY	AREAS OF DAMAGE	COMMON SYMPTOMS
Anterior inferior cerebellar	Lateral Pontine syndrome	
	Vestibular nuclei	Vertigo, nystagmus, nausea, ipsilesional falling
	Cochlear nucleus	Ipsilateral tinnitus and deafness
	Trigeminal nucleus	Ipsilateral sensory loss to face; ipsilateral paresis of muscles of mastication (dysarthria, dysphagia)
Posterior inferior cerebellar	Wallenberg syndrome (lateral medulla)	
	Cerebellum/peduncles	Ipsilateral limb and gait ataxia
	Vestibular nuclei	Vertigo, nystagmus, nausea
	Cr N IX	Dysphagia
	Cr N X	Dysphonia
	Horner's syndrome	
	Postganglionic sympathetic neuron damage	Ipsilateral ptosis, miosis, and anhidrosis
	Cr N V – sensory portion	Ipsilateral facial sensory loss
	2nd order spinothalamic neurons	Contralateral loss of pain and temperature in extremities
Superior cerebellar	Cerebellum/peduncles	Ipsilateral ataxia (mild trunk, severe limb and gait), vertigo/dizziness, nausea, vomiting, dysarthria, dysmetria, optokinetic nystagmus
	Medial lemniscus/spinal lemniscus (midbrain)	Contralateral sensory loss (touch, pain and temperature)
	Corticospinal fibers (pons)	Contralateral paresis

*Strokes of the anterior cerebral artery are uncommon, most likely due to the redundancy of circulation from the right and left systems.

**Damage to both areas results in Global aphasia (both expressive and receptive).

***A (Reproduced, with permission, from Afifi AK, Bergman RA. *Functional Neuroanatomy*. 2nd edition. New York, NY: McGraw-Hill; 2005, Fig 28-2, pg. 361.)

****B (Reproduced, with permission, from Afifi AK, Bergman RA. *Functional Neuroanatomy*. 2nd edition. New York, NY: McGraw-Hill; 2005, Fig 28-1, pg. 360.)

FIGURE 10-5 A–E. Brainstem circulation and stroke syndromes. Ascending syndromes A–E, from the medulla (A) to the midbrain (E), illustrate the complexity of structures damaged with lateral and medial stroke syndromes at each level. Damage to the corticospinal tracts, medial lemniscus, and spinothalamic tract result in loss of function contralateral to the lesion; damage at the level of the lower medulla often results in bilateral loss of corticospinal and medial lemniscal function because of the decussation of these fibers at this level. Typically cranial nerve, spinocerebellar or cerebellar peduncle or medial longitudinal fasciculus symptoms are ipsilateral to the lesion. Thus, brain stem syndromes often present with contralateral or bilateral changes in the limbs, ipsilateral or bilateral changes in balance/proprioception, and ipsilateral or bilateral changes in cranial nerve function. (Reproduced with permission from Hauser SL (ED) *Harrison's Neurology in Clinical Medicine* 3rd Ed, New York, NY: McGraw-Hill; 2013. Figures 27-10-14, pp 280 – 284.)

(uncrossed) corticospinal fibers or disruption of bilateral cortical networks, associated with motor planning and control. Also, loss of cortical projections from the lesioned hemisphere to the non-lesioned hemisphere results in lowered inhibition of the intact motor cortex that may disrupt fine motor control.

Notably, the literature has included a number of terms to describe the extremities contralateral to a unilateral lesion post-stroke, including terms like "affected/more affected," "involved/more involved," and "paretic" with the limbs ipsilateral to the stroke referred to as "non-affected/lesser affected," "noninvolved/lesser involved," or "non-paretic." Since paresis best characterizes the contralesional extremities and has not been found in the ipsilesional extremities post-stroke, this chapter will use that label; the term non-paretic will be used to refer to the ipsilesional extremities. It should be noted that this does not mean there is no change in function, only that there is no paresis.

Sensory Dysfunction

Sensory dysfunction post-stroke is complex, involving multiple areas of the parietal and frontal lobes, and often goes undiagnosed because of that complexity. Sensory function includes touch perception, vibration, proprioception, pain, and discrimination of hot/cold, texture, weight, and shape. Often clinical evaluation of sensation focuses on touch, pain, and proprioception only. These may be impaired post-stroke on the limbs, face, and trunk contralateral to the lesion, sometimes referred to as **hemianesthesia**. This term is misleading, in that it suggests complete loss of sensation, yet sensation is rarely completely absent. It is much more common to have diminished sensation of varying degrees in different parts of the hemiparetic side. Sensory discrimination is less likely to be evaluated but more likely to be impaired; further, the sensory networks supporting sensory discrimination abilities are bilateral and include areas in the parietal and frontal cortices. Thus, sensory discrimination abilities are likely to be impaired bilaterally, especially when sensory discrimination loss ipsilesionally is moderate to severe.

There are also two complex conditions associated with sensory disruption post-stroke: pusher and neglect syndromes. **Pusher syndrome** (contraversive pushing) is a confusing condition, in which the patient pushes forcefully with his non-paretic extremities toward the paretic side, to the point of pushing himself completely over. Contraversive pushing can occur with damage to either hemisphere. When it occurs with right hemisphere damage, it is frequently associated with neglect syndrome. When it occurs with left hemisphere damage, it is commonly associated with aphasia; thus, there has been much confusion about the origin of this disorder. However, the common site of damage seems to be the ventral posterolateral nucleus of the thalamus,[4] which is a synapsing site for vestibular neuron projections. The consequence of this damage seems to be an impaired sense of upright; when tested, clients with pusher syndrome feel "upright" when shifted 18–20 degrees away from midline, so in pushing, they are really trying to "right" themselves. **Neglect syndrome** is also a complex disorder, characterized by failure to attend to things to one side of the body. It is much more common with right stroke but can occur with left; when it occurs on the left, it is typically less severe. In the event of a right CVA, the client may completely ignore objects in the left environment, including his own body

parts (the paretic arm and leg); plus, there is complete unawareness of this deficit. Diagnosis can be easily made by paper and pencil tasks such as target cancellations tests or the clock drawing test; in both of these, the client will fail to complete the task on the impaired side (see Figure 10-6).

Although the exact nature of the lesion that produces this deficit continues to be evaluated, it appears to be related to loss of superior longitudinal fasciculus fibers between the parietal lobe and the dorsal frontal cortex. These fibers are key components of the attention network.[5]

Visual Field Disruption

The visual system disruption with an MCA stroke can result in a visual field loss. Mr. Brown presents with a **homonymous hemianopia**, which refers to the loss of the visual field contralateral to the lesion (or in his case, to the right) and results from damage to the optic fibers (radiations) at some point after they

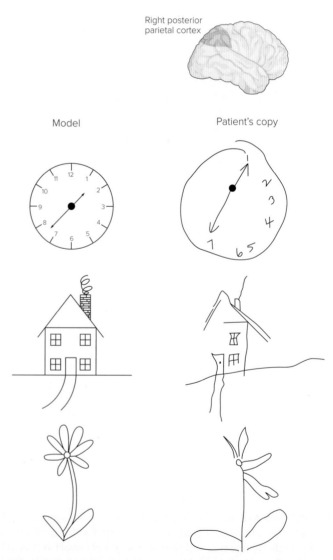

FIGURE 10-6 Unilateral spatial neglect syndrome paper and pencil testing outcomes. (Reproduced with permission from Bloom F, Lazerson A: *Brain, Mind and Behavior*, 2nd ed. New York: Freeman; 1988.)

leave the optic chiasm. **Quadrantanopia** is the loss of a quadrant, or quarter, of the visual field; again, this occurs contralateral to the side of the lesion. When only the parietal fibers are damaged, the superior retinal fibers are disrupted, resulting in loss of the lower visual field; when Meyer's loop in the temporal lobe is damaged, the inferior retinal fibers are disrupted, resulting in loss of the upper visual field. It is important to remember that visual fields are projected to both eyes and that the upper part of our visual field projects to the lower part of the retina, subsequently projecting to the occipital lobe through Meyer's loop in the temporal lobe, while the lower part of the visual field projects to the upper part of the retina and then to the occipital lobe through the parietal lobe. See Figure 10-7 for an illustration of these visual field deficits.

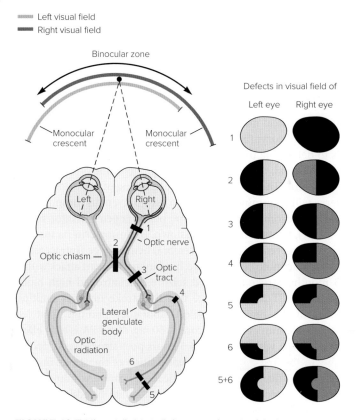

FIGURE 10-7 Visual field deficits associated with damage to visual projections. 1 = Unilateral blindness associated with optic nerve damage; 2 = bitemporal hemianopia due to damage of crossing nasal fibers at the optic chiasm; 3 = homonymous hemianopia due to optic tract damage; 4 = superior contralateral quadrantanopia due to damage of Meyer's loop; 5 = superior contralateral quadrantanopia with preservation of the macular vision duplicated in the parietal radiations; 6 = lower contralateral quadrantanopia due to damage of the parietal radiations with sparing of the macular vision due to duplication in Meyer's loop fibers; 5+6 = homonymous hemianopia, typically with macular sparing, which results from the large representative area for central vision in the occipital lobe that is rarely completely disrupted with a posterior cerebral artery occlusion. (Reproduced with permission from Kandel ER, Schwartz JH, Jessell TM, Siegelbaum SA, Hudspeth AJ. *Principles of Neural Science*, 5th ED, New York, NY: McGraw-Hill; 2013. Figure 25-5, p. 561.)

Language Dysfunction

Mr. Brown also presents with expressive aphasia or the absence/disruption of verbal expression. **Aphasia**, which refers to language impairment, presents primarily in three forms: expressive, receptive, or global. Since the language centers are in the left hemisphere in most individuals, aphasia is usually associated with a left MCA stroke. In **expressive aphasia** (also called non-fluent aphasia), there is damage to **Broca's area** in the frontal lobe and the dorsal stream, as described in Chapter 7, that impedes the ability to form words. Patients will understand what is said to them and often can produce single words or simple phrases but not complete sentences (syntax disruption). Frustration often occurs, since they are aware of what they want to say but unable to say it. Often writing ability is intact but limited because of the associated hemiparesis. Expressive aphasia should not be confused with **dysarthria**, which is associated with paresis of the oral musculature secondary to damage to the primary motor cortex, resulting in speech that is difficult to understand because of poor oral musculature control. **Speech apraxia** can also result in poor speech formulation due to disruption of the motor planning process to produce speech but results from premotor cortex damage and not damage to Broca's area. **Receptive aphasia** (fluent aphasia) is associated with damage to **Wernicke's area** in the temporal lobe and the ventral stream; it is an impairment of not only the ability to understand what is said but also in the ability to create and monitor the verbalizations that are uttered. When we talk, we first must determine what we want to say and then listen to monitor the accuracy of what is verbalized. In receptive aphasia, the ability to select the right words and monitor one's speech is impaired, so although speech can be produced, it is likely gibberish. Plus, the survivor is unable to monitor their speech, so they are unaware that their utterance doesn't make sense. They also don't understand the listener's confusion with their statements. Frustration is, again, common. Finally, large strokes that impact both Broca's and Wernicke's areas or both the ventral and dorsal streams can result in a devastating loss of the function of both, referred to as **global aphasia**. Survivors of such a stroke are unable to understand or produce speech. A less common speech anomaly is **conductive aphasia**, which presents as an error in putting the syllables of words or the words within a phrase together (a phonological error). An example of such an error would be facemat or plantmat for placemat; the client is likely to make multiple attempts to select the right combination of syllables or words. This deficit has been historically thought to result from disruption of the arcuate fibers, connecting Wernicke's area with Broca's area; however, overlapping lesions within a small posterior aspect of the parietal lobe (posterior temporal region), which is a sight for sensory integration, may be the primary location of this aspect of speech (Figure 10-8).[6] Other abilities, associated with language, including writing (**agraphia/dysgraphia**) and reading (**acquired dyslexia or alexia**) can also be disrupted post-stroke. When the dysgraphia and dyslexia occur together, they are usually associated with damage to the left parietal lobe and can also be associated with aphasia. When alexia occurs without agraphia, it is most commonly associated with occipital lobe damage. It is always important to distinguish true agraphia and alexia from the consequences of aphasia.

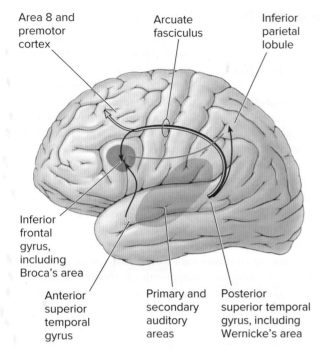

FIGURE 10-8 Areas of the cerebral hemisphere supporting language function. Regions of the temporal, parietal, and frontal lobes are linked via the arcuate fasciculus to support the complex components of language function, typically in the left hemisphere. (Reproduced with permission from Martin JH. *Neuroanatomy Text and Atlas*, 4th ED. New York, NY: McGraw-Hill; 2012, Figure 8-11 Left Side, p 195.)

Cognitive Dysfunction

Cognitive dysfunction is common post-stroke with an estimated incidence of 10–82%[7]; the incidence is greater in older survivors, and the outcome confounded by concurrent neural degeneration from Alzheimer's disease or other dementia (i.e., multi-infarct).[8] Specific cognitive deficits relate closely to the size and location of the lesion; however, the disruption of memory post-stroke appears to be much more complex. First, damage in the area of the hippocampus within the temporal lobe rarely occurs with any of the common stroke syndromes; however, this temporal region is highly connected to many other areas of the brain to support memory function. A decreased level of activity in the medial temporal lobe has been found to be associated with impaired short-term memory; it is thought that this change likely relates to a disruption of the networks of projections to that area, since no lesions were present in the temporal lobe. **Working** or **episodic memory**, which is important for many daily activities, including sensory discrimination, is most commonly affected.[9] Cognitive impairment post-stroke can be categorized as mild (subjective awareness of minor issues but with no effect on activities or participation), moderate (affects complex activities but not ADLs or routine activities), or severe (difficulties in all aspects of daily living). Despite the frequency of post-stroke cognitive deficits, they often go undiagnosed, and therefore, untreated due to the complexity of the post-stroke symptoms and the focus on recovery of sensorimotor function and activities of daily living. Even survivors that score within

the normal range on the Mini Mental exam© (a common test of orientation and memory) have been found to have some level of cognitive deficit when more comprehensive testing is conducted. Yet, early cognitive impairment has been found to persist with little improvement; in severe cases progression to dementia is likely.[8] Therapists should be aware of this and watch for the ability of clients to follow directions and retain information from one session to the next. If a problem is noted, referral to a psychologist for evaluation and treatment may be beneficial. Restructuring of the treatment sessions, focusing more on procedural rather than declarative knowledge, may facilitate the relearning of motor skills in those with severe cognitive dysfunction. However, there is a paucity of information on treatment methods that facilitate learning in those with post-stroke cognitive deficits, but therapists should borrow from the literature on Alzheimer's disease to structure their treatment activities.

● ACUTE MEDICAL MANAGEMENT OF STROKE

Ischemic Stroke

Initial medical management of stroke must include a comprehensive history; the most important component of this history is to determine the last moment that the client was neurologically normal, or in other words, to pinpoint the onset of stroke symptoms. This, along with careful clearing of exclusionary criteria, will determine the ability to use intravenous thrombolysis, such as recombinant tissue-type plasminogen activator (rTPA or TPA), to assist in clot breakdown. Exclusion criteria for TPA include current or previous cerebral hemorrhage (intracerebral or subarachnoid); prior stroke, head injury, or heart attack within 3 months; stroke associated seizure; uncontrolled high blood pressure; CT/MRI evidence that the stroke involves multiple lobes of the brain; and select laboratory findings (platelets ≤ 100,000 mm³; blood glucose ≤ 50 mg/dL). TPA is only effective if given within the first 4.5 hours post-stroke onset, preferably in the first 3 hours, so identification of the stroke onset is crucial for determining that critical application window. A CT or MRI is required to rule out intracranial bleeding prior to application; ischemic changes are typically not evident until at least 6 hours post-onset, so imaging at admission may not allow visualization of the hypoperfusion, characteristic of ischemic stroke. Sonothrombolysis (ultrasound facilitated thrombolysis) has been found to enhance the effects of TPA without increased risk and may be administered in some stroke centers. Since stroke and cardiac events often occur together, a 12-lead electrocardiogram (ECG) is recommended. When TPA is applied, antihypertensive control is delayed unless the systolic pressure exceeds 220 mmHg, and then, it is very slowly reduced by no more than 15% in the first 24 hours.[10]

Hemorrhagic Stroke

Brain hemorrhage is associated with a pooling of blood (hematoma) that results in cerebral edema and potentially hydrocephalus as debris and blood infiltrate the ventricles and impede/impair CSF flow and production. Loss of consciousness and breathing impairment are much more common with hemorrhagic stroke; therefore, it is more likely that intubation and mechanical ventilation are needed on ER admission. Post-stroke hypertension is also common with hemorrhagic stroke; again, the control of this hypertension remains controversial but is typically done in a conservative fashion with careful monitoring of intracranial pressure, mean arterial blood pressure, and systolic blood pressure. Elevated intracranial pressure frequently accompanies brain hemorrhage; thus, careful monitoring is also critical. Methods to reduce intracranial pressure, associated with hemorrhage, include elevation of the head of the bed by 30 degrees, administration of analgesics or sedatives, or hyperventilation (increasing CO_2 levels to 30–35 mmHg). Hemorrhage frequently occurs in individuals already receiving anticoagulant therapy and, thus, necessitates a reversal of the effect of the anticoagulant medications; although this includes discontinuation of the medication, other pharmacologic interventions are required to hasten the reversal of the anticoagulating effects.[11]

Measuring Stroke Severity

Physicians commonly assess stroke function in the acute period with the **NIH Stroke Scale (NIHSS)** or its modified version, the **mNIHSS**. The modified version was developed to eliminate components that were redundant or had demonstrated poorer reliability; it also rescaled the sensory component.[12] Both are used in the clinic (Table 10-3). On both scales, a zero is associated with normal function, and therefore, a lower total score is associated with better (more normal) function. It should be noted that survivors with very different stroke symptoms can obtain equivalent total scores, so the individual component scores will provide better clarity.

Other scales that may be used by medical professionals to describe stroke outcome include the Modified Rankin Scale and the Glasgow Outcome Scale. Both characterize outcomes, based on the level of disability. The **Modified Rankin** is a 6-point scale: 0 = no symptoms and 6 = death; the magnitude of disability is ranked in the intermediate scores (1 = symptoms with

TABLE 10-3	NIHSS versus mNIHSS Scales
NIHSS	**mNIHSS**

1. Consciousness
 	
    1a. General (0–3); alert – unresponsive
 	
    1b. Responds to 2 questions (0–3)
 	
        What month is it?
 	
        How old are you?
 	
    1c. Responds to 2 commands (0–3)
 	
        Open and close eyes
 	
        Grip and release with non-paretic hand
	Eliminated 1a; 1b and 1c are the same.

2. Gaze (0–3): normal, palsy, forced deviation	Gaze – Same
3. Visual (0–4): normal, partial hemianopia, complete hemianopia, bilateral hemianopia	Visual – Same
4. Facial palsy (0–3): normal – complete paralysis	Facial palsy – Excluded

5. Motor arm:
 	
    5a. – Left (0–4) Normal – no movement
 	
    5b. – Right (0–4) Normal – no movement
	Motor arm – Same

6. Motor Leg:
 	
    6a. – Left (0–4) Normal – no movement
 	
    6b. – Right (0–4) Normal – no movement
	Motor leg – Same

7. Limb ataxia (0–2): absent, 1 limb, 2 limbs	Ataxia – Excluded
8. Sensory (0–2): normal, mild–moderate, severe	Sensory modified (0–1): normal, abnormal
9. Best language (0–3): normal, mild–mod, severe, mute	Language – Same
10. Dysarthria (0–2): normal, mild–mod, severe	Excluded
11. Neglect (0–2): none, inattention, profound hemi-inattention	Neglect – Same
Total score = 0–45	Total score: 0–35

no significant disability, 2 = slight disability, 3 = moderate disability, 4 = moderate disability, and 5 = severe disability). The **Glasgow Outcome Scale** (GOS) is a similar 5-point scale: 1 = good recovery, 2 = moderate disability, 3 = severe disability, 4 = persistent vegetative state, 5 = death. Obviously, these are somewhat subjective ratings, and therefore, don't provide a clear picture of the individual stroke survivor.

Initial Stroke Outcomes

Of those admitted to an acute care hospital with a diagnosed stroke, about 20% will die from the initial event or a complication, and another 20% will return home. Of those returning home, some will have had a very mild stroke that won't require rehabilitation; others will require varying levels of care (nursing, therapy) either in the home or an outpatient facility. The remaining 60% will require admission to a second facility, either a skilled nursing facility (SNF) or an inpatient rehabilitation hospital or unit. Medicare policy designates that transfer to a rehabilitation unit can only be made if the survivor will soon be able or is able to participate in 3 hours of therapy (OT, PT, Speech) per day, 5–6 days per week, to qualify for coverage; other health insurance has largely adopted this policy as well. If the survivor is medically unstable or progressing too slowly for this level of treatment, transfer to a skilled nursing facility or home, with nursing and therapy at a lesser frequency, occurs. Subsequent admission to a rehabilitation facility can occur, if the survivor's stamina and recovery progresses to the level of meeting the 3 hours/day of treatment with further improvement likely. Inpatient rehabilitation typically lasts 15 days for post-stroke rehabilitation in the United States.[13] It should be noted that rehabilitation services (PT, OT, ST) are also provided in a SNF with a frequency that may approach that of a rehabilitation unit/hospital; however, the frequency and duration of treatment is matched to the tolerance level of the individual client.

● ACUTE NEUROPLASTICITY POST-STROKE

How does the Brain Try to Heal Itself in the First Hours/Days Post-stroke?

Neurologic insult, such as stroke, induces a cascade of events aimed at neural repair and return to homeostasis, often referred to as **spontaneous reorganization**. The initial impact of stroke is a loss of blood flow to the impacted areas with a central portion of cell death (**necrosis**), surrounded by an area of cell dysfunction known as the **penumbra**. Early reorganization focuses on reperfusion of surviving tissue in the penumbra, often through **angiogenesis** (small blood vessel or capillary proliferation), and an infiltration of inflammatory cells to begin the healing process; if reperfusion is unsuccessful, due to extensive blood vessel damage, there will be a spread of necrotic tissue into the penumbra. However, successful reperfusion is associated with removal of necrotic tissue, a decrease in edema, and receding inflammation infiltrates. There is a gradual stabilization of remaining functional neuronal networks. Yet, neuronal loss at the infarct site results in disruption of networks distant from the

actual infarct site, both those that project to the site and those to which the site projects. Thus, this cascade of events necessitates a dying back of lost neuronal axons as well as a change in synaptic organization at local and distant projection areas. These synaptic changes can include the unmasking of latent synapses; a proliferation of synaptic receptors, axon terminals, and dendritic branches; changes in membrane excitability; and changes in neurotransmitter production, release, reuptake, and/or degradation, resulting in enhanced or diminished activity within a synapse. It should be remembered that there are usually competing influences (excitatory or inhibitory) at any synapse. Reorganization is dependent on the activity of surviving neurons; thus, if only inhibitory neurons survive, these changes may result in exaggerated inhibition at a given synapse. Obviously, the opposite can occur in the presence of the survival of only excitatory projections. Optimal recovery is most likely dependent on a balance in remaining systems between inhibitory and excitatory projections.

● PHYSICAL THERAPY MANAGEMENT IN THE ACUTE CARE FACILITY

General Concepts

Mr. Brown is in the acute stage of recovery from stroke and the primary focus is on medical and physical issues related to saving his life. The therapy staff serves a dual role, in this early time point, focused on assessment and treatment for the acute phase of stroke as well as prevention of common complications that might impede full potential for recovery. The initial hospitalization for stroke typically lasts 24–72 hours with subsequent discharge to a skilled nursing facility, inpatient rehabilitation hospital/unit, or home.

It is important to keep the goals for long-term rehabilitation in mind even in the acute period. Studies have shown that early intervention is a key to long-term improvement. In addition, this focus on rehabilitation prevents **learned nonuse**. This concept originated from Taub's work (1994) with sensory deafferentation in monkeys, achieved through severing the dorsal roots to one upper limb. Following this procedure, he noted that the monkeys failed to use the limb despite the fact that their motor function remained intact; he coined the term "learned nonuse" for this phenomenon. Their initial clumsy movements, without sensory input, were unsuccessful in achieving the goal of the movement; as a result, the monkeys stopped using the limb. Taub hypothesized that this was similar to people post-stroke, when not only sensory input but also motor control is impaired; thus, when stroke survivors initially try to move, they are met with failure, and even as their motor ability improves, they may fail to use the arm in meaningful ways. To prevent learned nonuse, it is critical to incorporate active movement of the paretic limbs in all activities; to do so, activities need to be well conceived and appropriate assistance be provided to assure success.[14]

In an environment focused on efficient care that optimizes use of funds, there is a great deal of pressure to return patients to the setting with the lowest level of care, and if possible, home as quickly as possible. This means that therapists, in the acute care setting, must focus on returning the client to the highest level of independent function possible as quickly as they can. This early focus on return to function can result in an emphasis on compensatory treatment techniques. **Compensatory treatment techniques** are those that encourage use of the non-paretic extremity to perform functional tasks independently, while allowing the paretic extremity to be ignored. Teaching the client to eat and dress with the non-paretic hand and providing tools that allow return to function with only one hand are compensatory techniques for the UE. The use of walking devices that promote minimal weight-bearing on the paretic LE allow a gait pattern that is essentially using only the non-paretic LE, and thus, is a compensatory technique. Transfers that are done with the majority of weight born through the non-paretic LE are also compensatory. Early compensation has been shown to lead to learned nonuse and failure to recover use of the limb to its full potential. Therefore, the therapist must strike a balance between rehabilitation for the long-term benefit of the client and speedy return to function to allow a return to home or lower level of care. The therapist should keep in mind that they are the professional who is responsible for advocating for client's long-term rehabilitation potential. Research provides evidence that therapy in the acute stage can lead to better outcomes at the 1-year mark. Treatment plans shown to be effective focus on the following key objectives:

1. Assessment
2. Early Intervention and Prevention of Complications
3. Task-Oriented Practice
4. Intensive Repetitive Practice

The Assessment

The neurologic assessment, outlined in Chapter 9, should be followed for the acute client post-stroke. When strength testing, fatigue should be avoided and position changes minimized by completing all testing possible in each position,

before changing positions. [This principle can be continued once treatment is initiated to minimize position changes.] See Table 10-4 for a description of ROM and exercise suggestions by positions. Strength testing is usually initiated at the level of 3/5, testing to see if the individual can move the joint through the ROM against gravity. If not, then that joint is tested in a gravity eliminated position. If the joint can be moved through the full ROM antigravity, then resistance is added to determine the strength grade. Many individuals with CVA are bound in synergy patterns. Strength testing should not be done within synergy patterns. If the only movement is within a synergy, then a description of the strength should be noted but a numerical grade cannot be given.

Case Example

After determining that Mr. Brown is able to hear and see the therapist as well as understand instructions, strength should be assessed in the bed starting with AROM. To optimize Mr. Brown's ability to follow instructions, the therapist should stand on his left side so that he can both see and hear the therapist without interference due to the hemianopia. If Mr. Brown does not exhibit active dorsiflexion in supine or side-lying, he should then be placed in supine with the head of the bed elevated so that he can see his foot. When asked to dorsiflex his foot, while flexing the hip and knee, the therapist notes whether the ankle moves into dorsiflexion. This would be documented as "able to dorsiflex through full ROM against gravity within the flexor synergy." At times, dorsiflexion may not be noted until the client attempts to ambulate.

In those clients, who do not exhibit any active dorsiflexion during strength testing, be sure to begin ambulation by encouraging dorsiflexion and have someone palpate and carefully

TABLE 10-4	Joint Motions by Position for Use in Testing AROM and Doing Bed Exercises in the Acute Care Setting	
POSITION	**MOVEMENTS GRAVITY ELIMINATED**	**MOVEMENTS AGAINST GRAVITY**
Supine	Hip abduction Hip adduction Hip external rotation Knee flexion Knee extension Ankle dorsiflexion	Hip flexion Hip internal rotation Knee extension (hip flexed and leg supported on a pillow) Ankle dorsiflexion
Side-lying	Hip flexion Hip extension Hip internal rotation Knee flexion Knee extension Ankle dorsiflexion	Hip abduction Hip adduction Hip external rotation
Prone		Hip extension Knee flexion Ankle plantarflexion

observe the ankle to note any activity. Also, keep in mind, during the evaluation and early treatment sessions, that motions such as dorsiflexion, finger and wrist extension, and shoulder protraction are not strong parts of any of the synergy patterns but are commonly resisted by hypertonic muscles, often leading to more difficulty in activating and regaining use of these muscle groups. Special attention to these muscles, during evaluation and treatment, will be critical to assure recovery of function in these muscle groups. Also, to minimize position changes, keep in mind what position Mr. Brown will be placed in at the end of therapy and plan the session to finish in that posture.

Standardized outcome measures are an integral component of the examination and should be utilized in the acute care setting. This can be challenging as there are limited measures available for this setting. Measures that have been recommended by the Neurology Section of the APTA's Stroke EDGE task force are the 6-minute walk, 10-m walk, Functional Reach, Orpington Prognostic Scale, Postural Assessment Scale for Stroke Patients, and the Timed Up and Go. Additional measures that are appropriate for this setting can be found on the neurology section website at http://www.neuropt.org/go/EDGE.

BOX 10-1	Borg Exertion Scale[17]	
EXERTION DESCRIPTION	**BORG RATING**	**ACTIVITY EXAMPLES**
None	6	Sitting
Very, very light	7–8	Washing hands
Very light	9–10	Washing dishes
Fairly light	11–12	Leisurely walking
Somewhat hard	13–14	Brisk walking
Hard	15–16	Maintained exercise to elevate heart rate
Very hard	17–18	Sustained activity at highest level possible
Very, very hard	19–20	Extreme burst of activity at maximum capacity

Data from Borg G.A. Psychophysical bases of perceived exertion. Medicine and Science in Sports and Exercise. 1982; 14:377–381.

Case Example

Mr. Brown is not yet able to ambulate without assistance, so the measure most appropriate for him would be the Orpington Prognostic Scale and the Postural Assessment Scale for Stroke Patients. Utilizing the Orpington Prognostic Scale will assist the therapist and other team members in developing discharge goals based on his prognosis. Trunk control and posture are expected to improve during the acute care stay. The Postural Assessment Scale is an objective measure of trunk control and will be valuable in providing an objective measure of therapy progress. Other tools to consider would be the Fugl Meyer and the Trunk Impairment scale.

Early Intervention and Prevention of Complications

Individuals who suffer complications during the acute and sub-acute stages of recovery tend to have lower functional status at 1 year post CVA. Early activity and upright posture (sitting or standing) can prevent complications such as deep vein thrombosis, pulmonary emboli, pneumonia, and falls.[15] In addition to these risk factors, progression of the lesion has been found to occur in 11% of patients,[16] after leaving acute care, and this is one of the major predictors of a change to a lower level of functioning or death after discharge. Monitoring vitals and systematic progression of activity is particularly necessary to ensure patient safety during the acute and sub-acute phases of rehabilitation.

Based on the evidence and these considerations, Mr. Brown's vital signs (blood pressure, pulse and respiration rate) should be evaluated by the therapist, before, during, and after each session for signs of any abnormal response to activity such as a rapid rise in pulse, abnormal rise or fall in blood pressure, or new arrhythmia. Therapy should be mildly exerting, consistent with the Borg exertion scale (e.g. <12) (Box 10-1). During the acute stage, the goal is to get Mr. Brown sitting upright and working on active movement without stressing the cardiovascular system. Cardiovascular fitness training is not initiated until the sub-acute phase of rehabilitation.

The acute period focuses on preventing complications, including contractures, infections such as pneumonia, thrombi in the extremities, skin breakdown, and postural hypotension. Clients should be encouraged to move all of their joints through the full ROM, three to five times a day, to maintain tissue extensibility and prevent contracture. One session per day of passive range of motion exercises with a therapist is minimally effective in maintaining normal tissue extensibility. Encourage the patient, family, and all health care workers to assist the client in moving his extremities on a regular basis and at least three times a day.

Skin breakdown is prevented through frequent position changes (at least every 2 hours), proper positioning to prevent pressure areas (see Table 10-5), and maintenance of healthy, dry skin. Thrombi and postural hypotension are also prevented through active movement and frequent changes in position. Use of an upright posture, as soon as is medically possible, can prevent the occurrence of postural hypotension. If upright postures are not feasible, then active muscle contraction of the lower extremities encourages blood flow and reduces the risk of thrombi and hypotension. Activities that encourage deep breaths and increase the respiratory rate will assist in maintaining air flow throughout the lung tissue and are an effective means of preventing pneumonia. When doing activities with patients in the acute care setting, take time to instruct them to breathe deeply and monitor them to ensure that they are filling their lungs fully. Position changes that include upright postures of the trunk also assist in lung motility and prevent infections of

TABLE 10-5	Positioning in Bed for CVA: Need Images, Supine Needs to Show Ankle Supported in Neutral and Not Plantarflexed		
SUPINE		**SIDE-LYING ON INVOLVED SIDE**	**SIDE-LYING ON UNINVOLVED SIDE**
Keys to positioning			
Involved shoulder should be in midline for abduction and flexion			
Involved elbow, wrist, and fingers in extension			
Involved forearm in neutral or supinated			
Hips and knees slightly flexed			
Hip neutral for rotation and slightly abducted			
Involved foot on foot board or in orthotic to maintain neutral ankle and prevent from going into plantarflexion			
Place pillows or padding at joints where there are bony prominences			

TABLE 10-6	Common Areas of Hypertonicity and Synergy Patterns after CVA		
	HYPERTONIC MUSCLE GROUPS	**FLEXOR SYNERGY PATTERN**	**EXTENSOR SYNERGY PATTERN**
Upper extremity			
Shoulder	Scapula retractors Adductors Internal rotators Extensors	Flexion Adduction Internal rotation	Extension Adduction Internal rotation
Elbow	Flexors	Flexion	Extension
Forearm	Pronators	Supination	Pronation
Wrist	Flexors	Flexion	Weak extension
Fingers	Flexors	Flexion	Weak extension
Lower extremity			
Hip	Flexors Adductors	Flexion Abduction External rotation	Extension Adduction Internal rotation
Knee	Flexors	Flexion	Extension
Ankle	Plantar flexors	Dorsiflexion	Plantarflexion Inversion

the lung. Having the patient perform AROM as well as position changes throughout the day allows for intensive repetition during the acute phase of rehabilitation. The use of intensive repetition as a key to successful rehabilitation post stroke will be discussed in more detail when the sub-acute and chronic phases of rehabilitation are discussed.

Hypertonicity of muscles may lead to contractures in these muscle groups (Table 10-6), and thus, positioning and ROM activities should focus on elongating potentially hypertonic muscle groups in order to prevent contracture and improve long-term prognosis, especially the ankle plantarflexors and hip flexors. Plantarflexors should be closely monitored for tone, and if increased tone is noted, the feet should be placed on a foot board, in an ankle contracture boot or static foot drop orthosis to prevent plantarflexion contracture and promote good ankle movement for transfers and mobility. Hip extension beyond neutral is a key component of normal gait. During the acute and sub-acute stages of rehabilitation, clients typically spend most of their day positioned in hip flexion, since they are sitting or lying down much of the day. Therapy should be designed to include PROM and AROM into hip extension. This can be done in side-lying or prone positions.

Case Example

Mr. Brown should be encouraged to actively participate in all movements whether he is able to do the movement or not. The therapist should provide assistance as needed and encourage Mr. Brown to look at the extremity, while it is moving, and to think about how it feels. Sensory stimulation of rubbing or a firm touch can also augment his ability to sense the extremity and better focus on activating the muscles. Imagery and visualization are effective means of improving motor control and should be utilized with Mr. Brown in the acute stage, when he is least able to tolerate rigorous exercise programs but can tolerate these types of therapeutic regimens.

Task-Oriented Practice

Therapy should be meaningful and encourage the use of activities or tasks to retrain motor control. Early acute therapy, in the bed, should include active-assistive ROM to increase strength and motor control as well as initial rolling from supine to side-lying. Since AROM exercises are performed in both supine and side-lying, therapy should start with supine exercises and then move to side-lying where more exercises will then be performed. Intermingling strengthening exercises with functional activities minimizes unnecessary position changes and the impact of fatigue on therapy. Evidence shows that early trunk exercises such as bridging, rolling in supine, and seated pelvic tilts, reaching and balancing activities on unstable surfaces leads to improvement in not only trunk function but also standing balance and mobility in acute and sub-acute stroke.[20]

Case Example

If on initiating therapy, Mr. Brown is in supine and is not able to move the right extremities through the ROM against gravity, he should be encouraged to perform gravity eliminated shoulder and hip abduction in supine. The therapist should provide him with a sliding board or assist to minimize friction between the extremity and the bed. In supine, he can also be assisted into a bridge position and to perform active bridging with the therapist helping to keep the pelvis level and to facilitate gluteal activation on the right, as needed. Facilitation of the gluteals is usually accomplished by applying a quick firm pressure into the lateral buttock with the finger tips.

Rolling/Bed Mobility

Rolling is an activity that can provide a great deal of benefit to the acute care client. It allows them to become more independent in pressure relief and position changes. Any independent movement is helpful in giving acute stroke clients a feeling of regaining control over their body and their lives and can be emotionally uplifting. When teaching bed mobility, the client should be encouraged to actively participate at all times, even if they aren't able to provide meaningful help. The therapist should

choose key points for hand placement that minimize therapist contact but allow optimal assistance to areas that are most impaired. Typically, placing the hands at the shoulders and hips is most helpful for bed mobility training. In addition, passive positioning can be used to preposition the client so that they are able to perform the transfer with minimal assistance from the therapist. It should be noted that handling always changes the motor output of the client and should be minimized in any way feasible, while keeping safety as a top priority.

Case Example

Mr. Brown has been lying in supine for 2 hours; therefore, he should be placed in side-lying at the end of therapy to prevent skin breakdown due to pressure, especially given his diagnosis of prediabetes. He wishes to read or watch TV after therapy and would be better able to utilize the call button and manipulate books and TV controllers, if placed on his right side with his stronger left side unimpeded. Therapy would then begin with Mr. Brown being taught to assist in rolling from supine onto his left side and then performing gravity eliminated activities with the right UE and LE such as shoulder, elbow, hip and knee flexion and extension. Mr. Brown should be encouraged to actively roll, and the therapist should not provide any more assistance than is absolutely necessary. Positioning can be utilized to help Mr. Brown to obtain success with less therapist assistance, such as making sure that the right arm is flexed so that it does not end up trapped under the body and assisting Mr. Brown to cross his right leg over his left leg for rolling. The therapist can then place hands at shoulder and pelvis and assist Mr. Brown to use momentum to rock two times and then roll over on the third try. He should also be encouraged to use his head by turning it with the roll for additional momentum. He can then practice rolling back to supine and then rolling to the right side where he should be instructed as to where the call button, bed controls, and TV controller are located. Verify that he understands how to use them and position him appropriately in side-lying at the end of the treatment session (Table 10-5). Nursing should be told the time of the position change and what position he was placed in so that they know to reposition Mr. Brown within 2 hours.

Upright Activities

Once the client is cleared to begin upright activities, including transfers and gait, and is feeling able to participate in these activities, therapy should immediately initiate them; this typically occurs by day 2, barring extensive medical complications. See Box 10-2 on the use of imagery to facilitate movement and Box 10-3 for transfer and early gait activities. Arm function can be addressed in supine, side-lying, and sitting. Eccentric activation may be the easiest place to start for clients with profound weakness. To perform a low-level eccentric exercise for the

BOX 10-2 Motor imagery

Motor imagery is done by instructing the individual to visualize how it feels to do a specific task. The therapist can have them focus on certain aspects of the task such as visualizing how it feels to place equal weight through the feet for a sit to stand transfer or to bend forward with "nose over toes" during sit to stand. Studies have shown that adding motor imagery to conventional therapy can improve outcomes in post-stroke clients.[18] In order to ensure efficacy, the Motor Imagery Questionnaire RS should be used to ensure that the client is able to utilize imagery.[19] Some clients with poor sensory function have been found to have difficulty imagining motor movements, and therefore, would not be expected to respond to a motor imagery intervention. The benefit of motor imagery, in the acute stage of therapy, is that it provides an opportunity for intensive practice without adding physiologic demands and requires no additional time from the therapy staff.

BOX 10-3 Techniques for teaching transfers and gait in the acute setting

Keys to working on transfers

- Encourage the individual to be an active participant.
- The therapist should not provide any more assistance than is absolutely necessary.
- Positioning of the extremities in positions that lead into the movement can be utilized to help obtain success.

Supine to side-lying

- Utilize passive positioning to minimize therapist assistance: make sure that the bottom arm is flexed so that it does not end up trapped under the body; if moving onto the non-paretic side, cross the paretic leg over non-paretic leg to position for rolling (the client should be encouraged to assist with this positioning, as able).
- The therapist can then place hands at shoulder and pelvis to assist the client to use momentum to rock twice and then roll over on the third try.
- Encourage head turning with the roll for additional momentum.

Side-lying to sitting edge of bed

- Roll to side-lying facing the edge of the bed, using the techniques above.
- Drop the legs off of the side of the bed, once in side-lying. Encourage the client to use the non-paretic leg to assist in getting the paretic leg off of the bed but with as much active movement of the paretic leg as possible.
- To make the move from side-lying to sitting easier, the head of the bed may be placed in a slightly elevated position.
- Instruct to push on the bed with both arms as the legs are dropped over the edge of the bed.
- The therapist should provide assistance at the shoulder and pelvis only as needed.
- If the paretic arm is "on top," the therapist may wish to assist by placing the hand in a weight-bearing position

- The therapist then places a hand on the client's hand to stabilize it in weight-bearing and places their other hand on the posterior aspect of the elbow to encourage active weight-bearing through the paretic arm.

Sit to stand from bed

- First, ensure that the feet are both flat on the floor with the hips and knees flexed to 90 degrees (or elevate the bed and place with hips and knees in a less flexed posture to make the transfer easier).
- Both arms should be placed in a position of weight-bearing during the transfer to encourage active movement and provide proprioceptive input in the early stages of recovery.
- The bedside table can be utilized to provide a stable surface for weight-bearing through bilateral arms. Bedside tables allow you to start with the table at a lower level and raise the table, as the client comes to standing, and then, provide a stable surface for standing activities that allows for use of both arms.
- If there is reasonable function in the paretic hand, then, the client can push off of the bed with bilateral UEs and then place the hands on a walker. Unilateral assistive devices should not be used for standing activities, as they encourage learned nonuse of the involved UE and LE and do not promote equal weight-bearing bilaterally.

Early Gait Activities: Acute Care

- Equal weight-bearing and use of the paretic leg should be a focus at this stage in rehabilitation.
- During gait, devices that allow for use of bilateral UEs post-CVA are parallel bars, wheeled walkers with arm trough attached, and the bedside table.
- Early gait and standing activities should focus on upright trunk control, encouraging use of the paretic limbs, during gait, and use of a step through pattern bilaterally.
- Therapist assistance with the paretic extremities can be provided, as needed, to advance the leg and brace the extremities for weight-bearing support.
- Regardless of ability, the client should attempt to actively take part in all movements to encourage recovery of movement, even in flaccid extremities.

elbow extensors, place the client in supine with the shoulder in 90 degrees of flexion and the elbow extended. The therapist supports the arm to prevent elbow flexion and instructs the client to slowly lower their hand to their mouth. The therapist provides assistance to slowly lower the hand and can provide sensory stimulation over the triceps to assist the client in developing an active contraction of this musculature. This activity allows the client to visualize the movement within a meaningful task; plus, the eccentric contraction, whichslows the descent of the arm, will typically be regained prior to the ability to perform concentric activation of the muscle. Once the client successfully achieves an eccentric contraction, it is likely that they would be ready to progress to gravity eliminated active movements.

Case Example (day 2)

The order of activities practiced should be based on where Mr. Brown is when therapy begins (lying or sitting in bed) as well as his goals. Transfer activities, including supine to sit and back, come to sit on the edge of the bed, and sit to stand, are initiated first and followed by early ambulation activities. In this case, we know that Mr. Brown has a wife to assist him at home and has set a goal of returning to his home. Therefore, assisted transfers and gait are reasonable goals for discharge from acute care. Given his moderate paresis of the arm and leg, he is likely to initially require moderate to maximal assistance for upright activities. Having a second person to assist, on the first day of upright activities, would allow for the incorporation of more challenging activities. Mr. Brown would begin this session by working on supine to sit on the edge of the bed (Table 10-7). To prevent learned nonuse, Mr. Brown should be instructed to try to use his right arm and leg for all activities. If he cannot use the extremity, the therapist should position it in weight-bearing and assist in holding the limb so that Mr. Brown uses it appropriately throughout all activities. Additionally, he should be directed to be aware of his paretic limbs through sensory inputs such as looking at the extremities and sensory cues such as light touch and/or pressure applied by the therapist.

Remember that during the acute stage of recovery, it is important to focus on preventing learned nonuse. This is accomplished by focusing on appropriate weight-bearing bilaterally, during all activities, and incorporating the paretic extremities into all activities. While canes and hemi-walkers provide the most viable assistance for functional ambulation on return to home, these devices do not function as the most appropriate assistive device for retraining a normal gait pattern. Utilizing devices that require or allow for bilateral UE support encourages equal weight-bearing and involves the paretic UE and LE in functional activities. During therapy, devices such as a wheeled walker with an arm trough, parallel bars, or the bedside table should be used to encourage use of bilateral UEs in equal weight-bearing. Discharge timing and location will determine when it is necessary to teach the individual to utilize a unilateral device, such as canes and hemi-walkers. These devices should not be introduced until it is necessary for return to independent function, such as a discharge to home, for a higher functioning client, as they utilize a compensatory method of gait training rather than rehabilitating the client to optimal long-term function. A short session with these devices at the end of each therapy session could be used to ensure that the client will be able to use a unilateral device for function, while focusing the majority of therapy time on bilateral UE weight-bearing with equal step length. The therapist should strike a delicate balance between the need to quickly move the client to independence in function and the need to rehabilitate for optimal neuroplasticity and full potential functional recovery. See Box 10-4 for key rehabilitation principles. The challenge for therapists is functioning within the health care environment, while focusing on what is in the best interest of the client, who is s/p CVA. Compensatory techniques achieve fast results for return to function but impede neuroplasticity and full recovery of function.

TABLE 10-7	Bed Mobility and Trunk Activities
POSITION	**ACTIVITY**
Supine: feet flat, hips and knees flexed	Bridging – if weak the therapist can assist on the weak side. Therapist can also provide sensory cueing to the gluteals to assist in activating the musculature. • Purpose: Strengthen trunk and hip musculature
Supine going to side-lying	Reach with arm in direction of roll • Purpose: Strengthens flexors of the trunk Pull on bedrail with UE • Purpose: Strengthens shoulder girdle musculature and biceps
Side-lying	Pelvic tilts • Purpose: Gravity eliminated trunk and hip musculature strengthening
Sitting edge of bed	Therapist pushes on the client at the shoulders while client works to maintain sitting balance. Therapist should provide pushes in the anterior, posterior, and side to side planes. • Purpose: Isometric coactivation of postural trunk musculature for stabilization Reaching up and down and side to side in front of body. Always have client reach for something such as a cup or other object as this encourages the neural system to activate the hand. • Purpose: Strengthens trunk musculature, reaching higher activates trunk extensors, reaching to the side activates the trunk rotators Reach laterally on bed • Purpose: Strengthens the muscles for trunk side-bending Place hand on ball and roll ball away from body and back toward body using either arm • Purpose: Provides support during trunk activities for individuals with balance problems or extremely weak trunk musculature

BOX 10-4 Keys to Rehabilitation of Function

1. Begin by making the task less physically demanding and within the ability level of the client by doing things such as
   a. Placing the extremity in a gravity eliminated position or raising seat heights for transfers
   b. Progression involves making the task more physically demanding until the client is doing the task as it occurs in the natural environment
   c. Adding variability to task practice will strengthen the learning process and make it more generalizable to "real-life" situations
2. Begin by using the task that demands the movement pattern you are training and does not allow for success with compensatory patterns, such as
   a. When training sit to stand with a focus on weight-bearing through the paretic leg, seating the client on an elevated surface will lower the physical demands and improve the likelihood of success; also, placing a soft object such as an egg carton under the **non-paretic** foot will further force weight-bearing through the paretic leg.
   b. To progress the task, change the set up to increasingly allow more choice by the client. For example: in the scenario above, the goal is to work on weight-bearing with the paretic leg by restricting the ability to weight bear through the non-paretic extremity. Progressions would allow the client more choice as to how much weight to bear through the paretic limb. One progression might be:
      i. Egg carton under non-paretic foot – forcing weight-bearing on paretic leg
      ii. Use of an assistive device such as a pole or table on the paretic side – forces the client to lean over the paretic side with some weight-bearing through the non-paretic leg
      iii. Use of an assistive device such as a pole or table in front of the client – allows the client to choose how much weight to bear on each leg. The goal is to have equal weight-bearing through the legs.

Assistance Levels

When documenting, it is important to accurately depict the amount of assistance required by the client during each activity. The appropriate method for identifying level of assistance is described in Chapter 9. The key to good therapy practice is to first and foremost set up the practice session in a way that ensures patient safety. A goal is to minimize the amount of help that the therapist has to provide and to optimize active involvement of the patient. For Mr. Brown to work on a sit to stand transfer it would be ideal to start from an elevated plinth with a firm surface. The plinth would be elevated to a level that enables Mr. Brown to do the sit to stand transfer with as little help as possible, ideally CGA. Since his right arm remains paretic, it should be incorporated into the transfer by placing it in a position of weight-bearing, both during the transfer and once standing.

Case Example

Mr. Brown comes to sitting on the edge of the bed with instruction and moderate assist of the therapist. He, then, works on his sit to stand transfer and standing balance using the bedside table for bilateral UE support. With a gait belt on and a wheelchair close at hand, he can attempt a few steps, using the bedside table as a wheeled walking device. The bedside table is beneficial for these activities, at this stage, because its height can be rapidly changed as Mr. Brown goes from sit to stand and returns to sitting from standing. Another option is the wheeled walker. Mr. Brown's hand can be placed on the walker and assisted to grasp by the therapist. He can then walk with the therapist helping to guide the walker and to advance his right leg. Ambulation should be initiated by having Mr. Brown take a step with his non-paretic (left) leg so that he immediately assumes weight-bearing on the paretic, right leg. This also places his right hip in extension, which will facilitate initiation of stepping (swing) on the right. The main peripheral drives for activating the gait pattern generator involve hip extension, during stance, and alternately loading and unloading the lower limbs. Since Mr. Brown is being discharged to a rehabilitation unit in 2 days, it is determined that ambulation with the wheeled walker is the most appropriate course of action for optimizing neuroplasticity and return to function. If he were returning home, gait training would be broken into two parts (1) gait with the walker to work on relearning an appropriate and functional gait pattern and (2) gait with a hemi-walker or cane to learn a functional gait for use in the home environment with his wife.

CASE A, PART II

Mr. Brown was transferred to the Rehabilitation Hospital on his fourth day post-stroke. His intake reveals mild spasticity developing in his ankle plantarflexors with 3/5 strength in quads, hams, and hip flexors, 2/5 strength in dorsiflexors, plantarflexors, and gluts. His arm has 1/5 strength in most muscles with moderate subluxation (grade 2) of the shoulder. Expressive aphasia persists, but he is able to utter single word responses to some questions. He is able to come to sitting at bedside, by rolling to his left and pushing up with left arm, and performs a standing pivot transfer into the wheelchair with minimal assistance. Weight-bearing is asymmetrical, but he is able to stand, using a quad cane, and walked 12' × 2 with moderate assist of 1, during his first treatment session.

Spasticity: What Is It and How Is It Medically Managed?

Spasticity is a sign of an upper motor neuron lesion and presents as both an increase in muscle tone (**hypertonia**) and exaggeration of tendon reflexes (**hyperreflexia**). Hypertonia in spasticity is a resistance to stretch that is velocity dependent, which means the faster you stretch, the greater the resistance to that stretch. This is referred to as the **tonic stretch reflex**. The cause of spasticity has received extensive research and is ongoing; however, there are multiple components at both the neurological and muscular levels. First, loss of corticobulbar projections results primarily in a loss of inhibitory control within the brainstem, creating some degree of unopposed excitation in remaining neural networks. This unopposed excitation has historically been referred to as a **release phenomenon**. The pontine reticular formation's descending pathway is known to facilitate upper extremity flexion (shoulder adductors and flexors, biceps, and wrist and finger flexors) and lower extremity hip flexors, hamstrings, and ankle plantarflexors. This facilitation is typically balanced by corticobulbar (cortex to medullary reticular formation) and corticospinal (cortex to the alpha motor neuron) inhibitory control and facilitation of opposing muscles via motor neurons in the spinal cord. Following stroke, corticospinal and corticobulbar fibers are often damaged. Thus, the reticulospinal fibers are "free" to produce unopposed excitation of the respective muscles in the extremities, leading to low-level muscle fiber contraction that is perceived as increased resting muscle tone. This hypertonia is accompanied by hyperreflexia of both the tonic and phasic stretch reflexes in spasticity. The **phasic stretch reflex** is the monosynaptic reflex, often referred to as a tendon reflex or tendon "jerk," and elicited by tendon tapping that activates Ia fibers from the muscle spindle that synapse directly on alpha motor neurons in the spinal cord, eliciting a quick responsive muscle contraction of the associated muscle. Hyperreflexia of the phasic stretch reflex also results from the loss of inhibitory influences, not in the brainstem, but in the synaptic junction between muscle spindle Ia fibers and alpha motor neurons. This allows the reflex activation to occur without descending inhibition (Figure 10-9). Whether or not spasticity develops and the magnitude of the spasticity, when it occurs, appears related to the location of the lesion and the degree of corticospinal and corticobulbar fiber damage; rehabilitation programming that focuses on recovery of isolated muscle function is important to maximize functional recovery and minimize spasticity development.[21]

Twenty to thirty percent of stroke survivors with hemiparesis will develop spasticity with onset typically in the first 3 months post-stroke.[18] In only about 4% of survivors is the spasticity severe. Spasticity is commonly measured by the original Ashworth Scale or modified Ashworth Scale as described in Chapter 9. Although changes in neuronal activity are a primary influence in spasticity development, spasticity is also associated with changes in the muscle. These changes include loss of sarcomeres, infiltration of the muscle with collagen, changes in muscle fiber type, especially the ratio of fast to slow twitch muscle fibers, and thereby, changes in the contractility and passive elasticity of muscle fibers. There is much debate over the relationship between the neurologic changes and the muscular changes, especially as to whether the neurologic changes induce the muscular changes, but this has yet to be determined. Neither the Ashworth nor the Modified Ashworth Scale effectively

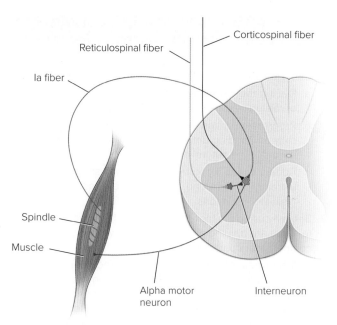

FIGURE 10-9 Illustration of hypertonia and hyperreflexia mechanisms. Loss of upper motor neuron fibers within the corticospinal tract removes inhibition from the reflex circuit within the spinal cord, creating increased excitability of the alpha motor neuron to Ia fiber activation. Further upstream, loss of corticobulbar fibers to the brainstem allows a net increase in facilitation to the monosynaptic reflex circuit from reticulospinal neurons, primarily through interneurons within the ventral horn. It should be noted that both inhibitory and excitatory interneurons are located within the ventral horn to modulate reflex activity. These interneurons are activated by many descending motor systems (corticospinal, reticulospinal, vestibulospinal), but when a stroke damages both corticospinal and corticobulbar fibers, the hypertonia that emerges seems driven by reticulospinal influences on alpha motor neurons to upper extremity flexors and lower extremity extensors. Secondary changes in muscle fibers emerge over time because of changes in innervation and contribute to the hypertonia and hyperreflexia seen, especially in more severe stroke.

distinguishes the neural contribution from the muscle contribution to spasticity.

PHYSICAL THERAPY MANAGEMENT IN THE REHABILITATION SETTING

During the first few days in the rehabilitation setting, clients are often still in the acute stage of recovery. This means that they remain medically fragile and easily fatigable, adding to the challenge of achieving optimal function in the short time frame that is reimbursable. Neuroplasticity remains a crucial element of the recovery process and must be considered alongside the pressures to regain independence in order to send the client to home or a lower level of care. Rehabilitation is focused on relearning functional tasks with impairments addressed within the practice of the functional tasks, when possible, and if not, then separately. It is often reasonable for clients to work on impairment level therapy tasks on their own, such as ROM and strengthening exercises.

Intensive Practice: Upper Extremity

Based on evidence from both basic science and clinical studies, learned nonuse is a negative outcome of poor rehabilitation of individuals post-stroke; it is recommended that early therapy encourage meaningful use of the paretic UE, which is often more impaired than the LE. Again, the paretic arm should be included in all activities and compensatory techniques should be avoided. In the case of a flaccid UE, the therapist should place it in a position of weight-bearing and then support it throughout transfers and gait so that weight is born as it would normally be, during all functional activities. In addition, the client should be encouraged to try to actively move the extremity during all PROM activities. An essential component of early therapy is to provide assistance as needed but no more than needed. In this way, the client experiences success in completing meaningful, active movement. Passive movement without actively engaging the client has not been shown to result in return of active movement to the paretic arm.

The intended use of the hand shapes the activation of the musculature throughout the UE. If a client is to perform a reaching task, they must have a meaningful end goal for the hand in order to appropriately shape UE movement. If the intent is to do an open handed push or slap, such as giving a high five, the activation patterns will be much different than if the end goal is to pull a thumbtack from a bulletin board. A high five involves hand and finger opening and primarily gross-motor control of the arm, while pulling out the thumbtack requires fine-motor control of the fingers and little to no finger extension. The force output and coordination required of these two tasks also differ with one being a highly coordinated, low force movement while the other allows for more error in both force production and aim of the hand. Clients who lack finger extension can benefit from performing reaching tasks with an end goal of grasping a large object that requires finger extension in order to grasp it successfully, such that hand opening is a natural goal of the movement. This encourages neural reorganization to recover the function of hand opening. The task should be relatively easy, and the therapist can assist with finger closing periodically to allow for positive reinforcement. A task-oriented approach focused on performance of normal daily activities with the paretic hand can be highly beneficial and encourages neuroplasticity as well as functional return. Tasks should be chosen that are meaningful to the client and that involve movements that are feasible for the client but have not yet been mastered. The physical demands can be altered to enhance performance, such as placing the hand on a smooth table to practice elbow flexion/extension, during a reaching task in a gravity eliminated position. This positioning also minimizes the degrees of freedom by supporting the arm such that the shoulder and trunk musculature do not have to provide this

---

BOX 10-5	**Keys to rehabilitation of the UE**

1. The hand shapes the activation of the entire UE
2. Use meaningful tasks
3. Lower physical demands by
   a. Placing the extremity in a gravity eliminated position for the key musculature
   b. Provide support to the trunk and proximal musculature to minimize degrees of freedom and focus on one joint motion
4. Choose functional tasks that will produce the movements that are the focus for that client's therapy session. Examples:
   a. For hand opening, have them reach for a 12-ounce soda can or small ball to encourage finger and wrist extension with a goal of lifting a relatively light object. This activity can also focus on the use of elbow extension in combination with shoulder flexion (moving out of synergy patterns).
   b. For coordination, have the individual reach for a small target and push on it.
   c. For fine motor control, have the client reach for a small object and remove it and then place it in another location. Example: remove thumbtack from bulletin board and place in small container for storage.

---

support. See Box 10-5 for a summary of the keys to rehabilitation of the UE.

Bilateral training is another method that is successful in returning function to the UE after CVA. This type of therapy involves performing the same task with both hands at the same time but independently. Both fine motor and gross motor tasks can be utilized during bilateral training.

This method is thought to normalize interhemispheric inhibition and improve lesioned hemisphere activity. Many tasks can be practiced in this manner, such as stacking blocks, erasing a blackboard, flipping cards. It has been found to improve both ipsilesional and contralesional arm function.[22,23]

The use of **functional electrical stimulation (FES)** has also been shown to be helpful. One study utilized the FES on the wrist extensors during bilateral wrist extension activities and demonstrated functional return of active wrist extension.[24] Similarly, **mirror activitie**s may benefit UE recovery. Mirror activities involve placing the non-paretic hand in a box with a two-way mirror and the paretic hand is placed alongside the mirror. The client moves the non-paretic hand, while looking at the mirror. The mirror makes it appear as though the paretic hand is moving. The key to all of these therapeutic activities is that they involve active participation of the client in attempting to move the paretic UE in a meaningful way.

Intensive Practice: Gait

As the client stabilizes, it now becomes feasible to focus on the concept of intensive practice for gait. Intensive practice is well supported by the literature and means a high number of repetitions are required to learn or relearn a skill. The literature on constraint induced therapy and treadmill training lead us to believe that the number of repetitions needed is in the range of hundreds to thousands. This number can be difficult to achieve using traditional therapy methods. Delivery that occurs only when the therapist is present limits the total time spent practicing the skill as well as the number of repetitions that can be feasibly accomplished. Therefore, clinicians and researchers have been investigating methods for providing practice opportunities on a frequent basis throughout the day. One very effective means of doing this is to utilize a team approach such that each team member knows how the client performs motor skills and activities of daily living. In this way, the client will be performing the learned tasks in the same manner, no matter who is with him, so that every repetition practices the correct and most beneficial means of doing the task. If the client is allowed to do tasks in an inappropriate manner, using poor motor control or only the non-paretic extremity, then, they will end up doing many more repetitions of the wrong technique than of the prioritized technique emphasized in therapy. Therefore, it is imperative that skills be practiced not only in therapy, but also when outside of therapy, in order to ensure that the number of repetitions of correct motor patterns exceeds the repetitions of incorrect motor patterns.

Another method of gait training that allows for intensive practice is **treadmill training** with a harness. Utilizing a treadmill with a harness can minimize therapist assistance and allow for gait training with fewer staff. The treadmill also allows for the consistent practice of a symmetrical gait over hundreds and thousands of repetitions. The harness can be used for body weight support (BWS), if the client has difficulty maintaining upright posture without assistance. Relatively few studies have examined the benefits of BWS treadmill training in the acute–sub-acute phase of recovery, for individuals who require assistance from a therapist to ambulate, but, in the few studies that have provided early body-weight supported treadmill training, a positive benefit has been reported.[25-27] Studies in spinal cord injury and stroke indicate that treadmill training should be augmented with or rapidly progressed to over-ground gait training due to the impact of task-specific training parameters (Box 10-6). The LEAPS trial provides evidence that, once an individual can ambulate independently with a device, it can be equally effective to train gait over-ground. In addition, studies into neuroplasticity indicate that the impact of treadmill training on neuronal changes differs between individuals in the acute stages and those further into the sub-acute stage of recovery. Combined, these findings further support the need to retrain a reciprocal and symmetrical gait pattern early in the recovery process.

Case Example

Mr. Brown is ambulating over-ground with a quad cane and moderate assist of one person. This does not afford him intensive practice of gait nor does it allow or promote a reciprocal gait pattern. It may be that Mr. Brown would be a good candidate for treadmill training to allow for more repetitions of a reciprocal gait pattern with less therapist support. He could continue to practice over-ground gait after each treadmill session, and as his gait and distance improves, he would be weaned off of the treadmill and onto a more task-oriented over-ground gait training program.

Both over-ground and treadmill training should focus on a reciprocal gait pattern that involves fully loading and unloading the paretic limb as well as taking a full step length; this will allow swing to be initiated from a position of hip extension. The treadmill is a very effective means of encouraging equal weight-bearing, symmetrical stepping, and the use of hip extension at terminal stance. Research has shown that the gait pattern generator is triggered when these components are present. When doing over-ground training, it is suggested that early in the training process these components can be facilitated by instructing the client to take the first step with the non-paretic limb. A step, large enough to place the non-paretic foot in front of the paretic foot, should be encouraged to facilitate loading of the paretic limb and an extended hip position just prior to swing. This would activate the gait pattern generator, which will further assist in achieving a reciprocal gait pattern. Any assistance provided should be kept to a minimum and faded as quickly as possible. FES can also be beneficial during gait training. It can be used to assist with any muscle group but is most commonly utilized on the tibialis anterior, often during both over-ground and treadmill-based gait training. Mr. Brown has significant weakness in his right dorsiflexors and would be a candidate for the use of FES on the tibialis anterior, during gait training.

Case Example

Clients should be encouraged to self-assess their performance and correct errors, based on this assessment. Mr. Brown has significant expressive aphasia, which would make it difficult for him to describe his performance to his therapist. This does not mean that he cannot perform self-assessment. He should be instructed to think about how the motor task felt and then asked some yes/no questions about his performance such as: "do you think you were putting equal weight on your right and left legs?" It may be appropriate to say something like, "that seemed to take a lot of effort, do you think you can do it in a way that would be less effortful?" If Mr. Brown indicates he is able to identify the difficulties in the activity, then, have him try again and watch

BOX 10-6	Parameters for Treadmill Training in the Post-stroke Population

- Start with an initial velocity of 0.25 m per second and 30% BW in non-ambulatory patients.[28]
- Treadmill speed should be increased incrementally as soon as possible
- Body weight support should be reduced incrementally as soon as possible

to see if he makes appropriate modifications. If he does not appropriately modify his movement, it would be appropriate to provide feedback as to what you are seeing and how to perform the activity in a way that will result in better overall coordination and motor control. A common example would be that Mr. Brown may be attempting to transition from sit to stand with most of his weight on his left leg, while reaching for the assistive device with his left hand. After self-assessing, he places his left hand on the chair and pushes off from the chair with this hand but continues to place most of his weight over the left leg. The therapist would then tell him, "that was good that you used your arm to push up from the chair, this time also use your right arm to push and try to also stand up on your right leg." Mr. Brown's communication could be augmented with the use of a writing pad and a picture board so that he can point to pictures, depicting common areas of communication, such as a restroom and food. If the client has receptive aphasia demonstration is the most appropriate method of instruction.

Another method, for enhancing time to practice, and therefore, intensity of practice, is the use of group therapy. This can be effective, if common pitfalls are avoided. The common pitfalls are allowing individuals to practice a task using poor technique or compensatory strategies and failure to adequately supervise for safety. It is important that the leader be trained to watch for and identify errors and to intervene, by pointing these errors out to the client and assisting him in correcting them. Group therapy should not replace individual therapy time, as clients require one on one time to develop the skills necessary to effectively practice skills before performing them in a group setting. Safety must be ensured for all clients in the group. If adequate staffing is not provided for the task practiced, this can result in unsafe situations or limited practice for members of the group that are unable to perform all skills, due to safety concerns.

Task-Oriented Therapy: Gait

Over-ground gait training should include training to maneuver around obstacles, walk on different surfaces (rough, smooth, soft, hard, sloping), change speeds, and perform dual tasks (talking, carrying something). The use of task-oriented gait training can assist in promoting a more normal gait pattern. This task-oriented approach works by encouraging the client to solve the motor problem while minimizing assistance and feedback from the therapist. It is also meaningful in that everyday tasks that the client wishes to perform, after returning home, are utilized for this training process. Suggested task-oriented activities for gait and transfers are given in Table 10-8 and an example therapy session is described in Box 10-7.

After UMN injury, it is common for individuals to have difficulty with dual-tasking, such as walking while talking. To reintegrate into the community, the individual needs to be able to not only walk and talk at the same time but also to walk while reading directions on a map or carrying and manipulating objects. Studies have noted that the ability to dual-task often remains impaired after formal rehabilitation has ended. To regain and improve this skill, therapy should incorporate activities that involve dual-tasking, such as carrying a cup of water while transferring and ambulating, walking and talking, and reading signs and navigating while walking. There are several outcome measures given in the appendix that are designed to assess dual-tasking skill, and these should be used to determine if there is a deficit in this area and to assess for mastery at the end of therapy.

Assistive Devices

The use of devices with wheels allows for a more normal step-through gait pattern. Studies utilizing treadmill training have demonstrated the importance of practicing gait with a step-through pattern to allow for the hip to go into extension just prior to swing. This positioning is a trigger to initiating swing, even in spinalized animals.

Case Example

If you are not able to keep Mr. Brown's hand on the walker, the use of a wheeled walker with a trough may be necessary. It may be sufficient to place his hand on the walker with the therapist's hand over it to hold it in place. The therapist can then assist in guiding the walker. Pushing the wheelchair can provide good support that is heavier and won't tip over.

Unilateral devices such as the cane and hemi-walker encourage a compensatory gait pattern with minimal weight-bearing and a shortened stance phase on the paretic side; usually, a step-to gait pattern is used. This pattern is not normal, and thus, could negatively impact neuroplasticity, during this early stage of recovery. The more time the client spends utilizing a gait pattern that encourages use of the paretic limb, the more likely the client is to recover to their full potential. If the client is able to use a unilateral device independently, they may do so in their room, but this does not preclude the use of bilateral devices during therapy to retrain gait with a more symmetrical gait pattern.

Another common issue is the lack of dorsiflexion and ensuing foot drop during gait. This can be successfully managed with an orthotic device. Caution should be used in providing an orthotic device too early in the rehabilitation process as this too could impede neuroplasticity and full recovery of function. If the ankle is fully supported in dorsiflexion, then the normal triggers to activate the dorsiflexors are removed, and this may result in learned nonuse of this muscle group. The use of an ace-wrap can provide a low-cost alternative that enhances safety and the ability to work on ambulation, while allowing normal sensory and neural inputs to the ankle musculature. Individuals, wearing ace-wraps to assist in maintaining dorsiflexion, still sense the need to activate the dorsiflexors and can still fire both the dorsi- and plantar-flexor muscle groups. An additional issue, related to orthotic prescription, is reimbursement. Once an orthotic has been purchased, the client is no longer eligible to receive insurance reimbursement for a new orthosis for an extended period of time (at present it is 2 years). It is highly likely that the client will continue to make rapid and meaningful changes in strength,

BOX 10-7 Circumduction Gait Pattern

One type of common gait deviation occurs when there is difficulty advancing the foot, typically due to a foot drop, resulting from lack of activation of the dorsiflexors. This often results in a circumduction gait pattern. If there is 2/5 or greater strength in the dorsiflexors and a 3/5 or greater strength in the hip flexors, the use of small obstacles can provide a means of eliciting dorsiflexion in stepping over the obstacle, rather than circumduction, and facilitating neural reorganization to achieve a more normal gait pattern. Another activity, to address circumduction, is to place a long low board in front of the client such that they have to step over the board with their involved LE, repeating for as many consecutive steps as necessary to change the pattern. The board should be long enough that it will block circumduction. The height of the board will encourage the use of hip, knee, and ankle flexion to clear the board. By using this technique the client has to problem solve how to get over the board and the task has been constrained in such a way as to block the use of abnormal movement patterns and only allow the motor pattern that the therapist wishes to retrain. Table 10-8 lists a number of common gait deviations and some examples of tasks that can be utilized to encourage use of a more functional and appropriate motor pattern for that task.

TABLE 10-8 Task-Oriented Approaches to Training Transfers and Gait Post-CVA

ACTIVITY	MOVEMENTS ENCOURAGED	MOVEMENTS DISCOURAGED
Transfers		
Transfer sit to stand with an egg carton or other "soft" object under the uninvolved LE	Weight-bearing on the paretic LE	Unilateral weight shift onto the non-paretic side
Transfer sit to stand with a bedside table in front and utilized for bilateral UE weight-bearing	Equal weight-bearing in bilateral UEs and LEs Forward weight shift for transfer initiation	Discourages posterior weight shift when straightening up to stand
Transfer sit to stand with a pole positioned in front and to the paretic side with both hands on the pole, non-paretic hand holding paretic hand on pole	Forward weight shift for transfer initiation Weight shift to the involved side Weight-bearing on involved LE Upright trunk, position hands high on pole to get upright trunk	Discourages posterior weight shift when straightening up to stand
Gait		
Walking while repetitively stepping with the paretic LE over a low board that extends 12" laterally	Swing with hip, knee, and ankle flexion Facilitates dorsiflexion	Swing with abduction as the primary means of advancing the leg
Walking up a slope	Hip flexion – to advance the leg Dorsiflexion – to clear the ground Muscle activity is increased in the hip, knee, and ankle extensors to propel the body uphill	Knee hyperextension
Walking down a slope	Knee extensors Encourages trunk extension to hold the person upright Requires eccentric gluteal activation and can increase strength in these muscles Also requires eccentric activation of the dorsiflexors to control for foot slap and can be used to strengthen these muscles	
Repetitively stepping over small objects with the non-paretic LE	Weight-bearing on the paretic LE	Decreased stance on the paretic LE
Walking with the paretic side next to a wall	Encourages the use of hip flexion for swing	Discourages circumduction for swing
Walking on uneven and soft surfaces	Encourages dorsiflexion Challenges balance	

ROM, tone, and function for weeks to months after discharge from the rehabilitation setting. This is likely to lead to the need to obtain a different orthosis than was indicated in the rehabilitation setting. Therefore, every attempt should be made to wait as long as possible to obtain a definitive ankle orthosis so that the client will be encouraged to make optimal progress in rehabilitation of this musculature and, thus, assure the appropriate insurance coverage to assist in purchasing their final, optimal orthotic that matches their long-term functional abilities.

Spasticity: Medical Management in the Chronic Phase

Chronic spasticity is a challenge to manage and may be unresponsive to physical therapy intervention. For those with localized spasticity in one or a few muscles/joints, they may benefit from **botulinum toxin** (**botox**) intramuscular injections; the most common type of botox used is Botulinum Toxin Type A,[29] which has several varieties. These injections are applied within the involved muscle and have a relatively localized effect; therefore, botox is not recommended when spasticity is widespread. Botox works by disrupting the release of acetylcholine, the neurotransmitter at the neuromuscular junction, which diminishes both tonic and phasic motor reflexes and, thereby, reduces spasticity. Changes in sensory neuron excitability, following injection, is thought to also have upstream implications, in the spinal cord and brainstem that may contribute to the decrease in spasticity observed. Enhanced physical therapy, following injection, is thought to improve function through its ability to strengthen opposing muscles and maximize functional use of the extremity, while the botox is active. The effect of botox is transient, lasting 12–20 weeks before spasticity returns; repeated injections, up to three applications, have been found to continue the effect. There is some concern that repeated injections might induce immunological resistance; however, no such reaction was found with three sequential injections, spaced 12–16 weeks apart.[30]

Widespread spasticity can be most effectively treated through **intrathecal baclofen** infusion. Baclofen is a GABA-β receptor agonist, which means that it functions like the inhibitory neurotransmitter, gamma amino butyric acid (GABA). When given orally, baclofen has trouble crossing the blood–brain barrier, and therefore, must be given in large doses to affect peripheral spasticity; these doses can also cause headaches, sedation, and lethargy, which limit its desirability as a treatment method. Other oral medications, such as diazepam, dantrolene, and tizanidine, are also sometimes used but similarly induce side effects of sedation and lethargy that limit their use post-stroke.[31] However, intrathecal infusion is applied directly into the subarachnoid space of the spinal column, between the arachnoid and pia maters, with much better focal spinal effects and fewer central effects such as sedation. It is most commonly applied via an implantable pump that can deliver continuous infusion or periodic boluses. Often a single bolus infusion will be tried to determine effectiveness prior to a pump implantation; the effect of a single bolus is relatively short (hours) but can give some idea of what change in tone might be expected. Implantation at the level of T2–T4 has been found to maximize effectiveness for those with both upper and lower extremity spasticity, compared to the typical site of implantation at T11–T12,[32] where the effect is maximal for lower extremity spasticity. Progression from a continuous infusion to a periodic bolus may optimize effectiveness. Physical therapy intervention after implantation is critical to maximize the effectiveness and minimize side effects, as tone decreases, with emphasis on increasing range of motion, strength, and function. Outcomes from baclofen infusion include not only decreased spasticity but also improved function, including mobility, walking speed, self-care, UE function, and work production; further, improvements have occurred years after stroke onset.[31,32] Initially, there was concern that baclofen infusion might result in diminished muscle strength on the non-paretic side due to the bilateral impact of baclofen infusion; however, this has not been documented in multiple trials. Notably, a common side effect is an initial decrease in function, following implantation. This results from the unmasking of weakness in spastic muscles or learned movement patterns that "use" the spasticity for function. Thus, this is a critical time for rehabilitation to address increasing strength and function. The methods for such rehabilitation are consistent with those described in the following sections.

CASE A, PART III

Mr. Brown returned home 4 weeks after his stroke and was referred to home health physical therapy and after 8 weeks to out-patient therapy. He is walking independently for short distances with a quad cane and right AFO. Stairs require the use of the railing and the quad cane and +1 min assist of his wife in a step-to pattern. He requires +1 mod assist to do curbs or walk on inclines or uneven surfaces. Transfers from firm surfaces at least 18 inches tall are independent but he requires assist for couches and standard height toilets. He uses a tub bench in his shower for bathing. Car transfers require +1 mod assist. He now has 2–3/5 strength in his elbow and shoulder muscles but limited hand movement. Spasticity in the fingers is noted, and the hand is partially fisted at rest; however, he can open the hand when reaching to touch a target. Grasp is facilitated by the spasticity, which makes release of objects difficult. He is using his left hand for all self-care activities; he has not resumed driving, due to the hemianopia. The aphasia is clearing with some continued word finding problems. Despite his significant progress, he is depressed at his inability to drive and return to work.

● PHYSICAL THERAPY MANAGEMENT IN THE HOME HEALTH AND OUT-PATIENT ENVIRONMENTS

Mr. Brown is now medically stable and has become proficient enough in his basic activities of daily living that he is able to return home with the assistance of his wife. He is dealing with the psychological impact of his life-altering experience, and once in his home environment, the changes in his bodily function and ability to participate are more evident to him and his family. It is at this time that many of our clients face issues of depression and anxiety as they are beyond the crisis and now face life-altering changes on a daily basis. Recovery has slowed at this point and improvements will now be more a function of Mr. Brown's work than natural recovery. He continues to have the potential to improve his mobility and upper extremity function and should be encouraged to choose realistic short-term goals and acknowledge the weekly gains that he will be making as he works toward his long-term goals. His depression should be assessed and monitored and appropriately followed by the team, which should, at a minimum, include his physician and any nursing staff involved in his care and may involve a psychologist or counselor.

In the home environment, an intensive task-oriented training program is the most feasible approach. Once Mr. Brown can be transported to out-patient therapy without undue fatigue or hardship, therapy moves to that environment. Home-based therapy has the advantage of allowing the practice of functional tasks in the environment in which Mr. Brown will be functioning, while out-patient therapy has the benefit of allowing the use of more equipment and encourages Mr. Brown to begin moving about in the community environment. The LEAPS trial has demonstrated that ambulation and lower extremity function will respond well to a home-based approach while other studies involving circuit training and constraint-induced movement therapy have supported the use of these out-patient based therapy programs.[33] Other issues to be tackled are Mr. Brown's increasing issues with spasticity and higher level functional activities.

Task-Oriented Training: Uneven Surfaces

Mr. Brown has achieved modified independence in ambulation but continues to have difficulties with uneven surfaces such as curbs and steps. Early step training is beneficial both functionally and as a way to work on underlying impairments. Use of a low step can strengthen the paretic leg both concentrically (when stepping up with the paretic leg) and eccentrically when stepping down with the non-paretic leg. Stepping with the non-paretic leg encourages weight-bearing on the paretic leg. This activity should be started as early as possible. Many individuals develop a compensatory step-to pattern on the stairs that does not utilize the paretic leg. In addition, this pattern of stair climbing is slow and does not return the individual to normal community function. While it may be beneficial for expediting independence for a return to home, this method does not promote long-term return to participation goals. Practice of a reciprocal stair climbing pattern should be initiated when step training is started and continued until it becomes functional. Use of the compensatory step-to pattern should be utilized sparingly and only when necessary for safety. If the client is too weak to do standard height steps, the task can be made less physically demanding by using lower step heights, railings, and FES.

Task-Oriented Training: Transfers Low Surfaces

Mr. Brown is having difficulty with transfers onto surfaces that are low and/or soft as well as those that require maneuvering in order to approach them (e.g. car). Clients who have difficulties with these types of transfers generally require work on underlying impairments, such as strength, as well as on motor control. Functional practice that progresses from higher to lower and firmer to softer surfaces and is initiated early in rehabilitation leads to the development of flexible strategies for transferring in many different situations rather than a rigid motor plan that limits the individual to transferring from only a firm seat with armrests. It may take longer to develop independence when utilizing this approach, but the payoff in the end is a higher level of functioning.

Intensive Task-Oriented Training: Other Paradigms

Once the client is able to transfer in and out of the car in a functional manner, out-patient therapy can be initiated. The benefit of out-patient therapy is the access to equipment such as FES, treadmills, and perhaps even robotics or virtual reality. In addition, this environment allows for the use of training paradigms such as circuit training and constraint-induced movement therapy (CIMT). Circuit training as well as standard and modified CIMT have been shown to be effective in rehabilitating both motor impairment and function.

Circuit Training

Circuit training is a method that involves setting up stations to practice specific skills or work on specific impairments. The client moves through a circuit, moving from station to station, and performing the activity or exercise at each station. The stations are set up such that the exercise or activity is individualized to each client as they move through that station. An example would be a station to work on sit to stand transfer training and lower extremity strengthening. At the station, there might be a standard height chair with a firm cushion or surface that can be placed in the chair to elevate the surface as well as a stool for a lower surface. Based on each client's physical capabilities and motor control, he/she would practice sit to stands from the chair that is appropriate for them. They would then progress, usually to the next lower surface, as their physical abilities and motor control improve. Progressions should challenge both motor control and physical limits. This training has been successfully utilized in an acute rehabilitation hospital setting (90-minute sessions, 5 days per week) and in sub-acute to chronic stroke in the out-patient setting. The stations can be supervised by staff or the clients can move through the stations in pairs. The use of pairs allows the partner to watch and give feedback on performance as well as document performance. Performance from the session is then used to motivate the individual at the next session. Examples of these programs can be found in the studies published by van de Port (out-patient)[34] and Rose (acute in-patient rehabilitation).[35]

Circuit training for Mr. Brown would need to focus on both arm and leg function with stations that encourage grasp and release as well as control of grip force. In addition, he should do stations for transfers to low surfaces and surfaces that require maneuvering (car seat) as well as stations that encourage work on gait speed and gait over uneven surfaces such as curbs, slopes, and rough terrain. Mr. Brown was an athlete and might enjoy working with a partner who is also s/p stroke as this would encourage teamwork that he has enjoyed in the past. He might also have enjoyed and seen the benefits of a strength training program, and so, might appreciate the incorporation of some traditional strength training equipment into his circuit work. Other clients may not respond well to traditional strength training with weights or other equipment and would then be encouraged to do a strength training program that is based on functional activities such as sit to stand for quads and gluteals or toe tapping for the dorsiflexors.

Strength training can be done with traditional weights or through the repetition of functional activities. If proper strength training protocols are followed (i.e., working to fatigue with 10 or fewer repetitions), then activities such as step-ups or sit to stand can be used to strengthen the hip and knee extensors. Tapping the foot to music may be sufficient to strengthen extremely weak dorsiflexors. The therapist has to set up the activity in a manner that works the key muscle groups to fatigue within the allotted number of repetitions, generally less than 10. The key to this therapy is the ability of the therapist to listen to the client and design an individualized program that incorporates meaningful activities for that client. This requires creative thinking skills as well as a strong understanding of the kinematics of movement across tasks and activities.

Constraint-Induced Movement Therapy (CI or CIMT)

CIMT, initially referred to as forced use, is a treatment paradigm focused on increasing use of the paretic hand after stroke. This technique was initially described by Taub,[36] from his work with monkeys, and first implemented by Wolf in a clinic population.[37] For the monkeys, Taub found that restricting movement of the intact arm "forced" the monkey to use the deafferented arm, and by 2 weeks, it was impossible to differentiate the function of the arm from its pre-surgical state. This work was translated into a clinical application by Wolf[37] that was then verified in a large multi-site clinical trial, known as the EXCITe (extremity constraint-induced therapy evaluation) trial (2006) in sub-acute and chronic post-stroke participants.[38]

CIMT has traditionally been applied as a 2-week intervention with 6-hour practice sessions daily, 5 days per week; participants wear a sling or mitt that precludes use of the non-paretic limb for most of their waking hours so that the client focuses on using their paretic limb for most daily activities. A behavioral contract, signed by the participants, outlines exceptions to the mitt wear as well as activities to practice at home. Treatment is focused on high-intensity repetition of tasks (massed practice) with the paretic limb, following motor learning principles and shaping strategies. In other words, tasks are used that challenge the individual's current level of performance but can be made incrementally more difficult. Practice is varied, and feedback is provided in a variable manner but includes both knowledge of performance and results.

Some tasks that are commonly used include stacking blocks, placing shapes in a shape sorter, erasing lines on a chalkboard, playing checkers, or completing dot-to-dot tracings. Some household tasks such as folding or hanging up clothes, ironing, or dusting may be included. Tasks can be chosen to emphasize shoulder or elbow motion, hand opening/closing, individual finger motion, or some combination of movements, based on the participant's needs. Obviously, this form of treatment requires the participant to have some degree of hand and arm function; in fact, initial participants were required to have 90 degrees of active shoulder and elbow flexion with at least 10 degrees of wrist and finger extension at each joint. More recently, this method has been used with individuals with less function but some degree of hand and arm function needs to be present.[39] Also, multiple clinical trials have demonstrated that CIMT can be provided with less time in the clinic (as little as two 30-minute sessions weekly) and improves hand mobility; however, the traditional methodology seems most effective in changing self-care and participation post-stroke, based on a recent meta-analysis.[40] Research needs to continue to evaluate alternative implementation methods, including telemedicine, to provide CIMT in a manner that more easily fits with insurance coverage and time for therapy post-stroke.

CIMT has also been administered to children with hemiparetic cerebral palsy from ages 18 months to the teenaged years. Restriction of the non-paretic arm has included using gloves or hand splints,[41] slings,[42] and casts[43] for 2 hours/day to 24 hours/day; the CIMT protocol has been provided in intervals of 2 weeks, consistent with the traditional model, to 6 weeks, and in doses of 9 hours per week to 6 hours per day. In one study, using a uni-valved cast for 3 weeks and comparing dosages of 3 hours to 6 hours per day, equivalent upper extremity improvements were found for both doses, suggesting that 3 hours per day is sufficient to achieve improvement in hand mobility and use in daily activities.[43] Similar to the adult protocol, massed practice of age appropriate play activities follows the principles of shaping and motor learning.

Sensory Training Post-stroke

Too often, sensory dysfunction, and its impact on motor recovery, is ignored. In the last decade, it has become evident that sensory dysfunction is much more common than previously thought, especially if sensory dysfunction across modalities (texture, weight, shape) is evaluated. Further, sensory function has been found to predict motor and quality of life outcomes, yet is rarely a focus of physical therapy intervention. There is some evidence that sensory function can be improved with high-intensity training protocols that are focused on sensory discrimination abilities.[44,45] There is also some suggestion that a training protocol that includes sensory discrimination activities that require active hand manipulation may improve motor function as well. It is recommended that this type of treatment use training parameters consistent with shaping and motor learning principles, as described for CIMT; occluding vision, through the use of a curtain or other obstruction, allows for hand manipulation of items in tasks designed for sensory discrimination. Too often, vision allows compensation for sensory deficits, and thus, practice with vision may not force use of the sensory discrimination neural network. Examples of tasks that can be used in sensory training are: finding all of the puzzle edge pieces in a cloth bag, placing items in a shape sorter behind a curtain, and matching a texture felt with the non-paretic hand by manipulating match objects with the paretic hand.[45] It should be noted that sensory discrimination dysfunction is often bilateral, so the non-paretic hand may not have intact sensation for these types of comparisons.

Robotics and Virtual Reality: Cochrane reviews and systematic reviews on robotics and virtual reality show that there is evidence to support further study of these interventions, but at this time, (2015) there is not sufficient evidence to state that they lead to improvements in daily function. Studies remain limited, small in scale, and diverse in methodology making it difficult to combine them for analysis across studies. Robotics has been used for rehabilitation of the arm and leg with the most promise in improving underlying impairments such as weakness and spasticity. This technique had the greatest impact on distal arm function (wrist and hand) and regaining ambulation in those who are non-ambulatory. Evidence for the use of virtual reality and video-games is positive but not yet sufficient to support changing clinical practice.

Neglect Syndrome and Pusher Syndrome

Rehabilitation of individuals, who have developed either the neglect or pusher syndrome, can be challenging. Both of these syndromes typically require a longer duration of rehabilitation to ensure safety and independence in daily activities.

Neglect Syndrome. The goal in rehabilitating this client is to assist the client to develop awareness of the paretic side and the environment on that side of their body. The first step is to assess the severity of the neglect and its impact on daily activities and function. Several outcome measures exist for this purpose, the line bisection test (illustrated in Figure 10-10), the Catherine Bergego Scale, cancellation tasks, and copying tasks. The line bisection, cancellation, and copying tests all give an indication of the side of neglect as well as the severity of the neglect. The Catherine Bergego Scale allows therapists to objectively assess the impact of neglect on functional activities such as grooming, eating, and navigating while walking.

Treatment involves the use of techniques that incorporate visual scanning, sensory awareness, and spatial organization training. Visual scanning involves visually engaging the client within the space where they are comfortable and then drawing their vision slowly to the neglected side. Once reaching the boundary keep the object to which they are visually engaged at the boundary and encourage them to maintain their focus on

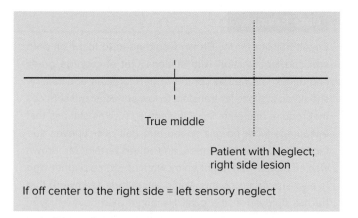

True middle

Patient with Neglect; right side lesion

If off center to the right side = left sensory neglect

FIGURE 10-10 Example of the line bisection test in an individual with neglect syndrome.

the object. This task is more engaging if the client has to interact with the visual target in some way such as having to read text. Sensory awareness training should involve both proprioception and the many cutaneous senses (touch, object recognition). Activities that include weight-bearing on the paretic side along with explicitly focusing the client's attention on the feeling of the weight-bearing are thought to be especially beneficial. It is also recommended that therapists provide sensory stimulation of different types (soft, rough, hot, cold) to the paretic limbs while having the client watch as the stimulus is applied and describe how it feels and where it is being placed. Studies have found that combining visual exploration with either TENS or vibration to the paretic upper trapezius are effective means of treating neglect syndrome.[46] The use of prisms combined with an active pointing activity has also been supported by research.[47] If the client is not eating well or otherwise severely impacted by the neglect, a compensatory technique is to turn the body so that the sternum faces the neglected space. The trunk is the internal representation of the body, and therefore, it appears that individuals with neglect are "neglecting" the space relative to the center of the trunk. If they are not eating food on the left side of the plate, turning their chair such that their sternum faces the left side of the plate will allow them to perceive the food from the left side of the plate to the right, and they will typically eat everything. This technique works well for seated activities but is typically not feasible for activities involving mobility. In addition, this technique is compensatory, and as such, does not aid in neuroplasticity nor resolution of the syndrome, so it should be used sparingly and only for issues where safety is a concern.

Pusher Syndrome. Individuals with pusher syndrome have a severely altered sense of their position in space. This results in their pushing strongly toward the paretic side in all positions and resisting any attempt at passive correction of their posture. Their head is turned to the non-paretic side and they are unable to relax their neck so that the head can be turned to the paretic side. They have a reduced ability to perceive stimuli coming in on the involved side and their tactile and kinesthetic sensation may be severely impaired. These individuals often do not see or hear things on the paretic side. They lack facial expression and have a monotonous voice. During movement, they tend to keep their weight on the non-paretic side, while pushing their center of mass over the paretic side. This results in their falling over, both in standing and sitting. Even after falling, you will note that they appear to continue to be pushing onto the paretic side. It is also common for these individuals to push backwards, and thus, appear to be resisting or fighting staff during transfers and gait training. In standing, the center of gravity is shifted to the paretic side, and they show no fear even when on the verge of falling. The legs are adducted and the paretic leg is flexed taking little weight with the non-paretic leg held in exaggerated extension. During stand to sit transfers, they often sit too soon, and they tend to talk a lot, offering lots of "explanations" for why things go wrong. These explanations are usually not appropriate to the situation. Due to the constant pushing motion, they are likely to develop skin breakdown and contractures. There is one objective measure of pushing, the Scale for Contraversive Pushing (SCP).[48] This scale allows clinicians to numerically rate the extent of the pushing behavior, and thus, have an objective means of tracking progress as the pushing resolves.

Treatment. The key to working with individuals who have pusher syndrome is to ensure they have visual information on vertical and use active movement to get vertical, followed by functional activities while in vertical. Patients who have contraversive pushing need to learn the following in sequential order:

1. Realize the disturbed perception of erect body position
2. Visually explore their surroundings and their body's relation to the surroundings. Use visual aids that give feedback about body orientation
3. Learn movements necessary to reach a vertical body position
4. Maintain vertical body position while performing other activities

Most of the treatments recommended here are most easily and safely performed with the therapist situated on the NON-paretic side of the client. This is a key element in the treatment as it facilitates the ability of the therapist to guard the client in a more effective manner. If the therapist were to sit on the paretic side, the client would be constantly pushing into the therapist, and the therapist would have to counteract this by pushing the client back to upright. In this situation, the therapist is in essence "fighting" the pushing. If the therapist guards from the non-paretic side, they can use a pulling motion to prevent the fall, and thus, use their own body weight to stabilize against the pushing. In addition, this situation allows the therapist to encourage the client to lean on them, and thereby, "break" the pushing behavior. The therapist is now having the client actively move out of pushing rather than fighting the client and resisting the pushing behavior.

The therapist should also structure the treatment such that there are visual cues available as to where vertical is situated. You might instruct the individual to look at a door frame, or you may put a stripe on a mirror in front of them. The key is to provide the client with a visual orientation to vertical. While utilizing the visual orientation, instruct the individual to actively move themselves into a more upright position. It is counterproductive to try to forcefully push them into upright. Rather, the therapist should provide activities that encourage actively moving out of the pushing posture. For example, have the client sit in front of a mirror. The therapist is on the non-paretic side and holds their hand up at shoulder level and instructs the client

to move their shoulder into the therapist's hand. This activity promotes the client actively move out of pushing and into the desired upright posture. [video-clip]

If the client expresses a strong fear of falling, which is common, the therapist could place a large Swiss ball on the mat on the non-paretic side of the client and place the client's non-paretic arm on the Swiss ball. The instruction is to push on the ball. Again, the client is in control and is actively moving out of the pushing behavior. By allowing the client to stay in control and providing appropriate support, they will have less fear of falling and be better able to work through the sense that they are falling, while moving out of the pushing behavior.

Standing activities can initially be quite difficult. Safety can be enhanced by placing a knee brace on the paretic limb, so it is in a position to assume weight-bearing. In addition, the non-paretic upper extremity should be in a position that does not allow pushing but does allow it to weight bear. This is best accomplished by keeping it in as much elbow flexion as possible. Use of a table that is at chest height can be helpful for standing activities as it allows the client to weight bear through the forearms, and thus, discourages pushing, while encouraging an upright posture and a very stable support surface. The therapist should once again guard from the non-paretic side. The hands can wrap around the pelvis, and the therapist can use their own body weight to counteract the pushing. Once again, the therapist would instruct the client to lean into them, cueing an active movement out of pushing. As the client progresses, reaching activities to the non-paretic side provide a means of practicing actively moving out of pushing. When gait is initiated, stepping over objects with the non-paretic leg encourages weight-bearing on the paretic side. Typically, devices that allow the client to use the non-paretic arm to push are discouraged. At times, the therapist may even hold the client's non-paretic arm in a position of shoulder adduction and internal rotation with full elbow flexion to prevent pushing. Once the pushing begins to subside, the therapist should wean away from preventing use of the non-paretic arm.

If the client has progressed to exhibiting a high level of cognitive functioning and good self-recognition of the pushing, the therapist can work on sitting by having the client close their eyes and assume what they perceive to be upright sitting. Then, ask the client to let you place them in true upright. This is followed by asking them to think about how this posture feels to them, while giving them feedback that they are truly in an upright posture. This is done with eyes closed because these individuals tend to stop resisting postural correction, when their eyes are closed.

• SUMMARY

All therapeutic techniques that lead to improved daily function for individuals who are post-stroke involved intensive, task-oriented practice of functional activities. Clinicians should focus on ensuring that their clients are provided opportunities to perform task-oriented practice that involves numerous repetitions of a functionally appropriate activity. Compensatory training may lead to a faster return to independence but ultimately negatively impacts neuroplasticity and results in poorer long-term functional outcomes and motor recovery.

Neuroplasticity: How does Treatment Induce Plasticity?

Neuroplasticity refers to the natural change in synaptic function that is associated with behavioral change, including learning new motor skills or a decrease in the amount of use of a given body part. Therefore, physical therapy interventions naturally induce neuroplasticity with long-lasting implications. Too often, early therapy focuses on improving function through use of the non-paretic limbs (i.e., lifting the paretic limb with the non-paretic limb). Therapists should keep in mind that limiting use of the paretic limb may result in loss of neural projections in the hand/arm or leg areas of the motor cortex; further, increased use of the non-paretic arm or leg will result in neuroplastic changes that expand the neuronal networks associated with these body parts. To preserve the neural networks and/or induce positive neural change within the lesioned hemisphere, it is imperative that therapy focus on increasing sensorimotor activity in the paretic limbs. Kleim outlined key principles that should guide physical therapy interventions to maximize neuroplasticity: (1) rehabilitation should focus on limb usage because failure to use the limbs will result in additional neural loss; (2) the plasticity induced will be specific to the treatment provided; (3) plasticity requires high intensity (rate and amount of practice) and many repetitions; and (4) early plasticity may improve or impede subsequent plasticity.[49] Too often, therapy sessions provide one or two repetitions of any given activity; it is unlikely that this is enough to produce plasticity or change unless the client is able to continually perform additional repetitions throughout the day. Home programs and involvement of family members or other health care professionals to encourage continuous activity is essential for assuring sufficient practice to induce plasticity.

What Kinds of Plasticity Are Found and How Are They Identified?

Plasticity, in vivo, has largely been evaluated using imaging methods such as anatomical and functional magnetic resonance imaging (fMRI), positron emission tomography (PET), or diffusion tensor imaging/tractography (DTI or DTT). Findings from anatomical imaging (MRI or CT) suggest that lesion location and volume, comparing different regions, are poor predictors of stroke outcome,[50] but when comparing the same vessel territory may be moderate predictors of outcome[51]; however, these methods do allow for the location of damage to be documented and measures of lesion volume as well as brain volume or specific brain components (i.e., cortex) to be analyzed. Further, high-intensity post-stroke training can increase cortex thickness in areas related to improved function,[52] as measured through MRI anatomical scanning methods. fMRI, which allows the visualization of changes in blood flow during a given activity (i.e., finger tapping), has shown that early motor recovery is often characterized by diffuse bilateral activation, compared to unilateral, typically contralateral, activation in non-stroke participants; however, good recovery is most often associated with a return to unilateral ipsilesional activation similar to non-stroke activation patterns. Plus, physical therapy training that is of high intensity can induce activation that is more similar to non-stroke activation, with the magnitude of activation

correlated with the magnitude of recovery. Post-stroke survivors with poorer sensorimotor recovery often maintain a bilateral and more diffuse activation pattern, suggesting that this pattern of activation is inconsistent with effective neuroplasticity. Diffusion tractography focuses on the evaluation of white matter projections and has revealed a strong relationship between the degree of white matter integrity, especially within the corticospinal projections, and functional motor outcomes.[53] However, the ability of training to increase white matter in the lesioned hemisphere has not been adequately evaluated.

Neuroplasticity within the sensory system appears to be more complex. First, although sensory perception, the ability to localize touch to a given body area, seems to be a unilateral process, involving the primary sensory cortex (S1) in the contralateral parietal lobe, sensory discrimination is a bilateral process, involving contralateral S1 and bilateral S2 (secondary sensory cortex) as well as bilateral areas of the prefrontal cortex. It is not surprising, then, that damage to this sensory discrimination network often results in a bilateral disturbance, which is greater in the contralesional hand. Sensory discrimination recovery seems to, in part, mirror motor recovery in that activation patterns that are similar to non-stroke patterns are associated with better recovery, suggesting that the best recovery is associated with plasticity within the S1 and S2 areas of the lesioned cortex. Further, it appears that the degree of integrity in the superior thalamic radiations (the sensory projections from the thalamus to the parietal cortex) is strongly related to the degree of sensory discrimination ability post-stroke.[50] However, there is some suggestion that the bilateral nature of sensory discrimination may allow for fairly effective sensory discrimination through increased use of the contralesional hemisphere. To date, there have been no studies that have evaluated the ability of sensory discrimination training to induce neuroplasticity within this bilateral network.

CASE B: BASILAR ARTERY ANEURYSM

Jennifer is a 36-year-old, Caucasian, female, who presented to the ER with what she termed was "the worst headache of her life." She complained of associated neck stiffness. CT scan revealed a large aneurysm at the basilar-vertebral artery junction that was leaking blood into the subarachnoid space. She was rushed to the OR and the aneurysm was successfully clipped. Post-surgery, she presents with complex symptomology, characterized by quadriparesis, right facial muscle paresis, diplopia, ptosis, nystagmus, vertigo, dysarthria, and dysphagia.

The symptoms described in this case most closely align with which stroke syndrome?

Basilar artery syndrome

Aneurysms: What are they? What causes them? And how are they medically managed?

An aneurysm is a weakening in a blood vessel wall that allows the wall to balloon out and presents a risk of rupture. Cerebral aneurysms are often asymptomatic and, therefore, undiagnosed with an estimated presence in 1–9% of the population; however, the occurrence of rupture into the subarachnoid space or surrounding brain tissue is about 1 in 10,000 people annually.[54] Up to 45% of those experiencing an aneurysm rupture die, often before getting to the hospital; the majority of those that survive will have some permanent neurologic deficit[55] consistent with the area of the rupture and damage to the surrounding tissue. Aneurysms are more common in women and with increasing age; although, pediatric occurrences are documented. Risk factors are similar to those for stroke and include hypertension, drug (especially cocaine) or excessive alcohol use, and smoking.

Aneurysms are most common in the junctions between the vessels within the Circle of Willis, especially in the anterior and posterior communicating arteries (see Figure 10-11). Other common sites are at the carotid bifurcation and the basilar artery tip (the point of bifurcation into the posterior cerebral arteries) as well as within the middle cerebral and posterior inferior cerebellar arteries.[55] Aneurysms are much more common in the anterior circulation with approximately 85% presenting there. Although most aneurysms are asymptomatic unless they rupture, some will present with neurologic symptoms, if they enlarge to the point that they are compressing the adjacent brain tissue. However, it is much more common for aneurysms to remain "silent" until a small leak or full rupture occurs. Small leaks may present with headache, cranial nerve changes, nausea, photophobia (sensitivity to light) or neck pain; these may precede an actual rupture by hours or days and are referred to as **sentinel hemorrhages**. Rupture commonly presents with what is known as a "thunderclap" headache, referring to a rapid onset severe headache, which results from blood flowing into the subarachnoid space or brain tissue. Consciousness may be lost as the bleeding progresses. Aneurysms can be detected by CT or MRI scans; however, cerebral angiograms are commonly used to confirm the diagnosis and guide treatment.

Medical management of an aneurysm that is leaking firsts focuses on stabilization of the patient and then prevention of a rupture; treatment is surgical, using coiling with or without a stent/balloon, or clipping. Coiling involves advancing tiny coils into the aneurysm to obstruct blood flow from the main vessel into the aneurysm; platinum coils are inserted via a catheter, typically guided through the femoral artery to the site of the aneurysm. A stent is a wire mesh tube that provides a shell for the coils and is more commonly used for fusiform aneurysms (those with wide oval openings). An alternative to a stent is what is known as a balloon, which is a small balloon catheter that is inserted with the coils to keep them in place. In some instances, repair requires a craniotomy and clipping of the aneurysm, which simply uses a small clip across the aneurysm's neck to prevent blood from entering the aneurysm. Treatment for an aneurysm rupture is the same as for one that is leaking; both coiling and clipping are used. The outcomes of aneurysm repair are dependent on the management of complications and the amount of brain damage, resulting from the initial bleed, if the aneurysm ruptured. Common complications after an aneurysm rupture and repair are hydrocephalus, vasospasm, and hyponatremia (low sodium). Each of these needs to be carefully managed.

Hydrocephalus may occur within 3 days of surgical repair or much later after discharge. In acute hydrocephalus, up to 40% spontaneously recover; therefore, early treatment may focus on monitoring. Progression of the hydrocephalus may require shunting to control cerebrospinal fluid buildup and further brain damage. This may be done by placement of an external ventricular drain (placed into the lateral ventricle and shunted externally), a lumbar drain, or repeated lumbar punctures. Of course, these treatments carry with them risk of their own complications, so initial monitoring is critical to assure the need for shunting.

Hyponatremia refers to a dramatic decrease in sodium in the brain. There is controversy over the cause of this condition post-aneurysm repair. However, treatment focuses on maintaining salt and fluid levels.

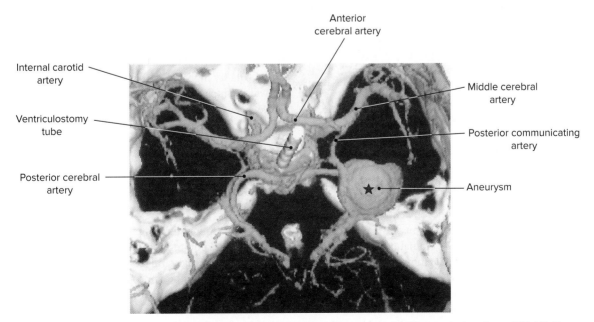

FIGURE 10-11 Illustration of aneurysm of the posterior cerebral artery. (Reproduced, with permission, from Afifi AK, Bergman RA. *Functional Neuroanatomy.* 2nd edition. New York, NY: McGraw-Hill; 2005, Fig 28-5, pg. 364.)

Vasospasm, post-aneurysm, can induce a subsequent CVA, so it is critical to prevent this complication. Notably, this complication is most common 5–14 days after rupture. Prevention has focused on pharmacologic management with the use of a calcium channel blocker, nimodipine, the most common method. Research is focused on identifying other, and perhaps better, medications to manage vasospasm.

Brainstem Stroke: Why Are the Symptoms so Confusing? What Is Locked-in Syndrome?

The brainstem is a complex structure that houses cranial nerve nuclei as well as the nuclei of the reticular and vestibular systems. In addition, it is an area of fiber passage for ascending sensory fibers, originating from all body parts and conveying sensory information to the thalamus and cortex, and descending motor fibers (corticobulbar, corticospinal), traveling to brainstem structures and the spinal cord. Therefore, damage within the brainstem can produce upper motor neuron syndrome, presenting with hemiparesis and spasticity, due to damage of corticospinal and corticobulbar fibers, or lower motor neuron syndrome, associated with damage of alpha motor neurons within the cranial nerve nuclei that innervate the muscles of the eyes, face, mouth, tongue, and palate. Further, symptoms can be ipsilateral, contralateral, or bilateral, depending on the structures damaged and the size of the respective lesion (Refer to Figure 10-5 and Table 10-2 for potential structures associated with brainstem levels and possible clinical presentations.)

Changes in sensory function similarly relate to the site of damage. Damage below the level of the cuneate and gracilis nuclei results in ipsilateral loss of somatosensory function, while damage at the level of these nuclei, as projection fibers cross, will produce bilateral somatosensory loss, and above this level will produce contralateral loss. Again, large lesions that impact both sides of the brainstem structures can also produce bilateral sensory loss. Since pain and temperature is conveyed in the anterolateral pathway's spinothalamic tract and not the dorsal column-medial lemniscal pathway, localized damage may result in the loss of one pathway and not the other below the merging of these sensory projections in the upper medulla. Damage to the lateral medulla is likely to disrupt the spinothalamic tract; while medial damage is likely to disrupt the medial lemniscal fibers. It should be noted that spinothalamic damage within the brainstem always yields contralateral dysfunction, so it is possible, but uncommon, to have ipsilateral loss of somatosensation and contralateral loss of pain and temperature with unilateral low-level medullary strokes. At the levels of the pons and midbrain, these projection pathways are collocated and damage will typically disrupt both, producing contralateral damage.

Cranial nuclei house the alpha motor neurons that innervate the muscles of the eyes (extraocular muscles), eyelids, face, tongue, and throat. Damage to motor cranial nerve nuclei produces ipsilateral lower motor neuron symptoms in the muscles innervated, presenting as weakness or flaccidity with hyporeflexia/areflexia. Similarly, the sensory cranial nerves receive ipsilateral projections from the eyes, ears, face, and oral structures, so damage to these nuclei results in ipsilateral loss of sensory function (somatosensory and pain and temperature).

There are four vestibular nuclei (lateral, medial, superior, inferior) located bilaterally in the upper medulla and lower pons that function with the inner ear and cerebellum to maintain the body's orientation in relation to the environment. Strokes that impact the medulla and pons will also disrupt the function of the vestibular nuclei, which include: (1) antigravity muscle control to maintain upright posture (lateral vestibulospinal tract); (2) reflexive control of head position with visual orientation (medial vestibulospinal tract); (3) vestibular-occular reflexes (nystagmus); and (4) integration of inner ear and cerebellar projections for motor control. The afferent and efferent projections of the vestibular nuclei are largely unilateral, so damage to these nuclei presents with ipsilateral symptoms. Similarly, cerebellar damage results in ipsilateral symptoms. It is difficult to differentiate the symptoms of vestibular nuclei and cerebellar damage, in part, because they often coexist. Nonetheless, damage within the vestibular network commonly results in ipsilesional nystagmus or ocular oscillations, vertigo, ataxia, or gaze paresis. When damage is localized to the vestibular nuclei, the ataxia produced is gravity dependent, absent when lying down but present in upright positions; due to the adjacency of the cochlear nucleus, vestibular damage also frequently presents with changes in auditory function (tinnitus, hearing loss). With cerebellar damage, ataxia is not gravity dependent and typically is associated with hypotonia, incoordination, and dysmetria (overshooting of intended targets).[56]

Locked-in Syndrome

Locked-in syndrome (LIS) is a phenomenon, most commonly associated with a basilar artery stroke and resultant ventral pons damage. It is characterized by quadreparesis and loss of bilateral cranial nerve function in cranial nerves V through XII, resulting in horizontal gaze palsy, the inability to speak (anarthria) or activate facial muscles. Control of vertical eye movement and the eyelids is typically maintained along with cognitive function. Communication can be achieved through vertical eye movement; however, the presence of nystagmus and other visual disturbances (diplopia, impaired accommodation) may complicate acquiring information through vision. For most, hearing remains intact. Recovery from LIS, from stroke, is poor and mortality high, yet outcome data are not well documented. However, intensive rehabilitation has been found to improve motor recovery and decrease mortality. The use of communication devices and other assistive technology is necessary to maximize function. Death, associated with LIS, most commonly results from respiratory complications.[57]

Assessment and Interventions Following Basilar Artery Aneurysm

Assessment, following basilar artery stroke, requires that the therapist incorporate more detailed examination of coordination, balance, visual, and vestibular function. Some outcome measures that may be appropriate include the Dynamic Gait Index, the Sensory Organization Test, Timed Up and Go, and the Dizziness Handicap Inventory. A full assessment of cranial nerve function should be conducted on anyone with a stroke in this region of the brain. In addition, coordination and balance assessment should be completed as outlined in the Evaluation (Chapter 9) and vestibular and cerebellar (Chapter 16) chapters.

Treatment for strokes that involve the posterior circulation typically requires that the therapist address the significant balance deficits that can result from damage to structures of the cerebellum and vestibular nuclei. These treatments are outlined in the chapter on vestibular and cerebellar disorders (Chapter 16). In addition to these issues, it is likely that these individuals may have damage to one or more of the cranial nerves and will require muscle reeducation for the facial, oral, and throat musculature. While physical therapists can make a valuable contribution to therapy for facial motor weakness, referral should be made to speech therapy, and the client should be managed with a team approach.

Functional retraining utilizing the motor learning concepts covered earlier in this chapter is also used after basilar artery stroke. These clients will also require that activities focus on postural control, balance, and coordination associated with vestibular system disruption. Examples of interventions for these conditions can be found in Chapter 16.

Case Example

Jennifer has diploplia, vertigo, and quadriparesis. An assessment tool that would give valuable objective outcomes for Jennifer and is valid in stroke and vestibular disorders is the Dynamic Gait Index.[58] Jennifer has a complex presentation, including many visual impairments. These will impede her ability to utilize vision for both balance and motor function feedback. Therapists should assess how her vision is interacting with her motor function and encourage her to learn to utilize her somatosensory feedback system for movement. In addition, objects that are used for functional training should be large and in strong, contrasting colors to simplify visual tracking. Vertigo secondary to cerebellar damage can be resistant to rehabilitation, but slow progress can be made through the use of accommodation exercises (see balance/vestibular chapter 16). Jennifer will likely need to work on gaze stabilization and accommodation exercises prior to being able to fully benefit from an intensive task-oriented approach. Once she has begun to accommodate to the changes in her vision and balance systems, she should respond to an intensive task-oriented approach as outlined earlier in this chapter. To accommodate her diplopia therapists should use large widely spaced print and simple line pictures for educational materials and home exercise programs. Jennifer's right facial paresis should respond to NMES and active exercise. Vision may be further impeded by the ptosis, and treatment focused on the levator muscle of the eye should be included in the therapy plan.

Therapy may involve interventions for lower and upper motor neuron injury. An appropriate therapy for both types of damage, as long as the lower motor neuron is intact, is the use of electrical stimulation. The unit can be set up for functional neuromuscular reeducation, or on flaccid muscles, may be set up to stimulate muscle activation in an attempt to promote neurologic recovery. If functional neuromuscular electrical stimulation (FES) is used correctly, it can help to promote neuroplasticity. The key is to encourage the use of visual and proprioceptive feedback, while using the unit to assist in movement. Use of FES assists in producing a more normal movement and can allow the individual to complete more repetitions. Thus, the individual can achieve intensive task-oriented practice of complicated movement patterns such as walking. A common use of FES is on the tibialis anterior during gait. The typical set up is to utilize a unit with a switch that goes under the heel in the shoe. As the individual walks, the switch triggers the stimulator to assist with dorsiflexion at the appropriate times during gait. The individual can then ambulate more steps with a proper gait pattern. There is also some evidence to suggest that use of electrical stimulation can slow or stop muscle fiber type conversion from type II to type I that is common following stroke. FES has been shown to be effective in rehabilitating hand, shoulder,[59,60] and ankle[60] function post-stroke.

Locked-in syndrome presents many challenges to the rehabilitation team. The key to a successful rehabilitation program is establishing communication with the individual. Initially, watching eye movements and asking yes/no questions may be utilized, but immediate referral to speech therapy should be made to acquire a communication device. Physical and Occupational therapists should focus on moving the limbs and encouraging active movement where possible. Electrical stimulation is suggested for use in this population to enhance motor recovery. Upright positioning remains important to prevent secondary complications and to promote interaction with the environment. Therapists should assess for and provide a chair for upright positioning.

CASE C: SICKLE CELL STROKE

Amelia is a 3-year-old, born of immigrant parents from Senegal, who was diagnosed with Sickle Cell disease at 9 months of age, following an initial episode of dactylitis (inflammation) of the 3rd digit of her right hand. She takes daily doses of folic acid and penicillin to manage her disease. She is rushed to the ED by her parents with slurring speech, listlessness, and mild left hemiparesis. CT identified an area of hypoperfusion in the right frontoparietal cortex. Sickle Cell disease is associated with abnormal red blood vessels that are more likely to clot and place the individual at risk for stroke as well as clotting within other organs (Figure 10-12 and Box 10-8).

What Are the Causes of Pediatric Stroke?

The causes of pediatric stroke are quite different than those for adult stroke. They include, but aren't limited to: congenital heart defects (septal defects such as patent foramen ovale), vascular

What is sickle cell anemia and why is it associated with stroke?

Sickle cell anemia (SCA) is an inherited autosomal recessive disorder that affects red blood cell formation, resulting in a sickle or crescent-shaped red blood cell (erythrocyte) instead of the typical circular shape (see Figure 10-12). This method of inheritance requires that both parents be carriers of the gene in order for a child to have the disorder. SCA is most commonly found in families with origins in Africa, the Mediterranean, Central and South America, the Caribbean, and the Middle East. The red blood cells are not only different in shape but are also weaker, more likely to rupture, and carry an abnormal hemoglobin protein, known as hemoglobin S, which is less effective in carrying oxygen. Remember, hemoglobin is the protein in red blood cells that carries oxygen.[64] Diagnosis of SCA can be made by a blood test, in which hemoglobin S can be identified.

The fragility of the sickle cell red blood cells in combination with the decreased amount of oxygen carried by hemoglobin S results in chronic anemia and subsequently, chronic fatigue. Notably, the red blood cells, in SCA, are also likely to stick together in clumps, thereby blocking smaller blood vessels throughout the body, including in the internal organs, extremities, and brain. When such a blockage occurs, especially in the internal organs, it results in severe pain, referred to as a "crisis" in SCA. The dactylitis, in Amelia's case, refers to a crisis occurring in the finger, creating pain and inflammation. Crises may occur with varying frequency in those affected. Organ damage, especially in the spleen, is common; spleen damage increases the chance of infection in those with SCA, which can, in turn, cause other problems.[64] Stroke is also a common problem in children with SCA, affecting 7–13% of those with the disorder, and is most common in those younger than 10 years of age.[65]

FIGURE 10-12 Sickle-shaped erythrocyte illustration. A single sickle-shaped red blood cell (erythrocyte) shown within a group of normal red blood cells.

anomalies in the cerebral vascular system (i.e., Moyamoya syndrome), infections (meningitis, encephalitis, human immunodeficiency virus), metabolic conditions (hyperlipidemia), and some genetic syndromes (neurofibromatosis, fibromuscular dysplasia, sickle cell anemia).

How do Pediatric Strokes Present?

In infants and young children, it is more common to see impaired consciousness or seizures than motor symptoms at stroke onset; sometimes irritability may be the initial symptom. Of course, it may be difficult to "see" early motor changes in a very young infant, and therefore, early signs may be overlooked. Thus, stroke may go undiagnosed in very young children. In older children, stroke appears, much like it does in adults, with changes in speech, coordination, or localized sensory or motor symptoms. Amelia, in the case description, presents with common symptoms of listlessness, mild hemiparesis, and slurring of speech. Diagnosis requires a complete history of symptom onset, blood work to rule out other causes and look for potential stroke causes (syphilis, encephalitis), and imaging. MRI scans provide a better likelihood of lesion identification than CT scans in young children with even better clarity at an earlier stage found with single photon emission computed tomography (SPECT), but MRI is more likely to be done. Sedation is often required to image young children and infants.[61,62]

Medical Management of Pediatric Stroke

The medical management of pediatric stroke is not that different from adult management. Early stabilization is critical. rTPA has not been approved for use in children, in part, because the onset of symptoms is rarely clear, and its effectiveness is maximal in the 3–4½ hour window after onset.[62] However, anticoagulants, such as heparin or warfarin, are used to decrease blood clotting. Inducing hypothermia has also been found to be neuroprotective in infants/young children and may be used. Also, antiepileptics may be used to prevent further brain damage secondary to post-stroke seizures.[63] Pediatric stroke, since it occurs during the developmental period, may have profound effects on subsequent development and acquisition of age appropriate milestones across domains – cognitive, emotional, sensorimotor. Physical therapy intervention will mirror that provided for children with cerebral palsy, and therefore, will be discussed in that chapter.

Treatment of SCA

Treatment of SCA is largely focused on prevention of crises and stroke, including monitoring for stroke potential, using transcranial Doppler ultrasound to identify potential areas of blockage, in which stroke could occur; chronic blood transfusions may also be given to replace the damaged blood cells. However, chronic blood transfusions are not without risk, including the complications of too much iron (iron overload), alloimmunity (an immune response to the transfused blood), and infection.[64] Other pharmacologic management may include: (1) folic acid to increase iron in the blood; (2) prophylactic antibiotics to minimize infections; (3) pain medications in the event of crisis; and (4) hydroxyurea to stimulate red blood cell formation.[64]

REFERENCES

1. Ahire A. Stroke Statistics and Stroke Facts. Available at: http://ezinearticles. com/?expert=Anne_Ahira.

2. National Stroke Association's Stroke 101 Fact Sheet. Available at: http:// www.stroke.org/site/DocServer/STROKE_101_Fact_Sheet.pdf?doc ID=4541. Accessed October 31, 2013.

3. Ng YS, Stein J, Ning M, Black-Schaffer, RM. Comparison of clinical char-acteristics and functional outcomes of ischemic stroke in different vascular territories. *Stroke*. 2007;38:2309-2314.

4. Karnath HO, Broetz D. Understanding and treating "pusher syndrome". *Phys Ther*. 2003;83:1119-1125.

5. Bartolomeo P, DeSchotten MT, Chica AB. Brain networks of visuospa-tial attention and their disruption in visual neglect. *Front Hum Neurosci*. 2012;6(article 10):1-10.

6. Buchsbaum BR, Baldo J, Okada K, Berman KF, Dronkers N, D'Esposito M, Hickok G. Conduction aphasia, sensory-motor integration, and phono-logical short-term memory – an aggregate analysis of lesion and fMRI data. *Brain Lang*. 2011;119:119-128.

7. Rasquin SM, Lodder J, Ponds RW, Winkens I, Jolles J, Verhey FR. Cognitive functioning after stroke: a one-year follow-up study. *Dement Geriatr Cogn Disord*. 2004;18:138-144.

8. Vakhnina NV, Nikitina YL, Parfenov VA, Yakhno NN. Post-stroke cognitive impairments. *Neurosci Behav Physiol*. 2009;39(8):16-21.

9. Snaphaan L, Rijpkema M, van Uden I, Fernandez G, de Leeuw FE. Reduced medial temporal lobe functionality in stroke patients: a functional magnetic resonance imaging study. *Brain*. 2009;132:1882-1888.

10. Barrett KM, Meschia JF. Acute ischemic stroke management: medical man-agement. *Semin Neurol*. 2010;30(5):461-468.

11. Elliott J, Smith M. The acute management of intracerebral hemorrhage: a clinical review. *Anesth Analg*. 2010;110:1419-1427.

12. Meyer BC, Hemmen TM, Jackson CM, Lyden PD. Modified national insti-tutes of health stroke scale for use in stroke clinical trials: prospective reli-ability and validity. *Stroke*. 2002;33:1261-1266.

13. Conroy BE, DeJong G, Horn SD. Hospital-based stroke rehabilitation in the United States. *Top Stroke Rehabil*. 2009;16(1):34-43.

14. Taub, E. Crago JE, Burgio LD, Groomes TE, Cook EW 3rd, DeLuca SC, Miller NE. An operant approach to rehabilitation medicine: overcoming learned nonuse by shaping. *J Exp Anal Behav*. 1994;61(2):281-293.

15. Meijer R, Ihnenfeldt DS, van Limbeek J, Vermeulen M, de Haan RJ. Prognostic factors in the subacute phase after stroke for the future resi-dence after six months to one year. A systematic review of the literature. *Clin Rehabil*. 2003;17(5):512-520.

16. Rocco A, Pasquini M, Cecconi E, et al. Monitoring after the acute stage of stroke: a prospective study. *Stroke*. 2007;38(4):1225-1228.

17. Borg GA. Psychophysical bases of perceived exertion. *Med Sci Sports Exerc*. 1982;14:377-381.

18. Zimmermann-Schlatter A, Schuster C, Puhan MA, Siekierka E, Steurer J. Efficacy of motor imagery in post-stroke rehabilitation: a systematic review. *J Neuroeng Rehabil*. 2008;5:8.

19. Gregg M, Hall C, Butler A. The MIQ-RS: a suitable option for examining movement imagery ability. *eCAM*. 2010;7(2):249-257.

20. Saeys W, Vereeck L, Truijen S, Lafosse C, Wuyts FP, Heyning PV. Randomized controlled trial of truncal exercises early after stroke to improve balance and mobility. *Neurorehabil Neural Repair*. 2012;26(3):231-238.

21. Sommerfeld DK, Gripenstedt UK, Welmer AK. Spasticity after stroke: an overview of prevalence, test instruments, and treatments. *Am J Phys Med Rehabil*. 2012;91(9):814-820.

22. Morris JH, Van Wijck F. Responses of the less affected arm to bilateral upper limb task training in early rehabilitation after stroke: a randomized controlled trial. *Arch Phys Med Rehabil*. 2012;93(7):1129-1137.

23. Wu C, Chuang L, Lin K, Chen H, Tsay P. Randomized trial of distributed constraint-induced therapy versus bilateral arm training for the rehabilita-tion of upper-limb motor control and function after stroke. *Neurorehabil Neural Repair*. 2011;24(2):130-139.

24. Chan MK, Tong RK, Chung KY. Bilateral upper limb training with func-tional electric stimulation iin patients with chronic stroke. *Neurorehab Neural Repair*. 2009;23(4):357-365.

25. Hesse S. Treadmill training with partial body weight support after stroke: a review. *NeuroRehabilitation*. 2008;23(1):55-65.

26. Lau KW, Mak MK. Speed-dependent treadmill training is effective to improve gait and balance performance in patients with sub-acute stroke. *J Rehabil Med: Official journal of the UEMS European Board of Physical and Rehabilitation Medicine*. 2011;43(8):709-713.

27. McCain KJ, Smith PS, Polo FE, Coleman SC, Baker S. Excellent outcomes for adults who experienced early standardized treadmill training dur-ing acute phase of recovery from stroke: a case series. *Top Stroke Rehabil*. 2011;18(4):428-36.

28. Hesse S. Treadmill training with partial body weight support after stroke: a review. *NeuroRehab*. 2008;23:55-65.

29. Olvey EL, Armstrong EP, Grizzle AJ. Contemporary pharmacologic treat-ments for spasticity of the upper limb after stroke: a systematic review. *Clin Ther*. 2010;32(4):2282-2303.

30. Bakheit AMO, Fedorova NV, Skoromets AA, Timerbaeva SL, Bhakta BB, Coxon L. The beneficial antispasticity effect of botulinum toxin type A is maintained after repeated treatment cycles. *J Neurol Neurosurg Psychiatry*. 2004;75:1558-1561.

31. Dvorak EM, Ketchum NC, McGuire JR. The underutilization of intrathecal baclofen in poststroke spasticity. *Top Stroke Rehabil*. 2011;18(3):195-202.

32. Schiess MC, Oh IJ, Stimming EF, Lucke J, Acosta F, Fisher S, Simpson RK. Prospective 12-month study of intrathecal baclofen therapy for poststroke spastic upper and lower extremity motor control and functional improve-ment. *Neuromodulation*. 2011;14:38-45.

33. Duncan PW, Sullivan KJ, Behrman AL, Azen SP, Wu SS, Nadeau SE, Dobkin BH, Rose DK, Tilson JK, Cen S, Hayden SK, LEAPS Investigation Team. Body-weight-supported treadmill rehabilitation after stroke. *N Engl J Med*. 2011;364:2026-2036.

34. Van de Port IGL, Wevers LEG, Lindeman E, Kwakkel G. Effects of circuit training as alaternative to ususal physiotherapy after stroke: randomized controlled trial. *BMJ*. 2012;344:e2672.

35. Rose D, Paris T, Crews E, Wu SS, Sun A, Behrman AL, Duncan P. Feasibilty and effectiveness of circuit training in acute stroke rehabilitation. *Neurorehabil Neural Repair*. 2011;25(2):140-148.

36. Taub E. Somatosensory deafferentation search with monkeys: implica-tions for rehabilitation medicine. In: LP Ince, ed. *Behavioral Psychology in Rehabilitation Medicine: Clinical Applications*. New York, NY: Williams & Wilkins; 1980:316-401.

37. Wolf SL, Lecraw DE, Barton LA, Jann BB. Forced use of hemiplegic upper extremities to reverse the effect of learned nonuse among chronic stroke and head injured patients. *Exp Neurol*. 1989;104(2):125-132.

38. Wolf SL, Winstein CJ, Miller JP, et al. Effect of constraint-induced move-ment therapy on upper extremity function 3 to 9 months after stroke: the EXCITE randomized clinical trial. *JAMA*. 2006;296(17):2095-2104.

39. Taub E, Uswatte G, Bowman MH, Mark VW, Delgado A, Bryson C, Morris D, Bishop-McKay S. Constraint-induced movement therapy combined with conventional neurorehabilitation techniques in chronic stroke patients with plegic hands: a case series. *Arch Phys Med Rehabil*. 2013;94:86-94.

40. Peurala SH, Kantanen MP, Sjogren T, Paltamaa J, Karhula M, Heinonen A. Effectiveness of constraint-induced movement therapy on activity and par-ticipation after stroke: a systematic review and meta-analysis of random-ized controlled trials. *Clin Rehabil*. 2011;26(3):209-223.

41. Eliasson AC, Shaw K, Berg E, Krumlinde-Sundholm L. An ecological approach of constraint induced movement therapy for 2-3 year old children: a randomized control trial. *Res Dev Disabil*. 2011;32:2820-3828.

42. Gordon AM, Chalres J, Wolf Sl. Methods of constraint-induced movement therapy for children with hemiplegic cerebral palsy: development of a child-friendly intervention for improving upper extremity function. *Arch Phys Med Rehabil*. 2005;86(4):836-844.

43. DeLuca SC, Case-Smith J, Stevenson R, Ramey SL. Constraint-induced movement therapy (CIMT) for young children with cerebral apalsy: effects of therapeutic dosage. *J Pediatr Rehabil Med*. 2012;5(2):133-142.

44. Byl NN, Pitsch EA, Abrams GM. Functional outcomes can vary by dose: learning-based sensorimotor training for patients stable poststroke. *Neurorehabil Neural Repair*. 2008;22:494-504.

45. Borstad AL, Bird T, Choi S, Goodman L, Schmalbrock P, Nichols-Larsen DS. Sensorimotor training induced neural reorganization after stroke. *JNPT*. 2013;37(1):27-36.

46. Pernet L, Jughters A, Kerckhofs E. The effectiveness of different treatment modalities for the rehabilitation of unilateral neglect in stroke patients: a systematic review. *NeuroRehabil*. 2013;33:611-620.

47. Fortis P, Ronchi R, Senna I, Perucca L, Posteraro L, et al. Rehabilitating patients with left spatial neglect by prism exposure during a visuomotor activity. *Neuropsych*. 2010;24(*6):681-697.

48. Baccini M, Paci M, Rinaldi LA. The scale of contraversive pushing: a reliability and validity study. *Neurorehabil Neural Repair*. 2006;20(4):468-472.

49. Kleim JA, Jones TA. Principles of experience-dependent neural plasticity: implications for rehabilitation after brain damage. *J Speech Lang Hear Res*. 2008;51:S225-S239.

50. Borstad A, Schmalbrock P, Choi S, Nichols-Larsen DS. Neural correlates supporting sensory discrimination after left hemisphere stroke. *Brain Res*. 2012;1460:78-87.

51. Schiemanck SK, Post MM, Kwakkel G, Witkamp TD, Kappelle LJ, Prevo AJH. Ischemic lesion volume correlates with long-term functional outcome and quality of life of middle cerebral artery stroke survivors. *Restor Neurol Neurosci*. 2005;23:257-263.

52. Gauthier LV, Taub E, Perkins C, Ortmann M, Mark VW, Uswatte G. Remodeling the brain: plastic structural brain changes produced by different motor therapies after stroke. *Stroke*. 2008:39(5):1520-1525.

53. Schaechter JD, Moore CK, Connell BD, Rosen BR, Dijkhuizen RM. Structural and functional plasticity in the somatosensory cortex of chronic stroke patients. *Brain*. 2006;129:2722-2733.

54. Dupont SA, Wijdicks EFM, Lanzino G, Rabinstein AA. Aneurysmal subarachnoid hemorrhave: an overview for the practicing neurologist. *Semin Neurol*. 2010;30(5):545-554.

55. Grobelny TJ. Brain aneurysms: epidemiology, treatment options, and milestones of endovascular treatment evolution. *Dis Mon*. 2011; 567:647-655.

56. Lee H. Neuro-otological aspects of cerebellar stroke syndrome. *J Clin Neurol*. 2009;5:65-73.

57. Schjolberg A, Sunnerhagen KS. Unlocking the locked in: a need for team approach in rehabilitation of survivors with locked-in syndrome. *Acta Neurol Scand*. 2012;125:192-198.

58. Available at: https://www.health.qld.gov.au/pahospital/biru/docs/vestibular_gait.pdf.

59. DeKroon JR, IIzerman MJ, Chae J, Lankhorst GJ, Zilvoid G. Relation between stimulation characteristics and clinical outcome in studies using electrical stimulation to improve motor control of the upper extremity in stroke. *J Rehabil Med*. 2005;37(2):65-74.

60. Daly JJ, Ruff Rl. Construction of efficacious gait and upper limb functional interventions based on brain plasticity evidence and model-based measures for stroke patients. *Sci World J*. 2006;7:2031-2045.

61. Steinlin M. A clinical approach to arterial ischemic childhood stroke; increasing knowledge over the last decade. *Neuroped*. 2012;43:1-9.

62. Fan HC, Hu CF, Juan CJ, Chen SJ. Current proceedings of childhood stroke. *Stroke Res Treat*. 2011;43:28-39.

63. Grunwald IQ, Kuhn AL. Current pediatric stroke treatment. 2011;76;6S:S80-S84.

64. Quinn CT. Sickle cell disease in childhood: from newborn screening through transition to adult medical care. *Pediatr Clin North Am*. 2013;60(6): 1363-1381.

65. Mazumdar M, Heeney MM, Sox CM, Lieu TA. Preventing stroke among children with sickle cell anemia: an analysis of strategies that involve transcranial Doppler testing and chronic transfusion. *Pediatrics*. 2007;120: e1107.

Review Questions

1. **You have your client in supine with hips extended and the feet turned outward. You are testing active range of motion. Which of the following motions is being tested with gravity eliminated in this position?**

   A. Ankle dorsiflexion

   B. Hip abduction

   C. Hip internal rotation

   D. Knee extension

2. **When providing range of motion in the acute care setting which of the following muscle groups should be a focus in the individual post-stroke who is developing typical patterns of hypertonicity through providing range of motion that moves the joint into _____**

   A. Elbow extension

   B. Forearm pronation

   C. Shoulder adduction

   D. Wrist extension

3. **Your client who is s/p CVA is having difficulty rolling from supine to side-lying. In order to work on this activity and improve his motor control and strength for the activity it would be advisable to:**

   A. Assist him to roll by placing your hands under his shoulder and hip and push him over into side-lying

   B. Cross his leg over the other leg in the direction he is rolling, then instruct him to use his arm and head to develop momentum and then roll over by flinging them to the side he is rolling onto

   C. Place a pillow between the legs to position them in abduction prior to initiating rolling

   D. Raise the foot of the bed and have him fling his arm and head side to side to develop momentum to move into the roll

4. **When rehabilitating for function the appropriate progression is to start with the task that is least physically demanding and use the task that**
   A. Allows for the most error in movement
   B. Avoids variability until the first form of the task is mastered
   C. Demands the movement pattern you are training
   D. Utilizes the non-paretic extremities to ensure the task is accomplished

5. **When working to retrain gait after a stroke the BEST choice of assistive device for the individual who continues to need a device during therapy sessions would be:**
   A. Parallel bars
   B. A quad cane or standard cane
   C. A standard walker
   D. A wheeled walker with arm trough

6. **Which of the following statements is true about best practice as related to the use of treadmill training with the individual post-stroke?**
   A. Is best used in the chronic stroke population
   B. Should be progressed to over-ground training
   C. Use 50% body weight support
   D. Use velocity set at 1.0 m/s or greater

7. **When training gait which of the following set ups would discourage knee hyperextension?**
   A. Stepping over small objects with the paretic extremity
   B. Transferring sit to stand with a soft object under the non-paretic foot
   C. Walking up a slope
   D. Walking while stepping with the non-paretic extremity

8. **Functional electrical stimulation (FES) can be used during gait to aid in dorsiflexion. Which of the following is a true statement regarding functional electrical stimulation?**
   A. At present there is insufficient evidence to support the use of FES
   B. Functional electrical stimulation can slow or stop muscle fiber type conversion
   C. The stimulation is applied to the dorsiflexors throughout the gait cycle
   D. The use of functional electrical stimulation impedes neuroplasticity

9. **In the client with "locked in" syndrome the key to successful rehabilitation is to:**
   A. **Establish a means of effective communication**
   B. Position the individual in upright to aid in breathing

C. Provide position changes at least every 2 hours
D. Provide sensory stimulation to assist in bringing them out of their coma

10. **When working with an individual who has developed "pusher syndrome" post-stroke it is important to:**
    A. Set up training to obtain effective weight-bearing on the side they are pushing toward
    B. Set up training to obtain effective weight-bearing on the side that is doing the pushing
    C. Set up the environment so that all visual stimuli are on the paretic side and force the gaze to that side
    D. Set up the environment so that all visual stimuli are on the non-paretic side and force the gaze to that side

11. **Which stroke syndrome is likely to produce lower extremity paresis without upper extremity paresis?**
    A. Anterior cerebral artery stroke
    B. Basilar artery stroke
    C. Middle cerebral artery stroke
    D. Posterior cerebral artery stroke

12. **Loss of the upper left visual field is likely to occur with damage to which component of the optic projections?**
    A. Left temporal optic radiations
    B. Left parietal optic radiations
    C. Right temporal optic radiations
    D. Right parietal optic radiations

13. **A patient presents with the ability to understand speech but can only produce a few single words. What type of aphasia would present like this?**
    A. Conductive aphasia
    B. Expressive aphasia
    C. Global aphasia
    D. Receptive aphasia

14. **Over activity of the pontine reticular formation is responsible for what post-stroke phenomenon?**
    A. Clonus
    B. Hyperreflexia
    C. Phasic stretch reflex
    D. Tonic stretch reflex

15. **Your patient is experiencing localized spasticity in the thumb abductor; what would be the most likely medical treatment to decrease his spasticity?**
    A. Intrathecal baclofen
    B. Injection of botulinum toxin type A
    C. Oral baclofen
    D. Oral diazepam

16. A patient presents with ipsilateral paresis of the facial muscles, ipsilateral sensory loss of the face, contralateral paresis of the trunk and extremities, and contralateral sensory loss in the trunk and extremities. A lesion of which area of the brain would produce these symptoms?

A. Cerebellum

B. Medulla

C. Midbrain

D. Pons

17. In infants, which symptom is most likely to be noticed at stroke onset?

A. Absent speech

B. Hemiparesis

C. Impaired consciousness

D. Sensory loss

Answers

1. B	2. D	3. B	4. C	5. D
6. B	7. C	8. B	9. A	10. A
11. A	12. C	13. B	14. D	15. B
16. D	17. C			

Traumatic Brain Injury and Brain Tumor

11

Deborah A. Kegelmeyer and Deborah S. Nichols-Larsen

OBJECTIVES

1) Differentiate the focal and diffuse injury and sequela associated with traumatic brain injury

2) Examine the medical management of the patient with traumatic brain injury

3) Differentiate the evaluation and treatment methods of those with traumatic brain injury from those for other neurologic conditions

4) Structure evaluations and treatment sessions appropriate to the cognitive recovery level described by the Ranchos Scale to promote both physical and cognitive gains

5) Manage various behaviors as they arise during a treatment session with particular emphasis paid to agitation

6) Screen for mild traumatic brain injury

7) Recognize family adjustment issues and provide appropriate education

8) Write goals with cognitive and behavioral qualifiers to the physical activities

9) Review the presentation, pathology, and medical management of brain tumor in adults and children

10) Discuss the role of physical therapy in the management of patients with brain tumor

CASE A, PART I

Aaron is a 22-year-old Caucasian male brought by ambulance to the Emergency Department, following a motor vehicle accident (MVA), in which he was driving without a seatbelt, struck an electric pole, and flew through the windshield. His blood alcohol level is .20, and he is unconscious with multiple fractures, including his right femur, right clavicle, right radius and ulna, multiple ribs and jaw. He has multiple contusions and a deep gash on the right side of his head, although the skull remains intact. He is not opening his eyes even to deep pressure on his palm or foot, is not verbalizing, and his intact left extremities are held in flexion.

● INTRODUCTION

Traumatic brain injury (TBI) is thought to affect up to 10 million people worldwide[1] and is a leading cause of long-term disability with 500,000 new cases[2] and an annual estimated cost of $17 billion dollars in the United States alone, yet that cost does not reflect the growing numbers of concussions (mild TBIs), for which medical attention is not typically sought.[1] It is more common in men, especially in the adolescent and young adult years (17–24), becoming more gender neutral in older adults. This commonly relates to the level of activity and degree of risk-taking displayed by boys/young men. The incidence of TBI has two peak time periods; the first is the 17–24 year range, and the second is at the 60–70 year range.

TBI can result from a blow to the head and/or sudden acceleration–deceleration of the head. As described in the case, many TBIs (often the most severe) occur as a result of a car accident, where the driver or passenger experiences a rapid forward movement of his body as the car hits an object or another car, stopped quickly by either the seatbelt, dashboard, or ground (acceleration–deceleration); in the worst situations, the car flips and there can be multiple head blows against the side window, roof of the car, and/or the dashboard along with rotational shear as the head and body roll, or the individual is thrown from the car with severe trauma to the head as it strikes the ground. Head injuries can be **open** or **closed**, referring to whether the skull is penetrated or intact. Penetrating injuries can arise from projectiles, like bullets, or are associated with skull fractures, where a piece of the skull itself penetrates the underlying brain tissue. Closed head injuries are much more common than penetrating injuries and result from MVAs, falls, and blows to the head from assaults as well as recreational activities, such as sports. Notably, falls are the most common cause of TBI, especially in young children and older adults. TBI is defined as mild, moderate, or severe, depending on the initial presentation and length of unconsciousness plus amnesiac period (see Table 11-1 and later section on amnesia), and this initial presentation is somewhat predictive of the potential outcome for the injury. Of note, some individuals with initially mild TBI have died and some with severe TBI recover and return to a normal level of participation and function. So, while these levels are somewhat predictive, they are not absolutely predictive, since site of injury, age, and co-morbidities also

TABLE 11-1   TBI Severity[1]

SEVERITY LEVEL	GLASGOW COMA SCORE	PERIOD OF UNCONSCIOUSNESS + AMNESIA	POTENTIAL OUTCOME
Mild (concussion)	13–15	<30 minutes	High likelihood of survival with minimal long-term disability
Moderate	9–12	30 minutes–24 hours	Good likelihood of survival but with some long-term disability
Severe	3–8	>24 hours	Poor likelihood of survival and high likelihood of long-term disability

impact outcomes. The Glasgow Coma Scale (Box 11-1) is used almost exclusively to document initial presentation; however, increasing use of sedation at the site of the accident is making its use more difficult by preventing the assessment of responsiveness, while improving outcomes. Other signs of TBI that may be evident on initial examination are noted in Box 11-2.

Based on the description of Aaron in Part I, how would he score on the GCS?

If you said 5, then you're correct.

BOX 11-1   Glasgow Coma Scale

The Glasgow Coma Scale (GCS) was developed in the 1970s and assesses eye movements, verbal responses, and motor behavior, looking for spontaneous versus responsive activity, with each scale recorded numerically as indicated here.

SCORE	EYE OPENING	VERBAL RESPON-SIVENESS	MOTOR BEHAVIOR
1	None	None	None
2	Opens in response	Makes sounds	Limbs in extension to deep pressure
3	Opens to verbal stimulation	Saying words	Limbs in flexion
4	Spontaneously opens	Confused but talking	Flexor withdrawal of limb to stimulus
5	N/A	Oriented	Localized response to stimulus
6	N/A	N/A	Moves to commands

Adapted with permission from Teasdale G, Maas A, Lecky F, et al: The Glasgow Coma Scale at 40 years: standing the test of time. *Lancet Neurol.* 2014 Aug;13(8):844-854.

BOX 11-2   Signs of Traumatic Brain Injury

1) Cerebrospinal fluid leaking from ears or nose
2) Confusion or agitation that may worsen
3) Dilated or unequal pupils
4) Headache
5) Nausea or vomiting
6) Positive neurologic signs – Babinski, decerebrate or decorticate posturing (see below)
7) Seizures

Decorticate posturing defines a condition of upper extremity flexion, including fisting of the hands, and lower extremity extension with toe extension that results from damage to the brain at the junction of the midbrain and diencephalon, resulting in dominant descending control by the medullary reticulospinal and rubrospinal tracts. In contrast, **decerebrate posturing** is characterized by excessive extension and internal rotation of the upper and lower extremities and extension of the trunk and neck secondary to damage at the level of the midbrain. Some patients will initially present in decorticate posturing that progresses to decerebrate posturing, which is an indication of lesion expansion or brain herniation.

● PATHOPHYSIOLOGY OF TBI

The typical TBI presents with two types of injury: focal and diffuse. **Focal injury** results at the area(s) of contact between the skull and the brain or from the projectile that penetrates the brain. In the typical acceleration–deceleration injury, there is a focal injury as the brain bumps into the skull as the body's momentum comes to a rapid stop, and then a **contra coup** (opposite side) injury as it "bounces back" into the opposite side of the skull. For example, Aaron's car hit an electric pole, causing his head to move rapidly forward, hitting the windshield on its way to the pavement and resulting in severe damage to the frontal lobe as the brain hit the anterior part of the skull; as he came to rest on the pavement, his brain would have quickly bounced back toward the posterior surface of the skull, creating a contra coup injury to the occipital lobe. The site of focal damage is characterized by (1) **contusions** – bruising of the brain surface, (2) **lacerations** – tearing of the pia or arachnoid matter or the brain tissue, and/or (3) **hematomas** – bleeding within the subdural or epidural spaces or within the brain tissue, referred to as **intraparenchymal**. These hemorrhages occur due to rupture of the blood vessels within these areas: (1) subdural – tearing of cerebral arteries or veins that bleed into the space between the dura and arachnoid matters, (2) epidural – tearing of meningeal arteries of the dura with bleeding into the space between the dura and the skull, and (3) intraparenchymal – tearing of the penetrating intracerebral arteries with bleeding into the brain tissue.

The **diffuse axonal injury** (DAI) results from the tearing of axons that comprise the white matter due to inertial or rotational forces as the brain "bounces" within the cranium (see Figure 11-1). MVAs are associated with the greatest amount of DAI[3]; however, even relatively minor concussions, as are seen in athletes, whether professional or amateur, from concussive events (e.g., helmet–helmet or head–head contact) have been shown to create axonal injury, and repeated concussions can produce permanent and significant damage (discussed later in this chapter).[2] DAI is most common in the white matter of the brainstem, corpus callosum, and parasagittal projections in the lateral hemispheres. It can be quantified as: **Grade 1** (mild) – microscopic changes noted in the white matter; **Grade 2** (moderate) – apparent damage to the corpus callosum; and **Grade 3** (severe) – damage to the corpus callosum and brainstem white matter.[2] Early imaging is used to determine the extent of the early damage; this is typically done with computed tomography (CT scan), which is effective in identifying hematomas or the location of projectiles or bone fragments in penetrating injuries. Later, magnetic resonance imaging (MRI) is used to better characterize the brain injury and may include diffusion tensor imaging (DTI) that can visualize white matter integrity; this can help in determining the potential prognosis.[4]

The consequences of TBI are dependent on the areas of focal damage and the degree of white matter damage. However, the initial trauma is followed by a cascade of secondary changes that result in further loss of neurons. First, damage to the axon disrupts the **axonal transport** conveying nutrients through the length of the axon, resulting ultimately in the loss of the distil segment of the axon. Second, there is a loss of ATP (adenosine 5'-triphosphate), disrupting the cellular mechanisms that maintain the sodium, calcium, and potassium cellular balance in the cell body and proximal axon, allowing calcium to rush into these components. At the same time, there is an overproduction of oxidants, generating oxidative stress, and exaggerated release of glutamate and free radicals, which further disrupt cellular function in damaged and adjacent neurons. **Anterograde degeneration** occurs early, resulting in the death of the distil segment; this is followed by **retrograde degeneration**, or a dying back, of the proximal axon segment and ultimately the cell body. These changes induce inflammation, trigger macrophages to invade the area, and further disrupt cellular function in adjacent neurons and glia.[2] Notably, the loss of neurons and white matter disruption seems to continue for a considerable time after the initial injury, resulting in additional general brain atrophy, white matter abnormalities, and secondary loss of function[1] that can occur months after the initial injury such that the individual demonstrates improvement to a point of plateau, followed by a subsequent loss of function.[5] These chronic changes, referred to as **negative or maladaptive plasticity**, appear related to amyloid and tau protein deposits and ongoing neuroinflammation, associated with reactive microglia (see Chapter 2).[5] Maladaptive plasticity may continue for years and is thought to result from the same processes that impact aging, including (1) decreasing activity levels within limited and often unstimulating environments; (2) disruption of sensory processing, referred to as noisy processing (see Chapter 17 on Aging), associated with decreased activity in the sensory cortices and less cognitive analysis of sensory information; and (3) decreased neuromodulation, stemming from lower levels of dopamine and acetylcholine that are critical for executive function and attention. Together these maladaptive plasticity changes result in further deterioration of those functions already disrupted by the initial injury.[5] The concept of maladaptive plasticity opens the door for physical therapists, along with the rehabilitation team, to address and potentially prevent negative plasticity.

● TBI CONSEQUENCES

Coma, Post-Traumatic Amnesia, and Executive Dysfunction

As should be evident from the earlier discussion of the GCS, the first consequence of a TBI is loss of consciousness; this can be so short that it goes unnoticed (seconds) or last for weeks. When the period of unconsciousness exceeds 6 hours, it is referred to as **coma**, characterized by a lack of responsiveness, volitional movement, and a sleep–wake cycle. Unlike in the movies, people

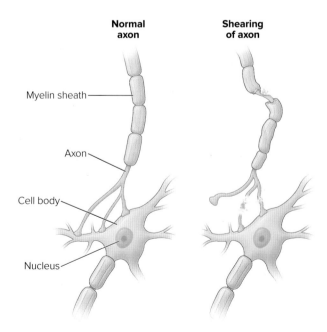

Normal axon

Shearing of axon

Myelin sheath

Axon

Cell body

Nucleus

FIGURE 11-1 Diffuse axonal injury: A. Normal neuron axon with connections to a postsynaptic neuron. **B.** Diffuse axonal injury is characterized by a twisting and tearing of the myelin and underlying axons; this will be followed by retrograde degeneration back to the cell body.

in coma do not just "wake up," they gradually emerge from the coma into a state of confusion; however, in those with mild injuries, this stage can last a minute or minutes, while in those with more severe injuries, it can last for many months, and for some, they never fully emerge from this state. Some survivors of severe TBI will enter what is known as a **vegetative state** (Stage II of the Braintree Scale – see Table 11-2), which is characterized by an emergence of a sleep–wake cycle and a generalized response to stimuli (Ranchos Scale – Level II, Table 11-2); when this condition is associated with an absence of cortical brain activity, it indicates a reliance on the brainstem centers that control the sleep cycle, respiration, and reflexive responsiveness and is, thereby, a permanent condition, in which patients can survive for many years (permanent vegetative state). Many move through this state to one of minimal consciousness, indicated by specific responses to stimulation (e.g., withdrawal of foot to touch of the sole) but no speech.

For those that emerge from coma, after a moderate to severe TBI, they progress through the vegetative state to a gradual reemergence of responsiveness and severe confusion, abnormal behavior (agitation, disinhibition, and altered mood), and memory disruption.[6] This period is referred to as **post-traumatic amnesia** (PTA), which disrupts memories prior to the accident as well as the formation of new memories, including the day-to-day activities within the hospital setting (see Box 11-3 for more information on amnesia). As PTA clears, the patient is left to deal with a myriad of deficits in multiple systems – sensory, motor, behavioral, and cognitive.[7] Ways to document recovery of behavior, memory, and responsiveness from TBI are the Ranchos Los Amigos Cognitive Recovery Scale,[8] Galveston Orientation and Amnesia Test (GOAT),[9] the Disability Rating Scale,[10] the JFK Coma Recovery Scale – Revised,[11] and the Braintree Scale of Neurologic Stages of Recovery from Brain Injury. The GOAT is principally used to identify the clearing of PTA and asks the patient a series of questions to determine orientation to person, place, time, and circumstance, including details of what is remembered about the accident and how he came to be at the hospital. Errors are scored and subtracted from a total of 100. Table 11-2 provides a comparison of some of these measures. It should be noted that recovery can stall at any level of these scales with no further progression or some delay (variable in length) between stage progressions.

Respiratory Distress Syndrome

Presentation

Respiratory compromise is associated with severe brain injury secondary to loss of consciousness and damage to medullary regions that control respiration. In addition, swallowing may be impaired, and facial and/or tracheal damage common with secondary bleeding or hematoma formation in the throat.[13] A secondary complication of TBI can be **acute respiratory distress syndrome** (ARDS), which occurs in up to 31% of TBI admissions, during their hospital course, and is characterized by inflammation of the lung lining, disruption of gas exchange, and hypoxia. This is a leading cause of death in those with TBI. ARDS occurs most commonly in association with other secondary complications (sepsis, renal or heart failure,

or hypertension).[14,15] There is no definitive test for ARDS, so it is diagnosed based on a combination of (1) a ratio of arterial oxygen partial pressure to inspired oxygen fraction that is <300 mm Hg, (2) a chest x-ray illustrating bilateral pulmonary edema, and (3) normal EKG (electrocardiogram).[14]

Treatment

In those with a GCS of ≤8, respiratory support is required either by intubation with an oropharyngeal, nasopharyngeal, or an endotracheal tube with ventilator support.[16] This is typically done at the site of the accident. Some patients with moderate TBI may also need ventilator support, if orofacial injuries are present, or they have disruption of respiratory function. For those that are able to breathe on their own, ventilation support, using continuous positive airway pressure (CPAP), provided through a mask, or positive pressure support, provided through a nasal cannula, may be enough.[4]

There is no definitive treatment for ARDS; in fact, the best treatment is prevention. Standard care for ARDS is to provide ventilator support that minimizes the stress on the lungs; this is typically done with what is termed **lung-protective ventilation**, which uses a lower inspiratory volume (tidal volume), to prevent over stretching the weakened alveoli, in combination with an increased respiration rate. For some, this will require additional sedation to prevent dyssynchrony between the patient and the ventilator.[15]

Intracranial Hypertension (ICH)

Presentation

Post-traumatic ICH arises from multiple causes. Initially, the presence of hematomas may create increased pressure, shifting the brain tissue across midline or caudally into the brainstem compartment. The latter can occur either (1) medially, producing bilateral compression of cranial nerve III with unresponsive pupil dilation or (2) laterally with herniation of the uncus of the temporal lobe, associated with unilateral pupil dilation (see Figure 11-2). Edema of the brain tissue, compromise of cerebrospinal fluid (CSF) circulation, and disruption of the autoregulatory mechanisms that maintain intracranial pressure (ICP) may further increase ICH days after the initial injury. Additionally, compromised blood flow may impede perfusion and, thereby, exacerbate ICH. Normally, ICP measures 10–15 mm Hg with cyclic increases and decreases, associated with cardiopulmonary rhythms; an increase to 20 mm Hg signals the need for treatment.[17] Signs of increased ICP include nausea, vomiting, papilledema (swelling around the optic disc) with retinal hemorrhaging, and drowsiness.

Treatment

First, ICP must be monitored in patients with severe TBI and any patient with an identified hematoma; this is typically done with a catheter placed in the epidural space or ventricle (less common) or a Richmond screw/bolt™ that is just screwed through the skull. The Richmond screw™ does not afford drainage of excessive CSF, which can be achieved through a catheter. Placement of catheters is done through a bur hole in the skull. Of course, placement of a catheter can cause additional brain trauma and potentially hemorrhage, especially when placed in the ventricle; it can also be a site for secondary infection, so careful monitoring for these issues

BOX 11-3 Amnesia

Amnesia is typically divided into two aspects: retrograde amnesia and anterograde amnesia. **Retrograde amnesia** is associated with a loss of memory for prior events; this likely results from an inability to retrieve those memories from our memory storage, which may relate to an inability to identify appropriate cues for memory retrieval. Since memory storage is not localized to a given area, damage in multiple areas can be associated with retrograde amnesia. **Anterograde amnesia** is an inability to form new memories, likely as a result of damage to the temporal or frontal lobes or the white matter connecting them; this impedes the consolidation of new memories. For those with a moderate to severe TBI, the consolidation of the memory of the accident is usually disrupted by the head injury, so most survivors do not remember the actual accident and may not remember a period of time leading up to the accident. This time period varies with the severity of the injury but can include just minutes, hours, or days. **Post-traumatic amnesia** is a period of both retrograde and anterograde amnesia in those with moderate to severe TBI. The retrograde amnesiac component may prevent patients from knowing their family members, friends, and information that defines who they are – occupation, likes/dislikes, etc. However, procedural and semantic memories (discussed in Chapter 7) are typically unaffected or more mildly affected. The anterograde amnesia component prevents new memory accrual, including memory for those providing the patient's care, the location of care, and the ability to verbalize what events or activities occurred previously (earlier in the day or over preceding days). However, procedural learning can occur even though the patient will not be able to verbalize the process. The clearing of PTA is an important stage for the patient, as

it indicates the ability to actively participate in their rehabilitation; early PTA recovery is characterized by the ability to remember the activities of the day and to begin to follow a schedule.

is critical.[4] The first step in treating ICH is sedation to minimize arterial hypertension, agitation, and the potential for fighting the rhythm of the ventilator, which can lead to increased ICH and dislodging of the catheter. However, sedation can have detrimental side effects, including depressed heart function and blood pressure and additional risk for infection. The second step involves administration of hyperosmolar agents (mannitol or hypertonic saline) to increase osmolarity in the blood and draw fluid out of the brain tissues into the circulation, reducing brain volume. Herniation into the brainstem, which can occur with hematoma expansion or excessive brain edema, is a medical emergency, requiring immediate treatment to relieve ICH and potentially necessitating surgical intervention. Large hematomas may also require surgical removal to minimize secondary brain damage and relieve ICH. In those, for whom sedation and hyperosmolarity treatment are ineffective, a decompression craniotomy may be performed to allow some brain expansion through the opening in the cranium. However, the benefit of this remains controversial.[17] Hyperventilation may also be used to increase cerebral perfusion to facilitate clearing of edema and hematomas.

Epilepsy

Presentation

Approximately 25% of patients with severe TBI will develop post-traumatic epilepsy (PTE) (see Chapter 19 for a description of epilepsy); this can occur within the first week of the incident

FIGURE 11-2 Brain shifts associated with traumatic hematoma: A. Frontotemporal hematoma compressing the lateral hemisphere with midline shift to the opposite side of center. **B.** Cerebral hematoma inducing herniation of the uncus and central white matter downward, compressing brainstem tissue.

TABLE 11-2 Measures of Recovery in TBI[1,2,8,10-12]

GLASGOW COMA SCALE SCORE[3]	JFK COMA RECOVERY SCALE – REVISED (SCORE)[11]	RANCHOS LOS AMIGOS COGNITIVE SCALE[8],*	BRAINTREE SCALE[12]	DISABILITY RATING SCALE[10],**
3	Unarousable (0); none responsive on all scales (0); may have abnormal posturing (1); total = 0–1	Stage I: Unresponsive	1. Coma – unresponsive	No response on any scale and totally dependent; total score = 29
4–8	Startles to auditory and visual stimuli (1 each); flexor withdrawal to noxious stimulus (2); reflexive oral responses (1); opens eyes to stimulation (1); no communication; total = 6	Stage II: Generalized response – whole limb or body response to touch, requires complete assistance	2. Vegetative state – begins sleep–wake cycle	Opens eye to pain (2); incomprehensible speech-groans/moans (3); extends (4) or flexes (3) limb to pain or withdraws (2); no awareness for feeding, toileting, grooming (3 each); totally dependent (5) and non-employable (3); total = 24–26
9–10	Localizes sound (1); object fixation – visual pursuit (2–3); localized response to noxious stimulus (3); vocalization/oral movement (2); intentional vocalizing (1); eye opening with or without stimulation (1–2); total = 10–12	Stage III: Localized response – moves part specific to site of touch/pinch, still requires total assistance	3. Minimally conscious – responds inconsistently, no speech	Opens eyes to speech (1) or spontaneously (0); incomprehensive speech (3); localized movement to stimulation (1); no feeding, toileting, or grooming (3 each); totally dependent (5); non-employable (3); total = 21–22
12–14	Moves to command inconsistently – consistently (3–4); reaches to object or recognizes object (4–5); object manipulation or automatic movement or functional object use (4–6); verbalizations understood (3); communication is functional (2); some attention to situation (3); total = 19–23	Stage IV: Confused and agitated, can be abusive and easily provoked, maximal assistance required Stage V: Confused with less agitation but still inappropriate behavior, requires maximal supervision	4. Post-traumatic amnesia	Spontaneous eye opening (0); confused speech (1); obeying commands to move (0); some awareness of feeding (2); some awareness of toileting needs (2); primitive ability to groom self (2); marked (4) assistance required; not employable (3); total = 17 Eye opening (0); confused speech (1); moving to commands (0); partial awareness of how to feed self, toileting and grooming (1 each); marked assistance all of the time (4); not employable (3); total = 10

(Continued)

TABLE 11-2 Measures of Recovery in TBI[2,8,10-12] (Continued)

GLASGOW COMA SCALE SCORE[3]	JFK COMA RECOVERY SCALE – REVISED (SCORE)[11]	RANCHOS LOS AMIGOS COGNITIVE SCALE[8],*	BRAINTREE SCALE[12]	DISABILITY RATING SCALE[10],**
15		Stage VI: Confused but more appropriate behavior; requires moderate supervision	5. PTA resolution, increased independence	Eye opening (0); oriented speech (0); obeying movement commands (0); full awareness of feeding, toileting, grooming needs (0 each); moderately dependent – needs supervision in the home (3); not employable (3) or able to work in sheltered workshop (2); total = 5 or 6
		Stage VII: Automatic appropriate – can complete ADLs and routine activities if physically able with minimal supervision/assistance, but still have memory problems and difficulty with problem-solving		
		Stave VIII: Purposeful, appropriate – independent in many tasks, understands limitations, still some behavioral problems, requires standby assistance	6. Increasing independence and social skills with return to community activity, work, etc.	Same as above but with increasing ability to perform independently with some supervision (1) and likely can work either in a sheltered workshop (2) or selected jobs (1); total = 2 or 3

*The Ranchos Scale actually has two more levels: IX that is associated with increasing ability to maintain focus and switch focus from one task to another but continued mild emotional/behavioral challenges that may require caregiver assistance to refocus; and X, which is associated with good goal directed function, the ability to multi-task, but still with some attentional challenges and the need for more time to complete some activities. Therapists rarely see patients that are at levels VIII–X.

**The Disability Rating Scale has a final category of functioning = independent in all skills (0) and work = unrestricted work ability (0).

(up to 16% of patients) or much later – a year or more post-injury. The incidence of PTE, following a moderate TBI is lower and rarely occurs in the late stages; in contrast, the incidence of PTE is much higher for those that experience a penetrating head injury at almost 53%.[18] Early PTE may exacerbate the original injury by contributing to the detrimental excitotoxicity that occurs post-injury; there is some suggestion that late PTE may also cause expansion of the initial brain tissue loss through a similar mechanism. The cause of these post-traumatic seizures remains elusive. One theory suggests that iron deposits left, as hematomas dissolve, trigger free radical formation that subsequently stimulates abnormal glutamate release and neuronal hyper-activation.[18] Another implicates pro-inflammatory cytokines in the development of lesion expansion and epilepsy onset.[19] The type of seizure is highly variable but includes generalized, focal, and focal that progress to generalized.[20] Focal seizures arise most frequently from the frontal or temporal lobes.[19]

Treatment

Most patients with severe TBI and some with moderate TBI will be placed on prophylactic antiepileptic medications, typically phenytoin, as soon as they are admitted to the hospital.[21] If the patient survives the first week without a seizure, this prophylactic application is weaned with careful observance for any indication of seizure emergence. There is some indication, however, that subclinical seizure episodes may take place without obvious symptoms, so even those that appear to be seizure free may, in fact, be having abnormal neuronal activation. Despite early administration of phenytoin, many TBI survivors will develop epilepsy either early or late. Long-term antiepileptic medications may control seizure activity with a variety of medications utilized (see Chapter 19 for potential medications). However, for those with focal epilepsy, surgical resection of injured tissue may be effective; this is more commonly possible with temporal than frontal epilepsy, as the area is more easily accessed and typically the seizure site is more focal.[19]

Inflammation: Systemic Inflammatory Syndrome and Multi-organ Dysfunction Syndrome

Presentation

CNS inflammation is a natural consequence of TBI; however, with severe injury there may be a systemic inflammatory response that can disrupt function in multiple organs. Systemic infection is characterized by cytokine diffusion through the blood–brain barrier (BBB) into the systemic circulation; this emergence of cytokines is accompanied by elevated plasma leukocytes plus alterations in circulating electrolytes, metal ions, excitatory amino acids, glucocorticoids, and free radicals.[22,23] Together, these changes trigger the liver to stimulate protein synthesis to achieve homeostasis, stimulate tissue repair, and decrease inflammation. However, with severe injury this acute response can be ineffective and transition to a condition known as **systemic inflammatory response syndrome** (SIRS) may occur; SIRS presents with fever, hyperventilation, and extreme elevation in white cell count that seems to result from injury-induced immunosuppression.[23] SIRS may damage not just the liver but also the lungs and kidneys, resulting in **multi-organ dysfunction syndrome** (MODS), which can ultimately lead to organ failure.

Treatment

At this time, there is no definitive treatment for MODS; multiple methods have been tried, including glucocorticoid and epoprostenol (a prostacyclin analogue) administration. Yet, none have been found to be more effective than standard medical care, which includes managing primary infections and treating ICH. Ultimately, approximately 10–20% of those that develop MODS will die.[22,23]

Hypermetabolism, Hypercatabolism, and GI Dysfunction

Presentation

Following a brain injury, the metabolic demand of the patient is elevated, referred to as hypermetabolism; this results from elevation in corticosteroids, epinephrine, norepinephrine, glucagon, and cortisol as well as increased circulating inflammatory mediators (e.g., cytokines).[24,25] Increased levels of epinephrine and norepinephrine disrupt the normal control of metabolism by the sympathetic nervous system that seems to be further exacerbated by a systemic inflammatory process with energy demands as high as 200% of normal.[24,25] In some cases, this hypermetabolism progresses to hypercatabolism, which involves exaggerated glucose utilization and the breakdown of body proteins (e.g., muscle – both skeletal and cardiac), leading to substantial loss of skeletal muscle.[25] The more severe the head injury (lower GCS), the greater the metabolic demand and likelihood of hypercatabolism.[25] The challenge of meeting the nutritional demands of the patient with a severe TBI can be exacerbated by orofacial injuries, dysphagia due to damage to the centers or cranial nerves that control swallowing, and disrupted gastrointestinal function. Gastrointestinal dysfunction is characterized by delayed or slower emptying of the GI tract and esophageal reflux secondary to diminished sphincter tone. The latter can result in aspirational pneumonia.[25]

A secondary complication of TBI is gastric stress ulcers. Multiple factors contribute to their development, including (1) the highly stressful nature of a severe head injury, impacting all major organ systems; (2) uninhibited parasympathetic activity, caused by damage to the hypothalamus and resulting in excessive gastric acid secretions; (3) diminished blood flow to the gastric mucosa, resulting from a cascade of post-traumatic changes; and (4) irritation or infection from enteral feedings.[26]

Treatment

Comprehensive nutritional support is critical to survival from severe brain injury. Initially, this is provided by IV, known as total parenteral nutrition (TPN); however, to meet the metabolic demands of the TBI survivor in coma or with severe orofacial injuries, enteral nutrition is commonly initiated within 24–48 hours of admission to the hospital. This requires placement of a nasogastric or orogastric tube.[24] If prolonged feeding support is required or orofacial injuries are severe, a percutaneous gastrostomy (PEG) tube is used, which is a tube placed directly into the stomach through the abdominal wall; when gastric dysfunction or reflux is severe or there is impaired gastric emptying, the tube may be placed into the jejunum (jejunostomy) to provide post-pyloric feeding.[25,27] To assist with ICH, a hyperosmolar formula is typically initiated early.[4] However, there remains uncertainty about the best other dietary components to provide, but there is some evidence to suggest a high-protein diet with zinc supplements and immune-enhancements may be beneficial.[24] Despite the controversy over the type of diet, it is critical to meet the high metabolic demand of the TBI survivor through appropriate nutrition therapy. As recovery progresses, it is also important to adapt the diet to meet the normalizing catabolic demand to prevent weight gain.

Dysautonomia/Paroxysmal Sympathetic Hyperactivation (PSH)

Presentation

Dysautonomia, more recently renamed PSH, is a dysregulation of autonomic function that presents in 10–12% of TBI admissions, especially in those with severe injury.[28] It is most common in those with fractures, infections, or prolonged ventilation that had significant DAI.[29] Although a definitive cause has not been identified, PSH likely results from damage to the connections between the cortex and hypothalamus, leading to a loss of inhibition and hypersensitivity to internal and external stimuli.[29] As a result, episodes of tachycardia, hyperpyrexia (fever), elevated blood pressure, extensor posturing (decorticate or decerebrate), and copious sweating occur, lasting a few minutes to hours. While most common when patients are in the ICU, this condition can persist into the rehabilitation phase, and when it does, is disruptive to recovery.

Treatment

Pharmacologic treatment is commonly used with a variety of medications attempted, including baclofen, beta blockers (e.g., propranolol), benzodiazepine, and morphine. Recently, intrathecal baclofen administration has been found to provide longer-term management; however, this may not be the first method of choice due to the need for surgical implantation of the administration catheter into the spinal epidural space.[28]

Neuropsychiatric Changes

Presentation

Perhaps the most debilitating consequences of TBI are the neuropsychiatric changes that ensue. Two common behavioral syndromes, experienced by many TBI survivors, are emotional and behavioral dyscontrol. **Emotional dyscontrol** manifests with agitation, irritability, restlessness, pathologic laughing/crying (pseudobulbar affect) and/or emotional lability. *Pathologic laughing/crying* appears as involuntary and sustained periods of these emotions that occur without provocation but disrupt function. In contrast, *emotional lability* is an exaggerated response to an appropriate trigger, so in this condition, there might be excessive crying to a somewhat sad situation (e.g., saying goodbye to a loved one that they will see again the next day). This condition is incredibly common and increases in frequency in the post-acute stages with up to 62% of survivors experiencing

it to some degree. **Behavioral dyscontrol** is characterized by disinhibition and sometimes aggression; this can result in the pulling out of IV lines and feeding tubes, fighting and swearing early in recovery as well as hyper-sexual behavior and excessive risk-taking in later recovery. Minor manifestations include poor social awareness and impulsivity; however, even these can have a profound impact on the long-term outcome of TBI, impeding social participation and employment. Notably, some TBI survivors will also experience other psychiatric conditions, of which depression is the most common; this will require careful monitoring and treatment but also must be distinguished from the more common emotional and behavioral dyscontrol.[30]

Treatment

The most critical treatment for the common neuropsychiatric consequences of TBI is careful and consistent behavioral management. This will be discussed within the physical therapy management section of this chapter but includes creating an environment to minimize excessive stimulation, maintaining a calm demeanor when working with clients, and preventing self-injurious behavior. In some cases, pharmacologic management is required; this can involve many forms but sedation to prevent self-injurious behavior early and antidepression medications to treat ongoing depression at later stages are common.[30]

Physical Therapy Management

The therapist, treating a client after a TBI, must manage three core problem areas: physical, cognitive, and behavioral. Just as in our case study of Aaron, many clients have been involved in some type of accident that has led to multiple trauma. In the physical area, there are findings similar to those discussed in Chapter 10 (CVA); though in the case of TBI, many of the problems may be bilateral and are often accompanied by musculoskeletal and peripheral nervous system injuries. Examination and treatment are conducted as outlined in Chapters 9 (Evaluation) and 10 with appropriate modifications for bilateral impairments. This chapter will discuss management of the cognitive and behavioral sequela of TBI.

Cognition/Memory

As discussed in Chapter 7, cognition is a complex function, involving the ability of the brain to process, store, retrieve, and manipulate information to solve problems. It includes:

- Attention – consists of selective attention, divided attention, and sustained attention.
- Memory – the ability to consolidate, store and retrieve facts, events, experiences, etc.
- Initiation – the ability to initiate action.
- Judgment – the ability to make considered decisions or come to sensible conclusions.
- Speed of processing – the rate at which directions can be processed into actions.

TBI may impact any of these areas; therefore, the physical therapy assessment includes careful examination of the domains of cognitive function, and treatment is based on these findings. Assessment of attention is typically done by observing the client's ability to stay focused on the task at hand, during the therapy evaluation. The client should also be observed in situations where there are distractions to determine if selective attention is impaired. Divided attention is intact, if the client can talk while carrying out a task (e.g., performing an exercise). Sustained attention is measured by the length of time the client can stay on task, during their work with the therapist.

Memory loss is common, after even mild TBI, and questions should be asked to assess the client's ability to retrieve old memories and acquire new ones. To identify the degree and recovery of retrograde amnesia, questioning about the period leading up to the injury, the time of the injury, and immediately after the injury will identify the window of memory loss. On subsequent therapy sessions, asking about events from the previous therapy session is a means to assess for the presence of anterograde amnesia. PTA, as described earlier in the chapter, is the inability to lay down memories reliably from one day to the next. This also includes orientation to time, person, place, and situation. The duration of PTA is a key indicator of injury severity and prognosis and is defined as the time from injury to regaining continuous memory for ongoing events (see Box 11-4).

For explanations of cognitive assessment for initiation, judgment, and speed of processing along with functional examples, see Table 11-3.

It is hypothesized that deficits in divided attention, executive function, and long-term memory are due to either impaired working memory or speed of processing deficits. A study by Ciarmelli et al. supports the hypothesis that deficits in these cognitive functions are primarily due to impairments in working memory.[32] Thus, progressively challenging working memory, during therapy, while allowing sufficient time to process information, should, hypothetically, lead to better functional outcomes.

Personality

The personality and behavioral changes that commonly occur after TBI have a significant impact on the individual's sense of self and can be quite debilitating for both the patient and their family and friends. Personality changes are most difficult for

CASE A, PART I

Differential assessment of Aaron's other cognitive abilities would be done as part of the physical therapy assessment as he is coming out of his coma. He is asked to wave good-bye to his mother. He is given time to respond, and it is noted that he waves after a 30-second delay. Also, during the evaluation, Aaron is asked to point to the red paper. After 2 minutes and a cue, he has not pointed to the paper. This assessment has shown that speed of processing is slow and that Aaron understands simple familiar commands, like "wave good-bye," but he is unable to cognitively process pointing to the red paper despite being given additional time to respond. Waving is limited by speed of processing, while the pointing task is limited by a higher level cognitive dysfunction.

individuals with mild TBI as they are cognizant of the changes and the impact of those changes on their friends and family. Therapists should acknowledge these changes, when working with the patient and family, and recognize the need to modify therapy based on mood and negative behaviors.

Recognizing cognitive and behavioral deficits is important as these are most closely associated with long-term disability.[33] Common behaviors that occur after TBI include agitation, confusion, perseveration, and apathy among others. See Table 11-6 for a description of each behavior and ways to manage those behaviors in the clinic. This text will address specific behavior-management techniques throughout the rest of the chapter based on the time since injury and the stage of recovery.

Motor Learning

Motor learning may be intact, depending on the areas of the brain impacted by the TBI, though it is common for some aspect of motor learning to be negatively impacted by TBI. Usually, procedural learning remains intact while declarative learning

TABLE 11-3	Cognitive Function and Assessment	
	HOW IT IMPACTS FUNCTION	**ASSESSMENT**
Initiation	Closely related to apathy though the two are separate and distinct entities. Individuals who lack initiative are capable of solving the problem but are unable to initiate the process. It can be difficult to separate issues with initiative from depression, apathy, or severe cognitive disability.	Need to rule out apathy and depression with input from psychology services. Observe the client's ability to generate a new conversation where he must choose the topic or engage in an activity that he is not specifically told to complete. Initiation often becomes a larger problem when the client returns home.
Judgment	Impairs safety	Ask the client to make decisions requiring them to judge safety in a controlled environment (e.g., ask the client when it is safe to cross a street in a mock set up or while under close supervision of therapy staff).
Speed of processing	There's a slowing of processing, but individuals with slow processing can solve the problem, if given enough time.	Allow time for processing during the examination to determine what time frame each client requires to process information. Once the time needed for successful processing is determined, future sessions can be conducted based on this measurement.

BOX 11-4 **Prognosis Based on PTA[31]**

Severity based on duration of PTA:

Mild = <1 hour

Moderate = >1 hour and <24 hours

Severe = >1 day and <7 days

Very severe = >7 days

Data from Nakase-Richardson R, Sepehri A, Sherer M, et al: Classification schema of posttraumatic amnesia duration-based injury severity relative to 1-year outcome: analysis of individuals with moderate and severe traumatic brain injury. *Arch Phys Med Rehabil*. 2009 Jan;90(1):17-19.

---

dural learning. For therapy tasks, such as sit to stand and transfer to walking with a rollator walker, TBI survivors often demonstrate intact procedural learning, but when asked to explain how to safely stand up, the client with a TBI is not able to explain the steps of the transfer. With repetition, these clients continue to demonstrate procedural learning to be safe while transferring. However, they are limited in their ability to apply this learning to new situations, requiring the therapy staff and family to teach the task in each environment, in which it will be performed.

Successful motor learning in individuals with cognitive, memory, or behavioral deficits requires many repetitions with consistent structure and feedback. A study by Kimberly et al. shows that the number of repetitions completed in studies that demonstrate neuroplasticity was far higher than that achieved in typical therapy. This highlights the need for therapists to be very cognizant of practice time and number of repetitions, if they hope to optimize neuroplastic changes after TBI.[34] To date, research in the area of motor learning and TBI is very limited due to difficulties in defining the population. One study demonstrated that gait adaptation to novel environmental demands is impaired in persons with chronic TBI, and therefore, may be an important skill to target in rehabilitation.[35] There is also evidence that some individuals with TBI can benefit from random (variable) learning methods, and that this type of learning improves transfer to novel conditions better than blocked practice, just as was found in non-TBI subjects.[36]

Early Management

Immediately following TBI, the focus of care is on saving the individual's life. Within the intensive care setting (ICU), therapists focus on determining the severity of the injury, preserving life, and prevention of further damage. As recovery progresses and the patient becomes more stable, therapy can be progressed to include mobility, strength, and range of motion. The initial PT assessment focuses on state of arousal, cognitive level as defined by the Ranchos Amigos Stages, and identifying injuries to the neuromuscular and musculoskeletal systems. The musculoskeletal and neurologic systems should be reevaluated periodically as it is easy to miss deficits in these systems in a comatose patient. Before standing and walking a client s/p TBI, the therapist must reassess the lower extremities for pain, ligamentous laxity, and signs of fracture. Minor injuries such as these can be missed in multi-trauma life and death situations. The therapist plays a critical role in monitoring the musculoskeletal system throughout the course of care.

CASE A, PART II

Aaron has been in the ICU for 10 days and remains in a coma. Physical therapy has been ordered, his ICP has normalized, and the intraventricular catheter has been removed and the skull closed. While performing ROM to the left UE, the therapist asks Aaron to help bend his arm into elbow flexion. On the third repetition, Aaron actively assists with elbow flexion. He is no longer posturing into flexion/extension and has been noted to open his eyes periodically, especially when his family is in the room. Aaron has a hard lump in his biceps muscle on the right and grimaces, during ROM to that arm. The therapist suspects that he has developed a heterotopic ossification (HO) in the biceps brachii (see discussion in latter section) and performs only active ROM to this muscle in the pain-free range to avoid further inflaming the tissue.

What coma level is Aaron in?

He is in Ranchos level III since he is responding to stimuli and following simple commands.

Is it safe for the therapist to begin to work on rolling side to side in supine?

Yes, the therapist could put Aaron in supine and work on side to side rolling with physician clearance, since his ICP is normalized. If his vitals make any notable changes or if he were running a fever, therapy should not proceed.

Contracture Prevention

In the ICU, therapists utilize position changes, range of motion exercises and splints to prevent contractures. The development of hypertonia often leads to severe contractures of the elbow and plantarflexors. Foot boards can be used to position the foot at 90 degrees but are only effective, if the client is consistently positioned correctly on the foot board and knee flexion can be avoided. The use of a padded boot that positions the ankle at 90 degrees is the most effective means of preventing contractures of the ankle. Contractures of the forearm, wrist, and hand are best prevented with splints that typically require an occupational therapy consultation for fitting and construction.

CASE A, PART III

Aaron should be positioned with pillows under both UEs such that his elbows are in slight flexion, his shoulder is slightly elevated and abducted, and the forearm is in neutral. His right wrist and fingers are in a cast for the forearm fracture, which should be supported by the pillow on the right and kept in slight flexion on the left. Padded semi-rigid boots are placed on his feet to position the ankles in 90 degrees of dorsiflexion.

In those individuals who develop contractures, the most common treatments are pharmacologic, stretching, dynamic splints, and serial casting. There is very little research examining the benefit of dynamic splints in individuals with hypertonia or those with TBI. Studies have shown improved range of motion in the elbow after dynamic splinting, when combined with botulinum toxin and stretching.[37] No studies were identified that examined the use of dynamic splinting of the LE in individuals with spasticity. Static stretching, using serial casting, has been shown to improve range of motion in individuals who are s/p TBI and is well tolerated.[38] A study comparing serial casting with dynamic splinting of the elbow found both modalities to be equally effective, but three individuals, assigned to the dynamic splinting group, requested to be changed to the static – serial casting group. Dynamic splinting is more likely to lead to complaints of discomfort or pain. In agitated individuals, a possible benefit of serial casting may be that the cast is more difficult for the patient to remove. Effective contracture reduction is difficult and maintenance of increased ROM appears to depend on the individual's ability to use that range of motion functionally.[39,40]

Dynamic splinting involves a splint that has a spring that provides a constant, low-level stretch. Dynamic splints favor the elastic response of tissue. It is easier to monitor skin status while using this type of splint, and it can be taken off to clean and to perform ROM exercises. Caution should be used in the presence of hypertonia, as this type of splint can aggravate hypertonia. Since these splints are also easily removed, they may not be effective in clients with agitation or poor cognitive function. Care should be taken to apply the splint exactly at the anatomic joint to avoid discomfort. This type of splint is also more likely to cause skin breakdown because it is not total contact.

Serial casting involves a prolonged low-level stretch that favors the plastic response of tissue and, thereby, results in a greater amount of permanent elongation with the least amount of trauma and weakening of tissue. When utilizing serial casting, the therapist performs range of motion to the joint, then, takes it to the end range but not into a stretch. The limb is casted in this position, and the cast remains on for 7–10 days. When the cast is removed, ROM and joint mobilizations are performed. The joint is then taken to end range but no further, and a new cast is applied. Casts are changed every week for 3–6 weeks. Serial casts are effective and safe and are associated with a lower risk of skin breakdown, as they are total contact. The limb must be monitored for circulation status distal to the cast and for signs of swelling.

Severe contractures that do not respond to therapy may be managed with **surgical release.** Typical sites of release are the heel cord (Achilles tendon), hamstrings, hip adductors, and the biceps brachii. Individuals undergoing lower extremity release are typically able to ambulate after the surgery. Not every patient, who exhibits toe walking or equino-varus, benefits from tendon lengthening surgery. Careful assessment should be performed to ensure that the individual is adopting this posture purely due to contracture. In some individuals, as discussed for the child with CP, tight muscles may provide stability for weight-bearing or to enhance stability in other joints of the leg. Therapists can provide valuable insight to the surgeon regarding the potential impact of tendon lengthening surgery on any given client.

Heterotopic ossification (HO) is the abnormal presence of bone in soft tissue and is most frequently seen with either musculoskeletal trauma, spinal cord injury, or central nervous system injury. Surgery to remove the bone cannot be done until the lesion is mature (typically 1.5 years) due to the high likelihood of recurrence.[41] Active motion is typically encouraged to minimize ROM loss. It remains controversial as to whether stretching leads to more inflammation and should be avoided. Until conclusive evidence is available, it is recommended that therapists provide active range of motion, in the pain-free range. If indicated, gentle passive range of motion can be undertaken, but stretching should be avoided.

Management of the Medically Stable Client S/P TBI

Once the client is medically stable, the task is to return them to society at the highest possible level of function. This is also the time when therapists may identify more minor musculoskeletal injuries that were not apparent during coma. At this time, the emphasis of management is based on level of cognitive functioning. One of the most common scales for cognitive and behavioral functioning after TBI is the Ranchos Los Amigos Levels of Cognitive Functioning (Ranchos Scale, as described in Table 11-2). This scale sets rules for the language all professionals use to communicate regarding the care of the client with TBI. It equips you to treat for physical, cognitive, and behavioral sequela of TBI. The Ranchos Scale provides a means to guide goal setting, based on the level of recovery. The recovery process from TBI is sequential, but as mentioned earlier, the patient's progress can stop at any level.

● ASSESSMENT AND MANAGEMENT BASED ON RANCHOS LOS AMIGOS LEVELS OF COGNITIVE FUNCTIONING (LOC)[42,43]

Coma Levels

The first three levels, Ranchos Los Amigos levels I, II, and III are often called the coma levels. In this stage of recovery, the individual is unresponsive and may be described as appearing to be asleep. In Stage I, the individual makes no response to stimuli, including painful stimuli. When the individual begins to make generalized responses to stimuli, they are said to be in Stage II. The responses in this stage are the same regardless of the type of stimulus presented. Responses may be physiologic changes, gross body movements, and/or vocalization. When the individual begins to withdraw from painful stimuli or blink when strong light crosses the visual field, they are making stimulus-specific responses and are said to be in Stage III. The individual may also follow simple commands like closing eyes or squeezing a hand. These responses are often inconsistent and may be delayed.

Management of TBI survivors, while in the stages of coma, focuses on maintaining the health of the individual with PT focusing on the musculoskeletal and neuromuscular systems. Learning is not possible while the client is in a coma. Proper positioning to prevent contracture is important and often must be done around tubes and wires. If the individual has elevated ICP, the head of the bed must be kept elevated to about 30 degrees[44] and should not be lowered until the physician clears the individual to go supine. Before performing any range of motion or positioning, the PT should check all lines and tubes and ensure that they are each out of the way for the intended movements. Specific positioning strategies are discussed in Chapter 10 (see Table 10-5).

It is important to talk to the person with TBI as you would talk to any other client. Studies have shown that individuals, who are in a coma, can hear, and it is believed that talking to them may help to arouse them and improve their responsiveness. In fact, a small study of ICU patients showed that time to arousal from coma was significantly shorter in individuals who spent 30 minutes a day listening to familiar auditory sounds on an MP3 player as compared to controls who did not.[45] The therapist should ask visitors for information about the person with TBI, and then, talk to him about topics that would be of interest to him as well as greeting him, before starting therapy, and explaining what you are going to be doing, during therapy. Carefully observe the client for any indication of a response to sensory stimulation. When feasible, rolling the person side to side can help to stimulate the vestibular system, while raising the bed into reverse Trendelenburg with a foot plate for weight-bearing can stimulate the autonomic nervous system and the somatosensory system. Additional sensory stimuli can be used clinically to stimulate the patient, including familiar odors to stimulate the olfactory system and touch with different textures to stimulate the somatosensory system. Multi-modal stimulation is an effective technique that involves health care professionals or the patient's family member(s) systematically applying stimulation to one or more of the patient's five senses, for the purpose of increasing patient responsiveness.[45] The rationale is that exposure to frequent and various sensory stimulation will activate the sensory systems and facilitate both dendritic growth and improved synaptic connectivity in those with damaged nervous systems[46,47] (see Box 11-5).

Motor examination becomes possible, once the individual enters Ranchos level IV. The examination and evaluation are conducted as outlined in Chapter 9 (Evaluation). The neurology section of the APTA convened a task-force in 2013 to determine the most appropriate outcome measures for use in the TBI population. Recommended measures are listed in Table 11-4.

BOX 11-5	Rules for Applying Multimodal Sensory Stimulation Program

- Before starting, check resting vital signs (heart rate, blood pressure, and respiratory rate). Monitor vitals throughout the treatment, and stop treatment if vital signs change in a significant manner.
- Avoid or minimize stimulation programs with patients that have a ventriculostomy, who still have unstable or high intracranial pressure (ICP) and/or cerebral perfusion pressure (CPP); monitor ICP and CPP during and after treatment.
- Control the environment to eliminate as many distractions as possible. The environment should be simple and uncluttered, with a limited number of people around the patient, and with the TV off and the door closed, during treatment.

- Make sure the patient is comfortable before starting.
- Present the stimuli in an orderly manner, and involve only one or two sensory modalities at a time. It is important to control how much and how often to provide stimulation, because patients can "habituate" or get used to the stimulation, in which case, the stimulation can become less meaningful.
- Explain to the patient what is happening before and while the stimuli are presented.
- Allow extra time for the patient to respond. Start by providing 1 or 2 minutes between stimulus presentations, until the length of response delay for that individual is established.
- Keep sessions brief – patients can usually tolerate 15–30 minutes.
- Conduct sessions frequently, allowing patients to respond several times daily, but alternating periods of stimulation with periods of rest.
- Select meaningful stimuli, such as the voices of family and friends, favorite music, smells of favorite foods, etc. Stimuli that have emotional significance to the patient are usually more likely to elicit a response.
- Provide verbal reinforcement for responses to increase the likelihood of getting responses in future sessions.

TABLE 11-4	TBI EDGE Recommendations[48]
Acute Setting	**In and Out-Patient Rehabilitation**
Agitated Behavior Scale Coma Recovery Scale* Revised Moss Attention Rating Scale Rancho Levels of Cognitive Function	High Level Mobility Assessment* Moss Attention Scale* 6-minute walk, 10-m walk, Berg Balance Scale Community Balance and Mobility Scale Disability Rating Scale Functional Assessment Measure Modified Ashworth Scale Patient Health Questionnaire Quality of Life after Brain Injury Rancho Levels of Cognitive Function
In-Patient Rehabilitation Only	**Out-Patient Rehabilitation Only**
Agitated Behavioral Scale Barthel Index Cog-Log and O(rientation)–Log Disorders of Consciousness Scale FIM (functional independence measure)	Action Research Arm Test Apathy Evaluation Scale Balance Error Scoring Scale Global Fatigue Index Sydney Psychosocial Re-integration Scale Community Integration Questionnaire Dizziness Handicap Inventory

*Highly recommended measures.
Data from American Physical Therapy Association. TBI EDGE outcome measures for in- and outpatient rehabilitation.

Ranchos Level IV: Confused and Agitated

The treatment strategy, for the Stage IV client, is a behavioral treatment strategy rather than a learning treatment strategy. For many therapists, this is a key philosophical shift. When employing a behavioral treatment strategy, the focus is on impairments and is more compensatory in nature. Cognitive learning requires that the individual can learn alternate ways to behave and can understand the consequences of their actions. The individual in this stage of recovery is not able to do either. To understand the consequences of one's actions, the individual must be able to discern between self and the environment, which individuals in Stage IV cannot. Cognitive learning first becomes possible in Ranchos Stage VI. The key to working with clients who are s/p TBI is to be calm and controlled, flexible, and consistent. Specific guidelines for setting up sessions with a client who has behavioral problems are listed in Table 11-5.

Motor learning is not dependent on cognitive learning and can occur starting in Ranchos Stage IV, or when the individual is able to actively move. The ability to motor learn is also dependent on which areas of the brain have been damaged and the severity of that damage. At this stage in recovery, any motor learning would be implicit and from repetitive practice of the movement.

CASE A, PART IV

Aaron is now 5 weeks post-accident and has been moved to an inpatient rehabilitation facility. He has become very agitated. He tries to get up out of the bed and has torn off part of the cast on his right arm. He tends to yell, but the statements he makes are not relevant to the situation. A net bed has been put in place, and the staff has been instructed to keep their hair tied back as he has been grabbing and pulling on staff member's hair and arms. He is also spitting, cussing, and masturbating. Aaron's mother is in tears as she exits his room.

Aaron is in Ranchos Stage IV, which features of his presentation tell us he is in this stage?

Agitation, tearing off the cast, trying to stand when he is unable to do so safely, inappropriate verbalizations, and the inability to recognize that staff and family member's hair and arms are not objects but belong to other people.

What should staff tell the mother when she becomes upset by his behavior?

Staff should explain that Aaron is in a state of confusion, in which he is being inundated with sensory stimuli but is unable to understand what is going on around him. His behavior is not aimed at any person, and he does not understand that his behavior is impacting other people.

Now that Aaron is in Ranchos Stage IV, his treatment will focus on reorienting him frequently, preventing self-harm and getting him to participate in activities that are meaningful, familiar, and automatic, such as walking. Aaron continues to have PTA and will not remember previous therapy sessions. Therapy activities should be short, and the therapist should come prepared with plans for multiple potential activities. Activities will have to be changed every few minutes, since Aaron will have a very short attention span. In addition, the therapist should become familiar with the signs that Aaron exhibits, when he is becoming agitated, so that activities can be changed at the earliest sign of agitation. Therapy should be highly structured, and it is best to have consistent staff work with Aaron to help him gain familiarity and comfort with his situation. Instructions

TABLE 11-5	Guidelines for Treating Clients —with Agitation
GUIDELINES	**STRATEGIES**
Provide a calm and controlled environment	• Treat the patient as an adult respecting them in your interactions even when they act childlike • Model calm and controlled behavior both verbally and physically
Be flexible in your planning and throughout the therapy session	• Redirect the patient physically and verbally rather than argue • Expect the unexpected • Plan several activities for each treatment goal and be willing to change activities when signs of agitation occur • End the treatment session on success for you and for the patient
Provide consistency from one session to the next	• Consistency occurs across all areas of care and requires interdisciplinary team management • Provide a structure and ensure that all members of the team will respond to behaviors in the same manner • Give as much control and responsibility as the patient can handle while maintaining that predictable and structured environment, as much as needed, to allow the patient to function optimally • Avoid over stimulation and chaotic stimulation as TBI patients are more sensitive to stress

should be simple and brief. Therapy should be conducted in a quiet environment with minimal distractions. Family members are asked to be part of therapy, whenever possible, to facilitate cooperation and to help keep the patient calm and comfortable. When agitation occurs, the activity is stopped, and the client is allowed to rest.

CASE A, PART V

Aaron is allowed to walk with weight-bearing, as tolerated. He is ambulated with two-person assist and a rollator walker with forearm support on the right side because of his fracture. Therapists place the walker in front of Aaron and stand on either side with the person on the left, helping to advance the left leg. Aaron's mother is asked to stand across the room and call to Aaron to come to her. Aaron responds to his mother by beginning to walk toward her. Midway across the room he begins to vocalize in a loud voice, the therapist recognizes that this is an early sign of agitation for Aaron and so his wheelchair is brought to them and he is told to "sit down" in a calm quiet voice. Aaron sits and continues to vocalize and pick at his cast on his right arm. His mother comes to him and talks to him in a quiet voice, while rubbing his shoulder, and he calms down. At this time, Aaron only tolerates 15 minutes of therapy, before he becomes severely agitated.

Examples of behaviors that typically indicate a client is becoming agitated are increased movements like wiggling or tapping the foot, vocalizations or a shortening of the attention span. Each client will have a unique presentation, and staff should learn to recognize each client's signs of oncoming agitation and respond to them by taking the client to a quiet place and allowing them to rest. When Aaron spits, he is told that this behavior is inappropriate in a calm and unemotional voice. The staff is told to be consistent, in managing this behavior, and to recognize that at this time Aaron is not able to learn to change the behavior. When he masturbates, staff tell him that this should be done in privacy, in his own room, and move him to his room. This is an example of an appropriate behavior in an inappropriate setting. As Aaron's cognitive skills improve, he will be taught to delay gratification, by asking him to stop behaviors such as masturbation, and wait a set amount of time until he goes to his room to engage in the behavior. The time to gratification is incrementally increased.

Agitation is a difficult behavior for staff and family. It can be very upsetting to family members to see their loved one acting inappropriately and out of character. For the individual in Ranchos Stage IV, agitation is the person reacting to their own internal confusion. In Ranchos Stages V–VIII, the individual is reacting to the environment. There are many misconceptions about agitation. Box 11-6 spells out some of these misconceptions and provides the correct explanation.

CASE A, PART VI

Aaron is now able to respond to simple commands fairly consistently. He requires external structure to function and to minimize agitation; thus, staff should follow the same schedule every day, and the same staff should work with him, whenever possible. He now demonstrates gross attention to the environment but is highly distractible and lacks the ability to focus his attention. He can converse on a social automatic level for short periods of time. For example, he will greet the therapist with "hello" and when asked "how are you?" he answers. If the conversation goes on too long, he becomes agitated and begins to hum loudly. His verbalizations are often inappropriate, and sometimes, he will make confabulatory statements such as saying he has pain in his leg because he was tackled, while playing football last week. His memory is severely impaired, and he has limited to no recall of previous therapy sessions. He is unable to learn new information at this time but demonstrates procedural learning improvements in therapy activities.

What Ranchos level is Aaron now in?

He is now in Ranchos level V. He remains somewhat agitated and has a short attention span, but he is able to converse in a social, automatic level.

During Ranchos level V, the staff work on extending the time that Aaron can stay on task and focus his attention. In physical therapy, they are working on walking without breaks for longer and longer periods of time. This serves to improve his endurance and his attention to task. When he begins to follow simple directions and demonstrates carryover of learning for tasks, such as dressing and sit to stand transfers, he is considered to have moved on to Ranchos level VI (the confused and appropriate stage). In level VI, he can complete goal-directed activities such as walk to the green chair and sit down, but he continues to require direction from staff to do the task safely. When asked what day it is, he answers incorrectly three out of five times, but he always answers with a day of the week, indicating his answers are appropriate to the situation. Aaron is still trying to remove his cast, but when staff explain that his arm is broken and he needs to leave the cast alone, he is compliant. He does require frequent reminders as he does not remember these instructions for more than a few hours.

In Ranchos Stages V and VI, individuals continue to exhibit agitation and other behaviors such as confusion, resistance to treatment, apathy, lack of initiation, inability to self-reflect, impulsivity, disinhibition, depression, perseveration, and confabulation. They may be resistant to treatment, and at this stage, are able to refuse. Often resistance is due to agitation and confusion. To manage resistance to treatment, the therapist can offer several choices for each activity to be practiced without any "yes/no" options. For these individuals, it is important to provide them with activity choices that offer a high likelihood of success and then provide positive feedback to reinforce their engagement in

---

BOX 11-6 | **Misconceptions Regarding Agitated Behavior and Its Management**

The person s/p TBI:

Is "mean" or angry at staff and visitors

    The person s/p TBI is confused and frightened.

    Agitation is a reaction to that fear and confusion.

Needs medication to "calm him down"

    Medication further reduces the person with TBI's ability to process stimuli and interpret what is going on around them, which compounds agitation and confusion.

    In addition, medications are often ineffective in calming the patient until the dosage is so high that the patient is lethargic and asleep.

Won't cooperate with treatment

    The person s/p TBI is cognitively unable to cooperate and is not capable of the motivation to participate.

Must be restrained at all times for everyone's protection

    Restraints result in increased agitation.

    People are calmer, if unrestrained.

Requires a large number of people to control them

    More people will increase agitation

Is yelling and should be yelled at to "be quiet"

    Usually there is something that is causing the client to get loud and yell; find out what it is and modify the environment accordingly.

Can't benefit from treatment

    Clients s/p TBI can benefit from treatment.

    Short treatment sessions are most effective.

Should be ignored until he calms down.

    Being alone in an unfamiliar environment increases fear and agitation.

    Human contact has a very calming effect.

---

therapy. See Table 11-6 for a description of each of these behaviors and suggestions for ways to manage these behaviors.

Return to employment is one of the major goals for adults s/p TBI, but up to 55% are not employed 3 years after injury.[50] The Functional Assessment Measure (FAM) was developed by clinicians to specifically address the major functional areas, including cognitive, behavioral, communication, and community functioning. The FAM consists of 12 items and is intended to be used in conjunction with the FIM (FIM+FAM). Scores <65 on the FAM are predictive of long-term unemployment.[50]

CASE A, PART VII

Aaron, at 10 weeks post-injury, is now behaving appropriately in the inpatient rehabilitation setting and is able to go through his dressing and self-care tasks independently. He does this very automatically and follows a set routine every day. He is able to learn new skills such as how to use a walker and how to use adaptive equipment to feed himself. He exhibits poor judgment when confronted with situations such as maneuvering in a room full of obstacles or crossing the street.

What Ranchos LOC is Aaron now in?

Aaron is in Ranchos Stage VII. He is exhibiting behaviors that are automatic and appropriate but lacks the judgment and abstract reasoning that are found in Ranchos Stage VIII.

It is important to note that, while Aaron has progressed through the Ranchos stages to level VII, progress can stop at any Ranchos level. Aaron has been in rehabilitation as long as his insurance will pay and his progress has slowed down substantially. At this point, he is discharged to home. He will continue therapy in the outpatient setting with a focus on community reintegration. Aaron may continue to progress through the Ranchos stages, or he may remain in Ranchos Stage VII. With his initial level of injury, his prognosis would indicate that he is unlikely to return to his previous level of functioning and could be expected to remain at a Ranchos Stage VII. In this stage, he is cognitively able to learn (see Box 11-7 for learning ability by stage of recovery). Aaron now has moderately decreased ability to learn and has carryover for new learning. He continues to require close supervision due to safety and judgment issues. Based on these difficulties, the recommendation is that he live with his parents. Were he to live on his own, it would need to be in a structured environment, and he would continue to require assistance with his finances, making appointments and getting to them, and any other higher level daily activity. Someone would need to be available to take him grocery shopping and to check on him frequently. An Assisted Living setting would also be appropriate for Aaron at this time. If Aaron continues to make progress he would first be appropriate for living alone with no supervision at Ranchos Stage VIII.

Agitation is no longer present on a daily basis but can be elicited, when Aaron is under a great deal of stress. In addition, he becomes impulsive, when he is with his old friends and/or in a highly stimulating environment. It is typical for individuals who are s/p TBI to continue to manifest behaviors that were present in earlier stages, when they are fatigued or under stress. Alcohol is very likely to intensify safety and judgment issues and should be avoided.

BOX 11-7 | **Ability to Learn Cognitively by Ranchos LOC**[8]

Stages I–V: absent

  Stage VI: severely impaired; some carryover for things relearned

  Stage VII: moderately decreased; some carryover for new learning

  Stage VIII: minimally impaired; good carryover for new learning with no supervision required for performance once learned

TABLE 11-6	Common Behaviors s/p TBI and Their Management[49]	
BEHAVIOR DESCRIPTION	**KEY TO MANAGEMENT**	**MANAGEMENT STRATEGIES**
Agitation is common s/p TBI and is defined as excesses of behavior. Typical agitated behaviors include restlessness, inability to focus or maintain attention, irritability and, at higher levels of agitation, combativeness.	Prevent escalation of agitation and modify the environment and staff behavior to avoid the use of both physical and medical restraints.	• Be calm both verbally and in your physical and nonverbal actions. • Treatment session goals should be flexible to allow adjustment to the level of agitation. • Treatment environment should be quiet with minimal external stimuli. • Be aware of tension building up in the client, stopping the external stimulation before agitation becomes combative. • Redirect the patient's attention and move them to a location with less stimulating or frustrating activities, until agitation is reduced. • Do not attempt to discuss agitation logically or elicit guilt for the behavior. • Do not leave the patient unsupervised or alone during agitation. • Try to maintain consistency in the personnel who interact with the patient so as to promote familiarity and decrease novel stimuli. • To the extent possible, permit moving about or verbalization during periods of increased agitation.
Confusion results from the inability of patients to recall minute-to-minute, hour-to-hour, or day-to-day events in their life. As a result, they are unable to understand their current situation in light of what has or what will occur. Associated problems include diminished attention, learning, and orientation.	Increase and even provide the external structure for the individual, particularly in regard to time, place, and activities.	• Place calendars in client's rooms with a schedule of daily activities posted in their room; also have one that they can take with them throughout the day. • Post the steps for them to follow for their ADLs in their room. • At the start of each treatment session, review your name, what day and date it is, what time of day it is, and where they are. Use calendars, clocks, name tags, and building signage to reinforce this information. • Maximize consistency and establish routines within and between treatment sessions • To increase client awareness, start each activity with a short and easy to understand explanation of what is expected of them. • At the end of the session, use the client's schedule to elicit from him or her the next activity, in which he/she will engage.
Impulsivity is a tendency to act without thinking. It is common in people s/p TBI and often seen along with agitation and confusion.	Provide consistency across caregivers and visitors, and have the client verbally rehearse strategies for each treatment activity.	• The entire team should attempt to use the same strategy with a patient; inconsistency will only create confusion. • Verbally review the steps for each activity, before allowing the patient to start. • Use a written list of steps that the patient reviews (out loud or to himself) before starting. • The patient verbally rehearses aloud the steps needed to complete the task. • The patient waits a few seconds, before beginning a task, and is instructed to think about how to complete the task, before doing it. • Aloud, verbal rehearsal should be consistently implemented, in all treatment sessions and throughout the day. As a patient demonstrates increased control, this can be gradually shaped into rehearsing to oneself and then simply pausing before starting the task.

(Continued)

TABLE 11-6   Common Behaviors s/p TBI and Their Management[49] (Continued)

BEHAVIOR DESCRIPTION	KEY TO MANAGEMENT	MANAGEMENT STRATEGIES
Disinhibition is an inability to stop oneself from acting on one's thoughts. *Sexually Inappropriate Behavior* is a special case of lack of inhibition.	Remain calm and provide concrete feedback about the behavior.	• Initially, focus on addressing simple situations that may be easiest for patients to learn to manage. • Identify the issue as "self-control" and use this as the key word for cueing the patient, when they need to be controlling their behaviors. • When delaying gratification is the issue, start with short increments between the behavior and the reward, lengthening the increment as the patient improves. Using a watch or timer for specific cueing may be helpful in this regard. • It is important to provide the patient with feedback on the inappropriateness of sexual behavior, in this situation, and not to regard its presence with negative attention. • Avoid emotional responses such as anger or embarrassment; this can reinforce the behavior. • Ignoring the behavior or passing it off with a humorous comment also may reinforce its presence and not provide the patient with the adequate information to understand that the behavior is inappropriate. • The best approach is an immediate, unemotional, straightforward expression of the inappropriateness of the behavior. Be certain the patient knows what behavior is being referred to, such as "your sexual hand gesture is inappropriate and won't be appreciated by most women/men."
Perseveration is a person's repetition of certain behaviors, either actions or verbalizations. Some individuals perseverate on a consistent theme, while others repeat external stimuli or their own immediately preceding responses.	Use cueing and pacing to interrupt the repetitive behavior and provide a stimulus to move on to the next step.	• Pace interactions with the client to allow disengagement from one activity before proceeding to the next. • Provide a highly structured environment. • Use cues to redirect the client from the perseverative behavior to the next step. • Do not attempt to use logic to "discuss away" a repetitive theme.
Confabulation is the creation of false memories and is frequent in confused patients, sometimes reflecting the inability to find another explanation for what is happening.	It is important to keep in mind that confabulation may be serving a purpose for the patient, including reducing anxiety.	• For lower functioning, more confused patients, ignore the confabulation and do not challenge its veracity. • For higher functioning patients, provide nonthreatening feedback on the inaccuracy of the memory; then, redirect attention to another task.
Inability to self-reflect is due to a lack of insight into the effects of ones behavior on others. The client is not aware of their capabilities or limitations and typically overestimates their ability to perform any given task. These patients will often blame others for their frustration and may exhibit paranoia.	Use concrete goals that are posted within easy access of the person with TBI, and note on the posted goal form as progress is made.	• Include the client in goal setting. • Goals should be concrete and progress should be recorded, where the client can monitor her own progress • Consistently attempt to elicit the client's insight into their deficits. Be nonjudgmental and express expectations that the deficit will be overcome. • Videotape can provide concrete feedback. • Only make the client aware of deficits that can be worked on in rehabilitation and for which you expect to see improvement. • Continual reinforcement is necessary, after insight is accomplished, to change the behavior.

TABLE 11-6	Common Behaviors s/p TBI and Their Management[49] (Continued)	
BEHAVIOR DESCRIPTION	**KEY TO MANAGEMENT**	**MANAGEMENT STRATEGIES**
Apathy can be differentiated from resistance by the presence of lethargy with a bland affect, an absence of agitation, and low motivation. *Depression* is sometimes evident as a patient's self-awareness improves. It may show itself in tears, but also may be evident in social withdrawal, self-degrading comments, anxiety, irritability, and catastrophizing.	Treatment should target choices and acknowledge accomplishments.	• Staff and family should encourage participation. • You may need to remind them of the consequences of their injury and the impact of the lack of participation in rehabilitation. • Graphs or other concrete ways of showing progress may be useful to elicit motivation. • Be firm in presenting activities and do not present yes/no choices. Offer two or more alternatives for a give activity. • Working in conjunction with other patients may be motivating. • Activities that the patient spontaneously shows interest in should be used to meet rehabilitation goals. • Ask the client to choose the activity to elicit motivation. • Identify short-term goals and be explicit about the relationship between therapy activities and these goals. • Review progress to date. • Redirect the patient's attention from catastrophic or anxious thoughts. • Inform the psychology staff of the nature of the patient's depressive or anxious thoughts.
Lack of Initiation differs from apathy in that the patient is motivated to perform an activity but is unable to determine how to carry it out. Lack of initiation may be evident in problems determining the correct sequence of steps or simply not knowing the first step. It is important to keep in mind that the patient is not always aware of this shortcoming and may provide other excuses for why an activity is not initiated or carried out.	Cueing at the start of or next step in an activity is the key to facilitating initiation.	• Cueing is the primary means of assisting a person who lacks initiation. Cues should be external. • Do not perform or passively assist them to initiate the activity. • Verbal cues should be used initially. Using the same word to cue the same behaviors will assist the patient in moving to the next step. • As independence increases, replace verbal cues with other external cues that do not require another person to present the cue. Examples of external cues are lists posted in the room for ADL routines. External cues should be succinct, readily visible, and free of distracting content. • Client's whose improvement continues should be weaned from external cues to simple verbal statements that can be said aloud or thought to oneself as the patient completes the activity. These self- reminders should be succinct and easy to learn. • While in the inpatient setting begin to train the patient and family in techniques for establishing a daily routine.

Goal Setting

When writing goals, it is important to include not only the functional or impairment level goal but also behavioral and cognitive modifiers. These modifiers allow the therapist to address all of the issues associated with the brain injury. In addition, cognitive deficits have a profound impact on learning and time to meet mobility goals. Consider what it takes to safely ambulate in the community. The individual must be able to walk independently but also be cognitively able to find their way and to determine safety (e.g., to cross streets). Problematic behaviors also interfere with successful therapy interventions and influence independence and safety in mobility. In order to engage in therapy, the individual must be able to maintain attention long enough to walk a set distance and to respond to requests to walk with the appropriate action. Box 11-8 provides examples of qualifiers that could be used when writing goals.

Family Adjustment

"a brain injury isn't like death. You're in limbo. After death, you eventually get on with your life. This TBI goes

BOX 11-8	Cognitive and Behavioral Goal and Documentation Modifiers

Appropriateness of Response: Does the individual's response fit in the correct category and do they use equipment appropriately.

- Aaron will lock his wheelchair and use his left hand appropriately on the arm of the wheelchair to come to standing on four of five attempts.

Attention: Describe the duration of time the individual is able to attend to a particular task (e.g., repetitions, distance, time).

- Aaron will be able to walk 30 feet × 3 within 1 minute without becoming distracted and with appropriate movement of the walker and standby assistance.

Body Awareness: Define neglect, the individual's attention to their hemiparetic side, their care of the non-weight-bearing body part.

- Aaron will note when his left foot has fallen off of the footrest and will place it back on the foot rest, using only self-cueing.

Carryover: Does the individual exhibit retention of repeated activities, and is there any evidence of new learning of skills, names, and places.

- Aaron will demonstrate carryover from the am session to the pm session of the sit–stand steps with only tactile cueing.

Cueing: Define the amount and type of cueing that is necessary to accomplish the task successfully (i.e., tactile, verbal, both).

- See above examples

Participation: Describe the number of activities, type of activity, is it easy or difficult, how long they participate in an activity, a treatment session, and will they participate in what you want them to do.

- Aaron was able to complete three consecutive activities within the am session without agitation or impulsivity, following single-step directions.

Orientation: Consider things like knowing the building, how to get to places, and how to get back, using a map, following a schedule, use of environmental cues (i.e., signs).

- Aaron is able to transport himself by wheelchair, using his right hand and foot for propulsion, on time, based on the schedule taped to his wheelchair tray.

Safety: This encompasses orientation skills, judgment, body awareness, environmental awareness, impulsivity, and carryover.

- Aaron is oriented × 2 (person and place) with improved awareness of avoiding weight-bearing on his broken arm and decreased attempts to remove his cast.

Social Interactions: Are they appropriate with peers and staff, sexually inappropriate, exhibit disinhibition, use effective communication.

- Aaron is greeting family and staff with appropriate "hi" and "good-bye" verbalization but is not remembering names from one meeting to the next.

on forever and you're dealing with it one stage or another for the rest of your life"

[family member[51, p3]]

"Almost all TBI survivors who have been comatose for more than a few days sustain irreversible alteration of some socially important aspect of psychological makeup"[52, p248]

At the time of injury, the family's energy is focused on their loved one's survival. As the patient comes out of coma, the family is confronted with all of the drastic changes that their loved one has undergone. Changes in personality and behavior are often the most difficult for family and friends to understand. Families, who do well, learn to "let go" of the person, who was there before the injury, and figure out a way to incorporate the "new person" into the family system. The therapist's role is to educate the family on how to physically assist the person s/p TBI but also on the effects of TBI on the entire person. Also, therapists are often in frequent close contact with the family and may be the person they first talk to about their feelings and their struggles to deal with this situation. Therapists play a key role in referring family members to local support systems.

Mild TBI and Concussion

Historically, concussion and mild TBI (mTBI) were considered separate entities; in fact, concussion was defined as a disturbance of brain function without permanent physiologic or structural damage, while mTBI involved a brief loss of consciousness with mild structural damage that could result in permanent disability. More recently it has been acknowledged that concussion is the mildest form of TBI that can result in microstructural damage that alters brain activity and connectivity that is not detectable through imaging methods and may involve loss of consciousness. Smaller axons are likely more susceptible to the overstretching thought to occur with a mild injury (rather than tearing) that, in turn, is followed by disruption of the sodium–potassium–calcium cellular balance and exaggerated metabolic cellular requirements with subsequent microstructural damage.[3,53] However, when multiple concussions occur, especially in close time proximity, they may have an additive effect on long-term cognitive ability, psychological health, and behavioral control (see later segment on second impact syndrome). Notably, in children, a relatively minor injury can result in significant, but often delayed, cerebral vasodilation and severe edema, referred to as juvenile head trauma syndrome.[53]

Brain injuries occur at an alarmingly high rate in athletes with sports-related TBI rates twice that of the TBI rates in the general population.[54] More alarming, concussions are increasingly common in adolescence, a time when the brain is still developing and potentially at greater risk for injury and/or poorer outcome from a mild injury. Of concern, is the indication that it takes a more severe blow to the head to induce symptoms in children/adolescents than it does in adults due to the structural differences in brain-skull size; thus, children that display symptoms have likely experienced a far greater force than an adult with comparable symptoms.[55] It also appears that symptoms in

TABLE 11-7	Symptoms of Concussion or mTBI[56]		
COGNITIVE	**PHYSICAL**	**EMOTIONAL**	**SLEEP**
Poorer concentration	Blurred vision	Irritability	Drowsiness/lethargy
Memory disturbance	Headache	Depression	Increased sleepiness
Slower processing	Nausea/vomiting	Hyper-emotionality	Insomnia
	Noise and/or light sensitivity	Anxiety	
	Poor balance/coordination		

children and adolescents take longer to recover and may still be undergoing neural recovery even after symptoms have dissipated and neurologic testing is normal.[55] Identification of individuals with mTBI can aid in primary prevention efforts, such as reducing risk for reinjury in high-risk groups. In addition, it can facilitate access to appropriate interventions that can reduce the long-term effects of mTBI. Table 11-7 provides details on early symptoms of mTBI/concussion. Notably, these may manifest some hours or even days after the initial injury.

In some athletes, repetitive mTBI has led to long-standing neural atrophy, especially in the frontal cortex.[54] Additionally, studies to date seem to indicate that executive functions are most sensitive to multiple mTBIs[53]; however, studies in this area are varied and often conflicting. Due to these worrisome findings, screening for mTBI has taken on a new urgency in athletics with more conservative management post-concussion or mTBI. Screening for mTBI includes tests of orientation, concentration, memory, external provocation, and neurologic integrity. Table 11-8 provides a detailed description of tests to be performed in each category. When an individual test is positive, the client should be removed from any heavy physical or athletic activity and not allowed to return, until they are cleared to do so by the physical therapist or physician.

Of note, there is also considerable controversy on how to treat someone, who has sustained a concussion, especially children and adolescents. Early recommendations for post-concussion treatment emphasized rest – both physical and cognitive – as well as normal neuropsychological testing prior to return to play for those sustaining an injury during sport. At least one study has found that a moderate level of physical activity (e.g., slow jogging) was associated with improved performance post-concussion on neuropsychological testing, while those with more intense physical activity (e.g., return to sports practice) performed worse.[56] Similarly, intense cognitive activity has been found to delay recovery, while more modest levels of cognitive activity have the same timeline for recovery than absolute rest.[57] Thus, while absolute rest may not be necessary for the recovery of the cognitive impairments from concussion, there is sufficient evidence to support recommendations for diminished level of both physical and cognitive activity for the first week or so after injury; in fact, this suggests that return to full activity (both cognitive and physical) may need to be delayed for some period of time after neuropsychological testing has

indicated a return to normal function . This is another opportunity for the physical therapist to contribute to the rehabilitation of those with mTBI by facilitating the introduction of moderate activities; there is also considerable need for research on what is the best way to rehabilitate the mTBI patient and when normal activity should be resumed.

TABLE 11-8	Screening Tests for Mild TBI
CATEGORY	**TESTS**
Orientation	Ask the athlete the time, place, name, and circumstances of injury
Concentration	Ask them to repeat a list of digits back to you in reverse order. For example if you say 9-3-5 they would repeat back "5-3-9": 3-1-7 4-6-8-2 5-9-3-7-4 Have them tell you the months of the year in reverse order
Memory	Ask the athlete names of teams from prior contests, names of the president, governor, other recent newsworthy events
Neurologic tests	Pupils – check for symmetry and reaction to light Coordination – have them perform finger to nose to finger and tandem walk Proprioception – have them perform finger to nose with eyes closed Romberg test – stand with feet together and eyes closed for 1 minute
External provocative tests	Have the athlete do a 40-yard sprint, 5 pushups, 5 sit-ups, 5 knee bends. A positive provocative test is the appearance of one or more associated symptoms: headache, dizziness, nausea, unsteadiness, photophobia, blurred or double vision, emotional lability, mental status change

For most individuals, a concussion resolves within a few weeks of the original injury. However, for up to 30%, symptoms persist much longer, resulting in what has been named post-concussive syndrome with domain symptoms similar to those for other TBI severity, including mild behavioral and executive function disruption.[53]

Long-Term Outcomes from TBI

As stated earlier, patients progress through the stages of recovery from TBI at different rates and may stall at any stage. For those that stall in a vegetative state (Ranchos II) for at least 1 month, about one-half will regain consciousness by 1 year, most of these within the first 3 months. After 1 year, it is unlikely that a patient will emerge from a vegetative state (VS). For those that stall at a Ranchos level III, there is a much better chance that they will recover with only minor disability than those that stall at level II, yet up to 40% will be severely disabled, if they remain in this minimally conscious state (MCS) for at least 30 days. For those with prolonged VS or MCS, about 50% have been reported to be discharged home and the other half to a skilled nursing facility at discharge from rehabilitation. Long-term follow-up for these patients found 25% improved to a level of mild or no disability; 25% continued to demonstrate severe disability; and the remainder (50%) displayed moderate disability, as rated on the Disability Rating Scale. Notably, 22% returned to work or school; however, about 5% of these, returned at a partial level.[12] Similarly, patient outcome has been found to relate to the length of time spent in prolonged PTA with those that returned to full or partial employment, school, or homemaking roles (productive) within 1 year distributed as follows: (1) moderate PTA (0–14 days) – 68% returned to productive lives; (2) moderately severe (15–29 days) – 41%; (3) severe (29–70 days) – 21%; and (4) extremely severe (>70 days) – 9%.[31] For many of those that fail to return to productivity, there is persisting behavioral (e.g., irritability/aggression, disinhibition/impulsivity) and executive dysfunction (e.g., impaired problem-solving, memory, and attention). Similarly, persisted problems with motor sequelae – balance problems, spasticity/dystonia – can impede function and return to productivity. In fact, tonal changes and balance deficits may worsen over time. This can be addressed by ongoing physical therapy to prevent contractures (splinting, stretching) and maximize function (therapeutic exercise, mobility training) long after the acute rehabilitation period. For some, medications may be required to control spasticity (e.g., baclofen or botulinum toxin).[58]

As mentioned in an earlier section of this chapter, the secondary neurologic consequences of TBI (e.g., inflammation, excitotoxicity) may continue in the post-TBI brain for a prolonged period after injury, resulting in secondary functional loss that may appear more than a year post-injury. Of interest, there is an increased incidence of both Alzheimer's and Parkinson diseases post-TBI; while these prolonged neurodegenerative processes have been implicated in the development of these diseases, other factors (e.g., environment and genetics) likely contribute to their occurrence.[18] Even in the absence of a degenerative disease, a moderate to severe TBI has been found to decrease a survivor's life expectancy for a variety of reasons. Ongoing seizures or respiratory issues can impact longevity with death associated with seizure activity or aspiration pneumonia, respectively. Further, younger TBI survivors are more likely to resume a high-risk lifestyle, including substance abuse that contributes to a higher mortality rate than non-injured controls.[59]

Interestingly, there are also multiple chronic changes that occur post-TBI that impact long-term survival. For one, up to 80% of survivors demonstrate a change in neuroendocrine function, resulting in **hypopituitarism** and secondary loss of circulating hormones, specifically growth, sex, and thyroid hormones. Loss of these critical hormones can result in diminished bone density/osteoporosis, exercise capacity/indurance, and muscle strength (weakness) that further limit the survivor's physical fitness.[58,59] Additionally, there is an increased occurrence of **metabolic syndrome** (obesity, hypertension, elevated blood lipids, and insulin resistance) in TBI survivors that likely stems from these hormonal changes in association with disturbance of the hypothalamic and thalamic satiety centers, limited mobility, and lack of initiation; in combination, these result in an inactive lifestyle, a propensity for weight gain, and risk of metabolic syndrome that increases susceptibility to heart disease, stroke, and diabetes.[58] Chronic hormonal changes along with the impact of loss of function, loss of income, and familial issues may contribute to the pervasiveness of **depression** and **anxiety** in TBI survivors, especially younger survivors. Further, depression is difficult to treat in this population because of the common side effects of antidepressants, including sedation, slowing mentation, and the possibility of inducing seizures. Also, up to 50% of survivors experience chronic pain, most commonly headaches, that can contribute to depression and affect quality of life. **Chronic pain** is also difficult to treat due to the high incidence of substance abuse in this population, and thereby, the need to avoid many pain medications.[58] This is an opportunity for the physical therapist with some success reported from biofeedback, TENS, ultrasound, and dry needling among others in treating the chronic pain conditions of TBI survivors.[58] Other chronic conditions that impact TBI survivors include **sleep disturbance**, most commonly insomnia and sleep–wake cycle disruption, with secondary **fatigue**.[59]

While mTBI or concussion by their very names indicate minimal or no apparent damage to the CNS, there is a growing body of evidence that multiple incidents of even mild head injury can result in permanent disability. First, there is **second-impact syndrome**, where a second mild injury in a close timeframe to the first, results in severe cerebral edema with potential brain herniation; this is thought to result from dysautoregulation

---

CASE A, PART VIII

For Aaron, he would likely fall into the severe group as described in the preceding paragraph as his coma lasted about 5 weeks and his PTA another 5 weeks (35 days). So, Aaron will likely return home, but it is relatively unlikely that he will be employed full-time 1 year post-injury.[31]

of cerebral blood flow and exaggerated catecholamine release that induce extensive cerebral edema. In almost all cases, this secondary injury is associated with sports participation (e.g., football, boxing, and hockey) in adolescent or young males. There is some indication that juvenile head trauma syndrome is, in fact, a secondary-impact injury manifestation.[53] For those that experience repetitive head injuries, there is almost a 20% likelihood of the development of a condition, known as **chronic traumatic encephalopathy**, previously known as pugilists dementia, as it was first diagnosed in boxers; however, in recent years it has been diagnosed much more pervasively in football players, who experienced numerous concussions. This condition initially manifests with emotional or behavioral changes but eventually develops into progressive memory and cognitive deficits (dementia). These changes are associated with a general cerebral atrophy and secondary expansion of the lateral ventricles.[53]

BRAIN TUMOR

CASE B, PART I

Alice is a 48-year-old woman, who was brought to the Emergency Department by the EMT, s/p grand mal seizure in her home within the last 30 minutes. Her daughter, aged 17, reports that her mother seemed fine immediately preceding the seizure and that to her knowledge this is the first such episode experienced by her mother. Her mother is postictal but the neurologic exam that could be completed is unremarkable – pupils are reactive and equal, reflexes are 2+, muscle tone is normal, and Babinski and Hoffman tests are negative. She is awaiting a CT scan.

Types of Primary Brain Tumors (PBTs)

PBTs are relatively uncommon with only about 200,000 people, around the world, diagnosed each year,[60] yet they are the most common tumors for children, secondary to only leukemia as the cancer cause of death in children.[61] The brain is also a common site for metastases in adults but not children; however, we will focus on PBTs within this chapter. Like tumors throughout the body, PBTs involve abnormal cell proliferation of neurons or glia within the brain or cells within structures of the brain – meninges (meningioma), vasculature, or pituitary or pineal glands.[60] PBTs are named for their cell type.

Based on the primary cells within the brain tissue, the most common tumor type in both adults (77% of adult PBTs)[59] and children (up to 50% of PBTs)[61] is the **glioma**. These can be further differentiated into *astrocytomas* (most common; from astrocytes), *oligodendrogliomas* (from oligodendrocytes), *ependymomas* (from ventricular lining ependymal cells), and *mixed gliomas*, which typically involve both astrocytes and oligodendrocytes. In addition, there are neuronal-glial tumors that involve both neurons and glia. Gliomas are staged progressively from relatively benign (Stages I and II) to malignant grades (Stages III and IV; see Table 11-9), based on their rate of growth, differentiation, and infiltration of the surrounding brain tissue. See Table 11-10 for tumor descriptions and staging. However, there is a tendency for some benign tumors to transition to malignant, so the initial staging may not reflect the ultimate stage. **Differentiation** is the ability to distinguish the cell types within the tumor under a microscope with better differentiation associated with more benign tumors. Increased severity is also associated with greater infiltration of the brain tissue. While **localized tumors** grow within the area of origin and are typically encapsulated, **infiltrating tumors** penetrate and become entwined with the surrounding neural tissue, making them much more difficult to remove. Yet, even localized tumors can damage surrounding brain tissue, resulting in permanent brain damage and even death, depending on their location. Other types of brain tumors have similar staging methods.[60,61]

Tumors are also distinguished by their location as (1) posterior fossa (infratentorial) – involving the cerebellum, vermis, or brainstem or (2) supratentorial (above the tentorium cerebelli) – involving the cerebrum, deep nuclei (basal ganglia), ventricular choroid plexus or ependymal cells (lining of the ventricles), optic track, hypothalamus, pituitary, pineal gland, or other structure.[60,61] Notably, children can present with a variety of tumors that are unique to the developing nervous system, of which the medulloblastoma is the most common with

TABLE 11-9	Staging of Glioma Tumors[60-62]	
STAGE	**CHARACTERISTICS**	**REPRESENTATIVE TYPES**
Stage I	Benign, localized, well differentiated, slowest growing, removable, good outcome	Pilocytic astrocytoma Gangliocytoma or ganglioglioma Giant cell astrocytoma
Stage II	Benign but may become malignant, slow growing, less differentiated than Stage I (look more abnormal), non-infiltrating, removable but may recur	Diffuse fibrillary astrocytoma Oligodendrogliomas
Stage III	Malignant, poor differentiation, infiltrating, faster growing, treated by surgery plus chemotherapy and/or radiation, likely to recur as Stage IV tumor	Anaplastic astrocytomas or oligoastrocytomas
Stage IV	Malignant, undifferentiated, faster growing with greater infiltration than Stage III, generate angiogenesis, very difficult to treat	Glioblastoma multiformis Medulloblastoma

TABLE 11-10	Tumor Locations and Characteristics	
TUMOR TYPE	**COMMON LOCATIONS**	**CHARACTERISTICS**
Ependymoma	Usually infratentorial but can be supratentorial (parietal or temporal lobe)	Arise from ventricular ependymal cells (lining of the ventricles); infratentorial tumors are typically Stage III while supratentorial tumors are typically Stage II.[61]
Gliomas	Anywhere	Arise from glial cells – astrocytes (astrocytoma), oligodendrocytes (oligodendrocytoma); can range from grade I to IV glioblastomas – Stage IV astrocytoma, stimulate abnormal angiogenesis, creating highly vascularized tumors. Prognosis is poor.[64]
Glioneuronal	Temporal or frontal lobes; cerebellum	Tumor comprised of both glial cells and neuronal components, arising from neuroepithelial tissues[62]; most common in temporal lobe. Associated with epilepsy that is pharmacologically resistant.[65]
Medulloblastoma	Cerebellum and vermis	Fast growing malignant posterior fossa tumor in children <7; associated with hydrocephalus.[61]
Meningioma	Arachnoid matter	Stages I–III (most are stage I); multiple genetic contributions; Stages I and II are effectively treated with surgery and radiation.[66]
Pituitary adenoma	Pituitary gland	Benign tumors of one of the six cell types of the pituitary, leading to abnormal secretion of the respective secretory hormones (adenocorticotropic, growth, prolactin, thyroid-stimulating, follicle-stimulating, and luteinizing) with associated symptomology. Tumor growth may disrupt pituitary function. Commonly treatable with gamma knife surgery.[67]
PNETs	Supratentorial – often within pineal gland	Metastasize easily so staged according to: 0 = no metastases; 1 = cells in CSF; 2 = supratentorial metastases; 3 = spinal metastases. Fatal in almost 50% (only 20% if in pineal gland), especially once metastasized. Treated with surgery and radiation, sometimes with chemotherapy.[63]

a 30% fatality rate; in the 70% that survive, there is often significant residual physical disability. These tumors occur in the posterior fossa, most commonly within the cerebellum, and are thought to develop from undifferentiated stem cells, originating in the germinal regions of the ventricular zone of the fourth ventricle.[60] Similarly, neuroectodermal tumors (PNETs) derive from neural crest cells (see Chapter 18 for description of neural tube development) and are, in effect, the same as medulloblastomas but occur supratentorially, rather than infratentorially.[63] See Table 11-10 for tumor types and staging.

CASE B, PART II

In the emergency department, once Alice was alert, a more complete history revealed frequent headaches of increasing severity over the last few weeks with associated nausea and some mild memory issues that Alice had attributed to insomnia. Alice underwent an unenhanced CT scan, which is typically the first type of imaging used to evaluate patients that present to the ED with initial seizure activity and can typically visualize the tumor and look for signs of hemorrhage or brain herniation. This was followed by an MRI the next day to more fully characterize the tumor. This diagnosed a Stage IV glioblastoma in the left temporal lobe with projections into the parietal lobe.

Tumor Symptoms

Although many tumor symptoms are site specific (e.g., ataxia with posterior fossa tumors), signs of increased ICP are often the first indications of the presence of a tumor. As with TBI, these include nausea, headaches, blurred vision secondary to papilledema and/or retinal hemorrhage, and drowsiness; as occurred with Alice, these symptoms may be attributed to other causes such as fatigue, stress, or a minor illness until they become more severe. In young infants, a tumor may present with irritability, sleep disturbances, protruding fontanelles, and poor feeding.[61] Also, many tumors induce seizures and ultimately epilepsy due to the irritation and eventual death of adjacent cells. Initial seizure activity is the first sign of the tumor in up to 50% of patients with brain tumors, and these can present as both generalized or partial seizures.[68] Seizure activity is most common in cerebral tumors, yet these are often the more treatable tumor types.[68] Memory or executive function changes are often associated with temporal or frontal lobe tumors; similarly, tumors of the posterior frontal/parietal lobe can present with contralateral sensorimotor disturbances similar to stroke. Of course, these tend to be mild at first and progress to more severe as the tumor grows. Tumors of the posterior fossa disrupt the cerebellum and brainstem; thus, they present with symptoms similar to a brainstem stroke or cerebellar disease, including incoordination, dizziness, ataxia, and cranial nerve disruption.

Adjacent area of edema

Tumor with enhancement of borders

FIGURE 11-3 CT scan of glioblastoma. In this T1-weighted image, the tumor appears dark with a surrounding area of high intensity that marks the border or external margin of the tumor. Also, infiltration of the surrounding area with edema appears as hyperintensity. (Reproduced with permission from Hauser SL: *Harrison's Neurology in Clinical Medicine*, 3rd edition. New York, NY: McGraw-Hill; 2013)

Tumor Diagnosis

Imaging is usually the only required diagnostic tool for tumor identification with **CT scanning** often the first method used, since it is readily available in most emergency rooms and offers a quick analysis. Tumors appear as areas of hypointensity (lighter) than the normal surrounding tissue, with those that are most dense and of higher grade appearing brighter on the scan. However, if a brain tumor is suspected, an MRI with and without gadolinium, which allows greater clarity, is the standard method for tumor identification. Gadolinium enhancement allows the determination of tumor characteristics, including cell differentiation, level of brain tissue infiltration, abnormal blood vessel development, and the degree of tissue necrosis and edema within and surrounding the tumor (see Figure 11-3). Depending on the MRI scan type, the tumor will appear either darker (T1 weighted) or lighter (T2 weighted) than the surrounding tissue. Additional imaging techniques, positron emission tomography (PET) can illustrate tissue metabolic activity, and MR spectroscopy can elucidate blood vessel proliferation/compromise and clarify tumor tissue composition. Sometimes, functional magnetic resonance imaging (fMRI) is used to clarify sensorimotor and cognitive regions prior to tumor resection to minimize damage to these areas.[61,69]

Tumor Pathogenesis

Some tumors, specifically gliomas and medulloblastomas, seem to arise from **abnormal neurogenesis**, which is the process by which neurons and glial cells are formed. While neurogenesis occurs in multiple areas during fetal development, in adults, only two areas of neurogenesis have been identified: (1) the subgranular zone of the hippocampus and (2) the subventricular zone of the lateral ventricles. Glioma formation is thought to result from abnormal cell differentiation, transforming normal stem cells into **tumor-producing stem cells**.[64] Similarly, medulloblastomas seem to arise from brainstem and fourth ventricle stem cells; since these neurogenic areas aren't active in adults, these tumors affect only children. While they may originate in the brainstem region, these tumor cells often enter the CSF and can, thereby, travel to areas of the forebrain or spinal cord.[70] Other tumor types seem to result from abnormal cell proliferation within the specified tissue (e.g., ependymoma – proliferation of ependymal cells).

So, what triggers this abnormal neurogenesis or cell proliferation? For normal neurogenesis, **transcription factors**, which are proteins that bind to DNA and control gene expression, promote or block cell proliferation. The abnormal neurogenesis, associated with tumor development, appears to result from a disruption of the natural neurogenic/gliogenic transcription factors. This disruption may be triggered by genetic anomalies, stemming from chromosome deletion or amplification.[70] Within our DNA, there exist genes, referred to as proto-oncogenes, that when mutated become **oncogenes** and trigger tumor development. Similarly, DNA includes natural **tumor suppressor genes** (TSGs; antioncogenes) that, when mutated, fail to suppress abnormal cell proliferation, thus, allowing tumor development via abnormal cell proliferation. While gliomas emerge from disruption of a natural cell proliferation process (neurogenesis of stem cells), other tumors appear to be the result of cell proliferation in normally non-replicating cells (e.g., meningioma). Oncogenes and the mutation of TSGs contribute to cell proliferation in most or all tumor types. Multiple genetic defects and changes in growth factors have been identified as triggers to these DNA changes with secondary changes in cell cycle regulation and cell metabolic processes identified. The cause of most types of brain tumors is likely multi-factorial and still under investigation. Further, environmental factors may contribute; however, only exposure to environmental radiation has been definitively linked to brain tumor development. In addition, immunosuppression, such as that associated with HIV infection, has been linked to brain tumor genesis.[60]

Medical Treatment of Brain Tumors

Brain tumors need to be aggressively treated to avoid secondary neural damage, resulting from their growth. Surgical resection and radiation therapy are the methods of choice for almost all tumor types. Stereotaxic radiosurgery (STR, gamma knife) is the use of high-dose radiation from multiple angles simultaneously, guided by imaging (CT or MRI) and stereotaxic (3 dimensional) coordinates. This is particularly useful when the tumor is located within the brainstem or deep within the cerebral hemispheres and surgical resection is not an option; however, it is also effective in benign tumors, such as meningiomas, either as the initial treatment modality or as a secondary treatment after initial resection.[71] Chemotherapy may also be implemented but is relatively ineffective for many tumor types. However, a combination of chemotherapy and STR, following primary resection of glioblastomas, has resulted in longer survival times.[71]

Other treatments that are receiving attention, include **gene-centered** treatments to correct the gene mutation, associated with the tumor growth; of course, identification of the appropriate genetic mutation will be key in developing these treatment methods. For glioblastomas and other progressive tumors that respond poorly to standard measures, some are examining the use of targeted **viruses**, which can kill tumor cells while leaving normal cells alone. This is an area of rapid growth but limited results at this time.[60]

Physical Therapy Management of the Patient with a Brain Tumor

CASE B, PART III

Alice underwent surgical resection, followed by stereotaxic radiation with chemotherapy. Following these treatments, she entered an inpatient rehabilitation unit with a diagnosis of profound sensory loss with secondary motor dysfunction, characterized by incoordination and apraxia. In addition, she presented with receptive aphasia and apparent memory loss.

As the case illustrates, damage from a brain tumor and the methods used to treat it can result in neurologic consequences similar to those of a stroke or focal brain injury. The damage is typically localized to the area of the tumor. However, more generalized effects of fatigue, cognitive dysfunction with impairments in processing speed, working memory or attention, and diminished respiratory capacity are also apparent after radiation therapy. Thus, a growing area for rehabilitation practitioners, especially physical therapists, is in the area of oncology rehabilitation. Therapy should focus on specific impairments and functional limitations as well as general physical conditioning. Early rehabilitation has been found to improve functional outcomes post medical treatment of brain tumors.[72] In addition, exercise post-radiation may ameliorate some of the devastating effects of this treatment, including fatigue, depression, and diminished physical conditioning, including muscle loss. Notably, there is some evidence from animal studies that exercise may also facilitate improved cortical gliogenesis, allowing repopulation of microglia that are lost with radiation treatments and, thereby, improve the microenvironment for neural function.[73]

CASE B, PART IV

For Alice, treatment focused on sensory retraining that included sensory stimulation with a variety of stimuli (e.g., hot/cold, textures, vibration, and electrical stimulation – TENS); this was progressed to sensory discrimination activities using manual manipulation with vision occluded by a curtain between handled objects and Alice. This allowed discrimination of temperature, texture, weight, and shape of objects, usually involving matching

to a target object. In addition, her treatment focused on many object manipulation tasks, whereby she had to place a block into a shape sorter or slot by orienting her hand to the orientation of the targeted slot. She also had impaired sensation in her leg/foot that resulted in tripping and exaggerated step height, so treatment focused on sensory stimulation to her foot and gait training to improve safety with ambulation on a variety of surfaces and often in bare feet to facilitate her "feeling" the surface. Initially, she demonstrated marked improvements and was discharged to outpatient care. On a follow-up visit, 6 weeks later, the therapist noted motor weakness in her left biceps and deltoid. Alice was referred back to her physician for evaluation, where recurrence of her tumor into her frontal lobe was diagnosed. Within a week, Alice was transferred to hospice, where she again received physical therapy. At this time, the focus of care was on minimizing pain and management of physical symptoms.

Physical therapy management of the terminal cancer patient is also a growing area of practice. Common treatments include exercise and range of motion (active, active assistive, or passive) to prevent painful contractures, transfer techniques and activities of daily living as function diminishes, management of edema, relaxation techniques, and/or massage to manage pain and muscle cramping.[74] In addition, physical therapists may be called upon to determine appropriate adaptive equipment – wheelchairs, ambulation aids – to maximize mobility for the terminal patient.

REFERENCES

1. Sundman MH, Hail EE, Chen NK. Examining the relationship between head trauma and neurodegenerative disease: a review of epidemiology, pathology, and neuroimaging techniques. *J Alzheimers Dis Parkinsonism*. 4. doi:10.4172/2161-0460.1000137.

2. Meythaler JM, Peduzzi JD, Eleftheriou E, Novack TA. Current concepts: diffuse axonal injury-associated traumatic brain injury. *Arch Phys Med Rehabil*. 2001;82:1461-1471.

3. Teasdale G, Maas A, Lecky F, Manley G, Stocchetti N, Murray G. The Glasgow Coma Scale at 4 years: standing the test of time. *Lancet Neurol*. 2014;18:844-854.

4. Pasquina P, Kirtley R, Ling G. Moderate-to-severe traumatic brain injury. *Semin Neurol*. 2014;34:572-583.

5. Tomaszczyk JC, Green NL, Frasca D, Colella B, Turner GR, Christensen BK, Green RE. Negative neuroplasticity in chronic traumatic brain injury and implications for neurorehabilitation. *Neuropsychol Rev*. 2014;24:409-427.

6. Sherer M, Yablon SA, Nakase-Richardson R. Patterns of recovery of post-traumatic confusional state in neurorehabilitation admissions after traumatic brain injury. *Arch Phys Med Rehabil*. 2009;96:1749-1754.

7. Andriessen TMJC, Jacobs B, Vos PE. Clinical characteristics and pathophysiological mechanisms of focal and diffuse traumatic brain injury. *J Cell Mol Med*. 2014;14(10):2381-2392.

8. Ranchos Los Amigos Cognitive Recovery Scale. Available at: https://www.jhsmh.org/LinkClick.aspx?fileticket=8hAd-OqTIQ0%3D&tabid=298. Accessed 3/5/2015.

9. Galveston Orientation and Amnesia Test (GOAT). Available at: http://scale-library.com/pdf/Galveston_Orientation_Amnesia_Test.pdf. Accessed 3/5/2015.

10. Disability Rating Scale. Available at: http://www.tbims.org/combi/drs/DRS%20Form.pdf. Accessed 3/5/2015.

11. Kalmar K, Giacino JT. The JFK Coma Recovery Scale – revised. *Neuropsychol Rehabil*. 2005;15:454-460.

12. Katz DI, Polyak M, Coughlan D, Nichols M, Roche A. Natural history of recovery from brain injury after prolonged disorders of consciousness: outcome of patients admitted to inpatient rehabilitation with 1-4 year follow-up. *Prog Brain Res*. 2009;177:73-88.

13. Keren O, Cohen M, Lazar-Zweker I, Groswasser Z. Tracheotomy in severe TBI patients: sequelae and relation to vocational outcome. *Brain Inj*. 2001;15(6):531-536.

14. Rincon F, Ghosh S, Dey S, Maltenfort M, Vibbert M, Urtecho J, McBride W, Moussouttas M, Bell R, Ratliff JK, Jallo J. Impact of acute lung injury and acute respiratory distress syndrome after traumatic brain injury in the United States. *Neurosurgery*. 2012;71:795-803.

15. Carlucci M, Graf N, Simmons JG, Corbridge SJ. Effective management of ARDS. *Nurse Pract*. 2014;39(12):35-40.

16. Franschman G, Peerdeman SM, Greuters S, Vieveen J, Brinkman ACM, Christiaans HM, Toor EJ, Jukema GN, Loer SA, Boer C, ALARM-TBI investigators. Prehospital endotracheal intubation in patients with severe traumatic brain injury: guidelines versus reality. *Resuscitation*. 2009;80:1147-1151.

17. Stocchetti N, Maas AIR. Traumatic intracranial hypertension. *N Engl J Med*. 2014;370:2121-2130.

18. Bramlett HM, Dietrich WD. Long-term consequences of traumatic brain injury: current status of potential mechanisms of injury and neurological outcomes. *J Neurotrauma*. 2015;32:1-15.

19. Gupta PK, Sayed N, Ding K, Agostini MA, Van Ness PC, Yablon S, Madden C, Mickey B, D'Abrosio R, Diaz-Arrastia R. Subtypes of post-traumatic epilepsy: clinical, electrophysiological, and imaging features. *J Neurotrauma*. 2014;31:1439-1443.

20. Lowenstein DH. Epilepsy after head injury: an overview. *Epilepsy*. 50(suppl 2):4-9.

21. Szaflarski JP, Nazzal Y, Dreer LE. Post-traumatic epilepsy: current and emerging treatment options. *Neuropsychiatr Dis Treat*. 2014;10:1469-1477.

22. Anthony DC, Couch Y. The systemic response to CNS injury. *Exp Neurol*. 2014;258:105-111.

23. Lu J, Goh SJ, Tng PYL, Deng YY, Ling EA, Moochhala S. Systemic inflammatory response following acute traumatic brain injury. *Front Biosci*. 2009;14:3795-3813.

24. Costello LAS, Lithander FE, Gruen RL, Williams LT. Nutrition therapy in the optimization of health outcomes in adult patients with moderate to severe traumatic brain injury: findings from a scoping review. *Injury*. 2014;45:1834-1841.

25. Pepe JL, Barba CA. The metabolic response to acute traumatic brain injury and implications for nutritional support. *J Head Trauma Rehabil*. 1999;14(5):462-474.

26. Biteghe-bi-Nzeng A, Wang Y. Cushings ulcer in traumatic brain injury. *Chin J Trauma*. 2008:11(2):114-119.

27. Acosta-Escribano J, Fernandez-Vivas M, Carmona TG, Caturia-Such J, Garcia-Martinez M, Menendez-Mainer A, Solera-Suarez M, Sanchez-Paya J. Gastric versus transpyloric feeding in severe traumatic brain injury: a prospective, randomized trial. *Intensive Care Med*. 2010;36:1532-1539.

28. Laxe S, Terre R, Leon D, Bernabeu M. How does dysautonomia influence the outcome of traumatic brain injured patients admitted in a neurorehabilitation unit? *Brain Inj*. 2013;27(12):1383-1387.

29. Hendricks HT, Heeren AH, Vos PE. Dysautonomia after severe traumatic brain injury. *Eur J Neurol*. 2001;17:1172-1177.

30. Arciniegas DB, Wortzel HS. Emotional and behavioral dyscontrol after traumatic brain injury. *Psychiatr Clin N Am*. 2014;37:31-53.

31. Nakase-Richardson R, Sepehri A, Sherer M, et al. Classification schema of posttraumatic amnesia duration-based injury severity relative to 1-year outcome: analysis of individuals with moderate and severe traumatic brain injury. *Arch Phys Med Rehabil*. 2009;90:17-19.

32. Ciaramelli E, Serino A, Di Santantonio A, Làdavas E. Central executive system impairment in traumatic brain injury. *Brain Cogn*. 2006;60(2):198-199.

33. Rabinowitz AR, Levin HS. Cognitive sequelae of traumatic brain injury. *Psychiatr Clin N Am*. 2014;37(1):1-11.

34. Kimberly TJ, Samargia S, Moore LG, Shakya JK, Lang CE. Comparison of amounts and types of practice during rehabilitation of traumatic brain injury and stroke. *J Rehabil Res Dev*. 2010;47(9):851-862.

35. Vasudevan EV1, Glass RN, Packel AT Effects of traumatic brain injury on locomotor adaptation. *J Neurol Phys Ther*. 2014;38(3):172-182.

36. Giuffrida CG, Demery JA, Reyes LR, Lebowitz BK, Hanlon RE. Functional skill learning in men with traumatic brain injury. *Am J Occup Ther*. 2009;63(4):398-407.

37. Lai JM, Francisco GE, Willis FB. Dynamic splinting after treatment with botulinum toxin type-A: a randomized controlled pilot study. *Adv Ther*. 2009;26(2):241-248.

38. Moseley AM The effect of casting combined with stretching on passive ankle dorsiflexion in adults with traumatic head injuries. *Phys Ther*. 1997;77(3):240-247; discussion 248-259.

39. Singer BJ, Jegasothy GM, Singer KP, Allison GT. Evaluation of serial casting to correct equinovarus deformity of the ankle after acquired brain injury in adults. *Arch Phys Med Rehabil*. 2003;84(4):483-491.

40. Moseley AM, Hassett LM, Leung J, Clare JS, Herbert RD, Harvey LA. Serial casting versus positioning for the treatment of elbow contractures in adults with traumatic brain injury: a randomized controlled trial. *Clin Rehabil*. 2008;22(5):406-417.

41. Shehab D, Elgazzar AH, Collier BD. Heterotopic ossification. *J Nucl Med*. 2002;43(3):346-353.

42. Gouvier WD, Blanton PD, LaPorte KK, Nepomuceno C. Reliability and validity of the Disability Rating Scale and the Levels of Cognitive Functioning Scale in monitoring recovery from severe head injury. *Arch Phys Med Rehabil*. 1987;68(2):94-97.

43. Flannery J. Using the levels of cognitive functioning assessment scale with patients with traumatic brain injury in an acute care setting. *Rehabil Nurs*. 1998;23(2):88-94.

44. Kose G, Hatipoglu S. Effect of head and body positioning on cerebral blood flow velocity in patients who underwent cranial surgery. *J Clin Nurs*. 2012;21(13-14):1859-1867.

45. Gorji MA, Araghiyansc F, Jafari H, Gorgi AM, Yazdani J. Effect of auditory stimulation on traumatic coma duration in intensive care unit of Medical Sciences University of Mazandarn, Iran. *Saudi J Anaesth*. 2014;8(1):69-72.

46. Cossu, G Therapeutic options to enhance coma arousal after traumatic brain injury: state of the art of current treatments to improve coma recovery. *Br J Neurosurg*. 2014;28(2):187.

47. Megha M, Harpreet S, Nayeem Z. Effect of frequency of multimodal coma stimulation on the consciousness levels of traumatic brain injury comatose patients. *Brain Inj*. 2013;27(5):570-577.

48. TBI EDGE outcome measures for in- and outpatient rehabilitation. Available at: http://www.neuropt.org/professional---resources/neurology---section---outcome---measures---recommendations. Accessed 3/5/2015.

49. Riedel D, Shaw V. Nursing management of patients with brain injury requiring one-on-one care. *Rehabil Nurs*. 1997;22(1):36-39.

50. Grauwmeijer E, Heijenbrok-Kal MH, Haitsma IK, Ribbers GM. A prospective study on employment outcome 3 years after moderate to severe traumatic brain injury. *Arch Phys Med Rehabil*. 2012;93(6):993-999.

51. Mitiguy, JS. Coping with survival. *Headlines*. 1990:228. In: Power PW, Dell Orto AE. *Families Living with Chronic Illness and Disability: Interventions, Challenges, and Opportunities*. New York, NY: Springer Publishing Company; 2004.

52. Lezak MD. Psychological implications of traumatic brain damage for the patient's family. *Rehabil Psychol.* 1986;3(4):241-250.

53. McKee AC, Daneshvar DH, Alvarez VE, Stein TD. The neuropathology of sport. *Acta Neuropathol.* 2014;127(1):29-51.

54. Karr JE, Areshenkoff CN, Garcia-Barrera MA. The neuropsychological outcomes of concussion: a systematic review of meta-analyses on the cognitive sequelae of mild traumatic brain injury. *Neuropsychology.* 2014;28(3):321-336.

55. McCrory P, Collie A, Anderson V, Davis G. Can we manage sport related concussion in children the same as adults? *Br J Sports Med.* 2004;38(5):516-519.

56. Mejerske CW, Mihalik JP, Ren D, Collins MW, Reddy CC, Lovell MR, Wagner AK. Concussion in sports: postconcussive activity levels, symptoms, and neurocognitive performance. *J Athl Train.* 2008;43(3):265-274.

57. Brown NJ, Mannix RC, O'Brien MJ, Gostine D, Collins MW, Meehan WP. Effect of cognitive activity level on duration of post-concussion symptoms. *Pediatrics.* 2014;133(2):e299-e304.

58. Murphy MP, Carmine H. Long-term health implications of individuals with TBI: a rehabilitation perspective. *NeuroRehabilitation.* 2012;31:85-94.

59. Bay EJ. Chartier KS. Chronic morbidities after traumatic brain injury: an update for the advanced practice nurse. *J Neurosci Nurs.* 2014;46(3):142-152.

60. Kheirollahi M, Dashti S, Khalaj Z, Nazemroaia F, Mahzouni P. Brain tumors: special characters for research and banking. *Adv Biomed Res.* 2015;4:4.

61. Koob M, Girard N. Cerebral tumors: specific features in children. *Diag Interv Imaging.* 2014;95:965-983.

62. Gilbert MR, Armstrong TS, Pope WB, van den Bent MJ, Wen PY. Facing the future of brain tumor clinical research. *Clin Cancer Res.* 2014;20(22):5591-5600.

63. Jakacki RI, Burger PC, Kocak M, Boyett JM, Goldwein J, Mehta M, Packer RJ, Tarbell NJ, Pollack IF. Outcome and prognostic factors for children with supratentorial primitive neuroectodermal tumors treated with carboplatin during radiotherapy. *Pediatr Blood Cancer.* 2015. doi:10.1002/pbc.25405.

64. Dubois LG, Campanati L, Righy C, D'Andrea-Meira I, Sporh RC, Porto-Carreiro I, Pereira CM, Balca-Silva J, Kahn SA, DosSantos MF, Oliveira MA, Ximenes-da-Silva A, Lopes MC, Faveret E, Gasparetto EL, Moura-Neto V. Gliomas and the vascular fragility of the blood brain barrier. *Front Cell Neurosci.* 2014;8(418):1-13.

65. Park CK, Phi JH, Park SH. Glial tumors with neuronal differentiation. *Neurosurg Clin N Am.* 2015;26:117-138.

66. Miller R, DeCandio ML, Dixon-Mah Y, Giglio P, Vandergrift WA, Blanik NL, Patel SJ, Varma AK, Das A. Molecular targets and treatment of meningioma. *J Neurol Neurosurg.* 2014;1(1):1-15.

67. Hasegawa T, Shintai K, Kato T, Iizuka H. Stereotactic radiosurgery as the initial treatment for patients with nonfunctioning pituitary adenomas. *World Neurosurg.* 2015. doi:10.1016/j.wneu.2015.01.054.

68. Giulioni M, Marucci G, Martinoni M, Marliani AF, Toni F, Bartiromo F, Volpi L, Riguzzi P, Bisulli F, Naldi I, Michelucci R, Baruzzi A, Tinuper P, Rubboli G. Epilepsy associated tumors. *World J Clin Cases.* 2014;2(1):623-641.

69. DeAngelis LM, Wen PY. Primary and metastatic tumors of the nervous system. In: *Harrison's Neurology in Clinical Medicine.* Chicago, IL: McGraw Hill; 2013.

70. Swartling FJ, Cancer M, Frantz A, Weishaupt H, Persson AI. Deregulated proliferation and differentiation in brain tumors. *Cell Tissue Res.* 2015;359:225-254.

71. Kondziolka D, Shin SM, Brunswick A, Kim I, Silverman JS. The biology of radiosurgery and its clinical applications for brain tumors. *Neuro-Oncol.* 2015;17(1):29-44.

72. Bartolo M, Zucchella C, Pace A, Lanzetta G, Vecchione C, Bartolo M, Grillea G, Serrao M, Tassorelli C, Sandrini G, Pierelli F. Early rehabilitation after surgery improves functional outcome in inpatients with brain tumors. *J Neurooncol.* 2012;107:537-544.

73. Rodgers SP, Trevino M, Zawaksi JA, Gaber MW, Leasure JL. Neurogenesis, exercise, and cognitive late effects of pediatric radiotherapy. *Neural Plast.* 2013; Article ID 698528, 12 pages.

74. Jensen W, Bialy L, Ketels G, Baumann FT, Bokemeyer C, Oechsle K. Physical exercise and therapy in terminally ill cancer patients: a retrospective feasibility analysis. *Support Care Cancer.* 2014;22:1261-1268.

Review Questions

1. **A young man experiences a closed head injury with a contusion of the right frontal lobe, from falling over the handlebars of his bicycle; the likely place for a contre coup injury would be:**

   A. Right temporal lobe

   B. Left temporal lobe

   C. Right parietal lobe

   D. Left occipital lobe

2. **A Grade 2 diffuse axonal injury typically involves damage to which structure(s):**

   A. Corpus callosum

   B. Corpus callosum and parasagittal projections

   C. Corpus callosum, parasagittal projections, and brainstem white matter

   D. Microstructural damage to the parasagittal white matter

3. **Chronic neurodegeneration (>1 year post-TBI) likely results from which mechanisms?**

   A. Anterograde degeneration

   B. Excitotoxicity

   C. Retrograde degeneration

   D. Negative plasticity

4. **Which assessment is commonly used to determine the clearance of post-traumatic amnesia?**

   A. Braintree Scale of Neurologic Stages of Recovery from Brain Injury

   B. Galveston Orientation and Amnesia Test

   C. JFK Coma Recovery Scale

   D. Ranchos Los Amigos Cognitive Recovery Scale

5. Amy is 14 weeks s/p a severe head injury; she does not remember anything about her accident. She is currently unable to remember what kind of job she held prior to the accident, anything about her 2 years of marriage to Matt, or details of her college years. She is able to remember her therapy schedules and transport herself to each session. Within sessions, she is able to remember some of the things learned from the preceding day and verbalize them. What kind of amnesia is Amy demonstrating?

A. Anterograde

B. Post-traumatic

C. Retrograde

6. A patient that is receiving PT in the ICU, following a severe TBI, begins to vomit. The therapist should be most concerned about:

A. Dysautonomia

B. Elevated intracranial pressure

C. Multi-organ failure

D. Seizure activity

7. A patient, recovering from TBI, is watching a TV show, where one of the characters dies; in response, the patient begins to cry and continues to cry for almost an hour. This is likely a sign of what condition?

A. Emotional dyscontrol

B. Emotional lability

C. Pathologic crying

D. Pseudobulbar affect

8. While assessing a client who is s/p TBI a therapist asks the client to demonstrate how to safely perform a sit to stand transfer. The client takes a long time to initiate the activity but then performs the activity in a safe and correct manner. When a nurse rushes the client to stand up from the dining room chair after dinner the client is unsafe and requires cueing. Based on this description the two transfers look different due to which area of cognitive function?

A. Loss of memory

B. Poor judgment

C. Slow speed of processing

D. Poor selective attention

9. To improve function that is impaired by deficits in divided attention and executive dysfunction the therapist should progressively challenge which area of cognitive functioning?

A. Working memory

B. Speed of processing

C. Selective attention

D. Initiation

10. In an individual with elevated intracranial pressure the head of the bed should be in what position?

A. Flat

B. Elevated to 10 degrees

C. Elevated to 30 degrees

D. In 5 degrees of Trendelenburg

11. An individual post-TBI who is in Ranchos LOC Stage IV and agitated has left hemiplegia and is doing repetitive sit to stand transfers in all therapies and with nursing. After a week he remains in Ranchos LOC IV and has improved his transfer from moderate assist to CGA with cueing. This improvement is due to:

A. Hypertrophy of the quadriceps

B. Explicit learning

C. Implicit learning

D. Improved memory

12. Multi-modal sensory stimulation programs should

A. Present stimuli in a random order

B. Include monitoring of vitals

C. Sessions can be up to 1 hour long

D. Use standardized stimuli with no emotional overlay

13. At which Ranchos LOC can you begin to expect explicit learning with carryover?

A. IV

B. V

C. VI

D. VII

14. In dealing with a client who is agitated which of the following is appropriate?

A. Restrain the individual to prevent self-harm and harm to others

B. Medication improves time to recovery from agitation and confusion

C. Be sure to bring at least three staff into the room to ensure that you can control the individual

D. Try to figure out what is causing them to be agitated and modify the environment and agitation can be decreased

15. For impulsivity which of the following is an appropriate intervention?

A. Use a written list of steps to be followed for each activity

B. Encourage task completion without rehearsal

C. Do not leave the client unsupervised

D. Provide calendars of daily activities

16. Which of the following is true regarding repetitive mild TBI
    A. Motor function is the area most sensitive to this damage
    B. External provocation is one means for screening for mild TBI
    C. Does not lead to neural changes such as atrophy
    D. Attention and concentration are not impacted

17. A teenage lacrosse player comes off the field after having been hit over the helmet with another player's lacrosse stick. The player says he feels fine and wishes to return to play. He can repeat digits back to you in reverse order and knows where he is and what happened. He is also able to tell you who they played a week ago and the score of the game. Pupils are symmetrical and reactive and finger to nose is normal. He is asked to sprint 40 yards and then to do five pushups. On the third pushup he vomits. Which of the following statements is true regarding his screen for mild TBI?
    A. The screening exam is negative and he can return to play
    B. The screening exam has a positive finding but it is only with provocation so he can return to play
    C. The provocation test was positive so he should be held from play

18. Recent research suggests that the best treatment for concussion is:
    A. Absolute rest
    B. Moderate levels of physical and cognitive activity are best
    C. Moderate physical activity with minimal cognitive activity is best
    D. High-level physical and cognitive activity are recommended.

19. For those with severe TBI, which long-term outcome is most likely?
    A. Complete return to work, school, or homemaking activity
    B. Return to supervised work and living environments
    C. No return to work but able to live independently
    D. Require total care at home and unable to work

20. A oligodendroglioma presents with fairly good differentiation, no infiltration, and is slow growing. This tumor would be staged as:
    A. Stage I
    B. Stage II
    C. Stage III
    D. Stage IV

21. Which tumor would correctly be classified as a glioma
    A. Astrocytoma
    B. Ependymoma
    C. Meningioma
    D. Pituitary adenoma

22. Which of the symptoms of a brain tumor is only found in young children?
    A. Irritability
    B. Fatigue/sleep disturbance
    C. Seizures
    D. Protruding fontanelles

23. For the patient, receiving radiation treatment for brain tumor, exercise should be avoided until treatment is complete?
    A. True
    B. False

24. In hospice, the primary focus of treatment should be?
    A. Increasing aerobic capacity
    B. Strengthening
    C. Pain management
    D. Walking endurance

Answers

1. D	2. A	3. D	4. B	5. C
6. B	7. B	8. C	9. A	10. C
11. C	12. B	13. C	14. D	15. A
16. B	17. C	18. C	19. B	20. B
21. A	22. D	23. B	24. C	

Spinal Cord Injury

12

D. Michele Basso

CASE A, PART I

Jane Roberts is a 45-year-old African-American woman who entered the Emergency Department via ambulance with a self-inflicted gunshot wound to the neck at C2–3. She was intubated in the field and placed on a respirator when admitted to the hospital. Her blood pressure, 98/62, and heart rate, 60, were low and continued to fall. Radiographs show a projectile near C2, a vertebral fracture of C2, and a bony fragment within the spinal canal. She has a history of depression and mild obesity but takes no medications for these conditions. Ms. Roberts presented in the Emergency Department with no volitional movement in any of the extremities. The plantar reflex was present, but deep tendon reflexes (DTRs) in all extremities were absent. She is not married, works in a parts-assembly factory, and lives alone in a two-story home.

● PATHOPHYSIOLOGY

What Is Spinal Cord Injury?

The spinal cord is protected by the surrounding bone of the vertebrae, but in severe trauma, the vertebrae fracture or dislocate. In fact, fracture, dislocation, and/or subluxation of the vertebrae are the most common causes of spinal cord injury (SCI). The damaged bony segments impinge the spinal cord and immediately cause a lesion. This direct damage to the spinal cord is called the **primary injury**. It is important to note that the spinal cord is almost never completely severed; some spinal cord tissue is usually spared. Commonly, the fractured or dislocated bone compresses the cord or only partially pierces it. In most cases, the primary injury begins in the gray matter of the cord, when the blood vessels shear and rupture, directly damaging neurons. There is frank hemorrhage at the injury site and small petechial hemorrhages away from the injury over the next couple of hours. White matter axons may also be directly lesioned with the primary injury. These initial events set off a complex secondary cascade that cause the lesion to expand in size, over a long distance and over a very long period of time.

The **secondary injury** events stem from a toxic environment created by the initial injury.[1] The opening of the blood–brain barrier allows red blood cells to flood the gray matter, and the iron and hemoglobin they contain are toxic to neurons that were not initially damaged by the trauma. As these bystander neurons die, they release neurotoxins and glutamate that go on to kill other neurons beyond the primary injury site. Other toxic substances are produced, including free radicals, reactive oxygen species, and peroxidases, which degrade cell membranes and cause further cell death. With this necrotic cell death, edema increases and the damaged blood vessels are sealed a few segments away from the primary injury, causing ischemia. Loss of oxygen results in expanding cell death, and even the cells that overcome this stress are often lost once blood flow returns to the area (reperfusion) as even higher levels of reactive oxygen species occur.

Another major contributor to secondary injury and lesion expansion is neuroinflammation.[1] Within the first few hours and days after the injury, resident microglia and infiltrating macrophages from the peripheral blood stream flood into the lesion center. Early on, they play an important beneficial role in sterilizing the wound and scavenging debris. However, the inflammatory response extends for very long periods of time, producing detrimental effects well away from the injury site. The activated microglia produce high levels of pro-inflammatory cytokines and chemokines, and these factors impair neuronal function up to 10 segments below the injury site. Additionally, oligodendrocytes are especially vulnerable to pro-inflammatory cytokines, leading to oligodendrocyte cell death and creating zones of demyelination many segments above and below the level of the injury. The notion that there is a localized site of SCI is being challenged, and it is important to start to understand that areas well away from the primary injury will also experience secondary lesion effects that will impact rehabilitation.

During this secondary injury phase, reactive astrocytes surround the primary lesion, creating a glial scar that acts as a physical barrier to regenerating axons. The astrocytes also produce chemical inhibitory barriers (i.e., chondroitin sulfate proteoglycans, known as CSPGs) that extend two or three segments above and below the primary injury. Reactive astrocytes extend well away from the injury site but are likely not creating a scar. Some ideas are that they are providing metabolic support and helping to control edema in these remote regions.

Importantly, these secondary injury pathways offer the best target for treatment after SCI. By quelling some or all of these pathways, the severity of lesion and resulting motor impairments can be greatly reduced. Thus, neuroprotection has been a major focus of scientific investigation. Regeneration, growth promotion, and cellular replacement therapies have also shown some promise in recent studies.[2,3] Any reduction of lesion size or effective cellular growth promotion will offer important substrates upon which to improve functional recovery after SCI.

Who has a Spinal Cord Injury?

Each year about 12,000 people have an SCI. The most common cause of SCI is trauma from car accidents (36%), falls (28%), violence (14%), or sports (9%).[4] Although sports-related injuries used to be the highest cause, it has steadily declined while vehicular accidents and falls continue to rise. The changes in injury patterns are also accompanied by an increase in age at the time of injury. In the 1970s, the average age at the time of SCI was about 27 years, but now, the average age is 42 years.[4] Still, about half of all SCIs occur in young people under the age of 30.[4] Spinal cord injuries also occur in men much more often than in women, at a rate of 75–80%.

Other causes of SCI include transverse myelitis, spinal stenosis, spinal abscess, or tumor. **Spinal stenosis** is the narrowing of the spinal canal and can be of such a large amount that the spinal cord becomes compressed. It most commonly occurs in the cervical or lumbar vertebrae. The narrow canal may not cause any neural symptoms until a minor trauma like a fall or neck hyperextension occurs. People with osteoarthritis are particularly at risk for hyperextension type SCI. With this otherwise minor trauma, the cord is greatly compressed resulting in a primary injury of the gray matter. We will discuss the specific type of SCI observed with spinal stenosis, called central cord syndrome, in a later section. Spinal stenosis-related SCI occurs in older individuals with a mean age of 64 years and effects women at a higher rate, about 40%, than in traumatic SCI.[5] The severity of the injury appears less than traumatic SCI in that paraplegia is more common than tetraplegia and rehabilitation is shorter.[5]

Transverse myelitis is pronounced inflammation across both sides of the spinal cord that typically occurs with a sudden onset over a few hours and worsens over a few weeks.[6] It isn't clear what initiates the inflammation, but viral infections are a strong candidate. Both children and adults can be affected with about 1400 people diagnosed each year with transverse myelitis. As in traumatic SCI, inflammatory cascades target oligodendrocytes and the resulting cell death produces regions of demyelination and axonal loss. The degree of recovery is highly variable with most individuals having long-term motor disabilities.[6] Recurrence is rare but not unheard of.

Differential Diagnosis – Could this be a Spinal Cord Injury?

Traumatic SCI is routinely diagnosed in the Emergency Department, but non-traumatic SCI is often misdiagnosed as a musculoskeletal condition; thus, physical therapists must be cautious when treating these conditions. In the case of abscess, tumor, or transverse myelitis, the primary symptom is back pain, which can be localized or radiating pain. Because this type of pain is common in both musculoskeletal conditions and non-traumatic SCI, a thorough neurologic examine is needed to rule out SCI. The best indicators of SCI are changes in reflexes below the level of pain, a positive Babinski sign, and/or difficulty voiding the bowel or bladder.

With SCI, there are two areas of neuropathology at the injury site – the neurons in the gray matter and the long ascending and descending white matter tracks. When the motor neurons in a segment or segments of the spinal cord are damaged, lower motor neuron (LMN) signs emerge. When white matter tracks are lesioned, upper motor neuron (UMN) signs occur. Most of the time, SCI results in both upper and lower motor neuron signs, since both gray and white matter are damaged.

Lower motor neuron signs include **areflexia** and **flaccid paralysis** early after injury and extreme **muscle atrophy** within weeks or months. These signs are directly related to death of motor neurons that innervate muscles at the level of the injury. Regions of flaccid paralysis and areflexia are used to determine the level of injury but are difficult to examine in the trunk where DTRs are not available for testing. Any LMN signs observed in people with musculoskeletal conditions, like low back pain, require immediate referral to a neurologist. The **Beevor sign** of the umbilicus may help to identify motor neuron loss within the thoracic region (T10–12). This is evident, when the upper rectus abdominus muscle is innervated but the lower part is poorly innervated and weak, so that only the upper rectus contracts forcefully. By raising the head from a supine position, the upper rectus pulls the umbilicus toward the head, identifying a lesion in the lower thoracic cord.

Upper motor neuron signs occur because information from the brain to the spinal cord is disrupted in the white matter tracks. **Hyperreflexia**, **spasticity**, **clonus**, and positive **Babinski** sign occur with UMN lesions (as described in Chapter 10 – Stroke), but unlike in stroke, these problems emerge because of damage to the axons of supraspinal neurons rather than to the neuron somas. Any person being treated for a musculoskeletal condition that demonstrates UMN signs must also be immediately referred to a neurologist.

● CLASSIFICATIONS OF SCI

Spinal cord injury is classified by the level and severity of the primary pathology using the **ASIA Impairment Scale** (AIS) and the **International Standards for Neurological Classification**

of SCI (ISNCSCI).[7] There is a free online training program to learn to administer the exam.[8] The level of the injury refers to the segmental location of the primary lesion, based on radiographic and clinical symptoms. The designated level is the most distal, uninvolved segment with normal function. A patient with a C4 level injury means that dysfunction and impairments occur below C4. Cervical injuries result in impairments of the upper and lower extremities, called tetraplegia. When SCI occurs in the thoracic or upper lumbar regions, the lower extremities are affected, which is known as paraplegia.

The severity of SCI is classified into four categories, AIS A to AIS D, ranging from complete to incomplete SCI (Table 12-1). The AIS/ISNCSCI system examines each sensory dermatome of the body for perception of sharp, dull, and light touch and assigns one of three scores – 0 = no sensation, 1 = altered sensation, which can be either hyper or hyposensitive, and 2 = normal sensation. Motor function is assessed using manual muscle testing (MMT) of five key muscle groups in each upper extremity and five muscles of each lower extremity. Traditional MMT scores ranging from 0 to 5 are used for each muscle group bilaterally, which yields a maximum score of 50 for upper extremity motor scores (UEMS) and 50 for lower extremity motor scores (LEMS).

There are several important clinical considerations for the AIS system. When the AIS classification is made at 72 hours after the injury, it can be a good predictor of whether people will go on to regain walking function. Some or intact pinprick sensation in the peri-anal region predicted ambulation in individuals with SCI.[9,10] During the first year after SCI, there is a high rate of AIS conversion to a higher classification.[11,12] This means that in the acute setting and during inpatient rehabilitation therapists should expect some sensory and motor recovery and use interventions that will encourage recovery. Traditionally, little change in AIS classification and motor scores have been reported between 1 and 5 years after SCI,[13] which has been used to focus rehabilitation within the first year of SCI. However, recent work has shown that walking-based programs on a treadmill for AIS C or D injuries greatly increased motor scores for both the upper and lower extremities in people with sub-acute to chronic SCI.[14] Conversion to higher AIS classification was greater than expected, and both people with tetraplegia and paraplegia improved with treatment.[13,14] These findings suggest that motor recovery after SCI is highly responsive to the type of rehabilitation administered, even at chronic time points.

While the AIS system is the most widely used classification system for SCI, it has several limitations. It does not measure motor function in the trunk that can be a clinically important indicator of the type of physical therapy treatment to deliver. The sensory score of 1 can mean that sensation is below normal (hyposensitive) or well-above normal (hypersensitive), thereby, making it a poor measure of neuropathic pain. An AIS A classification means the injury is *clinically complete* but postmortem studies of human SCI by Richard Bunge found that anatomical sparing occurred in a large number of AIS A cases.[15,16] Recently, Harkema and colleagues implanted epidural stimulators below the level of SCI in people with AIS A or AIS B injuries.[17] These individuals had no voluntary control of lower extremity muscles, prior to implantation, but on the first day of stimulation, each individual demonstrated voluntary movement of the leg, foot, or toe. Taken together with the work of Bunge, these studies indicate that even when AIS A complete classifications are assigned, anatomical sparing is highly likely. This sparing may be an important substrate for recovery of function, when task-specific training is delivered.

A new assessment tool, the **Neuromuscular Recovery Scale** (NRS), has been developed specifically to classify SCI relative to normal, pre-injury motor performance. It uses 14 items or tasks for trunk, upper extremity, and lower extremity motor control. The items range from coming to sitting, sitting, coming to stand, walking, and unimanual and bimanual manipulation. An overview of the NRS with video examples of the testing items is available.[18] The performance is scored in four broad phases (Phases 1–4) with higher phases reflecting greater return of normal movement. Each of these phases is further subdivided into three categories (A, B, or C) to better differentiate functional performance. The overall classification is designated by the Phase and subclassification (i.e., Phase 1A, Phase 4B, etc.) and reflects the lowest threshold of pre-injury function. The NRS can also be used to measure recovery of function by assigning one point for each subphase that is performed at a pre-injury level. A total of 161 points are available. The psychometrics of the NRS has been tested on people with AIS A–D SCI, in both the outpatient and inpatient rehabilitation settings. It has shown high interrater and test–retest reliability,[19,20] strong validity,[21] and better sensitivity to functional improvement over time than most other SCI outcome measures, including ISNCSCI motor and sensory scores, 10-m walk test, 6-minute walk test, Berg Balance test, and modified functional reach.[22] Because normal, pre-injury function is the basis of the scale, the NRS classification system enables the therapist to identify areas of function that are lagging behind and target treatment interventions to these areas.

Relationship between Injury and Clinical Presentation

To effectively treat SCI, it is important to understand the relationship between the injury and the clinical presentation. Some aspects of the injury result in permanent loss of function while others may have the potential to recover. Distinguishing between these can be accomplished by diagramming the lesion.

TABLE 12-1	Classification of SCI
AIS A	Complete; no sensory or motor function below the level of the injury
AIS B	Incomplete; no motor function but some sensation below the injury, including in the anal sphincter region (S4–5)
AIS C	Incomplete; some sensory and motor function below the injury but most of these muscles score below 3 on MMT
AIS D	Incomplete; sensory and motor function with at least half of the muscle groups scoring 3 or higher on MMT
AIS E	Normal motor and sensory function

A Brown-Sequard pattern of sensory loss   **B** Hyperreflexia in the weak leg   **C** Extradural compression at T8

Decreased pain and temperature

Weakness and decreased joint position and vibration sense

2+ 2+   2+ 2+

2+   2+

2+   3+

2+   4

FIGURE 12-1 Brown-Sequard pattern of injury. The primary symptoms of a BS pattern are ipsilesional motor and somatosensory dysfunction with contralesional loss of pain and temperature (**A**); hyperreflexia in the ipsilesional leg (**B**); and a lesion confined to one side of the spinal cord (**C**). (Reproduced with permission from Kandel ER, Schwartz JH, Jessell TM, Siegelbaum SA, Hudspeth AJ. *Principles of Neural Science*, 5th Ed, New York, NY: McGraw-Hill; 2013. Figure B-5, p. 1545.)

Brown-Sequard injury is an injury to primarily one side of the cord leaving the other side relatively intact (Figure 12-1). This type of injury can occur with fracture or dislocation but is most commonly seen after a penetrating injury from broken glass, a knife, or gunshot. The clinical presentation is motor impairment on the side of the lesion, loss of gross touch and vibration on the side of the lesion, and impairment of pain and temperature on the opposite side of the injury. Hyperreflexia as measured by brisk tendon reflexes and an upward Babinski response occurs below the lesion on the side of the injury (Figure 12-1B). Sweating, piloerection, and flushed face which are signs of autonomic dysfunction occur on the same side of the injury.

Central cord syndrome is caused by a lesion of the center core of the gray matter and occurs with trauma, tumors, or syrinxes and presents with LMN signs (flaccidity and muscle atrophy) of the upper extremities with less severe impairments of the lower extremities (Figure 12-2). Often the loss of hand function is pronounced and permanent, while the legs retain or regain a great deal of function sufficient to support walking with relatively stable balance. The lesion is primarily localized to the gray matter of the cervical cord, leaving most of the descending motor systems intact. In this way, there are lower motor signs at the level of the injury due to loss of motor neurons, while descending input from the brain can initiate central pattern generators (CPGs) for locomotion, which are intact below the injury.

Anterior spinal cord syndrome is a lesion of the anterior two-third of the spinal cord and is caused by damage or infarction of the anterior spinal artery (Figure 12-3). Interruption of blood flow through the artery can occur due to a blood clot and

is commonly referred to as spinal stroke. Other causes are bony fragments either blocking or cutting the artery, hyperflexion of the spinal column that compresses the artery, or clamping the

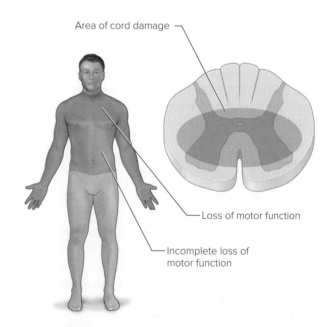

Area of cord damage

Loss of motor function

Incomplete loss of motor function

FIGURE 12-2 Central cord syndrome. This shows a lesion in the central gray matter, sparing a peripheral rim of white matter (right). The shaded areas (left) show the regions with complete loss of motor function (dark) and incomplete, mild loss of motor function (light).

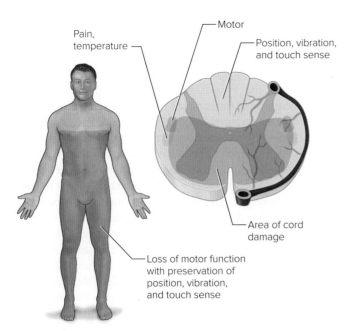

FIGURE 12-3 Anterior spinal cord injury. The lesion location in the ventral gray and white matter is shown on the right image of the cord. The shaded regions on the left show loss of motor function and pain and temperature sensation. Vibration and position sense remain.

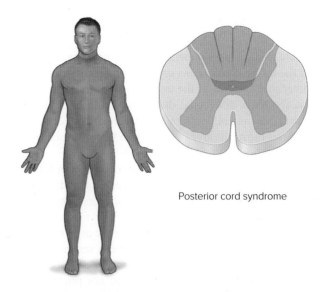

FIGURE 12-4 Posterior cord syndrome. The shaded region depicted in the right image of the cord shows the lesion located in the dorsal columns. The affected body regions are shown on the left which have loss of vibration and position sense.

descending aorta for abdominal surgery, which causes a delayed ischemic/reperfusion injury in up to 40% of surgical patients.[23] With anterior spinal cord syndrome, there is complete loss of volitional movement at and below the level of injury because the anterior and lateral corticospinal tracts are within the damaged area. Other descending motor systems, such as the vestibulospinal and reticulospinal tracts, also occupy these regions, resulting in a motor complete SCI. The ascending sensory tracts for pain and temperature also travel in the anterolateral white matter and are impaired at and below the level of the injury. However, the dorsal columns receive their blood supply from the dorsal spinal artery, so vibration and proprioception remain intact. This injury pattern is an example of an AIS B type of SCI. Depending on the level of SCI, autonomic impairments may also occur.

Posterior spinal cord syndrome (Figure 12-4) – The posterior part of the spinal cord can be lesioned by a penetrating wound to the back or hyperextension that fractures the vertebral arch; however, this is a rare type of SCI but has a classic presentation. Proprioception and vibration sense are lost while pain and temperature sensation remain intact. Motor function is also intact.

Conus medullaris (Figure 12-5) – The injury to the conus medullaris occurs at the L1 vertebral level, which is where the spinal cord tapers to an end. Nerves that originate from this part of the cord and nerves that travel through this space are affected by the injury. These nerves control legs, genitals, bladder, and bowel. The most common symptoms are: deep aching pain in the low back and numbness in the groin, thigh, leg, or foot. Urine retention, bowel dysfunction, and sexual impotence may also occur. These problems have a sudden onset and usually a bilateral presentation.

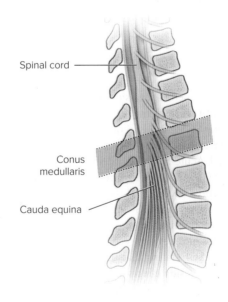

FIGURE 12-5 Conus medullaris and cauda equina injuries. The conus medullaris injury damages the distal portion of the spinal cord at L1; the cauda equina injury damages the spinal nerves, located in the spinal segments below the end of the cord.

Cauda Equina syndrome – The term cauda equina means horses tail and is named for the nerves that travel in the terminal spinal canal (Figure 12-5). It is difficult to differentiate Cauda Equina syndrome from a conus medullaris lesion because the nerves traveling down to their foramenal exit are often injured in both conditions. The location of the cauda equina injury will be below the L2 vertebral level. With a cauda equina injury, back pain is typically severe and stabbing (radicular) along dermatomal patterns, and the symptoms will likely be unilateral.

● MEDICAL MANAGEMENT

The acute medical management of SCI begins in the community when the injury is traumatic, or in the emergency department for other forms of SCI. If the injury is not of traumatic origin, then a thorough differential diagnosis should be undertaken with particular attention given to bowel and bladder function and reflexes below the area of concern so that someone with an abscess or tumor isn't sent home.

An early decision will be made as to whether spinal decompression and stabilization surgery is needed. Conditions that necessitate surgery include: progressive worsening of neurological symptoms, dislocated or locked facets, epidural abscesses, or cauda equina syndrome. The use of spinal decompression and stabilization surgery has been inconsistent and has not been considered standard of care for SCI because the level of evidence to support surgery was not prospective or randomized.[24,25] Recently, such a controlled surgical trial was conducted and found that 20% of people that receive decompression within about 14 hours of SCI regained two AIS grades or more at the 6-month follow-up.[26] In contrast, this level of improvement occurred in only 9% of people who had delayed surgery (2 days after SCI). Thus, spinal decompression and stabilization surgery within the first day after SCI should become more routine. As this surgical approach becomes widely adopted, physical therapists can expect greater gains in sensory and motor function in about half of the individuals who receive this surgery.

The other early medical decision will be whether to administer steroids. Until recently, the use of steroids within 8 hours of non-penetrating SCI was the recommended standard of care in the United States, based on three randomized controlled trials called National Acute Spinal Cord Injury Studies (NASCIS I, II, and III).[27,28] High-dose methylprednisolone improved motor and sensory scores on the AIS/ ISNCSCI exam in both people with complete or incomplete SCI. However, questions about scientific design, randomization, and data analysis emerged. Many physician groups have revised recommendations for steroid use for treatment of SCI, stating that any clinical gain may be heavily offset by serious side effects such as sepsis or pneumonia.[29] This means that the physical therapist will need to be a diligent member of the care team in any patient that receives methylprednisolone by checking for signs of sepsis, pneumonia, or other infections.

Once an SCI has been identified, the medical treatment focuses on several key factors that will continue to be carefully monitored throughout all phases of rehabilitation. Across the SCI treatment continuum, the physical therapist functions as part of a team. They are an extra set of eyes and hands to prevent life-threatening conditions, so it is important that the medical consequences and symptoms be familiar. Five areas of critical concern for the SCI team acutely, and thereafter are: (1) Cardiovascular changes, (2) Hypotension, (3) Bladder and Bowel Dysfunction, (4) Respiration, and (5) Skin Integrity. Hypotension and other cardiovascular complications result from autonomic dysfunction. These systems demand close attention because they represent life-threatening conditions if unmanaged.

Autonomic Dysfunction

Neuroanatomical Relationships and Normal Function

As introduced in Chapter 1, the autonomic nervous system is comprised of the sympathetic and parasympathetic systems that are responsible for complex reflex integration between the central nervous system (CNS) and vital organs. Excitatory sympathetic signals from receptors in the heart, arteries, and skeletal muscles are sent to the solitary nucleus in the brainstem. Parasympathetic input from Barrow receptors in the carotid artery, aortic arch, and other vessels inhibit the solitary nucleus via cranial nerves IX and X. Control of the heart is provided by two regions in the brain – the hypothalamus and the paraventricular nucleus surrounding the third ventricle. The hypothalamus increases sympathetic activity in the heart and other organs. Sympathetic vasomotor drive to the medulla raises blood pressure, and input to the raphe nucleus increases heart rate. The paraventricular nucleus sends axons to the spinal cord to also increase heart rate and regulate the sympathetic system in the lower thoracic cord.[30]

Effects of SCI

Cardiac and Vasomotor Changes – Injury at T6 or above interrupts supraspinal sympathetic control to the cardiac system, leaving the only control of the heart to parasympathetic innervation through the vagus nerve. Without sympathetic drive, the heart slows (**bradycardia**) and may beat at a fluctuating rate (**arrhythmia**). Problems with vasomotor responses also develop, including a decrease in vascular tone, which allows blood to pool in the vessels and organs thereby lowering blood pressure (**hypotension**). This sympathetic loss has been termed **neurogenic shock** and should not be confused with spinal shock described later. These cardiac and vasomotor effects last at least 5 weeks or longer. In lower SCI below T6, vasomotor control and cardiac responses remain normal.

Deep vein thrombosis – Loss of supraspinal sympathetic drive to the liver, spleen, and bone marrow may also contribute to the development of deep vein thrombosis (DVT). While stasis is one important factor in DVT, changes in blood platelets and fibrinogen have also been found in individuals with SCI who developed DVTs.[30] Another factor that likely contributes to DVT development is damage to the blood vessel itself due to additional trauma at the time of injury.

Autonomic dysreflexia (Figure 12-6) – This condition develops when the SCI is above T6. It is defined by a pronounced increase in blood pressure and rapid heart rate along with observable sign of sweating, piloerection (goose bumps), and facial flushing as well as symptoms of headache, blurred vision, and/or stuffy nose.[30] An important part of autonomic dysreflexia to remember is that the resting blood pressure is well below normal levels with SCI, so a serious increase, due to dysreflexia, may not appear out of "normal" range. Autonomic dysreflexia is a life-threatening condition, in which strong but not necessarily noxious sensory input below the level of the injury ascend in the cord (Figure 12-6A) and trigger a large sympathetic surge from the splanchnic nerves (Figure 12-6B). These signals cause vasoconstriction and hypertension.

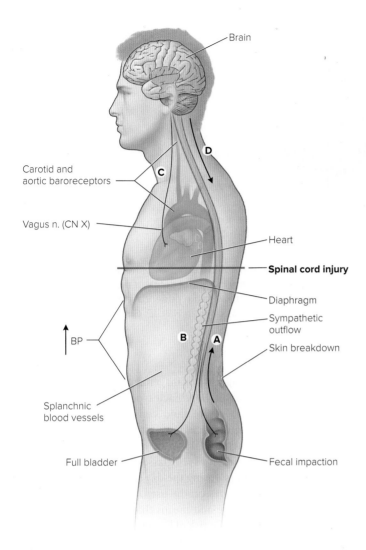

FIGURE 12-6 Autonomic dysreflexia. Autonomic dysreflexia occurs when stimuli below the injury cause an elevated blood pressure that cannot be inhibited because descending input from the brain is blocked by the injury.

TABLE 12-2	Cause of Autonomic Dysreflexia
Bladder	Full bladder
	Bladder kidney stones
	Blocked catheter
	UTI
Gastrointestinal tract	Bowel impaction
	Bowel distention
Integumentary system	Tight clothing or shoes
	Pressure ulcers
	Blisters, burns, bug bites
Reproductive system	Intercourse
	Ejaculation
	Labor
Other	Fracture
	DVT
	Heterotopic ossification

Baroreceptors in the neck signal the brain of this hypertensive crisis (Figure 12-6C) via cranial nerves IX and X, and two different reflexes are elicited to solve the problem (Figure 12-6D). First, greater descending sympathetic inhibitory drive is sent to the cord to stop the surge, but the signals are blocked by the injury. Second, parasympathetic input to slow the heart is conveyed through the vagus nerve, but the modest lowering of the heart rate does not compensate for the massive vasoconstriction. If left unchecked, seizures, pulmonary edema, myocardial infarction, stroke, and death can occur. Some of the potential causes of autonomic dysreflexia are shown in Table 12-2.

Bladder Dysfunction

Neuroanatomical Relationships

The bladder is made up of smooth muscle and retains fluid with two urethral sphincters – external and internal. The **detrusor**

muscle forms the wall of the bladder and the internal sphincter at the bladder neck. The bladder wall and internal sphincter are innervated by the **hypogastric nerve** (T11–L2), which is the post-ganglionic branch of the sympathetic nervous system and inhibits muscle contraction, while the bladder is filling (Figure 12-7). Of the two sphincters in the bladder, the **external urethral sphincter** is a true sphincter because it is comprised of striated muscle, innervated by the pudendal nerve (S2–4), and is under voluntary control. It is located at the urethral opening. The pudendal motor neurons are tonically active, which keeps the external sphincter closed and prevents bladder emptying until the time and place are appropriate. The internal sphincter is considered a functional sphincter that contracts or tightens in response to increased pressure of urine within the bladder, which means it is under reflex rather than voluntary control.

Normal Function

To void the bladder, contraction of the bladder muscles must be precisely timed with sphincter opening. It requires the integration of parasympathetic, sympathetic, and somatic nervous systems. Parasympathetic fibers control bladder emptying while the sympathetic fibers are active in bladder filling. Under normal conditions, the internal and external sphincters are closed and the urine collects in the bladder. When the bladder is full, bladder afferents in the wall send signals to the sacral spinal cord and to the micturition center in the brainstem. The brainstem sends inhibitory input to pudendal and hypogastric motor neurons, which allows the external and internal sphincters to relax. At the same time, the parasympathetic fibers in the pelvic nerve cause the detrusor muscle to contract, and urine is expelled.

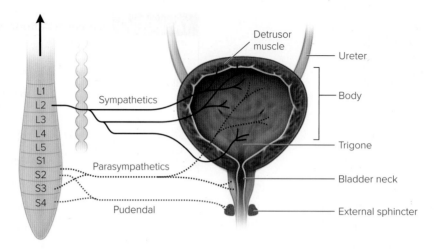

FIGURE 12-7 Sympathetic and parasympathetic innervation of the bladder and urethral sphincters. Sympathetic fibers promote relaxation of the bladder for filling and closure of the internal sphincter; parasympathetic fibers control detrusor muscle contraction and opening of the internal sphincter. The external sphincter is kept closed by the tonic activity in the pudendal nerve. For bladder emptying, this activity must be inhibited from higher brain centers. (Reproduced with permission from Hall JE: *Guyton & Hall Textbook of Medical Physiology*, 13th edition. Philadelphia, PA: Elsevier; 2016.)

Effects of SCI

With SCI, the ascending signal to the brainstem is typically impaired or lost completely and the response of the bladder walls become either hyper or hyporesponsive. A **spastic bladder** means that the sacral reflex is overactive, causing the bladder to contract regardless of the amount of urine in the bladder. A **flaccid bladder** occurs when the reflex response is blunted or absent entirely, and urine is not expelled from the bladder. With poor or absent afferent input to the brainstem, the coordinated control of the sphincters is lost, resulting in **sphincter dyssynergia**. This common problem occurs when the bladder contracts but the external sphincter does not open, which causes the bladder to distend. Pressure within the bladder becomes quite high, preventing the kidney from draining, so urine backs up in the kidneys, which is known as reflux. Reflux damages the bladder, ureters, and kidneys and can be life threatening. **Renal calculi** can also pose life-threatening conditions by blocking urine flow and damaging the kidneys. Stones form from calcium and other waste products that are not fully emptied from the bladder. About 20% of individuals with SCI develop renal calculi early and years after SCI.[31] Fewer people develop bladder calculi, about 14%, and typically this occurs within the first 3–6 months of injury.[31] The recurrence rate is quite high with 72% recurring within 2 years.[32] Risk factors for calculi development include tetraplegia, history of bladder infection, and high calcium concentrations in the blood.[32]

The most important goal of the bladder management program is to remove urine and prevent high pressures within the bladder. Another objective of bladder management is to prevent renal or bladder calculi (stones). There are several methods to accomplish these objectives, and the selection of the best bladder management depends on residual hand function, amount of support care available to the individual, and complications such as urinary tract infections and autonomic dysreflexia. In the acute stage of SCI, an indwelling catheter will be the most common method of removing urine from the bladder, and the transition to a long-term management program will occur during inpatient rehabilitation. Each type of management will require different amounts of fluid consumption in order to reduce the risk of calculi formation and infection.

Intermittent catheter – Moderate but not high water consumption of about 2 quarts (8–10 glasses) per day and catheterization every 4–6 hours during the day should occur. Sterile or "clean, aseptic" techniques can be used. Sterile catheter equipment has a one-time use and means that the insertion tube is not touched. It reduces the risk of bacteria entering the bladder. Clean technique has a multi-use catheter that must be cleaned after each use. Insurance coverage may limit or prevent the use of sterile catheters.

Indwelling catheter – High water consumption of about 3 quarts (15 glasses) per day should be maintained in order to reduce the risk of bladder or kidney stones.

Foley – a urethral catheter that is held in place by a partially inflated balloon. It is typically changed monthly. This type of catheter may inhibit or impede sexual function.

Suprapubic – a surgically inserted tube through the abdominal wall and into the bladder. This type of catheter is often selected by females because it does not have the problem of urine leakage like a urethral catheter. It also does not interfere with sexual function in males or females.

Condom catheter for males – Water consumption should be about 2 quarts (8–10 glasses) per day. It should be changed daily or every other day. There is no version of this system for females. This type of catheter is less effective if bladder contraction is weak or sphincter dyssynergia limits voiding.

Botulinum toxin (Botox) injection into the urinary sphincter – Growing evidence suggests that Botox injection is becoming more widely used to improve bladder voiding and overcome sphincter dyssynergia, after SCI. Botox induces muscle paralysis of the sphincter, allowing urine to pass more easily. It loses its effectiveness over 3–6 months. A recent systematic review suggests that voiding improved 30 days after Botox injection in people with SCI and other conditions[33]; however, evidence was limited and the need to reinject Botox were drawbacks. While surgical options exist (see below), use of Botox may be the best first step, since the effects are reversible.

Urethral stents – A mesh tube is inserted through the lumen of the sphincter so that it is held open, and urine will flow continuously. Risks include migration of the stent into the bladder, becoming encrusted or causing pain and autonomic dysreflexia.[33] Stents can be removed, if needed. A condom catheter is used to collect urine, making this procedure unavailable for women.

Sphincterotomy – Surgical cutting of the external sphincter is an irreversible but effective way to treat dyssynergia. It is often restricted to males and used after all other treatment options have failed. A condom catheter is used to collect urine. This procedure is not typically done for women because it causes continuous leakage of urine and poses a serious risk of skin ulcers (see below).

Reflex and manual techniques – These techniques apply pressure over the bladder to either stimulate afferent drive and elicit detrusor contraction or push the urine through a flaccid sphincter. The **Crede method** involves pressing down on the lower abdomen and, thereby, the bladder. **Suprapubic tapping** provides intermittent pressure over the bladder. **Valsalva maneuver** creates pressure by bearing down and/or leaning forward to empty the bladder.

Pharmacological agents are also part of bladder management. Failure to store urine can be treated with anticholinergics to reduce detrusor hyperreflexia and alpha-adrenergics to promote greater sphincter control. For difficulty emptying the bladder, cholinergics (bethanechol) increase bladder reflexes, alpha-adrenergic blockers aid in sphincter relaxation, and CNS depressants, like valium and baclofen, reduce dyssynergia.

Urinary Tract Infections

One of the most common complications of bladder dysfunction after SCI is urinary tract infection (UTI). Such infections will have elevated white blood cells and bacteria in the urine as well as some of the following symptoms: fever, chills, sweating, nausea, headache, greater spasticity, and autonomic dysreflexia in people with SCI at T6 or above. Treatment with antibiotics and immediate medical referral will be needed, if a UTI is suspected. Most people with SCI have bacteria in the bladder that is carried in from the skin or urethra during catheterization. For some individuals, these bacteria "colonize" the bladder and eventually do not initiate an infection. For other individuals, frequent symptomatic infections occur each year.[34]

A presumed cause of UTI was intermittent catheterization with clean but not sterile catheters, but until recently, there was no evidence to support this idea.[35] In this international study, individuals that reused catheters had four times the number of UTIs compared to individuals that never reused catheters. Due to cost and availability, single-use catheters were reused on average 34 times, but some individuals reused the catheter over 200 times. Thus, patient education to avoid catheter reuse may be an effective way to reduce UTIs. The incidence of UTIs was higher with indwelling catheterization than clean intermittent catheterization.[36]

Pulmonary Complication and Respiratory Dysfunction

Neuroanatomical Relationships

Respiration relies on descending neurologic drive from rhythm-generating neurons in the medulla. Both inspiratory and expiratory bulbar neurons reside in the medulla and send projections via the bulbospinal tract to the phrenic nucleus in the spinal cord. Some of the descending bulbospinal axons cross in the medulla, but the majority project ipsilaterally. The phrenic nucleus is located from C3 to C5 and innervates the diaphragm (Figure 12-8). The primary muscles of inspiration are the diaphragm and the scalenes, which are innervated from C2 to C7. Secondary muscles of inspiration are the sternocleidomastoid, innervated from C2 to C3 and the accessory cranial nerve, and intercostals, innervated from T1 to T11. Expiration is typically done passively, but the abdominal muscles, innervated by T7–L1, play an important role in forceful expiration (e.g., during coughing). Based on these innervation patterns, an SCI above C5 will impair most of the primary and secondary muscles for inspiration and expiration. Even lower injuries in the mid-thoracic region will reduce pulmonary function.

Normal Function

Typically, contraction of the diaphragm causes it to flatten out and pull the thorax down, while the scalenes, intercostals, and sternocleidomastoids contract to raise the thorax. In this way,

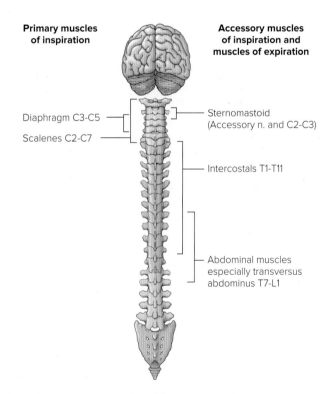

Primary muscles of inspiration

Accessory muscles of inspiration and muscles of expiration

Diaphragm C3-C5

Scalenes C2-C7

Sternomastoid (Accessory n. and C2-C3)

Intercostals T1-T11

Abdominal muscles especially transversus abdominus T7-L1

FIGURE 12-8 Levels of innervation for the primary and secondary respiratory muscles. The primary respiratory muscles (diaphragm and scalenes) and the sternomastoid (secondary muscle) are innervated from cervical spinal levels. Intercostal and abdominal muscles are secondary muscles, innervated from thoracic levels.

the thorax expands pulling air into the lungs. The secondary muscles become active only with greater ventilatory demand, as during running or exercise. When the diaphragm relaxes, the lungs and muscle tissue recoil, which passively pushes air from the lungs and causes expiration. Strong contraction of the abdominal muscles also helps drive air out of the lungs.

Effects of SCI

The degree of respiratory dysfunction, after SCI, depends on the level of the injury with the most severe effects occurring with high cervical SCI, but even low thoracic SCI can impair respiration. Partial or complete loss of neural drive to respiratory muscles is the most common cause of respiratory dysfunction and is termed **restrictive ventilator impairment** which includes:

- paralysis of the diaphragm due to lesion of bulbospinal axons, loss of phrenic motor neurons, or damage to the phrenic nerve. Cough is absent. This occurs with complete cervical SCI at C4 or above and requires a ventilator. Complete paralysis of the diaphragm results in a **paradoxical breathing** pattern, in which the abdomen retracts on inspiration and protrudes during exhalation. This pattern is caused by poor intercostal activation and weak abdominal contraction.

- paresis of the diaphragm due to incomplete injury of bulbospinal tract, phrenic motor neurons, or phrenic nerve. Cough is weak and ineffective. This occurs with incomplete cervical SCI from C2 to C4/5. A ventilator may be required, if vital capacity, inspiratory pressure, or CO_2 levels worsen.

- paralysis/paresis of intercostal and abdominal muscles. Cough is weak especially with upper thoracic injuries above T5. This occurs with complete or incomplete SCI from C5 to T11. A ventilator is typically not required unless complications arise.

Restrictive impairment also occurs in acute SCI of traumatic origin when the chest wall or lungs are injured at the same time. This damage can be a serious complication with long-lasting effects.

Obstructive ventilator impairment also contributes to SCI-related respiratory problems. Acute SCI, at T6 or above, causes autonomic dysfunction as described above. For the lungs, this means that excessive bronchial secretions and mucus are produced. Impaired sympathetic input allows unopposed parasympathetic drive, which causes bronchial spasm, vascular congestion, and ineffective ciliary activity to clear the mucus. The excess mucus builds up in the lungs, the cilia do not move the mucus out of the lungs and, although the cough reflex may be intact, the cough itself is weak and ineffective. These conditions place the patient at risk for **atelectasis** (collapse of alveoli), pneumonia, and respiratory failure.[37]

In individuals with tetraplegia, who do not require a ventilator, body position will effect respiration. In a seated posture, the weak or flaccid abdominal muscles allow the abdominal contents to protrude forward, which flattens the diaphragm and holds the thorax in an expanded position. With the inspiratory muscles already weak from the SCI, they are ineffective at overcoming this mechanical disadvantage. However, if the patient is placed in a supine position, gravity pulls the abdominal contents back, allowing even weak contractions of the diaphragm to expand the thorax and create inspiration. Greater respiratory capacity typically occurs in a supine position, during acute SCI, because the abdominal contents do not protrude and the diaphragm mechanics are more effective.

Use of an abdominal binder to compensate for abdominal laxity can produce immediate improvements in respiratory function, for people with tetraplegia. Increased lung volume and cough mechanics have been reported in an upright position when binders are used.[38]

Pressure Ulcers and Skin Integrity

Neuroanatomical Relationships and Normal Function

The skin is the largest organ of the body, serving as a protective barrier and maintaining thermoregulation. To cool the body, blood passes through vascular networks just below the skin surface. On cold days, receptors in the skin help to raise the body temperature by constricting the vessels near the surface. The autonomic nervous system controls blood flow and, thus, contributes to temperature regulation. The outer layer of the skin is the epidermis, where cells sluff off and new cells replace them. The dermis lies below and contains sensory receptors, sweat glands, lymphatic vessels, and blood vessels. Below the dermal layer, lie an adipose layer, muscle layer, and bone.

Effects of SCI

After SCI, light touch, pressure, and thermal sensation from areas below the injury are impaired, so signals to the brain telling you to move and relieve pressure are lost. Also, the neural control of blood flow is disrupted, making it difficult for people with SCI to control body temperature in extreme cold or heat conditions. A pressure ulcer develops when prolonged pressure is applied to the skin, usually over a bone, and injures the skin and deep tissues. The amount of pressure and the length of time the pressure is in place will increase the severity of the wound. High pressures for short periods and low pressures for long periods can both cause a pressure ulcer. The pressure crimps small blood vessels and prevents oxygen from reaching tissues under the area of pressure. Ischemia and cell death occur within the deeper tissues, while the superficial layers and skin may only show changes in skin blanching, initially. The wound begins below the skin and expands upward creating a pyramid shaped lesion with a small wound at the skin and a wide lesion at deeper levels.

There are several systems to stage the type and severity of pressure ulcers, but newer recommendations are to categorize rather than stage the wound. Staging implies that the wound develops and heals sequentially through each level (i.e., Stage 1 to Stage 2 to Stage 3 and the reverse with healing), but this isn't necessarily the case. An international panel of experts has developed a universal system that combines all of the different staging systems (Table 12-3).[39] Important assessment factors include color, depth of the wound, and presence of **slough**, which is stringy, soft moist tissue that is light in color, ranging from yellow, white, or green. **Eschar** is thick, hard tissue that is dark brown or black and attached to the wound bed or edges.

TABLE 12-3	Category of Pressure Ulcer
CATEGORY/STAGE	**DESCRIPTION**
Category/Stage 1	Non-blanchable erythema • Intact skin • Localized non-blanchable redness • May be painful, firm, soft, warmer, or colder than surrounding tissue • May be difficult to detect in individuals with dark skin tones
Category/Stage 2	Partial thickness • Shallow open wound with a red pink wound bed • No slough • May also be a closed or open fluid filled blister • No bruising
Category/Stage 3	Full thickness skin loss • Subcutaneous fat may be visible but bone, muscle, and tendon are not. Bone or tendon is not directly palpable. • Slough, if present, doesn't obscure tissue loss • May have undermining or tunneling • Shallow ulcers and deep ulcers can occur depending on body location and the amount of adipose tissue. Areas without adipose tissue will be shallow.
Category/Stage 4	Full thickness tissue loss • Bone, tendon, or muscle is exposed or directly palpable • Slough or eschar may be present • Undermining or tunneling likely • Depth varies by location • Ulcer may invade muscle, fascia, tendon, etc. likely leading to osteomyelitis or osteitis
Unclassified/Unstageable	Full thickness skin or tissue loss – Depth unknown • Depth obscured by slough or eschar and can't be determined until enough can be removed to see the wound bed • On the heel, stable eschar that is dry, adherent with no erythema is a good protective covering and should not be removed
Tissue injury	Suspected deep tissue injury – Depth unknown • Purple/maroon area of intact skin • Blood-filled blister from shear or pressure • Prior to discoloration/blister, area may be painful, firm, mushy, boggy, warmer, or cooler compared to intact tissue. • Evolution may be rapid and may have a blister covering a dark wound bed

At-risk Areas

Areas of the body with little or no adipose tissue overlying bony prominences have the highest risk for pressure ulcers. The most common locations for ulcers, after SCI, are the sacrum/coccyx, ischium, heels, and trochanters. Other areas that are at risk include the back of the head, scapula, elbows, knees, and ears as these locations will be exposed to pressure in some positions, when lying in bed.

The risk factors for pressure ulcers in the acute stage of SCI are related to medical conditions and medical procedures that restrict changing body positions. The risk of pressure ulcer is much higher for patients with: a tracheostomy, prolonged recovery following surgical decompression, or low arterial blood pressure when arriving in the emergency room.[40] Factors that restrict mobility before arriving at the hospital, also increase risk, including the length of time spent on the backboard, placement of a neck collar, and length of transportation time to the hospital.[40] Urinary incontinence poses less risk acutely because of the routine placement of an indwelling catheter in the emergency department. Risk factors, during inpatient rehabilitation, have not been well-studied and are confounded by a relatively high rate of pressure ulcers coming from acute hospitalization, estimated to be 30% or higher.[40,41] At chronic time points after SCI, many factors have an impact like socio-demographic, behavioral, neurological, and medical issues.[42] Perhaps the most concerning is a history of a previous ulcer. Estimates suggest that up to 90% of people with an ulcer will go on to have another, and the new ulcer may not be in the same location (i.e., recurrence).[43] A recurrence means that pathological tissue changes from the initial ulcer pose a serious risk. However, when the recurrent ulcer occurs in a new location, it suggests that systemic factors may pose the greatest risk.

Pressure Ulcer Prevention

To prevent pressure ulcers, during acute hospitalization, the patient's position must be changed every 2 hours, the heels should be raised off the bed, and the head of the bed should not be elevated above 30 degrees. Higher elevations of the head increase pressure over the sacrum, a high risk region. The heels need to float above the bed by placing a pillow under the calf. Be sure the knee is slightly flexed to avoid risking a DVT (see below). The important thing to remember about changing the position of the patient in bed is to avoid damaging the skin. Never drag the body across the surface as shear forces and friction can cause skin damage. Use any available assistive system to turn the patient such as sheets, grab bars, and/or overhead lift systems. Placing the person at a 30-degree tilt in side-lying, allows the greatest blood flow and produces lower pressures over the trochanters than a 90-degree side-lying position. Pillows and foam, rather than towels, should be used to maintain each position because towels create greater pressure rather than reducing pressure on the skin. Be mindful that pillows or foam should be placed between body parts that rest on each other. If angled side-lying cannot be used because of surgical precautions, then reposition the patient every 2 hours from side-lying to supine and then side-lying on the opposite side. In some facilities, special beds to reduce pressure may be available, and new bedside pressure mapping systems are emerging technologies that may help with prevention, during acute hospitalization.

A critical part of ulcer prevention during inpatient rehabilitation and thereafter will be pressure relief and checking the skin regularly. Inspecting the skin for redness, swelling, hardness or injuries like blisters, over at-risk areas, should be done daily. These areas include the sacrum, coccyx, ischial tuberosities, greater trochanters, heels, elbow, knee, ankle, and foot. Weight shifts, while seated in a wheel chair, should occur every 15 minutes, continue for 60 seconds, and the patient should be as independent as possible (Table 12-4).

To prevent pressure ulcers across the treatment continuum, several factors should be monitored and avoided.[44] Poor nutrition is a major risk factor in pressure ulcer development and makes healing of ulcers difficult. It is important that good dietary habits be in place not only to prevent pressure ulcers but also to ensure optimal participation in physical therapy. While there is no single nutritional factor that is associated with pressure ulcer, protein, albumin, and hemoglobin levels are commonly monitored after SCI as indicators of malnutrition. With insufficient protein consumption after SCI, the body catabolizes protein, resulting in poor collagen formation and a loss of lean body mass. A second factor is prolonged moisture on the skin. Two of the most common sources of moisture are sweating, in areas with skin-to-skin contact, and incontinence. Because urine and feces have high acidity, it is important to wash the exposed skin as quickly as possible, before the skin becomes irritated. Regular, long-term exposure to moisture causes skin maceration or break down. A third factor is smoking because nicotine limits cutaneous blood flow and reduces tissue oxygenation. Because pressure ulcer risk and prevention involves the interaction of many complex factors, greater emphasis is being placed on adopting a healthy lifestyle rather than focusing on patient education for unweighting techniques alone (i.e., weight shifts, cushions).[45] Therapists should encourage good nutrition, regular exercise, and smoking cessation at all stages of rehabilitation. These lifestyle changes will not only impact the risk of pressure ulcers but also cardiovascular conditions and other complications.

Neurogenic Bowel

Neuroanatomical Relationships

The colon extends from the small intestine to the anal sphincters at the end of the rectum (Figure 12-9). There are two sphincters: (1) an internal anal sphincter, made up of the inner, smooth muscle of the colon and (2) the striated, external anal sphincter which is under voluntary control. The internal sphincter is innervated by the hypogastric nerve (S2–S4), and the external sphincter is supplied by the pudendal nerve (S2–S4). The puborectalis muscle, innervated by roots from S1 to S5, encircles the rectum to hold it in a bent position, and along with the two sphincters, these three structures ensure fecal continence.

TABLE 12-4	Pressure Relief Techniques for SCI Levels	
SCI LEVEL	**METHOD**	**DIFFICULTY**
C4, C5, C6	Lateral Trunk Lean Hook the arm around the push handle of the wheelchair for balance and lean away to unweight the ischial tuberosity	Easiest to perform; requires less trunk control than other methods
C6 and below	Forward Lean Walk the hands down the legs to the floor if possible so the tuberosities are clear of the seat.	More difficult; requires more trunk control and balance
C6 and below	Wheel Chair Push Up Place the hands on the arm rests or wheels and push down until the buttocks are lifted off the seat	Most difficult; person must have the strength to lift their own weight
C4	Tilt the Back Rest Be sure the legs are elevated to unweight the pelvis as much as possible	In a manual wheelchair assistance required; in a power chair, may be done without help

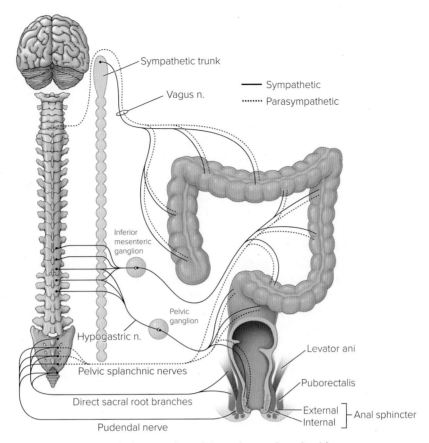

FIGURE 12-9 Sympathetic and parasympathetic innervation of the colon and anal sphincters.

While neural control of the colon includes the somatic and autonomic nervous systems, its primary innervation is the enteric nervous system, also called the intrinsic nervous system. The enteric nervous system is very interesting because it can function independently of the brain and autonomic nervous system and contains so many neurons that it is called the brain of the gut. This means that even after SCI and loss of communication with the brain, many of the functions of the colon remain intact. The enteric system is made up of: (1) the myenteric plexus (Auerbach's), located between muscle layers of the colon and (2) the submucosal plexus (Meissner's plexus), lying between the mucosa and the inner layer of muscle. The parasympathetic system, acting through the vagus and pelvic (S2–4) nerves, causes contraction of the colon. The sympathetic system, through the mesenteric (T9–12) and hypogastric (T12–L2) nerves, produces relaxation of the colon and decreases motility through the gut. Excitatory enteric reflexes are inhibited and the sphincters contract.

Normal Function

The role of the colon is to extract water and nutrients while forming food products into stool and propelling it to the rectum and anal sphincters. Reflex contractions of smooth muscle in the wall of the colon helps to mix the contents and then move the stool forward through an action called **peristalsis**. Stretch of the colon wall activates the myenteric plexus above the dilation, and the smooth muscle contracts, pushing the stool forward. At the same time, the plexus causes the muscles below the dilation

to relax, allowing the stool to move into the space. This motility occurs with only the enteric system and doesn't require brain or autonomic input. The gastrocolic reflex can also act solely through the enteric nervous system and initiates peristalsis in the small intestine and colon within minutes of food being eaten. These activities, driven by the enteric system, are coordinated with increased sympathetic drive to the internal anal sphincter, which increases tone, but once the rectum begins filling with stool, inhibition of the internal sphincter occurs. Sacral parasympathetics and the pelvic nerve add to the enteric activity to induce defecation. Stool in the rectum initiates stretch of the puborectalis muscle and the smooth muscle of the rectum. Defecation is under voluntary control and occurs when inhibition from the brain causes the external anal sphincter and puborectalis to relax. During coughing or valsalva maneuver, increased neural drive to the EAS and puborectalis prevent incontinence. Normal transit time of stool through the colon is 12–30 hours.[46]

Effects of SCI

After SCI, the autonomic and brain input is impaired or lost, but the enteric nervous system remains functional. This means that some motility will be present but control of the sphincters, especially the EAS will be greatly impaired. The transit time of stool is greatly prolonged to 80 hours or more,[47] which means greater extraction of water resulting in dry, hard stool. The location of the SCI will produce either UMN or LMN bowel dysfunction[48] (Table 12-5).

TABLE 12-5	Type of Bowel Dysfunction According to SCI Location		
SCI LOCATION	**TONE**	**TYPE OF DYSFUNCTION**	**CLINICAL PRESENTATION**
UMN – Injury above Conus medullaris	Hyperreflexic Spastic	Increased colonic wall tone Unable to relax EAS due to loss of supraspinal input; IAS relaxation remains intact with SCI above T12	Fecal retention, constipation with some reflex incontinence
LMN – Injury at conus medullaris and cauda equina	Areflexic Flaccid	Decreased motility due to loss of autonomic and supraspinal input Flaccid EAS; flaccid puborectalis muscle	Fecal incontinence, constipation

Bowel dysfunction presents major challenges to health and quality of life for individuals with SCI. The decline in motility, fecal retention, and constipation lead to a plethora of GI problems including: pain, abdominal distention, bloating, hemorrhoids, nausea, poor appetite, and gastroesophageal reflux. These complications can be even more severe, when the level of injury is above T6, because they elicit autonomic dysreflexia, a life-threatening condition as discussed earlier. Other serious complications include perianal abscess, stercoral perforation (a rupture of the intestinal wall), and intestinal obstruction.

Even more disabling to individuals with SCI are the anxiety, depression, and inability to maintain activities and lifestyle, caused not only by bowel dysfunction but also by the bowel management program.[49,50] The health problems and limitations to quality of life are preventable by creating an individualized bowel management program.

Bowel Management Program

The goal of the program is to achieve predictable, effective evacuation of stool in order to prevent unplanned elimination and reduce GI complications. For UMN hyperreflexic dysfunction, the objective of the program is to enable stool evacuation through rectal stimulation and formation of soft stool. For LMN areflexic dysfunction, the objective is to reduce incontinence by increasing stool firmness, so it is retained in the rectum and can be manually evacuated. To individualize the bowel program, the following parameters must be identified: pre-injury bowel habits, type of bowel dysfunction (spastic, flaccid), hand function, upper extremity strength and proprioception, sitting balance, spasticity and spasms, risk or presence of pressure ulcers, transfer skills, and feasibility of moving the program to the home

setting. Nutritional intake and food preferences, fluid consumption, and medications must also be tracked as they all influence bowel function. The bowel program will begin in the acute hospital setting. By adopting a routine time of day, regular intervals, and consistent preparatory procedures, it may be possible to "train" the enteric nervous system and associated reflexes to improve evacuation.

The role of the physical therapist in the bowel management program is to align the physical function of the individual with the type and location of the bowel program. Adaptations to the program will be required as recovery of function returns. The ability to perform the bowel program in sitting rather than lying in bed depends on good sitting balance, low severity and frequency of spasticity/spasms, ease of transfers, and low risk of pressure ulcers. A seated program can make use of the toilet, roll-in shower/commode chair, or padded commode seat. While a seated program improves evacuation and clean-up, it is difficult to access the anal region and poses pressure ulcer risk because of the long time spent sitting. The physical functions associated with the level of injury can help determine the role of the individual in bowel management and the need for assistance (Table 12-6).

Bowel programs require a multifaceted approach that make use of spared function, modulate fluid and food intake, and carefully consider the impact of medications on bowel function. In what seems counterintuitive, a high-fiber diet can actually reduce motility and lengthen colon transport time in individuals with SCI, thereby, requiring careful titration of fiber for each individual. Medications that can negatively impact bowel function by decreasing motility and increasing constipation include: antidepressants, anticholinergics, anti-spasticity

TABLE 12-6	SCI Level and Functional Support for Bowel Care	
LEVEL OF SCI	**FUNCTIONAL PERFORMANCE**	**ASSISTANCE**
C1–5	Dependent in clothing management, transfers, bowel program	Care attendant required
C6–7	May need assistance but is not dependent in clothing management, transfers, bowel program	Care attendant required for some assistance
C8–L2	Independent with clothing, transfers, and bowel program	No care attendant needed if seated

drugs, and narcotics. Most conservative approaches to bowel care will combine the gastrocolic reflex, digital stimulation of the colon, abdominal massage, and a stool softener or enema to aid in evacuation.[48] Digital stimulation involves insertion of a gloved finger into the rectum and moving it in a circular motion to elicit peristaltic waves via the enteric nervous system. Eating a meal also triggers peristalsis via the gastrocolic reflex, and using digital stimulation after a meal has an additive effect on motility. Suppositories such as dulcolax, glycerin, and polyethylene glycol reduce the time and support needed for the bowel program.[48]

Bowel management programs are usually conducted either daily or every other day. A successful program should be completed in 1 hour or less, but as many as 14% of those living with SCI report taking well beyond this time frame.[50] Other major problems with bowel management programs is a lack of flexibility when the program must be implemented, the interference of the program with other life activities such as work and recreation, lack of attendant care, as well as loss of autonomy and privacy.[50,51] About 20% of individuals require full assistance with their bowel care program, and these individuals have lower life satisfaction. Women with SCI report more problems with bowel function and have more symptoms of distension, pain, constipation, and unplanned evacuations.[50]

If conservative management proves ineffective, then oral medications and surgery may be necessary. Oral medications that stimulate intestinal motility and gastric emptying include metoclopramide, prucalopride, fampridine, neostigmine, and glycopyrrolate. Use of these pharmacological interventions has improved expulsion after SCI.[48] If complications continue after pharmacological treatment, then surgical interventions would include colostomy or ileostomy. This procedure opens the colon or intestine so stool flows into an external collection device, bypassing the rectum and anus. While these surgical procedures are often considered a failure in rehabilitation, people that elect to have a colostomy or ileostomy report high satisfaction and the desire to have had the procedure even earlier.[52] Individuals with a colostomy no longer perceived their bowel program as a problem, and the time to complete the program was significantly shorter.[53]

From a physical therapy perspective, bowel function benefits from increased activity and less bed rest after SCI. Both standing activity and electrical stimulation have been shown to improve bowel function, although the level and amount of evidence is limited.[54-57] Electrical stimulation has been used in two different approaches after SCI – to compensate for lost voluntary activation of abdominal muscles[55,56] or to induce neural plasticity in sacral spinal cord segments.[57] Two studies used the compensatory, electrical stimulation approach and induced abdominal muscle contraction to enhance abdominal pressures during defecation. In both studies, improved motility and reduced colonic transport time occurred.[55,56] In one study, an abdominal belt with embedded electrodes was applied at the level of the umbilicus during six bowel sessions.[55] Stimulation was randomized to be on during three sessions and off during the other three. Individuals did not know when the stimulation was turned on. In individuals with tetraplegia, the time for administering the bowel program was significantly lower,

when abdominal muscle stimulation was used.[55] In a second study, individuals with complete abdominal paralysis had eight stimulating electrodes placed over the external obliques and the rectus abdominus muscles. Stimulation intensity was sufficient to produce visible muscle contraction and occurred for short durations (25 minutes/day) over 8 weeks. Greater motility, faster transit time, and enhanced satisfaction with the bowel program occurred in individuals with stimulation compared to controls. Taking a neuroplasticity approach, a small study of two individuals with incomplete SCI and fecal incontinence applied electrical stimulation to the posterior tibial nerve in order to activate sacral sensory and motor fibers (S1–3), which form the nerve.[57] Stimulation (30 min/day) occurred every other day for 4 weeks and then every 2 months. Improvement in rectal sensation, pudendal motor function, quality of life, and lower severity of incontinence occurred. Each of these studies supports the role of physical therapy in improving bowel dysfunction by using noninvasive electrical stimulation. Although the studies are small, they hold good promise for improving bowel dysfunction either through compensation or facilitating neuroplasticity.

Unfortunately, there is almost no evidence of the role of motor activity provided during physical therapy, on bowel function. One study showed benefits to individuals with SCI of standing upright in a standing frame,[58] but dynamic activities have not been studied. In healthy individuals, running or cycling exercise dramatically increased bowel motility,[59] suggesting that exercise performed as part of physical therapy such as treadmill training, robotic training, arm ergometry, and other therapeutic interventions may improve bowel function after SCI. Exercise has also been implicated in improving incontinence and constipation.[60] In a pilot study of immobile patients, fecal incontinence was reduced by a combination of exercise and abdominal massage.[61] However, because exercise was not tested alone, it is unclear if it was the mediating factor.[61] Given the importance of exercise on gastrointestinal health in uninjured individuals,[60] it is critical to establish whether activity-based interventions, after SCI, can promote greater bowel function.

● PHYSICAL THERAPY IN THE ACUTE SETTING

During acute hospitalization, the patient will have most, if not all, of these medically challenging conditions that will impact the type of and tolerance for therapeutic interventions. All rehabilitation interventions will need to be performed without worsening these medical conditions. At this stage of rehabilitation, the physical therapist must anticipate the type of functional recovery that is likely given the level and severity of the SCI. It will be important to assure that the current rehabilitation interventions facilitate the next phases of therapy, in the inpatient and outpatient settings. Keep in mind that the next therapists shouldn't have to spend valuable treatment time undoing deleterious factors like joint contractures. The role of physical therapy is to assess motor and sensory function, prevent complications, incorporate spared muscles into rehabilitation, and continually monitor for return of motor and sensory function.

The Physical Therapy Assessment

Use the standardized neural assessment, described in Chapter 9. If no ISNCSCI /AIS exam has been performed, you will need to complete a full exam. If an exam has been completed by the physician, then a quick confirmation of the below-lesion muscle and sensory effects should be done. Remember, that we expect some return of sensorimotor function, and an early return may lead to more extensive recovery and better long-term prognosis. Perhaps the most attention should be directed at checking for trace muscle contractions, since it means that the motor neuron pool is not completely lost. Attention should also be focused on muscle groups not included in the ISNCSCI exam like shoulder abduction, shoulder depression, gluteus maximus and medius, hamstrings, and great toe extensors. These muscle groups are important for future actions like transfers, unweighting, and gait training. In the acute phase, the absence of muscle response or reflexes may not necessarily indicate the severity or location of the injury due to spinal shock.

Within minutes of SCI, widespread depression of neural activity in the spinal cord occurs and reflexes below the injury are absent or very weak (hyporeflexic). This pattern is called **spinal shock** or diaschesis. Spinal shock means that neurons and reflexes not directly damaged by the injury cease to function and over time return.[62] A classic example of spinal shock is early paralysis of both limbs after a unilateral hemisection or Brown-Sequard type injury. After a few days, motor activity returns in the contralateral limb. The return of uninjured function takes place over days, weeks, and months and progresses from hyporeflexia to hyperreflexia.[62] Reflexes appear in a sequential order: delayed plantar response, bulbocavernosus, cremasteric, ankle DTR, Babinski sign, and knee DTR[62] (see Table 12-7).

Many neurorehabilitationists consider the end of spinal shock to be when the cremasteric reflex returns, but keep in mind, that this reflex may be abolished by an SCI at the level of the conus medullaris or cauda equina. Some resolution of spinal shock will likely occur in the acute setting. As spinal shock resolves, not only do reflexes return but also expect to see spared voluntary movement return. For a physical therapist, it is often impossible to tell whether gains in function are due to treatment or to resolution of spinal shock especially because the time period of shock can be up to a year after SCI.

Few physical therapy assessment tools for SCI are available for the acute hospital phase after SCI. The APTA (EDGE) Task Force highly recommends six outcome measures for the 0–3 month acute period after SCI. However, within this time-frame, both acute and inpatient rehabilitation will occur. Only two measures would be feasible in the acute hospital setting, the AIS/ ISNCSCI exam described previously and handheld myometry. Handheld myometry uses a force transducer to objectively quantify muscle strength and has shown high reliability and greater sensitivity than manual muscle testing within the first week after SCI.[63,64]

TABLE 12-7	Sequential Resolution of Spinal Shock	
REFLEX	**ACTION**	**HYPO-HYPERREFLEXIA**
Delayed plantar response (L5–S2)	Strong deep pressure from heel along lateral border of sole of foot and across 3rd, 4th, 5th MT heads produces slow plantar flexion	Emerges within hours and worsens over first week; declines/absent after 1 week
Bulbocavernosus (S2–S4)	Squeezing glans penis or clitoris causes anal sphincter contraction	Emerges by 3 days; modest hyperreflexia develops within 4 weeks–1 year
Cremasteric (L1–L2 genitofemoral nerve)	Stroke of inner, upper thigh pulls up ipsilateral testicle	Emerges by 3 days; modest hyperreflexia develops within 1–12 months
Ankle Stretch reflex (S1–S2)	With foot dorsiflexed, tap of Achilles tendon causes plantarflexion	Emerges by 3 days; modest hyperreflexia develops within 1–12 months
Babinski (Corticospinal tract)	Pressure on sole of foot curving from heel up to MT heads causes big toe to lift, other toes to fan out; replaces delayed plantar response	Emerges by 3 days; modest hyperreflexia develops within 1–12 months
Flexor withdrawal (L2–S1)	Pinprick of sole of foot causes flexion of LE joints	Emerges by 3 days; modest hyperreflexia by 4 weeks, pronounced hyperreflexia by 1–12 months
DTRs Knee (L2–4) Biceps (C5–6) Triceps (C7–8) Brachioradialis (C6)	Tendon tap below the level of the injury causes brisk response	Emerges by 3 days; modest hyperreflexia by 4 weeks, pronounced hyperreflexia by 1–12 months

Ms. Roberts had an AIS/ISCNSCI completed 5 days after SCI, which confirmed the level of SCI at C2. The UEMS was 5 and the LEMS was 8. The motor scores were asymmetrical with higher motor scores on the left versus the right (Table 12-8). The pinprick scores were also asymmetrical with higher scores on the right versus the left. The S4-5 pinprick sensation appeared intact. The injury was classified as AIS C – Brown-Sequard injury due to the greater strength and impaired pain sensation contralateral to the major portion of the lesion. The poor pain sensation over the lower half of the body places her at high risk for pressure ulcers, so a regular skin inspection and turning schedule must be followed. Some pain sensation, although impaired, has returned in the neck and shoulder region which may help protect her scapulae from developing ulcers. Spine stabilization surgery was not performed, and the neck was immobilized with a cervical collar. Ms. Roberts had the ventilator removed on day 6.

TABLE 12-8	ASIA Motor Scores	
ASIA KEY MUSCLES	**RIGHT**	**LEFT**
C5 elbow flexors	0/5	2/5
C6 wrist extensors	0/5	1/5
C7 elbow extensors	0/5	2/5
C8 finger flexors	0/5	0/5
T1 finger abduction	0/5	0/5
L2 hip flexors	0/5	2/5
L3 knee extensors	1/5	2/5
L4 ankle dorsiflexors	0/5	0/5
L5 long toe extensors	0/5	0/5
S1 ankle plantar flexor	1/5	2/5

What other test should be performed by the physical therapist to diagnose Brown-Sequard syndrome?

Proprioception should be tested.

Babinski sign

What would you expect the results of the test to show in order to confirm Brown-Sequard syndrome?

Greater proprioceptive deficits on the right than the left side

Positive Babinski on the right foot only

Acute Physical Therapy Management

Prevent Complications

The most common medical complications at the acute stage include: pneumonia, pressure ulcer, and DVT. The physical therapist will reinforce the training provided to the patient and family for assisted coughing techniques, add breathing exercises to each treatment session, improve chest wall mobility through range of motion (ROM) of the trunk, and place an abdominal binder on all patients with SCI above T12.

Individuals with tetraplegia are at risk for future shoulder and elbow pain and injury. Careful positioning in the bed and a ROM program can help to prevent joint contractures or injuries. Avoid placing the arms on the abdomen or chest because the elbow flexors, shoulder abductors, and external rotators will be in a shortened position, creating a new, restrictive resting length. After SCI, hip and knee flexion contractures are quite common because of all of the time spent sitting. If there are no surgical or medical precautions, place the individual prone as part of the rotation to protect the skin. Prone position will maintain hip and knee extension, which will be critical if walking or standing becomes possible in the future.

Range of motion is a key determinant of function throughout rehabilitation and for return to home and full participation. In some muscle groups and joints, greater ROM will allow better function. However, in some muscles, shortened ROM will be beneficial. The optimal ROM for specific joints will enable independence in daily activities in the future, as provided in Table 12-9. The ROM activities will initially be largely passive due to spinal shock but should rely on active-assistive or active ROM for any voluntary muscle actions that the individual can produce.

TABLE 12-9	Physical Requirements for Functional Mobility
OPTIMAL JOINT ROM/ MUSCLE LENGTH	**ASSOCIATED FUNCTIONS**
Full elbow extension, full supination and 70–90 degrees wrist extension	WC propulsion; weight shifts; dressing; transfers
Neutral ankle dorsiflexion	Placing/maintaining feet on WC foot rest; important for future standing/walking
Hip and knee 90-degree flexion	Optimal WC use; dressing; transfers
Full external rotation and hip abduction	Dressing; putting on shoes and socks
Shortened finger flexors	A C6 SCI requires tight flexors to allow a grasp by extending the wrist – tenodesis grip
Long hamstrings	Attains 100+ hip flexion with knee extension; prevents falling backward in long sitting; must avoid stretching low back muscles
Shortened low back extensors	Improves stability in sitting

Incorporate Spared Muscles into Rehabilitation

Muscle activation will fall into one of three categories: (1) unimpaired and fully activated; (2) partially innervated and weak activation; (3) no activation. An unstable medical condition is typical, during this phase, so the individual will be unable to tolerate strenuous strength training activities. In addition, resistance might be contraindicated for muscle groups attaching to or crossing a vertebral fracture. At this stage, active exercise of muscle groups with full or partial innervation is important to reduce the risk of contracture and secondary complications. This exercise should be done as part of meaningful tasks like moving in the bed, whenever possible, in order to facilitate new skill learning, ensure better carry over to daily activities, and improve endurance.

CASE A, PART III

Ms. Roberts had passive ROM applied to all joints except the long finger extensors. Wrist extension was passively stretched with the fingers flexed in order to allow for the potential for a tenodesis grip in the future. She was encouraged to actively move each joint during the ROM exercise, and the therapist palpated for any muscle contraction. The ventilator connections restricted movement of the shoulder so ROM of the shoulders was coordinated with changing her position in bed to protect the skin. When she was lying on her right side, ROM of the left shoulder was completed. Once the ventilator was removed, Ms. Roberts was encouraged to perform deep breathing exercises, given an abdominal binder, and passive trunk rotation exercises were added.

Most individuals do not tolerate upright sitting early after SCI due to the cardiovascular changes and hypotension described earlier. Using heart rate, blood pressure, and medical concerns as your guide, individuals will begin a sitting program in the acute setting. Issues that would limit or prevent starting a sitting program include: an erratic heart rate or blood pressure, an unstable fracture or dislocation, and existence or risk of a pressure ulcer over the sacrum or ischial tuberosities. An abdominal binder and compression stockings at the legs will help reduce dizziness by preventing blood pooling in the legs. Raising the head of the bed will improve tolerance by adjusting the head angle near the threshold of dizziness for the patient and staying in that position for a few seconds to a few minutes, before lowering the head slightly. Each session will attempt to move the threshold higher with a goal of tolerating a 60 degree incline, at which point the individual can begin to use a reclining wheelchair (WC) with leg rests. The back can be lowered and the legs raised to compensate for dizziness or other symptoms. Once a WC can be used, pressure relief must be incorporated into the sitting program, by using different cushions and beginning to train the individual to perform components of weight shifts. Most people will not be able to perform weight shifts at this early stage of rehabilitation but educating them to adjust position every 15 minutes and increasing their tolerance of common positions, used for unweighting, will facilitate the transition to independent weight shifts in the future.

CASE A, PART IV

Ms. Roberts was restricted from starting a sitting program for the first week in the hospital, while evaluation of the fracture site and attempts to stabilize an erratic heart rate were made. Because individuals with cervical SCI will have abnormal breathing patterns when the head is elevated, the abdominal binder was applied to improve diaphragm and chest wall mechanics. Raising the head of the bed from horizontal caused an increase in respiration, abnormal breathing patterns, and drops in blood pressure and heart rate at about a 20-degree incline, during the first session. Reducing the angle stabilized the symptoms, and she tolerated up to 30 seconds per bout. Over the next 5 days, the head of the bed was raised to 45 degrees, and she maintained this position for up to 60 seconds. Ms. Roberts will be discharged to inpatient rehabilitation now that her medical condition has stabilized. The fact that she progressed from complete paralysis to some motor and sensory function within 5 days of injury suggests that some of the effects of spinal shock are resolving and greater return of muscle function may occur during inpatient rehabilitation. The presence of S4–5 pinprick sensation also points to further motor recovery over the next months. She also weaned from the ventilator in less than 7 days, which reduces the risk of complications and avoids long-term muscle weakness including the diaphragm.

MANAGEMENT OF THE PATIENT IN THE IN-PATIENT REHABILITATION SETTING

CASE A, PART V

Ms. Roberts transferred to inpatient rehabilitation 16 days after her SCI. The ASIA/ISCNSCI exam was performed within 3 days of admission to the rehabilitation hospital. Scores of the key muscle groups are shown in Table 12-10.

Testing for non-ASIA muscle groups had 2/5 strength for left shoulder abductors, 2/5 for the erector spinae and upper part of the rectus abdominus. Gluteus medius and maximus were 2/5 on the left and 1/5 on the right. The hamstrings were 3/5 on the left and 1/5 on the right. Proprioception on the left side was absent from C2 and below. DTRs were present for the biceps, brachioradialis, patella, and Achilles tendon bilaterally. The Babinski reflex was positive on the right and negative on the left. The delayed plantar response was absent. Tolerance of upright sitting had improved to 55 degrees. Ms. Roberts is dependent in all transfers, bed mobility, and daily activities, including dressing and eating.

TABLE 12-10	ASIA Motor Scores		
ASIA KEY MUSCLES		**RIGHT**	**LEFT**
C5	elbow flexors	0/5	4/5
C6	wrist extensors	0/5	3/5
C7	elbow extensors	0/5	2/5
C8	finger flexors	0/5	0/5
T1	finger abduction	0/5	0/5
L2	hip flexors	1/5	3/5
L3	knee extensors	1/5	3/5
L4	ankle dorsiflexors	0/5	1/5
L5	long toe extensors	0/5	0/5
S1	ankle plantar flexor	1/5	3/5

Impaired pinprick sensation was noted on the left but intact on the right

General Approach

The focus of inpatient and outpatient rehabilitation is moving beyond a compensatory approach and seeks to promote neuroplasticity and recovery. Compensation in SCI uses functional body parts, braces, or equipment to replace the impaired actions. There is a delicate balance between these approaches. Some compensatory techniques will likely be needed during periods of spinal shock or absent muscle activation in order to accomplish daily activities, like eating or dressing. However, reliance on compensation reduces the drive to those inactive neuromotor systems, thereby, providing an opportunity for maladaptive plasticity to emerge. After SCI, spontaneous reorganization in the nervous system occurs by filling synaptic sites vacated by the damaged systems. Animal and some human studies show that activity-based therapies can induce functional neuroplasticity.[65,66] Another reason to place greater emphasis on activity-dependent plasticity, instead of compensation, is because compensatory techniques can always be added, after plasticity and recovery have plateaued. However, if you start with these techniques, then it may be difficult to overcome maladaptive plasticity.

Three factors are important in using a neuroplasticity approach for rehabilitation. **First**, the individual should use maximal attention and effort in trying to perform the tasks. This will demand a level of stick-to-itiveness because there will be a high rate of errors or lack of response early on. **Second**, the training must allow errors to be made in order for skill learning to occur. An interesting study performed in rodents with SCI proved this point very well.[67] After SCI, a robot was used to move the leg in a stepping pattern using precise control of the movement with no errors in one group and less control that allowed movement errors in the other group. When the robot was turned off and the groups generated stepping on their own, the error-free group demonstrated poor walking and greater disability. **Third**, a high number of repetitions will be needed in order for training effects and recovery to emerge. In a rodent SCI model, a training dose of 100 steps during a treadmill

session was compared to 1000 steps per session.[68] Only the high-repetition training paradigm improved walking, showing that the benefits of rehabilitation depends on thousands of trials.

Spasticity versus Flaccidity

After spinal shock has resolved, spasticity and hyperreflexia develop in muscles supplied by motor neurons that have lost their descending motor drive (i.e., UMN lesion). **Spasticity**, as discussed in other chapters, is defined clinically as an increase in the velocity-dependent stretch of muscle.[69] The DTRs below the level of the injury will also be hyperexcitable, meaning they are easier to elicit and have a more robust response. Reflexes above the injury will be normal. Spasticity is a combination of limited or lost descending drive from the brain and greater input from the sensory afferents. Changes in the muscle fiber, collagen, and tendon also contribute to greater muscle tone.[70] When the motor neurons, the peripheral nerve, or the ventral root is damaged as part of the injury, the muscle and the reflex will be **flaccid**. This is considered an LMN injury. Most SCIs below T11 will have an LMN injury because the motor nerves are damaged and are referred to as conus medullaris/cauda equina SCI.

The most common treatment for spasticity and hyperreflexia is baclofen, a CNS inhibitor. It can reduce spasticity and flexor spasm, when given orally, but it carries many limiting side effects that can impede rehabilitation. These side effects include: drowsiness, dizziness, weakness, and ataxia.[71] To overcome these side effects and enable higher doses, baclofen can also be administered in an intrathecal pump directly over the spinal cord. It is important to note that use of baclofen will likely inhibit neural activation and limit the therapist's ability to promote activity-based neuroplasticity.

Physical therapy procedures have been used to reduce spasticity either alone or in combination with pharmacological agents. These activities include passive stretch/ROM, passive cycling, proprioceptive neuromuscular facilitation (PNF), hippotherapy, and passive standing in a frame; however, these produce conflicting effects on spasticity.[71] In contrast, functional electrical stimulation (FES) cycling and walking generally decreased spasticity.[71] Thus, activity-based physical therapy appears more likely to reduce spasticity than passive stretch/ROM, if even for short periods of time, after treatment. Notably, there is a chance that long-term direct electrical stimulation of the muscle over the motor nerve insertion may increase spasticity.[72]

A new training approach seeks to inhibit spasticity and hyperreflexia by changing underlying neuroplasticity. Wolpaw and colleagues have shown, in animal models of SCI, that the activity of spinal reflexes of leg muscles can be lowered through training.[73] The training involves providing a reward to the animal when the muscle EMG is sustained in a lower range for several seconds. The muscle activation is a read-out of motor neuron excitability, and evidence shows that training promotes greater inhibitory synapses on the motor neurons. Importantly, down-training the reflexes in animals with SCI promoted better locomotion and fewer movement impairments. These studies support the idea that, with focused attention and biofeedback, people with SCI can be trained to modify neuroplasticity and reduce spasticity and hyperreflexia. Studies of reflex down training in individuals with chronic SCI showed similar gains in function along with reductions in hyperreflexia and improvements in walking speed and motor control of the knee and ankle.[74]

Heterotopic Ossification

Heterotopic ossification (HO) is pathological bone formation within muscle and soft tissue and occurs in 10–78% of individuals with SCI.[75,76] It usually develops within the first 2 months of injury and is associated with other factors, including spasticity, pneumonia, smoking, and UTI.[77] While the mechanisms that cause HO are not fully understood, evidence shows that stem cells differentiate into bone forming cells rather than muscle, ligament, or fat cells.[78] The signals that drive the stem cells down an osteogenic path are unknown, but once the process has started, calcification occurs within a few weeks.[78] In the initial stages of HO, nonspecific signs of inflammation may appear. When it has more fully developed, the primary clinical symptoms will be joint and muscle pain with swelling in the region and a low fever. When the SCI is above T6, HO can cause autonomic dysreflexia, so HO must be considered when dysreflexia with an unknown cause emerges. The presence of HO severely limits ROM and can result in ankyloses (fixation) of the joint that can prevent daily activities, such as dressing, transfers, and WC use, if the joint/muscle length is severely limited. Prevention of HO may be possible by nonsteroidal anti-inflammatory drugs, prescribed early after SCI, before HO has started.[75] Once HO is diagnosed, surgical resection is considered in order to restore the lost ROM, but some individuals do not sustain long-term gains, possibly due to recurrence of HO.[79]

Osteoporosis

Within a few days after SCI, bone resorption begins, which results in high levels of calcium in the urine. This resorptive process continues for months and years and may continue throughout the life of the individual. It results in bone mineral loss of up to 50%, especially in the hip and knee. The primary cause appears to be prolonged bed rest, absence of muscle function, and no weight-bearing activities.[80] These mechanisms suggest that adding weight-bearing and muscle contraction activities can quell the bone loss, but a systematic review of FES cycling, treadmill training, electrical stimulation, and standing concluded that effects were limited or modest.[80]

The frank bone loss increases the risk of fracture. The following factors predict a fracture: under the age of 16 years, high alcohol use, low body mass index, SCI of 10 years or more, being female, motor complete SCI, paraplegia, prior fracture, family history of fractures, and use of anticonvulsants, heparin, or opioids.[81] The presence of five or more of these factors reflect a high fracture risk. The use of bisphosphonates, like tiludronate, clodronate, and etidronate, appears to prevent bone loss, if they are administered early during the acute phase of SCI.[80]

Physical Therapy Management in the Inpatient Rehabilitation Setting

The level and the completeness of SCI provide a guide for the expected function that will be available once spinal shock has resolved (Table 12-11). It is important to remember that these characteristics are a general guideline, and often individuals with SCI show unique recovery patterns. This means the physical therapist must be vigilant in checking for atypical gains and incorporate these into interventions. Given the short length of stay for inpatient rehabilitation, about a month, the primary goal is to prepare the individual for the next transition, typically to home. The individual will need to be able to manage bowel and bladder care, transfers, skin protection, components and use of the WC. The priorities of this phase of rehabilitation are:

- gain appropriate strength, mobility, balance, and endurance for expected functions;
- educating the patient and caregivers to perform functional tasks in bed mobility, transfers, pressure relief, and WC use;
- assess the home, work, and social environments in which the individual will live after discharge from rehabilitation.

Most patients will have a goal of returning home, when discharged from inpatient rehabilitation. To determine the focus of physical therapy interventions in this phase, the team will determine or predict the realistic living arrangements. Factors that are associated with a return to home include being married, high participation in physical therapy, and the ability to use equipment effectively.[82] People that are unmarried, older, black or Hispanic with a more severe SCI were more likely to be discharged to a nursing facility or location other than home.[82]

Little is known about which physical therapy interventions are most effective in individuals with SCI because of the complexity of the injury. Neurorehabilitationists developed a physical therapy taxonomy to begin to examine the most effect treatments.[83] The treatment focus for SCI and the rehabilitation disciplines that perform them is listed in Table 12-12. To increase strength, endurance, and skill learning, simpler tasks should be mastered, before moving to more difficult tasks. Recent evidence shows that the more time spent on musculoskeletal treatments (e.g., ROM/stretching, upright activities) was associated with greater reliance on others for motor function (i.e., lower FIM motor scores[82]). Therefore, the physical therapist will want to progress to functional tasks like bed mobility, transfers, and WC mobility as soon as possible. Gait training, during inpatient rehabilitation, is performed routinely in people with AIS D injury but occurs in only about 25% of individuals with AIS A, B, or C injuries.[84]

Bed Mobility

The importance of good bed mobility can't be underestimated because dressing, bowel management, and skin protection are performed within this environment. Activities on mat surfaces will be easier than in the bed, and a hospital bed is easier than a bed in the home. Transitioning to bed surfaces will be necessary in order to promote greatest functional attainment by the individual with SCI or the caregiver. People with high cervical SCI will depend on care attendants for bed mobility, and the role of the therapist will be to educate the patient and caregiver.

Independence in bed mobility will require skills in rolling and moving in and out of different positions. People with injuries at the lower cervical and thoracic levels should be able to achieve independence with equipment. Mat and bed activities can be structured to promote activity-dependent plasticity or for compensation (Table 12-13). The choice of which to use will

TABLE 12-11	Prediction of Mobility and Outcomes by Level of SCI		
SCI LEVEL	**EXPECTED ACTIVE MUSCLES**	**POTENTIAL FUNCTIONAL OUTCOME**	**REQUIRED EQUIPMENT**
C1–4	Neck and facial muscles Diaphragm – C4	*Bed mobility*: dependent *Transfers*: dependent *Pressure relief*: independent with power WC *Eating*: dependent *Dressing*: dependent *Grooming*: dependent *Bathing*: dependent *WC propulsion*: independent with power WC *Standing*: dependent *Walking*: not expected	Hospital bed Transfer board and/or lift Tilt or recliner WC; WC cushion – – – Rolling shower/commode chair Tilt table; standing frame ventilator
C5	Muscles listed for C1–4 Biceps, brachialis, brachioradialis Deltoid Infraspinatus Subscapularis	*Bed mobility*: min–mod assist *Transfers*: min assist *Pressure relief*: independent with power WC *Eating* : min assist *Dressing*: dependent *Grooming*: min assist *Bathing*: dependent *WC propulsion*: independent with power WC *Standing*: dependent *Walking*: not expected	Hospital bed Transfer board; lift Tilt or recliner WC; WC cushion Splints and equipment to assist eating, dressing, and grooming Rolling shower/commode chair Tilt table; standing frame
C6	Muscles for C1–5 Extensor carpi radialis Serratus anterior	*Bed mobility*: min assist *Transfers*: min assist *Pressure relief*: independent with power WC *Eating*: independent *Dressing*: independent upper body; min–mod asst lower body *Grooming*: independent *Bathing*: independent upper body; min–mod asst lower body *WC propulsion*: independent with power WC; manual: independent indoors; min–mod asst outdoors *Standing*: dependent *Walking*: not expected	Hospital bed Transfer board; lift Tilt or recliner WC; WC cushion Splints Splints Splints Rolling shower/commode chair Tilt table; standing frame
C7–8	Muscles for C1–6 Triceps, flexor carpi ulnaris, finger extensors Finger flexors C8	*Bed mobility*: independent *Transfers*: independent *Pressure relief*: independent with power WC *Eating*: independent *Dressing*: independent *Grooming*: independent *Bathing*: independent upper body; min asst lower body *WC propulsion*: manual independent indoors and outdoors *Standing*: min asst *Walking*: not expected	Hospital bed or standard bed With or without Transfer board WC cushion Adaptive devices Adaptive devices Adaptive devices Shower/commode chair Tilt table; standing frame
T1–9	Muscles for C1 to level of injury; Intrinsics of hand Intercostals Erector spinae Abdominals T6	*Bed mobility*: independent *Transfers*: independent *Pressure relief*: independent *Eating*: independent *Dressing*: independent *Grooming*: independent *Bathing*: independent *WC propulsion*: manual independent *Standing*: independent *Walking*: not functional	Standard bed With or without transfer board WC cushion Shower/commode chair Standing frame

(Continued)

TABLE 12-11	Prediction of Mobility and Outcomes by Level of SCI (Continued)		
SCI LEVEL	**EXPECTED ACTIVE MUSCLES**	**POTENTIAL FUNCTIONAL OUTCOME**	**REQUIRED EQUIPMENT**
T10–L1	Muscles C1 to level of injury; Intercostals, external and internal obliques; Rectus abdominus; L1 partial hip flexor	*Bed mobility*: independent *Transfers*: independent *Pressure relief*: independent *Eating*: independent *Dressing*: independent *Grooming*: independent *Bathing*: independent *WC propulsion*: manual independent *Standing*: independent *Walking*: functional; independent to min assist	Standard bed WC cushion Padded tub bench Standing frame Walker, forearm crutches, braces
L2–S5	Muscles C1 to level of injury; Iliopsoas; quadratus lumborum; priformis; obtruators	*Bed mobility*: independent *Transfers*: independent *Pressure relief*: independent *Eating*: independent *Dressing*: independent *Grooming*: independent *Bathing*: independent *WC propulsion*: manual independent *Standing*: independent *Walking*: functional; independent to min assist	Standard bed WC cushion Padded tub bench Standing frame Forearm crutches, braces

TABLE 12-12	Treatment Focus	
Bed mobility – PT and OT	Precedes transfer activities	
	Required for dressing, skin care, bowel care	
Transfers – PT and OT	Required for reintegration into daily activities	
WC mobility – PT and OT	Provides skeletal support with appropriate alignment, ensures skin integrity; improves or restores functional mobility	

depend on the anticipated functional outcomes for the SCI level (Table 12-13), time since injury, and completeness of the injury. If the SCI is low cervical or below and incomplete, task-specific training should be part of the training program in order to promote neural drive and plasticity.

CASE A, PART VI

Ms. Roberts is now able to perform some trunk muscle activation on the left side, but it is minimal and inconsistent. Part of treatment will be spent on strengthening these muscles and incorporating them in bed mobility. Ms. Roberts should be placed in side-lying. Rolling out of side-lying is the easiest form of rolling. She should be encouraged to initiate rolling using the shoulders and pelvis. Initially, she will have little success, so angling slightly out of side-lying will allow her to use gravity to assist the movement. Moving out of side-lying into supine will enable a transition to hook-lying – where the knees are bent and the feet are flat on the mat. Attempts to press down on the feet will try to recruit gluteal muscles and erector spinae. Lying prone on a wedge is an effective way to stretch the hip flexors. As upright tolerance improves, incorporate short and long sitting. She will require assistance when coming to short sitting and maintaining it with proper body alignment. Long sitting is important in order to enable dressing, and hamstring flexibility will be needed. In both sitting positions, therapy should progress from having the hands behind the pelvis, to out to the sides to in front. Add dynamic activities, like lifting one hand slightly to add difficulty, and strength and endurance training. Continue to encourage active use of the right upper extremity. It may take thousands of attempts before any muscle activation occurs, so be persistent and consistent.

Transfers

Transfers refer to moving between two surfaces. Skill attainment will depend on balance, arm strength, ability to manage equipment, and body type/size. Skill progression will move from an assisted transfer to independent performance and also move from easier to more difficult types of transfers. Transfer difficulty will progress from using a transfer board to seated transfers without a board to standing transfers, if feasible for the anticipated functional outcome (Table 12-11). The appropriate transfer type will pose the least risk to skin shearing, while allowing

TABLE 12-13	Bed Mobility Training Designed for Plasticity or Compensation	
FUNCTION	**TASK-SPECIFIC PLASTICITY**	**COMPENSATION**

Rolling
  Log rolling
  Segmental
	• Focused attention
	• Begin in side-lying and encourage pre-injury pattern
	• Structure for success by allowing gravity to assist the movement
		• Flex neck when moving supine to prone
		• Extend neck when moving prone to supine
		• Rocking or swinging extended arms to create momentum and carry pelvis over

Prone on elbows		• Use for stretching hip flexors • Used for changing position in bed
Prone on hands		• Stretch into hip and low back hyperextension • Prepare for gait

Short sitting
  Hips and knees
  flexed, feet on the
  floor
	• Use overhead lift or active assist to sit up from an incline or from supine
	• Train for success by starting nearly upright
	• Use mirrors to help correct body alignment if proprioception is impaired
	• Discourage using upper extremities
		• Use hands behind, at the side or in front of pelvis to increase stability
		• Use upper extremities to assist in maintaining an upright trunk

Long sitting
  Hips flexed,
  knees straight out
  on the mat
	• Use overhead lift or active assist to sit up from an incline or from supine
	• Train for success by starting nearly upright
	• Use mirrors to help correct body alignment if proprioception is impaired
		• In tetraplegia, use shoulder hyperextension to passively extend the elbow
		• Side-to-side weight shifts on elbows in supine and shoulder hyperextension to assume long sitting

as much independence as possible. As in bed mobility, the type of surface presents further difficulty, and training will need to emphasize the surfaces the individual will encounter at home such as WC to sofa, bed, toilet, tub/shower, floor, and vehicle. For individuals with high cervical SCI, lift equipment may be necessary for the home to protect the caregiver from injury.

CASE A, PART VII

With the return of upright tolerance, Ms. Roberts will need to begin to incorporate strength gains into functional tasks. To promote neuroplasticity, structure the tasks to allow trial and error as well as success. While breaking the task into its parts may be helpful for some, shortening the range or allowing gravity to assist the movement may improve skill learning. For transfer training, use of a ceiling mounted support system with adjustable levels of assistance will allow Ms. Roberts to practice the whole task. For each type of transfer, the level of support can be set to a range that allows her to move the weakest areas. To address her weak abdominals and erector spinae, use of the support system will allow Ms. Roberts to work against gravity in these tasks: moving from supine to sitting and back, forward leaning and back in the WC, and trunk rotation and reaching in all directions while sitting at the edge of mat. Progression through these tasks will be based on her ability to maintain good alignment of the head and body and then by adding challenges via lowering the support provided and/or adding arm movements. Moving from sitting to standing and back

can also be progressed by using a ceiling support system. Initially, the seat height should be elevated and the level of assistance increased to allow her to attempt and complete the whole task, that is, leaning forward and putting weight through the legs and standing. Through trial and error, she will learn where her center of gravity is and how to control it during all components of standing without the risk of falling.

WC Mobility

Two overall types of WCs will be used after SCI – a power WC, for individuals who do not have sufficient arm strength or function to propel themselves, and a manual WC, for those that do have such strength and funtion. The minimal physical criteria for propelling a manual WC, using standard push rims, include normal strength of the shoulder abductors, elbow flexors, and wrist extensors bilaterally. For individuals with less arm function, upper extremity pain, or poor endurance, power-assisted push rims will be beneficial. Power-assisted push rims boost the propulsion while requiring less shoulder muscle activity.[85] A hierarchy of WC mobility skills, from easiest to hardest, starts with propulsion over level surfaces, maneuvering in small spaces, mobility in crowded areas, moving over uneven terrain, moving up and down ramps/inclines, negotiating ridges and curbs, and descending stairs. Completing a formal WC skills training program, which moves through these progressive tasks, improves skills at least three times more than typical rehabilitation.[86] Importantly, the skill training program requires a total of only 2 hours over four sessions. To ensure that WC skills required for daily living are adequate, a new assessment

TABLE 12-14	Limitations and Seating Support According to Level of SCI	
LEVEL OF SCI	PHYSICAL LIMITATIONS	SEATING SUPPORTS
High cervical C1–4	No active balance Unable to use arms for support	Need extensive external support to have upright posture
Lower cervical C5–8 and high thoracic T1–T8	Uses arms for sitting support Kyphotic posture when both arms raised	Posterior and lateral supports to allow bimanual hand function
Low thoracic T9–12	Maintains upright trunk when arms raised Changes sitting postures frequently	Low back support may help

tool was developed: the **Wheelchair Skills Test**. This test is reliable, valid, and has normative values for SCI at different levels.[87] Additionally, training for the safe use of each component of the WC by the patient (when capable) or caregiver will be needed.

WC seating must reduce the risk of pressure ulcers, while maintaining good body alignment and promoting better function.[88] With weakness of trunk muscles, gravity will pull the head and upper body forward, pulling the spine into a C-shape or exaggerated kyphosis.[88] A posterior pelvic tilt and flattened lumbar spine also occur. This posture creates greater pressure over the sacrum, limited diaphragmatic breathing, and hyperextension of the neck to maintain gaze on the environment. Angling the seat backward slightly allows gravity to extend the spine and reduces these risks. Goals for seating support differ for level of injury and associated physical limitations (Table 12-14). Asymmetrical spasticity or strength causes deviation from good body alignment. Strengthening for the weak side is a therapeutic objective to allow for greater functional mobility and less risk of pressure ulcers. If asymmetry persists, then supports will likely improve seated posture.

CASE A, PART VIII

Early WC skills will focus on learning to manage the components of the WC using only the left arm and hand. WC mobility training will focus on propulsion using the left upper limb and left leg as muscle strength of the hamstrings returns to 3 or higher and elbow extensors reach 4/5. For pressure relief, she will need to start using the lateral weight shift techniques because she doesn't have enough trunk control to perform forward leaning or bilateral arm strength to lift the body.

Care of the Upper Limb

Individuals with tetraplegia consider hand function to be as important or more important as sexual function or bowel and bladder management.[89-91] While treatment of the upper limb is the focus of occupational therapy, it is expected that physical therapists will also care for the upper extremity. It is a fundamental part of most mobility functions after SCI such as transfers, WC use, pressure relief, and ambulation. The primary rehabilitation objectives for the upper extremity are to prevent complications, optimize function within the expected limits of the SCI, and restore function when possible. These objectives

will be addressed early, in the acute phase and through inpatient and outpatient rehabilitation. Here, we will discuss both the inpatient and outpatient approach since the greatest difference will be in progression of difficulty.

The physical capacity of the upper limb and the ability to withstand fatigue will be addressed by strength training with high repetitions. Because overall prognosis depends on the ability to perform physical activity, gains in strength are likely to allow better engagement in activity-based rehabilitation, especially since less is spent in rehabilitation. The theory is that an increase in the capacity to do work will translate in improvements in performing daily tasks, hand function, and gait. Strength training can utilize gravity or active-assistance with electric stimulation.

New approaches that are directed at increasing neuroplasticity have shown good effects and suggest that compensatory interventions might be able to be delayed or omitted entirely, in the future, for some people with tetraplegia.[92-94] Field-Fote and colleagues combined motor learning theory and somatosensory stimulation to augment afferent drive to the spinal cord. The theory is that the afferent stimulation will increase neural activity and the intensive massed practice will shape the plasticity into long-term functional plasticity, rather than maladaptive plasticity. Individuals with incomplete SCI, who completed this combined treatment, had significant gains in pinch strength, movement speed, and hand function. They outperformed individuals that completed massed practice alone or somatosensory stimulation alone.[93] Additionally, sensory perception improved and cortical excitability increased, supporting the idea that greater neural activation occurred with this treatment approach.

Splinting is a standard approach in individuals with tetraplegia to compensate for lost function and enable greater independence. The role of splinting is to prevent contractures, support and protect a weak joint, reduce the risk of pain and overstretching.[95] Splints for the hands and at the elbow to prevent flexor contracture, due to denervated triceps, are common.

One of the most serious and common long-term complications after SCI is the development of severe shoulder pain, which has been called "WC user's shoulder."[96] Shoulder pain can be seen within the first year of SCI but has been found in up to 100% of long-term WC users.[96] Elbow injuries are less common while carpal tunnel injuries lie in between.[95] These injuries are likely due to a combination of overuse and poor biomechanics, when performing tasks. Therefore, improving body position, during all mobility tasks, may limit the severity or delay the onset of shoulder and upper limb injuries. Joint resting strategies might also be helpful, but be mindful, that as one joint is protected the joints nearby may develop overuse injuries. Consider changes to equipment to improve ergonomics or better match current functional capacity and changes in body weight. Avoid or reduce transfers to non-level surfaces. Assess and change strengthening, stretching, and conditioning exercises.

TABLE 12-15	ASIA Motor Scores		
ASIA KEY MUSCLES		**RIGHT**	**LEFT**
C5	elbow flexors	0/5	4/5
C6	wrist extensors	0/5	3/5
C7	elbow extensors	0/5	2/5
C8	finger flexors	0/5	0/5
T1	finger abduction	0/5	0/5
L2	hip flexors	3/5	4/5
L3	knee extensors	3/5	5/5
L4	ankle dorsiflexors	1/5	3/5
L5	long toe extensors	1/5	1/5
S1	ankle plantar flexor	3/5	5/5

CASE A, PART IX

Ms. Roberts might benefit from an FES program for the right upper limb, since most of the muscles cannot be volitionally activated. The FES may help to facilitate muscle activity and strength, but it might also become an electrical splint that compensates for lost function. It will be important to have her attempt functional tasks with and without the FES system in order to promote skill development and reduce the risk of compensation so early after SCI. Once upper limb motor control begins to return, use of somatosensory stimulation and massed practice may be more beneficial to long-term recovery. The tasks used for massed practice should be functional and graded for difficulty, so the training can progress as greater control develops. The therapist would expect to see functional gains and improvement in sensation using somatosensory stimulation and massed practice, which would benefit her, since proprioception is impaired on the right.

CASE A, PART X: INPATIENT REHABILITATION DISCHARGE SUMMARY

Ms. Roberts made gains in strength, especially on the left (Table 12-15). Strength in non-ASIA/ ISNCSCI muscle groups also improved by one muscle grade for left shoulder abductors, erector spinae, left gluteus maximus, hamstrings, and the emergence of trace movement of the great toe extensors bilaterally was noted. Spinal shock continued to resolve and with that bowel and bladder function returned. Spasticity increased during inpatient rehabilitation with hyperreflexia noted in the DTRs of the patella, Achilles, and biceps bilaterally. There was no clonus, but the Babinski continues to be positive on the right.

Neuropathic pain developed in the right cervical region, which limited her ability to participate in her rehabilitation. Problems with focus emerged, and inconsistency in functional performance was noted. The motor scores of the right upper extremity likely do not reflect her true functional capacity. While she was unable to produce any muscle activation during the ASIA exam, later in the evaluation she was observed moving the right arm and hand. Despite a progressive return of function, she was lethargic, unable to focus, and having difficulty engaging in rehabilitation. Depression interfered with her progress during inpatient rehabilitation, and concern for her current and future well-being warranted inpatient treatment for depression in a psychiatric hospital.

PHYSICAL THERAPY MANAGEMENT OF THE PATIENT IN THE OUTPATIENT REHABILITATION SETTING

In this phase of rehabilitation, the emphasis will be to promote as much recovery as possible and to optimize functional performance to attain the highest level of independence possible. During this phase, things like neuropathic pain, hyperreflexia/spasticity, and sexuality become more prominent. Depression is also a concern. The greatest change in motor ability occurs within the first year after SCI, and the first 6 months see the sharpest rate of improvement.[12] This is the period when spinal shock is largely resolved and the opportunity to induce functional neuroplasticity should not be missed.

Chronic Complications of SCI

Neuropathic Pain – How Is It different from Acute Pain Related to Tissue Damage?

Pain is a complex problem that includes emotional, cognitive, physiological, and neural components and plays an important role in preventing serious, lasting body injury by alerting the individual to the noxious event. The traumatic nature of most SCI means that body tissues will be damaged as part of the trauma and will create pain. This type of acute pain is a natural part of the injury and healing process, and typically goes away. However, after SCI, pain responses can become quite abnormal in intensity, and this change can become permanent. This type of pain is called **neuropathic pain**.

Neuropathic pain develops due to direct trauma to the somatosensory system. This means that the spinal cord injury itself changes the remaining nervous system and produces neuropathic pain. Neuropathic pain is described as burning, stabbing, shooting, and crushing. It often emerges several months or years after the injury and interferes with the daily lives of individuals just as they are moving on from their SCI and returning to a more normal lifestyle. The prevalence of neuropathic pain is more than 80% one year after SCI.[97] Two types of neuropathic pain exist. **Allodynia** is intense pain to a normally innocuous stimulus like the wind blowing on the skin or clothing softly touching the skin. **Hyperalgesia** is exaggerated pain to a noxious stimulus like hot water or a sharp poke. The body regions affected by neuropathic pain can be quite far reaching and can occur below, above, and/or at the level of the injury.[98] While the causes of neuropathic pain are not well defined, there is mounting evidence that inflammation, microglial activation, and astrocytic reactivity play a role. There is also evidence of structural neuroplasticity within the dorsal horn of the spinal cord and within pain processing centers in the brain.[99]

Treatment for neuropathic pain after SCI is largely ineffective.[100] Gabapentin has shown some efficacy in reducing below-level neuropathic pain, but the negative side effects of drowsiness, constipation, nausea, loss of balance, and dizziness often outweigh its usefulness.[100] Minocycline which inhibits microglia has reduced below-level pain in rodents[101], but clinical efficacy in people has been questioned, based on a clinical trial for radicular nerve pain.[102] Exercise has shown promise in normalizing sensation in experimental SCI.[65,103] Importantly, individuals with SCI report the most effective treatment for pain is physical therapy.[104]

If effective treatments are going to be identified, it is critical that the complexity of neuropathic pain is carefully assessed and tracked. This means that the common numerical rating pain assessment scale is inadequate. A group of experts developed an assessment system specifically for pain due to SCI.[105] The pain basic data set classifies musculoskeletal, visceral, and neuropathic pain for the three worst pain problems.[106] The location, intensity, and duration of these pain problems are gathered. Importantly, the psychosocial and emotional impact of these pain problems are also assessed by measuring the degree to which pain interferes with daily activities, overall mood, and sleeping at night.

Sexual Function

A return to home and integration back into their social environment will shift priorities to resumption of sexual activities for both men and women. Sexuality is a major contributor to an individual's identity and sense of self. One of the first concerns after SCI is sexuality. As early as is feasible, an open discussion regarding sexual function should take place and continue at each stage of rehabilitation. Although this section is placed in the outpatient rehabilitation section, it is important to continually address sexuality. An open, direct, and nonjudgmental approach will be needed in order to allow the individual to feel comfortable communicating fears and problems. Resuming sexual function will depend on the level of SCI and completeness of the injury (Table 12-16).

Treatment to improve erectile dysfunction in men relies on phosphodiesterase type V inhibitors, like Viagra. If these are not effective, then, injectable intracavernosal medications, vacuum devices, and penile implants may be used. Achieving orgasm is more likely in incomplete SCI than when the injury is complete or in the sacral region. In men, who infrequently or do not ejaculate, vibration or electrical stimulation methods can be used to obtain semen to be used in fertilization technologies like in vitro fertilization. Smoking may have a negative effect on sexual function. Erection and lubrication depend on effective circulation and blood flow; smoking is known to reduce both of these.

Limitations in sexual function, for women, often include poor arousal and impaired orgasm. For the first 4 or 5 months after SCI, women will not have a menstrual cycle, but it returns within the first year. There are no apparent impairments in fertility or carrying a baby to term for women. However, pregnancy can worsen complications of SCI like spasticity, autonomic dysreflexia, bladder problems, and mobility.

The role of the physical therapist will be to assist the individual with SCI in finding safe, effective positions for sexual activity. High pressures should not occur on any body parts, during sexual activity, due to risk of fracture, dislocation, or ligament damage. Contractures may require support with pillows to reduce pressure. The therapist will also need to recommend positions, while keeping in mind the contraindications for the injury site.

Depression

Depression is a serious complication of SCI and occurs at high rates, not only in individuals with SCI, but also their caregivers. It has been estimated to be as high as 42% after SCI.[107] Depression is a constellation of symptoms of such frequency and severity to negatively affect functioning of the individual. Symptoms include: weight loss, insomnia, near daily fatigue or lethargy, feelings of worthlessness, difficulty thinking or concentrating, and recurring thoughts of death. Because many of these symptoms can also be caused by pain, medications, and the injury itself (sleep, weight changes), identifying depression is difficult, making it likely that many individuals with depression go untreated. Depression may be due, at least in part, to continual challenges that the individual with SCI must face and attempt to overcome, not the least of which are environmental barriers, social difficulties, and health problems.[108] Although these represent complex issues, they are all modifiable, which suggests that depression can be limited or prevented, using holistic approaches to the well-being of the individual with SCI.

TABLE 12-16	Limitations in Sexual Function After SCI	
SEXUAL FUNCTION	**MALE**	**FEMALE**
Cauda equina Conus medullaris	• No reflex erections • Occasional ejaculation	• Absent vaginal secretions • Fertility usually intact
Thoracic/cervical	• Short duration reflex erections • Occasional ejaculation	• Vaginal secretions present • Fertility intact • Absent sensation of labor pain

CASE A, PART XI

Ms. Roberts suffered her SCI as part of a suicide attempt, which is a definitive sign of depression. Her mental health will need to be monitored closely, during each phase of rehabilitation. Mood elevators were part of her medical care, beginning in the acute setting. Her physical rehabilitation was prioritized so that she could better participate in psychotherapy and group therapy treatments in the near future. In order for her to participate in group therapy, she will need to regain the ability to be upright, have good endurance, and other functions.

Physical Therapy Management

Gait Training

Perhaps the greatest divergence between training approaches occurs when considering whether to use a compensatory or plasticity-based approach for gait training. The classic gait training approach uses assistive devices and bracing to compensate for lost muscle function. In contrast, a body-weight support program minimizes bracing and allows stepping without assistive devices. There is considerable animal and human evidence that this type of training promotes greater muscle activation and restores complex firing patterns even in individuals with AIS A complete SCI.[66,109,110] Factors that promote this improvement include walking at a normal walking speed of 2.0 m/s on a treadmill, reducing the load across the legs by 50% or less, and requiring active participation by the individual rather than passively using a robot.[111] Evidence in animal studies shows remarkable cellular plasticity associated with task-specific training.[112,113] Therefore, implementation of a **body-weight support** program for gait training takes the approach that such training produces gains in neuroplasticity, muscle activation, and recovery of function that otherwise would be difficult or impossible to attain.

A compensatory approach takes the view that no further recovery is possible and that walking will only be restored through the use of technology, bracing, and/or assistive devices. In addition to conventional training (described below), other compensatory walking systems include implantable FES devices and new, FDA-approved exoskeletons.

Implantable FES systems supply electrical stimulation to key muscle groups for standing and walking. A computer controls the pattern of stimulation. The primary drawback of these systems is that energy costs and fatigue are quite high, while the walking speed is very slow. A non-implantable FES system provides stimulation over the skin and has been most widely used to perform cycle ergometry rather than walking. The surface FES system is used for strengthening, conditioning, and to reduce muscle atrophy.[114]

Engineers have been designing robotic devices with the hope of creating lightweight robots to perform stepping. The **Lokomat system** is a robotic treadmill training system, in which the patient's lower limbs are passively moved. Another form of robotic stepper is a **computer-controlled exoskeleton**, which allows the wearer to move freely in the environment. The software uses kinematic variables of the user to individualize the stepping pattern as well as movements from sit to upright and standing. At least one device has received FDA approval, the **ReWalk**, and is being used in rehabilitation facilities for gait training. The drawbacks of these systems are the high cost and users must have a high level of function and be able to stand with crutches.

Epidural stimulation may be a hybrid between activity-dependent training approaches and conventional compensatory techniques. An implantable stimulator is placed over the dura and delivers continuous electrical pulses to the dorsal root afferents, where they enter the cord.[17] When this stimulation is combined with task-specific training to stand or to step on a treadmill, individuals with complete SCI are able to voluntarily control leg movements. However, these new skills could only be performed when the stimulator was turned on. The epidural stimulator may compensate for loss of neural drive from the brain, but it facilitates learning plasticity.

Conventional Compensatory Gait Training

The focus of this rehabilitation will be to strengthen available arm and trunk muscles, stretch the hip to allow hip extension, and then progress to working with braces, the FES system, or exoskeletons. The physical characteristics required for conventional gait training include:

- Absence of hip flexion contracture. Ideally, hip range of motion into hyperextension would be present because this position activates the CPG and initiates the swing phase of locomotion.
- Absence of knee flexor contractures or plantar flexor contractures. Poor limb alignment will decrease stability and prevent balance.
- Good strength in shoulder depressors and ability to support full weight through the arms without pain. This facilitates the use of crutches or a walker.
- Low levels of spasticity or well-controlled spasticity. High tone restricts movement and spasms or clonus can cause loss of balance or falls.
- Good trunk control. For people with LMN injury, the lower extremity will be advanced using momentum created by trunk and pelvic rotation. Trunk control will also be required to maintain dynamic, upright balance, during walking.
- Dynamic balance in standing. This allows assistive devices and the lower extremities to be lifted and moved.
- Low risk of fracture. Osteoporosis is highest in complete SCI and at long periods after injury.
- Non-erratic blood pressure. Standing upright will challenge the cardiovascular system more than a seated upright position. This will be compounded by high physical exertion needed to stabilize with the arms and advance the legs.
- Highly motivated. Gait training is a strenuous activity demanding significant practice in order to develop the skill.

The individual will need to be able to don, doff, and manipulate the braces. The type of brace will depend on the impairments, related to the level of SCI (Table 12-17). Braces will be needed if knee hyperextension occurs and if ankle dorsiflexion

TABLE 12-17	Types of Braces for Different Levels of SCI
BRACE TYPE	**PURPOSE**
Reciprocal gait orthosis (RGO)	SCI T5–7 Facilitates hip flexion on one side simultaneously with hip extension on the opposite side
Hip-knee-ankle-foot orthosis (HKAFO)	SCI T5–7 Stabilizes the hip
Knee-ankle-foot orthosis (KAFO)	SCI T8–12 Used if quadriceps strength is less than 3/5; stance controlled knee joints are triggered by heel contact
Ankle foot orthosis (AFO)	SCI any level Provides toe clearance and helps with knee control
FES for dorsiflexion	SCI any level A cuff placed around the upper shank that delivers electrical impulses to the tibialis anterior at the appropriate point in the step cycle to produce dorsiflexion and then shuts off
Supra-malleolar orthosis (SMO)	SCI any level To control roll over of the ankles

is weak or absent. Braces protect the joint and also prevent leg collapse, when weight is placed on the limb. The initial phase will take place in the parallel bars, while wearing the braces. Activities that emphasize trunk balance with and without hand support, transfers and walking will allow the therapist to determine the safety and feasibility of progressing to working outside the parallel bars. Once free of the parallel bars, the individual will work on mobility skills, such as transferring from the WC, walking with different assistive devices, and negotiating rough terrain, inclines, and stairs. Conventional gait training may be the best option for individuals that have failed to respond to other forms of gait training.

Task-dependent Training for Locomotion

Use of body-weight supported locomotion has been extensively used in the clinic over the last 10 years or more. Three different types have been used: (1) Lokomat robotic system, (2) manually assisted training, generally referred to as Locomotor Training, and (3) a ceiling-mounted support system for overground training. While these systems have received great scrutiny of late, a randomized clinical trial in subacute SCI (inpatient and outpatient rehabilitation) established that Locomotor Training was as effective at improving gait speed and function as an overground gait training program matched for intensity.[115] A trial comparing the Lokomat Treadmill Training system found no difference from conventional therapy.[116] In chronic individuals with SCI, there have been at least 10 studies that compared functional performance before and after a treadmill training program and 5 randomized controlled trials. Across all studies, about 70% of patients improved following treatment.[114] Some studies show that Locomotor Training increased strength, balance, gait speed, and gait distance,[14,117] while others report the greatest gains to be with body weight support, FES, and overground rather than treadmill training.[111] Importantly, Lokomat training had no benefit compared to other types of training.[111] Factors that appear to predict a good training effect and improved gait speed include: shorter time since injury, lower levels of spasticity, voluntary bowel and bladder voiding, and walking speed before training.[118] In other words, individuals with greater capacity prior to training are the most likely to become fast walkers.

Locomotor Training Objectives

When using task-dependent techniques, encourage as much active movement as possible and provide as little assistance as needed. Walking is likely mediated by CPGs in the lumbar spinal cord that produce rhythmic, symmetrical stepping[119-121] (see Chapter 4 for description of CPG function). The CPG responds to afferent input from the limbs and integrates descending input from the brain to produce purposeful walking. After SCI, descending control is minimal, making the role of the afferent input more important. Training emphasizes sensory cues that induce stepping.[122]

- Use normal walking speeds of 2.0 m/s or higher.
- Maximize tolerable load on the stance limb without the knee buckling, typically no greater than 50% of the body weight is unloaded.
- Maintain good upright alignment of the head and body.
- Reproduce normal movements of walking with the hip, knee, and ankle.
- Synchronize hip extension of one limb with loading of the other. Hip extension induces swing so the contralateral limb must be in or near stance when extension is reached.
- Avoid weight-bearing through the upper limbs because it inhibits EMG activity in the lower extremities.[123]
- Produce synchronized symmetrical coordination between the limbs by using equal step lengths, swing times, arm swing.
- Reduce abnormal sensory stimulation, when assisting the movement. For stance, place the hands on extensor surfaces to increase extensor afferent cues. To assist swing, place hands on the flexor surfaces to increase flexor afferent cues.

Trainers are positioned at the pelvis, each leg, and the computer/treadmill controls. There are two components of training: (1) on the treadmill and (2) overground training. The retraining component uses manual assistance to reproduce normal stepping, as closely as possible. The trainers will adapt their assistance from step to step as they move the legs and pelvis/trunk. The second component is adaptability training, which requires the individual with SCI to reproduce the normal kinematics of stepping with as little assistance as possible. Adaptability training allows trial and error and places more emphasis on proximal trunk control, before reducing assistance at the lower joints. Retraining and adaptability components are used for stepping and standing, while on the treadmill, and the treatment session is typically 1 hour.

Overground training translates the skills developed on the treadmill to daily activities, transfers, and mobility. During this training, it is important to avoid abnormal sensory cues. Things like braces and certain assistive devices may inhibit activity and should be avoided, during treadmill and overground training sessions. Assistive devices that encourage weight-bearing through the arms and a forward leaning trunk prevent the hip from extending and reduce the signals to initiate swing. During overground training, assistive devices should promote an upright trunk and allow higher gait speeds (e.g., a high, rolling platform walker for individuals that need greater support). For individuals with more motor control, a rolling walker that is elevated to minimize weight through the arms will better reinforce normal body position and allow faster speeds than a standard walker.

Assessment

Gait speed, assessed via the 10-m walk test or the 6-minute walk test, reflects functional performance and a return to participation in the community.[124] The minimal gait speed threshold for individuals with SCI to become community ambulators is 0.44 m/s, which is lower than has been reported for stroke. This threshold was first defined in Europe[125] and later confirmed in the United States.[124] Therapists can use this benchmark for treatment progression. Also, there is value in collecting gait speed, using both walking tests rather than the traditional 10-m walk test alone.[124] In chronic SCI, the 6-minute walk test appears to reflect endurance (the ability to sustain gait speed); whereas the 10-m walk test might translate to a short burst of speed. The **Walking Index for Spinal Cord Injury II** is a highly recommended measure of walking recovery; however, it is based on the use of braces, which task-dependent training tries to avoid.[126] The **Spinal Cord Independence Measure III** is a patient report tool that assesses activities of daily living, coordination, eating, functional mobility, respiration, and incontinence.[127] High SCIM scores are associated with better balance, upper limb control, muscle strength, and ambulation.[128] Because the SCIM was specifically designed for SCI, it offers more detailed and appropriate assessment of functional independence than the more general Functional Independent Measure (FIM).

CASE A, PART XII

Because Ms. Roberts is showing continual gains in muscle activation and strength, her gait training program should start with a task-dependent neuroplasticity approach and wait to add compensatory components until recovery has plateaued. A Locomotor Training program, using a treadmill and body-weight support, would best match her current

---

functional abilities. An overground body-weight support program might be feasible, in the future, as greater trunk control returns and her ability to manage assistive devices with her hand improves. The initial focus during adaptability training will be to independently maintain the head and shoulders over the pelvis during standing and walking. In retraining, the focus will be to improve her endurance and tolerance of being upright. Hypotension, pain aggravation, and fatigue are likely for her because the level of her SCI is so high. Spasticity may worsen initially and then improve, due to greater time spent upright and weight-bearing. Avoid increasing spasticity medications and try to reduce them, if possible, in order to promote greater neuroplasticity from training. Progression will include reducing body-weight support and increasing treadmill speed. As the ability to take volitional steps returns and improves, stepping over obstacles, placed on the moving treadmill belt, can be added. During overground training, stepping without braces will help translate skills from the treadmill. Therapists will initially need to provide manual assistance, but as recovery occurs, Ms. Roberts should be encouraged to reproduce the stepping patterns from the treadmill.

Lifelong Considerations

Syringomyelia

Syringomyelia is the formation of a cerebrospinal fluid-filled cyst within the center of the spinal cord. It develops within months to many years after traumatic SCI and can be devastating because as the lesion expands it takes away important motor functions.[129] The symptoms of late-onset syringomyelia will be: a change in sensorimotor function like radicular pain, sensory loss, segmental weakness, gait ataxia, and increased spasticity.[130] Of serious concern, is the development of syringomyelia within the cervical region because it threatens diaphragm innervation and respiration. The most typical treatments for this condition include placing a shunt to remove the CSF from the cyst to slow its progression or untethering the cord, which is a procedure that removes the scar adhesions between the cord and the dura. The role of the physical therapist, in this condition, is to differentiate the cause of any loss of function. Because the cyst is slow growing, the rate of functional loss will be slow rather than sudden, making it more difficult to recognize. A small loss of function across more than one system (e.g., sensory and motor) warrants a closer examination for syringomyelia.

Cardiovascular Deconditioning

Cardiovascular disease (CVD) is the term used to capture problems of the heart and blood vessels. It is present in 30–50% of individuals with SCI[131, 132] and increases to 60–70%, when asymptomatic disease is included.[133] Unfortunately, death due to CVD is higher in people with SCI than able-bodied individuals.[131,132] Causes of CVD are a combination of loss of adrenergic control, poor diet, and physical inactivity. Adrenergic dysfunction is related to the level of the SCI and directly impacts cardiac function.

- T1: No supraspinal sympathetic control
- T1–T5: Partial preservation of sympathetic control
- Below T5: Full supraspinal sympathetic control

Because SCI lesion level cannot be changed, efforts to reduce CVD must focus on modifiable factors such as physical activity. The role of the physical therapist is to promote a healthy lifestyle and create a long-term fitness program for individuals with SCI. The prevalence of CVD suggests that after SCI, daily activity using a WC and other assistance is insufficient to maintain cardiovascular health. Several physical therapy interventions have proven effective in improving cardiac function:[134]

- Treadmill training with body weight support
- FES leg cycling of moderate to high intensity several times a week
- FES leg cycling combined with arm ergometry
- Aerobic arm cycling of moderate intensity several times a week

---

CASE A, PART XIII

Following her inpatient rehabilitation, Ms. Roberts spent time in a psychiatric hospital and then lived with friends for several months, while she participated in outpatient physical therapy. She ultimately returned to living in her own home, during her outpatient rehabilitation. Following 9 months of rehabilitation, Ms. Roberts was discharged with the ability to ambulate independently, using a straight cane. Right toe dragging, due to plantarflexor spasticity and weak dorsiflexors, required compensation with a walkaid electrical stimulator. She was able to ascend and descend stairs, using a handrail on the left. Upper limb function recovered extensively on the left, and gains in right hand function, as well as sensation occurred, with somatosensory stimulation and massed practice. A home fitness program, including stationary cycling, strengthening, and stretching was implemented. Neuropathic pain was controlled by gabapentin. Her depression was being medically managed, and she no longer attended group therapy. She was unable to return to work because of the physical demands and hand skills it requires.

REFERENCES

1. Profyris C, Cheema SS, Zang D, Azari MF, Boyle K, Petratos. Degenerative and regenerative mechanisms governing spinal cord injury. *Neurobiol Dis*. 2004;15:415-436.

2. Kanno H, Pearse DD, Ozawa H, Itoi E, Bunge MB. Schwann cell transplantation for spinal cord injury repair: its significant therapeutic potential and prospectus. *Rev Neurosci*. 2015;26(2):121-128. doi:10.1515/revneuro-2014-0068.

3. Lee-Kubli CA, Lu P. Induced pluripotent stem cell-derived neural stem cell therapies for spinal cord injury. *Neural Regen Res*. 2015;10:10-16

4. www.uab.edu/nscisc

5. McKinley WO, Tewksbury MA, Mujteba NM. Spinal stenosis vs traumatic spinal cord injury: a rehabilitation outcome comparison. *J Spinal Cord Med*. 2002;25(1):28-32.

6. West TW. Transverse myelitis – a review of the initial presentation, diagnosis, and initial management. *Discov Med*. 2013;16(88):167-177.

7. Burns S, Biering-Sørensen F, Donovan W, et al. International standards for neurological classification of spinal cord injury (revised 2011). *Top Spinal Cord Inj Rehabil*. 2012;18(1):85-99.

8. http://www.asia-spinalinjury.org/elearning/elearning.php

9. Crozier KS, Graziani V, Ditunno JF, Herbison GJ. Spinal cord injury: prognosis for ambulation based on sensory examination in patients who are initially motor complete. *Arch Phys Med Rehabil*. 1991;72(2):119-121.

10. Waters RL, Adkins RH, Yakua JS, Sie I. Motor and sensory recovery following incomplete tetraplegia. *Arch Phys Med Rehabil*. 1994;75(3):306-311.

11. Spiess MR, Müller RM, Rupp R, Schuld C, EM-SCI Study Group, van Hedel HJ. Conversion in ASIA impairment scale during the first year after traumatic spinal cord injury. *J Neurotrauma*. 2009;26(11):2027–2036.

12. van Middendorp JJ, Hosman AJ, Pouw MH, EM-SCI Study Group, Van de Meent H. ASIA impairment scale conversion in traumatic SCI: is it related with the ability to walk? A descriptive comparison with functional ambulation outcome measures in 273 patients. *Spinal Cord*. 2009;47(7):555–560.

13. Kirshblum S, Millis S, McKinley W, Tulsky D. Late neurologic recovery after traumatic spinal cord injury. *Arch Phys Med Rehabil*. 2004;85(11):1811-1817.

14. Buehner JJ, Forrest G, Schmidt-Read, M, White S, Tansey K, Basso DM. Relationship between ASIA exam and functional outcomes in the NeuroRecovery Network Locomotor Training Program. *Arch Phys Med Rehabil*. 2012;93:1530-1540.

15. Bunge RP, Puckett WR, Becerra JL, et al. Observations on the pathology of human spinal cord injury: a review and classification of 22 new cases with details from a case of chronic cord compression with extensive focal demyelination. *Adv Neurol*. 1993;59:75-89.

16. Bunge RP, Puckett WR, Hiester ED. Observations on the pathology of several types of human spinal cord injury, with emphasis on the astrocyte response to penetrating injuries. *Adv Neurol*. 1997;72:305-315.

17. Angeli CA, Edgerton VR, Gerasimenko YP, Harkema SJ. Altering spinal cord excitability enables voluntary movements after chronic complete paralysis in humans. *Brain*. 2014;137(pt 5):1394-1409.

18. www.NRS.com

19. Basso DM, Velozo C, Lorenz D, Suter S, Behrman A. Inter-rater reliability of the Neuromuscular Recovery Scale for spinal cord injury. *Arch Phys Med Rehabil*. 2015;96(8):1397-1403.

20. Behrman A, Velozo C, Suter S, Lorenz D, Basso DM. Test-retest reliability of the neuromuscular recovery scale. *Arch Phys Med Rehabil*. 2015;96(8):1375-1384.

21. Velozo C, Moorhouse M, Ardolino E, Lorenz D, Suter S, Basso DM, Behrman A. Validity of the Neuromuscular Recovery Scale: A measurement model approach. *Arcch Phys Med Rehabil*. 2015;96(8):1385-1396.

22. Tester NJ, Lorenz D, Suter S, et al. Responsiveness of the Neuromuscular Recovery Scale during outpatient activity-dependent rehabilitation for spinal cord injury. *Neurorehabil Neural Repair*. 2015, epub (Sept) pii:1545968315605181.

23. Wan IYP, Angelini GD, Bryan AJ, Ryder I, Underwood MJ. Prevention of spinal cord ischaemia during descending thoracic and thoracoabdominal aortic surgery. *Eur J Cardiothorac Surg*. 2001;19(2):203-213.

24. Mirza SK, Krengel WF 3rd, Chapman JR, Anderson PA, Bailey JC, Grady MS. Early versus delayed surgery for acute cervical spinal cord injury. *Clin Orthop Relat Surg*. 1999;(359):104-114.

25. Gaebler C, Maier R, Kutscha-Lissberg F, Mrkonjic L, Vecsei V. Results of spinal cord decompression and thoracolumbar pedicle stabilisation in relation to the time of operation. *Spinal Cord*. 1999;37(1):33-39.

26. Fehlings MG, Vaccaro A, Wilson JR, et al. Early versus delayed decompression for traumatic cervical spinal cord injury: results of the surgical timing in acute spinal cord injury study (STASCIC). *PLoS One.* 2012;7:e32037.

27. Bracken MB, Shepard MJ, Hellenbrand KG, et al. Methylprednisolone and neurological function 1 year after spinal cord injury. Results of the National Acute Spinal Cord Injury Study. *J Neurosurg.* 1985;63(5):704-713.

28. Bracken MB, Shepard MJ, Holford TR, et al. Administration of methylprednisolone for 24 or 48 hours or tirilazad mesylate for 48 hours in the treatment of acute spinal cord injury. Results of the Third National Acute Spinal Cord Injury Randomized Controlled Trial. National Acute Spinal Cord Injury Study. *JAMA.* 1997;277(20):1597-1604.

29. Anderson P. New CNS/AANS guidelines discourage steroids in spinal injury. *Medscape Medical News.* March 28, 2013. Available at: http://www.medscape.com/viewarticle/781669. Accessed April 7, 2013.

30. Furlan JD, Fehlings MG. Cardiovascular complications after acute spinal cord injury: pathophysiology, diagnosis and management. *Neurosurg Focus.* 2008;25(5):e13.

31. Hansen RB, Biering-Sorensen F, Kristensen JK. Urinary calculi following traumatic spinal cord injury. *Scand J Urol Nephrol.* 2007;41(2):115-119.

32. DeVivo MJ, Fine PR. Predicting renal calculus occurrence in spinal cord injury patients. *Arch Phys Med Rehabil.* 1986;67(10):722-725.

33. Utomo E, Groen J, Blok BF. Surgical management of functional bladder outlet obstruction in adults with neurogenic bladder dysfunction. *Cochrane Database Syst Rev.* 2014;5:CD004927.

34. Edokpolo LU, Stavris KB, Foster Jr. HE. Intermittent catheterization and recurrent urinary tract infection in spinal cord injury. *Top Spinal Cord Inj Rehabil.* 2012;18(2):187-192.

35. Krassioukov A, Cragg JJ, West C, Voss C, Krassioukov-Enns D. The good, the bad and the ugly of catheterization practices among elite athletes with spinal cord injury: a global perspective. *Spinal Cord.* 2015;53:78-82.

36. Singh R, Rohilla RK, Sangwa K, Siwach R, Magu NK, Sangwan SS. Bladder management methods and urological complications in spinal cord injury patients. *Indian J Orthop.* 2011;45(2):141-147.

37. Vazques RG, Sedes PR, Farina MM, Marques AM, Velasco MEF. Respiratory management in the patient with spinal cord injury. *Biomed Res Int.* 2013;2013:12. Article ID 168757. doi:10.1155/2013/168757.

38. Julia PE, Sa'ari MY, Hasnan N. Benefit of triple strap abdominal binder on voluntary cough in patients with spinal cord injury. *Spinal Cord.* 2011;49:1138-1142.

39. NPUAP. Available at: http://www.npuap.org/wp-content/uploads/2012/02/Final_Quick_Prevention_for_web_2010.pdf

40. Gélis A, Dupeyron A, Legros P, Benaïm C, Pelissier J, Fattal C. Pressure ulcer risk factors in persons with spinal cord injury part 1: the acute and rehabilitation stages. *Spinal Cord.* 2009;47:99-107. doi:10.1038/sc.2008.107.

41. DiVita MA, Granger CV, Goldstein R, Niewczyk P, Freudenheim JL. Risk factors for development of new or worsened pressure ulcers among patients in inpatient rehabilitation facilities in the United States: data from the uniform data system for medical rehabilitation. *Phys Med Rehabil.* 2015;7(6):599-612. doi:10.1016/j.pmrj.2015.01.007.

42. Gélis A, Dupeyron A, Legros P, Benaïm C, Pelissier J, Fattal C. Pressure ulcer risk factors in persons with spinal cord injury part 2: the chronic stage. *Spinal Cord.* 2009;47:651-661. doi:10.1038/sc.2009.32

43. Niazi ZB, Salzberg CA, Byrne DW, Viehbeck M. Recurrence of initial pressure ulcer in persons with spinal cord injuries. *Adv Wound Care.* 1997;10(3):38-42.

44. Consortium for Spinal Cord Medicine Pressure ulcer prevention and treatment following spinal cord injury: a clinical practice guideline for healthcare professionals. *J Spinal Cord Med.* 2001;24(Suppl 1):S40-101.

45. Krause JS, Vines CL, Farley TL, Sniezek J, Coker J. An exploratory study of pressure ulcers after spinal cord injury: relationship to protective behaviors and risk factors. *Arch Phys Med Rehabil.* 2001;82:107-113.

46. Spinal Cord Medicine Consortium. Clinical practice guidelines: neurogenic bowel management in adults with spinal cord injury. *J Spinal Cord Med.* 1998;21(3):248-293.

47. Nino-Murcia M, Vincent ME, Vaughan C, Fee WE, Goode RL, Robbins AH, Zboraiske FF. Esophagography and esophagoscopy. Comparison in the examination of patients with head and neck carcinoma. *Arch Otolaryngol Head Neck Surg.* 1990;116:917-919.

48. Krassioukov A, Eng JJ, Claxton G, Sakakibara BM, Shum S. Neurogenic bowel management after spinal cord injury: a systematic review of the evidence. *Spinal Cord.* 2010;48:718-733.

49. Glickman S, Kamm MA. Bowel dysfunction in spinal-cord-injury patients. *Lancet.* 1996;347:1651-1653.

50. Coggrave MJ, Norton C, Wilson-Barnett J. Management of neurogenic bowel dysfunction in the community after spinal cord injury: a postal survey in the United Kingdom. *Spinal Cord.* 2009;47:323-330.

51. Burns AS, St. Germain D, Connolly M, Delparte JJ, Guindon A, Hitzig SL, Craven C. Phenomenological study of neurogenic bowel from the perspective of individuals living with spinal cord injury. *Archive Phys Med Rehabil.* 2015;96(1):49-55.

52. Rosito O, Nino-Murcia M, Wolfe VA, Kiratli BJ, Perkash I. The effects of colostomy on the quality of life in patients with spinal cord injury: a retrospective analysis. *J Spinal Cord Med.* 2002;25(3):174-183.

53. Hansen RB, Staun M, Kalhauge A, Langholz E, Biering-Sorensen F. Bowel function and quality of life after colostomy in individuals with spinal cord injury. *J Spinal Cord Med.* 2015. epub March. doi: http://dx.doi.org/10.1179/2045772315Y.0000000006

54. Korsten M, Singal AK, Monga A, et al. Anorectal stimulation causes increased colonic motor activity in subjects with spinal cord injury. *J Spinal Cord Med.* 2007;30:31-35.

55. Korsten MA, Fajardo NR, Rosman AS, Creasey GH, Spungen AM, Bauman WA. Difficulty with evacuation after spinal cord injury: colonic motility during sleep and effects of abdominal wall stimulation. *JRRD.* 2004;41:95-99. .

56. Hascakova-Bartova R, Dinant J-F, Parent A, Ventura M. Neuromuscular electrical stimulation of completely paralyzed abdominal muscles in spinal cord-injured patients: a pilot study. *Spinal Cord.* 2008;46:445-450.

57. Mentes BB, Yuksel O, Aydin A, Tezcaner T, Leventoglu A, Aytac B. Posterior tibial nerve stimulation for fecal incontinence after partial spinal injury: preliminary report. *Tech Coloproctol.* 2007;11:115-119

58. Hoenig H, Murphy T, Galbraith J, Zolkewitz M. Case study to evaluate a standing table for managing constipation. *SCI Nurs.* 2001;18:74-77.

59. Oettle GJ. Effect of moderate exercise on bowel habit. *Gut.* 1991;32:941-944.

60. Peters HPF, DeVries WR, Vanberghe-Henegouwen GP, Akkermans LMA. Potential benefits and hazards of physical activity and exercise on the gastrointestinal tract. *Gut.* 2001;48:435-439.

61. Resende TL, Brocklehurst JC, O'Neill PA. A pilot study on the effect of exercise and abdominal massage on bowel habit in continuing care patients. *Clin Rehabil.* 1993;7:204-209.

62. Ditunno JF, Little JW, Tester A Burns AS. Spinal shock revisited: a four-phase model. *Spinal Cord.* 2004;42:383-395.

63. Schwartz S, Cohen ME, Herbison GJ, Shah A. Relationship between two measures of upper extremity strength: manual muscle test compared to hand-held myometry. *Arch Phys Med Rehabil.* 1992;73(11):1063-1068.

64. Herbison GJ, Isaac Z, Cohen ME, Ditunno JF. Strength post-spinal cord injury: myometer vs manual muscle test. *Spinal Cord.* 1996;34(9):543-548.

65. Hutchinson KJ, Gomez-Pinilla F, Crowe MJ, Ying Z, Basso DM. Three exercise paradigms differentially improve sensory recovery after spinal cord contusion in rats. *Brain.* 2004;127:1403-1414.

66. Hubli M, Dietz V. The physiological basis of neurorehabilitation – locomotor training after spinal cord injury. *J Neuroeng Rehabil.* 2013;10:5-8.

67. Ziegler MD, Zhong H, Roy RR, Edgerton VR. Why variability facilitates spinal learning. *J Neurosci.* 2010;30(32):10720-10726.

68. De Leon RD, See PA, Chow CH. Differential effects of low versus high amounts of weight supported treadmill training in spinally transected rats. *J Neurotrauma.* 2011;28(6):1021-1033.

69. Lance, JW. Symposium synopsis. In: Feldman RG, Young RR, Koella WP, eds. *Spasticity: Disordered Motor Control.* Chicago, IL: Year Book Medical Publishers; 1980:485-494.

70. Dietz V, Sinkjaer T. Spastic movement disorder: impaired reflex function and altered muscle mechanics. *Lancet Neurol.* 2007;6:725-733.

71. Hsieh JTC, Wolfe DL, McIntyre A, et al. Spasticity following spinal cord injury. In: Eng JJ, Teasell RW, Miller WC, et al., eds. *Spinal Cord Injury Rehabilitation Evidence*; 2012. Available at www.scireproject.com.

72. Robinson CJ, Kett NA, Bolam JM. Spasticity in spinal cord injured patients: 2: initial measures and long-term effects of surface electrical stimulation. *Arch Phys Med Rehabil.* 1988;69(10):862-868.

73. Chen XY, Chen Y, Wang Y, Thompson A, Carp JS, Segal RL, Wolpaw JR. Reflex conditioning: a new strategy for improving motor function after spinal cord injury. *Ann N Y Acad Sci.* 2010;1198(suppl 1):E12-E21.

74. Thompson AK, Pomerantz F, Wolpaw JR. Operant conditioning of a spinal reflex can improve locomotion after spinal cord injury in humans. *J Neurosci.* 2013;33(6):2365-2375.

75. Banovac K, Williams JM, Patrick LD, Haniff YM. Prevention of heterotopic ossification after spinal cord injury with indomethacin. *Spinal Cord.* 2001;39:370-374.

76. van Kuijk AA, Geurts AC, van Kuppevelt HJ. Neurogenic ossification in spinal cord injury. *Spinal Cord.* 2002;40:313-326.

77. Citak M, Suero EM, Backhaus M, Aach M, Godry H, Meindl R, Schildhauer TA. Risk factors for heterotopic ossification in patients with spinal cord injury: a case-control study of 264 patients. *Spine.* 2012;37(23):1953-1957.

78. Pape HC, Lehmann U, van GM, Gansslen A, von GS, Krettek C. Heterotopic ossifications in patients after severe blunt trauma with and without head trauma: incidence and patterns of distribution. *J Orthop Trauma.* 2001;15:229-237.

79. Garland DE, Orwin JF. Resection of heterotopic ossification in patients with spinal cord injuries. *Clin Orthop Relat Res.* 1989;242:169-276.

80. Craven BC, Lynch CL, Eng JJ. Bone health following spinal cord injury. In: Eng JJ, Teasell RW, Miller WC, et al., eds. *Spinal Cord Injury Rehabilitation Evidence.* Version 5.0. Vancouver; 2014:1–37. Available at www.scireproject.com.

81. Craven BC, Roberston LA, McGillivray CF, Adachi JD. Detection and treatment of sublesional osteoporosis among patients with chronic spinal cord injury: proposed paradigms. *Top Spinal Cord Injury Rehabil.* 2009;14(4):1-22.

82. Teeter L, Gassaway J, Taylor S, et al. Relationship of physical therapy inpatient rehabilitation interventions and patient characteristics to outcomes following spinal cord injury: the SCIRehab project. *J Spinal Cord Med.* 2012;35(6):503-526.

83. Natale A, Taylor S, LaBarbera J, et al. SCIRehab Project series: the physical therapy taxonomy. *J Spinal Cord Med.* 2009;32(3):270-282.

84. Taylor-Schroeder S, LaBarbera J, McDowell S, et al. Physical therapy treatment time during inpatient spinal cord injury rehabilitation. *J Spinal Cord Med.* 2011;34:149-161.

85. Lighthall-Haubert L, Requejo PS, Mulroy SJ, Newsam CJ, Bontrager E, Gronley JK, Perry J. Comparison of shoulder muscle electromyographic activity during standard manual wheelchair and push-rim activated power assisted wheelchair propulsion in persons with complete tetraplegia. *Arch Phys Med Rehabil.* 2009;90(11):1904-1915.

86. MacPhee AH, Kirby RL, Coolen AL, Smith C, MacLeod DA, Dupuis DJ. Wheelchair skills training program: a randomized clinical trial of wheelchair users undergoing initial rehabilitation *Arch Phys Med Rehabil.* 2004;85(1):41-50.

87. Lemay V, Routhier F, Noreau L, Phang SH, Ginis KA. Relationships between wheelchair skills, wheelchair mobility and level of injury in individuals with spinal cord injury. *Spinal Cord.* 2012;50(1):37-41.

88. Minkel JL. Seating and mobility considerations for people with spinal cord injury. *Phys Ther.* 2000;80(7):701-709.

89. Anderson KD. Targeting recovery: priorities of the spinal cord-injured population. *J Neurotrauma.* 2004;21:1371-1383.

90. Hanson RW, Franklin MR. Sexual loss in relation to other functional losses for spinal cord injured males. *Arch Phys Med Rehabil.* 1979;57:291-293.

91. Snoek GJ, Ijzerman MJ, Hermens HJ, Biering-Sorensen F. Survey of the needs of patients with spinal cord injury: impact and priority for improvement in hand function in tetraplegics. *Spinal Cord.* 2004;42:526-532.

92. Beekhuizen KS, Field-Fote EC. Massed practice versus massed practice with stimulation: effects on upper extremity function and cortical plasticity in individuals with incomplete cervical spinal cord injury. *Neurorehabil Neural Repair.* 2005;19:33-45.

93. Beekhuizen KS, Field-Fote EC. Sensory stimulation augments the effects of massed practice training in persons with tetraplegia. *Arch Phys Med Rehabil.* 2008;89:602-608.

94. Hoffman LR, Field-Fote EC. Cortical reorganization following bimanual training and somatosensory stimulation in cervical spinal cord injury: a case report. *Phys Ther.* 2007;87:208-223.

95. Connoly SJ, McIntyre A, Mehta S, Foulon BL, Teasell RW. Upper limb rehabilitation following spinal cord injury. In: Eng JJ, Teasell RW, Miller WC, et al., eds. *Spinal Cord Injury Rehabilitation Evidence.* Version 5.0. Vancouver; 2014:1–74.

96. Nichols PJ, Norman PA, Ennis R. Wheelchair user's shoulder? Shoulder pain in patients with spinal cord lesions. *Scand J Rehabil Med.* 1979;11:29-32.

97. Cardenas DD, Bryce TN, Shem K, Richards JS, Elhefni H. Gender and minority differences in the pain experience of people with spinal cord injury. *Arch Phys Med Rehabil.* 2004;85:1774-1781.

98. Bryce TN, Biering-Sorensen F, Finnerup NB, et al. International Spinal Cord Injury Pain Classification: part I. Background and description. *Spinal cord.* 2012;50:413-417.

99. Finnerup NB, Baastrup C, Jensen TS. Neuropathic pain following spinal cord injury pain: mechanisms and treatment. *Scand J Pain.* 2009;51:S3-S11.

100. Cardenas DD, Jensen MP. Treatments for chronic pain in persons with spinal cord injury: a survey study. *J Spinal Cord Med.* 2006;29(2):109-117.

101. Hains BC Waxman SG. Activated microglia contribute to the maintenance of chronic pain after spinal cord injury. *J Neurosci.* 2006;26(16):4308-4317.

102. Vanelderen P, Zundert JV, Kozicz T, et al. Effect of minocycline on lumbar radicular neuropathic pain: a randomized, placebo-controlled, double-blind clinical trial with amitriptyline as a comparator. *Pain Med.* 2015;122:399-406.

103. Detloff MR, Smith EJ, Quiros Molina D, Ganzer PD, Houle JD. Acute exercise prevents the development of neuropathic pain and the sprouting of non-peptidergic (GDNF- and artemin-responsive) c-fibers after spinal cord injury. *Exp Neurol.* 2014;255:38-48.

104. Widerstrom-Noga E, Turk DC. Types and effectiveness of treatments used by people with chronic pain associated with spinal cord injuries: influence of pain and psychosocial characteristics. *Spinal Cord.* 2003;41:600-609.

105. http://www.iscos.org.uk/international-sci-pain-data-sets

106. Widerstrom-Noga E, Biering-Sorensen F, Bryce TN, et al. The international spinal cord injury pain data set. *Spinal Cord.* 2008;46(12):818-823.

107. Krause JS, Kemp B, Coker J. Depression after spinal cord injury: relation to gender, ethnicity, aging and socioeconomic indicators. *Arch Phys Med Rehabil.* 2000;81:1099-1109.

108. Kemp B, Mosqueda L. *Aging with Disability: What the Clinician Needs to Know.* Boston, MA: John Hopkins University Press; 2004.

109. Harkema SJ, Hurley SL, Patel UK, Requejo PS, Dobkin BH, Edgerton VR. Human lumbosacral spinal cord interprets loading during stepping. *J Neurophysiol.* 1997;77(2):797-811.

110. Edgerton VR, Roy RR. Activity-dependent plasticity of spinal locomotion: implications for sensory processing. *Exer Sport Sci Rev.* 2009;37(4):171-178.

111. Field-fote EC, Roach KE. Influence of a locomotor training approach on walking speed and distance in people with chronic spinal cord injury: a randomized clinical trial. *Physical Ther.* 2011;1(1):48-60.

112. Tillakaratne NJ, de Leon RD, Hoang TX, Roy RR, Edgerton VR Tobin AJ. Use-dependent modulation of inhibitory capacity in the feline lumbar spinal cord. *J Neurosci.* 2002;22(8):3130-3143.

113. Martinez M, Delivet-Mongrain H, Leblond H, Rossignol S. Recovery of hindlimb locomotion after incomplete spinal cord injury in the cat involves spontaneous compensatory changes within the spinal locomotor circuitry. *J Neurophysiol.* 2011;106(4):1969-1984.

114. Lam T, Wolfe DL, Domingo A, Eng JJ, Sproule S. Lower limb rehabilitation following spinal cord injury. In: Eng JJ, Teasell RW, Miller WC, et al., eds. *Spinal Cord Injury Rehabilitation Evidence.* Version 5.0. Vancouver; 2014:1–73. Available at www.scireproject.com.

115. Dobkin B, Apple D, Barbeau H, et al. Weight-supported treadmill vs over-ground training for walking after acute incomplete SCI. *Neurology.* 2006;66:484-493.

116. Hornby GT, Campbell DD, Zemon DH, Kahn JH. Clinical and quantitative evaluation of robotic-assisted treadmill walking to retrain ambulation after spinal cord injury. *Top Spinal Cord Injury Rehabil.* 2005;11:1-17.

117. Harkema SJ, Schmidt-Read M, Lorenz DJ, Edgerton R, Behrman AL. Balance and ambulation improvements in individuals with chronic incomplete spinal cord injury using locomotor training-based rehabilitation. *Arch Phys Med Rehabil.* 2012;93:1508-1517.

118. Winchester P, Smith P, Foreman N, Mosby J, Pacheco F, Querry R, Tansey K. A prediction model for determining over ground walking speed after locomotor training in persons with motor incomplete spinal cord injury. *J Spinal Cord Med.* 2009;32:63-71.

119. Bussel B, Roby-Brami A, Neris OR, Yakovleff A. Evidence for a spinal stepping generator in man. Electrophysiological study. *Acta Neurobiol Exp (Wars).* 1996;56:465-468.

120. Bussel B, Roby-Brami A, Yakovleff A, Bennis N. Late flexion reflex in paraplegic patients. Evidence for a spinal stepping generator. *Brain Res Bull.* 1989;22:53-56.

121. Calancie B, Needham-Shropshire B, Jacobs P, Willer K, Zych G, Green BA. Involuntary stepping after chronic spinal cord injury. Evidence for a central rhythm generator for locomotion in man. *Brain.* 1994;117:1143-1159.

122. Behrman AL, Harkema SJ. Locomotor training after human spinal cord injury: a series of case studies. *Phys Ther.* 2000;80(7):688-700.

123. Visintin M, Barbeau H. The effects of body weight support on the locomotor pattern of spastic paretic patients. *Can J Neurol Sci.* 1989;16:315-325.

124. Forrest GF, Hutchinson K, Lorenz DJ, Buehner JJ, Vanhiel LR, Sisto SA, Basso DM. Are the 10 meter and 6 minute walk tests redundant in patients with spinal cord injury? *PLoS One.* 2014;9(5):e94108. doi: 10.1371/journal.pone.0094108. eCollection 2014.

125. van Hedel HJ, Dietz V, European Multicenter Study on Human Spinal Cord Injury (EM-SCI) Study Group. Walking during daily life can be validly and responsively assessed in subjects with a spinal cord injury. *Neurorehabil Neural Repair.* 2009;23(2):117-124.

126. Ditunno PL, Ditunno JF. Walking index for spinal cord injury (version II) scale revision. *Spinal Cord.* 2001;39:654-656.

127. Iztkovich M, Gelemter I. The spinal cord independence measure(SCIM) version III: reliability and validity in multicenter international study. *Disabil Rehabil.* 2007;29:1926-1933.

128. www.rehabmeasures.org

129. Ko HY, Kim W, Kim SY, Shin MJ, Cha YS, Chang JH. Factors associated with early post traumatic syringomyelia. *Spinal Cord.* 2012;50:695-698.

130. Brodbelt AR, Stoodely MA. Post-traumatic syringomyelia. A review. *J Clin Neurosci.* 2003;10:401-408.

131. Myers J, Lee M, Kirati J, Jaramillo J. Cardiovascular disease in spinal cord injury: an overview of prevalence, risk evaluation and management. *Am J Phys Med Rehabil.* 2007;86:142-152.

132. Myers J, Kirati J, Jaramillo J. The cardiometabolic benefits of routine physical activity in persons living with spinal cord injury. *Curr Cardiovasc Risk Rep.* 2012;6:323-330.

133. Bauman WA, Raza M, Chayes Z, Machac J. Tomographic thallium-201 myocardial perfusion imaging after intravenous dipyridamole in asymptomatic subjects with quadriplegia. *Arch Phys Med Rehabil.* 1993;74:740-744.

134. Warburton DER, Krassiokov A, Sproule S, Eng JJ. Cardiovascular health and exercise following spinal cord injury. In: Eng JJ, Teasell RW, Miller WC, et al., eds. *Spinal Cord Injury Rehabilitation Evidence.* Version 5.0. Vancouver; 2014:1–48. Available at www.scireproject.com.

Review Questions

1. **An individual with a spinal cord injury classified as AIS C will have the following functions below the level of the injury:**
   A. Complete motor paralysis only
   B. Spared motor function with complete sensory loss
   C. Complete sensory loss only
   D. Spared motor and sensory function

2. **An injury at C8 will likely produce the following impairments:**
   A. Autonomic dysreflexia
   B. Weak cough
   C. Kyphotic "C" sitting posture
   D. Weak finger abduction
   E. All of the above

3. **A central cord injury will typically have the following type of dysfunction**
   A. Loss of pain and temperature sensation only on one side of the body
   B. Severe atrophy of the hands and good motor control of the legs
   C. Paralysis of the legs and good proprioception in the legs
   D. Poor proprioception in the legs and good motor control of the legs

4. **Complete paralysis during the first week of injury means there will be no motor recovery.**
   A. True
   B. False

5. **Deep vein thrombosis is caused by which of the following:**
   A. Hypertension
   B. Spasticity
   C. Spinal shock
   D. Bed rest

6. **Which of the symptoms of autonomic dysreflexia are most likely to indicate a serious life-threatening problem:**
   A. Pounding headache
   B. Sweating
   C. Piloerection
   D. Facial flushing

7. **A flaccid bladder causes urine retention.**
   A. True
   B. False

8. **A urinary tract infection will interfere with physical therapy treatment because it:**
   A. Increases spasticity
   B. Causes nausea
   C. Triggers autonomic dysreflexia
   D. All of the above

9. **In the acute stage of cervical SCI, loss of sympathetic drive to the lungs causes:**
   A. Spasticity
   B. Hypotension
   C. Excessive bronchial secretions
   D. Damage to the cilia

10. **A patient with C6 tetraplegia has low blood oxygenation levels when sitting in an upright body position. This is most likely due to:**
    A. Abdominal protrusion that expands the thorax
    B. Greater mucous secretions
    C. Vasomotor constriction
    D. Loss of phrenic motor drive

11. **To prevent pressure ulcers at any stage of rehabilitation after SCI, the following factors should be modified:**
    A. Eliminate nicotine
    B. Perform pressure relief every 15 minutes while sitting
    C. Change positions in bed every 2 hours
    D. Avoid urinary incontinence
    E. All of the above

12. **An individual with a T8 SCI and upper motor neuron signs below the injury would be most at risk for which bowel dysfunction:**
    A. Fecal incontinence
    B. An areflexic bowel
    C. Fecal retention
    D. Poor motility

13. **For the patient described above with T8 SCI, the therapist will need to monitor for which of the following bowel conditions:**
    A. Abdominal distention and pain
    B. Autonomic dysreflexia
    C. Orthostatic hypotension
    D. Urinary tract infection

14. **An individual with a C5 complete SCI upon entry into inpatient rehabilitation will be expected to:**
    A. Exhibit no further recovery and remain AIS A
    B. Require a ventilator

C. Use a manual wheel chair
D. Have active shoulder muscles

15. **Heterotopic ossification poses a major problem for individuals with SCI because:**
    A. Joint range of motion becomes severely restricted and prevents dressing
    B. Of low recurrence rates
    C. Stem cells prevent autonomic dysreflexia
    D. Frank bone loss occurs

16. **In general, an individual with SCI would be expected to attain independent hand function if the SCI occurs below:**
    A. C2
    B. C4
    C. C6
    D. C8

17. **You are evaluating an individual with incomplete cervical SCI. What upper extremity muscle groups must have good strength in order for the individual to manually propel a wheel chair?**
    A. Deltoids
    B. Elbow extensors
    C. Finger extensors
    D. Erector spinae

18. **The upper extremity requires specific interventions as early as possible. The role of the physical therapist will be to:**
    A. Deliver passive stretching only
    B. Inform the occupational therapist of strength-related concerns
    C. Apply somatosensory stimulation and massed practice to improve motor control
    D. All of the above

19. **Neuropathic pain represents a major challenge for people with SCI because:**
    A. The late onset interferes with integration into social and daily routines
    B. Current treatments are ineffective
    C. Normally soft stimuli are perceived as severely painful
    D. All of the above

20. **A return to sexual function is expected for all individuals following SCI. The role of the physical therapist will be to:**
    A. Allow the nurse to discuss sexual function with the individual
    B. Assume that sexual drive will be lost due to the SCI
    C. Refer individuals who are bisexual or homosexual to the neuropsychologist
    D. None of the above

21. **Which of the following complications is most likely to occur for any individual with SCI regardless of lesion severity or location?**
    A. Urinary or bladder calculi
    B. Pneumonia
    C. Pressure ulcer
    D. Depression
    E. All of the above

22. **Gait training for individuals with complete SCI at T6 will most likely require:**
    A. A reciprocal gait orthosis
    B. A hip, knee, ankle orthosis
    C. An ankle foot orthosis
    D. A supra-malleolar orthosis

23. **Gait training with body weight support may benefit individuals with which of the following types of SCI**
    A. T1 SCI classified AIS B
    B. T9 SCI classified AIS A
    C. C6 SCI classified AIS C
    D. C2 SCI classified AIS D
    E. All of the above

24. **The long-term consequences of a spinal cord injury include:**
    A. Osteoporosis
    B. Cardiovascular disease
    C. Shoulder pain and dysfunction
    D. Syringomyelia
    E. All of the above

Answers

1. D	2. E	3. B	4. B	5. D
6. A	7. A	8. D	9. C	10. A
11. E	12. C	13. A	14. D	15. A
16. D	17. A	18. C	19. D	20. D
21. D	22. A	23. E	24. E	

Multiple Sclerosis Case

Anne D. Kloos and
Deborah A. Kegelmeyer

13

OBJECTIVES

1) Describe the demographics, risk factors, etiology, pathophysiology, common symptoms, and diagnosis of multiple sclerosis (MS)

2) Differentiate between the general progression and prognosis of the different types of MS

3) Discuss the medical management of MS

4) Design a physical therapy intervention program with appropriate goals and outcomes for the individual with MS

CASE A, PART I: MULTIPLE SCLEROSIS

Sheila Dillman is a 37-year-old white female. She came to Neurology Clinic for evaluation of her long-term neurologic complaints. Ms. Dillman relates that for the last 2 years she has noticed some strange symptoms, particularly heat intolerance which precedes the onset of difficulty with walking. She admits to several near falls and describes her gait during these episodes as a "stumbling gait." She also relates that over the last 2 years she goes through periods where her vision is blurry. Two months ago she underwent a divorce and moved to her own apartment. At this time she got sick with the flu and her condition worsened. At that time, she could not hold objects in her hands and had severe exhaustion. She also had several falls and intermittent joint pain on the left side of her body that was spread diffusely across multiple joints. More recently, her chart indicates that she abruptly developed a left hemisensory deficit. The MRI scan was performed at that time and revealed a multifocal white matter disease – areas of increased T2 signal in both cerebral hemispheres. Spinal tap was also done which revealed the presence of oligoclonal bands in CSF. Visual evoked response testing was abnormal with slowed conduction in optic nerves.

Findings on exam: She remains weak and numb on the left side; has impaired urinary bladder function, requiring multiple voids in the mornings and nocturia at times. She has become incontinent and now has to wear a pad during the day. She also has ongoing balance problems with some sensation of spinning, continuous tinnitus with mild hearing loss, and she is extremely fatigued. She complains of impaired short-term memory and irritability.

WHAT IS MULTIPLE SCLEROSIS?

Multiple Sclerosis (MS) is a chronic, progressive, inflammatory disease that affects neurons in the central nervous system. Jean-Martin Charcot is credited with the first comprehensive description of the disease in 1868. He described its clinical and pathological features and outlined the symptom triad known as Charcot's triad: intention tremor, nystagmus, and scanning speech.

EPIDEMIOLOGY/RISK

The incidence of MS is 30–80 per 100,000 population; about 400,000 people are affected with the disease in the United States. It is one of the most common causes of neurologic disability in young adults and typically affects individuals between the ages of 20 and 50, with the mean age of onset being 32 years. Children (≤18 years) and adults over the age of 50 are rarely affected. MS is two to three times more common in women than men. Whites of European ancestry have higher rates of MS than those of African, Asian, and Hispanic/Latino ancestry. Certain populations such as Alaskan Inuit, Norwegian Lapps, Australian Aborigines, and New Zealand Maoris almost never have MS. The incidence of MS increases the farther one travels from the equator, with the highest prevalence rates found in Scandinavian countries, northern Europe, northern United States, southern Canada, New Zealand, and southern Australia. Migration studies indicate that individuals who move before puberty from one geographic area to another tend to take on the risk level, either higher or lower, of the area to which they move. However, those who move after puberty tend to retain the risk level of their birthplace. Outbreaks or "epidemics" of MS have been reported, most notably in the Faroe Islands off the coast of Scotland when they were occupied by British soldiers during World War II, but the cause and significance of these outbreaks are not known.

Other factors associated with increased risk of MS are smoking and low blood levels of vitamin D. Epidemiological studies showed that smokers had a 40–80% increased risk of developing MS, and were greater than three times more likely to develop secondary progressive MS, if they presented with relapsing-remitting MS compared to nonsmokers.[1] Lower vitamin D levels caused by less sunlight (ultraviolet) exposure have been proposed to explain the higher incidence of MS the further the distance from the equator. A large prospective study of nurses in the United States found that women who used supplemental vitamin D, largely from multivitamins, had a 40% lower risk of MS than women who did not use vitamin D supplements.[2]

PATHOPHYSIOLOGY/ PATHOGENESIS

The exact cause of MS is unknown, but exposure to environmental agents, particularly viruses, is believed to trigger MS in genetically susceptible individuals. Although no particular virus has been confirmed to trigger the onset of MS in humans, a host of viruses including measles, human herpes virus-6 (HHV-6), human T-lymphotropic virus 1 (HTLV-1), and Epstein–Barr virus have been implicated as causative agents. Of these viruses, the Epstein–Barr virus is the most promising candidate.[3] No genes have been directly linked to MS, but specific human leukocyte antigen (HLA) genes located on chromosome 6 are strongly associated with the development of the disease. These genes encode proteins that are important for regulating immune cell functions. In addition, researchers have identified over 50 non-HLA genes that increase a person's risk of MS, the majority of which encode immune system-related molecules.[4] These genetic findings lend support to the idea that MS is primarily an immune-mediated disease. The risk of developing MS in the general population is 1:750, but rises to 1:40 in anyone who has a close relative (parent, sibling, child) with the disease. Twin studies have shown that the identical twin of a person with MS has about a 30% risk of developing the disease while the risk for fraternal twins is around 3%.[5]

The disease involves an immune system attack against the central nervous system mediated in part by activated T-cells (and perhaps B cells) that migrate through the blood–brain barrier into the CNS and initiate an immune response that results in inflammatory damage to the myelin covering as well as the axons themselves (Figure 13-1).

The damage to myelin and axons slows or interrupts the conduction of nerve impulses, resulting in symptoms specific to the damaged neurons. Reduction of inflammation and its associated edema along with compensatory remyelination by oligodendrocytes and/or axonal plasticity are thought to be responsible for the remission of symptoms (Figure 13-1 and Box 13-1). Over time, the oligodendrocytes die and remyelination is not possible. Demyelinated areas become filled with fibrous astrocytes that form scar tissue (sclerosis) or so-called sclerotic plaques that are pathologic hallmarks of the disease. The damaged axons become transected and undergo retrograde degeneration and eventually cell death. In addition to white matter, plaques are also found in cortical (temporal and frontal cortex, including motor areas) and subcortical (thalamus, basal ganglia, and cerebellum) gray matter and are also related to physical disability and cognitive impairments.[6] Recent studies suggest that gray matter pathology is, in part, independent of white matter lesions and may precede development of the white matter pathology.[7] Inflammatory and neurodegenerative

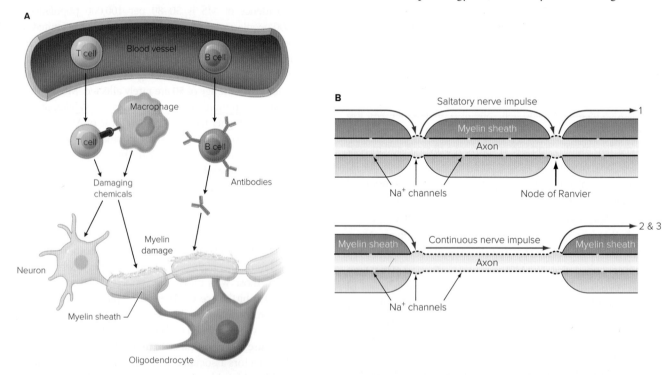

FIGURE 13-1 A. Autoimmune Process of Myelin Damage: Activated T cells and potentially B cells, followed by macrophage activity, induce myelin inflammation that can damage the myelin. During the inflammatory phase, conduction is impaired, producing symptoms associated with the involved axons; as inflammation recedes, recovery of symptoms occurs if remyelination is achieved. **B.** Schematic representation of demyelination and axonal degeneration in MS. 1) schematic of normal neural function in a myelinated axon; 2) in acute demyelination, action potentials can't cross the open space due to low numbers of voltage-gated sodium channels in the internodal axonal regions and stop; 3) in a demyelinated axon, conduction can take place if voltage gated sodium channels are added to the axon membrane through neuroplasticity. but is much slower; 4) with further loss of myelin, axon degeneration occurs (not shown). (B, Reproduced with permission from Hauser SL (ED) Harrison's *Neurology in Clinical Medicine* 3rd Ed, New York, NY: McGraw-Hill; 2013, Fig 39-1 , pg. 475.)

processes combine to eventually induce neuronal loss and brain atrophy. Axonal destruction occurs early and can be detected on MRI even before individuals are diagnosed with MS.

WHY DO SOME PEOPLE WITH MS SEEM TO GET SICKER AND THEN BETTER OVER TIME?

BOX 13-1 Types of MS

The clinical disease course varies widely and is unpredictable from person-to-person and within a particular person over time. However, there are four main subtypes that describe the most frequent clinical course for MS (Figure 13-2).

Relapsing-Remitting MS

Most individuals (about 85%) diagnosed with MS are initially diagnosed with relapsing-remitting MS (RRMS). People with RRMS have clearly defined relapses, also called attacks, flare-ups, or exacerbations, during which neurologic function worsens. These relapses are followed by remissions, defined as periods during which the disease does not progress and individuals experience complete or incomplete recovery of neurologic function. Incomplete recovery leads to incremental worsening of disability over time. Relapse rates for untreated RRMS are about one to two relapses a year and are correlated with disability.[8]

Secondary Progressive MS

Following an initial period of RRMS, many people develop a secondary-progressive (SPMS) disease course, in which the disease steadily worsens, with or without notable relapses and remissions or plateaus. Approximately 50% of people with RRMS developed SPMS within 10 years of diagnoses before the advent of disease-modifying medications. Long-term data are not yet available to determine if this transition is delayed in treated individuals.

Primary Progressive MS

Primary progressive MS (PPMS) affects approximately 10% of people and is characterized by slowly worsening neurologic function from the time of diagnosis with no distinct relapses or remissions. The rate of progression may vary over time, with occasional plateaus and temporary minor improvements. Individuals with PPMS tend to be older (i.e., around 40 years old) at the time of onset.

Progressive-Relapsing MS

Progressive-relapsing MS (PRMS) includes about 5% of people with MS who experience steadily worsening disease from the beginning, with superimposed relapses followed by no or little recovery along the way. In contrast to RRMS the disease continues to progress and disability increases even during the time between relapses.

In rare cases individuals with MS experience a very mild disease course called benign MS in which full neurologic function is preserved 15 years after disease onset. On the other extreme, some individuals experience a very rapid disease course called malignant MS (Marburg disease) leading to death within a short time of onset.

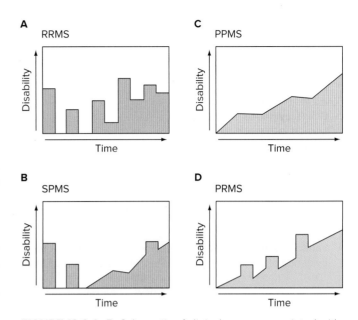

FIGURE 13-2 A–D. Schematic of clinical course associated with MS subtypes. (Reproduced with permission from Hauser SL (ED) *Harrison's Neurology in Clinical Medicine*, 3rd Ed, New York, NY: McGraw-Hill; 2013, Figure 39-2, pg. 479.)

Question: What type of MS is Sheila most likely exhibiting?

Sheila's past history describes a pattern of intermittent flare-ups of neurological symptoms that occurred suddenly and that resolved over time with periods of stable function between episodes, consistent with RRMS. More recently, her symptoms appear to be progressively worsening over time with evidence of multiple sclerotic lesions on the MRI, suggesting that she might be going into secondary progressive MS.

HOW IS MS DIAGNOSED?

Early diagnosis is important as early treatment may slow or prevent worsening of disability. However, due to the heterogeneity of symptoms and the lack of a definitive diagnostic test, it may take years before the diagnosis of MS is established. The diagnosis of MS remains a clinical diagnosis based on history and neurologic examination findings of evidence of at least two episodes of neurologic symptoms referable to myelinated regions of the CNS that are separated in space (i.e., cerebral white matter, brainstem, cerebellar tracts, optic nerves, spinal cord) and time. Many physicians use the *2010 Revised McDonald Diagnostic Criteria for MS* (Table 13-1) to make the diagnosis. All diseases that present with similar symptoms must be ruled out before the diagnosis of MS is made.

Imaging and Other Diagnostic Tests

Important lab and diagnostic tests that support the diagnosis of MS are MRI, cerebrospinal fluid (CSF) analysis, and evoked potential testing including visual, somatosensory, and brainstem

TABLE 13-1	2010 Revised McDonald Diagnostic Criteria for Multiple Sclerosis
CLINICAL PRESENTATION	**ADDITIONAL DATA NEEDED FOR MS DIAGNOSIS**
≥2 attacks[a]; objective clinical evidence of ≥2 lesions or objective clinical evidence of 1 lesion with reasonable historical evidence of a prior attack[b]	None[c]
≥2 attacks[a]; objective clinical evidence of 1 lesion	Dissemination in space, demonstrated by: ≥1 T2 lesion in at least 2 of 4 MS-typical regions of the CNS (periventricular, juxtacortical, infratentorial, or spinal cord)[d]; or Await a further clinical attack[a] implicating a different CNS site
1 attack[a]; objective clinical evidence of ≥2 lesions	Dissemination in time, demonstrated by: Simultaneous presence of asymptomatic gadolinium-enhancing and nonenhancing lesions at any time; or A new T2 and/or gadolinium-enhancing lesion(s) on follow-up MRI, irrespective of its timing with reference to a baseline scan; or Await a second clinical attack[a]
1 attack[a]; objective clinical evidence of 1 lesion (clinically isolated syndrome)	Dissemination in space and time, demonstrated by: For DIS: 1 T2 lesion in at least 2 of 4 MS-typical regions of the CNS (periventricular, juxtacortical, infratentorial, or spinal cord)[d]; or Await a second clinical attack[a] implicating a different CNS site; and For DIT: Simultaneous presence of asymptomatic gadolinium-enhancing and nonenhancing lesions at any time; or A new T2 and/or gadolinium-enhancing lesion(s) on follow-up MRI, irrespective of its timing with reference to a baseline scan; or Await a second clinical attack[a]
Insidious neurological progression suggestive of MS (PPMS)	1 year of disease progression (retrospectively or prospectively determined) plus 2 of 3 of the following criteria[d]: 1. Evidence for DIS in the brain based on ≥1 T2 lesions in the MS-characteristic (periventricular, juxtacortical, or infratentorial) regions 2. Evidence for DIS in the spinal cord based on ≥2 T2 lesions in the cord 3. Positive CSF (isoelectric focusing evidence of oligoclonal bands and/or elevated IgG index)

Reproduced with permission from Polman et al. Diagnostic criteria for Multiple Sclerosis: 2010 Revisions to the McDonald Criteria, *Ann Neurol* 2011 Feb;69(2):292-302.

If the Criteria are fulfilled and there is no better explanation for the clinical presentation, the diagnosis is "MS"; if suspicious, but the Criteria are not completely met, the diagnosis is "possible MS"; if another diagnosis arises during the evaluation that better explains the clinical presentation, then the diagnosis is "not MS."

[a]An attack (relapse; exacerbation) is defined as patient-reported or objectively observed events typical of an acute inflammatory demyelinating event in the CNS, current or historical, with duration of at least 24 hours, in the absence of fever or infection. It should be documented by contemporaneous neurological examination, but some historical events with symptoms and evolution characteristic for MS, but for which no objective neurological findings are documented, can provide reasonable evidence of a prior demyelinating event. Reports of paroxysmal symptoms (historical or current) should, however, consist of multiple episodes occurring over not less than 24 hours. Before a definite diagnosis of MS can be made, at least 1 attack must be corroborated by findings on neurological examination, visual evoked potential response in patients reporting prior visual disturbance, or MRI consistent with demyelination in the area of the CNS implicated in the historical report of neurological symptoms.

[b]Clinical diagnosis based on objective clinical findings for 2 attacks, is most secure. Reasonable historical evidence for 1 past attack, in the absence of documented objective neurological findings, can include historical events with symptoms and evolution characteristics for a prior inflammatory demyelinating event; at least 1 attack however, must be supported by objective findings.

[c]No additional tests are required. However, it is desirable that any diagnosis of MS be made with access to imaging based on these Criteria. If imaging or other tests (for instance, CSF) are undertaken and are negative, extreme caution needs to be taken before making a diagnosis of MS, and alternative diagnoses must be considered. There must be no better explanation for the clinical presentation, and objective evidence must be present to support a diagnosis of MS.

[d]Gadolinium-enhancing lesions are not required; symptomatic lesions are excluded from consideration in subjects with brainstem or spinal cord syndromes.

MS, multiple sclerosis; CNS, central nervous system; MRI, magnetic resonance imaging; DIS, dissemination in space; DIT, dissemination in time; PPMS, primary progressive multiple sclerosis; CSF, cerebrospinal fluid; IgG, immunoglobulin G.

auditory evoked responses. CSF that is positive for oligoclonal immunoglobulin G (IgG), an antibody that protects the body from infection, supports the diagnosis of MS. Evoked potential testing showing slowed conduction of sensory signals through the CNS is thought to reflect demyelination.

MRI is useful for detecting plaques or lesions even before clinical symptoms are evident, identifying areas of active inflammation, and establishing dissemination in time (how old the plaques/lesions are) (Figure 13-3).

MS lesions can be found anywhere in the CNS white matter, yet 15–37% are located in the gray matter.[8] Plaques located near or around the ventricles, called periventricular lesions, and in the corpus callosum are highly suggestive of MS. Gadolinium is attracted to areas of inflammation and is used as a contrast medium in T1-weighted MRI scans to identify newly active lesions. T2-weighted MRI scans provide information about axonal loss and disease progression in terms of the total amount of lesion area and brain atrophy.

MS SIGNS AND SYMPTOMS: WHY ARE THE SYMPTOMS SO VARIABLE IN DIFFERENT PATIENTS WITH MS?

Signs and symptoms vary considerably, depending on the location of lesions within the CNS but can include sensory, motor, cognitive, emotional, and autonomic manifestations. A first neurologic event in which a person experiences single or multiple symptoms that last at least 24 hours is often referred to as a clinically isolated syndrome (CIS). The most common early symptoms of MS are sensory, including numbness and

FIGURE 13-3 A–D. MRI findings in MS. Arrows point at areas of high intensity consistent with lesions. (Reproduced with permission from Hauser SL (ED) Harrison's *Neurology in Clinical Medicine*, 3rd Ed, New York, NY: McGraw-Hill; 2013, Figure 39-3, p 481.)

paresthesias (pins and needles sensation), or visual disturbances (e.g., blurred vision in one or both eyes, double vision, or diminished acuity/loss of vision). Common symptoms of MS are presented in Box 13-2. Symptoms typically develop rapidly over the course of minutes or hours but can develop slowly over weeks or months. They are unpredictable and vary from person to person, and from relapse to relapse in the same person.

When primary symptoms are poorly managed, secondary symptoms develop such as infections, falls, injuries, contractures, and pressure sores that contribute to disability and decreased quality of life. As the disease progresses, individuals experience tertiary symptoms such as loss of job, loss of intimacy, role changes, family disruption, social isolation, dependency, loss of self-esteem, and all possible consequences of chronic disease.

Sensory Dysfunction

Sensory disturbances affect the majority of individuals with MS and typically include paresthesias, tingling, and numbness affecting the face, body, or extremities. The distribution of sensory loss can be localized to a single cranial nerve or spinal nerve root distribution, a single limb (monoanesthesia), a single side of the body (hemianesthesia), as is the case for Ms. Dillman, or multiple areas (e.g., cranial nerves plus hemianesthesia). Disruption of touch, pressure, pain, temperature, and proprioception sensations can interfere with performance of functional activities and in severe cases lead to injuries from secondary wounds, burns, or falls. Complete loss of sensation (anesthesia) is uncommon.

Pain

Pain is a common complaint for individuals with MS and negatively impacts their daily activities and quality of life. Several different types of neuropathic pain can occur as a result of nerve damage including dysesthesias, optic or trigeminal neuritis, and/or Lhermitte's sign. Dysesthesias, the most common pain in MS, are achy, burning sensations that affect the limbs or around the trunk. They can be acute (sudden and spontaneous onset) or chronic and may worsen after exercise or with exposure to hot environments. In severe cases, individuals experience discomfort or pain from a light touch or pressure stimulus to the skin, including clothing. Trigeminal neuralgia is a severe, stabbing pain in the face related to damage of the trigeminal nerve. Lhermitte's sign, a brief electric shock-like sensation down the spine that occurs with neck flexion toward the chest, is often related to dorsal column damage in the cervical spinal cord (Figure 13-4). Musculoskeletal pain due to muscle or ligament strain can arise from mechanical stress, abnormal postures or movements, or joint immobility caused by muscle weakness, severe spasticity, and tonic muscle spasms.

Visual Disturbances

Visual disturbances occur in approximately 80% of individuals with MS. The most common problems are decreased or blurred vision (optic neuritis), double vision (diplopia), and involuntary eye movements (nystagmus). Optic neuritis refers to inflammation of the optic nerve and causes an acute blurring or graying

---

BOX 13-2 Common Symptoms of MS

Sensory Symptoms
Hypoesthesia, numbness
Paresthesias

Pain
Dysesthesias
Optic or trigeminal neuritis
Lhermitte's sign
Chronic pain

Visual Symptoms
Blurred or double vision
Diminished acuity/loss of vision
Scotoma
Internuclear Ophthalmoplegia
Nystagmus

Motor Symptoms
Weakness or paralysis
Fatigue
Spasticity
Impaired balance
Ataxia and intention tremor
Impaired gait and mobility
Impaired speech and swallowing

Cognitive Symptoms
Decreased information processing speed
Short-term memory problems
Decreased attention and concentration
Executive function problems
Impaired visual spatial processing
Impaired verbal fluency

Emotional/Behavioral Symptoms
Depression
Pseudobulbar affect
Euphoria
Lack of insight
Adjustment disorders
Obsessive–compulsive disorders

Cardiovascular dysautonomia

Bladder and Bowel Symptoms
Urinary urgency, frequency
Nocturia
Urinary hesitancy, dribbling
Constipation
Diarrhea
Incontinence

Sexual Symptoms
Erectile and ejaculatory dysfunction
Decreased vaginal lubrication
Decreased libido
Decreased ability to achieve orgasm

A Optic neuritis

1 Testing pupillary response

2 Fundoscopic examination of affected eye shows pallor of the optic disc

3 Localization of lesion

Normal eye   Affected eye

Retrobulbar (optic nerve)

B Internuclear ophthalmoplegia

1 Testing eye movement

2 Localization of lesion

Midbrain

III

MLF

Pons

Ponto-medullary junction

VI

C Additional signs

L'hermitte's sign

Babinski sign
3+

FIGURE 13-4 **Common intermittent symptoms of MS. A.1:** A light shown in the non-involved eye, produces constriction bilaterally but a light to the involved eye produces dilation, indicating a de-afferented pupil. **A.2:** Fundoscopic exam illustrates a blurring or elevation of the optic nerve. **A.3:** in the absence of a hemianopia, the lesion can be isolated to the optic nerve. **B.1:** When following a finger across the visual field, the involved eye fails to adduct (top and middle illustrations demonstrate this for either eye). Convergence to a finger pointing at the nose illustrates normal adduction., demonstrating CN III and nucleus integrity. **B.2:** Lesion is localized to the MLF. **C.** Demonstration of testing position for L'hermitte's sign. (Reproduced with permission from Kandel ER, Schwartz JH, Jessell TM, Siegelbaum SA, Hudspeth AJ. *Principles of Neural Science*, 5th ED, New York, NY: McGraw-Hill; 2013. Figure B-2, p. 1539.)

of vision or even blindness in one eye that is often accompanied by acute pain behind the eye. It is likely that Ms. Dillman was experiencing optic neuritis, during her episodes of blurred vision.

Scotomas or dark spots within the visual field can occur but often go unnoticed by the patient. Neuritis generally resolves within 4–12 weeks. A *Marcus Gunn pupil* can develop after neuritis, which is caused by impaired optic nerve function. Testing for the Marcus Gunn pupil is done using the swinging-flashlight test; when positive, the person's pupils dilate when a bright light is swung from the unaffected eye to the affected eye, instead of constricting. Shining the light in the unaffected eye causes both pupils to constrict (normal function); when the light is moved quickly to the affected eye, the pupils abnormally dilate due to poor light perception in the affected eye (Figure 13-4).

Diplopia occurs when eye movements are not coordinated so that the brain is getting two slightly different pictures simultaneously. This typically occurs when MS affects the brainstem, where the coordination of eye movements is controlled. *Internuclear ophthalmoplegia* (INO) is a common cause of double vision in MS. INO can be identified by impaired horizontal eye movement with gaze away from the affected eye, characterized by weak adduction of the affected eye and abduction nystagmus of the contralateral eye; it creates double vision because of this loss of coordination of the two eyes, resulting from a lesion in the medial longitudinal fasciculus (MLF) in the pons or the midbrain (Figure 13-4). Individuals with MS may also develop double vision from brainstem lesions affecting cranial nerves III, IV, or VI, each of which innervate specific eye muscles; disruption of eye control due to muscle weakness also alters coordinated eye movement, resulting in double vision. *Nystagmus* is characterized by involuntary rhythmic movements of the eye(s), either horizontally (back and forth) or vertically (up and down) and is a natural response to spinning. Lesions of the cerebellum or central vestibular pathways cause pathologic nystagmus, which is induced by looking to the sides or vertically (gaze-induced nystagmus) or by head movement. When working with a person with MS, therapists should assess to see what the effects of impaired vision are on the person's balance and mobility.

Motor Dysfunction

Motor impairments including weakness, fatigue, spasticity, and balance and coordination problems that lead to gait and mobility limitations and falls that negatively impact an individual's participation in work, school, home, and recreational activities and decrease quality of life.

Weakness

Weakness can be the result of motor cortex loss, cerebellar damage, or secondary changes in muscle, related to denervation or diminished use. As described in Chapter 5, force generation is associated with corticospinal projections, emanating from M1; therefore, damage to corticospinal neurons can disrupt force production within specific muscles, typically activated by the damaged neurons. Generalized muscle weakness, called *asthenia*, can result from cerebellar lesions and is associated with complaints of a sense of heaviness, excessive effort for simple tasks, and early onset of fatigue. The cerebellum plays a key role in baseline muscle tone, via its connections with the medial

descending system (vestibulospinal and reticulospinal tracts), and when disrupted by MS, there is a loss of this baseline tone, resulting in asthenia. Finally, inactivity can cause secondary muscle weakness from disuse, contributing to both weakness and fatigue; changes in muscle can include decreased oxidative capacity, impaired metabolic responses of muscles to load, and impaired excitation–contraction coupling. Notably, weakness can vary from mild to severe, and involve one or all extremities as well as the trunk.

Fatigue

Fatigue is one of the most common symptoms of MS, occurring in 75–95% of people. It occurs at all stages of the disease and is not related to the severity or to the duration of MS. Nearly half of patients with MS describe fatigue as the most disabling symptom of their illness. At least 65% of individuals with MS experience fatigue every day, usually during the afternoons. Fatigue is defined by the Panel on Fatigue of the MS Council for Clinical Practice Guidelines as "a subjective lack of physical and/or mental energy that is perceived by the individual or caregiver to interfere with usual or desirable activities." Fatigue, in MS, appears to be distinctly different from fatigue seen in healthy individuals or people with other neurological diagnoses.

The cause of fatigue is unknown but is most likely multifactorial (Figure 13-5).

Fatigue may be directly related to the disease mechanisms (primary fatigue) or may be secondary to non-disease-specific factors. Primary fatigue may be the result of inflammation, demyelination (i.e., slowing and desynchronization of nerve transmission or partial or complete conduction block), or

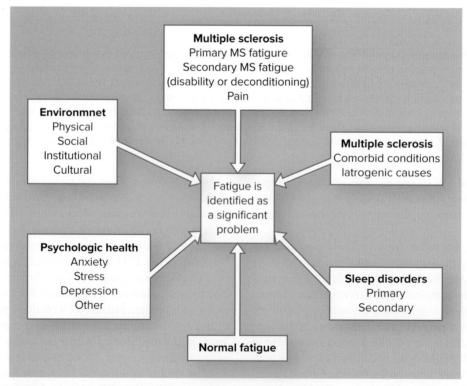

FIGURE 13-5 Multifactorial causes of fatigue. (Adapted with permission from Braley TJ, Chervin RD: *Fatigue in multiple sclerosis: mechanisms, evaluation, and treatment*, Sleep. 2010 Aug;33(8):1061-1067)

axonal loss.[9] Central fatigue develops because of failing central motor drive to spinal alpha motor neurons, which also contributes to weakness. Inactivity, as described in a preceding section, leads to muscle changes that may occur independently of CNS damage and also contribute to fatigue. Other secondary contributing factors include heat intolerance, depression, sleep disorders, side effects of medications (i.e., anti-inflammatory agents, antidepressants, analgesics, and others), medical conditions (i.e., hypothyroidism), secondary complications of MS (infections, respiratory impairment), and physical, social, and cultural aspects of the environment, in which the person lives and works.

Spasticity

Spasticity occurs in approximately 75% of people with MS. Those experiencing greater severity are typically males, older persons, or people with longer duration of MS. Spasticity, associated with MS, results from sclerosis and subsequent dysfunction or death, of upper motor neurons (UMN) contributing to the corticospinal pathways (see spasticity description in Chapter 10: Stroke). As with other conditions that impact UMNs, this damage produces a pattern of signs and symptoms, including paresis, spasticity, hyperreflexia and clonus, involuntary flexor and extensor spasms, exaggerated cutaneous reflexes, and Babinski's sign (see Chapter 10: Stroke), also referred to as spastic paresis. Ultimately, voluntary movement is disrupted and associated with poor muscle activation, synergistic movements, and abnormal co-contraction of muscles. When severe, MS spasticity can lead to abnormal posturing and joint immobility that results in pain, contractures, and difficulty in maintaining skin integrity. Hypertonia in the lower extremities increases the effort required for walking, which in turn, may decrease gait quality and the ability to walk long distances. Common gait deviations associated with spastic paresis include toe drag or foot drop, associated with either anterior tibialis and extensor digitorum weakness, spasticity in the gastrocnemius or both, and induces compensatory techniques of hip hike, trunk lean, circumduction of the leg to the side, and "vaulting" (raising the heel on the stronger leg to more easily swing the weaker leg through).

Balance and Coordination

Dizziness and problems with coordination and balance are among the most common mobility problems for people with MS. Dizziness arises from demyelinating lesions affecting the cerebellum (flocculonodular lobe) or central vestibular pathways. People with MS may report feeling off balance (disequilibrium), being lightheaded, or having the sensation that they or their surroundings are spinning (vertigo). Lesions affecting the cerebellum and cerebellar tracts produce symptoms of ataxia, tremors (postural and intention), hypotonia, truncal weakness, and general asthenia as described earlier in association with weakness. Ataxia consists of decreased coordination that is characterized by *dysmetria* (impaired ability to estimate distance in muscular action), *dyssynergia* (inability to coordinate voluntary muscle movements), and *dysdiadochokinesia* (inability to perform rapid, alternating movements). Postural tremors are observed as shaking, back-and-forth oscillatory movements

during sitting or standing. Intention or action tremors are rhythmic, shaking movements that occur with volitional movements, such as reaching for an object or moving the foot to a specific location. Severe tremors can interfere with functional activities, especially eating, speaking, writing, personal hygiene, and walking. Numbness of the feet, secondary to damage to the dorsal column medial lemniscal pathways, can also contribute to balance and walking difficulties (sensory ataxia).

Gait and Mobility

About 80% of individuals with MS have difficulty walking during the course of their disease. A variety of impairments including weakness, fatigue, spasticity, impaired sensation, vestibular symptoms, including ataxia, and visual deficits contribute to gait issues. Gait is often characterized by staggering, uneven steps, uncoordinated limb movements and improper foot placement, and frequent loss of balance. These symptoms result from damage to multiple areas of the nervous system, as described for the individual symptoms.

Speech and Swallowing Dysfunction

Speech and swallowing are affected by weakness, spasticity, tremor, and ataxia. Up to 40% of people with MS may have speech problems at some time during their disease. Individuals may exhibit dysarthria (slurred or poorly articulated speech) and dysphonia (changes in vocal quality, such as harshness, hoarseness, breathiness, or a hypernasal sound). Scanning dysarthria, speech in which the normal "melody" or speech pattern is disrupted, with abnormally long pauses between words or individual syllables of words, is often associated with MS. Swallowing problems, or dysphagia, can be due to poor coordination of tongue and oral muscles. Signs of swallowing difficulties include excessive chewing duration, difficulty holding food and liquid in the mouth, inability to swallow food, and coughing during or after meals. Chronic swallowing problems can lead to dehydration, poor nutrition, or aspiration pneumonia due to food particles or liquids entering the lungs while eating. Poor posture and respiratory control also contribute to speech and feeding problems.

Cognitive and Emotional/Behavioral Dysfunction

Cognitive Dysfunction

About 50% of individuals with MS have cognitive dysfunction secondary to the disease. Emerging evidence suggests that inflammation and atrophy within the gray matter may be more responsible for cognitive dysfunction than subcortical white matter damage. The cognitive areas that are most affected in MS include information-processing speed, short-term memory, attention and concentration (especially alternating and divided attention), executive functions (abstract reasoning, problem-solving, planning, and sequencing), visual spatial processing, and verbal fluency. In general, cognitive deficits tend to increase with worsening physical disability, disease duration, and a more progressive disease course.[10] Cognitive dysfunction can have a negative impact on an individual's employment status, family roles, social interactions, and independence with daily activities even when motor function is adequate.

Emotional/Behavioral Dysfunction

Emotional/behavioral symptoms and impairments such as depression, aggression, apathy, euphoria (exaggerated feelings of well-being and optimism that are incongruent with the person's level of disability), lack of insight, adjustment disorders (inability to adjust to or cope with a particular stressor), and obsessive–compulsive disorders (anxiety disorder characterized by intrusive thoughts that produce uneasiness, apprehension, fear, or worry) are prevalent in individuals with MS.[11] The mechanisms underlying these changes are thought to be due to white matter dysfunction within frontotemporal neuronal networks that modify a person's behavior, but maladapting coping responses that can occur in chronic illnesses with unpredictable functional decline may also contribute. Depression is the most common neuropsychiatric symptom in MS, with prevalence rates of 50%. Individuals with MS are at high risk for suicide ideation and attempts. *Pseudobulbar affect* (PBA), a neurologic disorder characterized by uncontrolled episodic crying or laughing without any apparent trigger, affects about 10% of individuals with MS. PBA may be related to corticobulbar tract lesions, leading to involuntary laughing and crying.

Autonomic Dysfunction

Cardiovascular Dysautonomia

Cardiovascular autonomic dysfunction has been reported to reach a prevalence between 10% and 50% in individuals with MS.[12] Pathologic findings have been highly variable with sympathetic pathology predominating in some individuals and

---

BOX 13-3   Autonomic Heart Control

Heart rate (HR) is a balance of the parasympathetic and sympathetic inputs to the heart. When there is an increase in parasympathetic input, heart rate decreases; when there is an increase in sympathetic input, heart rate increases. Changing position from sitting to supine is typically associated with an increase in parasympathetic influence with an associated decrease in HR, and coming to standing, conversely, is associated with an increase in sympathetic influence and a slight increase in HR. Similarly, blood pressure (BP) is modulated by the autonomic systems with vasoconstriction increased with sympathetic activation, raising BP, and vasodilation created by parasympathetic activation, lowering BP.

---

parasympathetic pathology in others. Dysautonomia appears more likely to occur in people who have more severe clinical disability. Sweating responses have been found to be decreased or absent in some individuals with MS. See Box 13-3 for a discussion of autonomic heart control.

Bladder Dysfunction

Bladder dysfunction is a frequent and distressing symptom of MS, affecting 80% of individuals intermittently and 96% of individuals who have MS for ≥10 years. Bladder dysfunction severity ranges from mild to severe. Table 13-2 outlines causes and symptoms of neurogenic bladder conditions.

Progressive declines in hand function and mobility (transfers and walking) also contribute to difficulties with personal hygiene and inability to toilet or manage bladder dysfunction.

TABLE 13-2   Bowel and Bladder Dysfunction

NEUROGENIC BLADDER

Types and Cause	Description	Symptoms
Hyperreflexic Spastic Bladder – UMN damage in spinal cord above sacral cord levels	Bladder is spastic; therefore, reflexively voids with minimal filling; bladder becomes smaller over time	Frequent urination; urgency with minimal bladder content
Hyporeflexive Bladder – LMN damage in sacral cord or cauda equina or pelvic nerve	Bladder becomes flaccid, loss of reflexive voiding	Hesitancy in initiating voiding; incomplete emptying (urinary retention); leakage between urination bouts
Detrusor Sphincter Dyssynergia (DSD) – UMN damage	Loss of coordination between bladder contraction and sphincter relaxation	Incomplete voiding with urinary retention, problems initiating voiding
Neurogenic Bowels		
Hypperreflexic Spastic Bowel – UMN lesions above the sacral cord levels	Intact defecation reflex; spasticity in the external sphincter and pelvic floor muscles	Constipation
Hyporeflexic Flaccid Bowel – LMN lesions of sacral cord, cauda equina or pelvic nerve	Disrupted defecation reflex; colonic slowing and internal anal sphincter dysfunction	Constipation or diarrhea; fecal incontinence

Large residual urine volumes increase the risk for urinary tract infections (UTIs) and kidney damage from frequent UTIs.

Bowel Dysfunction

Bowel problems are common, affecting 80% of people with MS. Neurogenic bowel types (Table 13-2) are a hyperreflexic spastic bowel or a hyporeflexic flaccid bowel, both of which are associated with constipation albeit from different neurologic causes. Other factors that contribute to constipation are inactivity, lack of adequate fluids, poor diet and bowel habits, and medication side effects. Fecal incontinence and diarrhea occurs with flaccidity of the external anal sphincter and pelvic floor muscles or secondary gastrointestinal problems (gastroenteritis, inflammatory bowel disease).

Sexual Dysfunction

Sexual dysfunction affects between 50 and 90% of individuals with MS and is a major cause of distress. The most frequent complaints are erectile and ejaculatory dysfunctions in men, uncomfortable sensory changes in the genitals and vaginal dryness in women, loss of sex drive, and difficulty in achieving orgasm in both genders.[13] These impairments may be directly related to demyelinating lesions in the CNS (see Chapter 12: Spinal Cord Injury for details), similar to those described for bowel and bladder dysfunction. Nonsexual physical changes such as fatigue, weakness, spasticity, incoordination, difficulty with mobility, bowel and bladder problems, numbness, pain or burning in nongenital areas, side effects from MS medications, and cognitive problems can also contribute to sexual dysfunction in MS. Psychological, social, and cultural factors that may affect sexual functioning in people with MS include negative self-image or body image, performance anxiety, changes in self-esteem, feelings of dependency, communication barriers with partner, depression, and family and social role changes or role conflict. Individuals with MS should be encouraged to talk with their neurologist or primary care physician if they are experiencing sexual problems so that they can be assessed for underlying causes and receive medical treatment or be referred to other health professionals as needed.

MS does not affect fertility or pregnancy outcomes, and pregnancy does not negatively impact the clinical course of the disease. Pregnant women with MS often experience decreased numbers of relapses, especially in the second and third trimester, due to the effects of pregnancy hormones on the immune system. Obstetric care, labor, and delivery is typically the same for women with MS as for women without MS. Use of disease-modifying immunomodulatory drugs are not approved for used during pregnancy and not recommended during breastfeeding. The risk of relapse increases after delivery and may be alleviated by breastfeeding, use of corticosteroids, or use of IMDs.

● MEDICAL MANAGEMENT

A team approach is needed to manage MS symptoms including but not limited to physicians, nurses, social workers, mental health professionals, and rehabilitation professionals (physical therapy, occupational therapy, and speech/language pathologists).

Long-Term Medical Management

Disease-modifying immunomodulatory drugs (IMDs) are the mainstay of treatment for MS. There are currently 10 US FDA-approved IMDs (Table 13-3) for long-term use with RRMS and relapsing forms of SPMS or PRMS. There are no FDA-approved IMDs to treat PPMS. IMDs have been shown to limit relapses, progression of disease, and new inflammatory lesions seen on MRI. Long-term studies of disease progression comparing patients who do not take IMDs versus IMD users have not been conducted. However, the National Multiple Sclerosis Society's (NMSS) National Clinical Advisory Board, in recognition of the influence of IMDs on the pathogenicity of the disease, recommends that IMDs be initiated as soon as possible and be continued unless there is a lack of clear benefit, intolerable side effects, or a better treatment is found. Most individuals with MS prefer to take an oral medication, as they experience both physical and psychological discomfort from repeated injections. Drug side effects and adverse reactions are common and may negatively affect adherence (Table 13-3).

Treatment of new symptoms depends on whether they are a relapse or pseudo-relapse. A relapse refers to new neurological symptoms or worsening of already existing symptoms that lasts at least 24 hours and that is separated from a previous attack by at least 30 days. Pseudo-relapses are temporary worsening or return of previously existing neurological symptoms. Many individuals with MS demonstrate heat intolerance such that any increases in ambient temperature (e.g., sun exposure, hot baths) or in internal body temperature (e.g., fever or vigorous exercise) can bring on a pseudo-relapse. For example, blurred vision associated with exercise is a pseudo-relapse. This phenomenon is named Uhthoff's symptom after a French neurologist in the 19th century who recognized that heat caused conduction block in demyelinated axons.

Management of Relapses and Symptoms

Acute relapses are usually treated with high-dose intravenous corticosteroids (methylprednisolone) for 3–5 days followed by a gradual tapering dose of an oral corticosteroid (prednisone, dexamethasone) for several days to weeks to reduce the severity of relapses and speed recovery. Adverse reactions of corticosteroid treatment include risk of infection due to immunosuppression, fluid retention, hypertension, hyperglycemia, electrolyte imbalances, and psychiatric/behavioral manifestations. Long-term risks are weight gain, cataracts, avascular necrosis, and osteoporosis.

Pain

Pain is managed according to its pathogenesis. Neuropathic pain from acute paroxysmal sensory symptoms (i.e., dysesthesias), trigeminal neuralgia, and Lhermitte's sign are often treated first with anticonvulsant medications including gabapentin, pregabalin, and carbamazepine (Table 13-4). In addition, the tricyclic antidepressant amitriptyline (Elavil) and the selective serotonin and norepinephrine reuptake inhibitor duloxetine (Cymbalta) are prescribed.

TABLE 13-3 Disease-Modifying Immunomodulatory Drugs

DRUG/INDICATIONS	TYPE	SIDE EFFECTS	ADMINISTRATION
Betaseron Indications: relapsing remitting and relapsing forms, CIS	Interferon beta-1b-immune system modulator with antiviral properties	Flu-like symptoms, injection-site skin reaction, blood count and liver test abnormalities	250 μg taken via subcutaneous injections every other day
Extavia Indications: relapsing remitting and relapsing forms, CIS	Interferon beta-1b-immune system modulator with antiviral properties	Flu-like symptoms, injection-site skin reaction, blood count and liver test abnormalities	250 μg taken via subcutaneous injections every other day
Axonex Indications: relapsing remitting and relapsing forms, CIS	Interferon beta-1a-immune system modulator with antiviral properties	Flu-like symptoms, injection site reaction	30 μg taken via weekly intermuscular injections
Rebif Indications: relapsing remitting and relapsing forms, CIS	Interferon beta-1a-immune system modulator with antiviral properties	Flu-like symptoms, injection-site skin reaction, blood count and liver test abnormalities	44 μg taken via subcutaneous injections three times weekly
Copaxone Indications: RRMS, CIS	Glatiramer acetate – synthetic chain of 4 amino acids found in myelin (immune system modulator that blocks attacks on myelin)	Injection-site reactions as well as occasional systemic reaction (chest pain, palpitations, dyspnea)	20 mg taken via daily subcutaneous injections
Tysabri Indications: monotherapy for relapsing forms; those with inadequate response to or inability to tolerate injectable agents	Natalizumab – a monoclonal antibody that inhibits adhesion molecules to prevent damaging immune cells from crossing the blood–brain barrier	Headache, fatigue, depression, joint pain, abdominal discomfort, and infection; associated with rare and fatal progressive multifocal leukoencephalopathy	IV infusion once every 4 weeks
Novantrone Indications: worsening RRMS, SPMS, PRMS	Mitoxantrone – antineoplastic drug (immune system modulator and suppressor)	Nausea, thinning hair, loss of menstrual periods, bladder infections, mouth sores; urine and whites of the eyes may turn a bluish color temporarily; seldom used due to risk for cardiac disease and leukemia	IV infusion once every 3 months (for 2–3 years maximum)
Gilenya Indications: relapsing forms of MS	Fingolimod – sphingosine-1-phosphate receptor modulator that blocks damaging T cells from leaving lymph nodes	Headache, flu, diarrhea, back pain, abnormal liver tests, cough, temporary slowing of the heart rate	0.5-mg capsule taken orally once per day
Aubagio Indications: relapsing forms of MS	Teriflunomide – interferes with pyrimidine synthesis to affect the production of T and B cells; may also inhibit nerve degeneration	Headache, elevations in liver enzymes, hair thinning, diarrhea, nausea, neutropenia, paresthesia (tingling, burning, or numbing sensation), birth defects if used during pregnancy	7- or 14-mg tablet taken orally, once per day
Tecfidera Indications: relapsing forms of MS	Dimethyl fumarate – immunomodulator with anti-inflammatory properties; may have neuroprotective effects	Flushing and gastrointestinal pain; reduced white-blood cell (lymphocyte) counts; elevated liver enzymes in small percentage of patients	240-mg tablet taken orally twice daily

TABLE 13-4	Symptomatic Medications	
MEDICATION	**MECHANISM OF ACTION**	**SIDE EFFECTS**
Neuropathic Pain Medications		
Gabapentin (Neurontin)	A gamma aminobutyric acid (GABA) analogue. *Note*: GABA is an inhibitory neurotransmitter	Dizziness, drowsiness, peripheral edema
Pregabalin (Lyrica)	Increases level of neuronal GABA by increasing glutamic acid decarboxylase (GAD), which facilitates GABA production	Dizziness, ataxia, somnolence, confusion, blurred vision, peripheral edema
Carbamazepine (Tegretol)	Potentiates GABA receptors	Diplopia, dizziness, hyponatremia, blood dyscrasias, lethargy; contraindicated with monoamine oxidase inhibitors (MAOIs) and bone marrow suppression
Antispasticity Oral and Injectable Medications		
Baclofen (Lioresal)	GABA receptor agonist	Fatigue, somnolence, weakness, dizziness, GI symptoms, bladder dysfunction
Tizanidine (Zanaflex)	Centrally acting alpha 2-adrenergic receptor agonist	Dry mouth, sedation, dizziness, orthostatic hypotension, edema, drug-induced hepatitis
Benzodiazepines: Diazepam (Valium) and clonazepam (Klonopin)	Enhances GABA with anticonvulsant, muscle relaxant, and anxiolytic properties	Drowsiness, cognitive impairment, agitation, loss of libido
Dantrolene (Dantrium)	Muscle relaxant that abolishes excitation–contraction coupling in muscle cells	CNS effects: speech and visual disturbances, depression, confusion, hallucinations, headache, insomnia, seizures, nervousness
Botulinum toxin (Botox)	Binds to presynaptic calcium docking protein and inhibits the release of acetylcholine at the neuromuscular junction	Weakness
Fatigue Medications		
Amantadine (Symmetrel)	Potentiates catecholaminergic/dopaminergic transmission	Hallucinations, confusion, insomnia, and dizziness
Modafinil (Provigil)	Activates the hypothalamus; increases release of norepinephrine and dopamine	Cardiac contraindications and reduction of BCP efficacy. Insomnia, anxiety, irritability, nausea, diarrhea, palpitations. SAE: Stevens–Johnson syndrome
Methylphenidate (Ritalin)	Increases dopamine and norepinephrine in the brain through reuptake inhibition of monoamine transporters	Angina, arrhythmias, palpitations, tachycardia, BP/HR changes, diaphoresis, dizziness, dry mouth
Depression Medications		
Fluoxetine (Prozac) and Sertraline (Zoloft)	Selective serotonin reuptake inhibitors (SSRIs); increases serotonin by blocking its reuptake from the synaptic junction	Anxiety, insomnia, increased appetite, tremors, GI symptoms, headaches, rash, and sexual dysfunction with decreased libido
Escitalopram (Lexapro) and Duloxetine (Cymbalta)	Selective norepinephrine reuptake inhibitors (SNRIs); increases both serotonin and norepinephrine in the brain	Same as SSRIs

(Continued)

TABLE 13-4 | Symptomatic Medications (*Continued*)

MEDICATION	MECHANISM OF ACTION	SIDE EFFECTS
Bupropion (Wellbutrin)	Dopamine and norepinephrine reuptake inhibitor	Anxiety, insomnia, weight loss; may lead to seizures at higher dosages
Imipramine (Tofranil) and Amitriptyline (Elavil)	Tricyclic antidepressants (TCAs); increases serotonin and norepinephrine in the brain by slowing the rate of reuptake	Dry mouth, urinary retention, constipation, BP/HR changes
Bladder Medications		
Oxybutynin (Ditropan), Tolterodine (Detrol), and Propantheline (Pro-Banthine)	Muscarinic acetylcholine receptor antagonists; block parasympathetic nervous system (PSNS)	Anticholinergic side effects: dry mouth, constipation, nausea, dysuria, abnormal vision, dizziness, somnolence
Tamsulosin (Flomax) and Prazosin (Minipress)	Alpha-1 adrenergic receptor antagonist; relaxes bladder sphincter	Dizziness, unusual weakness, drowsiness, insomnia, sexual issues, orthostatic hypotension
Sexual Dysfunction Medications		
Sildenafil (Viagra), Vardenafil (Levitra), and Tadalafil (Cialis)	Phosphodiesterase type 5 inhibitor (PDE5); prolongs phosphodiesterase (PDE) activity, causing vasodilation	Abnormal vision, diarrhea, flushing, headache, nasal congestion, urinary tract infection: contraindicated in history of cardiac disease

Data from Ben-Zacharia AB. Therapeutics for multiple sclerosis symptoms, Mt Sinai J Med. 2011 Mar-Apr;78(2):176-191.[14]

Spasticity

Therapeutic approaches to the management of spasticity are varied. Because spasticity varies so much from person to person, treatment must be tailored to the individual and involves a close partnership between the person with MS and health care professionals to achieve optimal dosing. Non-pharmacological treatments may include stretching and strengthening exercises, bracing and casting, assistive device prescription, and changes in daily activities. First-line medications for spasticity include baclofen and tizanidine (Table 13-4). Therapists should be aware that spasticity can be used to enhance function (i.e., extensor spasticity used to assist in sit-to-stand transfer), and therefore, significant reductions in spasticity might cause loss of function in some people. For severe cases of spasticity or intolerance to oral medications, a baclofen pump may be implanted to administer baclofen into the CSF of the lumbar spine. Improvements in spasticity reduction are usually greater in the lower extremities and trunk than the upper extremities with a baclofen pump. Other oral medications include gabapentin, benzodiazepines (diazepam and clonazepam), and dantrolene. Botulinum toxin type A (Botox) can be injected into affected muscle groups to promote stretching and muscle relaxation. Effects reach their peak in 1–2 weeks and last up to 3–4 months. Injections are then repeated. Botox treatment in combination with physical therapy may improve positioning and mobility and alleviate pain. When all antispasticity medications have failed, surgical procedures such as tendon transfer or selective dorsal rhizotomy may be considered (see Chapter 19: Cerebral Palsy).

Fatigue

Fatigue can be managed with non-pharmacological and pharmacological approaches. Non-pharmacological interventions include aerobic exercise and energy-conservation techniques. Spacing and pacing activities throughout the day, doing strenuous activities early in the morning, prioritizing tasks, taking rest breaks, and maintaining realistic expectations can conserve a person's energy. Pharmacological interventions include medications to increase energy level, such as amantadine, selective serotonin reuptake inhibitors (SSRIs), modafinil, and less commonly used, amphetamines like methylphenidate.

Ataxia and Tremor

Management of ataxia and tremor includes coordination exercises and task-specific training. Medications that have had modest success include clonazepam (Klonopin), propranolol (Inderal), buspirone (Buspar), ondansetron (Zofran), primidone (Mysoline), and topiramate (Topomax). Surgical interventions such as deep brain stimulation to the thalamus may be warranted for certain people.

Walking

Medical management for walking involves the medication dalfampridine (Ampyra), a potassium channel blocker that enhances conduction in damaged nerves. It is appropriate for individuals with all types of MS, who do not have a history of seizures or renal disease. Studies showed that individuals with MS taking dalfampridine had significantly increased walking speeds compared with those taking placebo.[14] Common side effects include dizziness, nervousness, and nausea.

Cognitive and Emotional Problems

Cognitive management in MS focuses on medical treatment, cognitive rehabilitation, and cognitive remediation programs. Evidence suggests that disease-modifying drugs may provide some modest benefit to cognition.[10] Acetylcholinesterase inhibitors, used to treat cognitive dysfunction in people with Alzheimer's disease, such as donepezil (Aricept), rivastigmine (Exelon), and galantamine (Razadyne) have shown some promising results in MS trials. Cognitive rehabilitation programs that aim to improve specific cognitive skills, using computer-based training and neuropsychological counseling, have shown some positive results in people with MS. Cognitive remediation programs that promote behaviors that optimize cognitive functioning such as avoiding smoking cigarettes, improving sleep, engaging in regular moderate exercise, and eating a balanced diet may also be beneficial for individuals with MS.

Management of depression includes medications, cognitive behavioral therapy (CBT), and psychotherapy. Antidepressant medications that are used include fluoxetine, sertraline, escitalopram, duloxetine, buproprion, imipramine, and amitriptyline (Table 13-4). Psychotherapy and CBT have proven to be efficacious for treatment of depression in MS.[14] Psychotherapy can help individuals with MS to accept and adjust to their illness; CBT can help people to improve their coping, social interaction, and problem-solving skills. Dextromethorphan hydrobromide and quinidine sulfate (Nuedexta) are used to treat pseudobulbar affect.

Bladder and Bowel Problems

Management of bladder dysfunction begins with a comprehensive urodynamic work-up to determine the cause of the problems. Treatment for a spastic bladder (storage problem) typically includes medications, dietary and behavioral modifications, and optional surgical procedures.[14] Anticholinergic medications (oxybutynin, tolterodine, propantheline) or tricyclic antidepressants (imipramine) are usually prescribed (Table 13-4). Dietary modifications include increasing fluid intake to eight glasses of water per day and restricting intake of caffeine, alcohol, foods high in acid (tomato or grapefruit), and spicy foods that irritate the bladder. Behavioral modifications to prevent accidents consist of contractions of pelvic floor muscles (Kegel's exercises) to improve bladder control, using relaxation techniques to delay voiding, and going to the bathroom on a regular schedule. Visual and auditory biofeedback can be used to train individuals how to perform Kegel's exercises. Some individuals may benefit from sacral nerve stimulation which involves implantation of a programmable stimulator subcutaneously at the S3 level that electrically stimulates the sacral nerve, causing contraction of the external urethral sphincter and pelvic floor muscles. Detrusor sphincter dyssynergia is managed with alpha-adrenergic blocking agents (tamsulosin, prazosin) and antispasticity medications (Table 13-4). A flaccid bladder (emptying problem) is managed by using techniques to facilitate voiding such as the Valsalva maneuver (squeezing the abdominal muscles to increase bladder pressure) and the Crede maneuver (applying manual pressure on the lower abdominal wall) or intermittent self-catheterization (ISC). In rare cases when bladder symptoms are not controlled with medication and/or ISC, continuous catheterization either with indwelling foley catheter insertion or with a condom catheter for men (Texas catheter) may be required. Surgical diversion of urine through a suprapubic catheter may be necessary for individuals who cannot perform self-catheterization.

Constipation can be treated with dietary changes including increased fluid intake, eating high-fiber foods (fruits, vegetables, whole grains), and/or adding bulking-forming supplements (Metamucil, FiberCon, Citrucel) or stool softeners such as sodium docusate (Colace). Incontinence is managed with avoidance of irritating foods (caffeine, alcohol, spicy foods) or addition of anticholinergic medications (tolterodine, propantheline). Bowel programs involve regular evacuation of bowels (daily or every other day) by stimulating the defecation reflex (spastic bowel) or by manual methods (flaccid bowel).

Sexual Dysfunction

Sexual dysfunction is managed with medications and counseling. Erectile dysfunction in men is treated with sildenafil, vardenafil, and tadalafil (Table 13-4). Lubricants and vibratory stimulation can relieve vaginal dryness in women. Health care professionals can counsel individuals with MS regarding transferring and positioning, and managing secondary symptoms that contribute to sexual dysfunction. Referral to a psychologist for discussions about intimacy, relationships, and communication may be beneficial.

Question: What medications would most likely be prescribed for Sheila?

Sheila will most likely be prescribed a disease-modifying IMD medication, most likely one of the interferon drugs or the oral medications. In addition, she may be treated symptomatically for her bladder dysfunction (i.e., spastic bladder) with anticholinergic medications, for her fatigue with amantadine or other fatigue medications, and for her short-term memory impairments with acetylcholinesterase inhibitors.

● PROGNOSIS

Life expectancy is typically normal or near-normal in the majority of individuals with MS, with 74% of individuals living 25 years after onset of symptoms. The majority of people with MS do not become severely physically disabled. At 15 years, it is estimated that 50% of individuals with MS will require the use of an assistive device to walk, and at 20 years, 50% will require a wheelchair. However, the numbers of individuals in the workforce 10 years after onset is low.

Although it is difficult to predict an individual's course with MS, there are several prognostic factors listed below that are identified in MS. These are only guidelines and do not apply to every individual.

- *Gender:* Women tend to do better than men, as men tend to develop MS at an older age and have the PPMS type.
- *Age:* Young age at onset is more favorable than onset after age 40, which is associated with a PPMS course and greater disability.
- *Symptoms:* Onset with only one symptom is a strong indicator of a favorable prognosis. Initial symptoms that affect

motor control, mental functioning, or urinary control or that affect multiple regions of the body have a less favorable prognosis.

- *Course of disease:* Benign and RRMS are associated with a better prognosis than PRMS and PPMS. Incomplete remissions, a short interval (<2 years) between the first and second attacks, and RRMS that becomes progressive shortly after onset indicate a poorer prognosis.
- *Neurological findings at 5 years:* Pyramidal and cerebellar signs with multiple areas involved at 5 years is a strong indicator of a worse prognosis and the possibility of severe disability.
- *MRI findings:* Low total lesion burden, low active lesion formation, and minimal myelin or axon loss are positive prognostic factors.

PHYSICAL THERAPY MANAGEMENT

Examination

Ms. Dillman is in an acute flare-up of her MS requiring precautions to avoid overwork during physical therapy activities. As noted earlier, MS affects nearly every system in the body, including visual, auditory, bowel and bladder, cognitive, psychological, and sensorimotor systems. Thus, a thorough systems review is performed to capture the impact on all systems and to develop a plan of care that is holistic and individualized. The neurologic assessment, outlined in Chapter 9, should be followed with adaptations made to include more detail in areas that are specifically impacted by MS. Motor control is highly dependent on sensory input, and MS affects both the motor and sensory systems; an examination of sensory function, strength, and motor control is typically performed by the physical therapist either independently or in conjunction with other team members such as an occupational therapist and/or neurologist. A thorough examination of the cranial nerves is highly recommended for individuals with MS to identify the extent of visual and auditory problems so that the therapy plan can be developed to accommodate for these losses and referrals can be made to the appropriate professionals. Assistive devices can be expensive to purchase; thus, waiting until remission to determine if a long-term assistive device is appropriate. CN assessment is also a means of identifying sensory and motor deficits in the face and neck such as Ms. Dillman's loss of sensation on the left side of her face.

CASE A, PART II

Ms. Dillman's CN assessment found no extraocular motor palsy and no difficulty with smooth pursuit (tracking of an object) or saccades (quick bilateral eye movements to orient to an object). This indicates that she will be able to utilize vision for navigation, during mobility tasks. If she were to have motor palsy in the extraocular muscles, she would have difficulties scanning for obstacles that could lead to falls and make driving difficult or even unsafe. In addition, impairments in smooth pursuit lead to difficulty tracking moving objects that can lead to mobility issues in a dynamic environment such as streets, stores, and the home. Since Ms. Dillman lives alone and has no pets, she is unlikely to experience difficulty related to smooth pursuit in the home environment. She has decreased hearing on the left, and her tongue movements are present and equal bilaterally. Ms. Dillman will be better able to hear instructions if therapy personnel stand on her right side and use visual cues that are large and stationary. Her speech has good volume and clarity, and the roof of the mouth elevates on testing; therefore, at present, there is no indication for a referral to speech therapy. Motor and sensory exam reveals intact strength in bilateral UEs except in the hands. She also has decreased finger dexterity bilaterally and *dysdiadochokinesia (difficulty with rapidly alternating movement)* on the left. There is mild strength loss in bilateral LEs. The reflex and sensory exams reveal +3 deep tendon reflexes at the ankles and knees, positive Babinski bilaterally, decreased light touch and pinprick on the left diffusely, and mild vibratory loss at bilateral halluces and medial malleoli. Functional testing indicates increased sway with narrowed base of support (Romberg position), loss of balance with tandem gait, and slow self-selected gait speed. *Question – Involvement of which cranial nerve would lead to difficulty looking down?* Damage to Cranial Nerve IV (trochlear nerve) would lead to impairments in looking down.

This system's review provides a fairly detailed description of Ms. Dillman's major impairments and indicates that she has some difficulties with gait as noted by her decreased gait speed. The systems review has also noted deficits in strength, sensation, and balance. A more detailed examination of these systems is indicated, based on the original review's findings, which will guide the choice of outcome measures. There are many factors to consider, including the patient's and therapist's goals for therapy, expected duration of therapy episode, and natural course of the disease. Box 13-4 lists outcome measures that are commonly utilized when working with individuals with MS and are recommended by the Neurology Section of the APTA along with G-Coding (functional limitation) categories. Given Ms. Dillman's fatigue, the examination is done with minimal position changes and using the fewest outcome measures possible.

CASE A, PART III

Ms. Dillman's short-term goal is to stop falling, and her long-term goal is to regain finger dexterity for typing and walking skill for golf. A referral to occupational therapy should be made. The physical therapist decides to focus on fall prevention until Ms. Dillman has stabilized. *Assessment:* To avoid fatiguing Ms. Dillman and to get a better understanding of the problems that she is encountering in her natural environment, the 12-item MS walking scale is chosen as one of the outcome measures. This is a self-assessment and does not require any activity, but it will give a sense of areas or situations that are most dangerous for her at this time. Other assessments that would be appropriate are: (1) the Dizziness Handicap Inventory to determine the impact of her dizziness on her function; (2) Timed 25-foot walk – to establish gait speed; (3) the 9-hole peg test – to establish a baseline for finger dexterity. *Findings:* The MS Walking Scale indicates that Ms. Dillman is holding onto objects and is very fearful when walking outdoors. She indicated that walking is very effortful for her and she cannot walk very far. It took her 7 seconds to walk 25 feet, which means her velocity is 1.0 m/s, and she was 2 standard deviations below the aged matched norm for her performance on the 9-hole peg test.

The outcome measures chosen give us an objective measure of Ms. Dillman's walking difficulties and will help guide treatment to improve safety and prevent falls. Additionally, they provide evidence that she has a slow gait and a significant impairment in dexterity. She should be educated about the benefits of occupational therapy to find ways to compensate through the use of assistive devices until she is out of the acute phase and then to rehabilitate her dexterity once she is in remission. Fatigue typically is one of the more common and disabling symptoms of

---

BOX 13-4   MS EDGE Highly Recommended Outcome Measures and G-Codes

12-Item MS Walking Scale[a,b]

6-Minute Walk Test[a]

9-Hole Peg Test[c]

Berg Balance Scale[b]

Dizziness Handicap Inventory[+ a,b,c,d]

MS Functional Composite[+ a,c]

MS Impact Scale (MSIS-29)[a,b,c,d]

MS Quality of Life (MS QoL-54)[a,b,c,d]

Timed 25 Foot Walk[a]

Timed Up and Go (TUG) with Cognitive and Manual[a,b]

MS EDGE Recommended Measures for Acute stage

Trunk Impairment Scale[b]

Maximal Inspiratory and Expiratory Pressure

VO_2 max and VO_2 peak

Modified Fatigue Impact Scale

+, Outpatient rehabilitation setting only; G-Codes – a, mobility: walking and moving around; b, changing and maintaining body position; c, carrying, moving, and handling objects; d, self-care.

MS and should be objectively measured. There are several measures available; however, the modified fatigue impact scale is recommended by the Neurology Section of the APTA. Given the impact that MS has on respiratory function, respiration should be observed and measured through maximum inspiratory and expiratory pressure and VO_2 max and VO_2 peak. If deficits are found in the respiratory system, a strengthening program should be included in Ms. Dillman's treatment plan. Objective and detailed evidence of all contributing impairments, including those from systems outside the neuromuscular system, is required to design, safely implement, and measure efficacy of therapy treatments.

Treatment

Therapy, for individuals with MS, is based on disease stage and areas of deficit, including fatigue, spasticity, sensory deficits, change in motor control, ataxia, and functional losses. Information in this chapter, regarding treatment of MS, is focused on the evidence for RRMS. Exceptions, for other forms of MS, are stated where appropriate. Few to no studies exist that examine the use of exercise or PT in individuals with secondary or primary progressive MS, so treatments must be based on what we know from RRMS and consideration of the underlying disease process.

Notably, treatment is very different for individuals who are experiencing an acute exacerbation. During an exacerbation, exercise is not recommended. The nerves are acutely inflamed and exercise could aggravate the inflammatory process. Additionally, individuals with MS are often prescribed high-dose corticosteroid treatment during exacerbations, which can lead to fluid retention, high BP, osteoporosis, and aseptic necrosis.

After an acute flare-up, therapists should check for swelling in the ankles and feet and be sure to monitor BP before starting exercise. Osteoporosis and aseptic necrosis (bone death secondary to vascular changes) leave the bones vulnerable to fracture. Caution should be taken to avoid high impact activities during and immediately after corticosteroid treatment. Aseptic necrosis most commonly impacts the head of the femur, so any complaint of hip pain should be taken seriously and fully investigated to rule out this condition. Individuals with MS should avoid performing exercise and daily living tasks in warm environments as they experience heat insensitivity and often become tired more easily when they are hot. Some individuals with MS experience Uhthoff's sign when they become warm. *Uhthoff's sign* is the worsening of neurologic symptoms, such as increased weakness, spasticity, or blurred vision, when the body gets overheated. These changes are temporary and indicate the need to rest and take measures to cool down. Use of lightweight, layered, and loosely fitting clothing is recommended during exercise to prevent overheating. Additionally, fans can be used during exercise to help keep temperatures cooler, and individuals with MS should be encouraged to drink cold drinks and take cool showers to help refresh and reenergize. For those with severe problems, there are cooling vests that can be prescribed.

Before considering exercise programs with an individual with MS, we must first ask ourselves; "is exercise safe and beneficial for this individual?" It has been determined that exercise does not trigger exacerbations[15]; rather, it has been found to improve muscle strength, aerobic capacity, walking performance, fatigue, balance, and quality of life in individuals with MS.[16-18] Although numerous studies demonstrate that exercise is safe and beneficial for individuals with MS, an additional question is whether the type of exercise matters? This question is difficult to answer at this time due to the paucity of studies. There are studies to indicate that the use of robot-assisted walking is no better than conventional over-ground walking programs to improve walking ability[19] and that whole-body vibration therapy does not yield consistent positive results for strength training. Comprehensive physical therapy programs, aerobic training, and strength training all have evidence in support of their use in MS. Preliminary data from early nonrandomized trials have indicated improved walking from hippotherapy, aquatic therapy, and the use of external focus of attention, which refers to focusing on results rather than the movement details. To summarize these findings, it appears that the type of exercise or therapy does matter, so the type of exercise or therapy chosen should be based on the specific impairments and functional losses to be addressed. Some types, such as strength training, are more effective for posture, while balance improves with a combination of balance, strength, and aerobic exercise. The mechanisms underlying the benefits of exercise in MS are not yet known, but evidence to date suggests that it may impact inflammation, neurodegeneration, cytokine levels, and central nervous system structure; however, the evidence is limited.[16,18,20]

Fatigue

As stated earlier in this chapter, fatigue is a severely disabling symptom of MS and can be challenging to treat. Additionally, it is difficult to determine whether central (changes in nervous system control) or peripheral factors (changes in the muscle or neuromuscular junction) are the primary cause of the fatigue. Peripheral fatigue is more easily treated through endurance activities such as riding a stationary bike or walking. Central fatigue also appears to respond to exercise but to a lesser degree.

Sensory Changes

Sensory changes in MS can be intermittent or chronic, leading to the need to frequently reassess sensation. Loss of sense of touch, pinprick, and localization are often in small areas and intermittent, but when they become chronic or lead to numbness, they can cause safety issues such as burns and pressure sores. The primary treatment for this is to teach the individual to modify their environment to prevent exposure to hot pipes or water and to be aware of the need to check positioning and the numb area of skin at least every 2 hours.

The other common sensory loss in MS is proprioception, which results in difficulty with balance and coordination. Treatment should focus on rehabilitation of the balance system and to teach safety measures when unable to rehabilitate the balance system. Therapy to improve sensory awareness of the limbs and joints focuses on weight-bearing activities that include changes in surface and base of support with or without alterations in vision. Box 13-5 has a list of exercises that can be performed to improve balance problems secondary to proprioceptive deficits. During each of these exercises,

---

BOX 13-5 | **Balance Exercises**

Static Balance Exercises

Narrowed base of support or Romberg – stand with feet together

Sharpened Romberg stance – stand with one foot in front of the other, with the heel of the front foot touching the toes of the back foot

Single limb stance – stand next to a bar or solid object and stand on one leg, 60 seconds is considered normal function

Dynamic Balance

Step front and step back – first step forward then back to neutral then step backwards with the same foot and back to neutral. Repeat with other leg.

Seesaw – swing arms side to side and move knees together and apart, both knees in and then both knees move out

Heel-toe walk – walk placing one foot directly in front of the other

Side stepping – step sideways using hip abduction and adduction

Braiding – lateral stepping, combined with forward and backward crossover steps

Backwards walking – practice walking backwards in a safe environment with a bar to grab if needed

Stairs – work on ascending and descending stairs with a reciprocal pattern

To increase difficulty also do each of these exercises with:

1. Soft surface – use dense foam such that the feet do not sink to the bottom of the foam
2. Uneven surface – walk over uneven ground outdoors
3. Alter vision – use dark sunglasses or place Vaseline on the lens of plastic glasses to distort vision
4. Remove vision – close eyes

instruction should be given to focus on being aware of how the feet feel and the sensation of each weight shift. Exercises are progressed incrementally by narrowing the base of support, changing the surface and altering vision. There is no difference in difficulty level between changing the surface and altering vision, but these should be added one at a time. Changes in vision and surface impact each individual differently and are dependent on the status of each individual's vestibular, somatosensory, and visual system (see Chapter 6 for a discussion of proprioception).

Sensory changes in the upper extremities are approached in the same manner with progressively more complex weight-bearing for the shoulder and elbow joints, which can be done in sitting or standing with arms on a table or in quadruped (hands and knees). Sensory loss in the hand is treated by setting up situations where the individual handles objects of different sizes, textures, and weights. To progress the activities, have the individual identify object characteristics while blocking their vision of the object. Another exercise is to place a small object in rice or something granular like rice and have them find it through the sense of touch.

Spasticity

Spasticity is difficult to treat, and the research in this area is sparse. There are many pharmacological treatments that have been covered in more detail earlier in this chapter. These come with the risk of side effects such as drowsiness, dizziness, confusion, nausea, and muscle weakness. Therefore, non-pharmacological treatment is still an important part of the management of spasticity. Physical activity including both active exercise and stretching on a daily basis can provide relief and is beneficial when done alone or in conjunction with pharmacological treatment. Ideally, the therapy would be initiated at the same time as the pharmacological treatment, and the person with MS is taught to perform the active exercises and stretches at home at least once a day. Choose active exercises that incorporate the spastic muscle groups as primary movers. **Example:** *have someone with spastic hamstrings walk backwards to use the hamstrings in an eccentric activity.* Repetitive transcranial magnetic stimulation has also demonstrated positive results.[21] Other treatments that have been tried but did not show benefit were TENS, vibration therapy, and rock climbing.

Ataxia

Ataxia, common in MS, is another condition that is very disabling and refractory to treatment. Physical therapy for this condition typically consists of exercises focused on relearning controlled and coordinated movements. The individual with ataxia is placed in a position so as to easily visualize the extremity to be exercised. While focusing on the extremity, they carefully move it to a target or goal with attention directed to creating a smooth movement and then return to the starting position. Some examples are given in Box 13-6.

Exercises to improve walking in individuals with ataxia are not specific to MS. The focus is on having the individual perform balance exercises where the base of support is progressively narrowed and vision is altered such as those listed in Box 13-5.

Additionally, practice with dual tasks, such as carrying a glass of water and walking while performing subtraction, are included in therapy sessions for ataxia in MS.[22] Improvements after treatment for ataxia are noted in dynamic balance but generally are not noted in static balance.

It is also somewhat common for therapists to try weighting the extremities or trunk to control ataxia and improve movement quality. There is some limited case-study evidence that this technique can work. Weighting is done with light weights to avoid unduly fatiguing the individual. Weighted vests are applied to control trunk stability and are believed to help provide a stable foundation for limb movements. Distal weighting is done by either wrapping small weights on the leg or arm, at the ankle and wrist respectively, or for the upper extremity, the object being lifted can also be progressively weighted. Feeding tools such as cups, forks, and spoons can be purchased that are heavier than is typical and with larger handle, which may improve coordination during feeding.

BOX 13-6 | **Extremity Exercises for Ataxia and Coordination**

Instructions: *I want you to copy the motion that I demonstrate, focusing on doing it slowly and smoothly.* Typically these are initially done with the individual in a position to watch what they are doing so that they can use visual feedback. To work on proprioception, they can be progressed to being done without visual feedback.

Upper Extremities

Alternate Flexion and Extension – Flex the right elbow while extending the left elbow and then reverse. Also do this with the wrist and shoulder.

Supination and Pronation – Alternately supinate and pronate the forearm. Difficulty is increased by first going progressively faster, supinating and pronating in sync, and then to make it even harder do it bilaterally and out of sync (i.e., the right forearm is supinated while the left forearm is pronated). You can also do this with shoulder external and internal rotation.

Finger Dexterity – Touch the 1st digit to the thumb and then extend, touch the 2nd digit to the thumb and extend, and continue to 3rd and 4th digits. Difficulty is increased by going progressively faster.

Rock, Paper Scissors – Make a pattern using the motions of fist to palm of opposite hand, palm to palm of opposite hand, and ulnar side of hand to palm of opposite hand. Start with a combination of two motions then progress to combinations of three motions. Have the individual with MS copy the pattern that you make. You can have them practice doing the pattern repetitively.

Lower Extremities

Flexion and Extension – While in supine slide the heel toward the buttocks and then straighten the leg back out slowly, alternately flexing and then extending the hips and knees. To make this more difficult, place the heel on the shin at knee level and trace the shin bone down to the ankle, then trace it back up. Focus on making a smooth motion.

Dorsiflexion and Plantarflexion – Alternate dorsi and plantar flexion of the ankle

Bilateral Ankle Dorsi and Plantar Flexion – While seated, first dorsiflex both feet (up on heel), then plantarflex both feet (up on toes) and repeat (See A above).

Alternate Dorsi and Plantar Flexion – While seated dorsiflex one foot (up on heel) while going into plantarflexion (up on toes) with the other foot and then reverse so that the feet are moving out of sync.

Tracing – While seated draw a circle on the floor using either the toes or heel of one foot, focus on making a smooth motion. A circle can be drawn on the floor and the individual is asked to trace the circle. Repeat with other leg.

Any pattern can be utilized and these can involve remembering and following increasingly complex patterns such as using a box diagram, created with tape on the floor (as shown below).

1	2
3	4

Instructions: "Please point your toes first to the 2 and then to the 3," followed by "please point your toes to the following numbers in the order given: 4, 1, 3, and 2." Any combination can be given and complexity and length can be progressed from simple to complex.

Functional Deficits: How Can Therapy Achieve Improved Function?

Treating functional losses in MS follows the same principles as in stroke and other neurologic diseases. Underlying impairments should be addressed and task-oriented practice implemented to improve function. Aerobic conditioning, strengthening programs, and balance exercises are all recommended as part of a comprehensive treatment plan for the individual with MS. Given the presence of significant fatigue, it is often necessary to incorporate aerobic and strength training into functional tasks such that underlying impairments are addressed at the same time that the individual with MS is relearning the functional activity.

CASE A, PART IV

Ms. Dillman's short-term goal is to stop falling, and her long-term goal is to regain finger dexterity for typing and walking skill for golf. The examination revealed that she has slow walking speed (1.0 m/s) and difficulties with coordination. In addition, she has left-sided weakness with strength grades in the left leg ranging from 2/5 in the dorsiflexors to 3+/5 in the knee and hip musculature. She complains of severe fatigue that is limiting her daily functions and causing her to be restricted to her house. During the acute stage, she is given an active range of motion program with stretching to select muscles to minimize loss of function during the exacerbation, and she is prescribed a 4-wheeled, swivel wheel walker (rollator) to improve safety during the acute phase. Once she is in remission, therapy should focus on improving strength, coordination, and independence in community ambulation. Initially, a circuit of exercises can be established with rest periods as needed. The activities should include sit to stand from a standard chair with repetitions guided by fatigue. For example, if she can do 6 before fatiguing, she should do 2 sets of 6, and as coming to standing becomes easier, the activity should be progressed by increasing the number of repetitions. Once she can do 10 repetitions, progression to a lower surface can be initiated; further progression to variable height and stability surfaces (e.g., stuffed chair, therapy ball) can also be initiated. Pulse and BP are monitored, and she should be worked to 60–65% of her VO$_2$ max as determined by the Karvonen formula: (220–age) × .65. Using this formula, she should be working at a heart rate of 101–119 bpm. During her treatment session, pulse should be monitored, and she should be encouraged to continue working until her heart rate reaches the appropriate range; then, she should continue to work, maintaining her HR in this range for aerobic training. She may initially need rest breaks every 10 minutes due to poor endurance but would slowly and progressively work up to 30 minutes of aerobic activity. See Box 13-7 for a summary of general principles of exercise progression in MS. Other activities that should be included in her therapy are the balance and coordination activities, described in Boxes 13-5 and 13-6, as well as walking. She should also perform stretching during her cool down period. Warm up might be done on a stationary bike, since use of the bike will not challenge her balance, as walking would. Finger dexterity should be included in her occupational therapy, and the team should also have her performing golf swings to provide active range of motion and strengthening to her shoulders.

As Ms. Dillman progresses and regains functional independence along with improvements in strength and endurance, she may initiate a strengthening program that involves weight lifting, and she may benefit from continued aerobic activity such as daily walking or use of the stationary bike to maintain fitness.

In addition to therapeutic exercise activities, Ms. Dillman, and others with MS, should be educated about energy-conservation techniques. Energy conservation and work simplification refer to completing tasks in the most energy-efficient way, in order to have enough energy for the activities enjoyed most. Box 13-8 lists principles of energy conservation and work simplification.

BOX 13-7 **Principles of Exercise Progression in MS**

1. Exercise should be prescribed on an intermittent basis with a pattern of a brief bout of exercise, followed by rest, and then another bout until desired exercise is completed. Training benefits using this type of exercise–rest pattern are similar to the outcomes of continuous exercise with an equal duration.

2. For resistance exercise, the rate of overload progression should be addressed with caution, and full recovery between training sessions should be allowed to prevent musculoskeletal overuse injuries.

3. Resistance can be safely increased by 2–5% when 15 repetitions are correctly performed in consecutive training sessions.

4. Cardiorespiratory and resistance programs should alternate training on separate days of the week, with 24–48 hours of recovery between training sessions.

5. Watch for Uhthoff's sign, and provide rest and cooling strategies when this occurs.

6. Given the impact of fatigue and weakness on performing activities of daily living, the exercise program progression should:
   - start by building up participation in activities of daily living;
   - progress to building in inefficiencies to normal daily tasks such as parking a little further away to increase walking distance;
   - move to participation in active recreation that the individual enjoys or typically participates in;
   - finally progress to a structured aerobic training program

---

BOX 13-8 **Energy Conservation and Work Simplification Techniques**

- Plan ahead, set priorities, and balance activities when planning a day. Keep in mind the tasks that must get done and the desired leisure activities. Plan the week ahead of time so that heavy and light tasks can be spread throughout the week.
- Make time for leisure activities.
- Pace activities by alternating rest breaks with activity. Limit each task performed so that fatigue doesn't prevent completion of the next task.
- If it is possible to sit while doing a task, it will save energy. Tasks like folding laundry and mixing up ingredients for cooking can and should be done seated. Keeping a bar stool in the kitchen provides a place to sit to work on projects at counter height.
- When possible, slide objects instead of lifting and carrying them.
- Use assistive devices to lessen the work load. Things like a rolling cart in the kitchen can save energy and enable completion of more daily activities.
- Arrange utensils, equipment, and work area to be efficient. Make sure the tools needed are in easy reach.
- Move heavy and frequently used objects to lower shelves or counter surface.
- Look for ways to make activities more efficient by sequencing activities in a more logical and efficient manner.
- Eliminate unnecessary tasks (e.g., let dishes air dry instead of towel drying them).
- Avoid doing activities in warm environments whenever possible. Do walking outdoors in the morning and evening hours, when it is coolest; use a fan during exercise; drink cold drinks; swim in pools with cooler water temperatures.
- Don't be afraid to ask for help.

Fitness

There is a growing body of evidence that aerobic fitness has a protective effect on parts of the brain that are impacted by MS,[23] including those involved with cognitive function. In addition, individuals with MS who exercise appear to have a slower rate of decline in function.[24] For individuals with MS, there are many barriers to participation in exercise programs, yet fitness is important for overall health and quality of life in these individuals. Barriers to exercise participation include fatigue and difficulty making time for exercise. Some individuals also express feeling uncomfortable working out in public due to the overt symptoms of their disease. Physical therapists can promote and assist in fitness programming by designing programs that are accessible for individuals with mobility deficits and safe to perform outside of therapy. Education is another key aspect of promoting fitness. Individuals with MS should be educated about the role exercise can play in decreasing fatigue and about energy-conservation techniques to help them deal with fatigue.

Exercise and Cognition

Emerging evidence points to possible benefits of exercise on cognitive function in the elderly and in those with neurodegenerative diseases. While this is a new field of study, exercise training to slow cognitive decline in individuals with MS is warranted based on evidence that (1) aerobic fitness, physical activity, and exercise training are associated with better cognitive function in older adults and (2) exercise training has comparable effects on mobility and quality of life outcomes in older adults and persons with MS. See Chapter 17: Aging for more information on cognition and exercise.

Treatment Strategies by Disease Stage

Early Stage

This chapter has gone through general treatment strategies, and Ms. Dillman initially presented in the early stage of her disease, allowing us to apply all of the previously discussed treatment methods to early stage individuals.

Middle Stage

As the disease progresses, individuals with MS typically experience declines in sensory and motor function. The severity of sensory decline has been poorly documented, since sensory function is not included in the Kurtzke EDSS; however, therapists should be careful to measure sensory function and consider its impact on motor function. Individuals, in the middle stage of the disease, develop more difficulty in ambulation and may require assistive devices such as walking aids and orthotics. Canes are the most typically used walking aids, providing additional input to the balance system and improving balance during gait. Canes do not provide adequate stability to prevent falls; individuals with a history of falling usually require the additional support provided by devices with a wider base of support. In choosing assistive devices, consider the impact each will have on the gait pattern and motor control. Devices such as canes and standard walkers lead to a step-to gait pattern, which is slower and more variable than the normal reciprocal pattern. Another consideration is dual-task demands. Individuals with MS walk slower. Double support time is further increased, when walking and performing a cognitive task in those with MS, a change not seen in age-matched controls.[25] These deficits in dual tasking may also make ambulation with assistive devices that require motor planning or cognitive control more difficult. The 4-wheeled, swivel wheel walker (rollator) promotes a reciprocal gait pattern and requires little motor coordination, since it is simply pushed, and thus, would be a low-level dual-task activity. Balance, gait pattern, and upper extremity function are other factors to be considered in device selection.

One of the more frequent problems associated with MS is foot drop. Common treatments for this include the use of ankle-foot orthotics (AFOs) and functional electrical stimulation (FES). Several case studies and small clinical trials have examined the benefits of AFOs in individuals with MS and produced variable findings. There is evidence that the spring-like AFO reduces the work of walking, but the impact of the AFO on spatiotemporal and kinematic aspects of gait is variable. Some studies report improvement in timed tasks with the AFO, and others report no change in time to perform the task. Another consideration in prescribing an orthotic is safety. This aspect has not been studied but is important. Some individuals with foot-drop are unable to compensate through increased flexion at the hip and knee, and so, experience tripping during gait. These individuals are likely to improve safety with an AFO whether they improve speed of movement or not.

Functional electrical stimulation to the peroneal nerve, triggered by a sensor in the heel of the shoe, is utilized in individuals with weak dorsiflexors and everters to produce foot clearance during gait. The FES produces an effect comparable to AFOs and can improve gait in individuals with MS. The benefits of AFOs in MS were less profound than in stroke.[26] There are indications that some individuals are able to regain adequate dorsiflexion/eversion strength to walk without the FES, after a period of FES use.

Late Stage

Ms. Dillman's MS will likely progress from RRMS to secondary progressive MS over time, and her impairments will become more disabling. It was previously believed that individuals in the later stages of neurodegenerative disease could not benefit from rehabilitative therapy. Recent studies have demonstrated that there is some ability to benefit from multidisciplinary rehabilitation, respiratory training, and cooling suits. These studies provide low-level evidence but suggest the need to further explore providing therapeutic interventions to non-ambulatory individuals with MS.

The muscles of respiration benefit from resistance training. A program of expiratory resistance training at 60% maximum expiratory pressure twice daily for 3 months can improve inspiratory and expiratory muscle strength and cough efficacy with improvements maintained after treatment is discontinued.[27,28] There are devices on the market to provide resistance training to the respiratory muscles that can be purchased at reasonable prices. In a study by Sapienza and Wheeler (2006)[28], the protocol was 4 weeks of training, 5 days per week, 5 times per day, and each session lasted 15–20 minutes. Functional improvement was seen in individuals with MS.

Along with disease progression, Ms. Dillman may experience difficulties in swallowing, cognitive dysfunction, and neurogenic bladder in addition to progression of her motor and sensory symptoms. Swallowing deficits can lead to aspiration that can lead to pneumonia. Ms. Dillman should be observed for any signs of swallowing deficits such as difficulty clearing food from her mouth or nonproductive cough; either warrants referral to speech therapy and/or a swallowing evaluation.

If mobility becomes severely limited, a wheelchair should be prescribed. Before purchasing a wheelchair, refer the individual with MS to a wheelchair clinic employing certified assistive technology professionals. Wheelchair prescription considers the individual's current needs and potential disease progression over time. Selection of the appropriate chair is complex. The first decision is whether the chair should be a manual or power chair. A power chair is prescribed when the individual lacks the muscle strength to self-propel a manual chair or they do not have adequate endurance to use a manual chair functionally. In addition, characteristics of the chair and the living environment need to be considered, including: (1) the ability of the user or their family to place the chair in and out of a vehicle, (2) the dimensions and size of the chair in relation to the dimensions of the home or anywhere the device will be used (e.g., workplace, shops, restaurants, parks, cars, and public transportation), and (3) whether the chair is appropriate for the individual's activities.

In summary the management of clients with MS is a complex and ongoing process that benefits from an interdisciplinary approach. Therapists should apply a holistic approach to examination and management of impairments and functional difficulties to improve participation.

REFERENCES

1. Hernan MA, Jick SS, Logroscino G, Olek MJ, Ascherio A, Jick H. Cigarette smoking and the progression of multiple sclerosis. *Brain.* 2005;128:1461-1465.

2. Munger KL, Zhang SM, O'Reilly E. Vitamin D intake and incidence of multiple sclerosis. *Neurology.* 2004;62:60-65.

3. Owens GP, Bennett JL. Trigger, pathogen, or bystander: the complex nexus linking Epstein-Barr virus and multiple sclerosis. *Mult Scler J.* 2012;18(9):1204-1208.

4. Gourraud P-A, Harbo HF, Hauser SL, Baranzini SE. The genetics of multiple sclerosis: an up-to-date review. *Immunol Rev.* 2012;248:87-103.

5. Hansen T, Skytthe A, Stenager E, Petersen HC, Brennum-Hansen H, Kyvik KO. Concordance for multiple sclerosis in Danish twins: an update of a nationwide study. *Mult Scler.* 2005;11:504-510.

6. Pirko I, Lucchinetti CF, Sriram S, Bakshi R. Gray matter involvement in multiple sclerosis. *Neurology.* 2007;68:634-642.

7. Horkova D, Kalincik T, Dusankova JB, Dolezai O. Clinical correlates of grey matter pathology in multiple sclerosis. *BMC Neurol.* 2012;12:10-20.

8. Maloni HW. Multiple sclerosis: managing patients in primary care. *Nurse Pract.* 2013;38:25-35.

9. Induruwa I, Constantinescu CS, Gran B. Fatigue in multiple sclerosis – a brief review. *J Neurol Sci.* 2012;323:9-15.

10. Messinis L, Kosmidis MH, Lyros E, Panathanasopoulos P. Assessment and rehabilitation of cognitive impairment in multiple sclerosis. *Int Rev Psychiatry.* 2010;22:22-34.

11. Rosti-Otajarvi E, Hamalainen P. Behavioural symptoms and impairments in multiple sclerosis: a systematic review and meta-analysis. *Mult Scler J.* 2012;19:31-45.

12. Merkelbach S, Haensch C-A, Hemmer B, Koehler J, Konig NH, Ziemssen T. Multiple sclerosis and the autonomic nervous system. *J Neurol.* 2006;253:1/21-1/25, online.

13. Celik DB, Poyraz EC, Bingol A, Idlman E, Ozakbas S, Kava D. Sexual dysfunction in multiple sclerosis: gender differences. *J Neurol Sci.* 2013;324:17-20.

14. Ben-Zacharia AB. Therapeutics for multiple sclerosis symptoms. *Mt Sinai J Med.* 2011;78:176-191.

15. Rietberg MB, Brooks D, Uitdehaag BM, Kwakkel G. Exercise therapy for multiple sclerosis. *Cochrane Database Syst Rev.* 2005;1:CD003980.

16. Motl RW, Smith DC, Elliott J, Weikert M, Diugonski D, Sosnoff JJ. Combined training improves walking mobility in persons with significant disability from multiple sclerosis: a pilot study. *JNPT.* 2012;36(1):32-37.

17. Paltamaa J, Sjogren T, Peurala SH, Heinonen A. Effects of physiotherapy interventions on balance in multiple sclerosis: a systematic review and meta-analysis of randomized controlled trials. *J Rehabil Med: Official Journal of the UEMS European Board of Physical and Rehabilitation Medicine.* 2012;44(10):811-823.

18. Pilutti LA, Greenlee TA, Motl RW, Nickrent MS, Petruzzello SJ. Effects of exercise training on fatigue in multiple sclerosis: a meta-analysis. *Psychosom Med.* 2013;75(6):575-580.

19. Vaney C, Gattlen B, Lugon-Moulin V, Meichtry A, Hausammann R, Foinant D, Anchisi-Bellwalkd AM, Palaci C, Hilfiker R. Robotic-assisted step training (lokomat) not superior to equal intensity of over-ground rehabilitation in patients with multiple sclerosis. *Neurorehabil Neural Rep.* 2012;26(3):212-221.

20. Courtney AM, Castro-Borrero W, Davis SL, Frohman TC, Frohman EM. Functional treatments in multiple sclerosis. *Curr Opin Neurol.* 2011;24(3):250-254.

21. Missaoui B, Thoumie P. How far do patients with sensory ataxia benefit from so-called "proprioceptive rehabilitation"? *Neurophysiol Clin/Clin Neurophysiol.* 2009;39(4-5):229-233.

22. Kalron A, Dvir Z, Achiron A. Effect of a cognitive task on postural control in patients with a clinically isolated syndrome suggestive of multiple sclerosis. *Eur J Phys Rehabil Med.* 2011;47(4): 579-586.

23. Prakash RS, Snook EM, Motl RW, Kramer AF. Aerobic fitness is associated with gray matter volume and white matter integrity in multiple sclerosis. *Brain Res.* 2010;1341:41-51.

24. Stuifbergen AK, Blozis SA, Harrison TC, Becker HA. Exercise, functional limitations, and quality of life: a longitudinal study of persons with multiple sclerosis. *Arch Phys Med Rehabil.* 2006;87(7):935-943.

25. Gosselink R, Kovacs L, Ketelaer P, Carton H, Decramer M. Respiratory muscle weakness and respiratory muscle training in severely disabled multiple sclerosis patients. *Arch Phys Med Rehabil.* 2000;81(6):747-751.

26. Taylor P, Humphreys L, Swain I. The long-term cost-effectiveness of the use of Functional Electric Stimulation for the correction of dropped foot due to upper motor neuron lesion. *J Rehabil Med: Official Journal of the UEMS European Board of Physical and Rehabilitation Medicine.* 2013;45(2):154-160.

27. Ray AD, Udhoji S, Mashtare TL, Fisher NM. A combined inspiratory and expiratory muscle training program improves respiratory muscle strength and fatigue in multiple sclerosis. *Arch Phys Med Rehabil.* 2013;94(10):1964-1970.

28. Sapienza CM, Wheeler K. Respiratory muscle strength training: functional outcomes versus plasticity. *Semi Speech Lang.* 2006;27(4):236-244.

Review Questions

1. **Which of the following questions is true regarding the epidemiology of MS?**

   A. There is an increasing prevalence of MS with increasing distance away from the equator

   B. There is an increasing prevalence of MS with decreasing distance away from the equator

   C. The prevalence of MS is equally distributed around the world

   D. The incidence of MS is highest in individuals of African and Asian descent

2. **The clear cause of MS is unknown, but which of the following factors are believed to be most important for the development of MS?**

   A. Environment, viruses, and genetics

   B. Ethnicity, diet, and antibiotic resistance

   C. Exercise, blood pressure, and sunlight

   D. Emotional health, diet, and smoking

3. **What pathophysiological process(es) in the CNS is/are involved in MS?**

   A. Inflammation and destruction of the myelin sheath

   B. Axonal degeneration

C. Formation of amyloid plaques

D. Both A and B

E. Both A and C

4. **Approximately what percent of patients with MS are diagnosed with relapsing-remitting MS?**

A. 15%

B. 60%

C. 85%

D. 95%

5. **For an episode of neurological symptoms to be called an MS relapse or exacerbation, the duration of symptoms and the time between the first and second episodes must be:**

A. 6 hours duration and 10 days separation

B. 12 hours duration and 20 days separation

C. 24 hours duration and 30 days separation

D. 48 hours duration and 60 days separation

6. **Which of the following factors is an indicator of a poor prognosis?**

A. Initial motor symptoms (tremor, ataxia, paralysis)

B. Female gender

C. Onset at an early age

D. Onset with only one symptom

7. **What is the most common, and often the most disabling symptom associated with MS?**

A. Spasticity

B. Pain

C. Depression

D. Fatigue

8. **What precaution in regards to exercise is specific to MS?**

A. Exercise can cause muscle atrophy in individuals with MS

B. Exercise is problematic due to breathing problems in individuals with MS

C. Exercise-induced increases in body temperature can cause temporary worsening or return of previously existing neurological symptoms

D. Exercise can induce emotional stress in individuals with MS

9. **Which of the following is currently the best medical treatment for the treatment of an acute relapse?**

A. Plasmapheresis

B. Interferon beta

C. Corticosteroids

D. Antibiotics

10. **Thomas and Sally are planning to start a family but Sally has MS. Which of the following statements is true about family planning and MS?**

A. The risk of relapses is higher during pregnancy

B. Certain methods of birth control are not effective for patients with MS

C. Fertility is unaffected in women with MS

D. Immunomodulatory drugs can be safely taken throughout pregnancy and postpartum

11. **Sally has MS and is complaining that she cannot make it through the day due to being tired. She is worried about her job and her ability to take care of her children after work. To objectively measure her fatigue you would use which of the following measures?**

A. Berg Balance Scale

B. 6-minute walk test

C. Modified Fatigue Impact Scale

D. Timed 25-foot walk

12. **Sally who has MS has been on high dose corticosteroid treatment immediately prior to starting therapy. During therapy she complains of hip pain that is constant and is worse with weight-bearing. Which of the following conditions should the therapist investigate and rule out before proceeding based on the history provided here?**

A. Aseptic necrosis

B. Bursitis

C. Joint instability

D. Radiculopathy

13. **Which of the following statements is true about exercise and multiple sclerosis?**

A. Exercise can trigger exacerbations

B. Exercise does not impact quality of life

C. Posture can be improved with strength training

D. Robot-assisted walking is better than over-ground walking

14. **Which of the following exercises can be done to improve static balance?**

A. Backward walking

B. Braiding

C. Sharpened Romberg stance

D. Step front and step back

15. **Sally who has MS has spasticity of the gastroc-soleus group. She should be prescribed stretching and which of the following exercises?**

A. Standing, go up on toes and slowly lower, repeat 10 times

B. Walk backwards at least 50 feet

C. Perform straight leg raises, repeat 20 times

D. Walk with toes up and weight on heels

16. **Therapy for ataxia in MS includes which of the following?**

    A. Perform balance exercises that focus on weight shifting

    B. Include dual task practice such as carrying a glass of water while walking

    C. Place forearm on table and concentrate on slowing spreading the fingers out and then bringing back together again

    D. Perform resistance strengthening to the involved extremities with weights

17. **Individuals with MS should be worked at what percent of the Karvonen formula (220–age) × _____?**

    A. Less than 40%

    B. Greater than 80%

    C. 60–65%

    D. The Karvonen formula should not be used in MS

18. **Sally who has MS is married with three children and lives in a two-story home. She works full time as an elementary teacher. She has fatigue and is being taught energy conservation and work simplification. Which of the following would be an appropriate modification for Sally?**

    A. Use a rolling chair or stool in the classroom so that she can roll from student to student when helping with assignments

    B. She needs to go to part-time at work

    C. Avoid attending her children's sports activities in the evening

    D. Do all strenuous activity in the morning then rest in afternoon and evening

19. **You are educating Sally about the role of exercise for fitness in individuals with MS. Which of the following statements is true about fitness and MS? Individuals with MS who exercise regularly:**

    A. Appear to have a faster rate of decline

    B. Have poorer quality of life

    C. Experience a protective effect on cognitive function

    D. Have poorer overall health

20. **In the late stage of multiple sclerosis which therapeutic programs are beneficial?**

    A. Balance training with an emphasis on narrowing the base of support

    B. Resistance training to improve walking

    C. Respiratory resistance training twice a day

    D. Robot-assisted gait training

Answers

1. A	2. A	3. D	4. C	5. C
6. A	7. D	8. C	9. C	10. C
11. C	12. A	13. C	14. C	15. A
16. B	17. C	18. A	19. C	20. C

Basal Ganglia Disorders: Parkinson's and Huntington's Diseases

14

Anne D. Kloos and Deborah A. Kegelmeyer

OBJECTIVES

1) Discuss the demographics and etiology of idiopathic Parkinson's (PD) and Huntington's diseases (HD)

2) Compare and contrast the pathological features and pathogenesis of idiopathic PD, PD plus syndromes, and HD

3) Differentiate between the diagnosis of idiopathic PD and HD

4) Compare and contrast typical signs and symptoms of idiopathic PD and HD

5) Describe the clinical course, prognosis, and medical and surgical treatment of idiopathic PD and HD

6) Discuss evidence-based examination of the client with PD and HD

7) Discuss evidence-based management of the client with PD and HD

8) Compare and contrast examination and management of early, middle, and late stage PD and HD

WHAT ARE PARKINSON'S AND HUNTINGTON'S DISEASES?

Parkinson's disease and Huntington's disease are progressive neurodegenerative disorders of the basal ganglia and its connections that profoundly impact motor, cognitive, and psychiatric functions of affected individuals. Parkinson's disease was named for James Parkinson, an English physician, whose work "An Essay on the Shaking Palsy" published in 1817 described six individuals with symptoms of the disease. Huntington's disease was named for George Huntington, an American physician, who published an article entitled "On Chorea" in 1872 that described the disease.

EPIDEMIOLOGY

Parkinson's disease (PD) is the second most common neurodegenerative disorder, after Alzheimer's disease, with an estimated 1 million Americans and 7–10 million people worldwide affected by the disease. There are approximately 60,000 new cases annually of PD in the United States.[1] The average age of onset is 60, and prevalence and incidence rates are very low in individuals under 40 years, increasing with age and peaking by age 80.[2] The disease is approximately 1.5 times more common in men than women. The incidence of PD was reported to be highest among Hispanics, followed by non-Hispanic whites, Asians, and Blacks in one study conducted in a multi-ethnic population in California.[3]

ETIOLOGY AND RISK FACTORS FOR PARKINSON'S DISEASE

Parkinsonism refers to a group of disorders with a variety of different underlying pathologies that can cause Parkinson's-like symptoms, including slowing movement (bradykinesia), tremor, rigidity or stiffness, and balance problems. PD, or idiopathic parkinsonism, is the most common disorder, affecting about 78% of individuals. **Secondary parkinsonism** results from identifiable causes such as toxins, trauma, multiple strokes, infections, metabolic disorders, and drugs. There are also conditions, called **parkinson-plus syndromes** that mimic PD in some ways but are caused by other neurodegenerative disorders.

IDIOPATHIC PARKINSON'S DISEASE

The exact cause of Parkinson's disease remains unknown,[4] but most scientists believe that it is caused by an interaction between genetic and environmental factors. Family history has been shown to be a strong risk factor for PD with a person's risk of developing PD 2.9 times greater if a first-degree relative had PD.[5] Twin studies have reported either no difference or higher concordance rates in monozygotic twins compared to dizygotic twins, when all ages were included, but among twins with PD diagnosed before age 50 the concordance rates were consistently higher in monozygotic twins.[4] These findings suggest that genetic factors play a more substantial role in early onset than late onset PD.

Mutations in various genes have been found in familial cases of PD, accounting for about 10–15% of diagnosed cases[4]; these include: (1) alpha-synuclein, leucine-rich repeat kinase 2 (LRRK2), (2) parkin RBR E3 ubiquitin protein ligase (PARK2), (3) phosphatase and tensin homolog (PTEN)-induced putative kinase 1 (PINK1), and (4) DJ-1. Epidemiological studies have identified several environmental factors that may increase the risk of developing PD, including long duration exposure to pesticides (e.g., rotenone, paraquat) or heavy metals (e.g., manganese, lead, copper), rural living, and well water drinking, which combined may account for higher rates of PD reported among some farmers, industrial workers, and miners.[4,6] Lifestyle factors that have been associated with a higher risk of later diagnosis of PD are previous head injury and taking beta-blocker drugs, whereas smoking, drinking coffee and tea (i.e., caffeine), physical activity, taking calcium channel blockers or nonsteroidal anti-inflammatory drugs (with exception of aspirin) are associated with a lower risk of PD.[6]

● SECONDARY PARKINSONISM

Toxic Parkinsonism

Carbon monoxide, mercury, and cyanide poisoning can lead to parkinsonism. MPTP (1-methyl 4-phenyl 1,2,3,6-tetrahydropyridine) is a chemical that can be produced accidentally during the manufacture of the recreational drug MPPP (1-methyl-4-phenyl-4-propionoxypiperidine), a synthetic heroin substitute. The neurotoxicity of MPTP was discovered in the early 1980s when drug addicts, who had consumed MPPP contaminated with MPTP, developed symptoms of PD within 3 days of ingestion. MPTP crosses the blood–brain barrier and is converted to a neurotoxin that selectively destroys dopamine cells in the substantia nigra.[4]

Post-Traumatic Parkinsonism

Severe or frequent head injuries can cause PD symptoms that are referred to as post-traumatic parkinsonism. This condition can also be associated with dementia. Boxers or other athletes, who have had multiple blows to the head or concussions, and people whose professions put them at increased risk for trauma to the head are susceptible to this condition.

● VASCULAR PARKINSONISM

Vascular (also referred to as "multi-infarct") parkinsonism is caused by one or more small strokes to the basal ganglia (BG). The onset of symptoms in a person with vascular parkinsonism can be sudden, or if strokes are very small, symptoms can progress gradually and resemble symptom progression for idiopathic PD. Symptoms of vascular parkinsonism often involve the lower extremities (e.g., gait and balance problems) more than the upper extremities. Notably, computerized tomography (CT) or magnetic resonance imaging (MRI) brain scans will show multiple minute or more extensive strokes.[4]

Infectious Diseases

Parkinsonism may occur as a result of different encephalitic conditions, most notably encephalitis lethargica, associated with a worldwide influenza epidemic between 1917 and 1926 that has not recurred. The book *Awakenings* by Oliver Sacks movingly describes the case histories of survivors of the 1917–1926 epidemic, most of whom developed parkinsonism many years after they were infected with encephalitis lethargica. Individuals with encephalitis secondary to human immunodeficiency virus (HIV), also known as HIV-associated dementia, can develop parkinsonism due to pathological changes in the BG.[4]

Metabolic Causes

In rare cases, parkinsonism can be caused by metabolic conditions that include thyroid disease (hypothyroidism, hyperthyroidism), end-stage renal disease, calcium metabolism disorders (hypoparathyroidism, hyperparathyroidism), liver failure (hepatocerebral degeneration), and inherited metabolism disorders (hereditary hemochromatosis, Gaucher's disease, phenylketonuria).[4]

Drug-Induced Parkinsonism

A variety of drugs commonly used in the treatment of other medical conditions may cause drug-induced parkinsonism by interfering with dopamine synaptic transmission (Table 14-1). The elderly are particularly susceptible to drug-induced parkinsonism; however, the parkinsonism symptoms typically resolves within a few weeks once the drug is discontinued.

● PARKINSON-PLUS SYNDROMES

Parkinson-plus syndromes are a group of neurodegenerative disorders that share many of the same symptoms as idiopathic PD due to neuronal damage in the substantia nigra, along with additional neurologic symptoms that are not characteristic of PD. These syndromes include progressive supranuclear palsy (PSP), multiple system atrophy (MSA; includes striatonigral degeneration [predominant parkinsonian symptoms categorized as MSA-P], olivopontocerebellar atrophy [predominant cerebellar symptoms categorized as MSA-C], and Shy–Drager syndrome [prominent autonomic symptoms]), cortical-basal ganglionic degeneration (CBGD), and dementia with Lewy bodies (DLB) (see Table 14-2). Clinical features suggestive of parkinsonism-plus syndromes include lack of or reduced response to anti-parkinsonian drugs such as levodopa, symmetrical signs at onset, lack of or irregular resting tremor, rigidity greater in the trunk than the extremities, early onset of dementia, frequent falls, or autonomic symptoms (e.g., postural hypotension, incontinence), visual signs (e.g., impaired vertical gaze, nystagmus), cerebellar signs, and motor apraxia.

TABLE 14-1	Drugs Associated with Drug-Induced Parkinsonism[7]	
ACTION	**DRUG TYPE**	**EXAMPLES**
Postsynaptic dopamine receptor blockers	Neuroleptics	Haloperidol (Haldol) Chlorpromazine (Thorazine) Risperidone (Risperdal)
	Antiemetics	Prochlorperazine (Compazine) Promethazine (Pherergan)
	Gastroprokinetics	Metoclopramide (Reglan)
Calcium channel blockers	Antihypertensives	Flunarizine Nifedipine (Procardia) Verapamil (Calan)
Presynaptic dopamine blockers		Reserpine Tetrabenazine Methyldopa (Aldomet)
Sodium channel blockers	Anticonvulsants	Phenytoin (Dilantin) Sodium Valproate (Depacote)
Noradrenergic uptake inhibitors	Antidepressants	Fluvoxamine (Luvox) Amitryptiline (Triavil) Trazodone (Desyrel)
Norepinephrine blocker/Serotonin facilitator	Mood stabilizers	Lithium

TABLE 14-2	Differential Diagnosis of Parkinson's Disease from Other Causes of Parkinsonism[8]	
TYPE OF PARKINSONISM	**CLINICAL FEATURES THAT DISTINGUISH CONDITION FROM PD**	**EXPECTED COURSE**
Vascular parkinsonism	Usually younger age at onset Parkinsonian-ataxic gait (short shuffling steps with wider base of support and variable stride length), leading to falls Lower extremity pyramidal signs (i.e., Babinski sign, hyperreflexia)	Usually shorter disease duration than PD.
Progressive supranuclear palsy	Vertical supranuclear gaze palsy (downward > upward) Axial rigidity more prominent than limb rigidity resulting in backward lean Frequent falls early in disease, especially backwards	Median survival 6.2 years (range 0.5–24 years).
Multiple system atrophy	Autonomic dysfunction (severe orthostatic hypotension, urinary and erectile dysfunction) Cerebellar signs (gait and limb ataxia, ataxic dysarthria, sustained gaze-evoked nystagmus)	Median survival 9.7 years; gait impairments occur early.
Corticobasal ganglionic degeneration	Early cognitive dysfunction with progressive dementia Marked limb apraxia and dystonia, predominantly in one upper extremity Alien limb phenomenon (involuntary motor activity of a limb along with feeling that limb doesn't belong to person)	Severe disability and death within 10 years.
Dementia with Lewy bodies	Progressive cognitive decline precedes parkinsonism Symmetric parkinsonian symptoms at onset Visual hallucinations Fluctuating cognition	Median survival 8 years after diagnosis.

OTHER NEURODEGENERATIVE DISEASES WITH PARKINSONISM

Other neurodegenerative diseases that are associated with Parkinson's-like symptoms include: (1) amyotrophic lateral sclerosis/parkinsonism-dementia complex (ALS/PDC) of Guam and the Kii island of Japan, (2) Alzheimer's disease with extrapyramidal signs, (3) the rigid variant of Huntington's disease, (4) neurodegeneration with brain iron accumulation (Hallervorden–Spatz disease) or copper (Wilson's disease) accumulation, (5) spongiform encephalopathies (e.g.,Creutzfeldt–Jakob disease, kuru), and (6) primary pallidal atrophy.

PATHOPHYSIOLOGY

The symptoms of PD are caused by degeneration of nigrostriatal dopamine-containing neurons whose cell bodies are in the **substantia nigra pars compacta** (SNpc) of the midbrain and project primarily to the putamen. These neurons also produce neuromelanin, giving them a dark appearance in brain specimens. As the dopamine neurons degenerate, they develop round cytoplasmic inclusion bodies called "Lewy bodies" that consist mostly of misfolded alpha-synuclein protein (see Chapter 17 for Lewy body dementia). Initiation and progression of PD is mediated by several cellular mechanisms, such as failures in the protein degradation machinery, mitochondrial dysfunction, oxidative stress, and continuous alpha-synuclein accumulation; these are driven through cell-to-cell interactions between glial cells and neurons that ultimately lead to cell death by apoptosis.[9]

Loss of nigrostriatal dopamine neurons in the substantia nigra results in **decreased dopamine levels in the striatum**, most notably in the putamen, which has important motor functions. Initially, the nervous system can compensate for this cell loss by adding axon collaterals. However, by the time symptoms are noticed, approximately 60% of the SNpc neurons have already been lost with almost an 80% reduction of dopamine in the putamen.[9] The effects of the loss of dopaminergic input from the SNpc to the striatum is a relative increased activity in the indirect motor pathway and decreased activity in the direct pathway due to the different actions of dopamine on these pathways (**refer to Figure 5-4 in Chapter 5**). These changes, in combination, lead to increased activity of the BG output nuclei, namely the globus pallidus (GPi) internal segment and substantia nigra pars reticulata, and thereby, produce increased inhibition of thalamocortical neurons and the pedunculopontine nucleus (PPN) of the midbrain. The result is a state of stiffness (rigidity) with difficulty both activating and relaxing muscles for isolated movements, leading to the lack of volitional and automatic movements that is characteristic of this disorder; thus, when the patient attempts to move, both agonists and antagonists are activated. Another consequence of BG dysfunction is slow movement (bradykinesia) and reduced movement amplitude (hypokinesia). In part, this may be a consequence of the excessive co-contraction and rigidity. But another factor seems to be an altered perception of movement velocity and amplitude. The person with parkinsonism thinks he is moving faster and farther than he really is.

Basal ganglia circuits are also connected to frontal and parietal lobe areas related to regulation and perception of sensation, so it is not unexpected that there would be some alterations in this system, as well. Loss of dopaminergic input to the striatum also affects associative, oculomotor, and limbic circuits, originating from dorsolateral prefrontal and anterior cingulate cortices, respectively, and contributing to cognitive, affective, and behavioral manifestations of PD (Box 14-1).[10]

BOX 14-1   Four Loops of the Basal Ganglia[10]

Although Chapter 5 detailed the two circuits of the BG (direct and indirect), there are actually four loops that integrate the basal ganglia to areas throughout the brain (see Figure 14-1); each loop begins in an area or areas of the cortex, projects to different components of the BG and then to the thalamus, and back to the originating area(s). The direct and indirect circuits from Chapter 5 make up the **motor** or **skeletomotor loop**. The **oculomotor loop** receives input from the frontal and supplementary eye fields along with the posterior parietal association cortex, an area of integration of visual information, and projects back to the prefrontal eye fields. This loop helps coordinate and modulate the speed of saccadic eye movements. Also, descending projections form the substantia nigra pars compacta to the superior colliculus contribute to the BG's control of saccadic eye movements and potentially impact the initiation of these movements. Disruption of this loop can result in involuntary saccades. The **associative loop** links the BG to the dorsolateral prefrontal and premotor cortices, which are areas of convergence for projections from multiple areas of the cortex, and contribute to executive function, including goal-directed behavior, especially movement planning, as well as problem solving, attention shifting, and dual-task performance – the ability to divide attention between two concurrent activities (e.g., talking while walking). Thus, executive dysfunction is often associated with PD; this is typically mild in early stages but present in up to 40% of patients and can proceed to dementia in later stages. Finally, the **limbic loop** links the anterior cingulate and medial orbitofrontal cortices to the BG and back to the anterior cingulate cortex and limbic association cortex through the mediodorsal thalamic nucleus. This loop contributes to behavioral motivation and emotional regulation. Psychological disorders in PD are common and include depression, anxiety, sleep disruption, and apathy. While these might seem like common reactions to a degenerative disorder, like PD, they often predate the onset of symptoms, leading some to describe a "PD personality"; this is likely due to early disruption of this loop.

A

1. Skeletomotor loop

2. Oculomotor loop

3. Associative loop

4. Limbic loop

FIGURE 14-1 Four basal ganglia loops. A. Illustrations of the four loops: (1) skeletomotor; (2) oculomotor; (3) associative; and (4) limbic. **B.** Cortical areas associated with the four loops. (Reproduced with permission from Martin JH. *Neuroanatomy Text & Atlas* 4th edition. New York, NY: McGraw-Hill; 2012. Figure 14-8, pg. 338–339.)

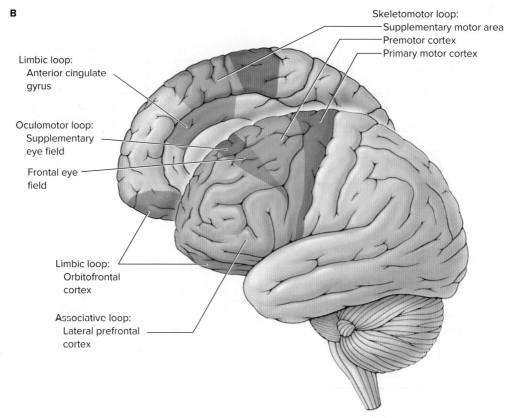

B

Limbic loop:
Anterior cingulate
gyrus

Oculomotor loop:
Supplementary
eye field

Frontal eye
field

Limbic loop:
Orbitofrontal
cortex

Associative loop:
Lateral prefrontal
cortex

Skeletomotor loop:
Supplementary motor area
Premotor cortex
Primary motor cortex

FIGURE 14-1 (*Continued*)

● CLINICAL PRESENTATION

Primary Motor Symptoms

Tremor

Tremor is the initial symptom for approximately 70% of individuals with PD and typically presents as an involuntary slow oscillation (4–6 cycles per second) of a hand or fingers on one side of the body. The tremor is a resting tremor because it is present at rest but usually stops with voluntary use of the body part. Many people initially exhibit a tremor between the thumb and index finger, often referred to as a pill-rolling tremor, but resting tremors may be seen in other body parts such as the forearm (pronation–supination), foot, jaw, or tongue. Stress and anxiety can exacerbate tremors, while relaxation and sleep will diminish them. As the disease progresses, tremors become more severe, of longer duration, and involve both sides of the body, which can interfere with a person's ability to do daily activities. Tremors in PD may be caused by cells within the ventral intermediate (VIM) nucleus of the thalamus that receive abnormal inhibitory inputs from the GPi, as surgical lesions to the VIM nucleus abolish the resting tremors.[11]

Bradykinesia

Bradykinesia, defined as slowness of voluntary movement, manifests as difficulty with initiation of movements and changing positions, such as arising from a seated position, plus involuntary slowing during movements. Hypokinesia, a reduction of movement amplitude, affects all movements and is a primary cause of reduced gait speed and step length. As the disease progresses, individuals may experience freezing episodes (akinesia), in which they have a sudden, temporary inability to move. To overcome the apparent inertia of the limbs, individuals with PD must concentrate intensely on doing even the simplest motor tasks. Movement initiation is particularly impaired when novel or unnatural movements are attempted, or when combining several movements concurrently (e.g., flexing the elbow while simultaneously squeezing an object with the same hand).[12] A proposed mechanism for bradykinesia is that motor cortical areas are inadequately activated by excitatory circuits that pass through the BG. Motor neuron pools in the spinal cord are not provided adequate facilitation, thereby affecting recruitment and discharge rates of motor units, resulting in small and weak movements. This hypothesis is supported by observations of seemingly "normal" movements in otherwise akinetic individuals with PD in response to certain situations (e.g., catching a ball thrown to them or being able to suddenly run when someone calls "fire"). Individuals with PD have impaired kinesthetic perception, such that distances are perceived to be shorter than normal, which may partially explain their hypokinetic movements.[13]

Rigidity

Rigidity affects proximal musculature early, especially the shoulders and neck, and later spreads to muscles of the face and extremities. The rigidity can be of two types: cogwheel and leadpipe. **Cogwheel rigidity** is a jerky, ratchet-like resistance to passive movement, caused by muscles alternately tensing and relaxing, while **leadpipe rigidity** is a more sustained resistance to passive movement. Individuals with PD often complain that their limbs feel "heavy" and "stiff" making it difficult for them to move. Active movement of the contralateral limb as well as mental and emotional stress can exacerbate rigidity. Rigidity of the neck and trunk (axial rigidity) can result in a loss of arm swing, and over time, contribute to a kyphotic posture. As rigidity worsens, it can interfere with a person's ability to turn over in bed, get in and out of chairs, and make turns during walking. Several mechanisms have been proposed to explain rigidity in PD, including abnormally high gain of long-latency muscle stretch reflexes, decreased inhibitory neuron activity in the spinal cord, and changes in elastic properties of muscles secondary to disuse.[11]

Postural Instability

Individuals with PD are typically not affected by postural instability in the early stages of the disease, but as the disease progresses, it becomes more prevalent and worsens. It is one of the most disabling symptoms of the disease because of its association with increased falls and loss of independence. Clinical and posturographic studies have contributed to significant advances in understanding the complex pathophysiology of postural instability in PD, but many questions still remain.

Abnormalities in balance control are a major factor contributing to postural instability in PD. These abnormalities include: (1) reduced limits of stability, (2) reduced magnitude of postural responses, (3) impaired postural adaptations, and (4) altered anticipatory postural adjustments. When standing still, the postural sway of individuals with PD tends to be larger, particularly in the mediolateral direction, and faster with more frequent corrections than in those without PD.[14] When individuals with PD are asked to lean as far as possible in different directions while standing, they move slower and are more fearful to reach their limits of stability, particularly in the forward direction.[15] In response to balance disturbances, individuals with PD demonstrate weak and insufficient postural responses, associated with an abnormal pattern of muscle cocontraction, that delays the return of the body center of mass to within the limits of stability.[16,17] Stepping responses to correct balance loss are late and smaller than normal in PD, requiring multiple steps to stop the movement.[17] In advanced stages, individuals with PD have no postural responses to perturbations and "fall like a tree." Individuals with PD have difficulty adapting postural responses to changing conditions (e.g., switching from an ankle to a hip strategy when going from standing on a large, firm surface to a narrow surface) and are unable to scale the size of postural responses appropriately to the size of balance disturbances.[16,18] Anticipatory postural adjustments (APAs) prior to voluntary movements are also altered in PD. In early stages of the disease, the magnitude of APAs for sit-to-stand transfers (i.e., hip flexion and forward displacement of the center of mass) was larger in individuals with PD relative to controls,[19] but as the disease progresses, individuals tend to have reduced APAs.[20,21] Reduced APAs for

self-initiated walking (i.e., weight shift to the opposite lower extremity in preparation for stepping) result in a longer time to initiate a step. Trembling of the knees that is observed in individuals with PD with freezing of gait (FOG) looks like multiple APAs in preparation for stepping, suggesting that there may be a problem in coupling the APA with voluntary movement (e.g., a step).[17]

Some studies have suggested that disordered sensory processing contributes to postural instability in PD. Proprioceptive deficits have been reported in individuals with PD[22] and may be related to impaired vertical body orientation in PD.[23] When individuals with PD were asked to stand upright on a tilting support platform in the absence of visual and vestibular information, they were unable to maintain a vertical trunk orientation as control subjects did.[24] Individuals with PD become increasingly dependent on visual cues for control of locomotion which may be an adaptive strategy to compensate for their proprioceptive deficits; while normal adults rely on dynamic visual information (i.e., the visual perception of motion of objects in the environment produced by a person's own movement) for ambulation only when balance is disturbed, individuals with PD are highly dependent on dynamic visual cues for the control of their gait speed, even under stable balance conditions.[25]

Over time, individuals with PD develop postural deformities. A stooped posture characterized by a forward head, rounded shoulders, and increased trunk, hip, and knee flexion commonly occurs and may contribute to postural instability by positioning the body center of mass closer to the forward limits of stability. The cause of the flexed posture is not clear but may be related to antigravity muscle weakness, increased flexor muscle tone, or an inaccurate sense of verticality.[17] Alternatively, the stooped posture may be a compensatory measure to prevent falls as individuals with PD become more unstable.[26] Other postural abnormalities associated with PD include **Camptocormia**, characterized by marked flexion of the trunk, and **Pisa syndrome**, which refers to a tilting of the trunk in the lateral plane, especially in sitting and standing.[24]

Falls are typically absent in the early stages, become more prevalent in the middle stages, and then taper off in the later stages as individuals become immobile. Approximately 70% of people living in the community with PD will have fallen in the previous year, and those who have fallen two or more times in the previous year are likely to fall again in the next 3 months.[26] The incidence of limb fractures from falls is significantly higher in individuals with PD, compared with age-matched controls, with about 27% of people experiencing a hip fracture within 10 years of diagnosis.[27] The cause of falls in people with PD is multi-factorial as illustrated in Figure 14-2. Prospective studies have identified disease severity, postural instability, FOG, and cognitive impairment as strong predictors of falls in PD.[28,29] A meta-analysis found that the best predictor of falling in people with PD was a history of two or more falls in the previous year (sensitivity 68%, specificity 81%).[30] "Fear of falling" in some individuals with PD with a history of falls can lead to a loss of self-confidence, activity avoidance, and increased dependence for mobility.

CASE A, PART I

Mr. Martin was first diagnosed with PD at age 60 when he noted that he had a persistent tremor in his right hand, especially when he was relaxing. He works as a vice-president of a large software company. At this time, the tremor is not interfering with typing or writing, but he feels it negatively impacts his image at work as it tends to be more noticeable when he is sitting in meetings. His wife and children also noticed that he was starting to slow down and walk more "like an old man." He continued to work and was started on therapy and medication at that time.

What symptoms is Mr. Martin displaying that suggest a diagnosis of PD?

Answer: His older age, resting tremor, and slowing of movements (bradykinesia) suggest a possible diagnosis of PD.

Secondary Motor Symptoms

Muscle Performance

Compared to neurologically normal adults, reduced muscle strength has been reported in individuals with PD across isometric, isokinetic, and isotonic modes of testing and across muscle groups of the upper and lower extremities.[31] Electromyography (EMG) studies of single motor units reveal multiple abnormalities, including delayed activation and relaxation of motor units, irregular and intermittent discharge patterns, a greater number of motor units recruited at low thresholds, and abnormal coactivation of antagonist muscles.[31,32] Possible explanations for the reduced ability to generate force in PD could be central imbalances in excitatory and inhibitory inputs to motor neurons, peripheral adaptations in motor neurons or muscles due to the disease or secondary disuse, or deviations in the normal aging process.[32,33] Weakness of the lower extremity musculature can compromise functional mobility and independence such as the sit-to-stand task, in which individuals with PD demonstrate reduced torques and rate of force development in the hip, knee, and ankle musculature that relate to their diminished ability to perform the task.[34] Strength changes appear to be related to the disease pathology as strength is improved in individuals who are "on" dopaminergic medications (i.e., levodopa) compared to when they are in the "off" state.

Gait

Gait disturbances are prevalent in middle to late stages of PD and contribute to falls, loss of independence, and institutionalization. Individuals with PD generally have slower gait velocity, shorter step lengths with increased forefoot loading at heel strike, increased step-to-step variability, and increased double support time.[35] Trunk rotation is reduced, resulting in decreased or absent arm swing and "**en bloc**" turning, in which individuals with PD require multiple small steps to accomplish a turn because they keep their neck and trunk rigid, rather than the usual twisting of the neck and trunk and pivoting on the toes. Heel-to-heel base of

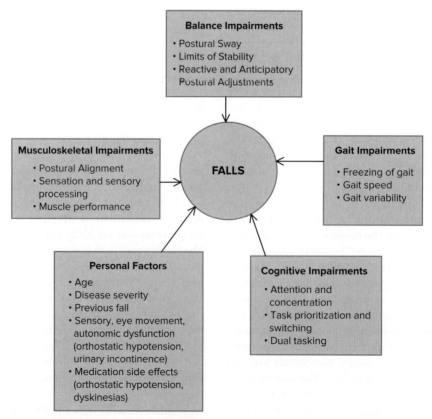

FIGURE 14-2 Fall risk factors in PD. Fall risk in PD is multifactorial, potentially stemming from musculoskeletal, balance, personal factors, gait impairments, and cognitive deficits.

support may be widened in early stages but typically decreases as the disease progresses. **Dystonia**, involuntary sustained muscular contractions that cause abnormal movements and/or postures, often affect the foot and ankle (mainly toe flexion and foot inversion), which can interfere with gait.[36] Increased gait variability is associated with increased fall risk in the elderly and in people with PD.[35] Other features of parkinsonian gait, specifically **festination** (i.e., acceleration and shortening of strides) and freezing (see next paragraph), may also predispose individuals to falls. A forward festinating gait (**anteropulsive**) in combination with a stooped posture leads to forward falls. Backward festinating gait (**retropulsive**) leads to backward falls.

Freezing of gait (FOG) is a manifestation of **akinesia**. When FOG occurs, individuals with PD describe feeling as if their feet are glued to the floor. Five subtypes of FOG have been described in PD: (1) start hesitation – as a person initiates walking, (2) turn hesitation – FOG during a turn, (3) hesitation in tight quarters, (4) destination hesitation – FOG as a person approaches a target, and (5) open space hesitation. FOG is significantly improved with levodopa therapy.[37] FOG in PD has been associated with cognitive and perceptual deficits due to changes in the frontal and parietal lobes.[38]

Dual-tasking (e.g., walking while counting backwards or talking) decreases gait speed and increases gait variability in PD and correlates with impaired executive dysfunction but not memory.[39] Healthy young adults and some older adults tend to prioritize motor over cognitive tasks, when multi-tasking, to avoid falls, referred to as the "posture first" strategy.[40] Studies have reported that non-demented individuals with PD have similar performance to control subjects, adopting the typical "posture first" strategy, during dual-task walking; however, when performing complex multiple motor and cognitive tasks they tend to prioritize the first task and then posture, which leads to greater numbers of errors (i.e., hesitations and motor blocks) on motor tasks compared to healthy young and older adults.[40] Difficulties with multi-tasking also manifest as difficulties prioritizing attention in complex environments. For example, individuals with PD walked significantly slower when navigating through an obstacle course while listening to music compared to without music, while healthy older adults showed no difference in gait speed in the music and no music conditions.[41]

Other Motor Symptoms

Speech disorders and dysphagia (impaired swallowing) due to bulbar dysfunction are frequently observed in patients with PD. These symptoms are thought to result from bradykinesia and rigidity of orofacial and laryngeal muscles. Individuals with PD exhibit **hypokinetic dysarthria**, characterized by reduced speech volume, monotone speech with little inflection in pitch, mumbled and imprecise articulation, and variable speaking rates (i.e., slow speaking rates with rushes of fast speech). Vocal quality is often described as breathy, hoarse, or harsh. Individuals with PD may have difficulties initiating speech, sometimes resulting in stuttering speech. At advanced stages, the person may only be able to whisper or may be unable to speak (**mutism**). Some individuals with PD complain of frequent word finding difficulties, referred to as "tip-of-the-tongue phenomenon." Dysphagia is usually caused by an inability to initiate the swallowing reflex

or by a prolongation of laryngeal or esophageal movement.[42] Dysphagia leads to choking, aspiration pneumonia, and impaired nutrition with weight loss. Excessive drooling (**sialorrhea**) may result from a decrease in spontaneous swallowing, can be particularly troubling during sleep or speech initiation, and can cause embarrassment in social situations.

Loss of automatic movements in PD can result in **hypomimia**, a combination of symptoms that includes reduced facial movements, slowed eye movements, slowed blinking, and reduced facial expression. The face of a person with hypomimia is often described as "mask-like" with a static mouth and unblinking eyes. Hypomimia can be one of the most frustrating symptoms of PD, as individuals who interact with the person with PD may falsely think that the person is emotionless, depressed, or uninterested. Educating family members and close friends about hypomimia can prevent or alleviate any confusion or distress they may be feeling.

Hand dexterity and finger coordination are affected in PD, even at early stages of the disease.[43] Individuals with PD have difficulty performing rapid, repetitive, alternating movements of the hand (finger taps, hand grips, hand pronation–supination) due to bradykinesia. Impaired fluency, coordination, and speed of fine motor movements negatively affects grasp and manipulation of objects, resulting in difficulties in performing tasks such as using a key or buttoning a shirt. **Micrographia**, a form of hypokinesia, is defined as abnormally small, cramped handwriting. Individuals with PD may demonstrate consistently small handwriting or they may start a writing segment with normal-sized handwriting and progress to continually smaller handwriting.

CASE A, PART II

At age 68, Mr. Martin complains that it is becoming very difficult for him to walk on the golf course and that he has fallen three times in the 6 months, since his previous visit to the neurologist. His medications were changed and he received a prescription for therapy.

What factors could be contributing to Mr. Martin's falls?

Answer: A variety of factors could be contributing to Mr. Martin's falls (see Figure 14-2). The fact that his medications were changed raises concerns about decreased drug effectiveness or possible side effects contributing to his falls which should be explored by the therapist.

Motor Learning

The striatum is involved in all stages of motor learning, and particularly, during consolidation of learned skills that consist of a sequence of movements. Studies have shown that learning of new motor skills or fine-tuning of skills is preserved in early stages of PD for those without dementia, but individuals with PD generally take longer to learn motor tasks than healthy controls. Deficits in motor learning have been documented for tasks that require multiple motor programs such as simultaneous movements (i.e., dual-tasks)[12,44] and sequential movements (i.e., switching from one movement to another).[45]

In addition, individuals with PD have impaired speed-accuracy learning or motor skill learning that involves the ability to make fast and accurate movements such as reaching.[46] Brain imaging studies found greater neural activity in individuals with PD in the cerebellum, premotor areas, parietal cortex, precuneus, and dorsolateral prefrontal cortex bilaterally, while performing well-rehearsed sequences of finger movements, suggesting that neural circuits for learning have reduced efficiency in PD.[44,45]

Motor learning in PD has also been shown to benefit from the use of external auditory or visual cueing, particularly with respect to gait.[47] Improved retention of motor learning has been found in individuals with PD when a slightly reduced frequency (66%) of augmented feedback (i.e., knowledge of results) is used rather than continuous feedback (100%),[48] and blocked practice has been found to be better than a random practice, which is the opposite of findings for control peers.[49] Additionally, motor learning appears to be more context-specific in individuals with PD with decrements reported when retention testing was done in conditions that differed from the practice conditions.[50] Advanced disease, dementia, and visual-perceptual deficits can ultimately degrade motor learning. Notably, motor learning may be improved when people with PD are "on" dopaminergic medications than when they are "off."

CASE A, PART III

At age 75, Mr. Martin, began falling again and reported that he was no longer able to enjoy golfing. His wife noted that he was rarely leaving the house, and he was falling daily. They also complained of sleep disturbances and changes in bowel and bladder.

● NON-MOTOR SYMPTOMS

Non-motor symptoms are common and may be more bothersome than motor symptoms for individuals with PD. These include autonomic dysfunction, cognitive/behavioral disorders, and sensory and sleep abnormalities (Table 14-3).

Autonomic Dysfunction

Autonomic dysfunction may be present in early disease stages[51] and is likely due to Lewy body pathology in the hypothalamus, intermediolateral nucleus of the spinal cord, sympathetic ganglia, dorsal motor nucleus of vagus, and the enteric nervous system.[52] Symptoms include orthostatic hypotension, thermoregulatory dysfunction (excessive sweating [**hyperhidrosis**], uncomfortable sensations of warmth and coldness), urinary symptoms (bladder urgency, frequency, and nocturia), and **sexual dysfunction** (erectile dysfunction, and problems with ejaculation in men and loss of lubrication and involuntary urination during sex in women); in rare instances, sexual dysfunction presents as **hypersexuality**, which is more common in men and in earlier onset, yet the cause is poorly understood.[53] Common skin problems that occur early in PD are **seborrhea** (increased oil secretion of the sebaceous glands) and **seborrheic dermatitis** (oily, chaffed, and reddened skin). Decreased gastrointestinal motility, reduced appetite perhaps secondary to loss of smell, and inadequate hydration in PD result in weight loss, constipation, fecal incontinence, gastroesophageal reflux, nausea, and vomiting.

Sympathetic denervation of the heart occurs early, progresses over time in most individuals with PD,[54] and may be associated with fatigue complaints.[55] Exercise capacity (maximal HR, oxygen consumption loads) in individuals with mild to moderate PD, exercising on a cycle ergometer was not significantly different from that of age-matched controls.[56,57] However, the individuals with PD demonstrated lower peak power and higher submaximal HRs and oxygen consumption rates.[56] Similar abnormalities of increased heart rate (HR) and blood pressure (BP) and decreased maximal oxygen consumption during exercise have been reported in individuals with moderate to severe PD.[58,59]

In advanced stages, individuals with PD may present with mild to moderate edema of the feet and ankles, due to circulatory changes, causing venous pooling, related to a sedentary lifestyle and prolonged sitting. This can be relieved by increasing physical activity or with elevation of the feet.

Orthostatic hypotension (OH) is a sharp drop in BP (drop of 20 mm Hg in systolic BP or 10 mm Hg in diastolic BP) that happens when a person gets up from bed or from a chair and can

TABLE 14-3	Non-motor Symptoms of PD		
AUTONOMIC	**COGNITIVE/EMOTIONAL/ BEHAVIORAL**	**SENSORY**	**SLEEP**
• Excessive sweating • Abnormal sensations of heat and cold • Seborrhea • Orthostatic hypotension • Urinary bladder dysfunction • Constipation • Sexual dysfunction • Respiratory disturbances	• Executive dysfunction • Working memory problems • Confusion/Dementia • Depression • Anxiety • Apathy • Obsessive–compulsive behavior • Fatigue	• Anosmia • Proprioceptive deficits • Visuospatial deficits • Sensory integration deficits • Paresthesias • Pain • Akathisia	• Excessive daytime somnolence • Insomnia • Rapid eye movement sleep behavior disorder • Restless legs syndrome • Periodic leg movement disorder • Sleep apnea • Nocturia

cause fainting or falls. Symptoms of OH can include lightheadedness, dizziness, weakness, difficulty thinking, headache, and feeling faint. The two primary causes of OH in PD are (1) insufficient HR increase with position changes due to autonomic abnormalities and (2) dopaminergic medications (carbidopa/levodopa [Sinemet®], bromocriptine [Parlodel®], ropinirole [Requip®], and pramipexole [Mirapex®]).[60] Additional causes of OH include use of diuretics, dehydration, cardiac disease, fever, and anemia.

Respiratory disturbances in individuals with PD typically occur in later disease stages and can be obstructive (difficulty with exhaling all of the air in the lungs) or restrictive (difficulty fully expanding the lungs with air).[61] The obstructive pattern may be related to rigidity, cervical arthrosis, or restricted range of motion in the neck; the restrictive pattern may be related to chest wall rigidity, decreased musculoskeletal flexibility, or a kyphotic posture. Respiration may also be compromised by respiratory dyskinesia, a side effect of levodopa therapy.[62] Pulmonary dysfunction can lead to reduced daily activity and cardiopulmonary deconditioning. A serious complication of respiratory dysfunction is pneumonia, which is a leading cause of death in individuals with PD.

Cognitive and Emotional/Behavioral Abnormalities

Cognitive impairment is present in about 25% of newly diagnosed individuals with PD. Affected cognitive functions in early stages of the disease include executive abilities (e.g., planning, decision making, concept formation, cognitive flexibility, switching between well-learned tasks), working memory (more retrieval than encoding deficits), visuospatial processing, psychomotor speed, and attention, whereas language is usually less affected.[63,64] Cognitive function may progressively decline over time, and some individuals will eventually develop dementia (called Parkinson's disease dementia [PDD]). Risk factors for early dementia in PD include older age, severe parkinsonism, and mild cognitive impairment.[65] Those with the postural instability-gait disorder (PIGD), a subtype of PD, are also at higher risk for dementia. An estimated 50–80% of individuals with PD eventually develop dementia within 10 years of diagnosis. **Bradyphrenia**, slowed thinking, is present at early stages in PD and is related to striatal pathology and depression.[66] Since it may take longer to process information with bradyphrenia, it can be frustrating to both the person and caregivers.

Depression, apathy, and anxiety are also common in individuals with PD. An estimated 30–45% of people with PD develop major depression, characterized by symptoms of depressed mood, loss of interest or pleasure in daily activities, fatigue, poor concentration and deficits in short-term memory, insomnia, and weight loss. Apathy can occur alone or in concomitance with depression in PD and is manifested by a lack of motivation or interest, reduced involvement in social aspects of life, reduced productivity, and reliance on others to structure daily activities.[67] Approximately 25–49% of individuals with PD have anxiety. Panic disorder (sudden and repeated attacks of fear), generalized anxiety disorder (chronic anxiety, exaggerated worry or tension, even when there is little

or nothing to worry about), and social phobia (social withdrawal) are the most common anxiety disorders reported. Symptoms of anxiety can include heart palpitations, shortness of breath, sweating, and trembling. Depression, apathy, and anxiety occur at all stages of the disease, including before onset of motor symptoms. They may be related to psychological and social worries experienced by individuals with PD as well as neurochemical changes involving dopamine, norepinephrine, and serotonin.[63]

In addition to mood disorders, many individuals with PD exhibit obsessive–compulsive and impulsive behaviors, such as binge eating and cravings (especially for sweets), compulsive foraging or shopping, hypersexuality, pathological gambling, and punding (i.e., intense fascination with repetitive handling, examining, sorting, and arranging of objects).[62] These behavioral symptoms have been associated with use of dopaminergic drugs, especially dopamine agonists.[68] Similarly, symptoms of levodopa toxicity include confusion, hallucinations, delusions, and psychosis.

Fatigue

Fatigue is a common symptom of PD and is one of the most disabling. Fatigue has been defined as an overwhelming sense of tiredness, a lack of energy, and a feeling of exhaustion. It manifests as difficulty in initiating and sustaining mental and physical tasks. Clinical studies using questionnaires have shown that fatigue is associated with motor as well as non-motor symptoms of PD.[69,70] Evidence supporting fatigue as a motor symptom of PD include its relationship with disease severity, motor complications (i.e., motor fluctuations experienced during levodopa therapy), prominent postural instability and gait symptoms, and physical deconditioning. Non-motor symptoms that have been associated with fatigue are depression, anxiety, excessive daytime sleepiness, and cardiovascular sympathetic dysfunction. Neuroimaging studies show that fatigue is associated with involvement of non-dopaminergic (i.e., serotonergic) or extrastriatal dopaminergic pathways.[70]

Sensory Abnormalities

Sensory symptoms that are common in PD include olfactory dysfunction, pain and paresthesias, akathesia, and visual disturbances (each will be discussed in the following sections). Individuals with PD frequently report a decline or loss of smell (**anosmia**) that typically occurs a few years prior to the onset of motor symptoms, making it an important symptom for diagnosis.[71] Loss of smell affects a person's ability to enjoy food, which may negatively impact food consumption and lead to weight loss. Olfactory dysfunction in PD has been associated with either neuronal loss in the amygdala or to decreased dopaminergic neurons in the olfactory bulb.

Pain and **paresthesias** (i.e., sensations of numbness, tingling, aching, burning) are reported by approximately 50% of individuals with PD. Pain in PD typically arises from the following five causes: (1) musculoskeletal problems related to rigidity and lack of spontaneous movements, poor posture, awkward mechanical stresses, or physical wear and tear; (2) radicular or neuropathic pain, often related to neck or back arthritis; (3) dystonia-related pain; (4) discomfort due to extreme restlessness (akathisia);

and (5) "central" pain, presumed to be due to alterations in central pain pathways.[72] One of the most common musculoskeletal complaints is shoulder pain or a frozen shoulder (i.e., adhesive capsulitis), which is sometimes the initial symptom of PD. Hip, back, and neck pain are all common complaints in PD. With prolonged immobility of a limb, contractures may develop, usually in the hands or feet. Radicular pain due to nerve root inflammation is often described as a burning pain that radiates in a dermatomal pattern. Dystonic spasms may cause painful foot equinovarus and toe curling, torticollis (abnormal, asymmetrical head or neck position), writer's cramp, oro-mandibular dystonia (dystonia of the face, jaw, or tongue), and blepharospasm (forced closure of the eyelids). Some individuals with PD experience discomfort from **akathisia**, a feeling of restlessness and a need to be in constant motion often manifested as rocking while standing or sitting, lifting the feet as if marching in place, and crossing and uncrossing the legs while sitting. Some people with parkinsonian akathisia are unable to sit still, lie in bed, drive a car, eat at a table, or attend social events. In rare cases, individuals experience "central" pain, described as bizarre unexplained sensations of stabbing, burning, and scalding, often in unusual body distributions such as the abdomen, chest, mouth, rectum, or genitalia. Pain complaints may be greater in people experiencing depression.

Visual disturbances in PD include impaired visual acuity, contrast sensitivity, color discrimination, visual fields, and motion perception. Abnormal saccadic and smooth pursuit eye movements have been reported in about 75% of people with PD. Saccadic (i.e., rapid) movements are slow and hypometric (i.e., undershoot their targets), while smooth pursuit movements have a jerky, cogwheeling appearance due to interruptions by small saccades. Convergent eye movements are associated with outward deviation of the eyes causing **diplopia** (double vision). Reduced eye blink can cause an abnormal tear film and dry, irritated eyes that itch and burn. Visual hallucinations are a chronic complication of PD, especially in people treated with levodopa and dopamine agonists. Anticholinergic drugs used in treatment of PD can cause blurred vision and sensitivity to light (photophobia). Visuospatial deficits have been identified in individuals using visual perception tasks involving spatial organization (i.e., line orientation, memory for spatial location, mental rotation [i.e., see an object and be able to rotate it mentally], object detection, and face recognition).[73] These alterations are hypothesized to play a role in FOG and in the development of visual hallucinations.

Sleep Disorders

Sleep problems may be an early sign of PD, even before motor symptoms have begun. Some of the common sleep problems for Parkinson's patients include: insomnia (problems with onset and maintenance of sleep), excessive daytime somnolence (sleepiness), nightmares, sleep attacks (a sudden involuntary episode of sleep), and sleep apnea (shallow or infrequent breathing during sleep). Rapid eye movement sleep behavior disorder (RBD) occurs in approximately one-third of individuals with PD and is a substantial risk factor for the development of PD. The disorder is characterized by violent dream content that the person "acts out" with talking, yelling, swearing, grabbing, punching, kicking, jumping, and other violent and potentially injurious activities that may involve the bed partner.[74] People with PD are also at higher risk for restless leg syndrome (i.e., throbbing, pulling, creeping, or other unpleasant sensations in the legs and an uncontrollable urge to move them) and periodic leg movement disorder (i.e., periodic rhythmic movements of the limbs that last a few minutes to several hours), two conditions that may seriously disrupt sleep. Nocturia (frequent nighttime urination) is another cause of interrupted sleep in PD.

In Part III, what non-motor symptoms is Mr. Martin exhibiting?

Answer: His sleep disturbances and autonomic dysfunction (bowel and bladder changes) are common non-motor symptoms of PD.

● MEDICAL DIAGNOSIS

Parkinson's disease is primarily a clinical diagnosis based on a physician's neurological examination findings. There is no test that can clearly identify the disease. Definitive diagnosis is only made at autopsy with pathological confirmation of the hallmark Lewy bodies. Diagnosis is typically based on history and clinical examination. Diagnostic criteria have been developed by the United Kingdom (UK) Parkinson's Disease Society Brain Bank[75] and the National Institute of Neurological Disorders and Stroke (NINDS) (Table 14-4).[76]

Differentiation of PD from other forms of parkinsonism is essential. The presence of extrapyramidal signs that are bilaterally symmetrical, lack of response to levodopa, early onset of dementia or postural instability, early autonomic signs, impaired vertical gaze, and motor apraxia are suggestive of Parkinson-plus syndromes. Essential tremor is differentiated from PD by the presence of bilateral, symmetrical low amplitude, high-frequency tremors that are mostly seen during voluntary movement and affect the head and voice in addition to the limbs. Increasingly, there has been an emphasis on identifying biomarkers to help diagnose presymptomatic disease. Early prodromal signs that may indicate PD-specific pathology prior to motor symptom onset have been identified as hyposmia (reduced ability to smell), constipation, mood disorders (i.e., depression, anxiety), RBD, reduced arm swing, and other mild motor function changes (e.g., trouble rising from chair, smaller handwriting, shaking of arms or legs, softer voice, less expressive face, shuffling or tiny steps, difficulty with buttons).[77,78] Neuroimaging (transcranial sonography, MRI [standard MRI and diffusion tensor imaging], and functional imaging using chemical markers to identify deficits in dopamine systems [positron emission imaging, PET; single photon emission computed tomography, SPECT; functional MRI]) can assist in the preclinical diagnosis of PD or in differentiating different parkinsonian syndromes. Elevated alpha-synuclein levels in the cerebrospinal fluid, blood, or saliva are being investigated as early biomarkers of PD.[79]

Due to frontal lobe dysfunction, some individuals with PD display primitive reflexes that can assist in the diagnosis of PD. These reflexes include the **glabellar reflex** (repetitive tapping to the glabellar region of the forehead induces eye blinks with each

TABLE 14-4	Diagnostic Criteria in the United Kingdom and the United States			
UK DIAGNOSTIC CRITERIA[75]		**US – NINDS DIAGNOSTIC CRITERIA**[76]		
Step 1	Slowing of movement (bradykinesia) Plus rigidity, resting tremor, or postural instability	**Group A features**	Asymmetry of symptoms Bradykinesia Resting tremor Rigidity
Step 2	Rule out causes of secondary parkinsonism	**Group B (features that indicate the need to look for an alternative diagnosis)**	Late symptoms that occur early (within 3 years of diagnosis) • Postural instability • Freezing • Hallucinations • Dementia • Supranuclear gaze palsy • Dysautonomia Documented cause of secondary parkinsonism
Step 3	Three of these symptoms: • Asymmetry/unilateral presentation • Resting tremor • Progression of symptoms • Response to PD meds for at least 5 years • Development of chorea with levodopa • Progression over 10 years	**Possible PD**	2–4 Group A features, one of which must be bradykinesia or tremor; no Group B features; and responsiveness to levodopa
		Probable PD	3–4 Group A features, none of the Group B features; and response to levodopa
		Definite PD	All Group A features plus autopsy evidence

tap that do not stop after a short number of taps), the **palmo-mental reflex** (stroking the palm causes contraction of the mentalis muscle on the chin), and the "**applause sign**" (tendency of some patients to continue clapping their hands in response to instructions to clap three times).

CLINICAL COURSE

The disease usually progresses slowly with a long subclinical period (without apparent symptoms) of about 5 years, followed by a gradual increase in symptoms for a mean duration of approximately 13 years. The rate of progression varies; individuals with young age at onset (<50 years) and those with tremor predominant PD typically have a slower rate of progression while those with PIGD, akinetic-rigid PD, and PDD generally have faster rates of decline.[80] Dementia and neurobehavioral disturbances are more common in individuals with PIGD and akinetic-rigid PD.[80] Progression is generally slower with levodopa therapy and mortality rates are improved. Death is usually due to pneumonia and cardiovascular disease.[81] The typical progression of symptoms across disease stages is shown in Table 14-5.

Two clinical measures that are widely used to measure disease progression and severity are the Unified Parkinson's Disease Rating Scale (UPDRS)[82] and the Hoehn–Yahr Classification of Disability Scale.[83] The original version of the UPDRS was modified by Goetz and colleagues in 2008 and was renamed the Movement Disorder Society-sponsored revision of the UPDRS

(MDS-UPDRS, Appendix A).[84] It consists of the following four parts: Part I – Non-motor Aspects of Experiences of Daily Living; Part II – Motor Experiences of Daily Living; Part III – Motor Examination; Part IV – Motor Complications. Items are rated on a five-point scale (0, normal or no problems; 1, minimal problems; 2, mild problems; 3, moderate problems; and 4, severe problems). The Hoehn–Yahr Classification of Disability Scale uses motor signs and functional status to stage the severity of the disease. Stage 1 indicates minimal disease impairment whereas Stage 5 indicates that a person is confined to bed or a wheelchair (Table 14-6). It was modified from its original version in 2004 by Goetz and colleagues with the addition of stages 1.5 and 2.5 to help describe the intermediate course of the disease.[85]

MEDICAL MANAGEMENT

Pharmacological Management

There is no cure for PD. Medical management aims to slow down the progression of the disease through neuroprotective strategies as well as treatment of motor and non-motor symptoms. A wide range of first-line medications is available for neuroprotective and symptomatic therapy (Table 14-7). The physician's choice of medications depends on many variables, including the person's age, symptom presentation, and other concurrent health issues. Starting medication early has been shown to slow disease progression. It is important for individuals with PD

TABLE 14-5	Progression of Symptoms Across Disease Stages in Parkinson's Disease (PD) and Huntington's Disease (HD)			
DISEASE	**PREMANIFEST**	**EARLY**	**MIDDLE**	**LATE**
PD	• Hyposmia • Constipation • Depression/Anxiety • Rapid eye movement (REM) sleep behavior disorder • Reduced arm swing • Mild motor function changes	• Unilateral tremor • Rigidity • Mild gait hypokinesia • Micrographia • Reduced speech volume	• Bilateral bradykinesia, axial and limb rigidity • Balance and gait deficits/Falls • Speech impairments • May need assistance toward end of stage	• Severe voluntary movement impairments • Pulmonary function and swallowing compromised • Dependence in mobility, self-care, and activities of daily living
HD	• Mild motor symptoms (rapid alternating movements, fine coordination, gait) • Difficulty with complex thinking tasks • Depression, aggression, irritability	• Mild chorea (mainly hands) • Mild balance problems (turns) • Abnormal extraocular movements • Mild visuospatial and cognitive deficits • Depression, irritability	• Chorea, dystonia • Voluntary movement abnormalities • Balance and gait deficits/Falls • Cognitive/Behavioral problems • Weight loss • Difficulties with self-care	• Bradykinesia, rigidity • Severe dysarthria, dysphagia • Chorea (may be less) • Global dementia • Psychosis • Dependence in mobility, self-care, and activities of daily living

TABLE 14-6	Hoehn and Yahr Staging of Parkinson's Scale[83]
STAGE (SEVERITY)	**DESCRIPTION**
1 (mild)	Ipsilateral symptoms, involving movement, facial expression, tremor, or posture but not limiting activities
1.5	Ipsilateral symptoms plus trunk impairment
2	Bilateral symptoms but no balance impairment
2.5	Mild–moderate; able to recover balance from posterior pull
Stage 3 (moderate)	Moderate disability affecting mobility and balance with bradykinesia
Stage 4 (severe)	Limited walking; requires caregiving assistance so can't live alone; diminishing tremor with increased rigidity and bradykinesia
Stage 5 (cachectic)	Unable to stand or walk; nursing care required

to take medications on a fixed schedule to maintain adequate levels of drugs in the bloodstream. According to the National Parkinson Foundation (NPF), three out of four individuals with PD do not receive medications on time in the hospital, resulting in serious complications. The Aware in Care kit found on the NPF website[86] can help patients, caregivers, and health professionals to avoid these complications.

Levodopa/Carbidopa (Sinemet®)

Levodopa (L-dopa) is the most potent treatment for PD, since it became widely available in the late 1960s. It is a dopamine precursor that is converted into dopamine by the enzyme dopa-decarboxylase within nerve cells in the brain. L-dopa administered by itself is almost entirely (99%) metabolized in the bloodstream before it reaches the brain, requiring administration of high doses that produce unpleasant side effects (i.e., nausea and vomiting). Therefore, it is combined with carbidopa, a decarboxylase inhibitor that prevents the peripheral metabolism of L-dopa, allowing therapeutic concentrations of L-dopa to enter the brain without unwanted side effects. The best known levodopa/carbidopa formulation is called Sinemet®. Sinemet tablets are available in many different ratios of carbidopa to levodopa (e.g., 10/100, 25/100, 50/200, and 25/250) and formulations, including short-acting immediate-release (IR) and long-acting controlled-release (CR) forms. There is also a formulation that dissolves in the mouth without water called Parcopa®.[88]

The primary effects of L-dopa therapy are to reduce motor symptoms of bradykinesia and rigidity, allowing increased speed of movement and strength. The effect of L-dopa on tremors is equivocal, with some individuals getting a reduction in tremor amplitude while others have little to no benefit. L-dopa's effects on postural instability have also been varied, with L-dopa causing improvements or worsening of postural sway in quiet stance, worsening of reactive postural adjustments, and

TABLE 14-7	Medications for PD[87]		
DRUG	**ACTION**	**SIDE EFFECTS**	**BRAND NAMES**
Levodopa/Carbidopa	L-dopa converted to dopamine in brain to restore DA levels.	Orthostatic hypotension, dyskinesias, hallucinations, sleepiness.	Sinemet, immediate and sustained release; Parcopa
Dopamine agonists	Directly stimulate postsynaptic dopamine receptors.	Nausea, sedation, dizziness, constipation, hallucinations. Linked to impulse control disorders (e.g., pathological gambling, compulsive shopping, hypersexuality).	Pramipexole (Mirapex), ropinirole (Requip), piribedil (Trivastal), rotigotine transdermal patch (Neupro), apomorphine (Uprima)
Anticholinergics	Block acetylcholine receptors and may inhibit dopamine reuptake in striatum.	Blurred vision, dry mouth, dizziness, and urinary retention; toxicity causes impaired memory, confusion, hallucinations, and delusions.	Trihexyphenidyl HCl (Artane), benztropine mesylate (Cogentin), procyclidine hydrochloride (Kemadrin)
Catechol-o-methyl transferase (COMT) inhibitors	Inhibits enzyme COMT to prevent degradation of dopamine.	Dyskinesia, nausea, vomiting, orthostatic hypotension, sleep disorders, hallucinations, diarrhea, liver damage with tolcapone	Entacapone (Comtan), entacapone and levodopa (Stalevo), tolcapone (Tasmar)
Monoamine oxidase B(MAO-B) inhibitors	Inhibits enzyme MAO-B to prevent degradation of dopamine.	Mild nausea, dry mouth, dizziness, orthostatic hypotension, confusion, hallucinations, insomnia	Selegiline hydrochloride (Eldepryl), rasagiline (Azilect)
Amantadine	Increases release of dopamine presynaptically; blocks acetylcholine receptors	Dizziness, nausea, and anorexia, livedo reticularis (i.e., purplish red blotchy spots on skin), leg edema, confusion, hallucinations	Amantadine hydrochloride (Symmetrel), Symadine

improvements in APAs and dynamic balance.[17] The decision about when to start levodopa/carbidopa is different for every person with PD and requires consideration of potential benefits, risks, and the availability of alternatives. Dramatic improvements in functional status are often observed with the initiation of levodopa therapy, and for a period of time (typically between 4 and 6 years), called the "honeymoon period," the drug provides sustained symptomatic relief with minimal side effects.

With increased dosing and prolonged use of L-dopa, individuals with PD experience a wearing-off state where the drug becomes less effective. At the same time, bothersome side effects of dyskinesia, dystonia, and motor fluctuations appear. **Dyskinesia** refers to uncontrolled, involuntary movements that typically present as **chorea** or **choreoathetosis** on the side most affected by PD, usually in the legs before the arms,[89] as discussed in Chapter 19 for cerebral palsy. **Chorea** refers to involuntary, rapid, irregular, purposeless, and unsustained movements that seem to flow from one body part to another. When writhing athetoid movements are superimposed on chorea it is called **choreoathetosis**. They may start as small movements in one area of the body and progress to large amplitude movements in multiple body parts. Dyskinesia typically involves the trunk, neck, head, and limbs; it is commonly seen at peak dose or when L-dopa levels are rising or wearing off, known as "**diphasic dyskinesia**." Individuals with young onset PD are more prone to getting dyskinesia. **Dystonia** among

people on dopaminergic therapy usually occurs during "off" periods (i.e., early in morning or between doses), typically involves dystonic inversion of the foot,[36] and is present at peak dose, affecting most often the neck and face. Diphasic dystonia can also occur and usually affects the leg and ipsilateral arm. Motor fluctuations include "on–off" phenomenon and wearing-off. The **on–off phenomenon** refers to periods when the medication unpredictably starts or stops working. Wearing-off refers to **end-of-dose deterioration**, a worsening of symptoms near the end of the timeframe when levodopa is expected to be effective. The underlying mechanisms of levodopa-induced dyskinesia (LID) and motor fluctuations are unclear but pulsatile dopamine stimulation (fluctuation of dopamine levels) of striatal postsynaptic receptors is important in its pathogenesis.[90] American Academy of Neurology practice guidelines for treating LID and motor fluctuations recommends administration of entacapone (Comtan) or rasagiline (Azilect) as firstline medications to reduce "off" time, amantadine to reduce dyskinesias, and deep brain stimulation to the subthalamic nucleus (STN) to reduce both.[91]

Dopamine Agonists

Dopamine agonists are often administered alone in individuals newly diagnosed, especially those younger than 60, because they can delay the need for levodopa and thus postpone the motor complications that occur with long-term levodopa therapy.

Dopamine agonists are also administered along with levodopa/carbidopa to reduce the amount of L-dopa needed and thereby prolong its effectiveness. In middle to late stages of the disease, dopamine agonists are often given, when (1) levodopa alone is not able to control symptoms and increasing the dose would cause excessive side effects or (2) the person taking levodopa is experiencing severe motor fluctuations. Agonists tend to be most effective for reducing bradykinesia and rigidity.

Apomorphine is an injectable, rapid-acting dopamine agonist that is usually effective within 10 minutes of injection and produces effects comparable to L-dopa for approximately 60–90 minutes. Because of its rapid effects it is used as a "rescue therapy" for individuals with PD, who are experiencing freezing episodes that are not relieved with L-dopa or other dopamine agonists.[87]

Anticholinergics

Interneurons in the striatum that release acetylcholine have antagonistic effects to dopamine on medium spiny striatal neurons that are part of the direct and indirect motor pathways through the BG; acetylcholine increases the excitability of neurons in the indirect pathway and inhibits neurons in the direct pathway.[92] There are also modulatory interactions between acetylcholine and dopamine in the striatum; acetylcholine triggers release of dopamine from nigrostriatal neurons while dopamine inhibits release of acetylcholine from striatal interneurons. Depletion of striatal dopamine, due to loss of nigrostriatal neurons in PD, causes increased excitability of cholinergic interneurons, thereby, causing a reduction in movement. Therefore, anticholinergic drugs that block the action of acetylcholine are used to treat PD. These drugs are most helpful to younger patients with PD, whose chief complaint is tremor, and for those individuals with dystonia that is not relieved with L-dopa.

Enzyme Inhibitors

Some anti-Parkinson drugs act by inhibiting enzymes that degrade dopamine, so that levels of striatal dopamine are enhanced. Two enzymes that break down dopamine are catechol-o-methyltransferase (COMT) and monoamine oxidase B (MAO-B). COMT inhibitors are always taken in combination with levodopa or with other anti-parkinsonian drugs. MAO-B inhibitors (e.g., selegiline and rasagiline) may have neuroprotective and neurorestorative effects and are usually used alone early in the disease to delay the need for levodopa.[93] In more advanced PD, they are combined with levodopa to decrease freezing episodes and motor fluctuations.

Amantadine

Amantadine was originally developed as an antiviral agent and was found in 1969 to reduce motor symptoms of PD. It can be used alone but typically is combined with other dopamine agonists and anticholinergics. It is beneficial for treating tremors and to treat dyskinesia that is unresponsive to conventional measures such as reduction of levodopa.

Physical Therapy Implications of Pharmacological Management

Physical therapists need to be aware of the medications that a person with PD is taking and their potential side effects.

Therapists should try to schedule their examination and treatments at a consistent time when the person is optimally dosed. If a person is experiencing motor fluctuations, the therapist should also assess the individual with PD during "off" times. Therapists need to monitor drug effectiveness on the person with PD's motor performance and functional status and communicate their observations and examination findings about any changes in functional status to the physician to assist in drug prescription.

CASE A, PART IV: PARKINSON DISEASE AT AGE 80

Mr. Martin requires care around the clock and is no longer ambulating. His wife reports that she has an aide that comes daily but she has injured her back transferring her husband, when the aide is not present. She is also concerned because Mr. Martin is having difficulty eating and taking his medication. She does not feel that the medication is helping him and reports that, when they increased the dosage, he developed "jerky movements" and was complaining that he could see snakes on the walls of the bedroom at night.

What is the cause of Mr. Martin's "jerky movements" and hallucinations?

Answer: He is most likely exhibiting dyskinesia and hallucinations due to long-term levodopa therapy.

In Part I, Mr. Martin is in the early stage of PD with a typical early presentation of resting tremor in the hand and bradykinesia. He continues to work, and therapy is focused on rehabilitation of his impairments and prevention of progression of motor symptoms. He is likely taking dopamine agonists and may not be on carbidopa–levodopa, at this time.

By Parts II and III of the case, he is likely to be on carbidopa–levodopa, and by Parts III and IV, he is likely having on/off episodes with his medication as well as unwanted medication side effects such as hallucinations, dyskinesia, or dystonia. Determining the medication schedule is particularly important for individuals who use carbidopa–levodopa because their ability to participate in therapy is best at peak dose, and some functional deficits are more likely to be evident at the end of their dose cycle. Therapists develop a plan of care to develop ways to maintain functional independence during both peak dose and end of dose times.

Nutritional Management

When foods with high protein content are ingested at the same time as L-dopa, they can interfere with the absorption of L-dopa. Therefore, individuals with PD may be advised to take L-dopa 30–45 minutes prior to meals and may also be prescribed a low-protein diet or protein redistribution, where most protein is eaten in the evening with the advice of a dietician. Individuals with PD should be encouraged to eat a healthy diet and may be advised to take food supplements for nutritional support, if they are losing weight or are underweight. Individuals with constipation are advised to drink more fluids and eat more fiber-rich foods. Occupational therapists help people with PD to improve upper extremity movements for feeding and recommend adaptive eating devices. Speech-language pathologists evaluate for dysphagia and recommend interventions to assist with swallowing dysfunction. A percutaneous endoscopic gastrostomy (PEG) may be necessary in advanced stages to maintain adequate nutrition.

Deep Brain Stimulation and Surgical Treatments

Deep brain stimulation (DBS) involves surgical implantation of a battery-operated medical device, called an implantable pulse generator (IPG), in the sub-clavicular area. This is connected by a thin wire that passes under the skin to electrodes that deliver high-frequency electrical stimulation to specific areas in the brain, thereby, blocking abnormal nerve signals that cause parkinsonian motor symptoms. DBS changes the brain firing pattern but does not slow the progression of the neurodegeneration. Areas that are typically stimulated in PD are the thalamus (Ventral Intermediate nucleus), subthalamic nucleus, globus pallidus internal segment and pedunculopontine nucleus. Following surgery, the physician adjusts the amount of stimulation provided by the device to best meet the individual's needs, thereafter, the person with PD can control the IPG's "on–off" switch externally, using a controller. The IPGs typically last 3–5 years, and the replacement procedure is relatively simple. DBS is presently used only for individuals whose symptoms cannot be adequately controlled with medications but are still responsive to levodopa to some degree; DBS is not effective for those who are no longer responding to levodopa. Many individuals experience a reduction of motor symptoms (i.e., tremors, rigidity, akinesia) with DBS and can reduce their medications, thereby, reducing side effects such as dyskinesia. Some improvements in gait disturbances and FOG have been observed with DBS of the STN with better effects from bilateral stimulation. DBS has equivocal effect on balance with both improvements or worsening reported, depending on the site of stimulation.[17] DBS does not improve cognitive symptoms in PD and may worsen them, so generally, it is not used when there are signs of dementia.

Palliative surgery to reduce parkinsonian symptoms includes pallidotomy and thalamotomy. **Pallidotomy** surgically destroys the GPi to reduce tremor, bradykinesia, rigidity, and LIDs. **Thalamotomy** destroys part of the ventral lateral nucleus of the thalamus to relieve tremors. Both surgeries can have serious complications and since DBS is available, are infrequently performed. **Restorative surgeries** to replace striatal dopamine or improve function of dopaminergic cells, such as fetal cell transplantation, gene therapy, and stem cell therapy are promising experimental treatments for PD. **Intrastriatal transplantation** of human embryonic mesencephalic dopamine rich tissue into individuals with PD has induced variable functional outcomes, with some, but not all, individuals showing significant improvements in motor symptoms.[94] Gene therapy for PD aims to surgically implant genetically modified cells that are incorporated into targeted cells in the striatum to produce enzymes that increase dopamine synthesis or decrease STN activity, to

deliver neurotrophic factors that protect dopamine neurons, or to alleviate genetic causes of PD.[95] Stem cell research in PD aims to create or find a renewable resource of dopamine-producing neurons for transplantation.

● EXAMINATION OF THE CLIENT WITH PARKINSON'S DISEASE

Client History

The client history involves gathering information regarding symptoms that are causing problems in daily life and elucidating the client's goals for therapy. In addition, it is important to know what medications the person with PD is taking as well as their dosing schedule. Some medications such as Sinemet® (carbidopa–levodopa) can have a significant impact on motor function, and therapy may need to be planned around the medication schedule. Falls are another issue that is common in PD and asking about fall history is an important component of the history. Typically, the fall history includes asking about a recent time frame as well as longer time frames such as falls in the last week and falls in the last 6 months. It is not uncommon for individuals with PD in Hoehn and Yahr stages 2.5, 3, and 4 to have frequent, even daily, falls.

Bodily Structure and Function

Neurologic System

The neurologic examination is carried out, as described in Chapter 9, with a focus on motor control and motor planning, since these are functions that are controlled by the BG. Sensation such as light touch, temperature, pinprick, and two-point discrimination are not usually altered by PD and so may be screened rather than evaluated in detail. Proprioception is typically impaired in PD with mild impairments appearing early in the course of the disease[96]; therefore, vibration and proprioception should be examined in more detail (see Chapter 9) The MDS-UPDRS[85] is an assessment that enables the clinician to examine impairments that are typical to PD, such as rigidity, tremor, and bradykinesia, as well as areas of common deficits (e.g., cognition and fatigue).

Cognitive Screen: Cognitive function impacts the ability to perform motor activities such as gait and transfers and is an important consideration when assessing safety. The Montreal Cognitive Assessment is a screen for dementia that is sensitive to mild cognitive impairment,[97] with demonstrated reliability and validity in PD[98] and is recommended for use by the Parkinson Disease Evidence Database to Guide Effectiveness (PDEDGE) taskforce of the Neurology Section of the APTA. It is quick and easy to administer, does not require special training and is free to use.

Fatigue: Fatigue is difficult to assess and to treat, but it is important to identify and document its impact on the client with PD. There is a Parkinson-specific measure called the Parkinson disease fatigue scale that is recommended for use in this population.[99]

Bradykinesia: To assess bradykinesia, the MDS-UPDRS includes finger tapping and toe tapping. For finger tapping, the client is instructed to repetitively touch the index finger to the thumb, opening the hand fully each time while the therapist observes speed, amplitude, including any decrement, hesitations, and halts on each side for 10 repetitions. It is scored as 0 (no problems), 1 (mild), 2 (moderate), 3 (severe), or 4 (cannot or can only barely perform task). Further descriptors for each category are included in the test. Bradykinesia of the lower extremity is assessed in a similar fashion via toe tapping, while keeping the heel on the floor.[85]

Balance: Postural instability is assessed with the Pull Test in the MDS-UPDRS. The patient is instructed to stand with feet shoulder-width apart and to do whatever they need to do to prevent falling. The examiner stands behind the patient and without warning grabs both shoulders and pulls backward quickly. The therapist should stand behind the patient at an arm's-length away with feet spread shoulder-width apart to prevent a fall. This test is scored from 0 to 4, with 0 being a normal response of 0–2 steps and no loss of balance, and 4 being unable to stand unassisted.[85]

Tremor: Tremor is described in terms of location (upper extremity, lower extremity, lip/jaw), amplitude and constancy (<25% of exam period, 26–50% of exam period, 51–75% of exam period, >75% of exam period). In addition, types of tremor (resting, postural, or kinetic) should be documented.

Dyskinesia: The assessment includes information about whether dyskinesias are present and if they are bothersome to the client or interfere with the client's ability to participate in the examination process in any way. If dyskinesias are present and bothersome, timing of medications is noted and considered as they may be a side effect of medications.

Freezing: Freezing and difficulty initiating movement are debilitating problems and a major cause of falls and disability in PD, but these symptoms can be difficult to elicit in the clinic. Freezing can be assessed in the clinic using a rapid 360-degree turn in both directions[100] or by observing gait in a confined space, such as walking into a corner and turning around. Yet, this will not always elicit freezing, even in individuals with severe FOG. To assess the impact on daily life, the therapist takes a history of frequency and typical triggers of freezing episodes. This may be augmented through use of the Freezing of Gait Questionnaire (FOGQ),[101] the only validated screening tool with excellent intra-rater reliability. On this questionnaire, there are six items on how freezing impacts the ability to walk during normal daily activities. The scale ranges from 0, which denotes normal movement, to 4, which indicates an inability to walk. The maximum score is 24, indicating more severe FOG. It has also been found to be a more sensitive measure of FOG than the freezing-while-walking item on the MDS-UPDRS, which simply asks the person to rate the freezing as none, rare, occasional, frequent, or frequent falls with freezing.[102]

Movement Scale: Size or scope of movement (movement scale) is assessed for both bradykinesia and coordination by having the person perform rapid, repetitive, thumb-to-index finger movement for 30 seconds (as described for bradykinesia). The therapist observes not only speed but any change in the amplitude of the movement. The hand should open fully with each motion before closing. For an individual with PD, finger-to-finger movements will get progressively smaller the longer the individual does the movement; the movements are slow, and in mid to late stage disease, irregular timing of the motions is noted.

Musculoskeletal System

Individuals with PD, like Mr. Martin, are often in late middle age or entering old age and commonly have musculoskeletal issues such as arthritis and disuse weakness. Functional loss of **strength** is not typically seen early in PD, and a manual muscle test is unlikely to pick up strength deficits caused by the disease, normal aging, or disuse until middle to late stages of the disease. Isokinetic testing, functional strength testing, or testing through the range of motion is recommended to detect early, subtle strength changes. Strength should be monitored throughout the disease process, including core strength. In addition, rigidity leads to stiffness, decreasing range of motion, and contracture; thus, assessment of **muscle length** and **joint range of motion** should also be monitored throughout the disease process. The muscle groups responsible for flexion and rotation (e.g., the pectorals, iliopsoas, hamstrings, and gastrocnemius muscles) are especially prone to shortening, so range of motion of the trunk and extremities is assessed periodically, with special attention paid to trunk extension, shoulder elevation/abduction, hip extension, knee extension, ankle dorsiflexion, and trunk and neck rotation. Moreover, **posture** is assessed for scoliosis and kyphosis as they typically occur in later stages of the disease.

Trunk rotation is the key to many functional activities such as walking with long strides and reaching. Trunk rotation can be safely assessed by examining the individual's ability to rotate, while seated with feet on the floor and arms crossed. The therapist instructs the individual to look back over his or her shoulder, and the therapist notes any side-to-side asymmetry. If a standard seat and location are used, rotation can be measured by placing numbers on the wall at 1-inch intervals and asking the individual to indicate the last number that can be read. Rotation can also be tested in standing (see Figure 14-3).

Functional Losses and Impact on Participation

Measurement and documentation of function provide the therapist with a means to document meaningful changes to improve the individual's ability to remain independent and active. In addition, the use of standardized measures improves communication by using a common language that allows comparison across therapists and clinics. The use of standardized measures also allows clinicians to better gauge the effectiveness of therapeutic interventions during and after therapy. Baseline measurements allow (1) quantification of any change in status throughout an episode of care, (2) documentation of disease progression, and (3) communication across different therapists and clinics.

The Neurology section of the APTA's PD EDGE taskforce recommends the use of a core set of measures across all stages

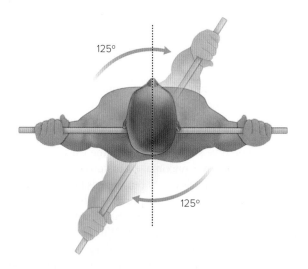

125°

125°

FIGURE 14-3 Overhead view of trunk rotation measurement method. A line is marked on the floor using tape, and a series of pairs of different colored points are marked on the tape, equidistant from the center mark on both the left and the right side. Clients stand (or sit) on the line with their feet shoulder-width apart, using the points as a guide to ensure that their feet are placed symmetrically on either side of the center mark. A wooden bar, approximately 4 feet long, is placed evenly across the subjects' shoulders and held in the subjects' hands, which rest as close to the shoulders as is comfortable. Clients are told to rotate as far as possible to the left or right, keeping the bar resting on their shoulders and not moving their feet. The therapist checks that the bar remains horizontal throughout the test. At the end of the rotation movement, a plumb bob or other weighted object on a string is attached to the left end of the bar for right rotation and the right end of the bar for left rotation. The bar is steadied by the rater and then the bob is allowed to drop to touch the floor. A nonpermanent marker pen is used to indicate where the plumb bob touches the floor. A long-armed goniometer is used to measure degrees of rotation. The axis of the goniometer is placed on the center of the line, and the stationary arm is placed along the line. A ruler or other lightweight long stick can be secured to the moving arm of the goniometer to reach the mark and allow for more accurate measurement. In a clinic that takes these measurements more frequently, a circle can be marked on the floor with the degrees marked along its arc at regular intervals; the therapist can simply take the measurement from the marks on the circle rather than use the goniometer every time. (Reproduced with permission from Evans KL, Refshauge KM, Adams R. Measurement of active rotation in standing: reliability of a simple test protocol. *Percept Mot Skills.* 2006:103(2):619-628.)

of the disease and across all clinics. These measures are grouped by the International Classification of Function (ICF) categories and are listed in Box 14-2.

Function and Activity Level Measures: Measures of gait, transfers, balance, falls screening, and participation do not differ significantly from those recommended in the evaluation chapter (9). Specific measures for use in PD can be found in Box 14-2.

BOX 14-2   PDEDGE Core Measures[103]

HIGHLY RECOMMENDED MEASURES		MEASURES RECOMMENDED FOR SPECIFIC CONSTRUCTS
Body Structure and Function		*Freezing of Gait*
MDS-UPDRS revision* – Part III	Montreal Cognitive Assessment	Freezing of Gait Questionnaire
		Fatigue
MDS-UPDRS – Part I		Parkinson's Fatigue Scale
Activity		*Fear of falling*
6-minute walk		ABC scale
10-m walk	Functional Gait Assessment (FGA)	*Dual-Task*
Mini BESTest		Timed Up and Go cognitive
MDS-UPDRS – Part II	Sit to stand 5 times	
	9-hole peg test	
Participation		
PDQ-8 or PDQ-39		

All measures in the highly recommended category are recommended for use in research and for students to learn to administer. *Recommend students exposed.

CASE STUDY A, PART V

Mr. Martin was initially evaluated (Part I) using the MDS-UPDRS revision, MoCA, 6 MWT, 10-m walk, Mini BESTest, FGA, Sit to stand 5 times, 9-hole peg test, and the PDQ-8; these are ideal for documenting baseline function and disease symptoms. At his visit at age 60 years (Part II), he reported having falls and difficulty walking outdoors. When repeating the core measures, the therapist noted that he scored in the high fall risk range on the Mini-BESTest and the FGA. Additionally, his score on the PDQ-8 had dropped, and he was walking slower and shorter distances (10-m walk test and 6 MWT). Using this data, the therapist and neurologist agreed that Mr. Martin should go through a course of individualized therapy to improve balance and walking and reassess his home exercise program. The use of the same measures allows justification for therapy and better tracking over time.

Mr. Martin moved to Florida at age 70 and at age 75 was referred for physical therapy for difficulty walking, inactivity, and falls. The therapist included the core measures in the examination, and having requested Mr. Martin's records, was able to compare his status with his last documented status, just 7 years previous. At this time, there was a marked drop in the 9-hole peg test, MoCA score, and the PDQ-8. The therapist was concerned about hand function, depression, and safety and made referrals to psychiatry and occupational therapy, based on these evaluative findings.

● MANAGING THE CLIENT WITH PARKINSON'S DISEASE

Bodily Functions

Range of Motion and Stretching

Work to maintain and improve joint and tissue flexibility begins as soon as a diagnosis is made with a focus on active extension and rotation. The hamstring muscles are particularly prone to contracture and should be stretched early in the disease process to maintain length and prevent contracture. If shortening and contracture occur, stretching is done 2–3 times a day, using a long slow stretch. Given the tendency for individuals with PD to develop a flexed posture and lack rotation during activities such as walking, therapy also focuses on trunk ROM into extension and rotation.

Strength

High-intensity exercise training results in myofiber hypertrophy of both type I and type II muscles, a shift to a less fatigable myofiber type profile, and increased mitochondrial complex activity.[104] In addition, strength training for greater than 8 weeks done at 60–70% of the single repetition max leads to significant improvements in the 6-minute walk test, stair descent time, and sit to stand.[105] There is no evidence that one type of exercise is superior to any other type, and both concentric and eccentric exercise are safe and well tolerated by individuals with PD.

However, it has been suggested that eccentric exercise might minimize oxygen consumption and maximize strengthening.[106]

Balance

Balance training is commonly recommended for individuals with PD. The balance exercises are individualized to the deficits noted in the assessment and must include exercises that are highly challenging for the individual.[107,108] There is evidence that repetitive step training with the use of a visual cue improves reaction time, maximal excursion of the limits of stability, and movement velocity,[109] but there is no evidence demonstrating that balance training prevents falls.[107,108] The use of home video games is popular and may improve compliance with exercise. For example, use of the Wii® fit board to practice weight shifts improved scores on the Berg Balance Scale but did not result in a minimal clinically important difference.[109] Whole body vibration is a new technique that is not yet supported by evidence.[110]

Activity

Mobility Training

Standard physical therapy typically involves task-oriented practice of gait and transfers. Practicing longer steps, turns, walking on uneven surfaces, and faster gait can lead to improved gait performance but is challenging to achieve as the individual must perform many repetitions of the correct movement pattern over a long period of time to bring about permanent changes in performance. Lasting benefits are achieved with 45–60 minutes of practice per session, 2–3 times per week for at least 8 weeks.[111,112] This level of intensity is difficult to achieve in traditional therapy due to limitations on the number of visits and reimbursement. Individualized physical therapy delivered at appropriate intensity for at least 1080 minutes leads to improvement in velocity, 2- or 6-minute walk test, step length, Timed Up and Go (TUG), Functional Reach Test, BBS, and clinician-rated motor UPDRS scores.[113]

FIGURE 14-4 Illustration of hamstring stretching methods. Instruction cues the individual to keep their head up and to focus on bringing their abdomen to their thigh to ensure that the stretch is done across the hip rather than overstretching the thoracic spine, which typically occurs when individuals try to put their face to their thigh. Due to balance issues it is best to perform stretches in sitting to better isolate the muscles to be stretched and allow the individual to perform the stretch without having to focus on maintaining their balance.

Treadmill training improves gait speed, stride length, endurance and leads to neuroplasticity in dopaminergic signaling.[114-116] Treadmill training for individuals with PD is equally effective without body weight support, and thus, the use of a harness is only recommended when needed to ensure safety. Treadmill training is started at the individual's comfortable walking speed or slightly slower and then increased in small increments. This is known as **speed-dependent treadmill training** and is an effective means of improving walking speed and stride length. It is important that training utilize walking and not running, as walking and running are not the same motor skill and training in one does not fully translate to improvement in the other. Training is done for 30–45 minutes, 2–3 times per week for at least 8 weeks and followed immediately by over-ground training to reinforce gains made on the treadmill. Cardiovascular fitness improves with both low-intensity and high-intensity treadmill training. Therefore, if a client needs to improve gait speed and fitness, a walking program on the treadmill that encourages walking at the fastest gait speed that can be achieved safely is likely to be most effective. Treadmill training does not improve strength or range of motion. Some facilities have robotic equipment to use during treadmill training. This equipment can decrease work for therapy staff but does not add any benefit for the PD client. Given that treadmill training is most effective for individuals with mild to moderate PD and does not typically require hands-on assistance by therapy staff, the use of robotics is not indicated in this population.[117]

Visual and auditory cueing: Individuals with PD respond well to cueing to increase movement amplitude and velocity.[118] Both visual and auditory cueing are effective. Typical methods for cueing include the use of visual cues on the floor to indicate appropriate step length, the use of lasers or other visual cues that move while walking, and the use of music or counting to set the step cadence. Placing tape or other visual stimuli on the floor is effective in improving step length but has the limitation of not being available in the natural environment, and it requires the individual to look down at all times, which increases the tendency to walk in a flexed posture. To alleviate these concerns, lasers are available to be attached to walkers and canes; also, there are special glasses that place a visual stimulus in front of the viewer. Both of these systems can increase step length, but the evidence on the lasers working in the natural environment is equivocal. Further, the glasses are typically bulky, and individuals are reticent to wear them in public. Auditory cueing is quite effective and has a strong body of evidence supporting its use, including improved scores on the dynamic gait index (DGI), the Tinetti mobility test (TMT), and the Freezing of Gait Questionnaire (FOGQ). The use of external auditory cues is also difficult in community environments, so attempts have been made to use internal cueing. Unfortunately, improvements from internal cueing were not maintained.[117] Cueing is a strategy that can be used, but to date, has not been shown to be optimal for long-term carryover and use in community environments. It remains one of the more effective means to assist individuals who have FOG.

Assistive devices are commonly prescribed to improve safety and decrease falls. Despite their common acceptance, little research has been done looking at their effectiveness and how best to prescribe them. Individuals with PD have difficulty with transitional movements (i.e., sit ↔ stand transfers), turning, and dual-tasking.[119] Of note, the use of an assistive device is a dual-task, and thus, could be theorized to be problematic for individuals with neurologic disorders that involve the BG, such as PD. Additionally, many assistive devices (canes, standard walker, two-wheeled walkers, and walking sticks) require the user to pick them up when turning and maneuvering, which creates a destabilizing force and removes the support or assistance from the user. Given these factors, devices that can be turned without lifting them from the ground would likely be safer for use, during turning activities. Four-wheeled rollator walkers allowed subjects with PD to achieve the highest walking velocity, least stumbles and falls during turning, and most consistent stepping.[120] Two-wheeled walkers led to difficulty and safety issues during turning and highly variable gait. Some individuals with PD tend to walk with a forward propulsive gait, resulting in their upper body moving forward of the lower body during gait. These individuals tend to respond well to a rollator walker with reverse brakes. Reverse brakes require the user to squeeze the hand brakes to release them and let go of the brakes to apply them. This system is helpful to many individuals with PD as it appears that they maintain better control of the walker while ambulating, and during a loss of balance, they tend to let go of the brakes rather than squeeze them anyway; thus, reverse brakes match their natural tendency. Rollator walkers are inexpensive to purchase, through a number of pharmacies and large retailers, and can be inexpensively converted to reverse-brake devices by personnel at bicycle and wheelchair repair shops. When prescribing an assistive device, community ambulation as well as home ambulation and the capabilities of the individual and their caregiver should be considered. Heavy devices may be difficult to place in a car, precluding use in the community, where they are most likely needed. Cost is also a consideration and may impede purchase of some devices. Insurance carriers have been reticent to provide coverage for assistive devices and may not cover devices such as the U-step walker, which has been designed for use by individuals with PD. Additionally, many devices are not useful on stairs and may even increase risk of falling on stairs. In the home, this problem can be alleviated by having a device on each level of the home so that one does not have to be carried up and down the stairs.

CASE STUDY A, PART VI

Mr. Martin benefited from the use of a cane, when his balance first began to decline to improve balance and signal other people in the environment to give him more space. Once he began to experience falls, a cane wasn't sufficient to prevent the falls, and he was given an individualized therapy program and prescribed a rollator walker. It is optimal for fitness, overall health and quality of life to encourage Mr. Martin to ambulate for as long as possible. When he began to exhibit a forward propulsive gait, his walker brakes were converted to reverse brakes with good success in decreasing his falls and improving his perceived safety. As he approached the later stages of his disease, he required assistance for ambulation, and his wife was unable to safely provide this assistance. He safely continued to walk with the Up and Go®, which is a device that partially supported his weight while walking but could also fully support his weight, during a loss of balance. It was used in the home environment to assist with ambulation while he could bear weight through his legs (Figure 14-5). The Merry walker® is a device that provides the opportunity for upper extremity support while walking with a rolling device and additionally has a harness that provides support if the individual experiences a loss of balance. The Merry Walker is large and only feasible for use in large hallways such as are found in nursing facilities.

Fall prevention is a common goal for our clients with PD but is one that is difficult to measure and to attain. We know that appropriate therapy can reduce fall risk scores on common fall risk assessment tools,[107] and at least one study found a trend that fall number was reduced.[121] A review, published by Canning et al. in 2014, found that (1) there is emerging evidence that group or individual supervised practice of challenging balance activities reduces falls; (2) home exercise programs have limited evidence of fall reduction/prevention; (3) mobility and physical activity can be improved without increasing falls;

and (4) interventions should be tailored to level of fall risk, history of falls (e.g., multiple or injurious), and presenting risk factors (e.g., cognitive impairment).[122]

It is clear that preventing falls requires individualized interventions that include balance training. Additionally, the interventions need to be based on each individual's unique impairments and situational factors. At this time, there are only three randomized clinical trials examining fall reduction, each demonstrated fall reduction using an individualized balance program with or without other interventions.[108,123,124] Many other studies have demonstrated that increasing activity and participation in exercise do not pose an additional fall risk for this population.

Transfer training is accomplished utilizing motor learning principles of task practice on varying surfaces to optimize carryover. Individuals with PD have difficulty getting their weight forward over their feet, and thus, have increasingly more difficulty as the surface that they are transferring from is lowered. It is critical to have the patient lean forward while keeping their head up to ensure that they will get a forward weight shift with an erect spine. Bending forward with a flexed spine increases the difficulty of straightening up at the end of the transfer and can result in the person with PD becoming stuck in a flexed posture. Use of the hands on the knees can help to encourage a forward weight shift as well as providing upper extremity assist for the transfer (Figure 14-6). When going stand to sit, placing the hands on the thighs and sliding them down to the knees encourages flexion at the hips to start the transfer and helps to maintain the body mass over the feet while providing upper extremity support.

FIGURE 14-5 Walkers for assisted gait. A. Up and Go® walker partially supports body weight, via a harness and a set of gas springs, while walking but fully supports body weight, during a loss of balance. **B.** Merry walker® provides the opportunity for upper extremity support, while walking with a rolling device that is weighted to prevent tipping and has a seat and strap, if the individual experiences a loss of balance, to prevent falls. The Merry Walker is large and only feasible for use in large hallways such as are found in nursing facilities.

FIGURE 14-6 Sit to stand transfer with hands on knees. Instruct the patient with PD to place their hands on their knees to encourage a forward weight shift as well as to provide upper extremity assist for coming to standing from sitting.

CASE STUDY A, PART VII

At age 80, Mr. Martin is requiring assistance with all transfers and mobility. His wife has reported a back injury from transferring him. In order to keep him at home, she is going to need assistance with transfers. She could do this by hiring round the clock aides, but this can be expensive. Additionally, she might be able to purchase a device to assist with transfers. There are a number of different options available. There are chairs that help lift the person up to a standing position called lift chairs (Figure 14-7). These are good for sitting in the living room area but are not helpful in areas such as the kitchen and bathroom. For these areas, there are powered sit to stand devices or lifts that can be independently used by Mr. Martin or can assist his wife to lift him (Figure 14-7B and C). These devices are also helpful to staff in nursing facilities.

Recreational Interventions

LSVT BIG is a technique based on the Lee Silverman Voice Treatment (LSVT) that requires intensive training over 16 sessions in 1 month. The training emphasizes the use of large amplitude movements and has been shown to improve amplitude of movement, walking speed, and performance on the TUG test, which is superior to a Nordic walking program and a standard home exercise program.[125,126] The key element of the program is repetitive, task-specific practice of large amplitude movements.

Music-based movement therapy is a promising intervention that is believed to result in improved compliance due to its fun and social nature. This therapy combines cognitive, cueing, and balance strategies with a physical activity. It also uses music as an auditory cue for movement. Several forms of dance have been investigated, including partnered tango dancing and non-partnered dancing. Both resulted in improved Berg balance scores and comfortable and fast-as-you can walking velocity that were maintained for a month.[127] Partner dancing participants expressed more enjoyment and a greater interest in continuing with the program than their non-partnered peers.

Video games are a popular activity and have been increasingly utilized in clinical environments. When these games involve appropriate movement strategies, they can improve balance and movement in individuals with PD. Individuals with PD have poorer performance on some of the video games and have been shown to have marked learning deficits on some games but not others. The ability of individuals with PD to play video games depends on the cognitive and motor learning demands of the game, requiring the therapist to carefully analyze the game to be prescribed and each individual's ability to play each game.[128] While video games may improve compliance due to their fun and engaging nature, they offer no additional advantages over more traditional balance training exercises.[129]

Writing and Hand Function

Micrographia is a common problem in individuals with PD, which has not been well studied. The standard recommendation for therapy is to practice large amplitude finger and hand movements to improve the amplitude of movement and to compensate through the use of lined paper. When using lined paper as a visual cue, individuals with PD are able to produce larger and more consistent handwriting.[130]

Fitness and Wellness

Individuals with neurologic diagnoses are often more sedentary and less fit than their peers. When asked why they don't

FIGURE 14-7 Devices to assist with sit–stand activities. A. Lift chair – motorized chair that slowly elevates the person to standing; **(B)** powered sit to stand device – allows person to come to standing with UE pull, harness around back to pull upward, and padded support to provide stability at calf; **(C)** full body lift device – uses a harness system for the caregiver to lift the patient to standing for transfer to bed, chair, or commode.

participate in community exercise programs, they report that they have low outcome expectations from exercise, lack time to exercise, and fear falling during exercise.[131] In order to improve compliance, therapists need to address these barriers. Education about the benefits of exercise and endorsements from their peers can help improve their expectations for benefit from exercise. Individualized exercise programs designed under the direction of a therapist can address the fear of falling, and if designed in partnership with the client, can address issues of time to perform exercise.

Evaluation and Treatment of Parkinson-Plus Syndromes

Vascular PD: The motor and sensory exam is based on impairments and focuses more on distal motor and sensory impairments. Treatment combines approaches for PD with those typically used for stroke rehabilitation, such as working on increasing stride length bilaterally, while also working on gait changes due to pyramidal signs such as muscular weakness or clonus (Table 10-8). Progress is typically slower than for those with either PD or CVA.

Lewy body dementia: Treatment is modified early on to accommodate for cognitive changes with a focus on teaching problem solving and ways to manage behaviors, related to poor problem solving. Due to issues with problem solving, there is an early focus on safety training before the cognitive issues become severe. In addition, motor learning is more severely impaired than in idiopathic PD, and therefore, therapists should employ a blocked practice schedule and avoid the use of random practice schedules. Progress will be slower than in idiopathic PD, and issues with attention will negatively impact some therapy sessions.

Progressive supranuclear palsy: The assessment includes an in-depth evaluation of eye movement. To assess ocular pursuit, have the client track an object up and down (vertical) and side to side (horizontal) and rate both vertical and horizontal movement using the following rating scale: (1) doesn't move to follow; (2) partial movement; or (3) complete movement. Early training should include a focus on balance activities and teaching to visually scan the environment for obstacles as well as to practice maneuvering around obstacles during gait. When choosing an adaptive device, consider the need to not only provide support, during episodes of lost balance, but to also provide a means to identify obstacles on the ground while also providing a means to maneuver around the obstacle. Canes are likely to allow for obstacle identification but will not prevent falls in individuals, who suffer loss of balance. Rollator walkers have been shown to provide for safe maneuvering around obstacles in both PD and HD and are, therefore, likely to work well for those with LBD.[120,132] No existing device meets all of the needs of this group of clients.

Multiple system atrophy: Since OH is prevalent and a significant problem in those with MSA, evaluation includes examination of BP during position changes. Treatment includes teaching the individual to transition slowly from supine to sit and sit to stand and to perform ankle pumps and other calf exercises before standing up. If coordination is impacted, include ataxia exercises in the treatment plan (Chapter 13, Box 13-3).

Corticobasal ganglionic degeneration: Coordination is typically more severely impaired in this condition, and deficits are noted early in disease progression. A thorough evaluation of coordination is conducted, and treatment to address coordination issues is implemented immediately. Coordination treatment includes the use of the ataxia exercises (outlined in Box 13-3 in Chapter 13) and work on coordination within function. Treatment of this disorder is challenging and requires the therapist to be flexible and creative. Table 14-8 provides a comparison of these Parkinson-plus syndromes to idiopathic PD.

TABLE 14-8	Parkinson-Plus Syndromes: Comparison to Idiopathic PD and Evaluation and Treatment			
	PROGNOSIS	**GAIT/BALANCE DESCRIPTION**	**OTHER SYMPTOMS**	**EVALUATION AND TREATMENT**
Vascular PD	Poor compared to idiopathic PD	More rapid decline	UPDRS scores higher (worse) at baseline	Motor and sensory exam Based on impairments
Dementia with Lewy bodies	8 years	Parkinsonian motor symptoms	Progressive cognitive decline, "fluctuations" in alertness and attention	Check cognition – MOCA Train safety as performance is highly variable
Progressive supranuclear palsy	Varies, choking leads to aspiration	Early postural instability with falls in first year	Vertical gaze paresis especially downward	Evaluate eye movement (UPDRS) Check for ability to visually scan environment and avoid obstacles
Multiple system atrophy	~9–10 years	Cerebellar dysfunction	Orthostatic hypotension	Examine for orthostatic hypotension Teach to deal with hypotension
Corticobasal ganglionic degeneration	~6–8 years	Bradykinesia – focal rigidity	Limb apraxia, dystonia	Eval coordination Look for apraxia Train coordination

HUNTINGTON'S DISEASE

Epidemiology

The prevalence of Huntington's disease (HD) in the United States is about 1 in every 10,000 people – about 30,000 people in all. There are another 250,000 Americans at risk of having HD. The onset is usually in midlife, between the ages of 30 and 50; although, about 5–10% of cases occur before the age of 20 (juvenile HD), and approximately 25% of cases occur after the age of 59 (late onset).[133] HD affects females slightly more than men and is more common in white people of Western European descent than in those of Asian or African ancestry.[134] Venezuela has the highest concentration of HD in the world, largely because of a family that lives along the shores of Lake Maracaibo. The original progenitor of this family lived in the early 1800s and left more than 18,000 descendants, of which approximately 14,000 individuals are still living.

Etiology and Risk Factors

HD is caused by an autosomal dominant mutation in either of an individual's two copies of a gene called *Huntingtin*, which was mapped to chromosome 4 in 1993. The DNA nucleotide triplet of cytosine, adenine, and guanine (CAG) is repeated many more times than in the normal gene (36–125 times compared to 11–30 times in normal genes). Individuals with CAG repeats ≥41 will develop the disease, those with 36–40 repeats may or may not develop the disease, and those with ≤35 repeats will not develop the disease. Any child of an affected person has a 50% chance of inheriting the disease.

There is a rough inverse correlation between the CAG repeat number and the age of onset of HD symptoms, such that individuals with early-onset HD tend to have longer repeat sizes. The number of CAG repeats can expand on replication, especially in males, which accounts for the occurrence of **genetic anticipation**, in which the age of onset of HD becomes earlier in successive generations, and the likelihood of paternal inheritance is greater in children with juvenile-onset HD. New-onset cases of HD in individuals with a negative family history can arise from an expansion of the gene in the borderline or normal CAG repeat range (28–35), most often coming from the father. CAG repeat number accounts for about 60% of the variation in age of onset, with the remainder of variability due to other genes and the environment. Although CAG number does not accurately predict what symptoms an individual will have, or how severe or rapid the course of the disease will be, some data suggest that the rate of progression might be faster with longer CAG repeats, particularly for individuals with juvenile-onset disease.[134]

The *Huntingtin* gene produces a protein that is also called *huntingtin (htt)* that is normally found in all cells throughout the body. The CAG triplet repeat in the gene codes for the amino acid glutamine. An increase in the size of the CAG segment in HD leads to the production of a mutant huntingtin protein with an abnormally long polyglutamine chain. The elongated protein is cut into smaller, toxic fragments that bind together and accumulate in neurons, disrupting their normal functions and, eventually, leading to neuronal death.[134]

CASE B, PART I

WD is a 42-year-old male with HD. Onset of motor symptoms was 1 year ago and his family notes that he has been easier to anger and clumsier for the last 3 years or so. WD's mother died of HD at age 60, after having been ill for about 20 years. WD has four siblings; his older sister has HD and an older brother has tested negative. He also has two younger brothers, one has been tested and was positive and the other has elected not to undergo genetic testing yet. WD has three children ages 16, 19, and 22. None of his children has undergone genetic testing. WD works as a pipe fitter in a local factory, and his wife works as a nurse's aide in a local nursing home. WD works day shift and his wife works 11 pm to 7 am. They live in a two-story home that they are renting with two dogs and a cat. The town they live in is small and in a very rural area.

What are the chances of WD's three children developing HD?

Answer: Because HD has an autosomal dominant inheritance pattern, each child has a 50% chance of developing the disease.

Pathophysiology

In HD, there is severe loss of neurons in the caudate and putamen nuclei of the BG. With the loss of cells, the head of the caudate becomes shrunken, and there is enlargement of the anterior horns of the lateral ventricles. Neuronal degeneration is also seen within the temporal and frontal lobes of the cerebral cortex and the Purkinje cells of the cerebellum.[134] Early HD is characterized by loss of striatal medium spiny enkephalin/GABA-containing projection neurons of the indirect BG pathway. The net result is relative disinhibition of the thalamus, which in turn excites the cortex, producing **hyperkinesia**, an increase in movements. In later stages of HD, all striatal projection neurons as well as cortical neurons degenerate, resulting in a relatively **hypokinetic** state that resembles parkinsonism.

Clinical Presentation

Symptoms usually evolve slowly and vary from person to person, even within the same family. Motor, cognitive, and behavioral functions can be affected. Some individuals may present with mild involuntary movements (chorea) and have more emotional/behavioral symptoms of HD while some have less emotional/behavioral symptoms with more chorea.

Motor Symptoms

Involuntary motor abnormalities in HD predominantly include **chorea** and **dystonia** (sustained muscular contractions resulting in abnormal postures or torsion movements), as described in Chapter 19 for cerebral palsy. Choreic movements initially give a person the appearance of being fidgety or restless, but as they progress, they affect the face, head, lips, tongue, and trunk, and cause flailing movements, called **ballisms**. The person with HD is often mistaken for being drunk due to the ataxic and "dancing" gait caused by chorea. Chorea in individuals with adult-onset HD initially worsens over time, but then, becomes less prominent in later stages in many with the emergence of parkinsonian symptoms (rigidity, bradykinesia). Although useful for diagnosis, chorea is a poor indicator of disease severity and typically does not interfere with functional task performance except in severe cases.[134] The most prevalent types of dystonia were reported to be internal shoulder rotation, sustained fist clenching, excessive knee flexion, and foot inversion.[135] Other involuntary movements that people with HD may display are **tics** (sudden, repetitive, non-rhythmic motor movement or vocalization, involving discrete muscle groups), **myoclonus** (brief, shock-like muscle contractions), and **tremors,** which may be present at rest, with posture, or with voluntary movements. Myoclonus and tremors are much more common in children and young adults with HD.

Voluntary motor impairments that impede performance of daily activities include bradykinesia and akinesia, as seen in PD, as well as **apraxia** (loss or impairment of the ability to execute complex coordinated movements without muscular or sensory impairment), **motor impersistence** (inability to maintain a voluntary muscle contraction at a constant level), diminished rapid alternating movements, and difficulties performing sequences of movements. Motor impersistence manifests as frequent dropping of objects and a "milkmaid's grip" during handshakes (alternating contraction and relaxation of the grip), an inability to hold the eyes closed, incomplete chewing, and inconsistent driving speeds. Motor impersistence is independent of chorea and is linearly progressive, making it a possible marker of disease severity.[134]

Musculoskeletal impairments in muscle performance, posture, and tone also occur in HD. Overall muscle strength is not initially a problem in HD, but strength can be diminished as the disease progresses, even before a loss of functional ability is apparent.[136] It is not known whether muscle weakness is a primary impairment of the disease process or secondary to decreased mobility and disuse atrophy. Studies in symptomatic individuals with HD and asymptomatic mutation carriers found delayed recovery of ATP levels in muscles after exercise due to mitochondrial dysfunction and abnormal staining for huntingtin in skeletal muscles, which may contribute to muscle weakness in HD.[137] Muscle tightness and postural changes may develop in people with HD due to poor postural habits, dystonic posturing, and immobility. In sitting, individuals with HD tend to adopt a slouched position with excessive thoracic kyphosis and posterior pelvic tilt. In later stages, patients often assume a more massed flexion posture. Deep tendon reflexes may be increased in HD. People with chorea may exhibit "**hung-up**" reflexes, in which after the tendon is tapped and the reflex action takes place, the limb slowly, rather than quickly, returns to its neutral position.

Motor impairments can negatively impact functional task performance. Hand dexterity and fine motor skills (e.g., finger tapping skills) are often impaired early in the disease and result in problems with writing, dressing, cutting food, and handling utensils.[136-140] Gait and balance disturbances can lead to

falls. Gait impairments begin early in HD and typically include slower gait speed, shorter and more variable stride length, a wider base of support, increased double support time, and increased trunk sway.[132,141-143] Balance deficits usually occur in the early to middle stages of the disease and manifest as delayed motor responses to unexpected balance disturbances and difficulties with tandem standing, single leg stance, and walking and standing with eyes closed.[143,144] Exaggerated movements, due to problems with force modulation control, may cause people with HD to lose their balance by reaching outside of their base of support or by vaulting up from a chair or out of bed. Problems with eccentric motor control can also cause falls, when people with HD sit down or descend stairs.

Speech and Swallowing Impairments

Speech disorders and dysphagia are symptoms of HD that develop over time. Individuals with HD demonstrate impaired speech performance characterized by abnormal articulation (production of speech sounds) and prosody (pitch, loudness, tempo, and rhythm in speech), a reduced speech rate with increased numbers of speech pauses, and marked difficulties with steadily repeating single syllables (e.g., /pa/, /ta/).[145] Studies of dysphagia, in individuals with HD with chorea, have shown numerous abnormalities, during all phases of ingestion: (1) oral phase – postural instability, hyperextension of the head and trunk, rapid and impulsive consumption of food, poor tongue control, uncoordinated swallow, repetitive swallow, and residual food remaining after the swallow; (2) pharyngeal phase – coughing, choking, and aspiration; and (3) esophageal phase – diaphragmatic chorea, slowed esophageal motility, and reflux.[146,147] The risk of aspiration is higher if the person engages in conversations while eating, due to exposure of the airway to food, when the vocal cords are open. Individuals with HD with rigidity and bradykinesia show mandibular rigidity, slow tongue chorea, delayed tongue transfer of food, prolonged swallow latency, and choking and coughing during meals.[147] Therapists should refer individuals with speech disorders and dysphagia to a speech-language pathologist for evaluation and treatment.

Motor Learning

Like individuals with PD, individuals with HD show deficits in motor sequence learning and speed-accuracy motor skill learning, presumably due to damage of frontostriatal circuits.[46] Some evidence suggests that explicit (conscious) motor sequence learning is impaired earlier (i.e., in premanifest stages) than implicit (unconscious) motor sequence learning, suggesting that explicit motor learning measures may be useful biomarkers of HD.[148,149] A study that examined the effects of motor imagery training on copying two Chinese letters twice in each of five sizes found that non-demented individuals with HD demonstrated a significant improvement in movement isochrony (increased speed with greater amplitude of movement), following the motor imagery training, that was not demonstrated in non-demented individuals with PD, suggesting that motor imagery is less affected in individuals with HD than those with PD and may enhance motor skill learning in this population.[150]

Cognitive Symptoms

Cognitive problems in individuals with HD occur early in the disease and include impaired perception of time, decreased speed of processing, impaired visuospatial perception, short-term memory decline, and executive function deficits.[151] In later stages, the cognitive deficits progress to global dementia. People with HD have problems estimating time early, with their spouses often complaining that their once-punctual spouse is frequently late and underestimates how long a task will take to complete. The speed of thinking and performance of motor skills such as finger tapping is slowed, making completion of ordinary cognitive and motor tasks tiring. Impaired visuospatial processing results in reduced awareness of body space and the environment and can lead to frequent bumping into objects. Individuals with HD have difficulties with learning new information and retrieving previously learned information, but in general, long-term memory is spared.[149] Executive functions are impaired, such as attention, planning, problem solving, decision making, sequencing, adapting to change, and cognitive flexibility (ability to switch between two different thoughts, and to think about multiple concepts simultaneously), all of which impede the acquisition of new motor skills. Individuals with HD often report difficulty with "multi-tasking", and studies have reported impaired dual-task performance, especially when a cognitive load is added to a motor task.[152] Notably, individuals with HD lack awareness of their own actions and feelings, often overestimating their competency in behavioral and emotional control and performance of activities of daily living.[153] Speech declines more rapidly than comprehension, although individuals with HD show difficulties with initiating conversations and comprehending what's heard and said, during conversations, due to slow cognitive processing.[151]

Emotional/Behavioral Symptoms

Emotional and behavioral symptoms are very frequently present in the early stage of the disease, often prior to the onset of motor symptoms. These symptoms not only negatively impact the person with HD's daily life, but they also adversely affect the person's family. Emotional and behavioral disturbances that are common in HD include depression, anxiety, apathy, irritability, disinhibition, impulsivity, obsessions, and perseveration.[154] **Depression** is the most common symptom and is difficult to diagnose because weight loss, apathy, and inactivity are also features of HD. Depression is usually associated with feelings of low self-esteem, guilt, and **anxiety**, which often occurs in relation to uncertainty about the start and/or the course of the disease. **Apathy** manifests as loss of energy and initiative, poor perseverance and quality of work, passive behavior, impaired judgment, poor self-care, and emotional blunting; it can be difficult to discriminate from depression. Apathy is related to disease stage, whereas depression and anxiety are not. **Irritability** is often the very first sign of HD, and its expression varies from rude or hurtful comments to serious disputes and physical aggression. People with HD with **disinhibition** and **impulsivity** may develop problem behaviors such as irritability, temper outbursts, sexual promiscuity, and acting without thinking. Individuals with obsessions and **perseveration** become "stuck" on one idea or activity, making it difficult for them to change from one activity or idea to another

or to deal with changes in routines. Other emotional/behavioral conditions found in individuals with HD are mania, bipolar disorders, and obsessive–compulsive disorders. Psychosis may occur in the later stages of the disease with delusions, paranoia, and hallucinations being the most frequent symptoms.[154] Sexual problems in HD are most commonly hypoactive sexual drive and inhibited orgasm, but hypersexuality can cause considerable problems in some individuals. The suicide rate for individuals with HD is estimated to be about 5–10 times greater than that of the general population (about 5–10%)[134] and occurs most frequently in premanifest gene carriers and early symptomatic individuals, especially around the time of gene testing or when independence diminishes.

Sleep Disturbances

Many individuals with HD experience insomnia. Electroencephalogram (EEG) studies have shown that individuals with HD show impaired initiation and maintenance of sleep, spend more time in non-rapid eye movement (NREM) sleep and less time in REM sleep, and have reduced total sleep time compared to controls. Individuals with HD also show increased awakenings, after sleep onset. The causes of insomnia may include depression and apathy, lack of daytime stimulation, disruptions of the sleep–wake cycle, medications, and involuntary movements.[155] Although choreic movements in HD tend to lessen during sleep, they may interfere with falling asleep or going back to sleep after a nighttime awakening. Poor sleep hygiene results in increased daytime somnolence. Apathetic individuals with HD often sleep excessively or spend large amounts of time in bed. Sleep studies are recommended for individuals with sleep problems.

Sensory Disturbances

Individuals with HD can experience musculoskeletal pain from dystonia, muscle imbalances, immobility, and injuries from falls or uncontrolled limb movements, which can cause a person to accidentally hit objects. There are some reports of people in late stages of HD with severe "central" pain presumably due to deafferentation from the disease process. Abnormalities in skin sensations have been reported in individuals in the later stages of HD, apparently due to disturbances in cortical processing of somatosensory information (deafferentation).[156] Studies that examined proprioceptive sensory function in people with HD found some deficits, but the extent to which these deficits affect active movements is unknown.[157] Patients with HD have eye movement abnormalities including delayed initiation of movements, slowed saccadic movements, and jerky smooth pursuit movements that begin early in the disease and may affect balance and walking performance.[158] In advanced stages, individuals may use head movements to initiate eye movement. Individuals with HD are able to detect smells, but have difficulty with identifying what smells are.[151]

Cardiovascular and Respiratory Function

Abnormalities in metabolic and physiologic responses to aerobic exercise have been reported in individuals with HD. Maximal exercise testing, using a cycle ergometer, of symptomatic individuals with HD found a normal cardiopulmonary response, with normal cardiac output and ventilation, but a reduced work capacity, lower anaerobic threshold (AT), and earlier increase in blood lactate compared to healthy controls.[159] During a submaximal aerobic exercise test, individuals with symptomatic HD did not achieve a steady-state HR, during the first phase of the cycling test with no resistance, and some individuals demonstrated a lower AT and were working anaerobically during the test.[158] Lower work capacity at a given HR may be due to reduced muscle strength or cardiorespiratory fitness levels, while the lower AT is hypothesized to be due to mitochondrial dysfunction or reduced capacity for gluconeogenesis in skeletal muscles of people with HD.[157,159]

Inactivity may lead to decreased cardiovascular endurance due to deconditioning in people with HD. Studies that investigated daytime activity levels, using activity monitors, reported significantly lower motor activity levels in people with HD compared to healthy controls[161] and significantly lower daily step counts in people with HD, who were recurrent fallers, compared to those who were non-fallers.[160] Lower daily activity levels were related to impaired voluntary movements, balance and gait disturbances, and reduced functional capacity.[161,162]

Respiratory function impairments may contribute to decreased endurance. People with HD exhibit obstructive and restrictive disorders of the respiratory system.[163] However, most people do not report respiratory symptoms until later stages of the disease. Pulmonary infections may contribute to morbidity and mortality in individuals with HD.

Falls

Falls are common in people with HD and often occur while the person is performing multiple tasks simultaneously, maneuvering around obstacles on the floor, turning, or climbing stairs.[142,161] Many factors likely contribute to falls, including involuntary movements (i.e., chorea, dystonia), voluntary movement impairments (bradykinesia, impaired force modulation, and eccentric motor control), musculoskeletal impairments (decreased muscle strength and endurance, poor posture), balance problems, gait impairments (especially bradykinesia, stride variability, and excessive trunk sway), cognitive deficits (decreased attention and ability to dual-task), behavioral changes (impulsiveness, impaired judgment leading to unsafe behaviors), visual disturbances, and visuospatial deficits.[164]

Weight Loss

Many individuals with HD experience considerable weight loss throughout all stages of the disease.[165,166] While the causes of weight loss are not well understood, multiple factors including dementia, depression, chewing and swallowing difficulties, orodental problems, motor disturbances, muscle atrophy from decreased activity, inadequate access to food, and side effects of medications have been found to contribute to weight loss in this population.[166] Referral to a dietician for nutritional counseling is advised for individuals with excessive weight loss.

Juvenile HD

Individuals with juvenile HD develop the same triad of motor, cognitive, and behavioral disturbances as in adult-onset HD, but there are some distinct differences in the symptomatology.[167,168] The most common presenting features of juvenile HD in the first decade of life are voluntary motor disturbances (i.e.,

abnormal gait, rigidity of limbs or trunk, slowed speech, swallowing problems, and drooling), cognitive deficits, behavioral disturbance, and seizures. Unlike adults who typically present with involuntary motor disturbances, chorea is uncommon in children with HD. Behavioral disturbances requiring medical or legal intervention or poor school performance may be the first symptom in an adolescent. Some children develop ataxia and other cerebellar signs and severe dystonia in later stages. Slowed saccadic eye movements with compensatory jerking of the head to look to the side is common. Seizures, usually of a generalized or myoclonic type, affect up to 25% of children.

CASE B, PART II

WD does not return to the clinic for 2 years, at which time he has marked deterioration in gait and balance; plus his wife reports that he has been fired from his work for behavioral issues as well as difficulty performing his job. WD states that he feels he was fine at work and expresses anger at being wrongly let go. When asked what he does during the day, he says that he watches TV. His wife reports that he is up at night, while she is at work, and that he tends to get on the computer or watch TV. During the day, when he is supposed to be taking care of the dog and doing household chores, he is sleeping. She has to either stay awake or frequently wake up to perform childcare duties and is experiencing high levels of fatigue. She also worries that he is going to fall and hurt himself, especially since he's beginning to have difficulty going up stairs, where he seems to catch his toe and trip.

What could be causing WD to trip on the stairs?

Answer: Factors that may be contributing to WD's tripping on stairs could include chorea, dystonia, bradykinesia, incoordination, lower extremity muscle weakness, anticipatory and dynamic balance problems, visual and visuospatial processing deficits, attention deficits and problems with dual-tasking, and going too fast due to impulsivity.

What could be causing WD's sleep to be disturbed?

Answer: WD's sleep might be disturbed by his chorea, depression and apathy, lack of daytime stimulation, and possibly disruptions of his sleep–wake cycle.

Diagnosis

Genetic testing can determine whether a person carries the HD gene. People with a positive test result risk losing health and life insurance as well as employment, which contributes to their psychological distress. For these reasons and because there is no cure for the disease, the majority of individuals "at risk" decide not to take the test. Those who undergo testing generally do so to assist in making career and family choices. Current protocols for genetic testing are designed to exclude testing for children or those with suicidal ideation, inform individuals of the implications of test results for relatives, identify subsequent sources of support, and protect confidentiality.[134]

If there is a positive family history of HD, the presence of typical motor signs and symptoms of HD are usually enough to confirm a diagnosis. A positive genetic test is cost effective and provides confirmation for individuals who have developed symptomatology consistent with HD, with or without a family history. Routine MRI and CT scans in middle to late stages of HD show a loss of striatal volume and increased size of the frontal horns of the lateral ventricles, but scans are usually unhelpful for diagnosis of HD in early stages. Functional neuroimaging (PET and functional MRI) can detect striatal atrophy in affected brains as much as 11 years before symptom onset and may be useful in diagnosing and tracking the progression of the disease.[134]

Clinical Course

The clinical course of HD can be divided into four approximate stages: premanifest, prediagnostic, early, middle, and late. The **premanifest** stage consists of a healthy period, when the person has no detectable clinical abnormalities, and a **prediagnostic** phase, when individuals may show subtle changes in personality, cognition, and motor control. Once individuals with HD have symptoms that are sufficiently developed for diagnosis, they are classified into early, middle, and late stages, based on their Total Functional Capacity (TFC) score.[169,170] The TFC is a 14-point scale that measures disability and participation restrictions in important life skills (work = 3 points, financial management = 3 points, family responsibilities/chores = 2 points) and activities of daily living (3 points), including where care is provided (home versus extended care facility: 3 points).

The disease usually progresses slowly with an average lifespan 10–20 years, after onset of symptoms. Progression of the disease tends to be more rapid in those diagnosed at an earlier age. Most people with HD die from complications of falls, malnourishment, infections, or pneumonia. The typical progression of symptoms across disease stages is shown in Table 14-9.

The Unified Huntington's Disease Rating Scale (UHDRS) is the standard assessment tool used to quantify disease severity and to track symptom changes over time.[171,172] It was developed as a clinical rating scale to assess four domains of clinical performance and capacity in individuals with HD: motor function, cognitive function, behavioral abnormalities, and functional capacity. The motor portion of the UHDRS includes 15 items each rated on a 0–4 scale (0 = normal). Scores can be calculated by summing questions from each section with higher scores indicating greater impairment. It has high reliability and validity[171]; however, it is intended to be performed only after extensive training and certification to administer the different components of the test.

CASE B, PART III

Eight years late, WD arrives at the clinic in a poorly fitted wheelchair with his wife and child. They report that they transfer him by "standing him up and turning him" and that he only walks when they walk him hand in hand with two-person assist.

Medical Management

Drug therapy in HD is directed toward motor, cognitive, and emotional/behavioral symptom management. Typical medications used for symptom management are summarized in Table 14-10. Therapists should be aware of the medications that individuals with HD are taking and any potential side effects. Surgical interventions such as deep brain stimulation, fetal cell transplantation, gene therapy, and stem cell therapy are in the experimental stages. Counseling can be helpful for affected individuals, their spouses, and individuals at risk for HD. Although few individuals take advantage of predictive or prenatal genetic testing, individuals with HD can benefit from frank discussions with health care professionals about family, financial, and career planning. Support groups are invaluable sources of information and insight that can help affected individuals and families deal with the difficulties of HD.

Physical Therapy Evaluation

Assessment of HD includes a standard neurologic assessment with the addition of chorea, eye movement, and motor impersistence testing. Eye movement and chorea are assessed using the UHDRS scale or the scale in Table 14-11. Chorea is observed while the individual sits quietly and during walking. The therapist observes all four extremities, the face, neck, and trunk.

TABLE 14-9	Total Functional Capacity Staging[169]	
STAGE	**TFC SCORES**	**DESCRIPTION**
Stage I (early)	11–13	No limitations in any area
Stage II (middle)	7–10	Some problems with work and financial capacity but still able to meet responsibilities at home and complete all ADLs
Stage III (middle)	3–6	Limited work ability, needs assistance with finances and home responsibilities; some difficulty with ADLs but still living at home.
Stage IV (late)	1–2	No longer working or able to take care of finances or home chores; increased difficulty with ADLs and may no longer be living at home.
Stage V (late)	0	Requires a total care facility and is unable to care for self

TABLE 14-10	Medications Used to Treat HD[173]	
SUBCLASS OF DRUG	**EXAMPLE MEDICATIONS**	**POTENTIAL SIDE EFFECTS**
Antichoreic Drugs		
Dopamine-depleting medication	Tetrabenazine (Xenazine)	Depression, extrapyramidal symptoms, drowsiness, akathesia
Atypical antipsychotics	Olanzapine (Zyprexa), Risperidone (Risperdal)	Extrapyramidal symptoms, drowsiness, akathesia
Neuroleptics (dopamine-blocking agents)	Haloperidol (Haldol), Fluphenazine (Prolixin)	Extrapyramidal symptoms, sedation, akathesia
Antidepressants (used for depression and sometimes for irritability and anxiety)		
Selective serotonin reuptake inhibitors (SSRI)	Fluoxetine (Prozac), Citalopram (Celexa), Sertraline (Zoloft), Paroxetine (Paxil)	Insomnia, gastrointestinal upset, restlessness, weight loss, dry mouth, anxiety, headache
Tricyclic antidepressant	Amytriptyline (Elavil), Nortriptyline (Pamelor)	Same as SSRIs
Other medications	Bupropion (Wellbutrin), Venlafaxine (Effexor)	Insomnia, headache
Antipsychotics (used for psychosis and sometimes for irritability or for chorea suppression)		
Atypical antipsychotics	Olanzapine (Zyprexa), Quetiapine (Seroquel), Ziprasidone (Geodon), Aripiprazole (Abilify)	Extrapyramidal symptoms, drowsiness, akathesia
Neuroleptics (dopamine-blocking agents)	Haloperidol (Haldol), Fluphenazine (Prolixin)	Extrapyramidal symptoms, sedation, akathesia

Motor impersistence is measured on the UHDRS by having the individual stick out their tongue and document ability to (1) fully protrude the tongue and (2) keep it out for 10 seconds. It is also important to assess for signs of motor impersistence during functional activities such as holding onto an object. This can be done by having the individual hold an object and walk to see if they drop the object or change their gait pattern. Another method is to have the individual hold onto an object while talking so that they aren't looking at their hand to see if they drop the object. Additionally, the presence of motor impersistence can negatively impact some assessment techniques. Manual muscle tests require that the person being tested hold an isometric contraction. In anyone with HD, failure to hold the isometric muscle contraction could be due to motor impersistence rather than inability of the muscle to develop and sustain contractile force. Also, some outcome measures require that the person perform balance or coordination activities with the eyes closed, which is difficult for someone with HD to maintain due to impersistence.

movement in both directions. The examiner observes all four extremities, the trunk, neck, and face, while he is sitting and when he walks, to rate his chorea. He has absent movement in the right arm and leg with constant mild movement in the face and intermittent mild movement in the trunk and the left arm and leg. The chorea remains evident during walking. On examination, using the UHDRS, WD holds out his tongue but pulls it back in, after only 8 seconds. Given the presence of early motor impersistence, the results of the MMT may be inaccurate, but WD is able to achieve normal scores in all four extremities for all major muscle groups. If he were to have any difficulty, the therapist would complete a functional examination of strength during activities that are important to WD, such as observing his ability to do sit to stand 5 times.

Individuals with HD have progressively more difficulty keeping their eyes closed on command due to motor impersistence. Verbal reminders can help them to keep their eyes closed. Testing a person with a blindfold is not the same as doing so with eyes closed and should not be substituted for the eyes closed condition. The neural system regulates according to whether or not the individual is trying to use vision, and therefore, it is important to ensure that vision is truly obscured, when testing balance without vision, and that vision is available but inaccurate when testing how well the system integrates sensory cues for balance.[174]

CASE B, PART IV

When WD started to present with symptoms, as described in Part I, he is referred for physical therapy evaluation. At his first visit, a full neurologic assessment including eye movement and chorea measures is completed. He is asked to follow a pen in the examiner's hand with his eyes both in the vertical and horizontal positions and has complete

TABLE 14-11	Suggested Rating Scale for Impairments Unique to HD

Ocular Pursuit (ability of the eyes to follow an object up and down [vertical] and side to side [horizontal])

Vertical	Horizontal
• Doesn't move to follow • Partial movement • Completes movement	• Doesn't move to follow • Partial movement • Completes movement

Chorea

Upper Extremities

Right		Left	
• Absent • Intermittent • Constant	• Mild (small movements, do not impede function) • Moderate (small- to medium-sized motions, may impede function) • Marked (medium to large size motions and impedes function)	• Absent • Intermittent • Constant	• Mild (small movements, do not impede function) • Moderate (small- to medium-sized motions, may impede function) • Marked (medium to large size motions and impedes function)

Lower Extremities

Right		Left	
• Absent • Intermittent • Constant	• Mild (small movements, do not impede function) • Moderate (small- to medium-sized motions, may impede function) • Marked (medium to large size motions and impedes function)	• Absent • Intermittent • Constant	• Mild (small movements, do not impede function) • Moderate (small- to medium-sized motions, may impede function) • Marked (medium to large size motions and impedes function)

Trunk

• Absent • Intermittent • Constant	• Mild (small movements, do not impede function) • Moderate (small- to medium-sized motions, may impede function) • Marked (medium to large size motions and impedes function)

Face

• Absent • Intermittent • Constant	• Mild (small movements, do not impede function) • Moderate (small- to medium-sized motions, may impede function) • Marked (medium to large size motions and impedes function)

*These ratings were created by D. Kegelmeyer.

CASE B, PART V

For WD, at his initial PT visit, there should be some determination of how his chorea, behavior, and cognition might be impacting his work. Since lack of insight is a common early symptom of HD, it is important to be detailed in the interview and to get family input, whenever possible. WD states that work is fine, but his wife reports that he has been disciplined twice in the last 6 months, once for poor work and once for an inappropriate verbal interaction with his supervisor. WD is referred to a social worker for counseling on impulse control and issues that may arise, when he is experiences stress at work. Therapy further assesses WD's fine motor control and makes a referral to occupational therapy, as the work-related issues, at this time, are related to declines in hand function. In addition, he is questioned in depth about his job requirements related to the need to walk in narrow spaces or on elevated surfaces. He does have to walk on catwalks, and this may become a safety issue in the near future. At this time, his therapy assessment shows that he can walk heel-toe without any stumbles, and his score on the TUG is 9 seconds, indicating that he is likely to be safe to continue with his activities at work. The therapist provides him with a home exercise program with an emphasis on balance activities involving narrowed stances. He is also encouraged to take up an activity that would improve overall fitness and provide him with stretching and relaxation.

Chorea is measured and documented objectively using the rating scale from Table 14-11. This allows for communication with the physician and close monitoring of the progression of the chorea. When chorea interferes with function, the therapist communicates with the neurologist to assist in the initiation of pharmacological management. While chorea is quite visible and can lead to declines in function, gait and balance deficits do not decline in parallel to the progression of chorea.[175] Rather than basing decisions about ambulation safety on visualization of chorea, a thorough and standardized assessment of gait and balance should be conducted to determine fall risk and provide a basis for safety recommendations. Outcome measures that are reliable and valid in HD include the TUG, TMT, and the BBS.[176]

CASE B, PART VI

Two years later at WD's next clinic visit (Case Study, Part II), WD is exhibiting significant functional loss along with changes in participation and in mood. A more thorough evaluation is warranted along with focused interdisciplinary care. WD now has a TUG time of 15 seconds and a TMT score of 19 and a BBS of 50. His ability to transfer and ambulate has declined, and he is at an increased risk of falling, according to the TUG and the TMT. Static balance, as measured by the BBS, is not yet severely impaired. Single limb stance time is now <5 seconds bilateral.

It is quite common for individuals with HD to exhibit significant deficits in single limb stance ability early in the disease process, which has implications for their ability to ambulate on uneven surfaces and to ascend and descend curbs and steps. Individuals with HD report that the majority of their falls occur while dual-tasking, avoiding an obstacle on the floor, or when ascending and descending stairs.[142]

● MANAGING THE CLIENT WITH HUNTINGTON'S DISEASE

Based on the findings, described in Part VI, WD needs social work for assistance in dealing with his job-related issues, since he has been fired from is job, and perhaps finding him a new job that is more appropriate, such as stocking shelves or bagging groceries. The physical therapy assessment reveals a TUG score of 20 seconds, inability to walk heel-toe or perform single limb stance and a TMT score of 18, indicating he is at high risk of falls and walking quite slowly. At this time, he would benefit from a formal physical therapy program. Evidence for physical therapy in HD is sparse but does include studies showing (1) that a 3-week inpatient PT program improves balance, as measured by the TMT, and physical performance scores[177]; (2) a gym program of stationary bike and strengthening exercises improved 6-minute walk test scores[178]; and (3) multi-directional stepping while playing Dance, Dance Revolution® improved ability to

maintain single limb stance for longer periods of time, during gait.[179] Areas to be addressed with therapy are determined based on identified impairments and functional losses; then, therapy is modified, based on the unique features of HD, such as chorea, cognitive changes, apathy, and dystonia. Methods of treatment are typically based on those used for PD and modified based on the unique characteristics of HD. The evidence for treatment efficacy for these methods such as strength training and treadmill walking is not yet established in HD, but given that it is also a result of damage to the BG, as is PD, similar treatment methods may be a good starting point for treatment planning.

In HD, apathy and lack of insight into their own deficits negatively impacts participation in activity and exercise programs. Apathy leads individuals with HD to lead a very sedentary lifestyle and withdraw from social activities that they previously enjoyed. It also has a negative impact on participation in community and physical therapy exercising. Apathy is best overcome through individualized rewards and setting up a daily schedule with short bouts of exercise/activity.

CASE B, PART VII

By his return to therapy after 2 years (part II), WD is very inactive and is showing signs of apathy, so his care plan includes 10 minutes of exercise daily with his wife or 16-year-old child at 3:00 in the afternoon. The use of a set, daily schedule improves compliance and minimizes arguments. WD also lacks insight into his impairments and functional losses. The therapist focuses on introducing an exercise that WD has done in the past and tells WD that it is good for his "HD" rather than trying to get him to recognize that his balance is poor and his walking is unsafe. When appropriate, concrete feedback, regarding WD's impairments, may be helpful in developing some insight into his limitations. For example, if he trips during therapy, the therapist would immediately point out that he lost his footing and instruct him that his therapy/exercise program will help him walk without losing his footing. Individuals with HD may also be limited in their ability to maintain or transfer this insight into new situations, due to their cognitive losses. In this situation, safety measures need to be taken to remove WD from unsafe situations and modify his environment(s) to provide improved safety.

Bodily Functions

Range of Motion and Stretching

These interventions would be the same as outlined previously in this chapter under PD.

Transfers

Individuals with HD tend to keep their weight shifted posterior, when going sit to stand, and to remain in a relatively extended posture, while shifting their weight posterior, when they go stand to sit, resulting in a fall into the seat. Additionally, they start to sit before they are aligned with the surface they plan to sit on. One method to encourage forward weight shift during transfers is to instruct the individual to place their hands on their thighs and push down through their legs, while going sit to stand and when going stand to sit, as described for PD (Figure 14-6). By doing this, the individual is forced to flex at the hips, keeping the center of mass aligned over the feet. In addition, it provides appropriate upper extremity support that facilitates, rather than hampers, proper body mechanics. Cueing with simple three-step instructions is used to encourage the individual to walk to the chair and turn, before lowering themselves onto the seat. Instruct the individual with HD to think and say "turn," "touch chair," and "now hands on legs and sit." Blocked practice of this task with many repetitions has been an effective way of teaching this transfer in our movement disorders clinic.

For those individuals who use an assistive device and cannot remember the cues, a cue card can be made and taped to the seat of their rollator walker. Caregivers are instructed to use a gait belt and to assist, by providing assistance at the hips. If chorea of the upper extremities is impeding caregivers during a transfer, the chorea can be minimized by instructing the individual with HD to "hug themselves."

Gait

Gait training is conducted, based on the impairments noted, and uses the techniques discussed in the PD section of this chapter. Research on walking devices and HD indicate that the rollator walker leads to the safest and smoothest gait.[132] As in PD, the rollator walker minimizes dual-task demands and provides a consistent source of stabilization, during turns. It is also easier to maneuver in small spaces.

Stairs

For individuals, who are still attempting curbs or stairs, the therapist should conduct a stair safety assessment. Individuals with HD report falls on stairs, while ascending and descending. They express that they have difficulty with foot placement. Observation of individuals with HD on stairs reveals a tendency to trip, while going up stairs, and to have uneven and unsafe foot placement, when going down stairs. Despite stating that they have fallen on stairs and knowing that they are not safe on stairs, individuals with HD continue to descend stairs rapidly without stopping at the top of the stairs and may not use a railing, even when it is present and needed. Therapy at this stage focuses on teaching the individual to: (1) stop, before starting the stairs and think about how to use the stairs safely; (2) grab the handrail; and (3) then, begin to ascend or descend. The individual with HD may also need to be taught to go slowly when descending the stairs. In the middle and late stages of the disease, the individual with HD has impaired short-term memory and cognition, resulting in an inability to cognitively learn the steps for safe stair use. They do remain able to motor learn and to learn new habits through repetition (implicit learning). If repeated frequently and done every time stairs are used, a new pattern for stair climbing can be learned in the middle stages of the disease. In the later stages of the disease, both cognitive and motor learning are severely impaired and unlikely to occur, so stair safety training is initiated early in the disease to ensure that it is a learned habit before they enter the later stages of the disease.

Caregivers are also taught to cue the individual to stop, think, and grab the handrail and encouraged to use a gait belt, when assisting someone on the stairs.

Late Stage Disease

In Part III of the case study, it has been 11 years since WD's diagnosis, and he is no longer ambulating. It is not unusual for clients to come to clinic having already purchased or borrowed a wheelchair. WD's wheelchair does not fit him and should be replaced with one that helps him sit upright and maintain independent mobility, if possible. Individuals with HD often slide out of their wheelchairs due to dystonic posturing and chorea. A seatbelt positioned at the pelvis keeps their hips back in the chair, enabling them to sit upright and remain functional. Additionally, individuals with HD are not able to use their arms to propel the wheelchair due to coordination deficits but are usually able to propel the chair using their feet. WD's wheelchair should be fitted so that he can keep his feet on the floor to propel the chair. It is recommended that the chair be fitted with elevating leg rests, as these can help to position the individual, keep them from sliding out of the chair, and will be needed as the individual becomes progressively less mobile.

WD's wife and children should be instructed on safe ways to perform transfers, including bending at the knees and using a gait belt to assist from the level of the hips. Additionally, family members are instructed that individuals with HD are slow to respond due to bradykinesia and difficulties with initiation. When the person with HD is instructed to do a task, the caregiver must allow extra time for the individual to respond. Caregivers often ask the person with HD to assist but do not give them time to respond, then, mistakenly believe that the person with HD is unwilling or unable to assist. Grab bars and other devices to assist with transfers must be firmly anchored in support beams as individuals with HD apply a great deal of shear force through objects, due to their chorea, and have been known to break furniture and grab bars, while trying to transfer.

Bathroom safety is a concern for individuals with HD, and falls are common in the bathroom and shower. Use of a tub or shower bench is highly recommended as many individuals with HD report losing their balance and falling in the shower, when they close their eyes. Furthermore, they fall when trying to climb over the edge of the tub. If the tub cannot be replaced with a shower, then, a bench should be placed in the tub. Toileting is another time when individuals are at high risk of falling. Grab bars or an elevated bedside commode placed over the toilet are helpful. Purchasing elastic waisted pants makes clothing removal safer and easier. Males may also need to be seated during all toileting as changes in balance can lead to falls.

In late stage disease, individuals with HD typically have significant chorea and dystonic posturing. These may even lead to falls from bed. The use of padded side rails, lowering the bed close to the ground, and/or moving furniture away from the bed helps to prevent injurious falls. Positioning in chairs eventually becomes quite difficult. In the home environment, recliner chairs are the safest option, as tilting the person back helps to prevent sliding out of the chair and provides head support. In long-term care facilities, the use of reclined chairs, with padding around the head, shoulders, and hips, helps to position the client and prevent

A Broda Chair   **B** Carefoam chair

FIGURE 14-8 Specialty chairs for seating the client with HD. (A, Used with permission of BRODA Seating, Kitchener, Ontario. B, Used with permission of CAREFOAM, Inc., Kitchener, Ontario)

injury, during choreic movements. At the time of this writing, there are two chairs on the market that fit the needs of the client with HD, the Broda® chair and the Carefoam® chair (Figure 14-8).

REFERENCES

1. Parkinson's Disease Foundation: statistics on Parkinson's. Available at: http://www.pdf.org/en/parkinson_statistics. Accessed June 3, 2014.

2. Parkinson's Disease Backgrounder. National Institute of Neurological Disorders and Stroke. Available at: http://www.ninds.nih.gov/disorders/parkinsons_disease/parkinsons_disease_backgrounder.htmed. Accessed July 3, 2014.

3. Van Den Eeden SK, Tanner CM, Bernstein AL, Fross RD, Leimpeter A, Bloch DA, Nelson LM. Incidence of Parkinson's disease: variation by age, gender, and race/ethnicity. *Am J Epidemiol.* 2003;157(11):1015-1022.

4. Wirdefeldt K, Adami H-O, Cole P, Trichopoulos D, Mandel J. Epidemiology and etiology of Parkinson's disease: a review of the evidence. *Eur J Epidemiol.* 2011;26:S1-S58.

5. Thacker EL, Ascherio A. Familial aggregation of Parkinson's disease: a meta-analysis. *Mov Disord.* 2008;23:1174-1183.

6. Noyce AJ, Bestwick JP, Silveira-Moriyama L, et al. Meta-analysis of early nonmotor features and risk factors for Parkinson disease. *Ann Neurol.* 2012;72:893-901.

7. Bondon-Guitton E, Perez-Lloret S, Bagheri H, Brefel C, Rascol O, Montastruc JL. Drug-induced parkinsonism: a review of 17 years' experience in a regional pharmacovigilance center in France. *Mov Disord.* 2011;26(12):2226-2231.

8. Poewe W, Wenning G. The differential diagnosis of Parkinson's disease. *Eur J Neurol.* 2002;9(S3):23-30.

9. Dauer W, Przedborski S. Parkinson's disease: mechanisms and models. *Neuron.* 2003;39:889-909.

10. Rodriguez-Oroz MC, Jahanshahi M, Krack P, Litvan I, Macias R, Bezard E, Obeso JA. Initial clinical manifestations of Parkinson's disease: features and pathophysiological mechanisms. *Lancet Neurol.* 2009;8:1128-1139.

11. Glendinning DS, Enoka RM. Motor unit behavior in Parkinson's disease. *Phys Ther.* 1994;74:61-70.

12. Benecke R, Rothwell JC, Dick JP, Day BL, Marsden CD. Performance of simultaneous movements in patients with Parkinson's disease. *Brain.* 1986;109:739-757.

13. Demirci M, Grill S, McShane L, Hallett M. A mismatch between kinesthetic and visual perception in Parkinson's disease. *Ann Neurol.* 1997;41(6):781-788.

14. Mancini M, Horak FB, Zampieri C, Carlson-Kuhta P, Nutt JG, Chiari L. Trunk accelerometry reveals postural instability in untreated Parkinson's disease. *Parkinsonism Relat Disord.* 2011;17(7):557-562.

15. Mancini M, Rocchi L, Horak FB, Chiari L. Effects of Parkinson's disease and levodopa on functional limits of stability. *Clin Biomech.* 2008;23(4):450-458.

16. Dimitrova D, Horak FB, Nutt JG. Postural muscle responses to multidirectional translations in patients with Parkinson's disease. *J Neurophysiol.* 2004;91(1):489-501.

17. Schoneburg B, Mancini M, Horak F, Nutt JG. Framework for understanding balance dysfunction in Parkinson's disease. *Mov Disord.* 2013;11:1474-1482.

18. Kim SD, Allen NE, Canning CG, Fung VS. Postural instability in patients with Parkinson's disease. Epidemiology, pathophysiology and management. *CNS Drugs.* 2013;27(2):97-112.

19. Inkster LM, Eng JJ. Postural control during a sit-to-stand task in individuals with mild Parkinson's disease. *Exp Brain Res.* 2004;154(1):33-38.

20. Latash ML, Aruin AS, Neyman I, Nicholas J. Anticipatory postural adjustments during self inflicted and predictable perturbations in Parkinson's disease. *J Neurol Neurosurg Psychiatry.* 1995;58(3):326-334.

21. Bleuse S, Cassim F, Blatt JL, et al. Anticipatory postural adjustments associated with arm movements in Parkinson's disease: a biomechanical analysis. *J Neurol Neurosurg Psychiatry.* 2008;79(8):881-887.

22. Khudados E, Cody FWJ, O'Boyle DJ. Proprioceptive regulation of voluntary ankle movements, demonstrated using muscle vibration, is impaired by Parkinson's disease. *J Neurol Neurosurg Psychiatry.* 1999;67(4):504-510.

23. Vaugoyeau M, Viel S, Assaiante C, Amblard B, Azulay JP. Impaired vertical postural control and proprioceptive integration deficits in Parkinson's disease. *Neuroscience.* 2007;146(2):852-863.

24. Vaugoyeau M, Azulay JP. Sensory information in the control of postural orientation in Parkinson's disease. *J Neurol Sci.* 2010;289:66-68.

25. Azulay JP, Mesure S, Ablard B, Blin O, Sangla I, Pouget J. Visual control of locomotion in Parikinson's disease. *Brain.* 1999;122(pt 1):111-120.

26. Ashburn A, Stack E, Pickering RM, Ward CD. A community-dwelling sample of people with Parkinson's disease: characteristics of fallers and nonfallers. *Age Ageing.* 2001;30:47-52.

27. Johnell O, Melton LJ, Atkinson EJ, O'Fallon WM, Kurland LT. Fracture risk in patients with parkinsonism: a population-based study in Olmsted County, Minnesota. *Age Ageing.* 1992:21:32-38.

28. Latt MD, Lors SR, Morris JG, Fung VS. Clinical and physiological assessments for elucidating falls risk in Parkinson's disease. *Mov Disord.* 2009;24(9):1280-1289.

29. Kerr GK, Worringham CJ, Cole MH, Lacherez PF, Wood JM, Silburn PA. Predictors of future falls in Parkinson disease. *Neurology.* 2010;75(2):116-124.

30. Pickering RM, Grimbergen YA, Rigney U, et al. A meta-analysis of six prospective studies of falling in Parkinson's disease. *Mov Disord.* 2007;22(13):1892-1900.

31. Falvo MJ, Schilling BK, Earhart GM. Parkinson's disease and resistive exercise: rationale, review, and recommendations. *Mov Disord.* 2008;23(1):1-11.

32. Glendinning DS, Enoka RM. Motor unit behavior in Parkinson's disease. *Phys Ther.* 1994;74(1):61-70.

33. Edstrom L. Selective changes in the sizes of red and white muscle fibres in upper motor lesions and parkinsonism. *J Neurol Sci.* 1970;11:537-550.

34. Inkster LM, Eng JJ, MacIntyre DL, Stoessl AJ. Leg muscle strength is reduced in Parkinson's disease and related to the ability to rise from a chair. *Mov Disord.* 2003;18:157-162.

35. Hausdorff JM, Cudkowicz ME, Firtion R, Wei JY, Goldberger AL. Gait variability and basal ganglia disorders: stride-to-stride variations of gait cycle timing in Parkinson's disease and Huntington's disease. *Mov Disord.* 1998;13(3):428-437.

36. Tolosa E, Compta Y. Dystonia in Parkinson's disease. *J Neurol.* 2006;253(suppl 7):VII7-VII13.

37. Schaafsma JD, Balash Y, Gurevich T, Bartels AL, Hausdorff JM, Giladi N. Characterization of freezing of gait subtypes and the response of each to levodopa in Parkinson's disease. *Eur J Neurol.* 2003;10(4):391-398.

38. Bohnen NI, Jahn K. Imaging: what can it tell us about parkinsonian gait. *Mov Disord.* 2013;28(11):1492-1500.

39. Ebersbach G, Moreau C, Gandor F, Defebvre L, Devos D. Clinical syndromes: parkinsonian gait. *Mov Disord.* 2013;28(11):1552-1559.

40. Amboni M, Barone P, Hausdorff JM. Cognitive contributions to gait and falls: evidence and implications. *Mov Disord.* 2013;28:1520-1533.

41. Brown LA, de Bruin N, Doan J, Suchowersky O, Hu B. Obstacle crossing among people with Parkinson disease is influenced by concurrent music. *JRRD.* 2010;47:225-232.

42. Potulska A, Friedman A, Krolicki L, Spychala A. Swallowing in Parkinson's disease. *Parkinsonism Relat Disord.* 2003;9:349-353.

43. Proud EL, Morris ME. Skilled hand dexterity in Parkinson's disease: effects of adding a concurrent task. *Arch Phys Med Rehabil.* 2010;91(5):794-799.

44. Wu T, Hallett M. A functional MRI study of automatic movements in patients with Parkinson's disease. *Brain.* 2005;128: 2250-2259.

45. Mentis MJ, Dhawan V, Feigin A, Delalot D, Zgaljardic D, Edwards C, Eidelberg D. Early stage Parkinson's disease patients and normal volunteers: comparative mechanisms of sequence learning. *Hum Brain Map.* 2003;20(4), 246-258.

46. Shabbott B, Ravindran R, Schumacher JW, Wasserman PB, Marder KS, Mazzoni P. Learning fast accurate movements requires intact frontostriatal circuits. *Front Hum Neurosci.* 2013;7:752.

47. Lim I, Van Wegen E, de Goede C, et al. Effects of external rhythmical cueing on gait in patients with Parkinson's disease: a systematic review. *Clin Rehabil.* 2005;19(7):695-713.

48. Chiviacowsky S, Campos T, Domingues MR. Reduced frequency of knowledge of results enhances learning in persons with Parkinson's disease. *Front Psychol.* 2010;16(1);article 226:1-6.

49. Lin CH, Sullivan KJ, Wu AD, Kantak S, Winstein CJ. Effect of task practice order on motor skill learning in adults with Parkinson disease: a pilot study. *Phys Ther.* 2007;87(9):1120-1131.

50. Nieuwboer A, Rochester L, Muncks L, Swinnen SP. Motor learning in Parkinson's disease: limitations and potential for rehabilitation. *Parkinsonism Relat Disord.* 2009;15(suppl 3):S53-S58.

51. Magalhaes M, Wenning GK, Daniel SE, Quinn NP. Autonomic dysfunction in pathologically confirmed multiple system atrophy and idiopathic Parkinson's disease – a retrospective comparison. *Acta Neurol Scand.* 1995;91(2):98-102.

52. Pfeiffer RF. Gastrointestinal dysfunction in Parkinson's disease (review). *Parkinsonism Relat Disord.* 2011;17(1):10-15.

53. Bronner G, Vodusek DB. Management of sexual dysfunction in Parkinson's disease. *Ther Adv Neurol Disord.* 2011;4(6):375-383.

54. Shen-Ting L, Dendi R, Holmes C, Goldstein DS. Progressive loss of cardiac sympathetic innervation in Parkinson's disease. *Ann Neurol.* 2002;52:220-223.

55. Nakamura T, Hirayama M, Hara T, Hama T, Watanabe H, Sobue G. Does cardiovascular autonomic dysfunction contribute to fatigue in Parkinson's disease? *Mov Disord.* 2011;26(10):1869-1874.

56. Protas EJ, Stanley RK, Jankovic J, MacNeill B. Cardiovascular and metabolic responses to upper- and lower-extremity exercise in men with idiopathic Parkinson's disease. *Phys Ther.* 1996;76:34-40.

57. Canning CG, Alison JA, Allen NE, Groeller H. Parkinson's disease: an investigation of exercise capacity, respiratory function, and gait. *Arch Phys Med Rehabil.* 1997;78:199-207.

58. Saltin B, Landin S. Work capacity, muscle strength and SDH activity in both legs of hemiparetic patients and patients with Parkinson's disease. *Scand J Clin Lab Invest.* 1975;35(6):531-558.

59. Carter JH, Nutt JG, Woodward WR. The effect of exercise on levodopa absorption. *Neurology.* 1992;42(10):2042-2045.

60. Senard JM, Brefel-Courbon C, Rascol O, Montastruc JL. Orthostatic hypotension in patients with Parkinson's disease: pathophysiology and management. *Drugs Aging.* 2001;18(7):495-505.

61. Shill H, Stacy M. Respiratory function in Parkinson's disease. *Clin Neurosci.* 1998;5(2):131-135.

62. Jankovic J. Parkinson's disease: clinical features and diagnosis. *J Neurol Neurosurg Psychiatry.* 2008;79;368-376.

63. Kehagia AA, Barker RA, Robbins TW. Neuropsychological and clinical heterogeneity of cognitive impairment and dementia in patients with Parkinson's disease. *Lancet Neurol.* 2010;9(12):1200-2013.

64. Barone P, Aarsland D, Burn D, Emre M, Kullsevsky J, Weintraub D. Cognitive impairment in nondemented Parkinson's disease. *Mov Disord.* 2011;26(14):2483-2495.

65. Docherty MJ, Burn DJ. Parkinson's dementia. *Curr Neurol Neurosci Rep.* 2010;10(4):292-298.

66. Rogers D, Lees AJ, Smith E, Trimble M, Stern GM. Bradyphrenia in Parkinson's disease and psychomotor retardation in depressive illness. An experimental study. *Brain.* 1987;110:761-776.

67. Santangelo G, Barone P, Cuoco S, et al. Apathy in untreated, de novo patients with Parkinson's disease: validation study of Apathy Evaluation Scale. *J Neurol.* 2014;261(12):2319-2328.

68. Weintraub D, Koester J, Potenza MN, et al. Impulse control disorders in Parkinson disease: a cross-sectional study of 3090 patients. *Arch Neurol.* 2006;63:969-973.

69. Fabbrini G, Latorre A, Suppa A, Bloise M, Frontoni M, Berardelli A. Fatigue in Parkinson's disease: motor or non-motor symptom? *Parkinsonism Relat Disord.* 2013;19:148-152.

70. Skorvanek M, Nagyova I, Rosenberger J, et al. Clinical determinants of primary and secondary fatigue in patients with Parkinson's disease. *J Neurol.* 2013;260(6):1554-1561.

71. Haehner A, Hummel T, Reichmann H. Olfactory loss in Parkinson's disease. 2011. doi:10.4061/2011/450939.

72. Ford B. Pain in Parkinson's disease. *Clin Neurosci.* 1998;5(2):63-72.

73. Caproni S, Muti M, Di Renzo A, et al. Subclinical visuospatial impairment in Parkinson's disease: the role of basal ganglia and limbic system. *Front Neurol.* 2014. doi:10.3389/fneur.2014.00152.

74. Ferini-Strambi L, Fantini ML, Zucconi M, et al. REM sleep behaviour disorder. *Neurol Sci*. 2005;26(S3):s186-s192.

75. United Kingdom Parkinson's Disease Society Brain Bank Clinical Diagnostic Criteria. Available at: http://www.ncbi.nlm.nih.gov/projects/gap/cgi-bin/GetPdf.cgi?id=phd000042. Accessed November 11, 2014.

76. Gelb DJ. Diagnostic criteria for Parkinson disease. *Arch Neurol*. 1999;56:33-39.

77. Lerche S, Seppi K, Behnke S, et al. Risk factors and prodromal markers and the development of Parkinson's disease. *J Neurol*. 2014;261:180-187.

78. Siderowf A, Lang AE. Premotor Parkinson's disease: concepts and definitions. *Mov Disord*. 2012;27(5):608-616.

79. Saracchi E, Fermi S, Brighina L. Emerging candidate biomarkers for Parkinson's disease: a review. *Aging Dis*. 2014;5(1):27-34.

80. Eggers C, Pedrosa DJ, Kahraman D, et al. *PLos One*. 2012;7(10):e46813. doi:10.1371/journal.pone.0046813.

81. Louis E, Marder K, Cote L, Tang M, Mayeux R. Mortality from Parkinson's disease. *Arch Neurol*. 1997;54:260-264.

82. Fahn S, Elton R. Members of the UPDRS Development Committee. In: Fahn S, Marsden CD, Calne DB, Goldstein M, eds. *Recent Development in Parkinson's Disease*. Vol 2. Florham Park, NJ: Macmillan Health Care Information; 1987:153-163, 293-304.

83. Hoehn MM, Yahr MD. Parkinsonism: onset, progression and mortality. *Neurology*. 1967;17(5):427-442.

84. Goetz CG, Tilley BC, Shaftman SR, et al., and Movement Disorder Society UPDRS Revision Task Force. Movement Disorder Society-sponsored revision of the Unified Parkinson's Disease Rating Scale (MDS-UPDRS): scale presentation and clinimetric testing results. *Mov Disord*. 2008;23(15):2129-2170.

85. Goetz CG, Poewe W, Rascol O, et al. Movement Disorder Society Task Force Report on the Hoehn and Yahr Staging Scale: status and recommendations. The Movement Disorder Society Task Force on Rating Scales for Parkinson's Disease. *Mov Disord*. 2004;19(9):1020-1028.

86. Aware in Care Kit. Available at: www.awarincare.org. Accessed 12/11/2014.

87. Faulkner MA. Safety overview of FDA-approved medications for the treatment of the motor symptoms of Parkinson's disease. *Expert Opin Drug Safety*. 2014;13(8):1055-1069.

88. Sinemet. Available at: www.drugs.com/pro/sinemet.html. Accessed 12/11/14.

89. Thanvi B, Lo N, Robinson T. Levodopa-induced dyskinesia in Parkinson's disease: clinical features, pathogenesis, prevention and treatment. *Postgrad Med J*. 2007;83(980):384-388.

90. Stocchi F, Jenner P, Obeso JA. When do levodopa motor fluctuations first appear in Parkinson's disease? *Eur Neurol*. 2010;63(5):257-266.

91. Pahwa R, Factor SA, Lyons KE, et al. Practice parameter: treatment of Parkinson disease with motor fluctuations and dyskinesia (an evidence-based review): report of the Quality Standards Subcommittee of the American Academy of Neurology. *Neurology*. 2006;66:983-995.

92. Benarroch EE. Effects of acetylcholine in the striatum. Recent insights and therapeutic implications. *Neurology*. 2012;79(3):274-281.

93. Riederer P, Laux G. MAO-inhibitors in Parkinson's disease. *Exp Neurobiol*. 2011;20(1):1-17.

94. Lindvall O, Bjorklund A. Cell therapy in Parkinson's disease. *NeuroRx*. 2004;1(4):382-393.

95. Coune PG, Schneider BL, Aebisher P. Parkinson's disease: gene therapies. *Cold Spring Harb Perspect Med*. 2010;2(4):a009431.

96. Zia S, Cody F, O'Boyle D. Joint position sense is impaired by Parkinson's disease. *Ann Neurol*. 2000;47(2):218-228.

97. Dalrymple-Alford J., MacAskill M, et al. The MoCA well-suited screen for cognitive impairment in Parkinson disease. *Neurology*. 2010;75(19):1717-1725.

98. Gill DJ, Freshman A, Blender JA, Ravina B. The Montreal cognitive assessment as a screening tool for cognitive impairment in Parkinson's disease. *Mov Disord*. 2008;23(7):1043-1046.

99. Brown RG, Dittner A, Findley L, Wessely SC. The Parkinson's fatigue scale. *Parkinsonism Relat Disord*. 2005;11(1):49-55.

100. Snijders AH, Haaxma CA, Hagen YJ, Munneke M, Bloem BR. Freezer or non-freezer: clinical assessment of freezing of gait. *Parkinsonism Relat Disord*. 2012;18(2):149-154.

101. Giladi N, Shabtai H, Simon ES, Biran S, Tal J, Korczyn AD. Construction of freezing of gait questionnaire for patients with Parkonsonism. *Parkinsonism Relat Dis*. 2000;6:165-170.

102. Giladi N, Azulay TJ, Rascol O, et al. Validation of the freezing of gait questionnaire in patients with Parkinson's disease. *Mov Disord*. 2009;24(5):655-661.

103. PD EDGE Core Measures. Available at: http://www.neuropt.org. Accessed 12/11/14.

104. Kelly NA, Ford MP, Standaert DG, et al. Novel, high-intensity exercise prescription improves muscle mass, mitochondrial function, and physical capacity in individuals with Parkinson's disease. *J Appl Physiol*. 2014;116(5):582-592.

105. Lima LO, Scianni A, Rodrigues-de-Paula F. Progressive resistance exercise improves strength and physical performance in people with mild to moderate Parkinson's disease: a systematic review. *J Physiother*. 2013;59(1):7-13.

106. Dibble LE, Hale TF, Marcus RL, Droge J, Gerber JP, LaStayo PC. High-intensity resistance training amplifies muscle hypertrophy and functional gains in persons with Parkinson's disease. *Mov Disord*. 2006;21(9):1444-1452.

107. Allen NE, Canning CG, Sherrington C, et al. The effects of an exercise program on fall risk factors in people with Parkinson's disease: a randomized controlled trial. *Mov Disord*. 2010;25(9):1217-1225.

108. Smania N, Corato E, Tinazzi M, et al. Effect of balance training on postural instability in patients with idiopathic Parkinson's disease. *Neurorehabil Neural Repair*. 2010;24(9):826-834.

109. Mhatre PV, Vilares I, Stibb SM, et al. Wii fit balance board playing improves balances and gait in Parkinson's disease. *PMR*. 2013;4(9):769-777.

110. Del Pozo-Cruz B, Adsuar JC, del Pozo Cruz JA, Olivares PR, Gusi N. Using whole-body vibration training in patients affected with common neurological diseases: a systematic literature review. *J Altern Complement Med*. 2012;18(1):29-41.

111. Ellis T, Motl RW. Physical activity behavior change in persons with neurologic disorders: overview and examples from Parkinson disease and multiple sclerosis. *J Neurol Phys Ther*. 2013;37(2):85-90.

112. Cholewa J, Boczarska-Jedynak M, Opala G. Influence of physiotherapy on severity of motor symptoms and quality of life in patients with Parkinson disease. *Neurol Neurochir Pol*. 2013;47(3):256-262.

113. Tomlinson CL, Patel S, Meek C, et al. Physiotherapy versus placebo or no intervention in Parkinson's disease. *Cochrane Database Syst Rev*. 2012;8:CD002817.

114. Fisher BE, Li Q, Nacca A, et al. Treadmill exercise elevates striatal dopamine D2 receptor binding potential in patients with early Parkinson's disease. *Neuroreport*. 2013;24(10):509-514.

115. Shulman LM, Katzel LI, Ivey FM, et al. Randomized clinical trial of 3 types of physical exercise for patients with Parkinson disease. *JAMA Neurol*. 2013;70(2):183-190.

116. Mehrholz J, Friis R, Kugler J, Twork S, Storch A, Pohl M. Treadmill training for patients with Parkinson's disease. *Cochrane Database Syst Rev*. 2010;(1):CD007830.

117. Picelli A, Melotti C, Origano F, Neri R, Waldner A, Smania N. Robot-assisted gait training versus equal intensity treadmill training in patients with mild to moderate Parkinson's disease: a randomized controlled trial. *Parkinsonism Relat Disord*. 2013;19(6):605-610.

118. Kadivar Z, Corcos DM, Foto J, Hondzinski JM. Effect of step-training and rhythmic auditory stimulation on functional performance in Parkinson patients. *Neurorehabil Neural Repair*. 2011;25(7):626-635.

119. Bloem BR, Grimbergen YA, van Dijk JG, Munneke M. The "posture second" strategy: a review of wrong priorities in Parkinson's disease. *J Neurol Sci.* 2006;248(1-2):196-204.

120. Kegelmeyer DA, Parthasarathy S, Kostyk SK, White SE, Kloos AD. Assistive devices alter gait patterns in Parkinson disease: advantages of the four-wheeled walker. *Gait Posture.* 2013;38(1):20-24.

121. Ashburn A, Fazakarley L, Ballinger C, Pickering R, McLellan LD, Fitton C. A randomised controlled trial of a home based exercise programme to reduce the risk of falling among people with Parkinson's disease. *J Neurol Neurosurg Psychiatry.* 2007;78(7):678-684.

122. Canning CG, Paul SS, Nieuwboer A. Prevention of falls in Parkinson's disease: a review of fall risk factors and the role of physical interventions. *Neurodegener Dis Manag.* 2014;4(3):203-221.

123. Li F, Harmer P, Fitzgerald K et al. Tai chi and postural stability in patients with Parkinson's disease. *N Engl J Med.* 2012;366(6): 511-519.

124. Goodwin VA, Richards SH, Henley W, Ewings P, Taylor AH, Campbell JL. An exercise intervention to prevent falls in people with Parkinson's disease: a pragmatic randomised controlled trial. *J Neurol Neurosurg Psychiatry.* 2011;82(11):1232-1238.

125. Farley BG, Koshland GF. Training BIG to move faster: the application of the speed-amplitude relation as a rehabilitation strategy for people with Parkinson's disease. *Exp Brain Res.* 2005;167(3):462-467.

126. Ebersbach G, Ebersbach A, Edler D, Kaufhold O, Kusch M, Kupsch A, Wissel J. Comparing exercise in Parkinson's disease – the Berlin LSVT®BIG study. *Mov Disord.* 2010;25(12):1902–1908. doi:10.1002/mds.23212. Erratum in: *Mov Disord.* 2010;25(14):2478.

127. Hackney ME, Earhart GM. Effects of dance on gait and balance in Parkinson's disease: a comparison of partnered and nonpartnered dance movement. *Neurorehabil Neural Repair.* 2010;24(4):384-392.

128. dos Santos Mendes FA, Pompeu JE, Modenesi Lobo A, Guedes da Silva K, Oliveira Tde P, Peterson Zomignani A, Pimentel Piemonte ME. Motor learning, retention and transfer after virtual-reality-based training in Parkinson's disease–effect of motor and cognitive demands of games: a longitudinal, controlled clinical study. *Physiotherapy.* 2012;98(3):217-223.

129. Pompeu JE, Mendes FA, Silva KG, Lobo AM, Oliveira Tde P, Zomignani AP, Piemonte ME. Effect of Nintendo Wii™-based motor and cognitive training on activities of daily living in patients with Parkinson's disease: a randomized clinical trial. *Physiotherapy.* 2012;98(3):196-204.

130. Oliveira RM, Gurd JM, Nixon P, Marshall JC, Passingham, RE. Micrographia in Parkinson's disease: the effect of providing external cues. *J Neurol Neurosurg Psychiatry.* 1997;63(4):429-433.

131. Ellis T, Boudreau JK, DeAngelis TR, et al. Barriers to exercise in people with Parkinson disease. *Phys Ther.* 2013;93(5):628-636.

132. Kloos AD, Kegelmeyer DK, White S, Kostyk S. The impact of different types of assistive devices on gait measures and safety in Huntington's disease. *PLoS One.* 2012;7(2):e30903.

133. Huntington's Disease Society of America's Fast Facts. Available at: http://www.hdsa.org/images/content/2/2/v2/22556/HDSA-FastFacts-2-7-14-final.pdf. Accessed 12/11/14.

134. Walker FO. Huntington's disease. *Lancet.* 2007;369:218-228.

135. Louis ED, Lee P, Quinn L Marder K. Dystonia in Huntington's disease: prevalence and clinical characteristics. *Mov Disord.* 1999;14(1):95-101.

136. Busse ME, Hughes G, Wiles CM, Rosser AE. Use of hand-held dynamometry in the evaluation of lower limb muscle strength in people with Huntington's disease. *J Neurol.* 2008;255:1534-1540.

137. Saft CS, Zange J, Andrich J, et al. Mitochondrial impairment in patients and asymptomatic mutation carriers of Huntington's disease. *Mov Disord.* 2005;20:674-679.

138. Wiesendanger M, Serrien DJ. Neurological problems affecting hand dexterity. *Brain Res Rev.* 2001;36(2-3):161-168.

139. García Ruiz PJ, Hernández J, Cantarero S, et al. Bradykinesia in Huntington's disease. A prospective, follow-up study. *J Neurol.* 2002:249(4):437-440.

140. Biglan KM, Ross CA, Langbehn DR, et al., PREDICT-HD Investigators of the Huntington Study Group. Motor abnormalities in premanifest persons with Huntington's disease: the PREDICT-HD study. *Mov Disord.* 2009;24:1763-1772.

141. Hausdorff JM, Cudkowicz ME, Firlion R, Wei JY, Goldberger AL. Gait variability and basal ganglia disorders: stride-to-stride variations of gait cycle timing in Parkinson's disease and Huntington's disease. *Mov Disord.* 1998;13(3):428-437.

142. Grimbergen YA, Knol MJ, Bloem BR, Kremer BP, Roos RA, Munneke M. Falls and gait disturbances in Huntington's disease. *Mov Disord.* 2008;23(7):970-976. doi:10.1002/mds.22003.

143. Rao AK, Muratori L, Louis ED, Moskowitz CB, Marder KS. Spectrum of gait impairments in presymptomatic and symptomatic Huntington's disease. *Mov Disord.* 2008;23(8):1100-1107.

144. Tian J, Herdman SJ, Zee DS, Folstein SE. Postural stability in patients with Huntington's disease. *Neurology.* 1992;42(6):1232-1238.

145. Skodda S, Schlegel U, Hoffmann R, Saft C. Impaired motor speech performance in Huntington's disease. *J Neural Transm.* 2014;121:399-407.

146. Heemskerk A-W, Roos RAC. Dysphagia in Huntington's disease: a review. *Dysphagia.* 2011;26:62-66.

147. Kagel MC, Leopold NA. Dysphagia in Huntington's disease: a 16-year retrospective. *Dysphagia.* 1992;7:106-114.

148. Feigin A, Ghilardi M-F, Huang C, et al. Preclinical Huntington's disease: compensatory brain responses during learning. *Ann Neurol.* 2006;59:53-59.

149. Schneider SA, Wilkinson L, Bhatia KP, Henley SMD, Rothwell JC, Tabrizi SJ, Jahanshahi M. Abnormal explicit but normal implicit sequence learning in premanifest and early Huntington's disease. *Mov Disord.* 2010;25:1343-1349.

150. Yaguez L, Canavan A, Lange HW, Homberg V. Motor learning by imagery is differentially affected in Parkinson's and Huntington's diseases. *Behav Brain Res.* 1999;102:115-127.

151. Paulsen JS. Cognitive impairment in Huntington's disease: diagnosis and treatment. *Neurol Neurosci Rep.* 2011;11(5):474-483.

152. Delval A, Krystkowiak P, Delliaux M, et al. Role of attentional resources on gait performance in Huntington's disease. *Mov Disord.* 2008;23(5):684-689.

153. Sitek EJ, Soltan W, Woeczorek D, et al. Unawareness of deficits in Huntington's disease. *J Int Neuropsychol Soc.* 2011;17:788-795.

154. Rosenblatt A. Neuropsychiatry of Huntington's disease. *Dialogues Clin Neurosci.* 2007;9(2):191-197.

155. Morton AJ. Circadian and sleep disorder in Huntington's disease. *Exp Neurol.* 2013;243:34-44.

156. Scherder E, Statema M. Huntington's disease. *The Lancet.* 2010;376:1464.

157. Seiss E, Praamstra P, Hesse CW, Rickards H. Proprioceptive sensory function in Parkinson's disease and Huntington's disease: evidence from proprioception-related EEG potentials. *Exp Brain Res.* 2003;148:308-319.

158. Hicks SL, Robert MP, Golding CV, Tabrizi SJ, Kennard C. Oculomotor deficits indicate the progression of Huntington's disease. *Prog Brain Res.* 2008;171:555-558.

159. Ciammola A, Sassone J, Sciacco M, et al. Low anaerobic threshold and increased skeletal muscle lactate production in subjects with Huntington's disease. *Mov Disord.* 2011;26:130-136.

160. Dawes H, Collett J, Debono K, et al. Exercise testing and training in people with Huntington's disease. *Clin Rehabil.* 2014. doi:10.1177/0269215514540921.

161. Van Vugt JP, Siesling S, Piet KK. Quantitative assessment of daytime motor activity provides a responsive measure of functional decline in patients with Huntington's disease. *Mov Disord.* 2001;16:481-488.

162. Busse ME, Wiles CM, Rosser AE. Mobility and falls in people with Huntington's disease. *J Neurol Neurosurg Psychiatry.* 2009;80:88-90.

163. Mehanna R, Jankovic J. Respiratory problems in neurologic movement disorders. *Parkinsonism Relat Disord.* 2010;16:626-638.

164. Quinn L, Busse M; On behalf of the members of the European Huntington's Disease Network Physiotherapy Working Group. Physiotherapy clinical guidelines for Huntington's disease. *Neurodegener Dis Manag.* 2012;2(1): 21-31.

165. Djousse L, Knowlton B, Cupples LA, Marder K, Shoulson I, Myers RH. Weight loss in the early stages of Huntington's disease. *Neurology.* 2002;59:1325-1330.

166. Aziz NA, van der Marck MA, Rikkert MG, et al. Weight loss in neurodegenerative disorders. *J Neurol.* 2008;255:1872-1880.

167. Kirkwood SC, Su JL, Connealy P, Faoroud T. Progression of symptoms in the early and middle stages of Huntington's disease. *Arch Neurol.* 2001;58:273-278.

168. Nance MA, Myers RH. Juvenile onset Huntington's disease – clinical and research perspectives. *Ment Retard Dev Disabil Res Rev.* 2001;7:153-157.

169. Shoulson I, Fahn S. Huntington's disease: clinical care and evaluation. *Neurology.* 1979;29:1-3.

170. Total Functional Capacity Staging. Available at: http://promoting excellence.growthhouse.org/huntingtons/monograph/pe5670.html. Accessed 12/11/14.

171. Huntington Study Group. Unified Huntington's Disease Rating Scale: reliability and consistency. *Mov Disord.* 1996;11:136-142.

172. Siesling S, van Vugt JP, Zwinderman KA, Kieburtz K, Roos RA. Unified Huntington's disease rating scale: a follow up. *Mov Disord.* 1998;13: 915-991.

173. Mason SL, Barker RA. Emerging drug therapies in Huntington's disease. *Expert Opin Emerg Drugs.* 2009;14(2):273-297.

174. Asslander L, Peterka RJ. Sensory reweighting dynamics in human postural control. *J Neurophysiol.* 2014;11(9):1852-1864.

175. Rao AK, Mazzoni P, Wasserman P, Marder K. Longitudinal change in gait and motor function in pre-manifest Huntington's disease. *PLoS Curr.* 2011;3:RRN1268.

176. Quinn L, Khalil H, Dawes H, et al. Reliability and minimal detectable change of physical performance measures in individuals with pre-manifest and manifest Huntington's disease. *Phys Ther.* 2013;93(7): 942-956.

177. Zinzi P, Salmaso D, DeGrandis R, et al. Effects of an intensive rehabilitation programme on patients with Huntington's disease: a pilot study. *Clin Rehabil.* 2007;21(7):602-613.

178. Busse M, Quinn L, Debono K, et al. A randomized feasibility study of a 12-week community-based exercise program for people with Huntington's disease. *J Neurol Phys Ther.* 2013;37(4):149-158.

179. Kloos AD, Fritz NE, Kostyk SK, Young GS, Kegelmeyer DA. Video game play (Dance Dance Revolution) as a potential exercise therapy in Huntington's disease: a controlled clinical trial. *Clin Rehabil.* 2013;27(11):972-982.

Review Questions

1. **Parkinson's disease is caused by loss of dopamine-containing neurons in the:**

   A. Substantia nigra pars reticulata

   B. Substantia nigra pars compacta

   C. Striatum

   D. Subthalamic nucleus

2. **A patient with Parkinson's Disease (Hoehn and Yahr Stage 3) who is taking Sinemet is receiving physical therapy for fall prevention. Which of the following impairments are most likely to contribute to the patient's balance problems?**

   A. Orthostatic hypotension, stooped posture, impaired postural reflexes

   B. Hypotonia, freezing of gait, orthostatic hypotension

   C. Chorea, stooped posture, festinating gait

   D. Stooped posture, dyskinesias, and motor impersistence

3. **A Parkinson-plus syndrome that is characterized by early postural instability and difficulty moving the eyes is:**

   A. Multiple system atrophy

   B. Corticobasal ganglionic degeneration

   C. Olivopontocerebellar atrophy

   D. Progressive supranuclear palsy

4. **A person with Parkinson's disease who is a good candidate for deep brain stimulation:**

   A. Has no response to levodopa

   B. Has never been treated with levodopa

   C. Has rigidity and dyskinesias that are no longer controlled with medications

   D. Has postural instability that is no longer controlled with medications

5. **A decarboxylase inhibitor carbidopa is given with levodopa (L-dopa) to:**

   A. Convert L-dopa to dopamine in the periphery so that it can cross the blood–brain barrier

   B. Aid in the uptake of L-dopa into nerve terminals

   C. Prevent the conversion of L-dopa to dopamine in the periphery

   D. Aid in the active transport of L-dopa across the blood–brain barrier.

6. **Which of the following neuropathological findings is characteristic of Huntington's Disease?**

   A. Degeneration of olfactory bulb neurons

   B. Atrophy of the caudate nucleus

   C. Demyelinating plaques surrounding lateral ventricles

   D. Lewy bodies in striatal neurons

7. **Early symptoms of Huntington's disease include:**

   A. Balance and gait disorders

   B. Depression and irritability

   C. Swallowing and speech impairments

   D. Dementia and hallucinations

8. **If a parent has Huntington's Disease, what is the chance of one of his or her children having HD?**

   A. 10%

   B. 25%

   C. 50%

   D. 75%

9. **When examining an individual with Huntington's disease, which of the following gait deviations are you MOST likely to observe?**

   A. Bilaterally shortened steps and reduced arm swing

   B. Decreased hip flexion with bilateral circumduction in the swing phase

   C. Bilateral Trendelenburg limp

   D. Wide-based gait with uneven step lengths

10. **In early Huntington's disease, involuntary movements like chorea are caused by damage to:**

    A. Medium spiny striatal projection neurons that are part of the indirect basal ganglia pathway

    B. Dopamine-containing nigrostriatal neurons

    C. Medium spiny striatal projection neurons that are part of the direct basal ganglia pathway

    D. Glutamate-containing subthalamic nucleus neurons

11. **A common method for assessing bradykinesia in Parkinson disease that is on the UPDRS.**

    A. Alternating pronation and supination

    B. Finger tapping

    C. Timed Up and Go

    D. The pull test

12. **Which of the following muscle groups is prone to shortening and contracture in individuals with Parkinson disease?**

    A. Ankle inverters

    B. Knee flexors

    C. Lumbar extensors

    D. Shoulder extensors

13. **Limited trunk rotation can lead to which of the following functional problems?**

    A. Ability to sit down on a chair

    B. Difficulty sleeping

    C. Tendency to fall posteriorly

    D. Walking with small steps

14. **Which of the following is one of the core measures recommended by the Neurology section PD EDGE taskforce for use when examining an individual with Parkinson disease?**

    A. Berg balance scale

    B. Mini-mental status exam

    C. Sit to stand 5 times

    D. Timed Up and Go

15. **Which of the following is a true statement regarding strength training individuals with Parkinson disease?**

    A. Eccentric exercise is contraindicated

    B. High-intensity strength training is not tolerated by individuals with PD

    C. Strength training leads to improvements in gait speed

    D. Strength training improves stair descent

16. **Balance training in individuals with PD leads to:**

    A. Faster reaction time

    B. Fewer falls

    C. Minimizes the limits of stability

    D. Slower movement velocity

17. **Treadmill training to improve walking speed should be done using**

    A. A harness to support partial body weight

    B. An aerobic training protocol

    C. Progressive increases in speed

    D. Speeds equivalent to running

18. **To alleviate freezing of gait the individual with PD should use**

    A. A gentle forward pull from the caregiver

    B. An assistive device

    C. Auditory cueing

    D. Rocking back and forth

19. **Which assistive device resulted in the fewest stumbles and lowest gait variability while maintaining gait speed?**

    A. A cane

    B. Front wheeled walker (2 wheels)

    C. Rollator walker (4 wheels, front two swivel)

    D. The U-Step walker

20. **A common reason that individuals with PD do not participate in community exercise programs is:**

    A. It costs too much

    B. They don't think it will help them

    C. They fear being made fun of

    D. They lack transportation

21. **An individual with Huntington's disease who has motor impersistence will demonstrate which of the following on examination:**

    A. A fall when a backward pull is applied to the shoulders

    B. Dance like involuntary movements

    C. Inability to move the eye side to side to follow the examiner's finger

    D. Inability to protrude the tongue and keep it there for several seconds

22. **In individuals with HD participation in activities is negatively impacted by which of the following psychological factors?**

    A. Agoraphobia

    B. Apathy

    C. Fear of falling

    D. Mania

23. **To overcome apathy the family and therapist should use which of the following techniques?**

    A. Use low-key and low-stimulation activities

    B. A set daily schedule

    C. New activities each day

    D. A quiet and soothing environment

24. **Individuals with HD often fall backwards into chairs, tipping the chair over, and sometimes breaking the chair. A method to improve safety of transfers is to teach the person with HD to:**

    A. Keep their eyes focused on the ceiling while sitting down

    B. Reach back for the chair before sitting in it

    C. Place hands on hips during the transfer and do a squat motion

    D. Place hands on thighs and slide the hands down while sitting

25. **When ascending and descending stairs individuals with HD exhibit which of the following problems?**

    A. Buckling of the knees

    B. Overuse of the railing

    C. Slow descent of stairs

    D. Uneven foot placement

Answers

1. B	2. A	3. D	4. C	5. C
6. B	7. B	8. C	9. D	10. A
11. B	12. B	13. D	14. C	15. D
16. A	17. C	18. C	19. C	20. B
21. D	22. B	23. B	24. D	25. D

Motor Neuron Disease and Neuropathies

Anne D. Kloos, Deborah A. Kegelmeyer, John A. Buford
and Jill C. Heathcock

15

OBJECTIVES

1) Describe the general approach to and interpretation of nerve conduction studies, including motor and sensory studies of peripheral nerves, and clinical electromyography

2) Describe the demographics, risk factors, etiology, pathophysiology, diagnosis, general progression and prognosis of Amyotrophic Lateral Sclerosis (ALS), Guillain–Barré Syndrome (GBS), Postpolio Syndrome (PPS), neuropathies, and brachial plexus injuries

3) Differentiate among signs and symptoms and impairments related to lower motor neuron pathology versus upper motor neuron pathology

4) Discuss the medical management of common symptoms found in individuals with motor neuron and neuropathy disorders

5) Design a physical therapy intervention program with appropriate goals and outcomes for the individual with motor neuron or neuropathy disorders

6) Discuss the current knowledge of degeneration and regeneration phenomena of nerve and muscle

● INTRODUCTION

This chapter focuses on diseases and disorders that affect neurons. Common to each of these disorders are changes in the way muscles are activated and nerves convey information. This may involve disruption in sensory afferents, lower or upper motor neurons, or all of these. Diagnosis of these conditions typically involves electrophysiologic testing, so we will begin this chapter with an introduction to these measures.

● ELECTROPHYSIOLOGIC TESTS

Electrophysiologic testing employs a variety of approaches to evaluate the function of the nervous system. This is also referred to as electrodiagnostic testing, but in a certain sense that is a misnomer. The results of these tests must always be correlated with other clinical findings and would never be diagnostic on their own. This is why the term electrophysiologic testing is more appropriate.

CASE A, PART I

Mr. Posner is a 40-year-old, married, father of two children, ages 7 and 9 who worked as the Chief Financial Officer at an insurance company. He was in good health until 6 months ago when he began to experience difficulty using his left hand for writing, typing on a computer keyboard, cutting food, handling utensils, and buttoning his shirts. He also noticed that his walking was slower and his legs sometimes felt "heavy and tired," after going up a flight of stairs. Mr. Posner went to a neurologist, who ordered a variety of tests, including electrophysiologic testing.

Usually, the focus of attention for electrophysiologic testing is on the peripheral nervous system, but there are approaches to measure central nervous system function, as well. **Nerve Conduction Studies** (NCS) in the peripheral nervous system are most useful for detecting reduced conduction velocity due to damage to the myelination of the nerves.[1] **Clinical Electromyography** (EMG) using needle electrodes within the muscles is the most reliable way to determine whether the axons themselves are injured.[1] Needle EMG can also allow for relatively specific testing of nerve root levels to aid in the diagnosis of radiculopathy.[2-5] Overall, the clinical reasoning used to interpret results from NCS and EMG studies mimics the clinician's reasoning using a combination of sensory testing and manual muscle testing. Findings are compared with known nerve root levels and peripheral innervations to identify the pathology. Electrophysiologic testing allows a greater degree of precision in grading the severity of the injury, provides the ability to distinguish myelin from axonal damage, and can be used to determine the chronicity of the pathology.

Nerve Conduction Studies (NCS)

Nerve conduction studies (aka Nerve Conduction Velocity Studies, NCV), are used to test the health and integrity of peripheral nerves. In general, the test is performed by using an electrical stimulator to depolarize a large number of axons in a single peripheral nerve. The response can be measured as an EMG (electromyographic) response, if the peripheral nerve innervates a muscle, or as the electrical potential created by action potentials traveling through another part of the nerve. If the nerve is damaged in some way that totally prevents transmission, the finding would be a total lack of response. Usually, however, there is partial damage. This will typically result in a response that is smaller than it should be, and conduction through the nerve that is slower than normal.

Motor Versus Sensory Tests

Motor Studies

In a motor test, the objective is to test the integrity of a nerve that innervates a muscle. There are a limited number of muscles that can be studied because there is not a motor test for every muscle in the body.[6] Typically, there is reason to suspect a problem with one or more peripheral nerves when a NCS is performed. The clinician would usually pick a particular peripheral nerve, such as the median, ulnar, or radial nerve in the forearm, and study one or two muscles innervated by that nerve to check for nerve function. For example, the ulnar nerve (Figure 15-1A) is usually tested with mm. abductor digiti minimi.[3,6] This ulnar-innervated muscle is easily accessible for surface EMG recording, and will typically be the first muscle in the hand to respond to ulnar nerve stimulation. For the median nerve, the mm. abductor pollicis brevis is used, and for the radial nerve, mm. extensor indicis proprius is used.[6] There will be a distal stimulation site and one or more proximal stimulation sites for most motor tests. For the median nerve, for example, the distal stimulation site is over the median nerve with a distance between the distal part of the stimulator and the proximal EMG electrode set to a standard of 8 cm.[6,7] From that point, the distance to more proximal sites must be measured, based on the individual, with a site in the antecubital fossa and another in the axilla used where the median nerve is accessible to stimulation. As an example in the lower extremity, the muscle studied for the deep fibular (peroneal) nerve would be extensor digitorum brevis in the foot.[6,8] The stimulation sites would be a point just lateral to the tibia 8-cm proximal to the EMG electrode, and a second point over the common fibular (peroneal) nerve by the fibular head.

The reason for having multiple stimulation sites along the length of the nerve is to be able to isolate a particular zone where nerve function is impaired.[1] In mild peripheral nerve injury, the injury mainly involves damage to the myelin sheath, with little or no actual loss of the axons themselves.[1] Because there are multiple Schwann cells that make myelin distributed along the length of the nerve, it is possible (and indeed, common) for a particular segment of nerve to sustain a **myelin injury**, while other parts of the nerve function normally. For example, consider an ulnar nerve injury at the elbow (Figure 15-1B). The conduction through the ulnar nerve from the distal forearm to the hand would be normal. The conduction from a forearm site just a few centimeters distal to the elbow could also be normal, but conduction impairment would be evident from a site just proximal to the elbow. It is important for the clinician to locate normal segments of nerve on either side of the damaged

segment, so with the ulnar nerve finding above, an additional stimulation site in the axilla would be required.[3,6] This would allow confirmation that segments of the ulnar nerve in the upper arm and in the forearm function normally, localizing the lesion to the elbow. To complete the picture, the clinician would want to confirm that the median nerve on the same side was normal, and that both the ulnar and median nerves on the other side were also normal.[3]

An important physiologic principle that allows motor testing to be done at multiple points along the nerve is the consistency in the sizes and conduction velocities of the alpha motoneuron axons. Alpha motoneuron axons do have a slight variation in size between the fibers going to slow oxidative versus fast glycolytic motor units, but compared to the whole range of nerve fiber sizes in a mixed peripheral nerve, the alpha motoneuron axons sizes and conduction velocities are relatively homogeneous.[1] A useful analogy is to think of an American football team running a 200-m sprint. The wide receivers and defensive backs will finish first. Running backs and linebackers will come in second. Defensive linemen will come in third, and offensive linemen will come in last. Individuals may vary, but as a rule, this would be the order of the groups. In this analogy, the very fastest group, the wide receivers and defensive backs, would be analogous to the large diameter sensory fibers. They are the fastest fibers in the nerve. The motor axons would be like the running backs and linebackers, who are still very fast. The linemen would be like the slower sensory fibers.

If we pick out the running backs and they all run 50, 100, or 200 m, they will still be bunched in a relatively tight pack for each distance. But if the whole team runs these various distances, then the farther the race, the greater the spread will be among the packs. In NCS, this spreading out of the arrival times of the action potentials is called **temporal dispersion**. Because the motor fibers are relatively homogenous in conduction velocity (temporal dispersion is low), stimulation at a variety of distances from the muscle will still result in a relatively synchronized arrival time for action potentials from all the stimulated axons, and hence, a relatively consistent size and duration of the EMG waveform recorded. This is the underlying physiology that allows testing for motor function at relatively long distances.

Sensory Studies

Sensory studies are more technically difficult to perform.[6] First, we do not have the luxury of recording an EMG response from a muscle. We must instead record the electrical potentials associated with action potentials traveling through the axons themselves. An EMG recording is actually produced by the action potentials and associated ionic currents in the muscle cells themselves, not the muscle nerves. Obviously, the muscle is much larger than a nerve, and there is much more current flow involved in a muscle action potential than a nerve action potential. The voltage from a muscle recorded through the skin is about 1000 times larger than the voltage that can be recorded through the skin from a nerve. Smaller voltages are harder to measure and are more susceptible to noise and technical error in the electrode placement and equipment setup, so this

FIGURE 15-1 Examples of motor and sensory studies for the ulnar nerve. In (**A**), the setup for measuring distal motor latency for the ulnar nerve is shown. In (**B**), additional proximal motor testing points are illustrated. With multiple points, the conduction velocities in the forearm, elbow, and arm segments can each be calculated. In (**C**), an antidromic sensory testing setup is illustrated. The stimulus is applied in a location similar to that used for the motor test. Recording electrodes around the small finger measure the SNAP as it passes antidromically through the digital nerves. **D** illustrates a sample ulnar nerve motor study in a case with mild slowing at the elbow. Arrows **o** and **p** indicate the onset and peak of each response. **E** illustrates a distal sensory antidromic study. Arrows **o**, **p**, and **t** indicate the onset, peak, and trough of each response. **F** shows the measures that would be obtained from D and E. For motor studies, the latency is based on the onset, and the amplitude is measured between the onset and peak. The segments are color coded, **D** for distal, **F** for forearm, **E** for elbow, and **A** for arm. To calculate conduction velocity for the proximal segments, the latency between responses from the two sites is divided by the distance between the sites. Normal conduction velocities should be faster than 50 m per second. Note the slowing at the elbow segment. Distal motor latency for the ulnar nerve at an 8 cm distance should be less than 4.2 msec and amplitude should exceed 2.5 mV. The values presented here should a normal distal motor result. For a sensory study at 14 cm, the latency should be less than 3.7 msec and the amplitude should exceed 15 μV. Sensory latencies are based on the time of the first peak, and the amplitude is measured from peak to trough. Again, this is a normal sensory study. The results are consistent with a mild myelin injury at the elbow. (A–C Adapted with permission from Centers for Disease Control and Prevention (CDC). Performing motor and sensory neuronal conduction studies in adult humans. NIOSH Publication No. 90-113, September 1990.)

makes sensory studies more difficult. Second, it is harder to be sure that the stimulating and recording electrodes are both in the proper location for a sensory study. For a motor study, we know the stimulation position is correct (if the muscle is intact) because we can see the muscle twitch, and with good knowledge of neuromuscular anatomy, it is not hard to find the muscles. In sensory studies, there is no corresponding response like a muscle twitch, and we cannot see or feel the nerve. We must know the anatomy and proper electrode positions to perform the test.

As noted above, there are also a wide variety of conduction velocities present among axons in a sensory nerve (temporal dispersion is high). As explained in the football team analogy above, this makes it hard to get accurate testing from long distances in sensory nerves. The arrivals of the action potentials are spread out, so the waveform is smaller and it can be hard to consistently measure its features. For this reason, there is usually only one distance, the most distal (shortest) segment, studied in a sensory test for a nerve conduction study. Additional distances can be tested, but this is not routine.

Motor and Sensory Studies Are Both Required

A complete nerve conduction study would include at least two sensory nerves and at least two motor nerves studied in the limb where there is a concern.[1,3,7-10] In addition, the same tests would need to be performed on the other side, and at least one of the other limbs should be studied (e.g., left arm, right arm, left leg). Additional tests would be added to rule in or rule out suspected conditions. Why include sensory tests when motor tests are easier? Sensory tests are more sensitive.[1] A pebble in the shoe of the wide receiver will make more difference (and be complained about for all to hear …) than a pebble in the shoe of the offensive lineman. The largest diameter axons are most sensitive to injury – even a slight myelin injury will notably reduce their conduction velocity. Hence, in mild forms of nerve damage, motor studies may be normal, but sensory studies will reveal the mild impairment. Thus, sensory and motor studies must both be done. Table 15-1 provides a list of nerves commonly tested in the upper and lower limbs for motor and sensory studies, including the stimulation and recording sites.

Measurements for NCS

The two most important measurements taken for NCS are latency (and where possible, conduction velocity) and amplitude.[6] From the most distal stimulation site to the recording location, we measure latency (the time between the stimulus and the response). Although it might be tempting to measure the distance and divide by time to calculate conduction velocity, this is invalid for the most distal site. When electrical stimulation is applied to a nerve, there is a series of events required to initiate an action potential. The capacitance of the tissue must be charged, voltage gated ion channels must open, and current must flow to depolarize the inside of the axon. This delay is called the **utilization time** and can take 0.5 msec or more.

In a motor study, there would be an additional synaptic delay of about the same duration at the synapse for the neuromuscular junction.[1] These delays may sound brief, but conduction velocities in human nerves are fast enough that the time taken to travel from the wrist to the finger might only be 2 msec, so these delays are substantial. Hence, for the most distal site, we measure the latency from the onset of stimulation to the response and record the number as a time without attempting to calculate velocity.

When there is more than one stimulation site on a nerve, as in a motor study, we can calculate the **conduction velocity** for the more proximal segments. Here, we take the difference in distance between the two stimulation sites and divide by the difference in latencies for the corresponding responses to calculate a conduction velocity local to the segment of nerve between the stimulation sites.[6] Whatever utilization time and synaptic delays might be present should not vary between stimulation sites, so as long as we focus on the relative times and distances, conduction velocity can be calculated. In the ulnar nerve example provided above, we would note a normal distal latency and normal conduction velocities in the forearm and upper arm segments, but a reduced conduction velocity in the segment at the elbow.[6,7]

Latency and velocity are the most reliable measures from NCS, but accurate readings require special care to use appropriate technique and to measure distances accurately.[6] Various studies have published normative values for distal latencies and segmental conduction velocities in the peripheral nervous system.[6,11] Modern testing equipment will typically have these values stored in software so that abnormal findings are automatically flagged.

The interpretation of prolonged latencies or reduced conduction velocities is that there is damage to the myelin.[1] In the race analogy above, we could imagine that there is a damaged section of the running track. The runners begin at normal speed, but

TABLE 15-1	Nerves and Sites for Electrophysiologic Testing[6]		
NERVE	**TEST**	**RECORDING**	**STIMULATION SITE(S)**
Median	Motor	Abductor pollicis brevis	Wrist, elbow, and axilla
Median	Sensory (antidromic)	Index finger	Wrist
Ulnar	Motor	Abductor digiti minimi	Wrist, below elbow, above elbow, axilla
Ulnar	Sensory (antidromic)	Small finger	Wrist
Radial	Motor	Extensor indicis proprius	Forearm, upper arm, axilla
Radial	Sensory	Thumb or dorsal wrist (antidromic)	Distal forearm
Deep fibular (peroneal)	Motor	Extensor digitorum brevis	Anterior leg, fibular head, popliteal space
Posterior tibial	Motor	Abductor hallucis	Distal leg above ankle, popliteal fossa
Sural	Sensory (antidromic)	Lateral foot	Posterior lower leg
Superficial fibular (peroneal)	Sensory (antidromic)	Dorsal foot	Anterolateral leg

slow down in the damaged section. Once past the damage, they return to normal speed. Myelin injury decreases the length constant of a myelinated nerve, which reduces conduction velocity.

In addition to latency and conduction velocity, the amplitude (size) of the response must also be measured. Due to individual variations in body composition and muscle and nerve location and size, there is more variation in amplitude. Nonetheless, amplitude must always be measured. In a motor study, for example, there will be multiple stimulation points along the length of the nerve. To ensure that the nerve was stimulated with equal effectiveness at all sites, we must attempt to achieve less than 10% variation in the amplitude of the responses.[1,6] Because temporal dispersion is low in motor nerves, this should be feasible if the nerve is normal.

If NCS reveals decreased amplitude and the test is done correctly, then this indicates a failure in conduction. Imagine in the running analogy that a section of track has totally failed; there is a giant pit. The runner cannot leave his lane, so he cannot finish the race. An action potential traveling along an axon can reach a point so severely damaged (by myelin loss or axonal injury) that conduction cannot continue. Just as the runner cannot switch lanes, the action potential cannot jump to another axon, so it ends. The result is fewer action potentials reaching the recording site, which results in a smaller amplitude of the response. With NCS, there is no way to distinguish between severe myelin and axonal injury; both will result in decreased amplitude.[1] Needle EMG does allow that distinction, so both NCS and EMG should be included in electrophysiologic testing.

Finally, in reading the results of NCS, there are some abbreviations commonly used that should be understood. In a motor study, the peripheral nerve is stimulated, the action potentials reach the neuromuscular junction, the muscle depolarizes, and twitches. What is being recorded is motor action potentials from all the motor units in the muscle that responded to the stimulus. The technical name for this is a **Compound Motor Action Potential**, and this is abbreviated as **CMAP**. So in motor studies for NCS, we record CMAPs. In sensory studies, we are also stimulating a large number of sensory axons and recording the combined voltage potential from them all as they pass under the recording site. We could call this a compound sensory nerve action potential, but the shorthand is simply **Sensory Nerve Action Potential**, and the abbreviation is **SNAP**. So in sensory studies for NCS, we record SNAPs.

Late Waves (F-Waves and H-Reflexes)

In certain locations in the body, a special kind of nerve conduction study can be performed to create a response that requires action potentials to travel from the stimulation site into the spinal cord and back out again. This can allow testing of the proximal nerve segments, including the brachial and lumbosacral plexus, when stimulation and recording sites are relatively inaccessible.

The H-reflex (named for the physician, Hoffmann, who described it) uses the circuits for the monosynaptic stretch reflex.[12] The peripheral nerve is stimulated to activate the Ia afferents from the muscle spindle. Action potentials travel along these fibers into the spinal cord, synapse monosynaptically on the alpha motoneurons, and cause them to make action

potentials. This volley of action potentials then travels out the alpha motoneuron axons to the muscles, resulting in a muscle twitch that can be measured with EMG.[1] Because of the long transit time required to the spinal cord and back, this is a type of late wave. The gamma motoneurons and actual muscle spindle proprioceptor organ are not involved in the H-reflex. The Ia afferent is stimulated directly, so no real muscle stretch is required.

Because the Ia afferents are among the largest, most heavily myelinated fibers in the nerve, they have the longest length constant and are therefore easiest to stimulate with electrical stimulation.[12] Hence, it is possible to stimulate a nerve with minimal current and elicit an H-reflex without directly stimulating the muscle. However, this is not a reliable approach to testing. If the nerve innervates the muscle appropriately, then it should be possible to stimulate a direct motor response in the muscle without waiting for the reflex, just as if this was a regular motor study. A reliable H-reflex test creates a small M-wave (the direct motor response) in order to establish effective and consistent stimulation (consistent M-wave size). This M-wave should not be full sized; it should be smaller than a full blown response. The measurement is the latency of the H-reflex that follows.[1] The latency is the only parameter used for the H-reflex. The objective is to elicit about 10 waves and demonstrate a consistent latency. If peripheral nerve tests are normal but the H-reflex latency is delayed, this is consistent with a nerve root impingement or nerve damage of some sort proximal to the most proximal stimulation site.

The F-wave also requires transmission through the proximal nerve to the spinal cord, but does not involve sensory fibers.[12] It was first described in the muscles of the foot, hence the abbreviation, F. Only the alpha motoneuron axons are involved in the F-wave. With stimulation of the motor axons, action potentials travel away from the stimulation site in both directions. The ones traveling toward the muscle in the normal direction (the **orthodromic** volley) produce a muscle twitch, whereas the ones traveling back toward the alpha motoneurons (the **antidromic** volley) would not be expected to do anything. However, due to special properties of motoneurons, a small subset of the motor pool will respond to the antidromic volley with depolarization sufficient to evoke an outgoing action potential. To observe this effect, maximal stimulation sufficient to produce a full blown M-wave is required. The exact latency of the F-wave will vary across trials because the exact set of alpha motoneurons participating is not always identical. Hence, 10–20 tests are performed, and the best latency is taken.[1]

H-reflexes can only be elicited from certain muscles. The only H-reflex used reliably in clinical testing is the soleus.[12] F-waves can be elicited from most distal muscles. Overall, late waves can be a useful adjunct in electrophysiologic testing, but they have limited sensitivity and specificity and would always need to be combined with other tests.[1]

Clinical Electromyography

There are many uses and applications of EMG, which is the recording and measurement of electrical potentials from the muscles. As described above, for example, CMAPs are used to measure motor responses to peripheral nerve stimulation. For studies in biomechanics and kinesiology, EMG is often used to discern how the muscles are activated in conjunction with movements like walking. For electrophysiologic testing, a different kind of EMG recording is used. A small needle is inserted directly into the muscle to record the electrical potentials in the immediate vicinity of the muscle cells themselves.

The purpose of this form of measurement is to study the activity of a single motor unit.[13] As noted in Chapter 4, a motor unit is comprised of one alpha motoneuron and all the muscle fibers it innervates. When the alpha motoneuron makes an action potential, all the muscle fibers in the motor unit should respond in a consistent manner. Wherever the needle tip happens to sit in the muscle, there should be a consistent and relatively synchronized pattern of ionic current flows each time a particular motor unit fires, and the consequence is a consistent voltage record in the recording.[13] A healthy motor unit should produce a wave form with an overall shape, duration, and amplitude that falls within general boundaries for the norm. The exact shape of each motor unit's waveform in the muscle will be unique, but factors such as the number of times the voltage goes positive and negative (baseline crossings) and the expectation that at least part of the waveform, usually the largest peak, should be negative (reflecting current going into the muscle cell) are hallmarks of normal motor unit waveforms.[1,13] Waveforms that are too brief, too long, too small, too large, or too complex with multiple baseline crossings can all be signs of specific pathologies.

Technically, a needle EMG study is easy to perform. The needle is smaller than most hypodermic syringes. A physical therapist is well aware of muscle location, function, and innervation, and this is the main knowledge needed to choose and study the muscles. In rare cases, there may be cause to study challenging muscles around the face or other sensitive locations. In this case, a responsible practitioner would refer out to someone more experienced, if necessary. The majority of studies are in the limbs and paraspinal muscles, where the risk of penetrating or damaging critical structures is low, and the physical therapist has more than adequate knowledge of the neuromuscular system. With appropriate training, needle EMG studies are well within the capacity of a physical therapist.[14]

In a typical test, a muscle is selected for study based on its innervation, including the peripheral nerve and the neurological segmental level from which it is controlled. The needle EMG is connected to a loudspeaker in addition to the recording circuit. With practice, the clinician can readily learn to hear the difference between normal and pathological waveforms in EMG. Again, the clinical reasoning mimics that used in selecting muscles to test, when there is suspected neuropathy or radiculopathy. The clinician should attempt to document the waveform and firing pattern for about 12 motor units from each muscle.[1] Studies indicate that this number provides the desired level of specificity and sensitivity. To do this, the pyramiding technique is usually employed. The needle is inserted into the muscle through the skin and recordings are made at three depths. Then the needle is withdrawn until it is not quite out of the skin, the angle is changed, and another set of three depths are studied. This is repeated two more times at differing angles, yielding 12 recording sites from one penetration of the skin.

From the first depth to the second and the second to the third in each electrode track, the needle is advanced rapidly to the next depth and then held still. In a denervated muscle, this mechanical irritation will evoke involuntary electrical activity in the muscle cells that cannot be suppressed. This is called **insertional activity**.[1] In a normal muscle, there will be a scratching sound while the electrode is advanced, but once the electrode is still, the muscle will be quiet. Therefore, significant insertional activity is abnormal and is a sign of axonal injury.

When the muscle fibers of a motor unit are first disconnected from the motoneuron, they will begin to atrophy and will begin making spontaneous action potentials in individual fibers of the motor unit.[13] Because only one myofibril fires at a time, these will be brief in duration and small in amplitude. Most importantly, they occur involuntarily while the patient is attempting to keep the muscle completely relaxed. These involuntary denervation potentials, also called **spontaneous potentials**, come in two distinct forms. One is called a **positive sharp wave**. These have a V-shaped appearance (by convention, positive is downward for EMG), and hence the name. The other waveform is a **fibrillation potential**. This is both positive and negative, but is extremely brief, much too brief to be a motor unit. For clinical interpretation, positive sharp waves and fibrillation potentials both mean the same thing; these spontaneous potentials are a highly specific sign of axonal injury.[13]

Another type of spontaneous potential is called a **fasciculation**. These are not always a sign of neuromuscular pathology and can be associated with fatigue, thyroid disorders, or excessive intake of stimulants. However, they also can result from peripheral nerve injuries or in lower motor neuron injuries. On EMG examination, a fasciculation looks like a normal single motor unit action potential. However, the fasciculation is involuntary. When a person is tired and the muscles around the eye twitch involuntarily, these are fasciculations. All people experience these from time to time, and they may not have any clinical significance. However, when they are widespread and cannot be explained by other common causes, and especially with accompanying signs of a primary neuromuscular disease, they become clinically significant.[15]

In a partially denervated muscle, over time, the motor units that remain innervated will be over worked to compensate. They will hypertrophy and be used even for low levels of effort. Hence, even with minimal effort, motor units with much larger than usual amplitude will be evident. These are called **giant potentials** and are an indication of relatively recent axonal injury.[13] The next stage in recovery would be for the alpha motoneuron axons, associated with these giant potentials, to develop collaterals and find ways to innervate the denervated muscle fibers nearby. The spontaneous potentials in these denervated fibers are a signal to the axon to find them. The motor unit that is composed of a combination of hypertrophied fibers as well as some recently reinnervated fibers will have a giant potential followed by some slower, smaller potentials called **satellite potentials**.[13] As the reinnervation proceeds, the satellite potentials will become stronger and somewhat earlier, but the motor unit in this case will not be able to reproduce the synchronous activation that would be found in a normal motor unit. The result is called a **complex polyphasic potential**, a waveform with multiple baseline crossings and a bizarre shape.[1,13] This would be the endpoint of the reinnervation process. Hence, EMG can be used to detect denervation, reinnervation, and the relative chronicity of the recovery process.

Normally, an individual should be able to gradually increase the recruitment of a muscle, adding in motor units according to the size principle.[13] Hence, with low effort, relatively small motor units are recruited at frequencies of 5–15 Hz. As effort increases, the frequency of the motor unit firing increases and more motor units are recruited. At moderate to full effort, the EMG recorded should become what is called a **full interference pattern**. So many motor units are firing that no single waveform can be distinguished, and the waveform is a chaotic assembly of up and down voltage changes. This is normal. The person should be able to reproduce this type of normal recruitment in any muscle on command.[1,13]

In muscular dystrophy, fewer and fewer muscle fibers over time will be functioning. The result can be that even when a person puts forth a full effort, it is still possible to observe individual motor units firing. This means there are so few motor units left that their waveforms cannot interfere with each other. In general, this type of waveform is called a **myopathic potential**.[1,15-16] There is also a phenomenon called **complex repetitive discharge**. In this condition, when a person begins to initiate light effort, a particular motor unit begins firing at an extreme rate, 50 Hz or more, and continues for several seconds, gradually reducing the rate, and then abruptly shutting off. **Myotonic discharge** is a similar phenomenon with a slightly different frequency profile. These are both considered relatively nonspecific findings that can occur in acute as well as chronic neuropathy or myopathy. A lack of complex repetitive discharges or myotonic discharge would be unexpected in myopathies, but their overall diagnostic utility is considered low.[17]

In sum, clinical EMG testing in any given muscle will involve the study of insertional activity, recording at rest to determine whether spontaneous potentials are present, recruitment through the range of efforts to determine whether myopathy is present, and then a systematic search to record resting activity and document motor unit waveforms from about 12 sites in the muscle.[1,13] If any abnormal findings are to be obtained, this number of sites should be sufficient to permit their observation.

RADICULOPATHY

In a suspected radiculopathy, the compression is at the nerve root. In this case, peripheral nerve conduction velocities may be relatively normal, and sensory tests may also be intact, even in the presence of altered sensation from sensory testing because the lesion may be proximal to the dorsal root ganglion. The H-reflex may be helpful in S1 radiculopathy, but in general late waves are not sensitive. The most important aspect of the examination in suspected radiculopathy will be the EMG. There are published clinical guidelines that recommend selected muscles in cases of suspected radiculopathy.[2,3] The general approach is to study muscles at various segmental levels, but not all on the same peripheral nerve, to provide a contrast between the nerve roots versus the peripheral nerves to correlate with the findings.[1] In addition, it is important to include paraspinal muscles. These proximal muscles, being close to the spinal cord, may show findings different than the limb muscles, and this can aid in determining the chronicity of the lesion.[4-5] Once a particular level is suspected for the radiculopathy, additional muscles are tested for that root level. The goal is to find two or more muscles from the same nerve root level but on different peripheral nerves that both show positive findings, but muscles from other root levels on the same peripheral nerve demonstrate normal findings.[1] This is not always possible, but the logic of the clinical reasoning for confirming radiculopathy should be evident.

PLANNING THE ELECTROPHYSIOLOGIC TEST

An electrophysiologic test may be ordered when neuropathy or myopathy is suspected, or in the examination for selected neurodegenerative diseases. Typically, there is a suspicion that a particular condition is present, such as carpal tunnel syndrome, a brachial plexus injury, etc., and the test will be designed around that expectation. As mentioned above, the clinician must always test both limbs (e.g., left and right arm) when a problem is suspected in one, and should also perform one test on the other extremity. For example, if a left arm problem is suspected, then the left and right arms should both be tested, and one leg should be tested, as well. This helps rule out central nervous system or systemic problems that could present as a peripheral nerve injury. The examination should include motor and sensory studies for NCS and EMG for selected muscles. In each limb, two motor tests and two sensory tests should be conducted to test different peripheral nerves. This helps differentiate nerve root levels from peripheral nerves. Finally, if radiculopathy is suspected, a set of muscles for EMG should be chosen to represent various spinal nerve root levels as well as various peripheral nerves. Late waves can be studied as well when the suspected pathology includes proximal nerve segments, as in plexus or nerve root injuries. To plan the electrophysiologic test, the clinician would review the suspected pathologies, consult the relevant clinical practice guidelines for that condition, determine which motor and sensory studies to conduct with NCS, and which muscles to study with needle EMG. In the limb with the impairment, the full set of muscles would be studied. In the limb(s) thought to be normal, EMG in key muscles would be recorded to confirm normal findings, but a full blown study might not be indicated. During the test, as findings unfold, the clinician would be guided by the results to selected additional tests to confirm or rule out the suspected condition(s). With this approach, electrophysiologic testing is a valuable part of the examination for the diagnosis of neuromuscular disorders (Table 15-2).

TABLE 15-2	Common Neuropathies and the Expected Findings from Electrophysiologic Testing
CONDITION	TYPICAL FINDINGS
Carpal Tunnel syndrome (median nerve mononeuropathy at the wrist)	Mild: prolonged distal latency in median sensory tests. Moderate: prolonged motor latencies, reduced SNAP and CMAP amplitudes. Severe: muscle atrophy, EMG + for denervation
Ulnar neuropathy at the elbow	Reduced conduction velocity across the elbow. Motor amplitude drops for stimulation above the elbow. Ulnar SNAP reduced (sensory fibers may have axonal injury). EMG + for denervation
Radial neuropathy at the axilla	Decreased SNAP and CMAP amplitudes if axonal injury. EMG + for denervation potentials, even in Triceps.
Radiculopathy	May have normal motor and sensory latencies, but reduced amplitude in the affected levels for CMAPs and SNAPs. EMG evidence of denervation in muscles at the affected level. Paraspinal muscles and limb muscles should both be examined.
Spinal stenosis	Presents like a multilevel, bilateral radiculopathy.
Plexopathies	NCS and EMG findings best explained by a particular part of the plexus rather than any one peripheral nerve of segmental level. CMAP and SNAP amplitudes reduced. EMG + for denervation.
Peroneal neuropathy at the fibular head	Tibial and sural nerve function intact, peroneal innervated muscles show positive findings, CMAPs and SNAPs reduced for peroneal motor and sensory NCS, reduced conduction velocity located at the fibular head, H-reflex normal, but F-waves impaired or absent.
Tarsal Tunnel syndrome	Prolonged distal motor latencies from tibial nerve in abductor hallucis and abductor digiti minimi pedis. Potentially prolonged latencies, reduced amplitudes, or both across the tarsal tunnel in the medial and lateral plantar nerves. Normal sural and peroneal nerve studies.
Diabetic peripheral neuropathy	Gloves and socks pattern of impairment, first noted in sensory studies, with motor findings indicating more severe impairment. Multiple nerves affected by distal slowing, not attributable to any particular nerve or segmental level.
ALS	Early signs would be EMG + for denervation potentials (with fasciculations considered significant) in multiple muscles at at least spinal levels and with varying degrees of chronicity (i.e., giant potentials as well as polyphasic potentials), but motor conduction velocities are normal. Reduced recruitment. Sensory testing would be normal unless there was some secondary problem (e.g., CTS).
Myopathies (limb girdle dystrophies)	Reduced recruitment levels, high frequency recruitment of motor units with minimal effort (early recruitment), small amplitude motor units, myotonic discharges.
Myasthenia gravis	Sensory studies normal. CAMP amplitude decrease by 10% or more in repetitive stimulation at around 3 Hz (2–5 Hz range acceptable). The decrement should be more pronounced after a short bout of exercise with the affected muscle.
Guillain–Barré syndrome	Combination of motor and sensory peripheral nerve involvement in upper and lower limbs. Motor symptoms are usually more severe than sensory in early stages. The LE sural nerve sensory test is often normal despite problems elsewhere ("sural sparing"), which is rare in other polyneuropathies. There is usually a distal onset with progression proximally. The principal signs are myelin injury (prolonged latencies with decreased amplitudes due to temporal dispersion) without axonal injury, but there can be axonal loss (EMG + for denervation) as a consequence of the myelin injury.

• AMYOTROPHIC LATERAL SCLEROSIS (ALS)

CASE A, PART II

Mr. Posner demonstrated abnormalities in both his motor NCS and the EMG studies, indicating a loss of motor axons and beginning muscle atrophy. Sensory studies in the upper and lower limbs were all normal. In the motor studies, CMAP latencies were normal (myelin intact), but amplitudes were reduced (axonal loss). EMG revealed spontaneous potentials (positive sharp waves and fibrillations) and polyphasic potentials in proximal and distal muscles of the upper and lower limbs. Recruitment was diminished, with failure to produce a full interference pattern in the muscles most affected. His neurologist diagnosed amyotrophic lateral sclerosis.

Epidemiology and Risk Factors

Motor neuron disease (MND) is the term given to a group of neurodegenerative diseases that selectively affect motor neurons. Amyotrophic Lateral Sclerosis (ALS) is classified as a rare disease, but it is the most common type of MND. It was first described in 1869 by French neurologist Jean-Martin Charcot, but since the beloved baseball player Lou Gehrig was diagnosed with it in 1939, the disease is commonly associated with his name in the United States. The number of new cases per year is generally two per 100,000 population, with the incidence increasing until age 80, above which there is a rapid drop in new cases.[18] The number of individuals living with ALS, within the United States, is estimated to be between five and seven cases per 100,000 population, which equates to 15,000–21,000 Americans living with ALS at any one time (based on US Census bureau population data from 2014).[18] Within the United States, non-Hispanic Caucasians are twice as likely as African American and Hispanic populations to develop ALS.[19]

Known risk factors for ALS include age, gender, family history, disease-causing mutations (in hereditary forms of ALS), and residence in geographic areas where clusters of patients with ALS have been reported. ALS primarily affects adults between the ages of 40 and 70 (mean age is 57) and is more frequent in men than women (1.56:1.00 ratio).[18,20] Although most patients with ALS have no family history of the disease (sporadic ALS, SALS), 5–10% of cases inherit the disease and are considered to be familial (FALS) cases. The Pacific island of Guam (US) and the Kii peninsula of Japan are two major regions of the world where an increased incidence of ALS with parkinsonism-dementia complex (PDC) has been observed. In addition, an almost twofold increased risk of ALS was found among military personnel deployed to the Gulf Region during the Gulf War.[21]

Some studies have reported links between lifestyle factors and ALS, including (1) cigarette smoking and alcohol intake; (2) having a body mass index in the normal to underweight range; (3) history of vigorous physical activity such as heavy manual labor, extreme athleticism; (4) physical trauma – skeletal fractures, electric shocks associated with unconsciousness or burns, or surgeries; and (5) dietary factors – eating high amounts of glutamate (i.e., protein) or saturated fat, low amounts of fiber or antioxidants. Similarly, environmental factors have also been linked to ALS, including (1) exposures to neurotoxins in agricultural chemicals (i.e., fertilizers and pesticides), (2) metals (i.e., lead, mercury, aluminum), (3) organic solvents (i.e., cleaning solvents and degreasers, alcohols and ketones, leaded gasoline fumes), and (4) repeated electric shocks. However, current evidence is not sufficient to definitively determine the influence of these factors on the risk of ALS.[18,22,23]

Pathophysiology

ALS is named for its pathophysiology. The term "amyotrophy" means atrophy of muscle fibers, which are denervated as their corresponding cranial and spinal motor neurons in the brainstem and ventral horns of the spinal cord (i.e., lower motor neurons) degenerate (Figure 15-2). Lateral sclerosis refers to hardening of the ventral and lateral columns of the spinal cord as corticospinal neurons (i.e., upper motor neurons) in these areas degenerate and are replaced by fibrous astrocytes (gliosis).

The etiology for most cases of ALS is unknown. The neurodegenerative process in ALS is thought to result from multiple mechanisms that individually or in combination result in neuron degeneration, neuron death, and finally ALS. These mechanisms include genetic mutations, glutamate excitotoxicity, mitochondrial dysfunction, neurofilament aggregation, neurotrophic factor deficits, ribonucleic acid (RNA) metabolism disorders, autoimmune reaction, and programmed cell death (apoptosis).[24,25] Mutations in superoxide dismutase 1 (SOD1), a gene on chromosome 21 that encodes the enzyme copper-zinc superoxide dismutase (CuZnSOD), are the most common cause of FALS.[25,26] The normal CuZnSOD enzyme functions to rid neurons of harmful free radicals.[24] The detrimental effects of the mutant SOD1 enzyme are thought to be mediated by a gain of one or more toxic functions, rather than the loss of normal function.[25] Sporadic ALS (SALS) has been linked to a variety of genetic mutations, including an SOD1 mutation that confers a susceptibility for the disease and/or modifies the age of onset and severity of the disease.[24,25] Elevated levels of glutamate, an excitatory neurotransmitter, have been found in individuals with SALS, which can be toxic to neurons.[25] The observation that the only effective medical treatment for ALS is riluzole, a drug that inhibits glutamate release, supports the excitotoxicity theory. Mitochondrial morphological abnormalities and/or evidence of mitochondrial dysfunction have been identified in the skeletal muscle, spinal cord, and frontal cortex of patients with SALS.[24] Abnormal aggregation of neurofilaments in the cell body and proximal axons of motor neurons is one of the most common pathological findings in ALS. Neurofilament aggregations are thought to disrupt axonal transport of proteins and organelles from cell bodies to axon terminal endings that are critical to neuronal function and survival. Deficits in growth factors (i.e., vascular endothelial growth factor [VEGF], ciliary

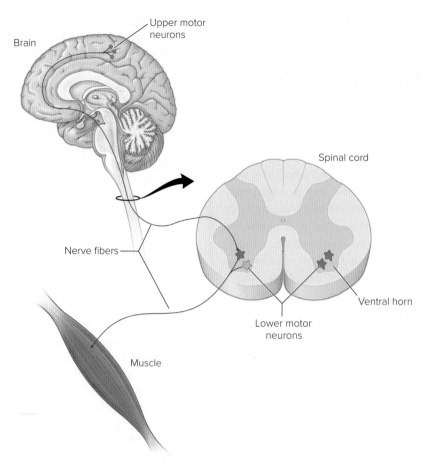

FIGURE 15-2 Pathophysiology of ALS. ALS affects upper motor neurons that arise from the cortex and brainstem as well as cranial and spinal lower motor neurons that arise from the brainstem and spinal cord.

neurotrophic factor [CNTF], insulin growth factor-1, glial cell line-derived neurotrophic factor [GBNF], and brain-derived neurotrophic factor [BDNF]) have been investigated and potentially implicated in the pathogenesis of ALS.[25,27] Genetic mutations of the RNA processing protein tar DNA-binding protein-43 (TDP-43) has also been associated with ALS.[7,8] There is also evidence for inflammatory damage of motor neurons caused by activated astrocytes and microglia, suggesting that ALS may have an autoimmune basis.[24,25] Motor neurons die in ALS through a programmed cell death mechanism similar to apoptosis that appears to be caused by activation of caspase pathways that break down essential cell proteins.[24,25]

The selective damage to motor neurons in ALS is hypothesized to be due to (1) their large size and long axonal length that require high mitochondrial activity and neurofilament content for energy and structural integrity and (2) the high content of SOD1 protein within them.[28] In addition, motor neurons appear to be especially sensitive to glutamate excitotoxicity.[28] Motor neuron loss is greater in large myelinated motor neurons than smaller ones and proceeds more rapidly in the early stages of the disease than later ones. Neuropathological and electrophysiological evidence indicates that neurodegeneration begins in the distal axon and proceeds in a "dying back" pattern toward the cell body; notably, cortical and spinal motor neurons degenerate independently of each other.[29,30] On biopsy, degeneration of motor axons with associated atrophy can be observed in the

ventral roots in the spinal cord and within the corticospinal tracts. In advanced cases, atrophy may be present in the frontal (i.e., primary motor and premotor cortex) and temporal lobes as well. As axons degenerate in the periphery, collateral branches of surviving axons in the surrounding area will sprout and reinnervate denervated muscle fibers, thereby compensating for the motor unit loss. However, once the motor unit loss exceeds about 50%, reinnervation cannot compensate for the degeneration and motor impairments develop. By the time most patients report weakness, they have already lost as much as 50% of their motor neurons in the areas of weakness.

Clinical Presentation and Progression

The classic presentation of ALS is slowly progressive, asymmetric muscular weakness and atrophy indicative of LMN involvement along with UMN signs of hyperreflexia. In 70–80% of patients, symptoms begin in the extremities (i.e., limb-onset ALS), while 20–30% of patients present with bulbar symptoms (i.e., bulbar-onset ALS) (Table 15-3). Distal extremity muscles (i.e., hands and feet) are often involved before proximal extremity muscles. As in Mr. Posner's case, patients with early leg involvement often complain of tripping, stumbling, or awkwardness, when walking or running; those with arm involvement may complain of dropping things and difficulty picking up small objects or buttoning shirts. Bulbar-onset ALS occurs more frequently in middle-aged women, and initial symptoms

TABLE 15-3	Motor Neuron Pathology and Associated Signs and Symptoms in ALS	
MOTOR NEURON TYPE	**AFFECTED NEURONS**	**ASSOCIATED SIGNS AND SYMPTOMS**
Upper motor neurons (UMN)	Pyramidal Betz motor neurons in the cerebral cortex, corticospinal and corticobulbar tracts	Loss of dexterity or the ability to coordinate movements; muscle paresis; spasticity; Hoffmann and Babinski reflexes; hyperreflexia; spastic dysarthria
Brainstem motor neurons (Bulbar)	Cranial nerve nuclei: V (trigeminal), VII (facial), IX (glossopharyngeal), X (vagus), and XII (hypoglossal)	Difficulty with chewing, Dysphagia; flaccid dysarthria/anarthria
Lower motor neurons (LMN)	Ventral horn cells in the spinal cord	Muscle paralysis and atrophy; fasciculations; flaccid tone; hyporeflexia; respiratory problems

include difficulty chewing, swallowing, and speaking. Tongue fasciculations (visible muscle twitches of the tongue) and atrophy as well as an increased jaw jerk reflex are common signs of bulbar-onset ALS. Despite the variability in symptom presentation, the course of the disease is similar in most patients with progressive spread of muscle weakness to other areas, leading eventually to total paralysis of spinal musculature and muscles innervated by the cranial nerves.

Clinical features that are atypical of ALS include sensory dysfunction, bowel and bladder impairment, autonomic dysfunction, abnormalities of eye movements, movement disorders, and cognitive dysfunction. Sensory pathways for the most part are spared in ALS, although studies have reported sensory deficits in some individuals.[31,32] Some individuals with ALS may complain of vague, ill-defined sensory symptoms of paresthesia or focal pain. Motor neurons at the second sacral level in the spinal cord (S2) that control the anal and external urethral sphincter muscles and muscles of the pelvic floor are also generally spared. However, some individuals do experience urinary symptoms, such as urgency, obstructive micturition, or both, suggesting that supranuclear control over sympathetic, parasympathetic, and somatic neurons may be abnormal in ALS. The oculomotor, trochlear, and abducens nerves that control external ocular muscles are also typically spared, until late

stages of the disease. Individuals who are maintained on long-term ventilation may develop ophthalmoplegia, a complete ocular paralysis and inability to tightly close the eyes due to degeneration of these nerves.

Longitudinal studies of the natural history of ALS have revealed that symptoms tend to progress in a contiguous manner, meaning that they spread from one focal region to an anatomically adjacent area.[33] For example, symptoms that start in one arm spread the fastest to the opposite arm, then to the ipsilateral leg, contralateral leg, and brainstem in that order. Thus, patients with initial unilateral arm or leg involvement often develop symptoms in spinal cord levels before they develop bulbar symptoms.

Diagnosis and Variants of ALS

Due to a lack of definitive diagnostic tests or biological markers, the diagnosis of ALS is made by clinical findings of a progressive course of weakness, with both UMN and LMN findings in four anatomically defined regions of the body: brainstem (bulbar), cervical, thoracic, and lumbosacral. Differential medical diagnosis includes exclusion of other musculoskeletal, neurologic, or systemic conditions. The El Escorial World Federation of Neurology criteria for the diagnosis of ALS (possible, probable, and definite) has been widely accepted for use in clinical practice, clinical trials, and research (see Table 15-4).[34]

TABLE 15-4	El Escorial Criteria for Diagnosis of ALS[34]	
ALS DIAGNOSTIC CATEGORY	**REQUIREMENTS**
Definite ALS	LMN and UMN signs in the brainstem and 2 spinal regions or in 3 spinal regions
Definite familial ALS	LMN and UMN signs in 1 region of the body plus laboratory-supported identification of gene mutation associated with ALS
Probable ALS	LMN and UMN signs in at least 2 regions with some UMN signs rostral to LMN signs
Probable ALS (laboratory supported)	LMN and UMN signs in only 1 region of the body, or UMN signs alone are present in 1 region, plus electromyographic evidence of acute denervation in 2 or more muscles in 2 or more limbs
Possible ALS	LMN and UMN signs in only 1 region of the body or UMN signs are found alone in 2 or more regions or LMN signs are found rostral to UMN signs, plus the diagnosis of probable ALS (laboratory supported) cannot be proven

ALS, amyotrophic lateral sclerosis; LMN, lower motor neuron; UMN, upper motor neuron.

Electrophysiological, muscle biopsy, and neuroimaging studies can be used to support the diagnosis of ALS and to rule out other diagnoses. NCS of peripheral sensory and motor neurons are usually normal or near normal in ALS. Electromyographic studies typically reveal signs of active denervation (i.e., fibrillation and fasciculation potentials, positive sharp waves) as well as chronic denervation (i.e., large or unstable motor unit potentials, reduced motor unit recruitment) (see Electromyography section). Muscle biopsy studies in ALS corroborate EMG findings, showing signs of denervation (i.e., atrophied muscle fibers) and reinnervation (i.e., fiber type grouping) (Figure 15-3). Degeneration of corticospinal tracts and altered cortical activation, during motor tasks, has been detected in patients with ALS, using conventional magnetic resonance imaging (MRI), transcranial magnetic stimulation (TMS), proton magnetic resonance spectroscopy (^{1}H-MRS), functional MRI (fMRI), and diffusion tensor MRI.[35] The sensitivity and specificity of neuroimaging techniques to diagnose ALS is currently under investigation.

There are several variants of SALS (primary lateral sclerosis, progressive spinal muscular atrophy, progressive bulbar palsy, and pseudobulbar palsy) that may evolve over time to become classical ALS (Table 15-5). **Primary lateral sclerosis** (PLS) is a slowly progressive disorder caused by damage of the corticospinal and sometimes corticobulbar pathways resulting in purely UMN symptoms. **Progressive muscular atrophy** (PMA) is an entirely LMN disorder that affects extremity muscles initially and only later affects bulbar and respiratory muscles. **Progressive bulbar palsy** (PBP) is due to degeneration of cranial motor neurons IX, X, and XII resulting in bulbar symptoms; it is more common in older women. **Pseudobulbar palsy** (aka spastic bulbar palsy) results from corticobulbar tract degeneration and is characterized by spastic dysarthria, dysphagia, dysphonia, impairment of voluntary movements of tongue and facial muscles, and emotional lability. Patients with PLS and PMA typically have a longer survival than classical ALS, while those with bulbar variants usually have a worse prognosis.

In addition to classical ALS, there are also variants of ALS that have additional features called **ALS-Plus syndromes**. It is now recognized that a subset of patients with ALS have cognitive and behavioral changes and some develop frontotemporal dementia (ALS-FTD) or Parkinsonism-dementia complex (PDC).[35-37] Neuronal loss in frontal and temporal lobes and degeneration of cranial and spinal motor neurons, with relative sparing of corticospinal and corticobulbar tracts, characterize ALS-FTD. Thus, patients with ALS-FTD show signs and symptoms of frontal and temporal lobe dysfunction along with LMN signs (i.e., weakness, muscle atrophy, and fasciculations). Individuals with ALS-PDC show additional signs of parkinsonism (i.e., bradykinesia, rigidity, tremor), related to neuronal degeneration in the substantia nigra. In addition, about a third of patients with ALS show mild cognitive (ALSci) and/or behavioral (ALSbi) impairments.[38] ALSci is characterized by early deficits in verbal (letter) fluency and a mild dysexecutive syndrome, while ALSbi is characterized by some criteria for FTD, especially apathy.[39-41] The clinical course is usually more rapid in patients with ALS-FTD, most likely because they typically have bulbar involvement and may be noncompliant with treatment recommendations due to lack of understanding or apathy. The mutated TDP-43 protein was found in the neuronal inclusions of patients with ALS and patients with ALS-FDT, suggesting that there may be a common mechanism underlying these variants.[42]

Medical Prognosis

ALS is a steadily progressive disease and does not usually have periods of remission; stable plateaus are rare. The rate of progression is usually consistent for each patient but varies widely

FIGURE 15-3 Muscle biopsy findings in ALS. Top left: Normal: muscle fibers with polygonal fiber shape; top right: ALS: atrophic, angulated muscle fibers (end of arrows); bottom left: normal muscle contains a random checkerboard-like interdigitation of Type I (cream) and Type II (brown) myofiber types. Bottom right: Fiber grouping seen in ALS: the left-hand side shows a field composed exclusively of Type II myofibers, stained purple. On the right side is a field of Type I myofibers, stained pink.

TABLE 15-5	Variants of Sporadic Amyotrophic Lateral Sclerosis	
TYPE	**UMN SIGNS AND SYMPTOMS**	**LMN SIGNS AND SYMPTOMS**
Amyotrophic lateral sclerosis (ALS)	Yes – brainstem and spinal regions	Yes – brainstem and spinal regions
Primary lateral sclerosis (PLS)	Yes – brainstem and spinal regions	No
Progressive spinal muscular atrophy (PMA)	No	Yes – spinal regions
Progressive bulbar palsy	No	Yes – brainstem region
Pseudobulbar palsy	Yes – brainstem region	No

UMN, upper motor neuron; LMN, lower motor neuron; brainstem region refers to involvement of bulbar (mouth, face, throat) muscles; spinal regions refers to involvement of respiratory and arm, leg, and trunk muscles.

TABLE 15-6	Prognostic Factors of ALS
POSITIVE PROGNOSTIC FACTORS	**NEGATIVE PROGNOSTIC FACTORS**
• Younger age at onset (<40 years old) • Limb versus bulbar onset • Longer interval between onset and diagnosis • Less severe involvement at the time of diagnosis • Predominant UMN signs at the time of diagnosis • Attendance at multidisciplinary ALS clinics • Better psychological well-being • Use of riluzole (2–3 months) • Use of ventilatory assistance • Primary lateral sclerosis (PLS) or progressive muscular atrophy (PMA)	• Cognitive abnormalities and dementia • Progressive bulbar palsy or pseudobulbar palsy • Respiratory symptoms at onset • Malnutrition

between individuals with disease durations ranging from a few months to 20 years. Death occurs on average 3–5 years from the time of diagnosis, primarily from respiratory failure.[18] Other frequent causes of death are aspiration pneumonia and malnutrition. Several factors are associated with a better prognosis in patients with ALS (Table 15-6).[43-45]

Medical Management

The clinical management of patients with ALS is complex and requires a comprehensive and multidisciplinary approach. Specialized centers or clinics that meet rigorous standards set by the Amyotrophic Lateral Sclerosis Association (ALSA) and the Muscular Dystrophy Association (MDA) are considered to be the most advantageous health care setting for the management of individuals with ALS. Studies, comparing a cohort of patients attending a multidisciplinary clinic versus those attending a general neurology clinic, reported that the median survival of the ALS clinic cohort was 7.5 and 10.2 months longer than for patients in the general neurology cohort, and the prognosis of bulbar onset patients was extended by 9.6 months.[46,47] These findings suggest that more active and aggressive management, including increased use of noninvasive ventilation, attention to nutrition, and earlier referral to palliative services enhances survival.

Although there is no cure for ALS, many clinical trials to evaluate medications for reducing mortality and treating symptoms are ongoing. At present, Riluzole® (Rilutec) is the only medication approved by the Food and Drug Administration to treat ALS. This drug is a glutamate inhibitor and delays disease progression modestly, extending survival for about 2–4 months.[48] The drug is usually well tolerated, but adverse effects include fatigue, weakness, nausea, vomiting, dizziness, and liver toxicity (requires discontinuation). In addition to riluzole, there are many medications and interventions that are used to treat symptoms (Table 15-7).[49,50] Recommendations and guidelines for the symptomatic care of patients with ALS were published by the American Academy of Neurology[51,52] and by the European Federation of Neurological Societies.[53]

Management of Respiratory Impairments

Weakness of the bulbar muscles that manage the upper airway and the spinal inspiratory and expiratory muscles leads to respiratory impairments that increase the patient's risk for respiratory tract infections. Infections can be prevented with yearly pneumococcal and influenza vaccinations,[18] avoidance of aspiration, and effective management of oral and pulmonary secretions. Supplemental oxygen is used very cautiously with patients with ALS because it can suppress the drive to breathe, thereby leading to worsening hypercapnia and respiratory arrest. It is recommended only for those with concomitant pulmonary disease and as a comfort measure for those who decline ventilatory support.

When forced vital capacity (FVC) decreases to 50% of predicted normal, **positive-pressure noninvasive ventilation** (NIPPV) is recommended.[51] NIPPV does not require placement of a tracheal tube and can be delivered by mouth, oralnasally, or nasally. **Bi-level positive airway pressure** (BiPAP) is a positive airway pressure system that delivers different pressures, during inspiration and expiration, and is well tolerated by many individuals with ALS. Most patients with ALS begin

TABLE 15-7	Symptomatic Treatment of Amyotrophic Lateral Sclerosis	
SYMPTOM TREATED	**MEDICAL MANAGEMENT**	**OTHER TREATMENTS**
Excessive watery saliva (sialorrhea)	Amitriptyline (Elavil); transdermal hyoscine (Scopolamine); atropine; injections of botulinum toxin into parotid and salivary glands; irradiation of salivary glands.	Home suction device; dark grape juice; sugar-free citrus lozenges; nebulization or steam inhalation.
Thick saliva and bronchial secretions	Mucolytics (N-acetylcysteine); beta-receptor antagonists (propranolol [Inderal], metoprolol [Toprol]); anticholinergic bronchodilators (ipratropium, theophylline).	Manually assisted coughing techniques; home suction device; mechanical insufflator–exsufflator cough machines; rehydration (jelly or ice); pineapple or papaya juice; reduced intake of dairy products, alcohol, and caffeine.
Dysphagia	Enteric feeding considered if there is more than 10% loss of baseline weight; percutaneous endoscopic gastroscopy (PEG) preferably before FVC falls below 50% predicted; radiologically inserted gastrostomy (RIG) for individuals with FVC ≤50%; nasogastric tube feeding and IV hydration as temporary measure or for patients who refuse PEG.	Referrals to nutritionist or registered dietician for dietary counseling and management and SLP for swallowing evaluation; PT/OT to address proper sitting posture and adaptive eating utensils; eating and swallowing strategies such as: taking smaller bites of food; modifications to texture and consistency of food (blending food, adding thickeners to drinks); nutritional supplements to increase caloric intake; "chin tuck" maneuver or performing a clearing cough after each swallow.
Respiratory impairments	Noninvasive positive pressure (NIPPV) ventilation (i.e., BiPAP) if FVC <50% predicted or there are respiratory symptoms; tracheostomy ventilation if NIPPV not tolerated or NIPPV is not able to compensate for respiratory impairment; morphine for relief from respiratory distress if ventilation is refused.	PT to provide: patient and caregiver education, breathing exercises, positioning to optimize ventilation, airway clearance techniques; prompt treatment of pneumonia and pulmonary infections, prevention by vaccination, avoidance of contact with people with colds or influenza; prevention and treatment of deep vein thromboses to avoid pulmonary emboli.
Dysarthria		Referral to an SLP; speaking techniques (exaggerate articulation or decrease the rate of speech); "Low-" to "high-tech" communication devices; referral to prosthodontist for palatal lift.
Muscle cramps	Levetiracetam (Keppra)	Stretching exercises; massage; hydrotherapy in heated pools; proper diet and hydration.
Spasticity	Lioresal (baclofen); tizanidine (Zanaflex); intrathecal baclofen for intractable spasticity; botulinum toxin type A.	PT/OT to provide: passive ROM, stretching exercises, postural and positioning techniques, splinting.
Muscle fasciculations	Lorazepam (Ativan)	Avoidance of caffeine and nicotine
Depression and anxiety	Depression medications: amitriptyline (Elavil), SSRIs, mirtazapine (later stages); anxiety medications: Bupropion (Wellbutrin), benzodiazepines (diazepam)	Increased physical activity; psychological support; referral to mental health professional for counseling
Pain	Simple analgesics; nonsteroidal anti-inflammatory drugs; narcotics for refractory pain.	PT to provide: ROM, joint mobilization, stretching exercises, pressure relief techniques (padding, seating cushions, air mattresses) and positioning, orthoses for joint support
Urinary urgency	Oxybutynin chloride (Ditropan); tolterodine tartrate (Detrol)	Pelvic floor (Kegel) exercises; timed voiding program; biofeedback
Constipation	Lactulose; Senna	Increased activity; hydration; increased fiber intake.

(Continued)

TABLE 15-7	Symptomatic Treatment of Amyotrophic Lateral Sclerosis (*Continued*)	
SYMPTOM TREATED	**MEDICAL MANAGEMENT**	**OTHER TREATMENTS**
Pseudobulbar affect	Amitriptyline (Elavil); fluvoxamine (Luvox); dextromethorphan and quinidine	Educate patient and family about the nature of emotional lability and that it is part of ALS, rather than the patient being inappropriate.
Insomnia	Amitriptyline (Elavil); mirtazapine (Remeron); zolpidem (Ambien)	PT to provide pressure relief techniques and positioning; assisted ventilation (BiPAP)
Fatigue	Modafinil (Provigil)	PT/OT to provide: aerobic exercise program (early to middle stages), education on energy-conservation techniques (frequent rest breaks, using wheelchair for long distances, taking elevator instead of stairs, adaptive equipment use, etc.)

Botox, botulinum toxin; BiPAP, bi-level positive airway pressure; FVC, forced vital capacity; SNP, sniff nasal pressure; CR, controlled release; ROM, range of motion; SLP, speech language pathologist; SSRI, selective serotonin reuptake inhibitor; PT, physical therapy; OT, occupational therapy.

using BiPAP at night while asleep. As ALS progresses, the number of hours of assisted ventilation will increase and may go up to 24 hours per day. Several studies have reported prolonged survival times from initiation of noninvasive ventilation, ranging from 7 to 15 months, and increased quality of life in patients with respiratory compromise or moderately impaired bulbar function, who used NIPPV compared to those who did not.[54-56] Eventually noninvasive ventilation will be ineffective, and a decision to either go on invasive ventilation (IV) with tracheostomy via surgical intervention or to go to hospice care must be made. Due to the emotional, social, and financial burden of IV, patients and families must be informed of the costs and benefits of this intervention. Survival rates after initiation of IV were 69% at 2 years and 33% at 5 years.[57]

Bronchial mucus plugging, exacerbated by weak cough function, is the chief precipitating factor of acute respiratory failure of individuals with ALS.[58] Manually assisted coughing techniques and use of a mechanical insufflation–exsufflation (MI-E) device can facilitate clearance of respiratory and oral secretions.[51,58] The MI-E device is usually set to deliver initial lung inflation with +40 cm H_2O and then a negative exsufflation cycle at −40 cm H_2O (adjusted for each person). A peak expiratory "cough" flow within normal range is achieved, which allows for the clearance of secretions.[59]

Physical Therapy Evaluation of Individuals with ALS

Due to the variety and various combinations of regions affected in ALS, therapists must conduct a careful and comprehensive examination of each patient to determine the extent of their primary, secondary, and composite impairments and determine how those impairments are related to their activity limitations and participation restrictions. Reexamination at regular intervals, using standard outcome measures, is necessary to determine the extent and rate of progression of the disease and to ensure that therapeutic interventions are administered in a timely manner (e.g., PEG placement before a patient's FVC is <50% of predicted vital capacity [VC]). The extent and timing of reexaminations may depend on whether the therapist

is part of an ALS multidisciplinary team or an independent, clinic-based therapist and the severity of the patient's disease. Therapists working as team members may have a more limited role, related to assessment of gross motor function and ADLs, while clinic-based therapists may need to carry out more comprehensive assessments that also examine bulbar and respiratory function, environmental barriers to independence, and caregiver demands.

Before the patient's first visit or at the first visit, the patient or caregiver should be asked to keep an activity log for several days that records the patient's activities in 15-minute time intervals, the position the activity is performed in (i.e., lying, sitting, standing, moving), the self-reported fatigue level (no fatigue = 0, extreme fatigue = 10), and the location and intensity (0-10) of pain. The therapist should review the patient's medical record and activity logs to obtain information about the time since diagnosis, the progression of symptoms to date, other health conditions that would affect the patient's course of therapy, and the patient's current activities and his/her tolerance for them. The subjective history should include questions related to the patient's lifestyle, ability to perform ADLs, employment, hobbies or interests, chief complaints, the patient's and family members' understanding of ALS and the likely progression and prognosis, and the patient's immediate concerns and goals for physical therapy. A standard systems review and neurological examination that includes vital signs at rest, communication status and ability to follow commands, skin and sensory integrity, muscle strength, joint range of motion, and postural alignment should be performed (see Evaluation - Chapter 9). The following tests and measures can be used to assess and evaluate an individual with ALS (Table 15-8). Therapists should refer to the World Federation of Neurology's *Guidelines for the Use and Performance of Quantitative Outcome Measures in ALS Clinical Trials* for a more detailed description of the standard test and measures used in clinical trials.[60] It is important to include participation tests and measures as they may be more positively impacted by physical therapy interventions than impairment and activity level measures due to the progressive nature of the disease.

TABLE 15-8 ALS Impairment, Activity, and Participation Assessments		
IMPAIRMENT LEVEL ASSESSMENTS	**ACTIVITY LEVEL ASSESSMENTS**	**PARTICIPATION LEVEL ASSESSMENTS**
• Cognitive screen (verbal fluency) • Psychological screen (ADI-12, BDI, CES-D, HADS, STAI, HDRS, HARS) • Pain (10-point rating scale, VAS) • ROM (muscle length versus joint limitations) • Muscle strength (MMT, strain gauge tensiometer) • Hand and upper extremity function (Purdue pegboard) • Reflexes (DTRs, Babinski, Hoffmann) • Tone (Modified Ashworth Scale) • Cranial nerve screen • Respiratory Assessment (VC, FVC, MIP, aerobic capacity and endurance testing) • Fatigue (FSS, MFI)	• ALSFRS, ALSFRS-R • Other functional measures (AALS, ALSSS, Norris Scale) • General Health (Schwab and England) • Balance (POMA, TUG, BBS, FRT) • Gait (Timed walk test) • Functional Status (FIM)	• ALSAQ-40 (ALSAQ-5) • ALSSQOL • Health-related QOL (SF-36, SEIQoL-DW, SIP)

AALS, Appel ALS Scale; ADI-12, ALS Depression Inventory 12; ALSAQ-40, ALS Assessment Questionnaire 40; ALSFRS(-R), Functional Rating Scale(-Revised); ALSSQOL, ALS-specific QOL instrument; ALSSS, ALS Severity Scale; BBS, Berg Balance Scale; BDI, Beck Depression Inventory; CES-D, Center of Epidemiologic Study-Depression Scale; DTR, deep tendon reflex; FIM, Functional Independence Measure; FRT, Functional Reach Test; FSS, Fatigue Severity Scale; FVC, forced vital capacity; HADS, Hospital Anxiety and Depression Scale; HARS, Hamilton Anxiety Rating Scale; HDRS, Hamilton Depression Rating Scale; MFI, Multidimensional Fatigue Inventory; MIP, maximum inspiratory pressure; MMT, manual muscle test; POMA, Performance Oriented Mobility Assessment; SEIQoL-DW, Schedule for Evaluation of Individual Quality of Life-Direct Weighting; SIP, Sickness Impact Profile; STAI, State-Trait Anxiety Inventory; TUG, Timed Up and Go; VAS, Visual Analogue Scale; VC, vital capacity.

Impairment Level Assessments

The therapist's examination of body structure/function impairments may include the following tests and measures:

Cognition: Several rapid cognitive screening tools that include tests of verbal fluency have been developed to identify patients with ALS with cognitive deficits.[61-63] Verbal (letter) fluency deficits are a sensitive measure of cognitive dysfunction in the ALS population.[39] If cognitive screens are abnormal, referral for a neuropsychological evaluation is indicated.

Psychosocial function: Depression and anxiety are common in patients with ALS as well as their caregivers.[64] Major depression is infrequent (around 10%), but depressive symptoms are reported by 44–75% of individuals with ALS.[65] Some studies have shown an association between greater functional impairment and the severity of anxiety,[66] but other studies have found no correlation.[67] General depression and anxiety assessments that have been used for patients with ALS in clinical trials include the Beck Depression Inventory (BDI),[68] the Center of Epidemiologic Study-Depression Scale (CES-D),[69] the Hospital Anxiety and Depression Scale (HADS),[70] the Spielberger State-Trait Anxiety Inventory (STAI),[71] the Hamilton Depression Rating Scale (HDRS),[72] and the Hamilton Anxiety Rating Scale (HARS).[73] The ALS Depression Inventory 12 (ADI-12) is an ALS-specific screening instrument for depression that excludes statements addressing activities that depend on an intact motor system.[74] Patients with ALS, who test positive on depression and anxiety screens, should be referred to a psychologist or psychiatrist for further evaluation.

Pain: People with ALS may experience muscle cramps and spasms related to upper motor neuron pathology, and pain is reported in up to 75% of patients, particularly in later stages.[65]

Musculoskeletal pain develops with increased muscle weakness and abnormal muscle tone that results in immobility, contractures and joint stiffness, and/or loss of integrity. Some patients may develop painful adhesive capsulitis of the shoulder (i.e., "frozen shoulder"). Pain should be assessed subjectively and objectively, either using a numerical rating scale (0 = no pain to 10 = the worst pain imaginable) or the Visual Analog Scale (VAS). A careful examination of the underlying causes of pain is required to determine whether it is a primary impairment of ALS (e.g., muscle sprain, ligament strains, traumatic injuries from falls) or if it arises from secondary impairments (e.g., decreased ROM, adhesive capsulitis) or composite impairments (e.g., joint malalignment secondary to spasticity or weakness).

Muscle performance: Muscle weakness is the primary deficit of ALS and leads to difficulties with performance of functional activities. Jette et al.[75] found that decreases in walking ability were precipitated by small changes in lower extremity muscle force; individuals with ALS (1) dropped from being independent community ambulators to needing assistance, when their mean percentage of predicted normal maximal isometric force (%PMF) of lower extremity muscles dropped below 54%PMF; (2) became in-home ambulators when strength dropped to 37%PMF; and (3) were no longer able to walk when strength dropped to approximately 19%PMF. Assessment of maximum voluntary isometric contraction (MVIC), using a strain gauge tensiometer system, is considered to be the most direct technique for investigating motor unit loss and has been used extensively in clinical trials.[60,76] Advantages of this method are that it produces highly reliable and sensitive data, accurately measures muscle strength in weak as well as strong muscles, is relatively safe, and does not induce fatigue in the majority of patients.

Disadvantages are that MVIC testing requires specialized equipment and extensive training to use. Alternative test methods are manual muscle testing (MMT) or electronic handheld dynamometer testing. One study that compared test reliability of MMT and MVIC scores in patients with ALS found that the tests had equal reproducibility, when administered by uniformly trained physical therapists.[77]

Upper extremity motor function: Hand and upper extremity function has been measured, using the Purdue pegboard test in clinical trials.[78] This test is sensitive to change over time, and normal values are published.[79,80] Initiation, modification, and control of movement patterns and voluntary postures can be assessed through observation.

Reflex integrity: Deep tendon reflexes, pathological reflexes (e.g., Babinski's and Hoffmann's signs), and muscle tone using the Modified Ashworth Scale should be assessed to discriminate UMN versus LMN involvement.[81]

Cranial nerve integrity: Dysphagia (difficulty swallowing liquids, foods, or saliva) and dysarthria (impairment in speech production) are some of the most distressing and problematic symptoms of ALS that negatively affect quality of life. With progressive weakness of the lips, tongue, palate, and mastication muscles, individuals with ALS experience swallowing problems that lead to choking, drooling, and increased risk for aspiration. Weakness of the muscles of speech (lips, tongue, larynx, and soft palate) and respiration results in compromised speech, characterized by hypernasality, slow speed and cadence, and reduced volume. Evaluation of bulbar function includes testing of cranial nerves III, IV, V, VI, VII, IX, X, and XII. Oral motor function, phonation, and speech production can be assessed through the interview and observation. Referral to a nutritionist and speech language pathologist for consultation is recommended.

Respiratory system assessment: Since respiratory failure is the major cause of death in ALS, respiratory status and function should be closely monitored. Assessment of pulmonary function includes (1) the patient's reports of respiratory symptoms, (2) inspection of the patient's respiratory rate, rhythm, depth, and chest expansion, (3) auscultation of breath sounds, (4) cough effectiveness testing, and (5) VC or FVC, using a handheld spirometer. Overnight oxygen saturation monitoring and maximal inspiratory pressure (MIP) are more effective in detecting early respiratory insufficiency than sitting FVC.[51] Supine FVC may predict diaphragm weakness better than sitting FVC.[51] Breathing is more difficult in supine because gravity is not able to assist in lowering the diaphragm. Sniff nasal pressure (SNP, a short, sharp, voluntary inspiratory maneuver) may be effective in detecting hypercapnia, and peak cough expiratory flow (PCEF) is a widely used measure of cough effectiveness.[51] Aerobic capacity and endurance may be assessed in earlier stages of ALS, using standardized exercise test protocols to evaluate and monitor responses to aerobic conditioning, and should be assessed during functional activities. Baseline measures of FVC or SNP are early predictors of survival.[82-84]

Fatigue: Fatigue is a frequent and sometimes debilitating symptom in ALS that may be caused by peripheral and central mechanisms.[85,86] No ALS-specific measures exist; the Fatigue Severity Scale (FSS)[87] and the Multidimensional Fatigue Inventory (MFI)[88] have been used in studies.

Integumentary system assessment: Skin integrity is usually not compromised in ALS, even in the late stage, because sensation is normally preserved. Skin inspection at contact points between the body and assistive, adaptive, orthotic, protective and supportive devices, mobility devices, and the sleeping surface should be performed regularly, especially when the patient becomes immobile. Swelling of the distal limbs due to a lack of muscle pumping action from weakened limbs should also be evaluated.

Activity Level Assessments

The therapist's examination of activity limitations may include the following tests and measures.

Balance: Although muscle weakness may affect dynamic balance, such as during gait, postural sway during static stance in ambulatory individuals with ALS is typically not different than control subjects despite significant weakness and spasticity, possibly due to intact sensation.[89] No ALS-specific balance test or measure exists; balance tests that have been used in other neuromuscular patient populations include the Tinetti Performance Oriented Mobility Assessment (POMA),[90] the Timed Up and Go (TUG) Test,[91] Berg Balance Scale (BBS),[92] and the Functional Reach Test (FRT).[93] Low total Tinetti Balance Test scores, indicating impaired balance, have been found to be moderately to strongly related to lower extremity muscle weakness and activity limitations, in individuals with ALS,[94] and one study suggests that the Tinetti Balance Test is a reliable measure for individuals in the early or early-middle stages of ALS.[95] Another study found that TUG times increased linearly over 6 months, were negatively correlated with MMT scores and functional measures, and predicted falls using a cutoff of 14 seconds in 31 patients with ALS.[96]

Gait assessment: Gait stability, efficiency, safety, and endurance with or without the use of orthotic and assistive devices should be assessed regularly. Timed 15-feet walk tests have been used to assess gait in clinical trials.

Functional status: Functional mobility skills, safety, and energy expenditure should be assessed. The Functional Independence Measure (FIM™) has been used to document functional status in clinical trials.[97] Basic and instrumental ADLs and the need for adaptive equipment may also be assessed by an occupational therapist.

Posture, body mechanics, and ergonomics: Static and dynamic postural alignment and position, ergonomics, and body mechanics, during self-care, home management, work, community, or leisure activities should be assessed. Caregivers should also be assessed in these areas, when the patient requires physical assistance from them.

Disease-specific measures: The ALS Functional Rating Scale (ALSFRS)[98] and the revised version which includes additional respiratory items (ALSFRS-R),[99] are used to measure functional status and change in patients with ALS. This instrument is available online.[100] The individual is asked to rate his/her function, for the 10–12 items, on a scale from 4 (normal function) to 0 (unable to attempt the task). Both scales have been found to be valid and reliable for measuring the decline in function that results from loss of muscular strength, either in person, in the clinic or via telephone interview, and to predict

9-month survival.[101] Other scales that measure disease severity include: the Appel ALS Scale (AALS),[102] the ALS Severity Scale (ALSSS),[103] and the Norris Scale.[104]

Activities of daily living: The Schwab and England Scale has been used in clinical trials to evaluate ADL function in individuals with ALS.[105] It is an 11-point global measure of functioning that asks the rater to report ADL function from 100% (normal) to 0% (vegetative functions only). The ALS CNTF Treatment Study Group found the scale to have excellent test–retest reliability, to correlate well with qualitative and quantitative changes in function, and to be sensitive to changes over time.[106]

Participation Level Assessments

The therapist's examination of participation may include the following tests and measures.

Environmental barriers: Environmental assessment should focus on the patient's home and work ergonomics and energy conservation as well as safety at current and future functional levels.

Quality of life (QOL): Generic health-related quality of life measures that have been evaluated in individuals with ALS include the SF-36,[107] the Schedule for Evaluation of Individual Quality of Life-Direct Weighting (SEIQoL-DW),[108] and the Sickness Impact Profile (SIP).[109] ALS-specific QOL measures include the ALS Assessment Questionnaire 40 (ALSAQ-40)[110,111] and the ALS-specific QOL instrument (ALSSQOL).[112] The ALSAQ-40 contains 40 items that assess five distinct areas of health: mobility (10 items), ADLs (10 items), eating and drinking (3 items), communication (7 items), and emotional functioning (10 items). Patients answer each question on a five-point Likert scale, based on their condition over the past 2 weeks, and a summary score is obtained, ranging from 0 (best health status) to 100 (worst health status). The validity, reliability, and amount of change over time for each of the five domains that is meaningful to patients has been reported.[110,111] The ALSAQ-40 was shortened to five items and was also found to be valid and reliable.[113] The ALSSQOL contains 59 items that assess psychological, support, existential, and spiritual domains, in addition to a physical domain. Patient's score each item on a 0–10 scale, with 0 the least desirable situation and 10 the most desirable. Thus, total scores range from 0 to 590. The test was found to have concurrent, convergent, and discriminant validity for the overall instrument and convergent validity for its subscales.[114]

Goal Setting and Exercise Prescription

Therapists may have difficulty setting physical therapy goals for patients with ALS due to the progressive nature of the disease and a common belief that, because there is no "cure" for the disease, it is kinder to avoid additional demands on the person with ALS, who is already coping with many functional losses. Others believe that exercise will accelerate the disease or give people false hopes that it can delay progression. However, the literature on ALS, and other neuromuscular diseases, suggests that individuals with ALS can benefit from individually tailored exercise and activity programs throughout all stages of the disease. Including patients in goal setting can increase their motivation to comply with exercise programs and may give them and their families a sense of control over the circumstances in which they find themselves.

The general overarching goals of physical therapy throughout all stages of ALS are to maintain optimal independence in daily living and a good quality of life. More specific physical therapy goals include (1) maintain safe and independent mobility and function; (2) maintain maximal muscle strength and endurance within the amount imposed by the disease; (3) prevent and minimize secondary impairments of the disease (e.g., contractures, disuse atrophy, decubitus ulcers, thrombophlebitis, aspiration); (4) prevent or manage pain; (5) educate on energy-conservation techniques to prevent unnecessary fatigue and respiratory discomfort; and (6) provide adaptive, assistive, and orthotic equipment to maximize functional independence.

When prescribing exercise and activity programs for individuals with ALS, therapists must carefully balance the level of activity to avoid disuse atrophy from low activity levels or, conversely, overwork damage from excessive activity. Fatigue and ambulation difficulties often lead to reduced activity levels in individuals with ALS that can compound already low activity levels, if they led a sedentary lifestyle prior to diagnosis. Inadequate levels of activity, in turn, lead to cardiovascular deconditioning and muscle disuse weakness that ultimately can affect functional performance. On the other hand, excessive exercise can cause undue fatigue that limits a person's ability to perform daily activities, during recovery periods, and/or cause overuse damage to muscles and tendons that results in pain and loss of strength.

Historically, general strengthening and endurance exercises have not been part of the standard care of individuals with ALS. Early studies recommended people with ALS should not exercise beyond their daily activities.[115] These recommendations were based on some epidemiological studies that suggested that high levels of physical activity may be associated with an increased risk of progression of the degeneration of the disease.[116] Other studies reported abnormal physiologic responses to exercise in people with ALS (i.e., increased lactate production, decreased anaerobic lactate threshold, decreased work capacity, increased oxygen cost of submaximal exercise, and abnormalities in plasma and muscle lipid metabolism),[117,118] which suggested that exercise might facilitate the pathogenic mechanisms of ALS (glutamate excitotoxicity, increased free radicals, excessive inflammation).[119] There was also evidence suggesting that high-intensity or highly repetitive exercise could increase muscle and motor neuron denervation in people with neuromuscular diseases. Anecdotal evidence from therapists and physicians, working with individuals during the poliomyelitis epidemics in the 1940s and 1950s, reported that patients, who exercised muscles with below fair grades either repeatedly or against heavy loads, often lost the ability to contract the muscle.[120] Testing of this observation, in rats, found similar findings; vigorous exercise caused muscle damage in denervated muscles (i.e., less than one-third of the motor units were functional), whereas it caused hypertrophy in muscles that had more than one-third of motor units functional.[121] In polio and ALS, there is collateral sprouting of intact axons to innervate "orphaned" (i.e., denervated) muscle fibers, following axonal degeneration, that results in a larger number of muscle fibers being innervated by a smaller pool of motor neurons. Studies using rat models of partial denervation of skeletal muscles have shown that exercise has a negative effect on the stability of these giant motor units.[122,123] After partial denervation of the rats' hindlimbs, enlarged motor units were found to decrease significantly in size over time, with high-intensity exercise further accelerating this loss of chronically enlarged motor units and reducing sprouting of intact axons in extensively denervated muscles.[122,123] Repeated maximal eccentric contractions such as hiking downhill in non-exercised individuals can result in muscle weakness for several weeks even in normal muscle fibers.[124] Although normal muscle can adapt to repeated eccentric exercise, it is uncertain whether this effect is possible in people with neuromuscular disease. Other potential mechanisms for exercise intolerance in people with ALS include mitochondrial dysfunction, abnormal muscle lipid metabolism, impaired muscle activation due to impaired excitation–contraction coupling, and central activation failure.[125,126]

Notably, there are researchers, who suggest that moderate exercise programs may be safe and possibly beneficial for people with ALS. Exercise adapted to each individual's exercise capacity that does not overload the nervous, muscular, and respiratory systems should avoid exacerbation of pathophysiologic mechanisms of ALS. Moderate exercise can improve neuronal plasticity (e.g., release of neurotrophic factors, dendritic restructuring, enhanced protein synthesis, strengthening of synaptic connections to target muscles, maintaining organization and firing of muscle fibrils, improving axonal transport) and enhance cardiovascular and peripheral circulation, which may positively affect free radical balance and oxidation of muscle fibers to modify the excitotoxic environment.[86] Evidence, supporting the safety and benefits of moderate exercise in individuals with ALS is accumulating. Lui and Byl[86] systematically reviewed research, related to moderate exercise, for maintaining independence without increasing disease progression in individuals with ALS. The human studies that were included in this review are summarized in Table 15-9. When outcomes were averaged across human studies, moderate intensity exercise was found to be beneficial for maintaining strength (mean weighted difference risk ratio [MWD risk ratio], 3.62), performance on the Norris ALS Scale (MWD risk ratio, 4.3), and function (i.e., ALS-FRS, FIM scores; MWD risk ratio, 3.12) in comparison to non-exercising controls. Moderate exercise also improved respiratory function in persons with ALS (MWD effect size, 1.2–1.39 [numbers over 0.8 are considered large]; MWD risk ratio, 1.66) compared to non-exercising controls. There were no reported adverse effects in any of the human studies; however, there was a large dropout rate over time. In animal models (i.e., transgenic mice with superoxide dismutase-1 ALS), moderate exercise increased survival (effect size = 1.39 in favor of exercise group) and delayed the time to reach a 50% decline in motor function (122 days exercise group versus 115 days control groups). The few negative effects in the animal models were associated with very high-intensity exercise (e.g., progressive treadmill training at 9–22 m/min for 20–45 minutes daily) and slow rate exercise (0.1 m/min on a running wheel for 6.7 hours a day), which was less activity than usual for animals with unrestricted activity.[86] Sanjak et al.[127] examined the effects of a moderate intensity body weight-supported treadmill training program in ambulatory individuals with ALS in the early to middle stages. Participants (n = 9)

performed 30 minutes of treadmill walking with up to 40% of their weight supported by an overhead harness in six intervals, of 5 minutes of exercise interspersed with 5 minutes of rest for 3 times per week, for 8 weeks. Treadmill speed was determined by each participant's own tolerated stepping pace, and rate of perceived exertion (RPE) was not to exceed level 12–13 (moderate) on the modified Borg perceived exertion scale. Following the 8-week intervention, participants showed significantly improved RPE, Fatigue Severity Scores, and walking distance during the treadmill and overground 6-minute walk tests, providing further support for the benefits of moderate exercise in the ALS population.[127]

Based on the evidence and current practice, general guidelines for prescribing strengthening and endurance exercises for individuals with ALS are in Box 15-1. Clinicians should monitor each person's response to exercise to determine whether the exercises are appropriate and safe and to adjust programs as the disease progresses. Possible signs and symptoms of muscle overwork include delayed onset muscle soreness, peaking between days 1 and 5 after activity; a reduction in maximum force production that gradually recovers and/or severe muscle cramping after exercise; a feeling of heaviness in the extremities; increased muscle fasciculations; or prolonged shortness of breath.[132] Patients should be advised not to carry out activities to the point of extreme fatigue (i.e., inability to perform daily activities following exercise due to exhaustion, pain, fasciculations, or muscle cramping).[133] If a patient shows signs of prolonged muscle weakness after starting an exercise program or reports persistent morning fatigue after exercise on the previous day, the clinician should carefully adjust the exercise program intensity to eliminate any further muscle overuse. While strengthening and endurance exercises may not improve the strength of muscles already weakened by ALS or change the course of the disease, they may have positive physiological and psychological effects for individuals with ALS, especially when implemented in the early stages.

Physical Therapy Treatment

Dal Bello-Haas proposed a three-stage model for the progression of ALS as a framework for physical therapy clinical management (see Table 15-10).[135] In the early stage, individuals are independent with mobility, ADLs and speech, despite mild to moderate weakness in specific muscle groups. The person may experience some difficulty with mobility and ADLs toward the end of the stage. During the middle stage, the person with ALS has severe muscle weakness in some groups and mild to moderate weakness in others. There is a progressive decline in mobility and ADLs, along with increasing fatigue and pain; together these result in some compensation or dependence on others. In the late stage, the person is totally dependent with mobility and ADLs, due to severe weakness of axial and extremity muscles. Dysarthria, dysphagia, respiratory compromise, and pain are all common features of this stage.

Three general approaches are used to direct physical therapy interventions across the disease stages: preventative, restorative, and compensatory.[135] Preventative interventions aim to minimize potential impairments (e.g., loss of ROM, aerobic capacity, strength) and activity limitations. Restorative interventions

TABLE 15-9 Controlled Exercise Studies in ALS

REFERENCE	SUBJECTS	DESIGN/TREATMENT	INTENSITY/DURATION	OUTCOME MEASURES	RESULTS
Aksu et al.[128]	26 subjects: Supervised + HEP group (n=13) HEP only group (n=13)	Prospective, convenience assignment to groups; E: PNF + strengthening+ stretching + functional mobility+ breathing exs. C: AAROM+ stretching + breathing exs.	E: 45–60 minutes, 3 times per week × 8 weeks (rehab hospital) then HEP up to 1 year at home C: 10 reps per exercise × 2–3 sets per day, walking "as tolerated" at home up to 1 year	• Modified Norris Limb Scale • Cumulative isometric muscle strength for 34 extremity muscles, trunk, and grip using handheld dynamometer • UE and LE joint PROM with goniometer	Supervised group had significantly greater joint ROM, trunk and hand grip strength, and Norris Limb Scale scores than controls at 8 weeks; Norris Limb Scale scores significantly greater than controls at 12 months.
Dal Bello-Haas et al.[129]	27 subjects (early stage) Resistance training group (n=13) Usual care group (n=14); 8 in the resistance group and 10 in the usual care group completed the study.	Randomized clinical trial; E: PT-prescribed UE and LE PREs + stretching exs. at home C: UE and LE stretching exercises only	E: PREs to muscles with grades ≥3 at moderate load (5 reps at full 6-RM, 5 reps at 75% 6-RM, 5 reps at 50% 6-RM) 3 times per week + stretching once daily C: 5 reps of each exercise once daily	• Cumulative isometric muscle strength in LEs using MVIC testing • ALSFRS total score • SF-36 • Fatigue Severity Scale	At 6 months, Exercise group had significantly greater ALSFRS, SF-36 Physical Function scores, and less decline in LE strength; no significant difference in fatigue; no adverse effects.
Drory et al.[130]	25 subjects (early to middle stages) Exercise group (n=14) Control group (n=11)	Prospective controlled; random assignment E: Active exercise (concentric contractions), trunk and limbs C: No additional activities besides daily routine	E: Moderate load (tailored to subject), 15-minute bouts twice per day for up to 6 months.	• ALSFRS total score • Cumulative strength of 20 muscles using manual muscle testing (MMT) • Fatigue Severity Scale (FSS) • Ashworth Spasticity Scale • Pain • SF-36	At 3 months, Exercise group had significantly less decline in ALSFRS as well as significantly less spasticity than controls; other measures not significant; at 6 months no significant differences on all measures.
Pinto et al.[131]	20 subjects Treadmill group (n=8) Control group (n=12)	Prospective controlled; random assignment E: Treadmill with BiPAP C: No additional activities besides daily routine with BiPAP	E: Treadmill training using Bruce or Naughton protocols; exercise to anaerobic threshold until stop parameters: subjective fatigue, leg pain, HR above 75% rest values, oxygen desaturation not correctible with NIPPV. Duration up to 12 months.	• Spinal and Bulbar Norris Scale scores • FIM • Barthel Scale • FVC	At 12 months, Treadmill group had significantly greater FIM scores, and had a slower spinal Norris score decline than controls; there was also a significant difference in the slope of FVC decline; no adverse events reported.

A/AAROM, active/active-assisted range of motion; C, control; E, experimental; HEP, home exercise program; PREs, progressive resistive exercises; RM, repetition maximum; PROM, passive range of motion; UE, upper extremity; LE, lower extremity; MMT, manual muscle test; MVIC, maximum voluntary isometric contraction; ALSFRS, Amyotrophic Lateral Sclerosis Functional Rating Scale; ASH, Ashworth Spasticity Scale; FSS, Fatigue Severity Scale; BiPAP, bilevel positive airway pressure; HR, heart rate; FIM, Functional Independence Measure; FVC, forced vital capacity; NIPPV, noninvasive positive pressure ventilation.

BOX 15-1	General Exercise Guidelines for Individuals with ALS

- Start exercise interventions when individuals are in the early stages of the disease so that they have sufficient strength, respiratory function, and endurance to exercise without excessive fatigue.[86]
- Strengthening exercise programs should emphasize concentric rather than eccentric muscle contractions, at moderate resistance and intensity (e.g., 1–2 sets of 8–12 reps or 3 sets of 5 reps), in muscles that have anti-gravity strength (i.e., >3 grade strength) exclusively.
- Endurance exercise programs should emphasize moderate intensity activities (50–80% peak HR, 11–13 RPE, 3 times per week) as tolerated without inducing excessive fatigue. Rest periods are recommended, especially if continuous activity goes beyond 15 minutes.
- Individuals with ALS should be advised to have adequate oxygenation, ventilation, and intake of carbohydrates and fluids before exercising.[134]
- Use available technology (e.g., assistive devices, body weight-supported systems) to optimize exercise program effectiveness without causing excessive fatigue.[86]
- Exercise compliance can be improved by integrating enjoyable physical activities along with the formal exercise program, providing opportunities for socialization, and providing rewards for accomplishment of goals.

TABLE 15-10	Amyotrophic Lateral Sclerosis Disease Stages and Common Intervention Strategies[135]	
STAGE	**COMMON IMPAIRMENTS AND ACTIVITY LIMITATIONS**	**INTERVENTIONS**
Early	• Mild to moderate weakness in specific muscle groups • Difficulty with ADLs and mobility toward the end of this stage	Restorative/Preventative: • Strengthening exercises[128,130] • Endurance exercises[127,131] • ROM (active, active-assisted) and stretching exercises[136] Compensatory: • Assess potential need for appropriate adaptive and assistive devices • Assess potential need for ergonomic modifications of the home/workplace • Educate patient about the disease process, energy conservation, and support groups
Middle	• Severe muscle weakness in some groups; mild to moderate weakness in other groups • Progressive decrease in mobility and ADLs throughout this stage • Increasing fatigue throughout this stage • Wheelchair needed for long distances; increased wheelchair use toward end of stage • Pain (especially shoulders)	Compensatory: • Support weak muscles (assistive devices, supportive devices, adaptive equipment, slings, orthoses) • Modify the workplace/home (e.g., install ramp, move bedroom to first floor) • Prescribe wheelchair • Educate caregivers regarding functional training Preventative: • ROM (active, active-assisted, passive) and stretching exercises[136] • Strengthening exercises (early middle)[128,130] • Endurance exercises (early middle)[127,131] • Assess need for pressure-relieving devices (e.g., pressure distributing mattress)
Late	• Wheelchair dependent or restricted to bed • Complete dependence with ADLs • Severe weakness of UE, LE, neck and trunk muscles • Dysarthria, dysphagia • Respiratory compromise • Pain	Preventative: • Passive ROM • Pulmonary hygiene* • Hospital bed and pressure-relieving devices • Skin care, hygiene* • Educate caregivers on prevention of secondary complications Compensatory: • Educate caregivers regarding transfers, positioning, turning, skin care • Mechanical lift

*May be restorative.

CASE A, PART III: EARLY STAGE

Mr. Posner was referred by his neurologist to outpatient physical therapy with a diagnosis of probable ALS, laboratory supported. At his initial physical therapy session, the patient reported a previous history of an old football injury of the left knee with a chronically torn meniscus. He complained that the weakness in his hands, which was worse on the left than the right, and the stiffness in his legs were interfering with his ability to walk, go upstairs, and play golf. He stated that he could not hit the golf ball as far as in years past. Other than golfing on weekends, when the weather was good, he stated that he did not engage in any regular exercise program. His medications included riluzole (50 mg twice daily), baclofen (10 mg twice daily), vitamin C (1000 mg once daily), vitamin E (800 units once daily), co-enzyme Q10 (600 mg once daily), and a multiple vitamin once daily. He had health care benefits through his job with 15 outpatient physical therapy visits allowed per year. The physical therapist's examination findings revealed the following impairments:

- Decreased flexibility of bilateral shoulder extensors and internal rotators, hip adductors, quadriceps, and gastrocnemius muscles on passive ROM
- Mild atrophy of the intrinsic hand muscles, left greater than right
- Decreased strength in cervical and distal extremity muscles with bilateral finger flexor and hand intrinsic muscles [Left = G (4) range; Right = G+ (4+)], ankle dorsiflexors [G (4)], neck extensors G (4), and neck flexors G+ (4+)
- Brisk reflexes (3+) at the jaw and all extremity joints; Babinski and Hoffmann's signs positive bilaterally; Modified Ashworth Scale scores were 1 in bilateral biceps and wrist flexor muscles and 1+ in bilateral hip adductors, hamstring, and gastrocnemius muscles
- Sitting FVC: 4.45 L (91% of predicted)
- Sitting posture demonstrated a forward head and rounded shoulder posture

The therapist's examination revealed the following activity limitations and participation restrictions:

- Balance (standing): Unilateral stance/eyes open, R=25 seconds; L=23 seconds
- Slow walking velocity (15-foot walk test = 12 seconds; no assistive device; stiff gait with bilaterally decreased hip and knee flexion during swing phase and foot flat initial contact)
- Mild ADL and mobility deficits as indicated by ALSFRS-R score: 41/48 and Schwab and England score: 90% (can do all chores but with some degree of slowness, difficulty, or impairment). See Table 15-13.
- Functional endurance deficits indicated by fatigue when going up stairs or prolonged LE activities

ALSFRS-R Assessment

Item	Score	ALSFRS-R Score Descriptor
Speech	4	Normal speech processes
Salivation	4	Normal
Swallowing	4	Normal eating habits
Handwriting (pre-ALS dominant hand)	3	Slow or sloppy; all words are legible
Cutting food and handling utensils (patients without gastrostomy)	3	Somewhat slow and clumsy, but no help needed
Dressing and hygiene	3	Independent and complete self-care with effort or decreased efficiency
Turning in bed, adjusting bed clothes	3	Somewhat slow and clumsy, but no help needed
Walking	3	Early ambulation difficulties
Climbing stairs	3	Mild unsteadiness or fatigue
Dyspnoea	4	None
Orthopnea	4	None
Respiratory insufficiency	4	None, e.g., no BiPAP at present

The therapist's diagnostic impression was that the patient's hand weakness was affecting his ability to perform ADLs and the spasticity and distal weakness in his legs was affecting his gait and stair climbing. His respiratory and LE impairments were mildly affecting his endurance for LE activities.

are targeted toward remediating or improving already existing impairments and activity limitations (e.g., strengthening, balance, and endurance exercises). Compensatory interventions are directed toward modifying activities, tasks, or environments to minimize activity limitations and disablement (e.g., orthotics, assistive devices, wheelchairs).

Individuals, in the early stage of ALS, such as Mr. Posner, should be encouraged to continue as many of their pre-diagnostic activities as possible. For example, Mr. Posner enjoys golfing and should be encouraged to continue playing as tolerated. If walking on the golf course is too fatiguing, the therapist can suggest that he use a golf cart, reduce the number of holes played, or hit balls at a driving range. If upper extremity weakness limits his golf swing for distance shots, he can play the greens or putting courses. He may benefit from adaptations to his club handles to prevent rotation of the club on impact through application of nonskid materials on club handles such as Dycem™[137] or a larger size grip. If Mr. Posner was leading a sedentary lifestyle before his diagnosis, he should be encouraged to increase his activity level. Walking, swimming, bicycling (three-wheeler or stationary bike, if needed), gardening, doing household chores, or working out to specific exercise routines are ways for individuals with ALS to keep active. Kamide et al.[138] reported that a combination of walking and ADL exercises significantly reduced functional decline in early stage patients with ALS. Therapists, family members, and caregivers should support individuals with ALS to engage in activities that are safe and enjoyable for them to do for as long as possible.

Mr. Posner is likely to need physical therapy care in the future due to the progressive nature of the disease. Therefore, the therapist should not use up all of the patient's allotted yearly physical therapy visits for this episode of care. Educating the patient on a home exercise program to maintain or improve his maximum functional capacity with ongoing therapist reevaluation were priorities of the patient's plan of care. The program included the following:

1. General exercise: neck and extremity strengthening exercises (isometric or isotonic with submaximal elastic band resistance or small weights), alternating LEs on one day and the UEs on the other; AROM and stretching exercises to tight musculature; and daily walking for 10 minutes or as tolerated.

2. Energy conservation strategies for fatigue prevention during ADLs and leisure activities (e.g., sitting down or taking a rest, when he starts to feel fatigued; doing strenuous activities during the time of day that he has the most energy; planning the week so that he doesn't have to do a lot of strenuous tasks in one day).

3. Referral to occupational therapy for evaluation of ADLs and recommendations for adaptive devices to assist with cutting food and using utensils and self-care.

4. Education on signs and symptoms of overwork fatigue and ALS resources and support groups available through the Amyotrophic Lateral Sclerosis Association (ALSA) and the Muscular Dystrophy Association (MDA).

5. Follow-up appointments every 3–4 months for reevaluations.

CASE A, PART IV: MIDDLE STAGE

One year after his diagnosis, Mr. Posner was again referred by his neurologist for outpatient physical therapy, now diagnosed with definite ALS and adhesive capsulitis. The neurologist's orders were for gait training and reduction of shoulder pain. The patient reported that he stopped working at the insurance company about a month ago and was placed on permanent disability. He stated that he missed going to work and talking with his coworkers and had felt very depressed about it. His main social contacts were with his family and friends from church. He also contacted the local ALS Association and had been attending support group meetings with his family. The patient's baclofen had been increased to 20 mg in the morning and afternoon and 40 mg at bedtime. He was also taking Paxil 20 mg once daily for his depression. He has dropped 30 pounds, since his diagnosis. The patient's chief complaints were as follows:

- Pain throughout his shoulders bilaterally, worse on the left side than the right side, especially with overhead activities; he described the pain as "a sharp ache deep in the shoulders."

- Neck pain, if he was sitting for long periods or riding in the car.

- SOB while walking, bathing, and dressing; some difficulty sleeping at night due to SOB, but not using more than two pillows; he was able to clear secretions with coughing.

He was able to do most ADLs by himself but very slowly and with much effort. He used a manual wheelchair for mobility in the community, due to fatigue when walking long distances; at home, he ambulated with the assistance of two people or a four-wheeled walker with attached forearm troughs, due to his hand grip weakness. He was no longer able to perform his home stretching program independently because of increased muscle tightness and decreased balance and muscle control. He had fallen backwards on several occasions, during the past 6 months, when ambulating without assistance; one occurred in his driveway and resulted in injury to his back.

The patient had a ramp installed at his home, and his bedroom was located on the first floor. Grab bars were installed in the shower and beside the toilet, and the patient had a raised toilet seat. The patient was no longer driving. He was able to transport his manual wheelchair and walker in the trunk of his car, when going places. The patient's health coverage was currently COBRA, but he was in the process of getting Medicare. He was concerned that Medicare would not pay for his riluzole and that he would not have enough money to pay for it. His goals for physical therapy were to have decreased shoulder and neck pain and increased overall flexibility to move and walk better and not fall.

The physical therapist's examination findings revealed the following body/structure impairments:

- Mild edema in his feet and marked wasting of the intrinsic muscles of both hands; ankles were in a slightly plantarflexed and inverted position at rest; some fasciculations noted in the tongue and upper extremities.

- Decreased bilateral shoulder AROM: abduction (63 degrees Left; 76 degrees Right); flexion (78 degrees Left; 83 degrees Right); external rotation (25 degrees Left; 35 degrees Right) and internal rotation (40 degrees Left; 43 degrees Right) with pain (8 out of 10 on the left and 5 out of 10 on the right), during movements; PROM of shoulders limited bilaterally by muscle spasticity and guarding to 50% of NL (normal limits) in all directions; mild to moderate decreased glenohumeral mobility in all directions with mild subluxation noted bilaterally; passive ankle dorsiflexion limited bilaterally to 5 degrees.

- Decreased strength of the neck and bilateral UEs and LEs on MMT: elbow flexors F+ (3+), elbow extensors G (4), finger flexors P+ (2+), and hand intrinsics T (1), hip flexors G (4), knee extensors G (3), ankle dorsiflexors F(3), and ankle plantarflexors, evertors, invertors G− (4−), neck extensors G− (4−), neck flexors G (4)

- Brisk stretch reflexes(3+), with 2–3 beating clonus in ankles bilaterally; Modified Ashworth Scale scores were 1+ in bilateral biceps and wrist flexor muscles and 2 in bilateral hip adductors, quadriceps, hamstring, and gastrocnemius muscles.

- Sitting FVC: 3.77 L (77% of predicted).

The therapist's examination revealed the following activity limitations and participation restrictions:

- Balance (standing): Unilateral stance/eyes open, R=10 seconds; L=8 seconds

- Speech was slightly decreased in volume, slow, and slightly hypernasal, after the patient spoke for a while, but articulation was good; mild facial weakness as shown by difficulty holding air in his cheeks against resistance; able to swallow all foods, but sometimes choked on his saliva or when drinking water or coffee.

- Transfers sit-to-stand were slow with standby assist.

- Slow walking velocity (15-foot walk test = 15 seconds using four-wheeled walker with attached forearm troughs and standby assist; narrow base of support and forefoot contact at initial contact bilaterally)

- Moderate ADL and mobility deficits as indicated by ALSFRS-R score: 28/48 and Schwab and England score: 60% (can do most chores but very slowly and with much effort; makes errors).

Item	Score	ALSFRS-R Score Descriptor
Speech	3	Detectable speech disturbance
Salivation	3	Slight but definite excess of saliva in mouth; may have minimal drooling
Swallowing	3	Early eating problems – occasional choking
Handwriting (pre-ALS dominant hand)	2	Not all words are legible
Cutting food and handling utensils (patients without gastrostomy)	2	Intermittent assistance or substitute methods
Dressing and hygiene	2	Intermittent assistance or substitute methods
Turning in bed, adjusting bed clothes	2	Can turn alone or adjust sheets, but with great difficulty
Walking	2	Walks with assistance
Climbing stairs	0	Cannot do
Dyspnoea	2	Occurs with one or more of the following: eating, bathing, dressing (ADL)
Orthopnea	3	Some difficulty sleeping at night due to SOB. Does not routinely use more than 2 pillows.
Respiratory insufficiency	4	None, e.g., no BiPAP at present

The physical therapist's diagnostic impression was that the patient was in transition from ambulation with an assistive device for short distances to dependence on a wheelchair for mobility. Pain and decreased ROM in bilateral shoulders was likely due to adhesive capsulitis secondary to immobility.

Shoulder Pain

As with Mr. Posner, shoulder pain may develop in people with ALS and can progress to significant restrictions of shoulder motions in a capsular pattern. Causative factors of pain may include (1) abnormal scapulohumeral rhythm secondary to spasticity or weakness, causing muscle imbalances that lead to impingement; (2) overuse of strong muscles; (3) prolonged immobility or reduced ROM; (4) marked shoulder weakness (in some cases "hanging arm" syndrome) and resultant gleno-humeral subluxation; or (5) a fall. Depending on the cause of the pain, interventions may include modalities, ROM and passive stretching exercises, joint mobilizations, and education about proper shoulder support (e.g., using arm rests on chairs or tabletop) and protection (e.g., avoid pulling the arms to assist a seated person with ALS to standing). Wearing a sling, similar to those used post-stroke, may benefit individuals with significant subluxation. Adhesive capsulitis has been managed successfully, in individuals with ALS, using intra-articular analgesic and anti-inflammatory cocktail injections, followed by a course of aggressive ROM exercises.[139]

Cervical Weakness

Mr. Posner is experiencing cervical muscle weakness that is a common problem for people with ALS.[140] Cervical extensor muscles are typically more affected than flexors. Initially people with ALS may complain that their necks feel stiff or they feel "heavy-headed," after reading or writing, or they may notice that they have difficulty holding their heads straight with unanticipated movements, such as during sudden accelerations while sitting in a car. The weakness progresses to the point where the head begins to fall forward, and at advanced stages, the neck becomes completely flexed with the head dropped forward. The forward head position causes cervical pain and impairs ambulation and eating. For mild to moderate cervical weakness, such as Mr. Posner is experiencing, a soft collar may be worn for specific activities such as riding in the car. For moderate to severe weakness, a semi-rigid or rigid collar is needed to provide adequate support. Collars such as the Philadelphia collar™,[141] Miami-J Collar™,[142] and Malibu Collar™[143] offer good support, but patients may feel confined or uncomfortably warm. The lightweight Headmaster collar™[144] has an open design that allows air circulation and is often well tolerated by individuals with ALS; it may be inadequate if rotation and lateral flexion weakness is also present.

Respiratory Weakness

Mr. Posner is experiencing shortness of breath with exertional activities and during sleep. Difficulty sleeping may be the first symptom of hypoventilation. The patient should be taught how to balance activity and rest so as not to become too fatigued. In addition, he and his family should be educated about signs and symptoms of aspiration; causes and signs of respiratory infection; management of oral secretions (oral suction device), positioning to avoid aspiration (upper cervical spine flexion ["chin tuck" maneuver] during eating), and the Heimlich maneuver, in case of choking episodes. Specific breathing exercises and positioning to maximize pulmonary ventilation and perfusion may be administered, but their effectiveness in ALS is currently unknown. One small double-blind, randomized study examined the effects of an inspiratory muscle training (IMT) program (10-minute sessions 3 times per day for 12 weeks) on nine individuals with ALS. Subjects in the IMT group showed trends toward better FVC, VC, MIP, and SNP values, compared to a control group that completed sham training; the gains in inspiratory muscle strength were partially reversed at an 8-week follow-up, after the training stopped.[145] Pinto et al.[146] examined the effects of IMT training (10-minute sessions twice daily for 4 months) in 26 individuals with ALS and found transient non-significant improvements in ASLFRS respiratory subscale scores and some respiratory function measures (SNP, peak expiratory flow, maximal voluntary ventilation), following the intervention.

LE Muscle Weakness and Gait Impairments

Mr. Posner is experiencing gait difficulties that are typical for individuals in the middle stage of the disease. Ambulatory assistive device prescription for individuals with ALS must take into account the patient's LE muscle strength or instability, UE function, extent and rate of disease progression, acceptance by the patient, and financial restrictions. At early stages, patients with ALS may benefit from use of a cane, but as the disease advances, wheeled walkers (i.e., four-wheeled walkers or front-wheeled walkers), which do not require the person to lift the device, are recommended. Mr. Posner is demonstrating bilateral ankle dorsiflexor weakness with resultant foot drop that may benefit from use of ankle-foot orthoses (AFOs). Given his good knee extensor strength with mild ankle strength deficits, articulated (hinged) AFOs that allow dorsiflexion may be a good choice for him. Solid AFOs should be considered for individuals with medial/lateral instability of the ankle and quadriceps weakness. If disease progression is rapid and a person will probably wear the AFO for a limited time, a commercially manufactured AFO may suffice.

Transfers and Mobility

Mr. Posner is having difficulty with sit-to-stand transfers due to LE weakness. Simple interventions include putting a firm cushion in a chair (2–3 inches) or elevating his chair with prefabricated blocks. Self-powered lifting seat cushions are portable and inexpensive, but the person needs adequate trunk control and balance for safe use. Recliner chairs with powered seat lifts may also help a person to rise from a seated position, but they are more expensive.

Once the individual is not able to stand, transfer boards may be used for transfers either independently, if arm strength and sitting balance is sufficient, or with caregiver assistance. Use of transfer belts can make transfers easier for the caregiver and prevent pulling on the patient's arms. Swivel cushions that swivel in both directions can make getting in and out of a car less difficult. When transfers become difficult, even with caregiver assistance, a hydraulic or mechanical lift such as the Hoyer lift™[147] is required. Use of hospital beds makes bed mobility and transfers easier for the patient and caregiver. Chair glides or stairway lifts are recommended for individuals, living in multilevel homes, that can't go up and down stairs. If insurance will not reimburse for stairway lifts, some medical supply companies may rent them, or the local ALSA or MDA chapter may have recycled lifts to loan.

Mr. Posner's muscle weakness and limited endurance necessitate that he use a wheelchair, when going long distances.

Since most insurance companies will only reimburse for one wheelchair, individuals in the early to middle stages of ALS are advised to rent a manual wheelchair or obtain a loaner from a local ALSA or MDA chapter. Manual wheelchair features that were preferred by patients with ALS include lightweight frame, small wheelbase, high reclining back and supports for the head, trunk, and extremities.[148] As the disease progresses, a power wheelchair customized to the patient's needs will be required. Desirable features for powered wheelchairs are (1) tilt-in-space/recline features with a high firm back and headrest that allow the patient to shift weight and rest, while in the chair, (2) easy maneuverability (smaller wheelbase and less heavy), (3) lumbar support, (4) air or gel-filled cushion, (5) adjustable leg rests, (6) removable armrests for ease of transfer, and (7) potential mounting area for portable respirator equipment if needed.[148]

Activities of Daily Living

Mr. Posner's UE and LE weakness is impairing his ability to carry out many of his ADLs. A large variety of adaptive equipment is available to help maintain function. Foam tubing to increase the size of utensil handles, modified handles or holders on utensils and cups, long-levered jar openers, plate guards, rocker knives, universal cuffs (for holding tools and instruments) and mobile arm supports can assist a person with feeding and eating. For self-care and bathing, bathing benches, bath tub seats, handheld shower heads, grab bars, shower commodes, raised toilet seats, bath mitts, long-handled sponges, electric toothbrushes or shavers, and strap-fitted hairbrushes are recommended. Zipper pulls, button hooks, Velcro clothing closures, and elastic shoelaces make dressing easier. Increasing the size of a pen/pencil with a triangular grip or cylindrical foam can make writing easier and more legible. Book holders, automatic page turners, and an adjustable angle table make reading easier. Other useful equipment includes key holders, doorknob adapters, personal alarm systems, switch-operated environmental controls for turning lights or the television on and off, and speaker phones with automatic dialing. Some of these may be too expensive for the patient and family to acquire.

Psychosocial Issues

Mr. Posner is mourning the loss of his friendships at work and of his standing as a competent Chief Financial Officer. Because of the progressive nature of the disease, individuals with ALS must cope with continuous losses of physical health and abilities, body image, work and family roles, identity, and family and social networks. The physical therapist must attend to the patient's ability to cope and adapt to these changes and be able to differentiate between normal grief reactions to changes in function and symptoms of fear, anxiety, and depression. Purtilo and Haddad[149] identified four major fears of individuals with a terminal condition: fear of isolation, fear of pain, fear of dependence, and fear of death itself. Mr. Posner's fear of isolation increased when he was no longer able to go to work. Fortunately, he has maintained contacts with family members, church friends, and support group members. Mr. Posner is also experiencing increased pain and discomfort that is causing him anxiety. With aggressive management of his pain, through medications and physical therapy, these anxieties may be relieved. His increasing dependence on others for driving, walking, and ADLs are similarly causing him to feel stressed because of the increased burden that he feels he is putting on his wife and children. His wife may feel stressed and anxious about having to take over her husband's responsibilities, and his children may be frustrated with the need to provide care to their father. Referral to a psychologist for individual and family counseling may be beneficial to improve communication and resolve conflicts. Therapists must be prepared to help patients, families, and caregivers find effective ways to cope with the emotional, social, and physical stress that accompanies living with ALS.

Medicare does not have caps on outpatient physical therapy visits for patients with ALS. Reduction of shoulder pain and improved shoulder ROM, family training in ROM exercises, and preparation for the patient's future mobility needs were the goals of the plan of care which included:

1. Therapeutic interventions for improved bilateral shoulder ROM and pain reduction;

2. Family training in passive UE and LE ROM and stretching exercises;

3. Interventions for LE edema control;

4. LE ankle-foot orthoses and power wheelchair prescription;

5. Referrals to occupational therapy for ADL evaluation, to a speech and language pathologist for speech and swallowing evaluation, to a dietician for dietary counseling, and a social worker for information on how to pay for his medications.

CASE A, PART V: LATE STAGE

Two years post diagnosis, home physical therapy is requested to assess caregiver demands and to make recommendations. Fourteen months after Mr. Posner's diagnosis, he underwent PEG placement due to problems with dysphagia and declining respiratory status. The patient's wife quit her teaching job to be able to care full time for the patient. She stated that she is feeling exhausted and stressed by the demands of taking care of her husband. She also stated that the children, who are now ages 13 and 11, are having a difficult time dealing with their fathers' declining physical capacity, had been angry and irritable with her at times, and their grades had dropped in school. The patient does not yet have advanced directives, but the wife states that she is afraid to talk to him about it for fear that he will become depressed. The patient takes baclofen 20 mg four times daily and tizanidine 4 mg at bedtime. He also takes lithium carbonate 300 mg twice daily, per his request, following the publication of an article that suggested that it might slow the progression of the disease. The patient purchased a minivan that is equipped to transport his power wheelchair for going to church or other community events and an electric hospital bed with an anti-pressure mattress. The patient's and wife's complaints were as follows:

- Wife is unable to put the AFOs on the patient's feet due to his limited ankle ROM, making transfers very difficult because the patient stands on his toes. She almost dropped the patient several times, during transfers, and wants to be able to transfer patient with less difficulty.
- Patient is SOB even when he is sitting at rest. He has started using BiPAP every night, and states that it helps him to breathe better even during the day. He can only sleep with his head raised at night. His cough is weak, and he has some difficulty clearing his secretions.
- Patient has constant bilateral shoulder pain, left greater than right, that decreases his function and quality of life; the patient wants to have decreased shoulder pain.
- Patient needs a significant amount of help for self-care and mobility.
- Patient is able to stand with help and take a few steps with difficulty but is unable to ambulate.
- Patient enjoys socializing with family and friends at children's school and sports events and at church but is having difficulty conversing with people due to speech deficits and fatigue.
- Patient feels "useless" and wants be less of a burden on his wife and family.

The physical therapist's examination findings revealed the following impairments:

- Marked atrophy and fasciculations in the tongue and all extremities.
- Alert and oriented times 3; some psychomotor slowing as shown by a slight delay in responses to questions.
- Two finger subluxation of both shoulders.
- Shoulder pain measures 4 out of 10 on the left and 2 out of 10 on the right at rest and increases during movement
- Minimal active movement in his UEs, and some antigravity movement in his LEs; shoulder PROM is 70% of NL in all directions due to spasticity, muscular tightness, and guarding; bilateral finger flexor and plantarflexor contractures
- Decreased strength throughout neck and bilateral UEs and LEs on MMT: UE muscles in the 0 to T (1) range, LE muscles in the P+ (2+) range proximally and 0 in the ankle dorsiflexors and plantarflexors, neck extensors P (2), neck flexors F− (3−).
- Brisk stretch reflexes (3+), with continuous clonus in bilateral ankles; Modified Ashworth Scale scores are 2 in bilateral biceps and wrist flexor muscles and 3 in bilateral hip adductors, quadriceps, hamstring, and gastrocnemius muscles
- FVC: 2.49 L (51% of predicted)

The physical therapist's examination findings revealed the following activity limitations and participation restrictions:

- Balance (standing): Unilateral stance/eyes open, unable to stand on one leg
- Speech is barely understandable with concentration; patient is on a soft mechanical diet and only uses the PEG for supplemental feedings and water; he occasionally chokes, when swallowing food and medications.

Item	Score	ALSFRS-R Score Descriptor
Speech	2	Intelligible with repeating
Salivation	2	Marked excess of saliva with some drooling
Swallowing	1	Needs supplemental tube feeding
Handwriting (pre-ALS dominant hand)	0	Unable to grip pen
Cutting food and handling utensils (patients without gastrostomy)	0	Needs to be fed
Dressing and hygiene	1	Needs attendant for self-care
Turning in bed, adjusting bed clothes	1	Can initiate, but no turn or adjust sheets alone
Walking	1	Non-ambulatory functional movement only
Climbing stairs	0	Cannot do
Dyspnoea	1	Occurs at rest, difficulty breathing when either sitting or lying
Orthopnea	2	Needs extra pillow in order to sleep (more than two)
Respiratory insufficiency	3	Intermittent use of Bi PAP

- Transfers sit-to-stand and sit-to-supine with maximal assist of 1.

- Stands with his feet plantarflexed due to increased tone and muscle tightness and with his legs close together; can move his legs a couple of steps for transfers but quickly fatigues.

- Severe ADL and mobility deficits as indicated by ALSFRS-R score: 14/48 and Schwab and England score: 20% (can do nothing alone; may be able to help a little in some tasks)

The physical therapist's diagnostic impression was that the patient was quadriplegic and was dependent on his wife for ADLs. His shoulder pain and decreased ROM were likely due to a combination of instability and immobility. The patient was likely to need hospice care in the near future.

Primary goals at this stage were to maintain the patient's comfort, prevent complications, and ease caregiving burden.

1. Instruct patient's wife in basic body mechanics to use during lifting and patient care activities, PROM exercises, assisted coughing techniques, the use of a Hoyer lift™ for transfers, and use of positioning devices for the lower extremities (e.g., L-Nard boots, hip abduction splints).

2. Referrals to a speech and language pathologist for speech and swallowing evaluations and recommendations for augmentative communication devices, and to a social worker for information on respite care for the wife, family counseling, and advanced directives.

● GUILLAIN–BARRÉ SYNDROME

CASE B, PART I

Mrs. Roberts is a 56-year-old registered nurse who awoke with "pins-and-needles" sensations and accompanying numbness in her hands. Upon arising, she became aware of mild incoordination and weakness of her lower extremities. The weakness progressed to involve her upper extremities, and she was hospitalized by her family physician 3 days later. She previously had been in excellent health with the exception of a 4-day hospitalization 2 weeks earlier for a flu-like syndrome, consisting of mild fever, swollen lymph nodes, general feeling of illness, and diffuse joint and muscle pains. A precise diagnosis had not been established, but her symptoms resolved. After performing an examination and ordering some tests her physician gave her a diagnosis of Guillain–Barré syndrome.

Guillain–Barré Syndrome (GBS) is a group of neuropathic conditions that affect the peripheral nervous system, causing motor neuropathy with progressive weakness and diminished or absent reflexes. Sensory and autonomic nerve involvement is also possible. In contrast to ALS, GBS has a good prognosis with most patients recovering to their prior functional status by 1 year after onset.

Incidence and Risk Factors

The annual incidence of GBS is about two per 100,000 persons, and an estimated 3000–6000 people develop GBS each year on average in the United States.[150] The incidence of GBS increases with age, and people over age 50 are at greatest risk for developing GBS.[150,151] The male-to-female ratio is 3:2.[151]

Etiology and Pathophysiology

Several infections are implicated in the development of GBS. About two-thirds of patients with GBS have respiratory and gastrointestinal symptoms that precede the onset of neurologic symptoms by 1–3 weeks. The strongest evidence implicates *Campylobacter jejuni* infection, but GBS has also been reported following infection with *Mycoplasma pneumonia*, cytomegalovirus, *Haemophilus influenza*, varicella-zoster virus (herpes), and Epstein–Barr virus (mononucleosis).[152] Stressful events and surgeries have also been associated with the disease.[152] Despite some reports of GBS developing after vaccinations (i.e., tetanus, hepatitis, and influenza), there is not sufficient evidence to support vaccinations as a cause of GBS.

There are at least two pathologies that result in a clinical diagnosis of GBS (see Figure 15-4).[153] The demyelinating variant of GBS (acute inflammatory demyelinating polyradiculoneuropathy [AIDP]; see Table 15-11) is characterized by damage to the myelin sheath, surrounding axons by white blood cells (T lymphocytes and macrophages). This process is preceded by antibodies, binding to myelin antigens that activate a group of blood proteins, known as complement, which in turn lead to the degradation of myelin. Macrophages subsequently act as scavengers to remove myelin debris (see Figure 15-4A). Axonal damage may also occur secondary to demyelination. In contrast, the axonal variant (acute motor axonal neuropathy [AMAN]; see Table 15-11) is mediated by immunoglobulin G (IgG) antibodies and complement acting directly against the cell membrane covering the axon without lymphocyte involvement (see Figure 15-4B).[153] In this form of GBS, various antibodies bind to gangliosides on the cell membrane of the axons at the nodes of Ranvier. Gangliosides are groups of substances found in peripheral nerves. The key four gangliosides, against which antibodies have been described, are GM1, GD1a, GT1a, and GQ1b, with different anti-ganglioside antibodies being associated with different subtypes of GBS (Table 15-11). The production of these

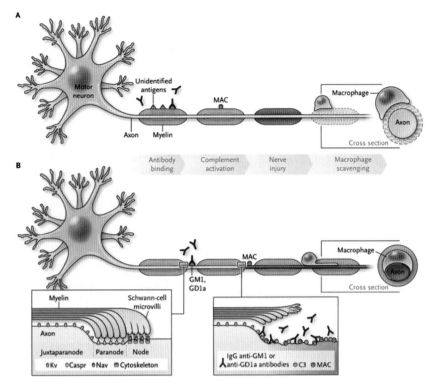

FIGURE 15-4 Possible Guillain–Barré pathologies.[151,152,154,155] **A.** Antibodies bind to mylin antigens and activate blood proteins (complement) that damage myelin; **B.** Immunoglobulin G antibodies bind to gangliosides on cell membrane of axons and activate complement that damages axons (Reproduced with permission from Rinaldi S. Update on Guillain–Barré syndrome, *J Peripher Nerv Syst* 2013 Jun;18(2):99-112.)

TABLE 15-11	GBS Subtypes		
TYPE	**PATHOLOGIC FEATURES**	**CLINICAL FEATURES**	**NERVE CONDUCTION STUDIES**
Acute inflammatory demyelinating polyradiculo-neuropathy (AIDP)	Multifocal peripheral demyelination Slow remyelination Probably both humeral and cellular immune mechanisms	Progressive, symmetrical weakness; hyporeflexia or areflexia Often accompanied by sensory symptoms, CN* weakness, and autonomic involvement	Demyelinating polyneuropathy
Acute motor axonal neuropathy (AMAN)	Antibodies against gangliosides GM1, GD1a/b, GalNAc-GD1a in peripheral motor nerve axons; no demyelination	Strongly associated with *Campylobacter jejuni* infection; more common in the summer, younger patients, and in eastern Asia Only motor symptoms; CN involvement uncommon Deep tendon reflexes may be preserved	Axonal polyneuropathy, normal sensory action potential
Acute motor and sensory axonal neuropathy (AMSAN)	Mechanism similar to AMAN, but with sensory axonal degeneration	Similar to those of AMAN, but with predominantly sensory involvement	Axonal polyneuropathy, reduced or absent sensory action potential
Miller Fisher syndrome	Antibodies against gangliosides GQ1b, GD3, and GT1a Demyelination	Bilateral ophthalmoplegia Ataxia Areflexia Facial, bulbar weakness occurs in 50% of cases Trunk, extremity weakness occurs in 50% of cases	Generally normal, sometimes discrete changes in sensory conduction or H-reflex detected
Pharyngeo-cervico-brachial variant	Antibodies against mostly gangliosides GT1a, occasionally GQ1b, rarely GD1a; no demyelination	Weakness particularly of the throat muscles, face, neck, and shoulder muscles	Generally normal, sometimes axonal neuropathy in arms

*CN, cranial nerve.

antibodies, after an infection, is probably the result of molecular mimicry, where the immune system reacts to the foreign infectious substance, but the resultant antibodies, in turn, attack tissues that are naturally in the body. For example, after a *Campylobacter* infection, some people will produce IgG antibodies against bacterial cell wall substances (e.g., lipooligosaccharides) that cross react with nerve cell gangliosides. The binding of antibodies to gangliosides causes activation of complement that, in turn, leads to detachment of portions of the myelin near the nodes of Ranvier and eventually axonal degeneration of motor fibers.[153]

Clinical Presentation

The first symptoms of GBS are weakness, numbness, tingling, pain in the limbs, or some combination of these symptoms.[152] The main symptom in individuals with **AIDP** is rapidly progressive, bilateral, and relatively symmetric weakness of the limbs. In up to 90% of cases with AIDP, symptoms begin in the legs and progress proximally. Respiratory insufficiency, due to weakness of respiratory muscles, requires mechanical ventilation for about 25% of hospitalized patients. Respiratory failure is more common in patients with rapid progression of symptoms, upper limb weakness, autonomic dysfunction, or bulbar paralysis.[152] Patients typically have generalized hyporeflexia or areflexia.[156] The weakness continues to progress up to 1–3 weeks after the onset of symptoms, followed by a plateau of variable duration before resolution or stabilization with residual disability.[156] Two-thirds of patients are unable to walk independently, when maximum weakness is reached, and among severely affected patients, 20% remain unable to walk 6 months after the onset of symptoms.[156]

Other symptoms that may be present in individuals with GBS include cranial neuropathies, sensory disturbances, pain, and autonomic disturbances. Involvement of cranial motor neurons can cause facial, oropharyngeal, and oculomotor muscle weakness, associated with facial paralysis, dysarthria, dysphagia, and visual problems (i.e., diplopia, ophthalmoplegia, and pupillary disturbances). Sensory disturbances, such as distal hyperesthesias, numbness, and paresthesias (tingling, burning), are common and usually have a glove and stocking pattern. Pain, especially with movement, is common (50–89% of patients) and is described as severe, deep, aching, or cramping (similar to sciatica) in the affected muscles and back (especially lumbar, intrascapular, and cervical regions).[152] The pain is often worse at night. Autonomic symptoms occur in about two-thirds of patients and include cardiac arrhythmias, orthostasis, blood pressure instability, urinary retention, constipation, and slowing of gastrointestinal motility.[152]

GBS generally follows a monophasic course and typically does not recur, but two or more episodes have been reported in 2–5% of patients. In one study, patients with recurrent GBS showed similar signs and symptoms, during every episode, despite having different types of symptoms, in the precipitating infection, suggesting that genetic or immunological host factors may play an important role in recurrent GBS. Recurrences occurred more frequently in patients under 30, with milder symptoms, and in patients with the Miller Fisher variant of GBS (see Table 15-11).[157]

Diagnosis

The diagnostic criteria for GBS include progressive, relatively symmetrical weakness with decreased or absent deep tendon reflexes.[152] Symptoms must reach maximal intensity within 4 weeks of onset and other possible causes must be excluded, for a diagnosis to be made. Table 15-12 includes features necessary for the diagnosis. As described in Table 15-11, this syndrome has several distinct subtypes. **Acute inflammatory demyelinating polyradiculoneuropathy** (AIDP) is the most common subtype and accounts for up to 90% of the GBS cases in the United States.[151] Specific changes in cerebrospinal fluid (CSF) and electrodiagnostic studies are strongly supportive of the diagnosis.[152] Diagnostic lumbar puncture findings include increased protein levels (albumin) and a normal white blood cell count in the CSF (see Table 15-12). The normal CSF white blood cell count helps differentiate GBS from other infectious, inflammatory, and malignant diseases.[152] NCS may show prolonged distal motor latencies, conduction slowing, conduction block, and temporal dispersion (loss of synchrony in the nerve action potentials) of compound muscle action potentials (CMAPs) with resultant decrease in CMAP amplitude in demyelinating cases (AIDP). In addition, F-waves and H-reflexes may be prolonged or absent. In **primary axonal damage** (AMAN variant), the findings include reduced amplitude of CMAPs without conduction slowing. In the acute phase, the only needle EMG abnormality may be abnormal motor recruitment, with decreased recruitment and rapid firing motor units in weak muscles. Fibrillations may be seen after 3–4 weeks, if some axonal injury occurs.

Other tests include blood tests and neuroimaging. Blood tests are generally performed to exclude the possibility of another cause of weakness (low potassium, Lyme disease, human immunodeficiency virus [HIV]). MRI is usually performed in GBS to rule out other potential causes of the clinical presentation, especially myelopathy.[153] A few small case series studies have looked at positive imaging findings that may be suggestive of GBS. The most often reported finding is greater gadolinium enhancement of the ventral compared to the dorsal roots of the cauda equina.[153]

Prognosis

Even in developed countries, the mortality rate from GBS is about 5%, mostly due to medical complications such as sepsis, pulmonary emboli, or unexplained cardiac arrest, possibly related to dysautonomia.[156] Recovery depends on the amount of remyelination and/or axonal regrowth. The process of remyelination occurs rapidly; however, regrowth of damaged axons, after Wallerian degeneration, is a slow process, with the rate of growth being about 1 mm/day.[158] Recovery from GBS is generally good. A large study of the literature on outcomes in individuals with GBS, who were appropriately treated, found that 82% of individuals were able to walk unaided at 6 months, and 84.1% walked unaided at 1 year, after the onset of GBS.[159] However, only 61% of individuals had full recovery of motor strength, 38% needed to change employment due to GBS, 66% of patients reported pain, and 14% were left with severe disability at 1 year.[159,160] The most common long-term deficits are

TABLE 15-12	Diagnosis of GBS[152]
FEATURE	**COMMENTS**
Required for diagnosis	
Bilateral symptoms	Usually begins in the legs
Decreased deep tendon reflexes	Complete areflexia often occurs in affected limbs
Subacute, weakness, and diminished/absent reflexes	Peaks within 4 weeks: peaks by 2 weeks in 50% of cases, and by 3 weeks in 80% of cases
Supportive of diagnosis	
Clinical features	
Autonomic involvement	Cardiac arrhythmias, orthostasis, blood pressure instability, urinary retention, slowing of gastrointestinal motility; absent in some subtypes
Cranial nerve involvement	Facial weakness occurs in 30–50% of cases; rarely an initial feature
Relatively symmetrical	Symptoms may not be absolutely symmetrical in affected limbs or face
Sensory involvement	Usually mild; absent in some subtypes, prominent in others (i.e., acute motor-sensory axonal neuropathy)
Symptom pattern over time	Peak by 2–4 weeks, with variable plateau, followed by recovery; permanent sequelae are possible
Cerebrospinal fluid findings	
Elevated protein levels	Levels may be normal early, but they are elevated by the end of the second week of symptoms in 90% of cases
Normal white blood cell count	Less than 10 per mm³ (10 × 10⁶ per L)
NCV findings	
Slowing (<60% normal velocity) or blockage of nerve conduction	Slowing of nerve conduction occurs in 80% of cases, but this make take weeks to develop

weakness of the anterior tibialis muscle and, less commonly, foot and hand intrinsics, quadriceps, and gluteal musculature. Some patients have long-term recurrences of fatigue and/or exhaustion, accompanied by pain and muscle aches, that can occur with the exertion of normal walking or working and can be alleviated by reduction of activity and rest.[161] Fatigue was independent of the severity of neurological deficits and was hypothesized to be due to post-infectious fatigue, dysautonomia, and psycho-sociological consequences of the disease.[161]

Moderate to severe sensory deficits (impaired response to pin-prick, light touch, proprioception, and vibration) were found in the arms of 38% and in the legs of 66% of 122 patients at 3–6 years, after recovery from acute GBS.[162]

The variations in the rate and extent of recovery in GBS make functional prognosis difficult. However, clinical scoring systems have been developed to aid in predicting individuals, who will need mechanical ventilation, and to predict long-term functional disability. Walgaard et al.[163] published a clinical prediction model that uses the number of days between the onset of weakness and hospital admission, the presence or absence of facial or bulbar weakness, and the severity of the limb weakness (Medical Research Council [MRC] sumscore; the sum of MRC scores [0–5] on six muscles bilaterally) to predict the likelihood that respiratory insufficiency will develop. Walgaard et al.[164] also published a clinical prediction model, called the Modified Erasmus GBS Outcome Scale, that uses the patient's age, the presence or absence of antecedent diarrhea, and severity of limb weakness (MRC sumscore) to predict whether a patient will be able to walk independently at 1, 3, or 6 months. Higher scores predict greater disability. Both scales are validated in the GBS population. Worse outcomes are associated with antecedent diarrheal illness, older age, more severe symptoms at their peak, rapid progression of symptoms, inability to walk at 14 days, and axonal involvement.[152]

Medical Management

Because of the unpredictable course and potential for death, patients with evidence of GBS should be hospitalized for intensive monitoring of cardiac, respiratory, bowel and bladder function, and provision of supportive care by a multidisciplinary team, until it has been established that there is no evidence of clinical progression. In patients with moderate to severe symptoms, respiratory compromise can develop rapidly, and mechanical ventilation may be required, if VC drops below 60% of predicted or less than 20 mL/kg.[152] Swallowing should be assessed to identify patients at risk for aspiration, necessitating the placement of a nasogastric tube. Subcutaneous heparin and compression stockings may be administered to decrease the risk of deep vein thrombosis, and patients with limited mobility should be monitored and positioned to prevent skin breakdown. If patients experience neuropathic pain, gabapentin (Neurontin) and carbamazepine (Tegretol) have been found to benefit patients with GBS, in intensive care units.[152] Increased skin sensitivity to touch may necessitate gentle handling and removal of irritating stimuli. Cardiac arrhythmia and extreme hypertension or hypotension, occurs in 20% of patients with GBS.[156] Bradycardia may be so severe that it causes asystole, necessitating the use of a temporary cardiac pacemaker.[156] Other possible complications include urinary retention and constipation, which may be addressed by bladder catheterization and the use of laxatives, respectively.

Specific treatments to speed recovery and/or eliminate symptoms of GBS include plasma exchange and intravenous immunoglobulin (IVIg). Plasma exchange (removal of plasma from withdrawn blood with retransfusion of the blood cells back into the blood with a plasma subsitute) removes damaging antibodies and complement and has been shown to improve the time to recover walking ability, minimize the need for mechanical ventilation, decrease the duration of ventilation, and result in greater muscle strength after 1 year, compared with placebo, in individuals with AIDP.[165,166] Optimal response is achieved when plasma exchange is performed within a week of symptom onset; those with mild GBS benefited from two sessions of plasma exchange, but more severely affected patients required at least four exchanges.[167] IVIg treatment (intravenous infusion of immunoglobulin preparation) has been shown to hasten recovery in non-ambulatory adults and children, compared with supportive therapy alone.[165] It is thought that immunoglobulin may act by neutralizing pathogenic antibodies and inhibiting complement activation, resulting in reduced nerve injury and faster clinical improvement. In general, IVIg has replaced plasma exchange as the treatment of choice, in many medical centers, because of its greater convenience and availability.[156] The standard treatment regimen is a total dose of 2 g per kilogram of body weight over a period of 5 days. The combination of plasma exchange, followed by a course of IVIg, is not significantly better than plasma exchange or immunoglobulin alone.[168] Neither prednisolone nor methylprednisolone can significantly accelerate recovery or affect the long-term outcome in patients with GBS.[169]

Physical Therapy Evaluation of the Individual with GBS

Physical therapy examination of the patient with GBS should start with a medical records review and history taking to obtain information about the time since diagnosis, recent illnesses or injuries, during the 4 weeks prior to GBS onset, the rate of progression and extent of symptoms, any preexisting neuromotor or medical conditions that might impact recovery, results of electrodiagnostic testing, and the patient's goals for physical therapy. A standard systems review and neurological examination should be performed with specific consideration to the following areas.

Motor System Function

Muscle weakness is a primary impairment of GBS and should be assessed to track progression of the disease initially and later to track recovery, to predict and prevent the development of contractures, and to determine the appropriate intensity of exercise interventions to implement. Therapists should visually inspect the patient to identify muscle atrophy and the presence of muscle fasciculations. Muscle strength in the neck and extremities can be directly assessed with MMT, dynamometry, or isokinetic testing, depending on the disease stage, or indirectly through functional testing. A cranial nerve screen should be conducted. Joint ROM may be initially assessed passively and, eventually, actively, using a goniometer. Foot and wrist drop are common and may require bracing or splinting to prevent contractures.

Depending on the MMT and ROM findings, balance, mobility (e.g., transfers, wheelchair propulsion, ambulation), self-care tasks (e.g., grooming, feeding, and dressing), and other functional tasks related to the patient's work and/or leisure activities should be assessed. The BBS, TUG, and Five Times Sit-To-Stand (5TSTS) test have been used to assess balance and mobility in individuals with GBS and other neurological disorders.[170-172] Gait speed has been measured with or without use of an ambulatory assistive device using a 10-m walk test.[170] Finger dexterity may be measured using a Nine Hole Peg Test (9HPT).[170] Therapists need to ensure that the patient with GBS is well rested, prior to mobility and functional testing. They should also ask the patient about and monitor for potential complications, related to weakness and immobility, such as falls and deep vein thromboses.

Three functional scales that have been used in clinical trials of individuals with GBS, include the Inflammatory Neuropathy Cause and Treatment (INCAT) group overall disability sum score (ODSS), the GBS Disability Scale (also called the modified Hughes functional scale), and the modified Rankin scale (see Table 15-13).

Respiratory failure, during the acute stage, results from progressive respiratory muscle weakness, involving both the inspiratory and expiratory muscles, and is a major complication of GBS, occurring in about 30% of patients.[177] Early signs of respiratory distress include tachypnea, tachycardia, air hunger, interrupted speech, use of accessory respiratory muscles, paradoxical breathing, and orthopnea; later signs include bradypnea, cardiac arrhythmias, loss of consciousness, and respiratory arrest.[177] Vital capacity and maximal inspiratory and expiratory pressures (MIP, MEP), assessed with a handheld spirometer, are measures of respiratory muscle strength that are frequently used to monitor the breathing status of the patient with GBS. In a retrospective study of 114 patients with GBS, a VC lower than 20 mL/kg, MIP lower than 30 cm H_2O, and MEP lower than 40 cm H_2O (the so-called "20/30/40 rule"), or a greater than 30% decrease from baseline of VC, MIP, or MEP was associated with impending progression of respiratory failure and need for mechanical ventilation.[178]

Fatigue is a common complaint in individuals with GBS. Patients can rate their fatigue, using a VAS, with "no fatigue" and "worst imaginable fatigue" as opposite extremes. Other fatigue scales that have been used in individuals with GBS include the FSS, the Checklist Individual Strength (CIS) fatigue subscale, the MFI, and the Fatigue Impact Scale (FIS).[161,179] Patients should not be tested to exhaustion, since recovery from fatigue can take some time and will delay the rehabilitation process.

Sensory System Function

Sensory function, including light touch, pressure, vibration, and pinprick, should be assessed frequently in patients with GBS to track the progress of reinnervation, to monitor muscle soreness and to avoid causing unnecessary pain during therapy. The INCAT sensory sum score is a sensory scale developed for patients with immune-mediated polyneuropathies that ranges from 0 ("normal sensation") to 20 ("most severe sensory deficit") and is the summation of pinprick and vibration grades (range 0–4) of the arms and legs and a two-point

TABLE 15-13	Functional Scales Used in GBS Disability Ratings	
FUNCTIONAL SCALE	**DESCRIPTION**	**SCORING**
Overall Disability Sum Score[173,174]	Patient report with arm and leg subscales. Arm = dressing (buttons and zippers), washing and combing hair, knife and fork use, turning a key in a lock Legs = walking and use of assistive devices	Total • 0 = no signs of disability • 12 = most severe disability score Individual items: Arms • 0 = normal • 5 = severe and bilateral Individual items: Legs • 0 = walking is not affected • 7 = restricted to WC or bed with no purposeful leg movements
GBS Disability Scale[174,175]	Describes functional status along 5-point scale	1 = able to run with minor signs/symptoms 2 = able to walk 10 m but not run 3 = able to walk 10 m with help 4 = unable to walk, in bed 5 = dead
Modified Rankin Scale[176]	5-point scale	0 = no symptoms 5 = severe disability (bedridden, incontinent, requiring constant nursing care)

discrimination grade (range 0–4) on the index finger.[180] Pain can be reported by the patient, using a VAS, with "no pain" and "unbearable pain" as opposite extremes.[170] Therapists should use a body chart to identify both the locations and specific types (paraesthesia, numbness, tingling, or hyperesthesia) of sensory loss or changes. It is also important for therapists to monitor for pressure sores and/or teach the patient to perform skin inspections in areas where skin sensation is diminished or absent.

Autonomic System Function

Autonomic dysfunction in GBS may cause extreme fluctuations of heart rate, blood pressure, and body temperature, as well as bowel and bladder problems. Therapists should monitor heart rate and blood pressure in resting and immediately after activity. If the patient reports dizziness, the therapist might consider obtaining a blood pressure and heart rate while supine and then standing to identify orthostatic hypotension. Therapists should also monitor patients for signs of abnormal body temperature, bowel and bladder control.

Psychosocial Systems

GBS is often a frightening and distressful experience to patients, especially to those who progress to complete paralysis and respiratory failure. Therapists should assess the patient's psychological and emotional health, coping strategies, and quality of life throughout all stages of the disease. Therapists can screen the patient for depression and anxiety using a variety of instruments (Table 15-14). Health-related quality of life measures that have been used in individuals with neuromuscular diseases are the Nottingham Health Profile, the SIP, and the SF-36.[179] It is also important to assess the caregiver and environmental

support that the patient has at home and determine what their needs may be after discharge.

A summary of the tests and measures that can be used to assess and evaluate an individual with GBS are found in Table 15-14. Based on the medical records review, subjective history, and examination findings, the therapist and patient should collaborate on setting physical therapy goals. General goals for physical therapy may include (1) facilitate respiratory, speech, and swallowing functions; (2) reduce pain; (3) prevent secondary complications (e.g., contractures, pressure sores, DVTs, and injury to weakened or denervated muscle); (4) initiate a graduated mobility program to obtain maximal function as reinnervation occurs; and (5) facilitate return to previous life roles and improved quality of life.

Physical Therapy Interventions

The evidence, regarding exercise and rehabilitation in people with GBS, is limited with only one randomized clinical trial identified in a systematic review paper of rehabilitation interventions published in 2012.[181] However, several studies support that high-intensity inpatient or outpatient multidisciplinary rehabilitation, including physical therapy, minimizes disability and improves quality of life in individuals with GBS.[182,183] The one randomized controlled trial, compared high-intensity outpatient multidisciplinary rehabilitation (i.e., 3 one-hour sessions of interrupted therapy/week, involving half-hour blocks of occupational, social, psychology, speech and physical therapy sessions 2–3 times per week for up to 12 weeks) with low-intensity rehabilitation (i.e., home-based program of maintenance exercises and education for self-management with a 30-minute physical program [walking, stretching] twice weekly and usual activity at home), for individuals in the chronic phase of

TABLE 15-14	GBS Impairment, Activity, and Participation Assessments		
IMPAIRMENT LEVEL ASSESSMENTS	**ACTIVITY LEVEL ASSESSMENTS**	**PARTICIPATION LEVEL ASSESSMENTS**	
• Cognitive screen (Mini-Mental State Examination) • Psychological screen (BDI, CES-D, HADS, STAI, HDRS, HARS) • Sensation (light touch, pressure, vibration, and pinprick) • Pain (10-point rating scale, VAS) • ROM (muscle length versus joint limitations) • Muscle strength (MMT, dynamometer, isokinetic testing, functional testing) • Hand and upper extremity function (Nine-hole peg test) • Reflexes (DTRs) • Tone (Modified Ashworth Scale) • Cranial nerve screen • Respiratory Assessment (VC, MIP, MEP, aerobic capacity, and endurance testing) • Fatigue (FSS, CIS fatigue, MFI, FIS)	• Balance (TUG, BBS, FTSTS) • Gait (10-m walk test) • Functional Status (Inflammatory Neuropathy Cause and Treatment group ODSS, modified GBS Disability Scale, modified Rankin scale, FIM, Barthel Index)	• Health-related QOL (Nottingham Health Profile, Sickness Impact Profile, SF-36)	

BBS, Berg Balance Scale; BDI, Beck Depression Inventory; CES-D, Center of Epidemiologic Study-Depression Scale; CIS, Checklist Individual Strength; DTR, deep tendon reflex; FSS, Fatigue Severity Scale; FIM, Functional Independence Measure; FIS, Fatigue Impact Scale; HADS, Hospital Anxiety and Depression Scale; HARS, Hamilton Anxiety Rating Scale; HDRS, Hamilton Depression Rating Scale; MEP, maximal expiratory pressure; MFI, Multidimensional Fatigue Inventory; MIP, maximal inspiratory pressure; MMT, manual muscle test; ODSS, overall disability sum score; STAI, State-Trait Anxiety Inventory; TUG, Timed Up and Go; 5TSTS, Five Times Sit-To-Stand; VAS, Visual Analogue Scale; VC, vital capacity.

GBS. Following the intervention, the individuals, in the high-intensity group, showed significantly greater improvement in function (FIM scores) than the low-intensity treatment group (68% versus 32%; p<0.0005).[183]

Acute/Progressive Stage

In the acute stages of GBS, patients may be in an intensive care unit (ICU) on ventilation with varying degrees of paralysis and sensory dysfunction. Physical therapy interventions in this stage typically include respiratory care, facilitation of speech and swallowing functions, pain management, bed positioning, ROM exercises, gentle stretching, massage, and initiation of functional activities in sitting and standing as tolerated. Depending on the facility, physical therapists may provide postural drainage, chest percussion, chest stretching, resistive inspiratory training, or assist with special protocols to prevent over fatigue of respiratory muscles, when weaning patients with GBS from a ventilator. Application of transcutaneous nerve stimulation (TENS) may be effective in reducing the pain of peripheral neuropathy in persons with GBS.[184,185] Therapists may manage and/or collaborate with speech pathologists and occupational therapists on dysarthria and dysphagia treatment programs. Patients with hypersensitivity to touch may benefit from a "cradle" that holds the sheets away from the body or by wrapping limbs snugly with elastic bandages. To prevent contractures and pressure sores, positioning, splinting, and ROM programs should be implemented.[186] Patients who are completely immobile should be turned at least every 2 hours. The skin over bony prominences, such as elbows and heels, should be protected, using foam or sheepskin pads. Application of ankle-foot and resting wrist and hand splints or a rolled cloth in the hand to provide prolonged positioning may help to maintain good alignment of the feet and hands. Passive ROM that includes accessory and physiological motions to the ends of normal range for all extremity joints, neck, and trunk should be performed at least twice daily. With proper instruction from the therapist, caregivers may be able to safely perform passive ROM exercises. If patients can move actively without pain or excessive fatigue, they can be instructed to perform the ROM themselves. If the patient can't complete a movement, the therapist or a well-trained caregiver can assist them to get the full range. To increase compliance, therapists should post the positioning, splinting, and ROM recommendations with diagrams as needed in a prominent location near the patients' beds. If tightness of muscles that span two joints (i.e., hamstrings, gastrocnemius) develops, gentle stretching at endpoint range for 10–30 seconds may alleviate the problem.[181] Swelling of limbs, due to prolonged immobility or concomitant cardiac conditions, may be treated with limb elevation and edema-specific massage. Upright activities can be started in the ICU, using a circle electric or standing bed or by initiating a sitting program as soon as tolerated. Patients who experience orthostatic hypotension may benefit from wearing an abdominal binder, foot-to-thigh compression stockings, and getting good hydration.

Mrs. Robert's weakness progressed to flaccid quadriplegia with complete cranial nerve involvement that required mechanical ventilation. While in the ICU, she received physical therapy interventions of chest stretching exercises, bed positioning, a passive ROM program, and application of ankle splints to maintain 90 degrees of dorsiflexion with neutral eversion–inversion. A positioning and ROM schedule with pictures of the positions and ROM movements was posted at her bedside. Due to her complaints of extreme hypersensitivity to touch, a cradle was placed on the bed to prevent sheets from touching her, and she was fitted with above-knee light pressure stockings. OT fabricated bilateral wrist and finger splints, a speech therapist helped her to relearn safe swallowing patterns, and a dietician ensured that she got proper nutrition.

Progression of her symptoms appeared to plateau at approximately 14 days after onset, followed by gradual return of respiratory functions. She was weaned from the ventilator after 25 days, which was a difficult process. Her PT provided instruction in breathing exercises, which she performed every 1 or 2 hours, that were vital to her ability to wean off of the ventilator. After weaning, she was transferred to a general floor and was brought to the PT department for her therapy. As her strength returned, she progressed to doing active assistive, active, and finally resistive trunk and extremity exercises. A mat program of rolling and supine to sit activities was implemented. Her therapist carefully monitored all of her activities to make sure that she was not overworking weak muscle groups.

Chronic/Recovery Stage

Once the weakness stops progressing, the plateau period may last only a few days to a few weeks, depending on whether only myelin or the axons themselves were affected. Strength will return over weeks to months and usually occurs in a descending pattern with arm function returning sooner than leg function. As strength begins to return, the therapist can slowly add active exercise, with frequent breaks, and monitoring for signs of fatigue.[181,187] Evidence suggests that excessive exercise, during early reinnervation, when only a few motor units are functioning, leads to paradoxical weakening rather than the expected hypertrophy.[187,188] Therefore, it is very important that exercise programs initially be non-fatiguing. Therapists should avoid putting any antigravity strain on muscles until strength reaches at least a 3/5 (Fair) MMT grade. Slings or adaptive devices (e.g., powder boards) that support the weight of the limb in a gravity-eliminated position will allow patients to perform active movements in muscles that lack antigravity strength. Exercises should be stopped at the first signs of fatigue or muscle ache. Any progression of resistance or repetitions of strengthening exercises should be monitored for 3–7 days for increased weakness, muscle spasm, or soreness, before progressing further.[188] If weakness or soreness follows exercise, it is best to not repeat the activity for several days and, then, reinitiate it at a lower level of resistance or number of repetitions and increase gradually. Low numbers of repetitions and high frequency of short periods of exercise are recommended initially.[158] Once reinnervation occurs and motor units are responsive, muscle reeducation can begin. To help patients to contract a muscle, the therapist must first demonstrate a movement and, then, teach the patient which muscle to contract to make the movement. As strength and exercise tolerance increases, resistive exercises that incorporate multi-joint and across-plane movements such as proprioceptive neuromuscular facilitation (PNF) patterns have been recommended.[158] Individuals with GBS have problems with fast-twitch muscle fiber recruitment for unknown reasons, which may benefit from practice of activities that push speed or rapid rises and falls in muscle force production (e.g., fast walking, jumping, quick changes in direction during walking and lunges).[158]

Most patients require a wheelchair for mobility, for several months, until their strength and endurance improves. Initially, they may need a wheelchair with a high, reclining back, but as strength improves, they may switch to a more lightweight and easily maneuverable chair. Deciding whether a patient with GBS should rent or purchase a wheelchair can be a difficult decision for a therapist to make, since it may be hard to predict how long the wheelchair will be necessary. When transitioning from wheelchair mobility to independent ambulation, patients may start in the parallel bars and progress to walking with a rollator walker with a seat to allow frequent rests. Eventually, they may progress to using lofstrand crutches or a cane. Since wheelchairs and ambulatory assistive devices are not always covered by insurance, therapists need to carefully consider the cost to the patient. Some individuals with GBS have residual weakness of the anterior compartment musculature that requires the use of an AFO.

Even when strength has returned, rehabilitation and exercise may need to continue to address fatigue. Cardiopulmonary fitness may be decreased in patients recovering from GBS, due to altered muscle function or sedentary lifestyle.[158,189] Several studies have reported positive effects of endurance training in individuals with GBS, not only improving cardiopulmonary function but also enhancing overall function, quality of life, and self-reported fatigue.[190,191] Tuckey and Greenwood[192] reported positive effects of partial body-weight support treadmill exercise for a 44-year-old male 6 months post-onset of severe GBS. If fatigue symptoms persist, the therapist may recommend work simplification and energy-conservation strategies.

Patients with GBS, who had prolonged ICU experiences, especially those who had respiratory failure and were on a ventilator, can have posttraumatic stress disorder (PTSD) and are likely to have increased incidence of anxiety, depression, and panic disorders years after discharge.[193] Although many people recover well from GBS, some patients report that they have had to make job changes, alter their leisure activities, and have had psychosocial changes due to their GBS.[194] Therapists must assess the patient's levels of fears and try to alleviate anxieties by talking with the patient and family members about their concerns. Therapists should refer patients to local GBS support groups, if they are available. If overwhelming anxiety and depression persist, a referral to a psychologist or psychiatrist is warranted.

CASE B, PART III

After 2 months of hospitalization, Mrs. Roberts was discharged home to return for daily outpatient rehabilitation. Her PT recommended an ultralight rental wheelchair, and she was fitted with prefabricated adjustable AFOs, for her bilateral foot drop, with the plan to order custom molded AFOs, after 4–6 months, if her dorsiflexor weakness persisted. Both the PT and OT visited her home with a social worker to determine what home adaptations and support services she and her husband needed. She continued to show gradual recovery over the next 1.5 years and progressed to a walker, then to lofstrand crutches, and eventually to independent ambulation. She used her AFOs at all times for the first 12 months and then was able to cut back to only wearing them for walking long distances or when prolonged eccentric activity was required (e.g., hiking downhill). She was able to do all of her previous activities but needed to pace her activities, during the day, to prevent excessive fatigue.

● POSTPOLIO SYNDROME (PPS)

CASE C, PART I

Megan is a 57-year-old female, who had polio at age 11 months, resulting in weakness of the left leg and right arm. She is a human resources manager in a large accounting firm. Six months ago, she began to have pain in her shoulders and left leg and states that she felt fatigued all day and began having trouble keeping up with work and other daily activities. Prior to this, she relates that she has always been able to walk independently but did have a "limp." Physician records indicate that her strength 2 years ago was F (3) in her left hip flexors and abductors, F+ (3+) in her left dorsiflexors and the rest of her left LE musculature was G (4). Her right UE strength was grossly F-G (3–4) with scapular winging on shoulder elevation. Her right grip strength was G− (4−). On examination at this time, she has P (2) strength in her left dorsiflexors and hip musculature and F+ (3+) strength in her right dorsiflexors. Right UE shoulder elevators are F− (3−), external and internal rotators are P (2), and grip strength is F (3). She has taken a family medical leave of absence from work, as she is too fatigued to put in a 40-hour work week, and states that once home, she mostly rests and no longer participates in social activities. Her shoulder pain is achy in nature and generalized across her shoulders and upper back. It is constant and keeps her awake at night at times.

Acute anterior poliomyelitis is a viral disease, in which the *poliovirus* enters the body by oral ingestion and multiplies in the intestine. The majority of infected individuals (95–99%) remain asymptomatic; but 1–5% of persons develop a fever, fatigue, headache, vomiting, stiffness in the neck, and pain in the limbs, similar to viral meningitis. It can strike at any age but affects mainly children under 3 (over 50% of all cases). It has largely been eradicated through vaccination programs, but there were 416 reported cases in 2013.[195] Polio leads to asymmetric, flaccid paralysis, with the legs more commonly involved than the arms. In 10–15% of all paralytic cases, severe bulbar weakness occurs. After the initial infection, the virus is shed in feces for several weeks and can spread rapidly through a community.

Pathology of the Polio Virus

The pathological findings consist of inflammation of meninges and anterior horn cells, with loss of spinal and bulbar motor neurons. Less common findings include abnormalities in the cerebellar nuclei, basal ganglia, reticular formation, hypothalamus, thalamus, cortical neurons, and dorsal horn.[196] Recovery begins in weeks and reaches a plateau in 6–8 months. The extent of neurological and functional recovery is determined by three major factors:

1. the number of motor neurons that recover and resume their normal function;
2. the number of motor neurons that sprout axons to reinnervate muscle fibers left denervated by death of motor neurons (i.e., collateral sprouting); and
3. the degree of muscle hypertrophy wherein muscle fibers may increase in size from 2 to 3 times normal size.

Due to collateral sprouting, a single motor neuron that normally innervates 100 muscle fibers might eventually innervate 700–2000 fibers. As a result, survivors of acute polio have a few, significantly enlarged motor units, doing the work previously performed by many units. Fiber type grouping occurs in the reinnervated muscle, and the normal mosaic interspersion of Type I and Type II fibers will be diminished or absent. Compensation by collateral sprouting and muscle hypertrophy may result in normal manual muscle tests even though more than half the original anterior horn cells are destroyed in some patients.

CASE C, PART II

Megan has residual involvement of the calf muscles in her left leg but was able to ambulate with only a mild limp.

If innervation of her tibialis anterior was severely compromised, how did she manage to dorsiflex her foot during gait? The tibialis anterior may have continued to work through reinnervation by surviving motor neurons. Also, she may have been using other muscles of the foot and ankle, such as the toe extensors, to substitute.

Postpolio Syndrome Presentation

Postpolio syndrome (PPS) is a condition that affects people who have had polio, followed by a period of neurological stability, and then, develop new or exacerbated symptoms several years after the acute poliomyelitis infection. The exact incidence and prevalence of PPS is unknown. According to the US National Health Interview Survey in 1987, there were an estimated 1 million polio survivors in the United States, with 443,000 reporting to have had paralytic polio. Accurate statistics do not exist today, as some polio survivors have died, and new cases have been diagnosed. Researchers estimate that the condition affects 25–40% of polio survivors. Factors associated with PPS development and typical signs of PPS are listed in Table 15-15.

Fatigue has been identified as the most common and most debilitating symptom of PPS.[196] Patients with PPS experience and can differentiate between fatigue, associated with new muscle weakness, and "central fatigue" that causes attention and cognitive problems, suggesting that fatigue in PPS may be caused by impaired brain function as well as degenerated motor units.[196] Fatigue in PPS may not appear at the time of the activity, and recovery may not occur with typical rest periods.[199] It is often described as overwhelming exhaustion that is sudden and completely wipes the person out and commonly occurs in the late afternoon or early evening.

Muscle weakness, in PPS, is most prominent in muscles that were severely affected in the initial infection, but it may also occur in clinically unaffected muscles.[200] The pattern of weakness is typically asymmetric but may be proximal, distal, or patchy[201]; it is primarily observed with repetitive and stabilizing contractions, rather than with single maximum contractions, possibly due to a decreased ability of muscles to recover rapidly after contracting.[202] New muscle involvement may also cause signs and symptoms such as muscle fasciculations, cramps,

atrophy, and elevation of muscle enzymes in the blood.[203] Individuals with previous poliomyelitis may have been able to maintain a high functional level for years, despite having only a few strong muscle groups, due to compensatory mechanisms, but late-onset muscle weakness of a significant muscle group can lead to disproportionately large functional losses, including reduced balance, increased falling, and the need to use assistive devices for walking or a wheelchair.[204,205]

Pain is a common complaint with PPS.[205,206] The pain intensity is high and is more often located in parts of the body that were previously affected by polio than in parts that were not.[205] Patients with PPS frequently report cramping pain in the legs (most often the upper leg musculature) and aching pain in the neck and shoulders.[205,206] Pain is most common in women, young patients, or patients who have had a long stable period.[205] Although the pain can have multiple causes, it is mostly associated with mechanical stress on muscles, tendons, and joints, from altered biomechanics, and is related to the amount of physical activity.[205] An EMG study of walking in people with PPS found overuse and substitution activity of the vastus lateralis, biceps femoris, and gluteus maximus muscles, when the soleus muscle is not functioning.[207] Over the long term, this substitution and overcompensation may lead to microtrauma of ligaments and joints and overexhaustion of motor units that results in pain. Similarly, pain may arise from overuse of muscles with use of assistive devices or propelling manual wheelchairs. The incidence of pain in 114 patients with PPS increased from 84%, in those who ambulated without orthoses, to 100% in those who used crutches or wheelchairs for locomotion.[206]

Diagnosis of PPS

The European Federation of Neurological Societies diagnostic criteria for PPS is shown in Box 15-2.[208] Diagnostic work up will be performed to exclude other conditions that might cause the health problems listed above. In addition the physician will do blood tests to see if creatine kinase is elevated which is consistent with PPS. Electromyographic testing will show abnormalities of chronic denervation. Muscle biopsy is done to see if there

TABLE 15-15	Factors Associated with PPS Development and Signs of PPS
FACTORS ASSOCIATED WITH PPS DEVELOPMENT[197]	**SIGNS OF PPS[198]**
Age greater than 10	New muscular weakness
Prior hospitalization for the acute illness	Fatigue
Ventilator dependency	Pain
Paralytic involvement of all four extremities	Onset or aggravation of muscle atrophy
Rapid return of functional strength following extensive initial involvement	Onset or aggravation of preexisting difficulties in accomplishing daily life activities
	Cold intolerance
	Sleep disorders
	Dysphonia or dysphagia
	Respiratory deficiency

BOX 15-2	European Federation of Neurological Societies Diagnostic Criteria for PPS[208]

- Confirmed medical history of poliomyelitis;
- Partial or almost complete neurological recovery after the acute period;
- A period of neurological stability that lasted for at least 15 years;
- A recent muscular weakness with a sudden onset and quick progressing deterioration;
- At least two new symptoms among the following ones:
  - Excessive fatigue
  - Muscle or joint pain
  - Muscle atrophy
  - Cold intolerance
- No other medical explanation.

is evidence of fiber type grouping due to chronic denervation/reinnervation or active denervation as shown by the presence of small angulated fibers that arise with terminal sprouting.

Does Megan show signs and symptoms of postpolio syndrome?

Yes, she has excessive fatigue, joint and muscle pain, muscle weakness, and atrophy. She previously had polio and had a stable period of recovery for >20 years. She now has new onset of symptoms that fit PPS.

Etiology of PPS

The cause of PPS is unknown, but experts have offered several theories. PPS is believed to be secondary to both peripheral and central nervous system changes. The denervation process leads to changes in muscle fiber type, typically from Type II to Type I – slow twitch; this change may lead to difficulty in adapting to the constraints, placed on that muscle, and eventually to overwork.[209] In addition, the energy production capacity of Type I muscle fibers in polio survivors is decreased, leading to greater fatigability.[209] Finally, there is instability in the long-term course of the reinnervation process, in which the enlarged motor units progressively lose their terminal axon sprouts. This process seems to be aggravated by overwork. Studies have demonstrated this effect in the tibialis anterior but not the biceps brachii muscle, leading to the hypothesis that muscle with intense, regular activity demands is subject to a more intense denervation–reinnervation process.[210] This may be due to several underlying factors. The giant motor units that are formed, during the initial recovery process, may not be able to sustain indefinitely the metabolic demands of all their sprouts; therefore, more pruning than sprouting occurs. There is also a proposed central mechanism as polio survivors exhibit an alteration of the motor cortex's capacity to command locomotor action, compared to controls.[209] Some evidence suggests that there may be genetic viral materials in the system that are able to stimulate and deregulate the inflammatory and immune system response. Notably, it has been shown that virus reactivation or persistent infection does not occur.[209]

Medical Management and Prognosis of PPS

There is no specific pharmaceutical treatment for the syndrome itself, but studies indicate that intravenous immunoglobulin may reduce pain, increase quality of life, and improve strength.[209] Prednisone has been used but has not been validated to improve fatigue or muscle strength. In a small, randomized clinical trial, supplementation with CoQ10 also did not provide additional benefit beyond resistance exercise by itself.[211] Joint deformities, arthrosis, and limb-length inequality may require surgery. Increased function can be achieved by arthrodesis, tendon transfers, and muscle transplantation.[205]

PPS is a very slowly progressing condition, marked by long periods of stability. The severity of PPS depends on the degree of the residual weakness and disability an individual has after the original polio infection. People who had only minimal initial symptoms and develop PPS will most likely experience only mild PPS symptoms, while those, who were left with severe residual weakness, may develop a more severe case of PPS with a greater loss of muscle function, difficulties in swallowing and/or breathing, and more periods of fatigue.

Physical Therapy Examination

Clients who have had poliomyelitis should undergo careful MMT of individual muscles to determine which muscles are weak. It is important to focus on individual muscles rather than muscle groups, in order to implement a focused treatment plan that is safe and avoids overworking affected muscles. In addition, endurance and fatigue are evaluated as they are two of the areas that negatively impact function, in individuals with PPS. Outcome measures that are reliable for assessing gait in PPS are the TUG, 6-minute walk test, and measurement of comfortable and fast walking speeds.

CASE C, PART III

Megan underwent strength testing, which demonstrated progressive weakness in previously affected muscles (left dorsiflexors, hip flexors and abductors; right shoulder elevators and grip strength) as well as some new muscles (left hip extension and adduction, right dorsiflexion). Additionally, her 6-minute walk test was 400 feet, which is well below age-matched norms and her comfortable walking speed was 1.0 m/sec, considered slow for her age. She filled out a fatigue questionnaire that indicated significant decline in function and participation due to fatigue. These examination findings indicated a need to work on endurance, strength in unaffected muscle groups, and fatigue to assist in improving function. She may also benefit from use of assistive devices.

Physical Therapy Management of PPS

Because fatigue is a major complaint in individuals with PPS, it should be a focus of physical therapy. Low to moderate intensity exercise programs, including aerobic (i.e., treadmill, bicycle, fast walking, swimming) and resistive exercises, have been shown to reduce fatigue in individuals with PPS.[198,212] Individuals should use the Borg rating of perceived exertion to determine appropriate exercise intensity for aerobic exercise. Graded exercise programs that are slowly progressed and include supervision, by a physical therapist, are recommended. A study by Oncu et al.[212] showed that individuals with PPS, who performed an exercise program under the supervision of a physical therapist in a rehabilitation clinic, demonstrated greater improvements in functional capacity, while the group doing the program as a home exercise program did not improve functional capacity. In addition, clients should be taught energy-conservation measures, including the use of handicap license plates to allow parking closer to establishment doors, balancing activity and rest throughout the day, sitting instead of standing, rearranging their home so that frequently used objects are in easy reach, and use of a scooter or similar motorized vehicle, when traveling a distance.

BOX 15-3	General Principles for Designing Exercise Programs

- Use a low to moderate exercise intensity.
- Slowly progress exercise, especially if muscles have not been exercised for a while and/or have obvious chronic weakness from acute poliomyelitis.
- Strengthening exercises should only be attempted with muscles that can move against gravity.[198]
- Pace exercise to avoid fatigue (intermittent periods of rest and exercise).
- Rotate exercise types, such as stretching, general (aerobic) conditioning, strengthening, endurance or joint range of motion exercises.
- Exercise should not cause muscle soreness or pain.
- Exercise should not lead to fatigue that prevents participation in other activities that day or the days following.

The key factor in prescribing exercise for individuals with PPS is to avoid overwork of weakened muscles, which can present as muscle aches or tenderness to touch. Some authors have recommended that strengthening exercises in PPS should only be done on muscles with at least antigravity strength or muscles with more strength in reserve than is required for minimum function.[197] To objectively measure if a muscle has enough reserve, the therapist can measure a person's muscle strength before and after walking for 1–2 minutes.[197] Strengthening programs should focus on (1) unaffected muscle groups that can take over some functions of the overworked muscles and (2) submaximal exercise to maintain strength and function in affected muscle groups. Halstead and colleagues established a limb classification system based on EMG evidence of anterior horn cell disease, remote and recent history, and formal physical examination to help guide exercise prescription in people with PPS.[213] The limb is classified into one of five classes, according to the most affected muscle in that extremity. Exercise guidelines have been recommended for each of the five classes.[197,213] See Box 15-3 for general principles for designing exercise programs. If muscle weakness is severe and/or overwork signs and symptoms persist, it may be necessary to prescribe assistive devices including orthoses, wheelchairs, and/or adaptive equipment. Modalities are also helpful for pain relief including heat, TENS, and massage.

Psychosocial Considerations in PPS

Psychological symptoms such as chronic stress, depression, anxiety, compulsiveness, and type A behavior have been described in polio survivors.[214] These symptoms may not only be distressful but may interfere with the individual's ability to make lifestyle changes to manage late-onset symptoms. Understanding the background and the social milieu that influenced their lives is beneficial to their care. During the polio epidemics in the 1940s and 1950s, fear of contracting polio was rampant. A coping strategy, at that time, was to encourage children to achieve high levels of physical performance. If a child contracted polio, the recommended treatment at that time was to hospitalize the person for months away from their families and friends, causing many children to feel abandoned and anxious. Polio patients were expected to be a "good patient," by working hard, and were not encouraged to talk about their disabilities. These acute experiences may have pushed survivors into lifelong patterns of type A behavior, making it difficult for them to cope with new postpolio symptoms, emerging years later.[214] Patients may have difficulty shifting from a philosophy of "no pain, no gain" to one of energy conservation and rest. Fear of loss of independence and prospects of role changing may cause the breakdown of the coping strategies that they have used for years. The therapist's sensitivity, support, and respect will play a major role in the patient's compliance with treatment. Conservative management that does not involve major lifestyle changes should be tried first. Therapists should also provide information about support groups in the community.

CASE C, PART IV

Megan is prescribed a submaximal, progressive aerobic program of pedometer walking to improve fatigue and endurance. She is also given strengthening for all muscles not previously affected by polio that have a strength grade of 3+ or greater. Additionally, she is prescribed ankle orthotics to assist with dorsiflexion and improve her gait pattern to be safer and more energy efficient. She performs her exercise program under the supervision of a therapist and is closely monitored before and after exercise for muscle pain or tenderness to ensure that she is not pushed to the point of overworking any muscle groups.

● PERIPHERAL NEUROPATHIES

Peripheral neuropathy is damage to nerves, leading to impaired sensation, movement, gland, or organ function. If the damage is isolated to one nerve, it is known as **mononeuropathy**, and if it involves more than one nerve it is **polyneuropathy**. When multiple nerves are affected but the pattern is not symmetrical, it is referred to as **multifocal mononeuropathy** or **multiple mononeuropathy**. Neuropathies are common, affecting 3–4% of those over the age of 55 with damage secondary to diabetes, being the most common cause of peripheral neuropathies.[215] It is estimated that 50% of individuals, diagnosed with diabetes (Type I and II), have peripheral neuropathy. Other causes of neuropathy are trauma, infection, autoimmune disorders, and inherited disorders (Table 15-16). When there is damage to nerves through any of these mechanisms, it is the large-diameter fibers that are more vulnerable than small-diameter fibers, meaning that light touch is the first sensation to be impaired followed by pain and temperature.

Classifications of Traumatic Nerve Injuries

Nerve injuries can be classified by the extent of injury and the chance of spontaneous recovery. The two most widely accepted

TABLE 15-16 | Causes of Peripheral Neuropathies

CATEGORY	MECHANISM OF NERVE DAMAGE	EXAMPLES
Trauma		
Stretch injury	Severance or tearing of the nerve due to a traction force	• Brachial plexus damage at birth (Erb's Palsy) • Radial nerve injury secondary to a humeral fracture
Lacerations, stab wounds, and penetrating trauma	Partial or complete severing of the nerve	• May be a clean cut (surgical incision, glass) or • Irregular (blunt instruments, knife stabbings)
Compression	Mechanical deformation and ischemia	• "Saturday night palsy" in which the radial nerve is compressed while sleeping either from a partner laying on the arm or from placement of the arm under the body. It is known as "Saturday night palsy" because it is thought to be more common when the person is impaired by alcohol. • Bone displacement from fracture • Hematoma • Compartment syndrome – swelling within the facial sheath following severe trauma
Repetitive stress injury	Repetitive flexing of a joint leads to irritation and swelling. When swelling is in a constricted area through which a nerve passes the nerve becomes compressed.	• Carpal tunnel is a well-known condition that is thought to be caused by repetitive stress such as typing or working with a jack hammer.
Systemic Disease		
Diabetes I and II	Most common form in the United States; mechanism is usually loss of peripheral blood flow leading to ischemia of the distal nerve endings.	• Usually a symmetrical distal polyneuropathy. • Sensorimotor neuropathy found in up to 50% of patients involves paresthesia, hyperesthesia, sensory loss of vibration, pressure, pain and temperature; presence of a foot ulcer may clue physician into diagnosis.[216] • Acute diabetic mononeuropathy (carpal tunnel, cranial nerves): common nerves compressed are the median at the wrist (carpal tunnel), ulnar at the elbow, peroneal at the fibular head, lateral cutaneous nerve of the thigh at the inguinal ligament. • Diabetic autonomic neuropathy is a widespread disorder of the cholinergic, adrenergic and peptidergic autonomic fibers that leads to dysregulation of one or more of the following systems: cardiac, sexual, gastrointestinal, sudomotor (sweating), pupillomotor (blurred vision), and bladder dysfunction.
Kidney disorders	Leads to high levels of ammonia in the blood	• Caused by uremic toxicity
Autoimmune diseases	Sjogren's syndrome Lupus Rheumatoid arthritis and other connective tissue disorders Acute inflammatory demyelinating neuropathy (Guillain–Barré syndrome) Chronic inflammatory demyelinating polyradiculopathy (CIDP) Multifocal motor neuropathy	• Immune system attacks the body's own tissues, leading to nerve damage. • Inflammation in tissues around nerves can spread directly into nerve fibers. • Over time, these chronic autoimmune conditions can destroy joints, organs, and connective tissues, making nerve fibers more vulnerable to compression injuries and entrapment. • Guillain–Barré can damage motor, sensory, and autonomic nerve fibers. • CIDP usually damages sensory and motor nerves, leaving autonomic nerves intact. • Multifocal motor neuropathy affects motor nerves exclusively; it may be chronic or acute.

(continued)

TABLE 15-16 Causes of Peripheral Neuropathies (*Continued*)

CATEGORY	MECHANISM OF NERVE DAMAGE	EXAMPLES
Vitamin deficiencies and alcoholism	Deficiencies of vitamins E, B1, B6, B12, niacin, thiamine Alcohol abuse	• Damage to the nerves associated with long-term alcohol abuse may not be reversible when a person stops drinking alcohol. • Chronic alcohol abuse also frequently leads to nutritional deficiencies (including B12, thiamine, and folate) that contribute to the development of peripheral neuropathy.
Vascular disease	Lack of blood to the nerves, most commonly the terminal nerve endings leads to ischemia	• Vasculitis leads to loss of distal blood supply and anoxic damage to distal nerve fibers
Cancers	Neuroblastomas, tumors, paraneoplastic syndromes	• Cancer can infiltrate nerve fibers or exert damaging compression forces on nerve fibers. • Tumors also can arise directly from nerve tissue cells. • Paraneoplastic syndromes can indirectly cause widespread nerve damage. • Toxicity from the chemotherapeutic agents and radiation used to treat cancer also can cause peripheral neuropathy.
Infections	Herpes varicella zoster (shingles), Epstein–Barr virus, West Nile virus, cytomegalovirus, and herpes simplex members of the large family of human herpes viruses. Lyme disease, diphtheria, and leprosy are bacterial diseases HIV, human immunodeficiency virus leading to AIDs Lyme disease, diphtheria, and leprosy	• The viruses can severely damage sensory nerves, causing attacks of sharp, lightning-like pain. Post-herpetic neuralgia is long-lasting, particularly intense pain that often occurs after an attack of shingles. • The bacterial infections are characterized by extensive peripheral nerve damage. • A rapidly progressive, painful polyneuropathy affecting the feet and hands is often the first clinically apparent sign of HIV infection. • Bacterial diseases characterized by extensive peripheral nerve damage.

Inherited neuropathies	Charcot–Marie–Tooth disease
	Mutations in genes that produce proteins involved in the structure/function of the peripheral nerve axon or the myelin sheath.
		Symptoms include:
		  • Extreme weakening and wasting of muscles in the lower legs and feet
		  • Foot deformities, such as high arches and hammertoes
		  • Gait abnormalities: foot drop and a high-stepped gait
		  • Loss of tendon reflexes and numbness in the lower limbs
		  • Decreased or increased sensation
		  • Dutonomic changes: decreased sweating; edema; uncontrolled BP, HR; bowel and bladder problems
		  • Motor changes: weakness or paralysis; muscle atrophy
		  • Trophic changes: shiny skin, brittle nails, neurogenic joint damage

Toxins		
Heavy metals and environmental toxins	Lead, mercury, arsenic, insecticides, and solvents	
Drugs	Anticonvulsants Antiviral agents Antibiotics Some heart and blood pressure medications Chemotherapy drugs	• In most cases, the neuropathy resolves when these medications are discontinued or dosages are adjusted. • About 30–40% of people who undergo chemotherapy develop peripheral neuropathy and it is a leading reason why people with cancer stop chemotherapy early. • The severity of chemotherapy induced peripheral neuropathy (CIPN) varies from person to person.

nerve injury classification systems were developed by Seddon and Sunderland (see Table 15-17).[217] Seddon classifies injuries as: Class I (neurapraxias) – segmental demyelination due to focal compression but the axon remains intact; Class II (axonotmesis) – the axon is damaged but the endoneurium remains intact; and Class III (neurotmesis) – a complete severance of nerve fibers and the supporting endoneurium.[218] With Class II and III injuries, there is degeneration of the fiber distal to the cell body that is called Wallerian degeneration.

In **neurapraxia** (Seddon's Class I Injury), there is a reversible blockade of nerve conduction due to mild or moderate focal compression. This may result in decreased strength, absence of DTRs, and loss of sensation (confined to large diameter fibers). There is usually no loss of autonomic nerve function and no permanent damage to the axon. Recovery is usually spontaneous and occurs within 3 months. **Axonotmesis** (Class II) is usually caused by crush injuries and results in a variable loss of sensory, motor, and autonomic nerve function. Damage is to the myelinated and unmyelinated fibers. Prognosis for effective regeneration is good because the integrity of the endoneurium is maintained but may be slow (several months to a year) as regeneration occurs at rate of 1–1.5 mm/day. **Neurotmesis** (Class III) are typically caused by stab wounds, high-velocity projectiles, or nerve traction that completely transects the nerve. Axonal regeneration may occur, but generally occurs with low fidelity (i.e., axon may not regrow to reconnect to the same end target) because the connective tissue layers are disrupted. Deficits may involve sensory, motor, and autonomic nerves and may be permanent. This type of injury has a high incidence of neuroma formation. A **neuroma** is a growth or tumor of nerve tissue that is most often benign.

Sunderland further refined Seddon's categories based on the realization that injuries had widely variable prognoses. **Neurapraxia** is equivalent to a Sunderland type 1 injury. In a Sunderland type 2 injury, the endoneurium, perineurium, and epineurium are still intact, but the axons are physiologically disrupted. Because the endoneurium is intact, the regenerating axons are directed along their original course, and complete functional recovery can be expected. The time for recovery depends on the level of injury, as the axon must regenerate distal to the end-organ. It can usually be measured in months, as opposed to weeks, for a Sunderland type 1 injury.

Sunderland's 3rd degree injury (Seddon's axonotmesis, Class II) involves disruption of the axon and endoneurium, but the perineurium and epineurium are intact. This injury can result in axon misdirection and potential debilitating consequences as recovery is incomplete in this grade of injury for a number of reasons. There is more severe retrograde injury to cell bodies, which either destroys neurons or slows their recovery, and without an intact endoneurium, fibrosis occurs, which hinders axonal regeneration. Finally, end-organs may undergo changes that impede full recovery.

Sunderland's 4th degree injury (Seddon's axonotmesis, Class II) involves disruption of all structures except the epineurium. Axon regeneration is disorganized, and surgical intervention is required to restore function. In both Seddon's Class II (Sunderlands 3rd and 4th) and III injuries, there is Wallerian degeneration, meaning a degeneration of the axon distal to the site of injury. The axon shrinks, fragments, and becomes irregular in shape. Schwann cells and macrophages that migrate to the area break down axonal fragments and myelin. Schwann cells also proliferate and form columns of cells, called bands of Bungner, that guide regenerating axons toward their original target tissue.

There are also changes in the nerve proximal to the site of injury, including retraction of the proximal stump, clot formation at the severed end, increased numbers of ribosomes around the nucleus (chromatolysis), and an enlarged and decentralized cell body. Axonal degeneration occurs in the proximal stump for a minimum of two to three nodes of Ranvier. The proximal stump sprouts many axons that grow toward the distal Schwann cell tube. The Schwann cells at the end of the proximal stump also proliferate and attempt to form a bridge between the proximal and distal stumps. As regeneration continues distally, axons may become re-myelinated and eventually connect with the target tissue (Figure 15-5).[219]

TABLE 15-17	Classification of Traumatic Nerve Injuries			
SEVERITY	**DESCRIPTION**	**RECOVERY PATTERN**	**RATE OF RECOVERY**	**SURGERY**
First: Neurapraxia	Local ion-induced conduction block or demyelination with restoration in weeks	Complete	Fast (days–12 weeks)	None
Second: Axonotmesis	Disruption of axon with regeneration and full recovery	Complete	Slow (3 cm/month)	None
Third: Axonotmesis	Disruption of axon and endoneurium causing disorganized regeneration	Varies	Slow (3 cm/month)	Varies
Fourth: Axonotmesis	Disruption of axon, endoneurium, perineurium, with intact epineurium and no regeneration	None	None	Yes
Fifth: Neurotmesis	Transection of the nerve	None	None	Yes

FIGURE 15-5 Class II peripheral nerve injury and recovery. (Reproduced with permission from Mescher AL (Ed). *Junqueira's Basic Histology*, 13ed. New York, NY: McGraw-Hill; 2013. Fig 9-30.)

Effects of Muscle Denervation

When muscles become denervated, they undergo several changes in structure, including atrophy of both Type I and II fiber types and proliferation of extra-junctional acetylcholine receptors, which are normally found only at the neuromuscular junction. When complete denervation of a muscle lasts longer than 21 days, the muscle becomes fibrotic, leading to a substantial decrease in the recovery of muscle mass and force production.

Surgical Repair

There are two basic types of surgical repair: (1) immediate (primary) repair, which is performed 8–12 hours after injury; and (2) early delayed (secondary) repair, performed 2–6 weeks after injury. Immediate repair is typically done with clean nerve transections (partial or full), while early delayed repair is done when major trauma and contamination are associated with the nerve damage. Surgical repair, involving nerve suturing, is most effective. In distal injuries, the entire nerve is sutured as a unit, using sutures placed in the epineurium. Funicular repair involves suturing of individual funiculi within the nerve trunk. This technique is used with proximal injuries.

Signs of Recovery Following Neurotmesis

When neurotmesis occurs, healing can occur if the proximal and distal stumps are sutured; axons in the proximal stumps will sprout and may regenerate connections to the target tissue. The axon regrowth typically proceeds at rate of 1 mm/day. Sensory recovery occurs before return of voluntary movement and is assessed by looking for the presence of deep pressure pain sensation, as this is the first sign of recovery. Deep pressure pain sensation is followed by superficial pain, then heat and cold, and finally, light touch and tactile discrimination. When motor nerves are affected, recovery is based on strength of contraction. For both sensory and motor recovery the Medical Research Council Grading System for Nerve Recovery is commonly used to assess and document recovery[220] (Table 15-18).

Nerve Grafts

When primary repair cannot be performed without putting undue tension on the remaining nerve, nerve grafting is required. **Autografts** (donor and recipient are the same biologic organism) remain the standard for nerve grafting material. **Allografts** (graft from a different species) have not shown recovery equivalent to that obtained with autogenous nerve and are still considered experimental. The most common source of autograft is the sural nerve, which is easy to obtain, the appropriate diameter for most surgical needs, and loss of this nerve, from its primary site, has minimal impact on function. Other graft sources include the anterior branch of the medial antebrachial cutaneous nerve, the lateral femoral

TABLE 15-18	Medical Research Council Grading System for Nerve Recovery[222]		
MOTOR RECOVERY		**SENSORY RECOVERY**	
M0	No contraction	S0	None
M1	Return of palpable contraction in the proximal muscles	S1	Deep cutaneous pain only
M2	Poor muscle grade activity in proximal muscles; palpable (trace) intrinsics	S1+	Deep and superficial pain
M3	Fair strength in proximal and distil muscles	S2	Superficial pain and some touch
M4	Good muscle strength, still weak intrinsics	S2+	As in S2, but with an exaggerated response
M5	Recovered strength in all muscles	S3	Disappearance of exaggerated response with >15 mm 2-point discrimination
		S3+	Better localization of stimulation with 7–15 mm of 2-point discrimination
		S4	Complete recovery

cutaneous nerve, and the superficial radial sensory nerve.[219] If an autograft is not feasible, then a **nerve conduit** (artificial nerve graft) is often used to provide a pathway for nerve regeneration to occur. Potential advantages of nerve conduits, over allografts, include absorbability, lack of donor-site morbidity, and lack of axonal escape.[221]

CASE D, PART I

Tina, a 50-year-old woman, was injured 2 days ago, when a load of lumber fell from a shelf, pinning her left forearm. The following signs and symptoms are noted on her left side:

- She does not feel pinprick, touch, temperature, or vibration on the medial hand, little finger, and medial half of the ring finger.
- Sweating is absent in the same distribution as the sensory loss.
- Radial wrist extension and flexion and finger extension strength are normal on manual muscle tests.
- She is unable to flex the middle and distal phalanges of the fourth and fifth digits, abduct or adduct her fingers, or adduct the hand.

What nerve is injured in this patient? Ulnar nerve

What is the most likely classification of this injury (i.e., Class I, II, or III)? Class II axonotmesis

Suppose that the nerve was crushed near the elbow, about 20 cm from her fingers. Approximately how long will it be before she regains the ability to abduct and adduct her fingers? 200 days

---

Diabetic and Related Neuropathies

Diabetic neuropathy is a frequent sequela of both Type I and II diabetes, occurring in 30–40% of those with diabetes and involves either motor or sensory nerves, or both (see Table 15-19). Individuals who smoke, are of older age, and have uncontrolled blood glucose levels are at higher risk of developing neuropathy as are those with a longer duration of diabetes. There are many types of diabetic neuropathy including (1) distal symmetric polyneuropathy, (2) autonomic neuropathy, (3) diabetic radiculoplexus neuropathy (DRPN; aka diabetic proximal motor neuropathy or diabetic amyotrophy), and (4) diabetic focal peripheral neuropathies (cranial mononeuropathy; aka diabetic ophthalmoplegia).

Diabetic distal symmetric polyneuropathy (DSP) is the most common type of diabetic neuropathy, presenting with foot pain and paresthesias that occur bilaterally and symmetrically in a stocking distribution in the distal legs. Large-fiber sensory nerve involvement results in tingling paresthesias and a perception that the feet feel "numb or asleep" along with distally impaired vibration, joint position, and touch-pressure sensation, and diminished or absent ankle reflexes.[223] If small sensory fibers are involved, the patient reports pricking, stabbing, and burning sensations. DSP may also be associated with motor weakness that leads to foot drop and reduced ankle reflexes. **Diabetic autonomic neuropathy** usually accompanies diabetic DSP, but in rare cases, it occurs alone. Autonomic symptoms and deficits are usually mild until late stages of disease. It potentially involves all organs that receive autonomic innervation. The pathogenesis of diabetic DSP is multifactorial and involves complex interactions between the degree of blood glucose level control, diabetes duration, age-related nerve loss, and other factors such as blood pressure, lipid levels, and weight.[223] These risk factors act together to activate biochemical pathways that damage nerves and small blood vessels.

Severe diabetic DSP may cause loss of sensation, extreme sensitivity to touch, including light touch (allodynia), loss of balance and coordination, and loss of reflexes and muscle weakness. These impairments lead to widening of the foot, foot ulcers, and gait changes. When the foot widens and structures shift, weight bearing occurs through structures that don't commonly bear weight and this leads to foot ulcers that can lead to

TABLE 15-19 Comparison of Diabetic Polyneuropathy and Subtypes[223]

FEATURES/SYMPTOMS/SIGNS	DSP	DRPN	CIDP	DMN
Symptoms				
Acute/subacute onset	No	Yes	Yes	At times
Progression rate	Years	Weeks/months	Weeks/months	Variable
Pain/allodynia	<20% (feet)	Yes	No	Yes (focal)
Numbness/tingling	Yes	At times	Yes	Yes (focal)
Weakness	Late	Yes	Yes	Motor nerve
Dysautonomia	Yes	Yes (about 50%)	No	No
Signs				
Decreased vibration, joint position	Yes	Variable	Yes	No
Decreased pain, temperature	Yes	Variable	At times	Yes (focal)
Weakness/atrophy	Late distal	Proximal, at times distal	Proximal and distal	Proximal and distal (at times)
Orthostatic hypotension	Mild	Yes	No	No
Anatomical pattern				
Symmetric	Yes	No	Yes	No
Proximal predominant	No	Yes	When severe	Variable
Stocking-glove	Yes	No	Yes	No
Prognosis				
Chronic/progressive	Yes	No	About 33%	Yes
Monophasic/resolution	No	Yes (partial)	Often	No
Pathophysiology	Metabolic/microvascular	Immune-mediated	Immune-mediated	Compressive/ischemic

CIDP, chronic inflammatory demyelinating polyradiculopathy; DMN, diabetic mononeuropathy; DRPN, diabetic radiculoplexus neuropathy; DSP, distal symmetric polyneuropathy.

amputation. Foot care and proper footwear should be initiated early in the disease to prevent these secondary complications. Wearing well-fitted shoes with good support and padding for the metatarsal heads and examining the feet daily can help prevent amputations.

Diabetic radiculoplexus neuropathy (DRPN) can affect cervical, thoracic, and/or lumbosacral regions but the most common is lumbosacral DRPN.[223] Lumbosacral DRPN typically affects middle-aged or older individuals with Type II diabetes. It presents with severe unilateral or asymmetric proximal pain, involving the back, hip, or anterior thigh, followed by asymmetric proximal leg weakness and profound atrophy.[223] The pain and weakness spread in a progressive or stepwise manner, over weeks to months, to nearby and contralateral segments with some people becoming wheelchair-dependent or developing asymmetric quadriparesis. Weight loss and dysautonomia are common with about half of patients experiencing orthostatic hypotension and changes in sexual, bladder, and bowel function. The pathogenesis of DRPN is an ischemic injury caused by an immune-mediated microvasculitis ,involving motor, sensory, and autonomic fibers. Recovery usually begins within 9–12 months, although recovery can be incomplete and last for many years.[223]

Some **focal peripheral mononeuropathies** (DMN), involving cranial, thoracic, or extremity nerves, are associated with diabetes.[223] Cranial mononeuropathy presents as isolated lesions of cranial nerves III, IV, or VI. Symptoms include unilateral headache, ptosis, and impaired extraocular movements, resulting in diplopia that develops over a few hours. Another common focal neuropathy of diabetes is a **unilateral truncal (thoracic) radiculopathy**, which presents as acute abdominal pain suggestive of an intra-abdominal process, herpes zoster, or a spinal process.[223] In addition, nerves that are susceptible to compression or cumulative trauma, including the median, ulnar, radial, lateral femoral cutaneous, fibular, and plantar nerves, are frequently injured in patients with diabetes.[223]

Chronic inflammatory demyelinating polyradiculopathy (CIDP), sometimes called chronic relapsing polyneuropathy, is an immune-mediated neuropathy that may be associated with diabetes. One study reported that patients with diabetes were 11 times more likely to have CIDP, compared with those without diabetes, but other studies have failed to confirm an increased risk.[223,224] The disorder causes demyelination of peripheral nerves, resulting in progressive weakness and impaired sensory function in the extremities. Young adults and men are more commonly affected. It often presents with symptoms of tingling or numbness (beginning in the toes and fingers), weakness of the arms and legs, areflexia, and fatigue. The course of CIDP varies widely among individuals. Some individuals may have a bout of CIDP, followed by spontaneous recovery, while others may have many bouts with partial recovery in between relapses. CIDP is closely related to GBS and is considered the chronic counterpart of that acute disease. Medical treatment for CIDP includes corticosteroids, such as prednisone, which may be prescribed alone or in combination with immunosuppressant drugs. Plasmapheresis (plasma exchange) and intravenous immunoglobulin (IVIg) therapy are also effective. IVIg may be used even as a first-line therapy.

Physical Therapy Assessment of Neuropathies

When assessing for neuropathy, both sensory and motor systems should be thoroughly examined. It is important to identify the cause of neuropathy so that appropriate treatment and prevention can be implemented. For instance, diabetic neuropathy tends to primarily involve the sensory system, and it is important to prevent further progression through tight control of blood glucose levels. In Guillain–Barré, the motor system is more involved. Sensory and motor findings are usually in a symmetrical glove and stocking distribution. Sensory and motor assessment are covered in Chapter 9 (Evaluation). When sensory neuropathy is suspected, a thorough examination, using monofilaments and other tests for all sensory modalities, is necessary to implement the most effective treatment plan.

In addition to these standard evaluation techniques, it is also helpful to obtain NCV and EMG testing (see the discussion at the beginning of this chapter). Another specialized test is Tinel's sign, in which you tap over the nerve; a positive sign is pain or tingling, in the distribution of the nerve, and indicates that the nerve is irritated. Assessment should be done systematically, noting the distribution of sensory and motor loss. Use of dermatomes and myotomes allows clinicians to identify the nerve(s) involved (see Figure 3.4 in Chapter 3 of this text for a dermatome map). Finally proprioceptive, kinesthetic, and vibratory testing are used to assess the dorsal column-medial lemniscus pathway. Of these tests vibratory testing is the most sensitive and valid.

Tests for Autonomic Neuropathy

Diabetes also impacts the autonomic nervous system and can lead to cardiovascular autonomic neuropathy (CAN), gastrointestinal neuropathy, and genitourinary neuropathy. CAN is present in about 20% of individuals with diabetes and increases to 35–65% in older diabetics.[225] It may contribute to myocardial infarction, arrhythmia, and sudden death. It also impacts

response to exercise. Gastrointestinal neuropathy can lead to gastroparesis (abnormal gastric emptying), and genitourinary neuropathy can cause neurogenic bladder and sexual dysfunction. Physical therapists must be acutely aware of the potential for CAN, when prescribing exercise for their clients with diabetes or other disorders that can damage the autonomic nervous system. Symptoms include exercise intolerance, early fatigue and weakness with exercise, resting tachycardia, abnormal blood pressure regulation, postural hypotension, dizziness, and syncope. Subclinical CAN has been detected in individuals with Type II diabetes 1 year after diagnosis and in those with Type I 2 years after diagnosis.[216] Physical therapists can screen for CAN by testing for orthostatic hypotension, taking pulse and noting any resting tachycardia; screening questionnaires developed to assess for symptoms of autonomic neuropathy are also available (Box 15-4). In subjects with well-controlled Type II diabetes, even with minimal evidence of CAN, altered cardiac autonomic balance is present and can be detected through an exercise-based assessment for CAN. The early post-exercise recovery period in diabetes is characterized by enhanced sympathoexcitation, diminished parasympathetic reactivation, and delay in heart rate recovery.[226] In addition, the squatting test is an active posture maneuver that imposes significant orthostatic stresses. In normal subjects, this maneuver does not lead to any symptoms, but in those with CAN, both the increase in blood pressure, during squatting, and the decrease in blood pressure, during standing, may be exaggerated and sustained, potentially leading to complaints and adverse events.[227] To do this screen, monitor pulse and blood pressure carefully, during the transition from standing to squatting, from squatting to standing, and for several minutes after the individual returns to standing. If the screen is positive with these position changes, the client should be referred for cardiovascular autonomic reflex tests, prior to instituting any significant aerobic exercise program.

Treatment of CAN involves cardiovascular risk reduction and lifestyle intervention. Exercise should be graded, with a slow progression, and should be supervised.[216] Resistance exercise may be beneficial, as a study demonstrated that low-intensity

---

BOX 15-4   Autonomic Screening

Ask the patient, if (s)he has experienced any of the following, scoring as (1 = never; 2 = occasionally; 3 = sometimes; 4 = often; 5 = frequently)

- Lightheadedness
- Dry mouth or eyes
- Blue, pale, cold, or sweating feet (more than the rest of the body)
- Absent sweating in feet, during exercise
- Sweating of the hands, more than the rest of the body
- Vomiting or bloating after eating
- Three bouts of diarrhea/day
- Constipation (<1 bowel movement/day)
- Any urine incontinence
- Males only – problems with achieving an erection

resistance training improved left ventricular function in rats with diabetes.[228] Low level, slowly progressive aerobic exercise is also beneficial for those with diabetes and CAN.[229] If the individual has resting tachycardia, beta-blocker medications may be used. Physical therapists can teach the individual with orthostatic hypotension to rise, from supine and sitting, in increments, resting after each position change. In addition, isometric contraction of the plantarflexors along with ankle pumps can help to improve blood flow from the lower extremities.

CASE E, PART I

RT is a 68-year-old obese male with history of hypertension, who retired from an office job with the government and presently, teaches part-time at a local business college. Approximately 3 months ago, he noticed some burning and tingling in his feet and was evaluated by his physician. Laboratory studies taken at that time revealed a fasting blood glucose of 146 mg/dL and his HbA$_{1c}$ was 7.2% (normal 4.0–6.0%). His physician referred him to physical therapy for difficulty walking, per the patient's self-report. RT's HbA$_{1c}$ indicates that he has not had good glycemic control over the last few months and is at increased risk for peripheral and autonomic neuropathy.

What type of neuropathy is RT at highest risk for developing? A symmetrical distal polyneuropathy

What tests and measures specific to neuropathy should be done with RT? Monofilament testing of the foot, for protective sensation, proprioceptive and vibratory testing to determine if his gait problems stem from issues in the dorsal medial lemniscal pathway.

Should he be tested for CAN? If so what tests should the PT administer? Tests for autonomic neuropathy should also be completed. A squatting test and an assessment of orthostatic hypotension during supine to stand should be administered.

If the screen for CAN is positive can RT begin an exercise program? If so what type? Yes, he can begin exercise if it is supervised and progressed slowly. He might benefit from both resistance exercise to improve left ventricular function and aerobic exercise to improve overall health, glycemic control, and cardiopulmonary function.

Physical Therapy Management of Individuals with Peripheral Neuropathies

Pain Management

The best treatment for peripheral neuropathies is prevention. In those with prediabetes and diabetes, long-term control of blood glucose levels through appropriate diet, oral drugs, or insulin injections is key to preventing tissue damage. Exercise can be an effective modality for prevention and treatment. In a mouse model of Type I diabetes, exercise delayed the onset of

mechanical hypersensitivity (independent of glucose control), reduced changes in calcium ion function to improve electrophysiological deficits,[230] and reduced myelin loss.[231] While the research was performed in diabetes, it demonstrates that exercise is an effective means of reducing oxidative stress, which is the underlying mechanism of nerve damage in many disorders. Another non-pharmaceutical treatment that is effective is TENS, which activates central mechanisms to provide analgesia.[232] Low-frequency TENS activates K-opioid receptors in the spinal cord and the brainstem, whereas high-frequency TENS produces its effect via C-opioid receptors. Deep heat can make pain worse and massage has not been shown to be effective.[232] Medications that are used to decrease neuropathic pain include tricyclic antidepressants (Elavil, Pamelor), anticonvulsants (Carbamazepine, Phenytoin), and analgesics (Vicodin, Capsaicin topical cream). These each have side effects and variable effectiveness.

Functional Training

In those with diabetic peripheral neuropathy, exercise improves balance,[233] trunk proprioception, strength,[234,235] 6-minute walk (6MW) distance, and habitual physical activity.[236] In a controlled clinical trial, individuals with CIDP, who performed an exercise program, had improved strength and quality of life (SF-36) as compared to no improvements in control subjects who did not exercise.[237] The exercise program was a relatively mild one, including body weight resistance exercises, active range of motion, some theraband exercises, and stretching (10 repetitions of each per day). In addition, they did a progressive walking and cycling program, 10–20 minutes daily, at 60–70% of maximum heart rate, or the "somewhat hard" Borg rating of perceived exertion.[237] Long-term aerobic exercise of brisk walking, 4 hours per week over 4 years, in individuals with diabetes, prevented the onset of or slowed the progression of motor and sensory neuropathies.[238] Exercise has also been shown to improve function in older adults with diabetic neuropathies as measured by the BBS, FRT, TUG, and the 10-m walk.[234]

CASE E, PART II

RT already has sensory changes and would benefit from a walking program. If he complains of pain, the most effective treatment would be TENS. He has been referred to therapy due to complaints of difficulty walking. The evidence shows that a multifactorial program of strengthening, balance training, and range of motion is likely to improve his balance and walking function.

Denervated Muscle

The effectiveness of electrical stimulation after axonotmesis has not been proven. For the patient who is expected to have nerve regrowth after complete denervation, electrical stimulation, using galvanic current to the denervated muscle, has been used to maintain the connective tissue mobility within the denervated muscle, with the goal of minimizing fibrosis and having a mobile end-organ, when reinnervation takes place. However, there is controversy in the literature about the use of electrical stimulation in denervated muscle, as it has been found to slow but does not prevent muscle atrophy. In an animal model of a crush injury, the addition of electrical stimulation slowed recovery compared to animals that did not receive electrical stimulation.[239] In addition, the longer pulse duration needed to cause a contraction in denervated muscle may be too painful for some people to tolerate. For partially denervated muscle, the recommended treatment is muscle reeducation. Available evidence does not support the use of electrical stimulation in partially denervated muscles.[239,240] Ohtake et al.[240] recommended deferring the use of electrical stimulation in individuals with Bell's palsy for 3 months because 64% of patients with Bell's palsy will have regained normal function within this time period. **In Case D, Tina has a recent compression injury of her ulnar nerve. Based on the evidence, she would not benefit from electrical stimulation but, instead, should be treated initially with rest, followed by muscle reeducation.**

Sensory Impairment

Treatment for sensory impairment is focused on teaching the client that they are at risk of injuring the limb, since they cannot feel it nor painful stimuli that might harm the limb. The therapist should teach the client to frequently check the position of the limb, observe the skin for any signs of irritation, and avoid tight or restrictive clothing and shoes. They will also need to learn to check water temperature and use extra caution around extremely hot or cold objects. **RT has sensory impairment of the feet and will need to select supportive shoes with good padding. He should also be educated to check his feet daily for redness or sores and to use caution, when initially wearing a new pair of shoes.**

● BRACHIAL PLEXUS INJURIES

CASE F, PART I

Jonathon was a full term, 9 lb, 10 oz, 22½ inch baby boy, born via vaginal delivery with no apparent complications, he was discharged home after 48 hours. At his 3-week pediatrician visit, his mother noted that he did not seem to move his left arm, as he does his right, and he frequently cries when being dressed as his left arm is maneuvered into shirts.

The brachial plexus, made up of spinal nerves from C5 to T1, makes up a large complex network of nerves (plexus) that run through the cervical-axillary canal. This plexus provides motor and sensory innervation to the upper extremity. The brachial plexus is at risk for some types of injury, typically accidental trauma, from traction to the arm or head that results in sheer,

stretch, compression, or tear of the peripheral nerve. As seen in Figure 15-6, the brachial plexus is described in roots, trunks, divisions, cords, and branches (nerves). As such, injury to a certain area of the plexus will present with common characteristics as the innervation path to the arm and hand can be traced. For example, if there is injury to the upper plexus, at the superior trunk, motor and sensory damage from C5 and C6 are expected, as is innervation through the lateral and posterior cords, and radial and ulnar nerves.

Brachial Plexus Palsy

Peripheral nerve injuries at the brachial plexus from a trauma are relatively common in pediatrics. The most common mechanism of injury is during an obstetric injury, when the head of the infant is pulled into lateral flexion as the baby is delivered or before the shoulders are delivered, causing stress on the brachial plexus; this is more likely with a larger baby, like Jonathon. During a breech birth (feet or bottom first) the arm(s) of the infant can be raised overhead, which can also result in stress on the brachial plexus during delivery; however, typically babies with breech presentation are now delivered by C-section, so this is less likely a cause of BPP in the United States. Risk factors for brachial plexus injury include shoulder dystocia (where the head has been delivered but the shoulder is stuck), prolonged delivery, difficult delivery, needing assistance such as forceps, and an infant greater than 4000 g. More than half of the cases of brachial plexus injury do not have these risk factors.[241] Accidental traction of the arm, during play, is also a common mechanism of injury to the brachial plexus in childhood.

Classification System

- Upper Palsy/Group I (Erb's Palsy) – C5 and C6 nerve roots (most common)
- Group II – C5, C6, and C7 nerve roots affected
- Lower Palsy/Group III (Klumpke's Palsy) – C8 and T1 nerve roots (rare)

Symptoms on the Injured Side

- Hypotonia of the arm and hand
- Muscle weakness; absence of antigravity movements
- Abnormal positioning of the shoulder, elbow (and especially) wrist, and hand
- Lack of sensation
- Less perspiration
- Lack of awareness of arm or hand
- Neglect
- Drooping eyelid
- Contractures of joints
- Pain
- Numbness or tingling
- Decreased girth
- Decreased grip strength
- Absent/weak Moro reflex
- Absent/weak protective reflexes

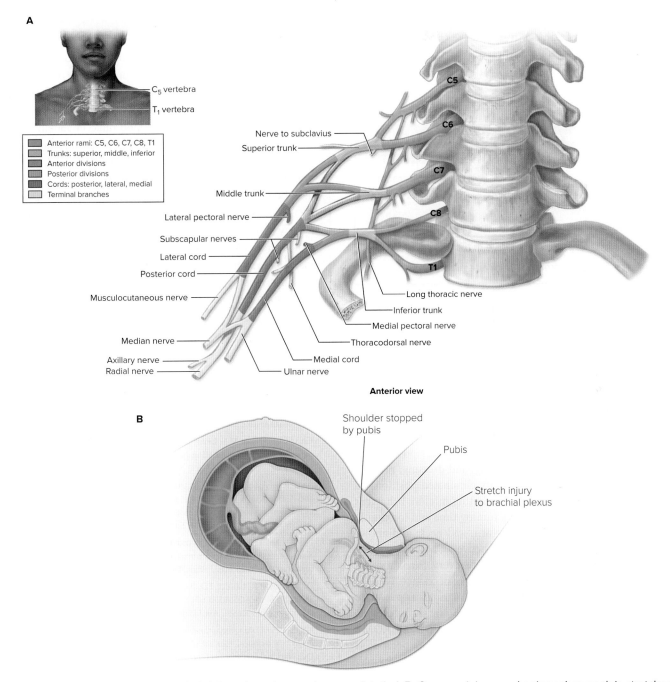

FIGURE 15-6 A. Brachial plexus with divisions, branches, and nerves detailed. **B.** Common injury mechanism when neck is stretched laterally to expel shoulder(s). (Part A: Reproduced with permission from McKinley M, O'Laughlin VD. *Human Anatomy* 3rd Edition. New York, NY: McGraw-Hill; 2012. Fig 16.9A, Pg. 498.)

CASE F, PART II

Jonathan demonstrates hypotonia of the left arm, especially at the shoulder and elbow (deltoids and biceps); when he's happy and kicking and moving his arms, he moves the left much less than the right. While he responds to tickling and pressure on his right arm and his left hand (except for the thumb), he does not respond to either on most of his left arm. He is diagnosed with Erb's Palsy (C5 and 6 brachial plexus injury).

Recovery

Spontaneous recovery happens in the majority of injuries to the brachial plexus. By 2 months of age, 60% of infants with brachial plexus injuries show no residual weakness, and at 4 months the percentage rises to 75% that spontaneously recover. The nerves may regrow or heal at 1 mm per day or 1 inch per month. Isolated elbow flexion, using the biceps, and spontaneous finger movement is a predictor of recovery at 3 months. After 4 months of age, only 4% of infants show any spontaneous recovery. Permanent damage remains in

10–18% of obstetric brachial plexus injuries, typically when there is more severe damage to the nerve (Box 15-5). These children will have residual weakness and permanent disability of the arm and hand.[242]

BOX 15-5	Types of Permanent Peripheral Nerve Injuries

Avulsion – Nerve root detached. Early surgery is recommended as the muscles are getting no nerve signal causing serious muscle wasting.

Axonotmesis – Nerve fiber injury, typically extensive

Neurotmesis – Ruptured/torn nerve in the middle

Scarring – Possible formation over a stretch or tear

Physical Therapy Intervention

Physical therapy for infants with a brachial plexus injury may begin immediately after the injury is identified, likely in the NICU, and continue when the infant goes home. First, a complete neurological examination should be completed to rule out central nervous system involvement and identify specific locations in the brachial plexus that are likely damaged. Intervention options include use of towels, rolls, and props for positioning; parent education for handling, bathing, and dressing; prevention of skin breakdown; using gravity eliminated positions to encourage some UE movement; promoting midline behaviors and avoiding neglect; encouraging tummy time and looking at both arms; avoiding stretch on the arm and neck; and allowing for rest and recovery. Passive and active ROM exercises will be prescribed after a period of rest and recovery. Facilitation of symmetry in fine and gross motor skills is necessary as there is some indication that infants with brachial plexus palsy are delayed in crawling, walking, and other motor skill development. Joint mobilization, common strengthening and ROMS exercises, taping, and electrical stimulation have all been used successfully in patients with brachial plexus injuries. Splints, casts, and Botox may be indicated for prevention of contractures. Recently, modified constraint induced movement therapy (CIMT), with the non-impaired arm restricted by a Velcro vest and repetitive movement training of the paretic arm, has been found to improve function in older children with brachial plexus palsy (see discussion in Chapters 10 – Stroke and 19 – Cerebral Palsy for details of CIMT therapy); it should be noted that this was a case series that also included botulinum toxin injections and that bracial plexus injuries are peripheral and all of the higher level evidence for CIMT is with central NS lesions and asymmetical CP.[243]

Surgical intervention is considered, if infants have not made spontaneous recovery in the first few months or for a known avulsion. For avulsion injuries and serious scarring, surgical interventions may be the only option. Surgical options include tendon, muscle, and nerve transfers; scar tissue removal (neurolysis), and nerve grafting.

CASE F, PART III

Jonathon's parents were instructed in a positioning program and passive range of motion to prevent loss of motion of the left arm. They were encouraged to stimulate reaching activities by (1) placing mobiles and toys on the left side of the crib; (2) placing a Velcro-strapped rattle in Jonathon's left hand to reinforce arm movement for short periods of time; and (3) encourganing midline movements and bilateral reaching and grasping by placing toys in midline on and above his chest. and (4) teaching cause and effect to link the movement of his left arm and hand to the movement of a toy (e.g. under direct supervision with a parent, attach a tether from his arm to an overhead mobile, for brief periods of time, so that arm movment makes the mobile move). By age 4 months, Jonathon's palsy had resolved, and he demonstrated full range of motion, typical antigravity movement, and equal use of his left arm in activities.

REFERENCES

1. Weiss L, Silver J, Weiss J. *Easy EMG*. 1st ed. Waltham, MA: Butterworth-Heinemann; June 10, 2004. ISBN 0750674318.

2. Cho SC, Ferrante MA, Levin KH, Harmon RL, So YT. Utility of electrodiagnostic testing in evaluating patients with lumbosacral radiculopathy: an evidence-based review. *Muscle Nerve*. 2010;42:276-282.

3. American Association of Electrodiagnostic Medicine (So YT, Weber CF, and Campbell WW). Practice parameter for needle electromyographic evaluation of patients with suspected cervical radiculopathy: summary statement. *Muscle Nerve*. 1999;22(suppl 8):S209-S211.

4. Dillingham TR, Lauder TD, Andary M, Kumar S, Pezzin LE, Stephens RT, Shannon S. Identifying lumbosacral radiculopathies: an optimal electromyographic screen. *Am J Phys Med Rehabil*. 2000;79(6):496-503.

5. Dillingham TR, Lauder TD, Andary M, Kumar S, Pezzin LE, Stephens RT, Shannon S. Identification of cervical radiculopathies: optimizing the electromyographic screen. *Am J Phys Med Rehabil*. 2001;80(2):84-91.

6. NIOSH. *Performing motor and sensory neuronal conduction studies in humans: a NIOSH technical manual (NIOSH) Publication No. 90-113*. Washington, DC: National Institute for Occupational Safety and Health; 1990.

7. AAEM (American Association of Electrodiagnostic Medicine Quality Assurance Committee, Campbell et al.). Practice parameter for electrodiagnostic studies in ulnar neuropathy at the elbow. *Neurology*. 1999;52:688.

8. American Association of Electrodiagnostic Medicine (Jablecki CK, Andary MT, Ball RD, Cherington M, Fisher MA, Phillips CH, So YT, Tulloch JW, Turk MA, Weichers DO, Wilbourn AJ, Wilkins DE, Williams FH, Ysla RGi.). Practice parameter for electrodiagnostic studies in carpal tunnel syndrome: summary statement. *Muscle Nerve*. 2002;25:918-922.

9. Marciniak C, Armon C, Wilson J, Miller R. Practice parameter: utility of electrodiagnostic techniques in evaluating patients with suspected peroneal neuropathy: an evidence based review. *Muscle Nerve*. 2005;31:520-527.

10. Patel AT, Gaines K, Malamut R, Park TA, Del Toro DR, Holland N. Usefulness of electrodiagnostic techniques in the evaluation of suspected tarsal tunnel syndrome: an evidence based review. *Muscle Nerve*. 2006;32:236-240.

11. AANEM. American Association of Neuromuscular and Diagnostic Medicine. Available at: http://www.aanem.org. Accessed March 29, 2015.

12. Barboi AC, Barkhaus PE. Electrodiagnostic testing in neuromuscular disorders. *Neurol Clin*. 2004;22(3):619-641.

13. Kraft GH. The electromyographer's guide to the motor unit. *Phys Med Rehabil Clin N Am*. 2007;8(4):711-732.

14. APTA (American Physical Therapy Association). Electrophysiologic Examination and Evaluation HOD P06-96-20-04. Available at: http://www.apta.org/uploadedFiles/APTAorg/About_Us/Policies/Practice/ElectrophysiologicExaminationEvaluation.pdf. Updated August 7, 2012. Accessed March 27, 2015.

15. De Carvalho M, Dengler R, Eisen A, et al. Electrodiagnostic criteria for diagnosis of ALS. *Clin Neurophysiol*. 2008;119:497-503.

16. Narayanaswami P, Weiss M, Selcen D, et al. Evidence-based guideline summary: diagnosis and treatment of limb-girdle and distal dystrophies. *Neurology*. 2014;83(16):1453-1463.

17. Fellows LK, Foster BJ, Chalk CH. Clinical significance of complex repetitive discharges: a case-control study. *Muscle Nerve*. 2003;28(4):504-507.

18. Amyotrophic Lateral Sclerosis Association. Available at: http://www.alsa.org/als-care/resources/publications-videos/factsheets/epidemiology.html. Accessed February 2, 2015.

19. Cronin S, Hardiman O, Traynor BJ. Ethnic variation in the incidence of ALS: a systematic review. *Neurology*. 2007;68:1002-1007.

20. Logroscino G, Traynor BJ, Hardiman O, et al., EURALS. Descriptive epidemiology of amyotrophic lateral sclerosis: new evidence and unsolved issues. *J Neurol Neurosurg Psychiatry*. 2008;79:6-11.

21. Horner RD, Kamins KG, Feussner JR, Grambow SC, Hoff-Lindquist J, Harati Y. Occurrence of amyotrophic lateral sclerosis among Gulf War veterans. *Neurology*. 2003;61:742-749.

22. Armon C. An evidence-based medicine approach to the evaluation of the role of exogenous risk factors in sporadic amyotrophic lateral sclerosis. *Neuroepidemiology*. 2003;22:217-228.

23. Armon C. Sports and trauma in amyotrophic lateral sclerosis revisited. *J Neurol Sci*. 2007;262:45-53.

24. Shaw PJ. Molecular and cellular pathways of neurodegeneration in motor neuron disease. *J Neurol Neurosurg Psychiatry*. 2005;76:1046-1057.

25. Rossi FH, Franco MC, Estevez AG. Pathophysiology of amyotrophic lateral sclerosis. In: Estévez AG, ed. *Current Advances in Amyotrophic Lateral Sclerosis*. 2013. doi:10.5772/56562.

26. Robberecht W, Philips T. The changing scene of amyotrophic lateral sclerosis. *Nat Rev Neurosci*. 2013;14(4):248-264.

27. Ekestern E. Neurotrophic factors and amyotrophic lateral sclerosis. *Neurodegener Dis*. 2004;1:88-100.

28. Shaw PJ, Eggett CJ. Molecular factors underlying selective vulnerability of motor neurons to neurodegeneration in amyotrophic lateral sclerosis. *J Neurol*. 2000;247(suppl 1):117-127.

29. Fischer LR, Lindsey R, Culver DG, Davis AA, Wang M, Castellano-Sanchez A. Amyotrophic lateral sclerosis is a distal axonopathy: evidence in mice and men. *Exp Neurol*. 2004;185:232-240.

30. Attarian S, Vedel J-P, Pouget J, Schmied A. Progression of cortical and spinal dysfunction over time in amyotrophic lateral sclerosis. *Muscle Nerve*. 2008;37:364-375.

31. Pugdahl K, Fuglsang-Frederiksen A, de Carvalho M, et al. Generalised sensory system abnormalities in amyotrophic lateral sclerosis: a European multicentre study. *J Neurol Neurosurg Psychiatry*. 2007;78(7):746-749.

32. Lulé D, Diekmann V, Müller HP, Kassubek J, Ludolph AC, Birbaumer N. Neuroimaging of multimodal sensory stimulation in amyotrophic lateral sclerosis. *J Neurol Neurosurg Psychiatry*. 2010;81(8):899-906.

33. Brooks BR. Natural history of ALS: symptoms, strength, pulmonary function, and disability. *Neurology*. 1996;47(suppl 2):S71-S81.

34. Brooks BR, Miller RG, Swash M, Munsat TL. El Escorial revisited: revised criteria for the diagnosis of amyotrophic lateral sclerosis. *Amyotroph Lateral Scler Other Motor Neuron Disord*. 2000;1:292-299.

35. Sanaya K, Douglas A. Neuroimaging in amyotrophic lateral sclerosis. *Amyotroph Lateral Scler Other Motor Neuron Disord*. 2003;4:243-248.

36. Neary D, Snowden JS, Gustafson L, et al. Frontotemporal lobar degeneration: a consensus on clinical diagnostic criteria. *Neurology*. 1998;51:1546-1554.

37. Kaji R, Izumi Y, Adachi Y, Kuzuhara S. ALS-parkinsonism-dementia complex of Kii and other related diseases in Japan. *Parkinsonism Relat Disord*. 2012;18(suppl 1):S190-S191.

38. Murphy J, Henry R, Lomen-Hoerth C. Establishing subtypes of the continuum of frontal lobe impairment in amyotrophic lateral sclerosis. *Arch Neurol*. 2007;64:330-334.

39. Abrahams S, Leigh PN, Goldstein LH. Cognitive change in ALS: a prospective study. *Neurology*. 2005;64:1222-1226.

40. Gibbons ZC, Richardson A, Neary D, Snowden JS. Behaviour in amyotrophic lateral sclerosis. *Amyotroph Lateral Scler*. 2008;9:67-74.

41. Witgert M, Salamone AR, Strutt AM, et al. Frontal-lobe mediated behavioural dysfunction in amyotrophic lateral sclerosis. *Eur J Neurol*. 2010;17:103-110.

42. Mackenzie IRA, Bigio EH, Ince PG, et al. Pathological TDP-43 distinguishes sporadic lateral sclerosis from amyotrophic lateral sclerosis with SOD1 mutations. *Ann Neurol*. 2007;61:427-434.

43. Czaplinski A, Yen AA, Appel SH. Forced vital capacity (FVC) as an indicator of survival and disease progression in an ALS clinic population. *J Neurol Neurosurg Psychiatry*. 2006a;77:390-392.

44. Magnus T, Beck M, Giess R, Puls I, Naumann M, Toyka KV. Disease progression in amyotrophic lateral sclerosis: predictors of survival. *Muscle Nerve*. 2002;25:709-714.

45. Mandioli J, Faglioni P, Nichelli P, Sola P. Amyotrophic lateral sclerosis: prognostic indicators of survival. *Amyotroph Lateral Scler*. 2006;7:217-220.

46. Traynor BJ, Alexander M, Corr B, Frost E, Hardiman O. Effect of a multidisciplinary amyotrophic lateral sclerosis (ALS) clinic on ALS survival: A population based study, 1996-2000 *J Neurol Neurosurg Psychiatry*. 2003;74:1258-1261.

47. Chiò A, Bottacchi E, Buffa C, Mutani R, Mora G, the PARALS. Positive effects of tertiary centres for amyotrophic lateral sclerosis on outcome and use of hospital facilities. *J Neurol Neurosurg Psychiatry*. 2006;77:948-950.

48. Miller RG, Mitchell JD, Lyon M, Moore DH. Riluzole for amyotrophic lateral sclerosis (ALS)/motor neuron disease (MND). *Cochrane Database Syst Rev*. 2007;1:CD001447.

49. Leigh PN, Abrahams S, Al-Chalabi A, et al., King's MND Care and Research Team. The management of motor neuron disease. *J Neurol Neurosurg Psychiatry*. 2003;74(suppl IV):iv32-iv47.

50. Radunovic A, Mitsumoto H, Leigh PN. Clinical care of patients with amyotrophic lateral sclerosis. *Lancet Neurol*. 2007;6:913-925.

51. Miller RG, Jackson CE, Kasarskis EJ, et al., Quality Standards Subcommittee of the American Academy of Neurology. Practice parameter update: the care of the patient with amyotrophic lateral sclerosis: drug, nutritional, and respiratory therapies (an evidence-based review): report of the Quality Standards Subcommittee of the American Academy of Neurology. *Neurology*. 2009a;73(15):1218–1226.

52. Miller RG, Jackson CE, Kasarskis EJ, et al., Quality Standards Subcommittee of the American Academy of Neurology. Practice parameter update: the care of the patient with amyotrophic lateral sclerosis: multidisciplinary care, symptom management, and cognitive/behavioral impairment (an evidence-based review): report of the Quality Standards Subcommittee of the American Academy of Neurology. *Neurology*. 2009b;73(15):1227–1233.

53. EFNS Task Force on Diagnosis and Management of Amyotrophic Lateral Sclerosis, Andersen PM, Abrahams S, Borasio GD, et al. EFNS guidelines on the clinical management of amyotrophic lateral sclerosis (MALS) – revised report of an EFNS task force. *Eur J Neurol*. 2012;19(3):360–375.

54. Kleopa KA, Sherman M, Neal B, Romano GJ, Heiman-Patterson T. BiPAP improves survival and rate of pulmonary function decline in patients with ALS. *J Neurol Sci*. 1999;164:82-88.

55. Bourke SC, Tomlinson M, Williams TL, Bullock RE, Shaw PJ, Gibson GJ. Effects of non-invasive ventilation on survival and quality of life in patients with amyotrophic lateral sclerosis: a randomised controlled trial. *Lancet Neurol*. 2006;5:140-147.

56. Lechtzin N, Scott Y, Busse AM, Clawson LL, Kimball R, Wiener CM. Early use of non-invasive ventilation prolongs survival in subjects with ALS. *Amyotroph Lateral Scler*. 2007;8:185-188.

57. Laub M, Midgren B. Survival of patients on home mechanical ventilation: a nationwide prospective study. *Respir Med.* 2007;101:1074-1078.

58. Hanayama K, Ishikawa Y, Bach JR. Amyotrophic lateral sclerosis. Successful treatment of mucous plugging by mechanical insufflation-exsufflation. *Am J Phys Med Rehabil.* 1997;76(4):338-339.

59. Bach JR. Amyotrophic lateral sclerosis: prolongation of life by noninvasive respiratory aids. *Chest.* 2002;122(1):92-98.

60. Brinkmann JR, Andres P, Mendoza M, Sanjak M. Guidelines for the use and performance of quantitative outcome measures in ALS clinical trials. *J Neurol Sci.* 1997;147:97-111.

61. Flaherty-Craig C, Brothers A, Dearman B, Eslinger P, Simmons Z. Penn State screen exam for the detection of frontal and temporal dysfunction syndromes: application to ALS. *Amyotroph Lateral Scler.* 2009;10(2):107-112.

62. Gordon PH, Wang Y, Doorish C, Lewis M, Battista V, Mitsumoto H, Marder K. A screening assessment of cognitive impairment in patients with ALS. *Amyotroph Lateral Scler.* 2007;8(6):362-365.

63. Woolley SC, York MK, Moore DH, Strutt AM, Murphy J, Schulz PE, Katz JS. Detecting frontotemporal dysfunction in ALS: utility of the ALS Cognitive Behavioral Screen (ALS-CBS). *Amyotroph Lateral Scler.* 2010;11(3):303-311.

64. Chen D, Guo X, Zheng Z, et al. Depression and anxiety in amyotrophic lateral sclerosis: correlations between the distress of patients and caregivers. *Muscle Nerve.* 2015;51(3):353-357.

65. Mitchell JD, Borasio GD. Amyotrophic lateral sclerosis. *Lancet.* 2007;369:2031-2041.

66. Oh H, Sin MK, Schepp KG, Choi-Kwon S. Depressive symptoms and functional impairment among amyotrophic lateral sclerosis patients in South Korea. *Rehabil Nurs.* 2012;37:136-144.

67. McElhiney MC, Rabkin JG, Gordon PH, Goetz R, Mitsumoto H. Prevalence of fatigue and depression in ALS patients and change over time. *J Neurol Neurosurg Psychiatry.* 2009;80:1146-1149.

68. Beck AT, Ward CH, Mendelson M, Mock J, Erbaugh J. An inventory for measuring depression. *Arch Gen Psychiatry.* 1961;4:561-571.

69. Radloff LS. The CES-D scale: a self-report depression scale for research in the general population. *Appl Psychol Meas.* 1977;1:385-401.

70. Zigmond AS, Snaith RP. The Hospital Anxiety and Depression Scale. *Acta Psychiatr Scand.* 1983;67:361-370.

71. Spielberger CS, Gorsuch RL, Lushene RE. *Manual for the State Trait Anxiety Inventory.* Palo Alto, CA: Consulting Psychologists Press; 1970.

72. Hedlund JL, Viewig BW. The Hamilton rating scale for depression: a comprehensive review. *J Oper Psychiatry.* 1979;10:149-165.

73. Hamilton M. The assessment of anxiety states by rating. *Br J Med Psychol.* 1959;32:50-55.

74. Kubler A, Winter S, Kaiser J, Birbaumer, N., Hautzinger, M. The ALS Depression Inventory (ADI): a questionnaire to measure depression in degenerative neurological diseases. *Z Klin Psychol Psychother.* 2005; 31:19-26.

75. Jette DU, Slavin MD, Andres PL, Munsat TL. The relationship of lower-limb muscle force to walking ability in patients with amyotrophic lateral sclerosis. *Phys Ther.* 1999;79:672-681.

76. Munsat TL, Andres P, Skerry L. Therapeutic trials in amyotrophic lateral sclerosis: measurement of clinical deficit. In: Rose C, ed. *Amyotrophic Lateral Sclerosis.* New York, NY: Demos Publications; 1990:65-76.

77. Great Lakes ALS Study Group. A comparison of muscle strength testing techniques in amyotrophic lateral sclerosis. *Neurology.* 2003;61:1503-1507.

78. Tiffin J. *Purdue Pegboard: Examiner manual.* Chicago, IL: Science Research Associates; 1968.

79. Desrosiers J, Hebert R, Bravo G, Dutil E. The Purdue Pegboard Test: normative data for people aged 60 and over. *Disabil Rehabil.* 1995;17:217-224.

80. Buddenberg LA, Davis C. Test-retest reliability of the Purdue Pegboard Test. *Am J Occup Ther.* 2000;54:555-558.

81. Bohannon RW, Smith MB. Interrater reliability of a modified Ashworth scale of muscle spasticity. *Phys Ther.* 1987;67:206-207.

82. Morgan RK, McNally S, Alexander M, Conroy R, Hardiman O, Costello RW. Use of sniff nasal-inspiratory force to predict survival in amyotrophic lateral sclerosis. *Am J Respir Crit Care Med.* 2005;171:269-274.

83. Czaplinski A, Yen AA, Appel SH. Amyotrophic lateral sclerosis: early predictors of prolonged survival. *J Neurol.* 2006b;253:1428-1436.

84. Schmidt EP, Drachman DB, Wiener CM, Clawson L, Kimball R, Lechtzin N. Pulmonary predictors of survival in amyotrophic lateral sclerosis: use in clinical trial design. *Muscle Nerve.* 2006;33:127-132.

85. Lou JS. Fatigue in amyotrophic lateral sclerosis. *Phys Med Rehabil N Am.* 2008;19(3):533-543.

86. Lui AJ, Byl NN. A systematic review of the effect of moderate intensity exercise on function and disease progression in amyotrophic lateral sclerosis. *J Neurol Phys Ther.* 2009;33(2):68-87.

87. Krupp LB, LaRocca NG, Muir-Nash J, Steinberg AD. The fatigue severity scale. Application to patients with multiple sclerosis and systemic lupus erythematosus. *Arch Neurol.* 1989;46(10):1121-1123.

88. Smets EM, Garssen B, Bonke B, De Haes JC. The Multidimensional Fatigue Inventory (MFI): psychometric qualities of an instrument to assess fatigue. *J Psychosom Res.* 1995;39(3):315-325.

89. Nardone A, Galante M, Lucas B, Schieppati M. Stance control is not affected by paresis and reflex hyperexcitability: the case of spastic patients. *J Neurol Neurosurg Psychiatry.* 2001;70(5):635-643.

90. Tinetti ME. Performance-oriented assessment of mobility problems in elderly patients. *J Am Geriatr Soc.* 1986;34:119-126.

91. Podsiadlo D, Richardson S. The timed "Up & Go": a test of basic functional mobility for frail elderly persons. *JAGS.* 1991;9:142-148.

92. Berg KO, Wood-Dauphinee SL, Williams JI, Maki B. Measuring balance in the elderly: validation of an instrument. *Can J Public Health.* 1992; 83(suppl 2):S7-S11.

93. Duncan PW, Weiner DK, Chandler J, Studenski S. Functional reach: a new clinical measure of balance. *J Gerontol.* 1990;45:M192-M197.

94. Kloos AD, Dal Bello-Haas V, Proch C, Mitsomoto H. Validity of the Tinetti Assessment Tool in individuals with ALS. In: *Proceedings of the 9th International Symposium on Amyotrophic Lateral Sclerosis/Motor Neuron Disease Conference.* Munich, Germany; 1998:149.

95. Kloos AD, Dal Bello-Haas V, Thome R. Cassidy J, Lewis L, Cusma T, Mitsumoto H. Interrater and intrarater reliability of the Tinetti Balance Test for individuals with amyotrophic lateral sclerosis. *J Neurol Phys Ther.* 2004;28(1):12-19.

96. Montes J, Cheng B, Diamond B, Doorish C, Mitsumoto H, Gordon PH. The Timed Up and Go Test: predicting falls in ALS. *Amyotroph Lateral Scler.* 2007;8:292-295.

97. Guide for the Uniform Data System for Medical Rehabilitation (Adult FIM™), version 4.0. Buffalo, NY: State University of New York at Buffalo; 1993.

98. Cedarbaum JM, Stambler N. Performance of the ALS Functional Rating Scale (ALSFRS) in multicenter clinical trials. *J Neurol Sci.* 1997;152(suppl):1-9.

99. Cedarbaum JM, Stambler N, Malta E, Fuller C, Hilt D, Thurmond B, Nakanishi A. The ALSFRS-R: A revised ALS Functional Rating Scale that incorporates assessments of respiratory function. BDNF ALS Study Group (Phase III). *J Neurol Sci.* 1999;169:13-21.

100. ALS Functional Rating Scale. Available at: http://www.outcomes-umassmed.org/ALS/alsscale.aspx. Accessed on March 30, 2015.

101. Kaufmann P, Levy G, Montes J, et al., QALS study group. Excellent inter-rater, intra-rater, and telephone-administered reliability of the ALSFRS-R in a multicenter clinical trial. *Amyotroph Lateral Scler.* 2007;8:42-46.

102. Appel V, Stewart SS, Smith G, Appel SH. A rating scale for amyotrophic lateral sclerosis: description and preliminary experience. *Ann Neurol.* 1987;22:328-333.

103. Hillel AD, Miller RM, Yorkston K, McDonald E, Norris FH, Konikow N. Amyotrophic Lateral Sclerosis Severity Scale. *Neuroepidemiology.* 1989;8:142-150.

104. Norris FH Jr, Calanchini PR, Fallat RJ, Panchari S, Jewett B. The administration of guanidine in amyotrophic lateral sclerosis. *Neurology.* 1974;24:721-728.

105. Schwab RS, England AC Jr. Projection techniques for evaluating surgery in Parkinson's disease. In: Gillingham J, Donaldson I, eds. *Third Symposium on Parkinson's Disease.* Edinburgh: Livingstone Ltd.; 1969:152-157.

105. The ALS CNTF Treatment Study (ACTS) Phase I-II Study Group. The amyotrophic lateral sclerosis functional rating scale: assessment of activities of daily living in patients with amyotrophic lateral sclerosis. *Arch Neurol.* 1996;53:141-147.

107. Ware JE Jr, Snow KK, Kosinski M. *SF-36(R) Health Survey: Manual and Interpretation Guide.* Lincoln, RI: QualityMetric Incorporated; 2000.

108. Hickey AM, Bury G, O'Boyle CA, Bradley F, O'Kelly FD, Shannon W. A new short form individual quality of life measure (SEIQoL-DW): application in a cohort of individuals with HIV/AIDS. *Br Med J.* 1996;313:29-33.

109. Bergner M, Bobbitt RA, Carter WB, Gilson BS. The Sickness Impact Profile: development and final revision of a health status measure. *Med Care.* 1981;19(8):787-805.

110. Jenkinson C, Fitzpatrick R, Brennan C, Bromberg M. Development and validation of a short measure of health status for individuals with amyotrophic lateral sclerosis/motor neuron disease: The ALSAQ-40. *J Neurol.* 1999a;246:16-21.

111. Jenkinson C, Fitzpatrick R, Brennan C, Swash M. Evidence for the validity and reliability of the ALS assessment questionnaire: the ALSAQ-40. *Amyotroph Lateral Scler Other Motor Neuron Disord.* 1999b;1:33-40.

112. Simmons Z, Felgoise SH, Bremer BA, et al. The ALSSQOL: balancing physical and nonphysical factors in assessing quality of life in ALS. *Neurology.* 2006;67:1659-1664.

113. Gołąb-Janowska M, Honczarenko K, Stankiewicz J. Usefulness of the ALSAQ-5 scale in evaluation of quality of life in amyotrophic lateral sclerosis. *Neurol Neurochir Pol.* 2010;44(6):560-566.

114. Jenkinson C, Fitzpatrick R. Reduced item set for the amyotrophic lateral sclerosis assessment questionnaire: development and validation of the ALSAQ-5. *J Neurol Neurosurg Psychiatry.* 2001;70:70-73.

115. Sinaki M, Mulder DW. Rehabilitation techniques for patients with amyotrophic lateral sclerosis. *Mayo Clin Proc.* 1978;53:173-178.

116. Chiò A, Benzi G, Dossena M, Mutani R, Mora G. Severely increased risk of amyotrophic lateral sclerosis among Italian professional football players. *Brain.* 2005;128:472-476.

117. Siciliano G, Pastorini E, Pasquali L, Manca ML, Iudice A, Murri L. Impaired oxidative metabolism in exercising muscle from ALS patients. *J Neurol Sci.* 2001;191(1-2):61-65.

118. Sanjak M, Paulson D, Sufit R, et al. Physiologic and metabolic response to progressive and prolonged exercise in amyotrophic lateral sclerosis. *Neurology.* 1987;37(7):1217-1220.

119. Longstreth WT, Nelson LM, Koepsell TD, van Belle G. Hypotheses to explain the association between vigorous physical activity and amyotrophic lateral sclerosis. *Med Hypotheses.* 1991;34(2):144-148.

120. Bennett RL, Knowlton GC. Overwork weakness in partially denervated skeletal muscle. *Clin Orthop.* 1958;12:22-29.

121. Reitsma W. Skeletal muscle hypertrophy after heavy exercise in rats with surgically reduced muscle function. *Am J Phys Med.* 1969;48:237-258.

122. Tam SL, Archibald V, Jassar B, Tyreman N, Gordon T. Increased neuromuscular activity reduces sprouting in partially denervated muscles. *J Neurosci.* 2001;21:654-667.

123. Tam SL, Archibald V, Tyreman N, Gordon T. Effect of exercise on stability of chronically enlarged motor units. *Muscle Nerve.* 2002;25:359-369.

124. LaStayo PC, Woolf JM, Lewek MD, Snyder-Mackler L, Reich T, Lindstedt SL. Eccentric muscle contractions: their contribution to injury, prevention, rehabilitation, and sport. *J Orthop Sports Phys Ther.* 2003;33(10):557-571.

125. Sharma KR, Kent-Braun JA, Majundars S, Huang Y, Mynhier M, Weiner MW, Miller RG. Physiology of fatigue in amyotrophic lateral sclerosis. *Neurology.* 1995;45:733-740.

126. Aboussouan LS. Mechanisms of exercise limitation and pulmonary rehabilitation for patients with neuromuscular disease. *Chron Respir Dis.* 2009;6:231-249.

127. Sanjak M, Bravver E, Bockenek WL, Norton J, Brooks BR. Supported treadmill ambulation for amyotrophic lateral sclerosis: a pilot study. *Arch Phys Med Rehabil.* 2010;91:1920-1929.

128. Aksu SK, Ayse Y, Yavuz T, Tan E. The effects of exercise therapy in amyotrophic lateral sclerosis. *Fizyoterapi Rehabilitasyon.* 2002;13:105-112.

129. Dal Bello-Haas V, Florence JM, Kloos AD, et al. A randomized controlled trial of resistance exercises in individuals with ALS. *Neurology.* 2007;68:2003-2007.

130. Drory VE, Goltsman E, Reznik JG, Mosek A, Korczyn AD. The value of muscle exercise in patients with amyotrophic lateral sclerosis. *J Neurol Sci.* 2001;191:133-137.

131. Pinto AC, Alves M, Nogueira A, et al. Can amyotrophic lateral sclerosis patients with respiratory insufficiency exercise? *J Neurol Sci.* 1999;169:69-75.

132. Mayadev AS, Weiss MD, Distad BJ, Krivickas LS, Carter GT. The amyotrophic lateral sclerosis center: a model of multidisciplinary management. *Phys Med Rehabil Clin N Am.* 2008;19:619-631.

133. Dal Bello-Haas V, Kloos AD, Mitsumoto H. Physical therapy for a patient through six stages of amyotrophic lateral sclerosis. *Phys Ther.* 1998;78:1312-1324.

134. Chen A, Montes J, Mitsumoto H. The role of exercise in amyotrophic lateral sclerosis. *Phys Med Rehabil Clin N Am.* 2008;19:545-557.

135. Dal Bello-Haas V. A framework for rehabilitation in degenerative diseases: planning care and maximizing quality of life. *Neurol Rep.* 2002;26(3):115-129.

136. de Almeida JP, Silvestre R, Pinto AC, de Carvalho M. Exercise and amyotrophic lateral sclerosis. *Neurol Sci.* 2012;33(1):9-15.

137. Dycem Non-slip products. Available at: www.dycem.com.

138. Kamide N, Asakawa T, Shibasaki N, et al. Identification of the type of exercise therapy that affects functioning in patients with early-stage amyotrophic lateral sclerosis: a multicenter, collaborative study. *Neurol Clinical Neurosci.* 2014;2:135-139.

139. Ingels PL, Rosenfeld J, Frick SL, Bryan WJ. Adhesive capsulitis: a common occurrence in patients with ALS. *Amyotroph Lateral Scler Other Motor Neuron Disord.* 2001;2(S2):60.

140. Gourie-Devi M, Nalini A, Sandhya S. Early or late appearance of "dropped head syndrome" in amyotrophic lateral sclerosis. *J Neurol Neurosurg Psychiatry.* 2003;74(5):683-686.

141. Philadelphia Cervical Collar Co., Thorofare, NJ 08086.

142. Miami-J Collar. Available from Jerome Medical, Moorestown, NJ 8057-3239.

143. Malibu Collar. Available from Seattle Systems, Poulsbo WA 98370.

144. Headmaster Collar. Available at symmetric Designs LTD, Salt Spring Island, BC, Canada ViK 1C9.

145. Cheah BC, Boland RA, Brodaty NE, Zoing MC, Jeffery SE, McKenzie DK, Kiernan MC. INSPIRATIonAL--INSPIRAtory muscle training in amyotrophic lateral sclerosis. *Amyotroph Lateral Scler.* 2009;10:384-392.

146. Pinto S, Swash M, de Carvalho M. Respiratory exercise in amyotrophic lateral sclerosis. *Amyotroph Lateral Scler.* 2012;13(1):33-43.

147. Hoyer Lift. Available from Sunrise Medical, Longmont, CO 80503.

148. Trail M, Nelson N, Van JN, Appel SH, Lai EC. Wheelchair use by patients with amyotrophic lateral sclerosis: a survey of user characteristics and selection preferences. *Arch Phys Med Rehabil.* 2001;82(1):98-102.

149. Purtilo R, Haddad A. *Health professional and patient interaction.* 7th ed. Philadelphia, PA: WB Saunders; 2007.

150. Center for Disease Control and Prevention. Available at: http://www.cdc.gov/h1n1flu/vaccination/gbs_qa.htm. Accessed February 28, 2015.

151. Sejvar JJ, Baughman AL, Wise M, Morgan OW. Population incidence of Guillain-Barré syndrome: a systematic review and meta-analysis. *Neuroepidemiology.* 2011;36:123-133.

152. Walling AD, Dickson G. Guillain-Barré syndrome. *Am Fam Physician.* 2013;87(3):191-197.

153. Rinaldi S. Update on Guillain-Barré syndrome. *J Peripher Nerv Syst.* 2013;18(2):99-112.

154. Uncini A, Kuwabara S. Electrodiagnostic criteria for Guillain-Barrè syndrome: a critical revision and the need for an update. *Clin Neurophysiol.* 2012;123(8):1487-1495.

155. Wakerley BR, Yuki N. Pharyngeal-cervical-brachial variant of Guillain-Barre syndrome. *J Neurol Neurosurg Psychiatry.* 2014;85(3):339-344.

156. Yuki N, Hartung H-P. Guillain-Barre syndrome. *N Engl J Med.* 2012; 366(24):2294-2304.

157. Kuitwaard K, van Koningsveld R, Ruts L, Jacobs BC, van Doorn PA. Recurrent Guillain-Barré syndrome. *J Neurol Neurosurg Psychiatry.* 2009;80:56-59.

158. Bassile CC. Guillain-Barré syndrome and exercise guidelines. *Neurol Rep.* 1996;20(2):198-203.

159. Rajabally YA, Uncini A. Outcome and its predictors in Guillain-Barré syndrome. *J Neurol Neurosurg Psychiatry.* 2012;83:711-718.

160. Ruts L, Drenthen J, Jongen JL, et al., Dutch GBS Study Group. Pain in Guillain-Barré syndrome: a long-term follow-up study. *Neurology.* 2010;75:1439-1447.

161. de Vries JM, Hagemanns MLC, Bussmann JBJ, van der Ploeg AT, van Doorn PA. Fatigue in neuromuscular disorders: focus on Guillain-Barré and Pompe disease. *Cell Mol Life Sci.* 2010;67(5):701-713.

162. Bernsen RA, Jager AE, Schmitz PI, van der Meché FG. Long-term sensory deficit after Guillain-Barré syndrome. *J Neurol.* 2001;248:483-486.

163. Walgaard C, Lingsma HF, Ruts L, et al. Prediction of respiratory insufficiency in Guillain-Barre syndrome. *Ann Neurol.* 2010;67:781-787.

164. Walgaard C, Lingsma HF, Ruts L, van Doorn PA, Steyerberg EW, Jacobs BC. Early recognition of poor prognosis in Guillain-Barre syndrome. *Neurology.* 2011;76:968-975.

165. Hughes RA, Wijdicks EF, Barohn R, et al. Practice parameter: immunotherapyfor Guillain-Barré syndrome: report of the Quality Standards Subcommittee of the American Academy of Neurology. *Neurology.* 2003;61(6):736-740.

166. Raphaël JC, Chevret S, Hughes RA, Annane D. Plasma exchange for Guillain-Barré syndrome. *Cochrane Database Syst Rev.* 2012;7:CD001798.

167. The French Cooperative Group on Plasma Exchange in Guillain-Barré Syndrome. Appropriate number of plasma exchanges in Guillain-Barré syndrome. *Ann Neurol.* 1997;41:298-306.

168. Plasma Exchange/Sandoglobulin Guillain-Barré Syndrome Trial Group. Randomised trial of plasma exchange, intravenous immunoglobulin, and combined treatments in Guillain-Barré syndrome. *Lancet.* 1997;349:225-230.

169. Hughes RA, Swan AV, van Doorn PA. Intravenous immunoglobulin for Guillain-Barré syndrome. *Cochrane Database Syst Rev.* 2014; 19(9):CD002063.

170. Forsberg A, Press R, Einarsson U, de Pedro-Cuesta J, Widén Holmqvist L, Swedish Epidemiological Study Group. Impairment in Guillain-Barré syndrome during the first 2 years after onset: a prospective study. *J Neurol Sci.* 2004;227:131-138.

171. Whitney S L, Wrisley DM., Marchetti GF, Gee MA, Redfern MS, Furman JM. Clinical measurement of sit-to-stand performance in people with balance disorders: validity of data for the Five-Times-Sit-to-Stand Test. *Phys Ther.* 2005;85(10):1034-1045.

172. Nordon-Craft A, Moss M, Quan D, Schenkman M. Intensive care unit-acquired weakness: implications for physical therapist management. *Phys Ther.* 2012;92(12):1494-1506.

173. Merkies IS, Schmitz PI, van der Meché FG, Samijn JP, van Doorn PA, Inflammatory Neuropathy Cause and Treatment (INCAT) group. Clinimetric evaluation of a new overall disability scale in immune mediated polyneuropathies. *J Neurol Neurosurg Psychiatry.* 2002;72(5):596-601.

174. Fokke C, van den Berg B, Drenthen J, Walgaard C, van Doorn PA, Jacobs BC. Diagnosis of Guillain-Barré syndrome and validation of Brighton criteria. *Brain.* 2014;137:33-43.

175. Hughes RA, Newsom-Davis JM, Perkin GD, Pierce JM. Controlled trial prednisolone in acute polyneuropathy. *Lancet.* 1978;2:750-753.

176. van Swieten, JC, Koudstaal, PJ, Visser, MC, Schouten, HJ, van Gijn, J. Interobserver agreement for the assessment of handicap in stroke patients. *Stroke.* 1988;19:604-607.

177. Orlikowski D, Prigent H, Sharshar T, Lofaso F, Raphael JC. Respiratory dysfunction in Guillain-Barré Syndrome. *Neurocrit Care.* 2004;1(4):415-422.

178. Lawn ND, Fletcher DD, Henderson RD, Wolter TD, Wijdicks EF. Anticipating mechanical ventilation in Guillain-Barre syndrome. *Arch Neurol.* 2001;58:893-898.

179. Féasson L, Camdessanché JP, El Mandhi L, Calmels P, Millet GY. Fatigue and neuromuscular diseases. *Ann Readapt Med Phys.* 2006;49:375-384.

180. Merkies I, Schmitz P, Van Der Meché F, Van Doorn P, for the Inflammatory Neuropathy Cause and Treatment (INCAT) group. Psychometric evaluation of a new sensory scale in immune-mediated polyneuropathies. *Neurology.* 2000;54:943-949.

181. Khan F, Amatya B. Rehabilitation interventions in patients with acute demyelinating inflammatory polyneuropathy: a systematic review. *Eur J Phys Rehabil Med.* 2012;48(3):507-522.

182. Khan F, Ng L, Amatya B, Brand C, Turner-Stokes L. Multidisciplinary care for Guillain-Barre syndrome. *Cochrane Database Syst Rev.* 2010;10:CD008505.

183. Khan F, Pallant JF, Amatya B, Ng L, Gorelik A, Brand C. Outcomes of high- and low-intensity rehabilitation programme for persons in chronic phase after Guillain-Barré syndrome: a randomized controlled trial. *J Rehabil Med.* 2011;43(7):638-646.

184. McCarthy JA, Zigenfus RW. Transcutaneous electrical nerve stimulation: an adjunct in the pain management of Guillain-Barré syndrome. *Phys Ther.* 1978;58(1):23-24.

185. Gersh MR, Wolf SL, Rao VR. Evaluation of transcutaneous electrical nerve stimulation for pain relief in peripheral neuropathy. *Phys Ther.* 1980;60(1):48-52.

186. Mullings KR, Alleva JT, Hudgins TH. Rehabilitation of Guillain-Barré syndrome. *Dis Mon.* 2010;56(5):288-292.

187. Herbison GJ, Jaweed MM, Ditunno JF Jr. Exercise therapies in peripheral neuropathies. *Arch Phys Med Rehabil.* 1983;64(5):201-205.

188. Bensman A. Strenuous exercise may impair muscle function in Guillain-Barré patients. *JAMA.* 1970;214:468-469.

189. Vajsar J, Fehlings D, Stephens D. Long-term outcome in children with Guillain-Barré syndrome. *J Pediatr.* 2003;142(3):305-309.

190. Pitetti KH, Barrett PJ, Abbas D. Endurance exercise training in Guillain-Barre syndrome. *Arch Phys Med Rehabil.* 1993;74(7):761-765.

191. Garssen MP, Bussmann JB, Schmitz PI, et al. Physical training and fatigue, fitness, and quality of life in Guillain-Barré syndrome and CIDP. *Neurology.* 2004;63(12):2393-2395.

192. Tuckey J, Greenwood R. Rehabilitation after severe Guillain-Barré syndrome: the use of partial body weight support. *Physiother Res Int.* 2004;9(2):96-103.

193. Simmons S. Guillain-Barré syndrome: a nursing nightmare that usually ends well. *Nursing.* 2010;40:24-29.

194. Bernsen RA, de Jager AE, Schmitz PI, van der Meché FG. Long-term impact on work and private life after Guillain-Barré syndrome. *J Neurol Sci.* 2002;201:13-17.

195. World Health Organization. Does polio still exist? Is it curable? Available at: http://www.who.int/features/qa/07/en. Accessed February 24, 2015.

196. Bruno RL, Sapolsky R, Zimmerman JR, Frick NM. Pathophysiology of a central cause of post-polio fatigue. *Ann N Y Acad Sci.* 1995;753:257-275.

197. McDonald-Williams MF. Exercise and postpolio. *Neurol Rep.* 1996;20(2):31-36.

198. Tiffreau V, Rapin A, Serafi R, Percebois-Macadré L, Supper C, Jolly D, Boyer FC. Post-polio syndrome and rehabilitation. *Ann Phys Rehabil Med.* 2010;53(1):42-50.

199. Berlly MH, Strauser WW, Hall KM. Fatigue in postpolio syndrome. *Arch Phys Med Rehabil.* 1991;72:115-118.

200. Halstead L. Assessment and differential diagnosis for post-polio syndrome. *Orthopedics.* 1991;14:1209-1217.

201. Jubelt B, Agre JC. Characteristics and management of postpolio syndrome. *JAMA.* 2000;284:412-414.

202. Rodriquez AA, Agre JC. Electrophysiological study of the quadriceps muscles during fatiguing exercise and recovery: a comparison of symptomatic and asymptomatic postpolio patients and controls. *Arch Phys Med Rehabil.* 1991;72:993-997.

203. Peach PE. Overwork weakness with evidence of muscle damage in a patient with residual paralysis from polio. *Arch Phys Med Rehabil.* 1990;71:248-250.

204. Lord S, Allen G, Williams P, Gandevia S. Risk of falling: predictors based on reduced strength in persons previously affected by polio. *Arch Phys Med Rehabil.* 2002;83:757-763.

205. Gonzalez H, Olsson T, Borg K. Management of postpolio syndrome. *Lancet Neurol.* 2010;9:634-642.

206. Smith L, McDermott K. Pain in post-poliomyelitis: addressing causes versus effects. In: Halstead L, Wiechers D, eds. *Research and Clinical Aspects of the Late Effects of Poliomyelitis.* White Plains, NY: March of Dimes Birth Defect Foundation. *Birth Defects Orig Artic Ser.* 1987;23(4):121–134.

207. Perry J, Burnfield JM. *Gait Analysis: Normal and Abnormal Function.* 2nd ed. Thorofare, NJ: Slack; 2010.

208. Farbu E, Gilhus NE, Barnes MP, Borg K, de Visser M, Driessen A, Howard R, Nollet F, Opara J, Stalberg E. EFNS guideline on diagnosis and management of post-polio syndrome. Report of an EFNS task force. *Eur J Neurol.* 2006;13:795-801.

209. Boyer FC, Tiffreau V, Rapin A, et al. Post-polio syndrome: pathophysiological hypotheses, diagnosis criteria, medication therapeutics. *Annal Phys Rehabil Med.* 2010;53:34-41.

210. Sandberg A, Stalberg E. Changes in macro electromyography over time in patients with a history of polio: a comparison of two muscles. *Arch Phys Med Rehabil.* 2004;85:1174-1182.

211. Skough K, Krossén C, Heiwe S, Theorell H, Borg K. Effects of resistance training in combination with coenzyme Q10 supplementation in patients with post-polio: a pilot study. *J Rehabil Med.* 2008;40(9):773-775.

212. Oncu J, Durmaz B, Karapolat H. Short-term effects of aerobic exercise on functional capacity, fatigue, and quality of life in patients with post-polio syndrome. *Clin Rehabil.* 2009;23(2):155-163.

213. Halstead LS, Gawne AC, Pham BT. National rehabilitation hospital limb classification for exercise, research, and clinical trials in post-polio patients. *Ann N Y Acad Sci.* 1995;753:343-353.

214. Bruno RL, Frick NM. The psychology of polio as prelude to post polio syndrome: behavior modification and psychotherapy. *Orthopedics.* 1991;14:1185-1193.

215. Said G. Diabetic neuropathy. *Handb Clin Neurol.* 2013;115:579-589.

216. Deli G, Bosnyak E, Pusch G, Komoly S, Feher G. Diabetic neuropathies: diagnosis and management. *Neuroendocrinology.* 2013;98(4):267-280.

217. Campbell WW. Evaluation and management of peripheral nerve injury. *Clin Neurophysiol.* 2008;119:1951-1965.

218. Seddon HJ. A classification of nerve injuries. *Br Med J.* 1942;27(12):237-239.

219. Lee SK, Wolfe SW. Peripheral nerve injury and repair. *J Am Acad Orthop Surg.* 2000;8(4):243-252.

220. Medical Research Council: Aids to the Investigation of Peripheral Nerve Injuries. London: Her Majesty's Stationary Office; 1943, revised, 1976.

221. Griffin JW, Hogan MV, Chhabra AB, Deal DN. Peripheral nerve repair and reconstruction. *J Bone Joint Surg Am.* 2013;95(23):2144-2151.

222. Rosenfield J, Paksima N. Peripheral nerve injuries and repair in the upper extremity. *Hop Joint Dis Bulletin.* 2002;60(3&4):155-161.

223. Albers JW, Pop-Busui R. Diabetic neuropathy: mechanisms, emerging treatments, and subtypes. *Curr Neuro Neurosci Rep.* 2014;473. doi:10.1007/s11910-0473-5.

224. Sharma KR, Cross J, Farronay O, Ayyar DR, Shebert RT, Bradley WG. Demyelinating neuropathy in diabetes mellitus. *Arch Neurol.* 2002;59(5):758-765.

225. Stables CL, Glasser RL, Feldman EL. Diabetic cardiac autonomic neuropathy: insights from animal models. *Auton Neurosci.* 2013;177(2):74-80.

226. Banthia S, Bergner DW, Chicos AB, et al. Detection of cardiovascular autonomic neuropathy using exercise testing in patients with type 2 diabetes mellitus. *J Diabetes Complications.* 2013;27(1):64-69.

227. Philips JC, Scheen AJ. Squatting test: a posture to study and counteract cardiovascular abnormalities associated with autonomic dysfunction. *Auton Neurosci.* 2011;162(1-2):3-9.

228. Mostarda CT, Rodrigues B, de Moraes OA, et al. Low intensity resistance training improves systolic function and cardiovascular autonomic control in diabetic rats. *J Diabetes Complications.* 2014;28(3):273-278.

229. Voulgari C, Pagoni S, Vinik A, Poirier P. Exercise improves cardiac autonomic function in obesity and diabetes. *Metabolism.* 2013;62(5):609-621.

230. Shankarappa SA, Piedras-Rentería ES, Stubbs EB Jr. Forced-exercise delays neuropathic pain in experimental diabetes: effects on voltage-activated calcium channels. *J Neurochem.* 2011;118(2):224-236.

231. Selagzi H, Buyukakilli B, Cimen B, Yilmaz N, Erdogan S. Protective and therapeutic effects of swimming exercise training on diabetic peripheral neuropathy of streptozotocin-induced diabetic rats. *J Endocrinol Investig.* 2008;31(11):971-978.

232. Akyuz G, Kenis O. Physical therapy modalities and rehabilitation techniques in the management of neuropathic pain. *Am J Phys Med Rehabil.* 2014;93:253-259.

233. Streckmann F, Zopf EM, Lehmann HC, et al. Exercise intervention studies in patients with peripheral neuropathy: a systematic review. *Sports Med.* 2014;44(9):1289-1304.

234. Song CH, Petrofsky JS, Lee SW, Lee KJ, Yim JE. Effects of an exercise program on balance and trunk proprioception in older adults with diabetic neuropathies. *Diabetes Tech Ther.* 2011;13:803-811.

235. Nardone A, Godi M, Artuso A, Schieppati M. Balance rehabilitation by moving platform and exercises in patients with neuropathy or vestibular deficit. *Arch Phys Med Rehabil.* 2010;91(12):1869-1877.

236. Mueller MJ, Tuttle LJ, LeMaster JW, Strube MJ. Weight-bearing versus nonweight-bearing exercise for persons with diabetes and peripheral neuropathy: a randomized controlled trial. *Arch Phys Med Rehabil.* 2013;94(5):829-838.

237. Ruhland JL, Shields RK. The effects of a home exercise program on impairment and health-related quality of life in persons with chronic peripheral neuropathies. *Phys Ther.* 1997;77:1026-1039.

238. Balducci S, Iacobellis G, Parisi L, Di Biase N, Calandriello E, Leonetti F, Fallucca F. Exercise training can modify the natural history of diabetic peripheral neuropathy. *J Diabetes Complications.* 2006;20:216-223.

239. Gigo-Benato D, Russo TL, Geuna S, Domingues NR, Salvini TF, Parizotto NA. Electrical stimulation impairs early functional recovery and accentuates skeletal muscle atrophy after sciatic nerve crush injury in rats. *Muscle Nerve.* 2010;41(5):685-693.

240. Ohtake PJ, Zafron ML, Poranki LG, Fish DR. Does electrical stimulation improve motor recovery in patients with idiopathic facial (Bell) palsy? *Phys Ther.* 2006;86(11):1558-1564.

241. Chauhan SP, Blackwell SB, Ananth CV. Neonatal brachial plexus palsy: incidence, prevalence, and temporal trends. *Semin Perinatol.* 2014;38(4):210-218.

242. Yang LJ. Neonatal brachial plexus palsy – management and prognostic factors. *Semin Perinatol.* 2014;38:222-234.

243. Santamato A, Panza F, Ranieri M, Fiore P. Effect of botulinum toxin type A and modified constraint-induced movement therapy on motor function of upper limb in children with obstetrical brachial plexus palsy. *Childs Nerv Syst.* 2011;27:2187-2192.

Review Questions

1. If a sensory study shows prolonged latencies but a motor study on the same peripheral nerve is normal, what does this typically indicate?

    A. Mild axonal injury

    B. Mild myelin injury

    C. Moderate axonal injury

    D. Moderate myelin injury

2. In a needle EMG study, why is it important to study insertional activity?

    A. To find evidence of axonal injury

    B. To find evidence of myopathy

    C. To study the neuromuscular junction

    D. To study the nociceptors

3. What is the difference between H-reflex testing and F-wave testing?

    A. Only F-wave testing requires normal motor neuron and motor axon function

    B. Only H-reflex testing is useful for detecting radiculopathy

    C. Only F-wave testing requires an intact nerve plexus

    D. Only H-reflex testing requires normal sensory axons

4. Death from amyotrophic lateral sclerosis (ALS) from the time of diagnosis occurs on average in:

    A. 6–12 months

    B. 1–3 years

    C. 3–5 years

    D. 5–7 years

5. A variant of sporadic ALS that features spasticity with only slight weakness of the extremities due to dysfunction of the corticospinal tract without lower motor neuron involvement is:

    A. Primary lateral sclerosis

    B. Progressive bulbar palsy

    C. Pseudobulbar palsy

    D. Progressive muscular atrophy

6. Which of the following impairments is relatively rare in people with ALS?

    A. Sensory deficits

    B. Dysphagia

    C. Weakness/paralysis of spinal muscles

    D. Fatigue

Questions 7 and 8 refer to the following scenario:

Mary Thomas is a 40-year-old female with familial ALS. She reports she has always been active prior to her diagnosis, playing tennis on the weekends and walking a mile every day with her dog. Mary complains that her left (L) toes have been catching on the floor when she walks quickly and that she has occasional mild cramping in her calf muscles, L greater than R. Otherwise, she has no other complaints and is independent with all mobility and ADLs. On physical examination, you note L DF strength is 3/5. Bilateral quads and hamstring strength = 4/5; bilateral plantarflexor strength = 4+/5.

7. Your best exercise prescription for Mary would be:

    A. Passive ROM exercises for the L foot and ankle

    B. High-intensity walking program

    C. Instructing Mary to take frequent rests when walking longer distances

    D. A lower extremity strengthening program for the proximal muscles

    E. All of the above

8. Which of the following findings would indicate a need to modify Mary's exercise plan?

    A. A Grade of 2 when you reevaluate the muscle strength of her lower extremities

    B. Increased incidences of calf cramping after exercise

    C. Reports of increased fatigue the day after exercise

    D. Increased fasciculations in the lower extremities with exercise

    E. All of the above

9. The tests that are most commonly used to diagnose Guillain–Barré syndrome (GBS) are:

    A. Lumbar puncture, somatosensory evoked potentials, magnetic resonance imaging (MRI)

    B. Blood tests, electromyography (EMG), magnetic resonance imaging (MRI)

    C. Lumbar puncture, electromyography (EMG), magnetic resonance imaging (MRI)

    D. Lumbar puncture, electromyography (EMG), positron emission tomography (PET)

10. In relation to the various subtypes of GBS, the most frequent subtype occurring in North America and Europe, which accounts for 90% of all GBS cases in these regions is:

    A. Acute motor and sensory axonal neuropathy (AMSAN)

    B. Acute motor axonal neuropathy (AMAN)

    C. Acute inflammatory demyelinating polyradiculoneuropathy (AIDP)

    D. Miller Fisher syndrome

11. Which of the following types of GBS has the worst prognosis?

    A. Acute motor and sensory axonal neuropathy (AMSAN)

    B. Acute inflammatory demyelinating polyradiculoneuropathy (AIDP)

    C. Chronic inflammatory demyelinating polyradiculopathy (CIDP)

    D. Miller Fisher syndrome

12. **Acute inflammatory demyelinating polyradiculoneuropathy (AIDP) attacks what part of the peripheral nerve?**

    A. Basement membranes surrounding Schwann cells

    B. Schwann cells

    C. Nodes of Ranvier

    D. Myelin sheath

13. **Which of the following immunotherapies has not demonstrated efficacy in the treatment of GBS?**

    A. Corticosteroids

    B. Plasma exchange

    C. Intravenous immunoglobulin

    D. All of the above have demonstrated efficacy in treating GBS

14. **Which of the following prognostic factors are associated with the WORST prognosis with GBS?**

    A. Progression of symptoms ≥7 days; did not require assisted ventilation; poor upper extremity muscle strength

    B. Progression of symptoms ≥7 days; respiratory muscle involvement requiring assisted ventilation; decreased amplitude findings on nerve conduction studies

    C. Progression of symptoms <7 days; did not require assisted ventilation; poor upper extremity muscle strength

    D. Progression of symptoms in <7 days; respiratory muscle involvement requiring assisted ventilation; decreased amplitude findings on nerve conduction studies

15. **The most appropriate initial exercise progression for a patient recovering from GBS with limb muscle strength ranging between P+ (2+) to F− (3−/5) strength is:**

    A. Functional based exercise → light progressive resistive exercise → active range of motion

    B. Passive range of motion→ active range of motion gravity-eliminated → active range of motion against gravity

    C. Active range of motion against gravity → light progressive resistive exercise → functional-based exercise

    D. Active range of motion gravity-eliminated → active range of motion against gravity → light progressive resistive exercise

16. **Which form of neuropathy affects motor and sensory and leaves autonomic nerves intact?**

    A. Chronic inflammatory demyelinating polyradiculopathy

    B. Diabetic peripheral neuropathy

    C. Guillain–Barré

    D. Multifocal motor neuropathy

17. **Which classification of nerve injury by Sunderland involves disruption of the axon and endoneurium with the perineurium and epineurium being left intact?**

    A. 1st degree

    B. 2nd degree

    C. 3rd degree

    D. 4th degree

18. **Which nerve is the most common source for autografts?**

    A. Brachial

    B. Femoral

    C. Radial

    D. Sural

19. **Tinel's sign is when you:**

    A. Put the nerve on a stretch and the distal limb goes numb

    B. Tap over the nerve and there is tingling in its distribution

    C. Compress the nerve and there is tingling in its distribution

    D. Tap over the nerve and the limb forcefully flexes

20. **A therapy client who is using the stationary bike as part of his therapy completes 20 minutes of pedaling and his heart rate is elevated to 110 bpm. After 5 minutes his heart rate is still 110 bpm. This response indicates:**

    A. A possible myocardial infarction (MI)

    B. Enhanced parasympathetic activation

    C. Possible cardiac autonomic neuropathy

    D. Orthostatic hypotension

21. **An appropriate intervention for diabetic clients to prevent or slow neuropathy is:**

    A. Brisk walking for at least 8 hours a week for 8 weeks

    B. Brisk walking for at least 4 hours a week as a lifelong activity

    C. Resistance training of major muscle groups at least 3 times a week

    D. Daily electrical stimulation to involved muscles

22. **In individuals who have recovered from polio which of the following is a true statement regarding the neuromuscular unit?**

    A. Type I fibers are disproportionately impacted

    B. Remaining muscle fibers are unable to hypertrophy

    C. Single motor neurons may innervate up to 2000 fibers

    D. Anterior horn cells may recover and regenerate to reinnervate the muscle

23. **Postpolio syndrome is diagnosed based on which of the following criteria?**

    A. There is a new onset of problems within 10 years of original infection

    B. There is onset of weakness in previously unaffected muscles years after the original infection

    C. Blood tests show low levels of creatine kinase

    D. Muscle biopsy indicates long-term denervation with no signs of reinnervation

24. True or False: It is believed that overwork plays a role in postpolio syndrome

A. True

B. False

25. A client with postpolio syndrome comes to therapy with foot drop. She wishes to regain walking without the use of an AFO or with the least intrusive AFO possible. On testing the tibialis anterior is graded 1/5 or trace strength. A recommended therapy would be to:

A. Prescribe resistance strengthening for the tibialis anterior

B. Prescribe a rigid AFO and discourage active dorsiflexion

C. Implement strengthening of the extensor hallicus longus and extensor digitorum longus muscles to perform dorsiflexion

D. Use a maximal exercise protocol working muscles to failure

26. Principles for designing exercise programs for individuals who have postpolio syndrome include:

A. Working to the point of fatigue and mild muscle soreness

B. Strengthening exercises for muscles with fair or lower strength grades

C. High intensity, brief exercise

D. Rotating exercise types such as aerobic and strengthening

27. The name of brachial plexus injury with only C5 and C6 involvement is:

A. Erb's Palsy

B. Klumpke's Palsy

C. Smith's Palsy

D. Class II Palsy

28. Spontaneous recovery for obstetric brachial plexus injury occurs:

A. Rarely

B. After surgery

C. In a majority of cases

D. With hypotonia

Answers

1. B	2. A	3. D	4. C	5. A
6. A	7. D	8. E	9. C	10. C
11. A	12. D	13. A	14. D	15. D
16. A	17. C	18. D	19. B	20. C
21. B	22. C	23. B	24. A	25. C
26. D	27. A	28. C		

Vestibular/Cerebellar Disorders

16

Anne D. Kloos

CASE A, PART I

Mrs. O'Hara, a 55-year-old woman, is experiencing episodes of "dizziness," beginning 2 weeks ago. She reports that her initial episode of "dizziness" occurred while she was rolling over in bed from her right to left side, and she describes feeling as if "the room was spinning." The episode lasted for a few seconds and went away by keeping her head completely still. She had mild nausea but no vomiting. The "dizziness" returned when she attempted to get out of bed to go the bathroom, lessened once she was upright, and worsened when she went to lie back down in bed. Mrs. O'Hara also noted that, over the last 2 weeks, the spinning sensations occurred when she looked up to reach for something in a cupboard in her kitchen or when she looked down to put on her shoes. While sitting, she has no symptoms. She notes that her symptoms started after she slipped on a patch of ice that caused her to fall and hit her head.

ANATOMY AND PHYSIOLOGY OF THE VESTIBULAR SYSTEM

The anatomy and physiology of the vestibular system and its role in the control of eye movements (via the vestibulo-ocular reflex) and postural stability (via the vestibulospinal reflex) are discussed in Chapter 6.

DISORDERS OF THE VESTIBULAR SYSTEM

Disorders of the vestibular system are common, especially among the elderly. One large epidemiological study estimated that as many as 35% of adults aged 40 years or older in the United States (approximately 69 million Americans) have experienced some form of vestibular dysfunction[1] with up to 65% of individuals older than 60 years of age experiencing dizziness or loss of balance, often on a daily basis.[2] Elderly individuals with dizziness also report memory problems and anxiety more frequently than non-dizzy elderly, which negatively impacts their quality of life.[3]

Vestibular disorders can be categorized by their location into peripheral and central vestibular disorders. Peripheral vestibular disorders involve the inner ear vestibular structures and/or the vestibular nerve. Central vestibular disorders primarily result from damage to the vestibular nuclei, the cerebellum, and the brainstem, including vestibular pathways within the brainstem that mediate vestibular reflexes (i.e., vestibulo-ocular reflex [VOR] and the vestibulospinal reflex [VSR]).

Peripheral Vestibular Disorders

Based on the anatomy, pathophysiology, and signs and symptoms, peripheral vestibular disorders can be further divided into the following three types: (1) acute unilateral vestibular hypofunction with the main symptom of acute onset rotatory vertigo; (2) bilateral vestibular hypofunction with the main symptom of postural imbalance; and (3) recurrent pathological excitation or inhibition of the peripheral vestibular system with the main symptom of recurrent attacks of vertigo.[4]

Unilateral Vestibular Hypofunction

Unilateral vestibular hypofunction (UVH) is characterized by a reduction or loss of peripheral vestibular function and can be caused by viral or bacterial infections (e.g., vestibular neuritis or neuronitis, labyrinthitis), head trauma, vascular occlusion, and unilateral vestibulopathy, following surgical procedures (e.g., labyrinthectomy and acoustic neuroma resections). Individuals with UVH experience (1) acute onset of severe rotational **vertigo** (a sensation of spinning), (2) **spontaneous horizontal-rotatory nystagmus**, beating toward the unaffected ear, (3) slight **oscillopsia** (perception that visualized objects are oscillating), when turning the head quickly to the affected side, (4) postural instability with a tendency to fall toward the affected side, and (5) nausea and vomiting. The symptoms of vertigo and nystagmus are produced by an imbalance of the tonic firing rates of the left and right sides of the vestibular system. At rest, vestibular afferents and their corresponding vestibular nuclei typically have a tonic firing rate of approximately 70–100 spikes per second. Damage to the vestibular system that decreases function unilaterally creates an imbalance between the two sides that results in the brain's misperception that movement of the head has occurred (in the direction of the more neutrally active healthy ear) and triggers the vestibulo-ocular reflex (VOR) in a corrective response.[5] Vision may become blurred with quick head movements to the affected side due to an impaired VOR. Imbalance, especially with head turns, results from decreased activation of the vestibulospinal reflex (VSR) on the affected side. Thus, a person with left UVH may experience sensations of spinning in a clockwise direction (i.e., toward the healthy right ear), spontaneous horizontal right-beating nystagmus (slow phase VOR eye movement to the left followed by fast saccades to the right), and blurred vision and loss of balance to the left side with head rotations to the left. With acute vertigo, excessive autonomic nervous system activity causes nausea, vomiting, pallor, and perspiration. Resolution of vertigo and spontaneous nystagmus usually occurs within 3–7 days in lit environments, as the patient is able to suppress the nystagmus with visual fixation, but spontaneous nystagmus may always be present in the dark. Resolution of the dynamic VOR and postural instability usually is slower to recover and may take up to a year.[6]

Vestibular Neuritis/Labyrinthitis

Vestibular neuritis (also called vestibular neuronitis) is the second most common peripheral cause of vertigo. It mainly affects individuals between 30 and 60 years, with peak incidence for women in the fourth decade and for men in the sixth decade.[7] Infection of the vestibular nerve results in nerve degeneration that is usually unilateral but can be bilateral.[8] Onset is often preceded by a viral infection of the upper respiratory or gastrointestinal tracts. Patients present with complaints of sudden, prolonged, severe vertigo that is worsened by head movements, associated with spontaneous horizontal-rotatory nystagmus, beating toward the good ear, postural imbalance to the affected side, and nausea. Hearing usually remains intact. Symptoms improve over a period of 48–72 hours and gradually return to normal over 6 weeks.[7] However, patients may continue to experience oscillopsia and impaired balance when rapidly turning the head to the affected side. Initially, vestibular suppressants (e.g., dimenhydrinate, scopolamine), antiemetic, and antinausea medications may be administered, and the patient may be put on bed rest. Use of high-dose steroids (i.e., methylprednisone) has been shown to hasten recovery;[9] however, once the symptoms diminish, the patient should start to ambulate, and vestibular suppressants are stopped to promote CNS compensation. Individuals with residual gaze instability and balance impairments may benefit from physical therapy.

Labyrinthitis is an inflammatory disorder of the membranous labyrinth, typically caused by viral and bacterial infections. The condition affects individuals of all ages, but viral labyrinthitis usually occurs in adults in their fourth to seventh decades of life.[8] The inflammation damages the vestibular and cochlear end organs, resulting in vestibular symptoms (vertigo, nystagmus, postural imbalance, nausea similar to vestibular neuritis) along with tinnitus (ringing in the ears) and/or hearing loss. Medical treatment aims to eliminate the infection and alleviate symptoms. As with vestibular neuritis, patients may experience chronic residual impairments that would benefit from physical therapy.

Vestibular Schwannoma (Acoustic Neuroma)

Vestibular schwannomas (VSs), historically called **acoustic neuromas**, are the most common intracranial tumors producing vestibular symptoms (Figure 16-1).[8] They are usually slow-growing, benign tumors that originate from the Schwann cells, lining the vestibular portion of the eighth cranial nerve, often within the internal auditory canal (IAC). The IAC also contains the facial nerve (cranial nerve VII). Early in the disease, when the tumor is small, patients may complain of vertigo, disequilibrium, tinnitus, and asymmetric hearing loss due to compression of the vestibulocochlear nerve. The slow growth of the tumor often allows for the brain to compensate, thereby, alleviating symptoms (see Figure 16-1). With continued growth, the tumor can compress the facial nerve within the IAC or the trigeminal nerve (cranial nerve V) at its root or ganglion, causing facial weakness and numbness, respectively. Eventually, the tumor grows to a size where it compresses the brainstem and cerebellum, causing difficulty in swallowing, impaired eye movements, gait ataxia, and possibly death. Treatment includes surgical excision and stereotactic radiation therapy (e.g., gamma knife).[8] With tumor removal, there is loss of vestibular nerve function, resulting in asymmetrical vestibular inputs. Ideally, physical therapy is started in the postoperative period to help relieve disequilibrium and oscillopsia symptoms, followed by outpatient treatment similar to treatment for UVH as needed).

Bilateral Vestibular Hypofunction

Bilateral vestibular hypofunction (BVH) or loss is most commonly caused by ototoxicity from taking certain classes of antibiotics (e.g., aminoglycosides gentamicin and streptomycin). Other possible causes include infections (meningitis, bilateral sequential vestibular neuritis), inner-ear autoimmune disorders, (e.g., Cogan's syndrome, ulcerative colitis, rheumatoid arthritis), bilateral Ménière's disease, bilateral tumors (acoustic neuromas in neurofibromatosis), and bilateral vestibulopathy due to aging. The prominent symptoms of BVH are disequilibrium, severe postural instability with resultant gait ataxia, and oscillopsia with head movement due to bilaterally impaired or absent vestibulospinal and vestibulo-ocular

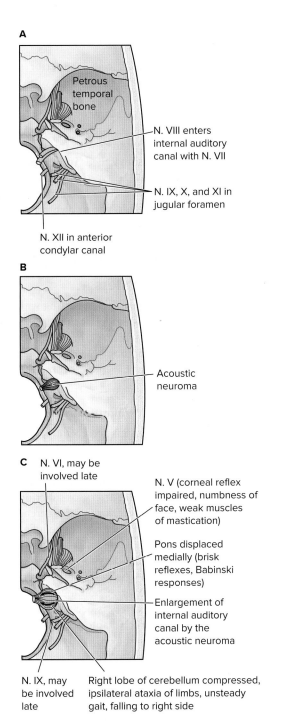

A

Petrous
temporal
bone

N. VIII enters
internal auditory
canal with N. VII

N. IX, X, and XI in
jugular foramen

N. XII in anterior
condylar canal

B

Acoustic
neuroma

C N. VI, may be
involved late

N. V (corneal reflex
impaired, numbness of
face, weak muscles
of mastication)

Pons displaced
medially (brisk
reflexes, Babinski
responses)

Enlargement of
internal auditory
canal by the
acoustic neuroma

N. IX, may
be involved
late

Right lobe of cerebellum compressed,
ipsilateral ataxia of limbs, unsteady
gait, falling to right side

FIGURE 16-1 Vestibular schwannoma (acoustic neuroma).
A. View of CN VII and VIII as they enter the internal auditory
canal in proximity to CN IX, X, and XI. **B.** Early stage acoustic
neuroma impinging on CN VII and VIII. **C.** Late stage acoustic
neuroma impinging on pons. (Adapted with permission from
Martin JH (Ed). *Neuroanatomy Text and Atlas*, 4th Ed. New York,
NY: McGraw-Hill; 2012. Fig 8-1, Pg 182.)

reflexes, respectively. Unless BVH is asymmetrical, individuals will not complain of nausea, vertigo, or nystagmus because there is no asymmetry of tonic resting firing rates of vestibular afferents. BVH symptoms are likely permanent, but people can return to high functional levels.

Recurrent Vestibular Disorders

Vestibular disorders that produce recurrent disruptions in vestibular function include benign paroxysmal positional vertigo, Ménière's disease (endolymphatic hydrops), and perilymphatic fistula. These disorders are characterized by intermittent periods of normal vestibular function with periods of abnormal function.[10]

Benign Paroxysmal Positional Vertigo

Benign paroxysmal positional vertigo (BPPV) is the most common peripheral vestibular disorder and is the cause of approximately 50% of dizziness in older people.[9,11] It typically affects women more than men, in their fourth and fifth decades of life. The condition occurs as a result of otoconia detaching from the otolithic membrane in the utricle and migrating into one of the semicircular canals (SCCs). BPPV can be categorized by the particular SCC involved and whether the detached otoconia are free-floating within the affected canal (**canalithiasis**) or attached to the cupula (**cupulolithiasis**). The most common form, accounting for 81–90% of all cases, is canalithiasis in the posterior SCC.[11] Because the otoconia have more than twice the density of the endolymph within the SCCs, the involved canal becomes gravity-sensitive. The shifting of otoconia with head movements causes deflection of the cupula, thereby sending abnormal input to the brain, resulting in the person's complaints of vertigo as well as an observable nystagmus. Other symptoms of BPPV may include disequilibrium, mild postural instability, and nausea. BPPV is typically unilateral; bilateral involvement is rare but can occur in association with head trauma. Activities that provoke symptoms vary across individuals, but they all involve rapidly changing the head's position with respect to gravity. With posterior SCC involvement, common problematic head movements include looking up, or rolling over and getting out of bed. The most common cause of BPPV in people <50 years is head injury, presumably due to a concussive force that displaces the otoconia. In people ≥50 years, the cause of BPPV is mostly unknown but is generally associated with age-related degeneration of the otolithic membrane. Physical therapy consisting of head maneuvers and vestibular rehabilitation exercises is the first choice of treatment for BPPV (see treatment section of this chapter). If the maneuvers and exercises are ineffective in controlling symptoms, a surgical procedure called posterior canal plugging may be recommended. Canal plugging stops the movement of particles within the posterior SCC with minimal impact on the rest of the inner ear. The surgery poses a small risk to hearing, but it has been found to be effective in 85–90% of individuals, who have had no response to any other treatment.[12]

Ménière's Disease

Ménière's disease is a disorder of the inner ear that is also known as **idiopathic endolymphatic hydrops**. It typically affects women more than men in their fourth and fifth decades of life.[8] The pathophysiology involves increased endolymphatic pressure within the inner ear possibly caused by malabsorption of endolymph in the endolymphatic duct and sac, leading to inappropriate nerve excitation. A typical attack is experienced initially as aural fullness (e.g., pressure, discomfort, fullness sensation in the ears), a reduction in hearing, and tinnitus (usually low-tone roaring), followed by rotational vertigo, postural imbalance, nystagmus, and nausea and vomiting after a few minutes.[7] The severe vertigo and disequilibrium may last from several minutes to up to 24 hours and can be debilitating. These symptoms gradually improve so that the person is usually able to walk within 72 hours. Hearing and tinnitus will also recover, but there may be residual permanent sensorineural hearing loss, particularly in the lower frequencies. With advanced disease, hearing does not return after the attack, and the symptoms of vertigo lessen in frequency and severity.

Medical treatment aims to reduce or prevent fluid buildup. Dietary restrictions of salt, caffeine, and alcohol are often advised but there is no proven evidence of their effectiveness. Pharmacologic treatments include vestibular suppressant, antiemetic, and antinausea medications during acute episodes and long-term use of betahistine (SERC; not currently FDA-approved but can be obtained by prescription at many compounding pharmacies in the United States) and diuretics to decrease endolymph volume.[13] In addition to medications, many patients with Ménière's disease require psychological counseling to cope with the changes to lifestyle and to manage stress brought about by the disease. In patients with disabling vertigo that does not respond to medications, surgical interventions to prevent fluid buildup (endolymphatic shunt placement) or to stop abnormal vestibular inputs, completed via vestibular nerve sectioning, chemical ablation with transtympanic gentamicin injection, or labyrinthectomy may be indicated; each of these result in complete hearing loss in the ear so are only performed in patients with preexisting hearing loss. Vestibular exercises are not recommended during acute attacks, but physical therapy may be beneficial for patients in treating the effects of chronic UVH or BVH, in the latter stages of the disease or in treating disequilibrium after destructive surgical procedures.

Perilymphatic Fistula

A perilymphatic fistula (PLF) is commonly caused by a tear or defect in the oval and/or round windows that separate the air-filled middle ear and the fluid-filled perilymphatic space of the inner ear. This small opening allows perilymph to leak into the middle ear. PLF is usually caused by head trauma (often minor), excessive intracranial or atmospheric pressure changes as in rapid airplane descent or scuba diving, extremely loud noises, objects perforating the tympanic membrane, ear surgery (stapedectomy), or vigorous straining as in lifting a heavy object. Patients report a "pop" in the ear, followed by the onset of sudden vertigo, hearing loss, and loud tinnitus.[7] Other symptoms may include postural imbalance, nystagmus, nausea, and vomiting. Some people experience pressure sensitivity, meaning that their symptoms may get worse with coughing, sneezing, or blowing their nose, as well as with exertion and activity. Medical treatment is bed rest with the head elevated for 5–10 days and avoidance of sneezing, coughing, or straining to allow spontaneous healing of the membrane. If symptoms persist longer than 4 weeks or hearing loss worsens, surgery to patch the fistulas can be performed. Physical therapy is usually not needed

for PLF, unless disequilibrium continues or UVH develops following surgery.

A particular variant of PLF, called **superior semicircular canal dehiscence**, occurs when a portion of the temporal bone that normally covers the superior (i.e., anterior) SCC is thin or missing, exposing the membranous SCC to stimuli that it normally does not receive (e.g., sound, changes in intracranial pressure, vibrations). Individuals with this condition often experience an unusual symptom called **Tullio's phenomenon** in which vestibular symptoms (i.e., vertigo, oscillopsia, nystagmus, ocular tilt reaction, and postural imbalance) are induced by auditory stimuli (e.g., loud noises, their own voice, or a musical instrument).

Table 16-1 summarizes the hallmark symptoms of the peripheral vestibular disorders discussed in this chapter.

Central Vestibular Disorders

Causes of central vestibular disorders occurring with dizziness are vertebrobasilar ischemic disease (including vertebrobasilar insufficiency and stroke), traumatic head injury, migraine-associated dizziness, and conditions that affect the brainstem and cerebellum (e.g., cerebellar degeneration, multiple sclerosis [MS], and tumors).

Vertebrobasilar Ischemic Stroke/Insufficiency

The blood supply to the brainstem, cerebellum, and inner ear is derived from the vertebrobasilar system (see Chapter 10). Occlusion of the subclavian, vertebral, or basilar arteries or their major branches, including the posterior inferior cerebellar artery, anterior inferior cerebellar artery, or superior cerebellar artery may result in vertigo. Posterior inferior cerebellar artery occlusion to the dorsolateral aspect of the medulla will result in Wallenberg's syndrome (lateral medullary syndrome). Lateral pontomedullary infarction secondary to occlusion of the anterior inferior cerebellar artery will result in lateral inferior pontine syndrome. Lateral superior pontine syndrome occurs when the superior cerebellar artery is occluded. For a description of these syndromes, refer to Chapter 10.

Vertebrobasilar insufficiency (VBI) is synonymous with a transient ischemic attack (TIA) of the vertebrobasilar system and is a common cause of vertigo in the elderly. Other associated symptoms of VBI include blurred vision or diplopia, drop attacks (sudden fall without loss of consciousness), syncope (fainting) or weakness, ataxia, and headaches. If left untreated, the disease process can progress to a stroke with long-lasting or permanent sequela. In fact, 29% of 84 patients with vertebrobasilar ischemic strokes had at least one episode of vertigo prior to their strokes.[14] Thus, it is important for clinicians to consider stroke in any person with acute vertigo and other concomitant neurologic signs and symptoms.

Traumatic Head Injury

Central vestibular disturbances are common, following head trauma secondary to diffuse damage to long white fiber tracts.[15] About 50–75% of individuals with mild traumatic brain injury may complain of vertigo that can persist for years, while almost all individuals with moderate brain injury complain of vertigo at some time.[16] Central vestibular lesions from head trauma

TABLE 16-1	**Symptomatology of Peripheral Vestibular Disorders**				
	UVH	**BVH**	**BPPV**	**MÉNIÈRE'S DISEASE**	**PERILYMPHATIC FISTULA**
Vertigo	+	−	+	+	+
Nystagmus	+	−	+	+	−/+
Duration of vertigo	Days to weeks	N/A	30 seconds–2 minutes	30 minutes–24 hours	Seconds to minutes
Nausea	+	−	−/+	+	−/+
Postural imbalance	+	++	+	+	+
Specific symptoms	Acute onset, tinnitus, hearing loss with labyrinthitis	Gait ataxia	Onset latency, adaptation	Fullness of ear, tinnitus, hearing loss	Loud tinnitus, Tullio's phenomenon
Precipitating event	Upper respiratory or gastrointestinal infection	Treatment with antibiotics (gentamicin, streptomycin)	Looking up, turning in bed		Head trauma, ear surgery, coughing, sneezing, straining
Outcome	Resolution of most symptoms by 1 year; dark vertigo may be permanent	Symptoms are typically permanent	Resolved with PT or surgery in most people	Vertigo severity diminishes but hearing loss is often permanent	Usually resolves in 4 weeks

Key: −, Absent; +, present; ++, very strong.

often result in vestibular symptoms of vertigo, nystagmus, and balance dysfunction that are accompanied by other neurologic signs such as hemisensory loss, hemiparesis, or ataxia depending on the CNS area involved.[16] The evaluation of individuals with head trauma is complicated because the peripheral vestibular system and the neck may also be injured. Peripheral vestibular injuries are often associated with temporal and/or facial bone fractures. Flexion-extension (i.e., "whiplash") injuries to the neck can also result in dizziness (see section entitled "Cervicogenic Dizziness").

Migraine-Associated Dizziness (Vestibular Migraine)

Migraine headaches affect approximately 10% of Americans, women more commonly than men, typically between the ages of 25 and 55.[17,18] People with a history of migraine headaches may experience episodic symptoms of vertigo, dizziness, imbalance, and motion sickness that can last minutes to hours.[19,20] About 50% of patients also experience cochlear symptoms (tinnitus, aural fullness, and hearing loss) with the vertigo.[20] In most patients, these symptoms are associated with a migraine headache and/or photophobia (intolerance to light) or phonophobia (intolerance to loud sounds), but some patients may experience these symptoms without a headache.[4] The diagnosis of migraine-associated dizziness (MAD) is complicated because it presents very similar to UVH, BPPV, or Ménière's disease. MAD should be considered in all patients who have migraine headache or a positive family history of migraine in the absence of other diagnoses. Patient report of a sense of imbalance in complex visual or motion environments is another clue to MAD.[21] Migraine headaches can be controlled with medications and lifestyle changes to avoid triggers for migraines (e.g., stress, diet, fluorescent lights). Vestibular rehabilitation may be beneficial for individuals with migraines that are controlled,[21,22] but exercises that stimulate the vestibular system can trigger migraines, if they are not controlled.[23]

Conditions Affecting the Brainstem and Cerebellum

Individuals with conditions that cause cerebellar degeneration (e.g., spinocerebellar ataxias, episodic ataxias, Friedreich's ataxia, cerebellar cortical atrophy, multiple system atrophy) may present with oculomotor deficits (abnormal ocular pursuit and improperly sized saccades), nystagmus (especially with downward and lateral gaze), incoordination of the extremities, a wide-based ataxic gait with uneven stride lengths, and inability to tandem walk.[21] Patients with disorders affecting the vestibulocerebellum may have difficulty with sensory integration, particularly visual-vestibular interaction, which may manifest as difficulty performing rapid head movements and maintaining balance while walking.[21] Demyelinating diseases such as MS may affect the vestibular nuclei, medial longitudinal fasciculus, and/or cerebellum, causing central vestibular dysfunction. Symptoms of vertigo, nystagmus (gaze-evoked and pendular), and disequilibrium are common in patients with MS.[15] Tumors in the brainstem and cerebellum may affect vestibular nuclei, central vestibular pathways, and the vestibulocerebellum.

● DIFFERENTIATING PERIPHERAL VESTIBULAR PATHOLOGY FROM CENTRAL VESTIBULAR PATHOLOGY

Table 16-2 delineates some of the characteristic features that can help distinguish patients with central vestibular pathology from those with peripheral vestibular pathology. Patients with central vestibular lesions more often complain of disequilibrium and ataxia rather than true vertigo. Often their inability to stand or walk distinguishes them from patients with peripheral lesions, who more commonly are able to stand or ambulate with assistance. Unlike peripheral lesions, nystagmus of central pathology changes direction with gaze, may be pendular (eyes oscillate at equal speeds), or may be purely vertical or torsional. Individuals with central vestibular lesions may have neurologic symptoms such as diplopia, altered consciousness, hemisensory loss, hemiparesis, and lateropulsion (tendency to fall to one side) that are not present with peripheral lesions. Peripheral vestibular lesions are more often associated with auditory symptoms.

● OTHER DIAGNOSES INVOLVING THE VESTIBULAR SYSTEM

Motion Sickness

Motion sickness is a common syndrome that occurs upon exposure to certain types of motion, such as passively riding in a car or airplane or viewing a 3D motion picture. Although nausea is the hallmark symptom, it is often preceded by pallor, malaise, drowsiness, and irritability.[24] Motion sickness is thought to be caused by conflict between the vestibular, visual, and other proprioceptive systems.[25] For example, consider the situation when you read in the car. Your eyes, fixed on the page, say that your head and body are not moving. However, as the car goes over bumps and accelerates/decelerates, your ears (i.e., vestibular system) disagree. This mismatch between what the visual and vestibular systems are telling you may explain why motion sickness is common in this scenario. Physical therapy has been successfully used to treat motion sickness.[26] Other treatments include cognitive-behavioral strategies (e.g., minimizing noxious motion, synchronizing the visual system with the motion by looking at the visual horizon, mentally rehearsing a trip route in advance), medications (i.e., scopolamine), and habituation exercises (gradually increasing the amount of motion).[24]

Cervicogenic Dizziness

Cervicogenic dizziness (also called cervical vertigo) is defined as symptoms of dizziness (including vertigo, disequilibrium, and light-headedness) arising from the cervical spine.[27] The main causes of cervicogenic dizziness are believed to be altered proprioceptive signals from the upper cervical spine, caused by disorders in vertebral segments C1–C3 and VBI (see above section entitled "Vertebrobasilar Ischemic Stroke/Insufficiency").[27] Similar to motion sickness, conflict between the vestibular, visual, and cervical inputs has been proposed to explain how cervical pain can lead to dizziness.[27] Inaccurate afferent inputs from inflamed or irritated cervical roots, proprioceptors of the facet joints, or the cervical musculature conflict with vestibular

TABLE 16-2	Common Symptoms Differentiating Central versus Peripheral Vestibular Pathology	
CENTRAL VESTIBULAR PATHOLOGY	**PERIPHERAL VESTIBULAR PATHOLOGY**
Uncommon to have hearing loss	Symptoms may include hearing loss, fullness in ears, tinnitus
Nystagmus direction is purely vertical or torsional.	Nystagmus is horizontal and torsional.
Pendular nystagmus (eyes oscillate at equal speeds)	Jerk nystagmus (nystagmus has slow and fast phases)
Nystagmus either does not change or reverses direction with gaze.	Nystagmus increases with gaze toward the direction of the fast phase (i.e., away from the side of the lesion).
Nystagmus either does not change or it increases with visual fixation.	Nystagmus is decreased with visual fixation.
Symptoms of acute vertigo not usually suppressed by visual fixation.	Symptoms of acute vertigo usually suppressed by visual fixation.
Nausea/vomiting more mild.	Nausea/vomiting usually severe.
Oscillopsia is severe.	Oscillopsia is mild unless lesion is bilateral.
Abnormal performance on smooth pursuit and/or saccades	Smooth pursuit tracking and saccade performance normal
If sudden onset, likely not able to stand and walk even with assistance (severe ataxia).	If sudden onset, can stand and walk with assistance (mild ataxia).
Other neurologic symptoms are present.	Other neurologic symptoms are rare.
Symptoms may recover slowly or never resolve.	Symptoms usually resolve within 7 days in people with UVH.

and visual inputs converging on brainstem nuclei (i.e., vestibular nuclei and reticular formation), resulting in altered oculomotor function and VOR, altered balance function, and perceptions of dizziness. Dizziness associated with neck pain is most common in patients with whiplash injuries, but also occurs in patients with cervical spondylosis and in those treated with cervical traction.[28] Physical therapy for cervical dysfunction and/or vestibular rehabilitation may be beneficial for these individuals.[28]

MEDICAL ASSESSMENT AND MANAGEMENT

Physicians use information from a person's medical history and findings from a physical examination as a basis for ordering diagnostic tests to assess the vestibular system function and to rule out alternative causes of symptoms.

Vestibular Function Tests

Electronystagmography/Videonystagmography

Electronystagmography (ENG) is a battery of eye movement tests that look for signs of vestibular dysfunction or neurological problems. During ENG, eye movements are recorded and analyzed, using small surface electrodes placed on the skin around the eyes. Alternatively, eye movements may be recorded by videonystagmography (VNG), using an infrared video camera mounted inside **Frenzel lenses** that the patient wears. Frenzel lenses consist of magnifying glasses and a lighting system that, when worn in a darkened room, allow the illuminated and magnified patient's eyes to be easily seen and prevent the patient from being able to suppress nystagmus by focusing the eyes. ENG/VNG tests includes measures of (1) oculomotor function (including gaze stability, and velocity, latency, and gain of smooth pursuit and saccadic eye movements) to identify pathology within the central oculomotor and vestibular systems, (2) positional testing (various head and whole body positions including the Dix–Hallpike maneuver) to determine positions that cause nystagmus, and (3) the caloric test (warm or cold water or air is circulated in the ear canal) to test horizontal SCC function (see Chapter 6: Special Senses for specifics on this test).[29] Eye movements for warm and cold irrigations in each ear are recorded, specifically, the peak slow component eye velocity (SCEV) is measured (i.e., slow phase of nystagmus); from this, a unilateral weakness percent (UW%), also referred to as the percent reduced vestibular response (%RVR), is calculated between the two ears. A difference of ≥26% is usually indicative of a clinically significant unilateral weakness in the ear producing the lesser responses.[29] The caloric test is considered the "gold standard" for identifying peripheral UVH and is particularly useful for determining the side of the deficit because each labyrinth is tested separately.[30]

Rotational Chair Testing

Rotational chair testing allows evaluation of both horizontal SCCs at head movement frequencies that are more physiologically natural (1–20 Hz) in contrast to caloric test (0.025 Hz). In individuals with normal vestibular function, rotational chair testing should induce nystagmus. Common rotational chair tests are the **sinusoidal harmonic acceleration test** (SHA) and the **step velocity test**. In the SHA, the patient is rotated in a pendular pattern (left/right) at various frequencies (0.01–1.28 Hz) while the peak chair velocity is typically fixed at 50–60 degrees/sec.[29] VOR parameters that are measured by this test include **gain** (ratio of slow phase eye velocity to head velocity [measured as chair velocity]) and **phase** (the timing relationship between the eye and head movement). The SHA test is the "gold standard" for identifying a bilateral vestibular weakness.[30] In the **step velocity test**, a stationary patient accelerates quickly to a predetermined peak velocity, continues to rotate in one direction at that velocity, and then is quickly stopped. The decay rate of nystagmus following both the abrupt angular acceleration and deceleration is measured and is called the **time constant**. The time constant is defined as the amount of time it takes for the slow phase velocity of the nystagmus to decline by 37% of its peak velocity, which typically takes 10–25 seconds (normal).[29] VOR phase and VOR time constant are measures of the same processes, namely transduction and velocity storage. Stimulation of hair cells by movement of the cupula generates a brief signal that lasts as long as the cupula is deflected. However, this response is sustained in the medial vestibular nucleus for longer than 10 seconds in individuals with normal vestibular function, supposedly as a means for the brain to detect low-frequency head rotation.[29] Lower velocity step rotations (about 60 degrees/sec) are used to determine the time constant and whether functional recovery of VOR gain has occurred from a chronic UVH, while higher velocity step rotations (>100 degrees/sec) are useful for detecting pathologically low VOR gains. Reduced gain, abnormal phase lead (i.e., eye movement is shifted slightly ahead of head movement), and shorter time constants are typically associated with peripheral vestibular pathology, while abnormally high gain, phase lag (i.e., eye movement is shifted slightly behind head movement), and longer time constants may indicate central (i.e., cerebellar) pathology.[29] Comparison of the VOR measures from rotations toward one ear with those from rotations to the opposite ear is used to determine whether weakness is present on one side.

Vestibular-Evoked Myogenic Potential

Otolith function (saccule and utricle) is tested with vestibular-evoked myogenic potential (VEMP). The two types of VEMP tests are the **cervical VEMP** (cVEMP) and **ocular VEMP** (oVEMP). Both types measure the latency, amplitude, and threshold of a muscle contraction, recorded by electromyography (EMG), to locate vestibular pathology.[31] The cVEMP is used to evaluate whether the saccule and the inferior vestibular nerve are intact and functioning normally. During cVEMP testing, headphones are placed over the ears and electrodes are placed over the contracted sternocleidomastoid (SCM) muscle. When sounds (i.e., loud clicks) are delivered to the ipsilateral ear in individuals with normal vestibular function, the electrodes record a transient inhibition of the ipsilateral contracted SCM muscle that occurs about 13 msec after the click.[29] This reflex is activated by sound stimulation of the saccular afferents that have ipsilateral disynaptic connections with the SCM muscle[29,31] The oVEMP is used to evaluate the function of the utricle and the superior vestibular nerve. In healthy individuals, loud clicks to the ear or bone vibrations to the forehead result in transient excitation of the contralateral inferior oblique (IO) eye muscle at a latency of 10 msec as recorded by electrodes placed under the eye.[29]

Computerized Dynamic Posturography

Computerized dynamic posturography (CDP) provides information about motor control or balance function under varying environmental conditions. It utilizes force plates to measure a person's center of pressure (COP) under challenging conditions. CDP is divided into sensory and motor components. The sensory portion, called the Sensory Organization Test (SOT), assesses an individual's ability to integrate visual, proprioceptive, and vestibular inputs to maintain balance. Patients are asked to stand still for 30 seconds for three trials under 6 increasingly difficult conditions with variations in reliable information provided by the visual and somatosensory systems (Figure 16-2). The SOT is not diagnostic, but it is useful in patients with postural instability to determine patterns of dysfunction produced by the 6 SOT test conditions (Table 16-3).[31] The motor portion includes the Motor Control Test (MCT) that assesses the latency, weight distribution, and amplitude of a person's postural responses to sudden displacements of the support surface, and an Adaptation Test (ADT) that assesses

FIGURE 16-2 Six testing conditions for the Sensory Organization Test (reprinted with permission from NeuroCom International). Vision is absent in Conditions 2 and 5. In Conditions 3 and 6, the surrounding wall sways with the person's body in the anterior/posterior (AP) direction, thereby reducing the accuracy of visual inputs for the perception of the body's motion relative to the visual field. In Conditions 4–6, the support surface sways along with the person's body, thereby, reducing the accuracy of somatosensory inputs for the perception of the body's AP motion relative to the support surface. (Reproduced with permission from Cavanaugh JT, Guskiewicz KM, Giuliani C, et al: Detecting altered postural control after cerebral concussion in athletes with normal postural stability, Br J Sports Med 2005 Nov;39(11):805–811.)

a person's ability to adapt to repeated perturbing stimuli (i.e., support surface tilts up or down at the same amplitude).

Visual Perception Tests

The **subjective visual vertical** (SVV) and **subjective visual horizontal** (SVH) tests are used to assess otolith function and the central pathways that convey gravitational information. The tests do not distinguish between saccular or utricular pathology. During these tests, patients are asked to align a dimly lit luminous bar (in a completely dark room) with what they perceive as being vertical (SVV) or horizontal (SVH). Individuals with normal vestibular function align the bar within ±2.0 degrees of true vertical or horizontal, while patients with either central or peripheral pathology align the bar with larger angular deviations. The direction of pathological SVV tilt is usually on the same side as the lesion (ipsiversive) in patients with unilateral peripheral vestibular neuritis and those with unilateral brainstem lesions that are lower than the upper pons.[32,33] With pathology of the cerebellum or unilateral brainstem lesions above the upper pons (i.e., midbrain, thalamus), the direction of SVV tilt is usually opposite to the side of the lesion (contraversive).[32,34]

Hearing Tests

Audiometry measures hearing function. Hearing evaluations are an important part of vestibular diagnostics. Several different audiometry tests, performed by an audiologist, may be completed. Individuals with vestibular disorders may have their hearing monitored at intervals over time, especially when there is evidence of tinnitus, hearing loss, or a sensation of fullness in the ears.

Neuroimaging

Magnetic resonance imaging (MRI) of the brain can reveal the presence of tumors, damage from strokes, and other soft-tissue abnormalities that might cause dizziness or vertigo. MRIs of structures in and around the inner ear may show problems such as an acoustic neuroma. Computerized axial tomography (CT) scans of the temporal bone (within which the inner ear resides) are often used to locate fractures.

Pharmacological Treatment

Treatment of Vertigo

Vestibular suppressant medications that are used for symptomatic treatment of acute vertigo, nausea, and vomiting are listed in Table 16-4. These drugs are not recommended for long-term use as they may inhibit central compensation and recovery of symptoms.

Treatment of Nystagmus

Several medications are used to suppress different forms of nystagmus. Pendular nystagmus, often associated with MS and brainstem strokes, can be suppressed with the anticonvulsant drug, gabapentin (Neurontin), or with memantine, a drug that blocks glutamate *N*-methyl-D-aspartate (NMDA) receptors.[35] Downbeat nystagmus, associated with cerebellar pathology, is effectively treated with potassium channel-blocking agents 4-aminopyridine (fampridine or dalfampridine) and 3.4-diaminopyridine (3,4-DAP).[35] Of the two, 4-aminopyridine

TABLE 16-3	Interpretation of Patterns of Responses for the Sensory Organization Test	
PATTERN	**ABNORMAL TEST CONDITION**	**INTERPRETATION**
Vestibular dysfunction or loss	5, 6	Suggests difficulty using vestibular input for stance; early falls seen with bilateral loss of vestibular function; falls late in the trial seen with reduced bilateral peripheral vestibular function and uncompensated loss of unilateral function.
Support surface dependence	4, 5, 6	Suggests abnormal reliance on foot support surface inputs for stance; person has difficulty using both visual and vestibular or vestibular inputs alone.
Visual preference	3, 6	Suggests that central adaptive mechanisms for suppression of conflicting visual input may be impaired.
Visual dependence	2, 3, 5, 6	Suggests abnormal reliance on vision for stance; person has difficulty using foot support surface and/or vestibular inputs for stance.
General sensory selection	3, 4, 5, 6	Suggests difficulty with balance control in conditions with any sensory conflict.

TABLE 16-4	Common Drugs Used to Treat Acute Vertigo and Associated Nausea and Emesis[35,36]				
MEDICATION	**CLASS**	**SEDATION**	**ANTIEMESIS**	**SIDE EFFECTS**	
Dimenhydrinate (Dramamine)	Antihistamine; phosphodiesterase inhibitor	+	++	Dry mouth, tinnitus, blurred vision, coordination problems	
Diphenhydramine (Benadryl)	Antihistamine	+	++	Tachycardia, urinary retention	
Promethazine (Phenergan)	Antihistamine; anticholinergic; phenothiazine	++	++	Dry mouth, constipation, blurred vision	
Meclizine (Antivert, Bonine)	Antihistamine; anticholinergic	++	+	Dry mouth, tiredness	
Prochlorperazine (Compazine)	Antihistamine; anticholinergic; phenothiazine	+	+++	Dry mouth, blurred vision, constipation	
Scopalamine (Transderm Scop)	Anticholinergic (nonselective muscarinic)	+	++	Dry mouth, dilated pupils, blurred vision	
Ondansetron (Zofran)	Serotonin 5-hydroxytryptamine$_3$ (5-HT$_3$) receptor antagonist		+++	Headache, constipation, blurred vision	
Lorazepam	Benzodiazepine	++	+	Addiction, effects increased with other sedative drugs	

+, Mild; ++, moderate; +++, prominent.

is more effective, has fewer side effects, and is available as a sustained-release preparation (Ampyra).[35] Other drugs that may be used to treat nystagmus are baclofen (Lioresal) and clonazepam (Klonopin).

● PHYSICAL THERAPY EXAMINATION

Medical and Subjective Histories

Physical therapists, treating individuals with complaints of dizziness and imbalance, must first take thorough medical and subjective histories and perform a systems review to sort out potential causes. The patients' current symptoms and past medical histories may assist the therapist to identify potential problems such as diabetes, heart disease, or neurological dysfunction that could negatively impact the patient's recovery. Patients should be asked about any medications that they are currently taking to determine if they are taking vestibular suppressant drugs (e.g., meclizine, scopolamine) that could delay recovery or might worsen their dizziness. For individuals taking vestibular suppressant drugs, the therapist should consult with the physician to see if they can be reduced or stopped. Therapists should also ask the patient or obtain from the medical record any diagnostic test reports, such as ENG/VNG, caloric, rotational chair, or VEMP tests.

Physical therapists must distinguish exactly what the patient is experiencing when feeling "dizzy" to be able to make appropriate clinical management decisions. Common types of dizziness symptoms and their possible causes are shown in Table 16-5. Notably, some patients, particularly patients with migraine, are chronically sensitive to motion, either of themselves or of the environment. Patient descriptions of their dizziness as an out-of-body experience, floating, or a spinning sensation inside of their head without accompanying nystagmus suggest a psychophysiological disorder (i.e., a combination of psychiatric factors and physiologic responses such as hyperventilation).

Information about the onset, frequency, duration, and intensity of symptoms, and what circumstances exacerbate and relieve the symptoms should be obtained. Examples of questions to ask patients with vestibular disorders are found in Box 16-1. Intensity of symptoms like vertigo, lightheadedness, disequilibrium, and oscillopsia can be quantified by a visual analogue scale (VAS). Patients are asked to answer a question (e.g., how intense is your vertigo right now?) by making a mark on a 10-cm line on a continuum from "none" at one end to "worst possible intensity" at the other to indicate the intensity of their symptoms at a particular moment. A fall history, including number of falls in the last 6 months, conditions under which falls occurred, whether the patient sought medical intervention as a result of a fall, and any lifestyle modifications made to prevent recurrent falls, should be obtained. The **Activities-Specific Balance Confidence**

Scale (ABC Scale) is useful for determining the patient's perceptions of his ability to balance.[37] The patient should be asked about previous and current functional status and activity level. Some patients will stay in their homes to avoid highly textured visual stimulation (e.g., light flickering through trees, walking down aisles in stores) or develop phobias such as fears of elevators and heights.[38] The **Vestibular Activities of Daily Living Scale** (VD-ADL) can assist therapists to identify current limitations in activity and participation.[39] Patients rate the effects of vertigo and balance disorders on their independence in performing 28 activities of daily living on a scale of 1–10 with 1 being "independent" and 10 being "too difficult, no longer perform."

The **Dizziness Handicap Inventory** (DHI) assesses a person's perception of the effects of a balance problem and the emotional, physical, or functional adjustments that he or she makes.[40] The questionnaire consists of 25 items that are divided into functional (9 items), emotional (9 items), and physical (7 items) subscales. Each item is assigned a value of four points for a "yes," two points for a "sometimes," and zero points for a "no." The inventory is reliable and DHI scores are highly correlated with scores on the impairment-based SOT.[41] Clinicians can administer the DHI (1) before a patient's initial exam to help determine the physical tests that should be performed and to establish a baseline and (2) after treatment to determine treatment efficacy.[42]

Therapists should ask patients about their functional goals for physical therapy and discuss with them whether they are

TABLE 16-5	Common Dizziness Symptoms and Possible Causes	
SYMPTOM	**DESCRIPTION**	**POSSIBLE CAUSES**
Vertigo (e.g., visualized spinning, tilting, dropping of the environment)	Illusion of movement, most commonly described as a feeling that they are spinning or that the room (environment) is spinning, often with nystagmus	Imbalance in tonic firing rates of left and right divisions of the vestibular system caused by unilateral peripheral (UVH, BPPV) or central lesions of vestibular nuclei.
Presyncope (near-faint)	Perception that he/she is about to faint; often associated with a buzzing sensation in the head, rubbery legs, constriction of the visual field, pallor, diaphoresis, and nausea.[5]	Diffuse decreased cerebral blood flow (i.e., cardiac arrhythmia, orthostatic hypotension)
Lightheadedness ("woozy")	Nonspecific type of dizziness that may be described as feeling "woozy" or disoriented	Decreased blood pressure (if accompanied by presyncope), hypoglycemia, drug intoxication, anxiety or panic disorders (associated with hyperventilation)
Disequilibrium (e.g., unsteadiness in standing and walking)	Feeling that a person is off balance. Patients typically do not experience disequilibrium while sitting or lying down but report unsteadiness upon standing or walking	Vestibular (BVH, chronic UVH), loss of lower extremity somatosensation, brainstem/ vestibular cortex lesions, cerebellar and motor pathway lesions.
Motion intolerance	Sensitivity to riding in a car or other moving vehicle	Sensory conflict (e.g., motion sickness), migraine headaches
Oscillopsia	Visual instability with head movement in which objects in the environment appear to move or bounce, often resulting in blurring or diplopia	Peripheral vestibular disorders (BVH, UVH, BPPV) and brainstem and cerebellar lesions
Out of body feeling, floating, spinning inside of head		Psychophysiological disorder (e.g., anxiety, conversion disorder, depression)

BOX 16-1   Questions to Ask People with Vestibular Disorders[38]

1. Do you have spells of vertigo (sensation of spinning)? If yes, how long do they last?
2. When was the last time the vertigo occurred?
3. Is the vertigo spontaneous (present at rest), caused by motion, or caused by position changes?
4. Do you feel like you are going to lose your balance? If yes, is the feeling of being off balance constant, spontaneous, caused by motion, caused by position changes, worse with fatigue, worse in the dark, worse outside, worse on uneven surfaces?
5. Do you feel off balance when you are lying down, sitting, standing, or walking?
6. Do you stumble, stagger, or side-step while walking?
7. Do you veer to one side while you walk? If yes, to which side do you veer?
8. At what time of the day do you feel best? worst?
9. How many times per day do you have symptoms?
10. Do you have hearing problems?
11. Do you have visual problems?
12. Have you been in an accident (e.g., motor vehicle)?
13. Do you live alone?
14. Do you have stairs in your home?
15. Do you smoke? If yes, how much per day?
16. Do you drink alcohol? If yes, how much per day/week?

---

realistic and attainable.[38] The **Vestibular Rehabilitation Benefit Questionnaire** is utilized clinically to assess the effectiveness of physical therapy interventions on an individual's symptoms and the impact of those symptoms on quality of life.[43] The 22-item questionnaire consists of items falling into three subscales: dizziness and anxiety (6 items), motion-provoked dizziness (5 items), and quality of life (11 items). The score for the entire tool ranges from 0 to 100%; zero percent indicates no deficit, and 100% indicates significant deficit as compared to the normal state.

Tests and Measures

Examination of the patient with dizziness includes assessment of eye movements (i.e., nystagmus, oculomotor, and vestibulo-ocular testing), positional testing, balance and gait assessment. These tests would be performed in addition to a systems review and standard neurological assessment that includes evaluation of somatosensation, pain, coordination, range of motion, muscle strength, and posture to identify concurrent impairments that might affect the patient's prognosis and treatment (refer to Chapter 9 – Neurologic Evaluation). To assess the contribution of vertebral artery occlusion to the patient's symptoms, a **seated vertebral artery test** can be performed, in which the patient performs in consecutive order: (1) rotation of the head opposite to the tested side as far as possible, (2) extension of the head, and then (3) a combination of head rotation and extension opposite to the tested side.[44] If the patient experiences symptoms such as dizziness, diplopia, dysarthria, dysphagia, drop attacks, nausea, vomiting, or sensory changes at any time the test is positive

and testing is stopped. A positive test may indicate VBI, but a negative test cannot rule it out.[44] If cervicogenic dizziness is suspected, a more detailed examination of the upper quarter, including cervical-thoracic mobility, tests for instability of the upper cervical spine, palpation of cervical spine musculature and facet joints, and segmental mobility testing of the cervical spine should be performed.[45] Testing procedures and interpretation of findings are as follows.

Spontaneous Nystagmus

Procedure: Ask the patient to fixate on a stationary target in neutral gaze position and observe for nystagmus or rhythmic refixation eye movements. Repeat with the patient wearing Frenzel lenses so that the person cannot suppress the nystagmus by fixating on an object.

Interpretation: If nystagmus is observed, the amplitude, direction, and effect of target fixation should be noted. Lesions of the labyrinth, vestibular nerve, and rarely the vestibular nuclei produce intense, horizontal-rotatory nystagmus that is enhanced under Frenzel lenses. In contrast, central lesions (e.g., brainstem, cerebellum, and cerebrum) cause less intense horizontal, vertical, torsional, or pendular nystagmus that is usually reduced under Frenzel lenses.

Gaze-Holding Nystagmus

Procedure: Ask the patient to gaze at a target placed 20–30 degrees to the left of center for 20 seconds. Observe for gaze-evoked nystagmus or change in direction, appearance, or intensity in spontaneous nystagmus. This should be repeated to the right.

Interpretation: The ability to maintain eccentric gaze is controlled by neural pathways in the brainstem and cerebellum, particularly the vestibulocerebellum. When these mechanisms fail to hold the eye in the eccentric position, the eye drifts toward the midline, followed by corrective saccades toward the target. Thus, central lesions produce direction-changing gaze-evoked nystagmus (i.e., the fast component of the nystagmus always beats in the direction of intended gaze). In contrast, acute peripheral UVH produces direction-fixed gaze holding nystagmus (the direction of the nystagmus is the same regardless of the eye-in-orbit position) and the nystagmus intensifies (i.e., the slow phase velocity of the nystagmus increases) when gazing in the direction of the fast phase.[38,46]

Smooth Pursuit

Procedure: Ask the patient to keep the head stationary, while following your finger with the eyes, as you slowly move it left and right, up and down.

Interpretation: Normal eye tracking of a slowly moving object generates a smooth eye movement that involves central pathways and cranial nerves III, IV, and VI. Smooth pursuit is abnormal if, during tracking, the patient repeatedly loses the target and then catches up with a small saccade. Abnormal smooth pursuit is consistent with a central lesion and is never a sign of peripheral vestibular impairment.

Saccades

Procedure: Ask the patient to look back and forth between two outstretched fingers held about 12 inches apart in the horizontal and vertical planes. Observe for latency of onset, speed, accuracy, and conjugate movement.

Interpretation: Saccadic eye movements are rapid eye movements that involve the frontal lobes, brainstem reticular formation, and cranial nerves III, IV, and VI. Healthy individuals can reach the targets with one eye movement or with one small corrective saccade. Abnormal saccadic eye movements are consistent with a central lesion and are never a sign of peripheral vestibular impairment.

Vestibulo-Ocular Reflex Cancellation (VORc)

Procedure: Ask the patient to voluntarily fixate on a moving target, while the patient's head is moved in the same direction.

Interpretation: The normal smooth pursuit system is able to override or "cancel" the VOR at slow head velocities, as a patient focuses his or her gaze on a target that moves simultaneously and in the same direction as the head moves. An abnormal response is observed when a patient's fixation on a target, moving synchronously with his or her head, is interrupted by saccades. An impaired VORc is consistent with a central nervous system disorder.[38]

Ocular Alignment

Procedure: Observe the seated patient for head tilt (associated with abnormal SVV), skew deviation (one eye being superiorly displaced in comparison with the other eye), ocular torsion (the superior pole of the eyes are rotated together in the frontal plane), or a combination of the three symptoms called the **ocular tilt reaction** (OTR).

Interpretation: In a healthy individual, the SVV is aligned with the gravitational vertical, and the axes of eyes and the head are horizontal and directed straight ahead.[47] The OTR indicates either a unilateral peripheral vestibular deficit (labyrinth or vestibular nerve) or a unilateral lesion of brainstem pathways. OTR from vestibular loss on the right side manifests as head tilts to the right, right eye drops down in the orbit, and both eyes statically rotate to the right.

Head-Thrust Test (HTT, also called Head Impulse Test [HIT])

Procedure: Ask the patient to fixate on a near target (e.g., the clinician's nose), grasp the patient's head, and apply a brief, small-amplitude (5–10 degrees), and high-acceleration (3000–4000 degrees/sec^2) head turn, first to one side and then to the other. When the head stops moving, the clinician looks to see if the eyes are still directed toward the target and watches for corrective saccades toward the target.

Interpretation: When the VOR is functioning normally, the eyes move in the direction opposite to the head movement and gaze remains fixated on the target during the head thrust. Observations of "catch-up" saccades, after a head thrust to one side, is a sign of decreased neural input from the ipsilateral horizontal SCC afferents or central vestibular neurons to the VOR because the contralateral vestibular afferents and central vestibular neurons are inhibited and cannot supply enough neural activity to stabilize gaze. Patients with unilateral peripheral or central vestibular pathology will not be able to maintain gaze on the target, when the head is moved quickly toward the side

of the lesion; individuals with bilateral loss of vestibular function will make corrective saccades after high-velocity head movements to both sides. Schubert et al.[48] reported that the HTT had a sensitivity of 71% for identifying UVH and 84% for BVH, and a specificity of 82% when the test was performed with the patient's head flexed forward 30 degrees and the head was moved unpredictably.[47]

Head-Shaking Induced Nystagmus Test (HSN)

Procedure: The patient is instructed to close his or her eyes. Tilt the head of the patient forward 30 degrees and oscillate the head in the horizontal plane at 2 Hz for 20 seconds. On stopping the oscillation, the patient opens the eyes and the clinician looks for nystagmus. The maneuver may be repeated in the vertical direction.

Interpretation: In individuals with normal vestibular function, nystagmus will not be present after the head shaking stops. An imbalance in the peripheral vestibular inputs to central vestibular nuclei can result in HSN. In cases of UVH, the patient may display nystagmus with the fast phase directed toward the healthy ear. Patients with complete bilateral vestibular function loss will not show HSN because there is no asymmetry between the vestibular inputs. Vertical nystagmus, following horizontal or vertical head shaking, indicates central pathology.

Dynamic Visual Acuity (DVA)

Procedure: Ask the patient to read the lowest (smallest) line possible on a wall-mounted acuity chart (Snellen eye chart or Lighthouse distance visual acuity test) with best corrected vision (glasses, contact lenses). Repeat the maneuver while passively oscillating the patient's head at 2 Hz, and record the number of lines of acuity "lost" during the headshake.

Interpretation: In normal individuals, visual acuity changes by one line in younger individuals and by two lines in older individuals.[38] If the person can only read lines more than 3 lines above the initial static visual acuity, he or she likely has vestibular dysfunction. Patients with bilateral vestibular loss, especially acutely, often lose 6–8 lines of visual acuity. A computerized version of the DVA has the benefit of being able to determine DVA for right and left head movements separately.[38]

Positional Testing

Static and dynamic position tests are performed to determine which head positions or movements provoke the patient's symptoms of vertigo, dizziness, nausea, and nystagmus. Static positions that are tested typically include (1) sitting with the head upright, (2) supine with head flexed forward approximately 30 degrees, (3) supine with the head turned right, and (4) supine with the head turned left. The Motion Sensitivity Test (MST) measures motion-provoked dizziness in patients using a series of 16 movements from least to most provocative (Table 16-6).[49,50] The severity and duration of the dizziness are recorded for each position and a cumulative score, the MST quotient, is calculated. A final score of 0–10 indicates mild motion sensitivity, with scores of 11–30 indicating moderate motion sensitivity, and scores of 31–100 indicating severe motion sensitivity.[38] The MST has been found to be reliable and valid.[51] Clinicians can use the results of static and

TABLE 16-6   Motion Sensitivity Test (Adapted from Smith-Wheelock et al.[49])

BASELINE SYMPTOMS	INTENSITY (A)	DURATION (B)	SCORE (A+B)
1. Sitting to supine			
2. Supine to left side			
3. Supine to right side			
4. Supine to sitting			
5. Left Dix–Hallpike test			
6. Return from left Dix–Hallpike test			
7. Right Dix–Hallpike test			
8. Return from right Dix–Hallpike test			
9. Sitting: nose toward left knee			
10. Return to sitting			
11. Sitting: nose toward right knee			
12. Return to sitting			
13. Sitting: head rotation (5 times)			
14. Sitting: head flexion and extension (5 times)			
15. Standing: 180-degree turn to right			
16. Standing: 180-degree turn to left			

Duration of dizziness: rated 0–3 (5–10 seconds = 1 point; 11–30 seconds = 2 points; ≥30 seconds = 3 points).
Intensity of dizziness: rated 0–5 (0 = no symptoms; 5 = severe dizziness).
Duration score + Intensity score = MST score (Maximum score for each position is 8 points; the total possible raw score is 128 [8 points × 16 positions]).
Motion sensitivity quotient: Number of symptom-provoking positions × MST score × 100 divided by 2048 (16 [total number of positions] × 128 [total possible MST score]).
Note: An MST quotient of 0 indicates no symptoms, whereas an MST quotient of 100 indicates severe unrelenting symptoms in all positions.
(Adapted with permission from Smith-Wheelock M, Shepard NT, Telian SA: Physical therapy program for vestibular rehabilitation, *Am J Otol* 1991 May;12(3):218–225.)

dynamic position tests to develop exercise programs for patients and to provide evidence of intervention efficacy.

Positional testing is used to identify whether a person has BPPV. Vestibular tests that identify BPPV, affecting the vertical SCCs (i.e., posterior and anterior SCCs), include the Dix–Hallpike Test (see Figure 16-3) and the Sidelying Test (Figure 16-4). The Dix–Hallpike Test has been considered the gold standard for diagnosing BPPV.[52] Starting from a long-sitting position with the head rotated 45 degrees to one side, the patient is moved to a supine position with the head extended 30 degrees below the horizontal and still rotated 45 degrees.

The clinician, then, observes the patient's eyes for nystagmus and asks if vertigo is being felt. The patient is then slowly brought back to the starting position, and the other side is tested. When the Dix–Hallpike Test is inapplicable, such as in individuals with neck and back problems or those with a positive vertebral artery test, the Sidelying Test may be used as an alternative. The patient is quickly moved from a seated position on the side of a plinth to sidelying with the head rotated 45 degrees in the opposite direction (Figure 16-4).[52] Horizontal SCC BPPV is diagnosed by the Roll Test (also called the Pagnini–McClure maneuver), in which the head is turned by about 90 degrees to each side while supine (Figure 16-5).

A positive test for BPPV from canalithiasis is characterized by (1) delayed onset of vertigo by 1–40 seconds after the person is placed in the provoking position; (2) presence of nystagmus with the same latency as the complaints of vertigo; and (3) increasing followed by decreasing intensity of vertigo and nystagmus that disappears within 60 seconds.[53] BPPV from cupulolithiasis is much less common than canalithiasis and is characterized by (1) immediate onset of vertigo when the person is moved into the provoking position; (2) nystagmus that appears with the same latency as the complaints of vertigo, and (3) persistence of the vertigo and nystagmus as long as the person's head is maintained in the provoking position.[53] The problematic SCC can be identified based on the characteristics of the observed nystagmus (Table 16-7). For the Dix–Hallpike and Sidelying tests, the posterior or anterior SCC that has BPPV is the side that reproduces nystagmus and vertigo. Determination of the affected horizontal SCC side with the roll test is more difficult because vertigo and nystagmus will be elicited in both the head left and head right positions. The clinician must carefully observe the nystagmus to determine whether the patient has the canalithiasis or the cupulolithiasis form of horizontal SCC BPPV. In the canalithiasis form of horizontal SCC BPPV, the nystagmus is **geotropic**, meaning that the fast phase beats toward the Earth and lasts <60

FIGURE 16-3 The Dix–Hallpike Test. (1) The patient long-sits on the examination table and the clinician turns the head horizontally 45 degrees, (2) the clinician maintains the 45-degree head rotation while bringing the patient quickly to a supine position with the neck extended 30 degrees beyond the horizontal. This figure shows testing for right posterior or right anterior semicircular canal BPPV. The corresponding illustrations demonstrate the orientation of the semicircular canals and location of the otolithic debris in the posterior canal (viewed from the patient's right side).

seconds.[53] In the cupulolithiasis form of horizontal SCC BPPV, the nystagmus is **apogeotropic**, meaning that the fast phase beats away from the Earth, and lasts >60 seconds.[53] The affected side is typically considered to be the more symptomatic side in canalithiasis and the less symptomatic side in cupulolithiasis.

Balance and Gait Assessment

Examination of balance and gait problems is important to determine the patient's functional status and fall risk. Testing should address static and dynamic balance, anticipatory postural control, reactive balance control, sensory and movement strategies, and balance during functional activities. Table 16-8 includes common static and dynamic balance tests and expected results in patients with specific vestibular disorders.

Static balance can be assessed by observing the patient's ability to maintain different postures. The **Romberg Test** tests the patient's ability to stand with the feet parallel and together with the eyes open and then closed for 30 seconds.[54] The **sharpened Romberg**, also known as the tandem Romberg, requires the patient to stand with the feet in a heel-to-toe position with arms folded across the chest and eyes closed for one minute.[54] The **Single-Leg Balance Stance Test** (SLB) asks the patient to stand on one leg without shoes with arms placed across the chest without letting the legs touch each other. Five 30-second trials are performed for each leg with a maximum possible score of 150 seconds per leg. Normal adults should be able to balance for 20–30 seconds on each leg.[55]

Dynamic balance control can be assessed by self-initiated movements and dynamic tests of balance. Observations of weight shifts performed in standing to the limits of stability in all directions, reaching tasks such as picking up objects off the floor or putting an object on a high shelf, or transitions from one position to another (e.g., supine-to-sit or sit-to-stand transfers) can be used to determine whether the patient moves efficiently, symmetrically, and safely. The **Five Times Sit-to-Stand Test** (FTSST) assesses the patients' abilities to balance while standing up and sitting down five times as quickly as possible from a standard armless chair.[56] The FTSST has been shown to be a reliable and valid measure in individuals with balance disorders.[56] The **Fukuda Stepping Test** (FST) is a dynamic test that

FIGURE 16-4 A–C. Sidelying Test. After seating the patient on the examination table, the clinician turns the head horizontally 45 degrees away from the involved ear. The clinician maintains the 45-degree head rotation while bringing the patient quickly to the side opposite to the head rotation. The corresponding illustrations demonstrate the orientation of the semicircular canals and location of the otolithic debris in the posterior canal (viewed from the front).

was originally developed as a test of vestibular function. The test is performed by having the patient stand with eyes closed and arms extended to shoulder height. The patient marches in place for 50 steps at the pace of a brisk walk. Progressive turning toward one side of 45 degrees or more is considered a positive test and suggests a unilateral peripheral or central vestibular deficit.[57] Honaker and Shepard[58] measured FST as a function of the patient's degree of caloric weakness on ENG and found that the FST was only sensitive in detecting individuals with severe weakness on ENG (>75% weakness).

Anticipatory postural control is evaluated by having the patient perform voluntary movements that require the development of a postural set to counteract a predicted postural disturbance. The patient's ability to catch or kick balls, open doors, lift objects of different weights, step over obstacles, and reach without losing balance is indicative of adequate anticipatory control. The **Functional Reach Test**[59] and the **Multi-Directional Reach Test**[60] require the patient to reach in different directions as far as possible without changing the base of support. Normative data are available, and the tests are reliable and valid.[59,60]

Automatic postural responses or reactive control can be assessed by the patient's response to external perturbations. Pushes (small or large, slow or rapid, anticipated and unanticipated) applied to the sternum, posterior trunk, or pelvis in different directions are widely used, but they are not quantifiable or reliable. The clinician subjectively rates the responses as

normal, good, fair, poor, or unable. The **Pull Test**,[61] **Backwards Release**,[62] and **Postural Stress Test**[63] are more objective and reliable measures of reactive postural control.

The **Clinical Test of Sensory Integration on Balance Test** (CTSIB), formerly called the "Foam and Dome" Test,[64] measures the patient's ability to balance under six different sensory conditions: (1) eyes open, stable surface (floor); (2) eyes closed, stable surface; (3) visual conflict (dome), stable surface; (4) eyes open, unstable surface (foam); (5) eyes closed, unstable surface; (6) visual conflict, unstable surface. The SOT is the computerized version of this test (see preceding section on posturography).[65] A modified version (mCTSIB) has the dome portion removed, using only four conditions of eyes open and closed while standing on the floor and then a dense piece of foam. Each condition is tested three times for 30 seconds. Interpretation of the results of the CTSIB and mCTSIB is the same as for the SOT (see Table 16-3). Patients lacking labyrinthine inputs become more dependent on accurate ankle proprioceptive and visual inputs to correctly organize their postural responses.[66] Inaccurate or distorted proprioceptive or visual inputs will often produce increased sway and falls in these individuals.[66] Giray et al.[67] demonstrated significant differences on the instrumented mCTSIB (NeuroCom Balance Master) between subjects with unilateral vestibular dysfunction who participated in a 4-week vestibular rehabilitation program and those who did not ($p < 0.05$) for all conditions and for the composite score.

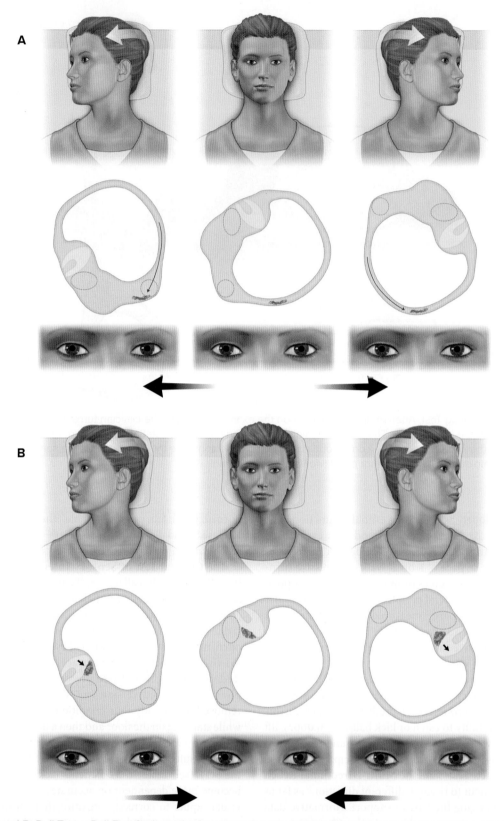

FIGURE 16-5 A and B. Roll Test – Roll Test for horizontal semicircular canal BPPV. The patient is positioned in supine with the head placed in 20-degree cervical flexion. The head is quickly turned about 90 degrees to each side. **A:** Canalithiasis. **B:** Cupulolithiasis. The corresponding illustrations demonstrate the location of the otolithic debris in the horizontal canal during each maneuver, and the direction of the induced nystagmus (arrows).

TABLE 16-7	Nystagmus Features by Canal Affected in BPPV
CANAL AFFECTED	**INITIAL RESPONSE IN DIX–HALLPIKE TEST**
Posterior	Upbeating and torsional (torsional toward affected ear)
Anterior	Downbeating and torsional (torsional toward affected ear)
Horizontal: canalithiasis	Geotropic (right-beating in head right position, left-beating in head left position)
Horizontal: cupulolithiasis	Apogeotropic (left-beating in right head position, right-beating in head left position)

During the functional evaluation of individuals with vestibular deficits the clinician should observe and document the patient's movement strategies in response to postural disturbances.[38] Horak and Nashner[68] described four movement strategies called ankle, hip, stepping, and suspensory strategies that healthy adults use to recover balance when standing on a surface that suddenly moves under them. In quiet stance and during small perturbations (i.e., slow-speed perturbations usually occurring on a large, firm surface), the **ankle strategy** acts to restore a person's center of mass (COM) to a stable position. The muscle activation sequence associated with the ankle strategy is a distal-to-proximal firing pattern of the ankle, hip, and trunk musculature. For rapid and/or large external perturbations or for movements executed with the COM near the limits of stability, a **hip strategy** is employed. The hip strategy uses rapid hip flexion or extension to move the COM within the BOS. The muscle activation sequence associated with the hip strategy occurs in a proximal-to-distal pattern. If a large force displaces the COM beyond the limits of stability, a forward or backward **stepping strategy** is used to enlarge the base of support and regain balance control. The **suspension strategy** is observed during balance tasks when a person quickly lowers his or her body COM by flexing the knees, causing associated flexion of the ankles and hips or a slight squatting motion. Horak et al.[69] found that patients with bilateral vestibular loss displayed normal ankle strategies in response to surface translations, but they did not use a hip strategy even when it was necessary to maintain balance while standing on a narrow balance beam. Clinicians should observe the patient's individual movement strategies to determine if they are sufficient and safe to achieve task goals.

Clinicians should assess the patient's gait through clinical observation, videotape analysis, or computerized gait or motion analysis systems. Observe patients walk at different speeds and directions, in crowded versus uncrowded settings, while moving the head, with interruptions of sudden stops, in obstacle courses, and with secondary motor or cognitive tasks to simulate activities that patients perform in their daily lives. Record whether specific activities increase their symptoms. Refer to Table 16-8 for common gait deviations found in patients with vestibular

TABLE 16-8	Common Balance Test Results for Vestibular Conditions			
TEST	**BPPV**	**UVH**	**BVH**	**CENTRAL LESION**
Romberg	Normal	Acute: abnormal Chronic: normal	Acute: abnormal Chronic: normal	Often normal
Tandem Romberg	Normal	Acute: cannot perform Chronic: abnormal, eyes closed	Abnormal; cannot perform with eyes closed	Abnormal
Single-legged stance	Normal	Acute: cannot perform Chronic: normal	Difficult to perform even during compensated stage, with EO	May be unable to perform
Gait	Acute: Normal or wide-based, slow, decreased trunk rotation Compensated: Normal	Acute: wide-based, slow, decreased trunk rotation; may need help initially Compensated: normal	Acute: wide-based, slow, decreased trunk rotation; cannot tandem walk EC Compensated: mild deviations	May be slow or shuffling, or marked ataxia
Turn head while walking	May cause slight unsteadiness	Acute: cannot keep balance Compensated: normal; some may slow cadence	Gait slows, BOS widens, step length decreases; may lose balance	May lose balance, increased ataxia

BPPV, benign paroxysmal postural vertigo; UVH, unilateral vestibular hypofunction; BVH, bilateral vestibular hypofunction; EO, eyes open; EC, eyes closed; BOS, base of support.

disorders. Individuals with peripheral vestibular disorders may adopt a stiff or robot-like gait pattern that limits movement of the head and trunk with excessive use of visual fixation.[38] A variety of gait disorders are seen with central pathology, but gait ataxia is usually associated with cerebellar dysfunction.

Functional tests are used to determine activity limitations and to identify tasks that a patient needs to practice. Three mobility scales Tinetti Performance-Oriented Mobility Assessment (POMA),[70] Timed Up and Go Test (TUG),[71] Berg Balance Scale (BBS)[72] and two gait scales (i.e., Dynamic Gait Index,[73] Functional Gait Assessment[74]) can be easily used to assess balance performance during functional activities. Most of these tests were designed to assess fall risk in the elderly, with the exception of the Functional Gait Assessment which was developed specifically for use with patients with vestibular disorders.

Clinicians should be alert to "red flags" that may appear during patient examinations. Examples of red flags are constitutional symptoms (i.e., unexplained weight loss, fever, fatigue, malaise), abnormal vital signs (orthostatic hypotension, dysrhythmia), undiagnosed CNS signs and symptoms (e.g., sensory impairments or loss, weakness, poor coordination, upper motor neuron signs [Babinski, spasticity, clonus], altered mental status, spontaneous nystagmus in room light after 2 weeks, vertical nystagmus without torsional component [not BPPV] in room light]), positive vertebral artery test, and cardiopulmonary distress. The clinician should report these symptoms to the referring physician or appropriate health care professional.

● PHYSICAL THERAPY TREATMENT

CASE A, PART II

Based on Mrs. O'Hara's complaints of episodic vertigo that was provoked by rolling in bed and commenced following a head injury, the therapist suspected a possible diagnosis of BPPV. A Dix–Hallpike test was performed with the patient wearing Frenzel lenses and identified a robust up-beating torsional nystagmus accompanied by worsening vertigo and nausea that occurred about 20 seconds after the patient was put in the test position (supine with her head extended over the exam table 30 degrees and rotated to the right 45 degrees) and disappeared 30 seconds later. Dix–Hallpike testing on the left side was negative. The clinician determined that the patient had canalithiasis BPPV involving the right posterior SCC.

Benign Paroxysmal Positional Vertigo

General physical therapy goals and expected outcomes for patients with BPPV are (1) removal of otoconia from the SCCs, (2) remission of vertigo with head movement, (3) improved balance, and (4) independence in all functional activities, involving head motions. Recommended treatment for BPPV utilizes particle repositioning head maneuvers that move the displaced otoconia out of the affected SCC. The three main maneuvers used to treat posterior and anterior SCC BPPV are the (1) Canalith Repositioning Maneuver, (2) Liberatory Maneuver, and (3) Brandt–Daroff Habituation Exercises. Evidence for the efficacy of these treatments to achieve remission of symptoms is strongest for the use of CRM for posterior SCC BPPV.[53] However, even with successful treatment with such maneuvers, BPPV recurs in about one-third of individuals after 1 year and in roughly 50% of all individuals treated by 5 years.[75,76]

The **Canalith Repositioning Maneuver** (CRM, also called the Epley maneuver) is based on the canalithiasis theory of free-floating debris in the SCC and is used to treat the canalithiasis form of posterior and anterior SCC BPPV.[11] CRM involves sequential movement of the head into five positions that will move the debris out of the SCC and into the vestibule (Figure 16-6).

The **Liberatory maneuver** (also called the Semont maneuver) is based on the cupulolithiasis theory of debris adhering to the cupula in the SCC and is used to treat cupulolithiasis of the posterior and anterior SCC BPPV. It can also be used as an alternative treatment for patients who do not tolerate or respond to the CRM. The Liberatory maneuver involves rapidly moving an individual from lying on one side to lying on the other (Figure 16-7). The rapid acceleration and deceleration of the movement from the initial sidelying position to the second (opposite side) sidelying position is presumed to dislodge debris adhering to the cupula of the SCC.[53] Elderly patients and those with back problems may not tolerate the quickness of movement required in this procedure.

Brandt–Daroff exercises consist of repeated movements into and out of positions that cause vertigo (Figure 16-8).[77] The mechanism by which they work is not entirely understood, but proposed mechanisms are: (1) habituation of the CNS to the provoking positions, (2) dislodging debris from the cupula, or (3) causing debris to float out of the SCC.[53] These exercises are typically prescribed for patients who continue to have persistent or mild vertigo even after the CRM and/or Liberatory maneuvers or do not tolerate those maneuvers. The exercises should be performed for 5–10 repetitions, three times per day until the patient has no vertigo for 2 consecutive days. Patients should be instructed that movements must be performed rapidly, which will probably provoke the symptoms. If vertigo is too severe, the number of repetitions can be reduced to three, performed three times per day. It is normal for patients to experience residual symptoms (i.e., disequilibrium and nausea) after doing the exercises, but these are usually temporary and should not prevent the patient from continuing the exercises.

Because of the relative rarity of horizontal SCC BPPV, there are no best practices established for treatment maneuvers. The canalithiasis form of horizontal canal BPPV can be effectively treated with either the Bar-B-Que Roll or the Casani (also known as the Gufoni) maneuvers.[78,79] The Bar-B-Que Roll maneuver entails moving the head through a series of 90-degree angles and pausing between each turn for 10–30 seconds (Figure 16-9). The Casani (or Gufoni) maneuver (Figure 16-10) is the primary treatment for the cupulolithiasis form of horizontal SCC BPPV.[80] For horizontal SCC canalithiasis BPPV that does not

FIGURE 16-6 Canalith Repositioning Maneuver. The patient is taken through five positions to move the debris through the canal: (**A**) long-sitting with the head rotated 45 degrees toward the affected side; (**B**) quickly moved to supine with head extended 30 degrees while maintaining the 45 degree rotation to the affected side, then maintained for 1–2 minutes; (**C**) turn head to the opposite side while maintaining extension over the end of the table; (**D**) roll to side without moving the head, again maintained for 1–2 minutes; (**E**) return to sitting on the side of the plinth.

FIGURE 16-7 Liberatory maneuver. The Liberatory maneuver is used to dislodge the debris within the cupula by (**A**) patient is initially in sidelying; (**B**) patient is rapidly brought to sitting on the side of the plinth; and (**C**) patient is rapidly brought to sidelying on the opposite side. This is done by a fluid movement from one side to the other.

FIGURE 16-8 Brandt–Daroff exercises. The patient begins by sitting sideways on the bed; then, quickly lies down on her side with her head turned 45 degrees toward the ceiling. She returns to upright and then quickly lies down on the other side, again with the head turned 45 degrees toward the ceiling.

FIGURE 16-9 Bar-B-Que Roll maneuver for the treatment of geotropic right horizontal SCC-BPPV. Turn head toward the involved ear while lying supine (**A**), then turn head 270 degrees toward the unaffected side through a series of stepwise 90-degree turns (**B–D**); then resume the sitting position (**E**). Each position should be maintained for at least 1 or 2 minutes, or until the induced nystagmus and vertigo are resolved. The corresponding illustrations demonstrate the orientation of the semicircular canals and the location of the otolithic debris in the horizontal canal.

FIGURE 16-10 Casani maneuver – for the treatment of horizontal SCC cupulolithiasis BPPV. In the Casani maneuver the patient moves quickly from sitting position (**A**) to sidelying on the affected side (**B**). The patient then quickly turns the head so that the nose points down 45 degrees (**C**) and remains in that position for 2–3 minutes before coming back to sitting. (Reproduced with permssion from Casani AP, Vannucci G, Fattori B, et al: The treatment of horizontal canal positional vertigo: our experience in 66 cases, *Laryngoscope* 2002 Jan;112(1):172–178.)

respond to head maneuvers, a home treatment called forced prolonged positioning may be recommended.[81] The patient goes to bed and lies in sidelying on the affected side (more symptomatic side) for 30–60 seconds and then slowly rolls over to sidelying with the unaffected ear down. The patient remains in this position all night, permitting the otoconia to gradually move out of the canal.

Originally, posttreatment instructions, following particle repositioning maneuvers, asked patients to keep their heads upright for 48 hours, including sleeping with the head elevated 45 degrees. The evidence does not support that sleeping upright after the CRM and Liberatory maneuvers is necessary.[82,83] After successful treatment with particle repositioning maneuvers, some patients may continue to experience residual disequilibrium and balance problems that may require further physical therapy interventions. Before discharging the patient, the physical therapist should teach the patient how to perform the appropriate techniques at home in case of recurrence.

CASE A, PART III

Based on Mrs. O'Hara's diagnosis of right posterior SCC canalithiasis BPPV, the patient was treated with the CRM (Epley) maneuver. Following treatment, the Dix–Hallpike test was performed again in the same position that had exacerbated her symptoms previously. The nystagmus had resolved and the patient reported marked improvement of her symptoms. The patient was given a BPPV education sheet, scheduled a follow-up in 2 weeks, and instructed to return to physical therapy as soon as possible if she experienced worsening symptoms. At the patient's follow-up, she reported complete resolution of symptoms and was able to lie flat in bed, roll over, and pitch her head up and down without causing vertigo.

CASE B, PART I

Mr. Huffman is a 65-year-old accountant who experienced a sudden onset of vertigo, nausea, vomiting, and imbalance 2 weeks after he had a flu-like illness. Ten days after the onset of his vertigo, he was referred to physical therapy for vestibular rehabilitation with a diagnosis of right UVH secondary to vestibular neuritis. Previous caloric testing reported a 35% weakness in the right ear. Oculomotor testing revealed a left-beating spontaneous vestibular nystagmus, which was suppressed in light. Gaze stability testing revealed an impaired VOR with a positive right head thrust test, and there was a change of visual acuity from 20/20 to 20/40 (i.e., 3-line decrement) on the DVA test. Mr. Huffman scored 15/24 on the DGI (score of <19 indicates increased risk of falls).[73] His mCTSIB results showed an impaired ability to maintain balance in the condition with his eyes closed and standing on foam (condition 6). His DHI of 40% indicated a moderate perception of handicap due to dizziness. The patient exhibited imbalance during the FGA, stepping outside a 12-inch wide path six times over a 20-feet long walkway. Mr. Huffman reported functional problems on the VD-ADL with scores of 4 (slower, cautious, more careful) on most activities. At the beginning of his evaluation, he rated his dizziness as 3/10 using a VAS. His self-rated dizziness increased to 7/10 during the evaluation, particularly with head turns.

Unilateral Vestibular Hypofunction

General physical therapy goals for individuals with UVH and expected outcomes are to (1) improve the patient's gaze stability to see clearly, during head movements, (2) decrease the patient's sensations of disequilibrium and oscillopsia with head motions, (3) improve static and dynamic postural stability, during functional tasks, and (4) return the patient to his or her previous level of activity and participation in society. Mechanisms that are involved in the recovery of function after unilateral vestibular loss include functional recovery of hair cells or vestibular nerves, spontaneous rebalancing of the tonic firing rate centrally, adaptive changes in the residual vestibular system, the substitution of alternative strategies, and habituation of unpleasant sensations.[84] Cochrane reviews in 2007 and 2011 on vestibular rehabilitation concluded that there is moderate to strong evidence that vestibular rehabilitation is a safe and effective treatment for patients with UVH or loss, and moderate evidence exists that vestibular rehabilitation is an effective treatment of patients during the acute onset of vestibular neuritis or after resection of VS.[85,86] Patients should expect improved function within 6 weeks, if they are compliant with vestibular rehabilitation exercises.[84]

Gaze Stability Exercises

Individuals with visual blurring and dizziness, when performing tasks that require visual tracking or gaze stabilization, can benefit from specific exercises. In patients with some vestibular function, adaptation of the VOR can be facilitated by exposing the patient to small amounts of **retinal slip**, which occurs when the image of an object moves off the fovea. The error signal that is generated by retinal slip stimulates vestibular adaptation within the brain. Exercises that are used to induce adaptation via retinal slip include having the patient maintain visual fixation of an object (i.e., thumb or business card) while the head is moving under the following two paradigms: (1) with the visual target stationary, the patient moves the head back and forth while maintaining visual fixation (X1 paradigm) and (2) the persons' head and the visual target move in opposite directions while the person keeps the target in focus (X2 paradigm) (Figure 16-11). These exercises can be progressed by (1) increasing the directions of head movements, (2) the duration and frequency of exercise bouts (e.g., start with 1 minute twice a day if tolerated

and progress to 2 minutes five times a day), (3) the speed of head movements, (4) the distance of the target (start with near target [3 feet] and progress to far target [8–10 feet]), (5) the size of the target (e.g., checkerboard, outdoors), or (6) changing body position (e.g., start sitting or standing, progressing to walking forward or backward, stepping up or down).[87]

In individuals with poor or no VOR, exercises that promote the use of saccadic and pursuit eye movements and central preprogramming are prescribed.[84] These exercises include (1) active eye movements followed by head movements between two horizontal targets and (2) visualization of remembered targets. In the eye followed by head movement exercise, two letters (e.g., X and Z) are placed on a wall about 2-feet apart (i.e., close enough that the patient can look at one of the targets and see the other target out of the corner of the eye). The patient is asked to look directly at the X, with the head rotated so that the nose is aligned with the X. Without moving the head, the patient shifts gaze to the other target. Then, the patient turns his/her head toward the second target, while maintaining fixation on the target during the head movement. The exercise is repeated to both sides multiple times. In the remembered target exercise, the patient starts by looking directly ahead at a target. Then the patient closes the eyes and turns the head, while attempting to maintain the eyes on the remembered target location. The patient opens the eyes and sees if he is looking at the target. This exercise may enhance use of cervical inputs to generate eye movements that keep the eye on target or cortical co-activation, producing the head and eye movement.[84]

Habituation Exercises (Motion Sensitivity)

Habituation exercises can be used to treat continual complaints of movement-provoked dizziness. These exercises are based on the concept that repeated exposure to provoking positions or movements causes a reduction in the response to the stimuli. The original habituation exercises were developed and studied by Cawthorne and Cooksey[88,89] (see Box 16-2), Norre and DeWeerdt,[90] and Dix.[91] In recent years, many clinicians use the Motion Sensitivity Quotient results (MSQ, see earlier section on

FIGURE 16-11 Gaze stability exercise. A. X1 Paradigm – Patient moves head back and forth while maintaining gaze on stable target. **B.** X2 Paradigm – Patient moves head back and forth while moving target in the opposite direction.

BOX 16-2   Cawthorne and Cooksey Habituation Exercises

The patient completes 4–5 repetitions of each exercise first slowly and then faster; many can be done initially with eyes open and then progressed to eyes closed[84,88,89]

Eye movements (sitting and standing):

- Holding the head still, looks up and down, to each side
- Looks at their finger as it moves closer to their eyes and further away

Head movement (sitting and standing):

- Alternately rotates head to the right and left
- Alternately moves head up and down

Body movement (sitting)

- Bends to the floor to pick up an object, returns to upright and lifts above head
- Circular shoulder movements
- Bends forward to retrieve object through their knees, returns to upright and then places back through knees

Coming to standing

- Rises to stand from sitting and returns (eyes open, eyes closed)
- Comes to standing and turns to right or left, returns to sitting (eyes open or closed)

Standing: can be done on firm surface and progress to soft surface

- Tosses a ball back and forth from one hand to another at waist level
- Tosses ball back and forth through knees while bent forward
- Single limb stance

Walking: can be done initially on a firm surface and progressed to a soft surface; can also progress to eyes closed

- Alternately turns head to right and left
- Tip toe walking
- Moves in a circle while therapist unexpectedly tosses a ball to them

TABLE 16-9   Progression of Habituation Exercises to Treat Patients with Unilateral Vestibular Hypofunction[93]

WEEK	HABITUATION EXERCISE
1	Large amplitude, rapid cervical movements (horizontal or vertical), consisting of 5 complete movements (cycles) performed 3 times in sitting
2	Large amplitude, rapid horizontal cervical rotation (seated) and standing pivots, or large amplitude, rapid vertical cervical movement (seated) and seated trunk flexion-extension, 3 sets of 5 cycles
3	Large amplitude, rapid horizontal and vertical cervical movements (seated) and standing pivots, or large amplitude, rapid horizontal and vertical cervical movements (seated) and seated trunk flexion-extension, 3 sets of 5 cycles
4	Large amplitude, rapid horizontal and vertical cervical movements (seated), standing pivots, and seated trunk flexion-extension, 3 sets of 5 cycles
5	Large amplitude, rapid horizontal and vertical cervical movements (standing), standing pivots, and seated trunk flexion-extension, 3 sets of 5 cycles
6	Large amplitude, rapid horizontal and vertical cervical movements (standing), standing pivots (180 degrees), seated trunk flexion-extension, Brandt–Daroff exercises (Figure 16-8), 3 sets of 5 cycles

testing) to determine provoking movements and to develop an individualized exercise program.[92,93] In this approach, up to four movements are chosen from the MSQ as the basis of the patient's exercise program. The patient repeats the movements three to five times, two to three times a day, with rests between movements to allow the symptoms to stop. The effectiveness of these exercises is improved, if the patient performs the movements quickly enough and through enough range to produce mild to moderate symptoms.[84] Whenever possible, the habituation exercises should be incorporated into the person's daily activities. In addition, a home exercise program (HEP) based on the provoking head movements, which may include Brandt–Daroff exercises, should be provided. Table 16-9 provides a progression of habituation exercises used to reduce dizziness in patients with UVH. It may take 4 weeks for symptoms to decrease.[84]

Postural Stability Exercises

Postural stability exercises aim to improve the patient's balance control and prevent falls. When developing an intervention program for balance impairments, clinicians need to consider their patients' impairments across all systems and decide which impairments can be rehabilitated and which require compensation or substitution. For example, individuals with vestibular deficits often experience postural instability, when performing activities with reduced visual and/or somatosensory inputs. Therefore, they may benefit from performing exercises and tasks that remove or alter visual and somatosensory cues to force them to utilize the remaining sensory inputs. Head movements should be included in exercises as many people with vestibular loss will decrease their head movement. Motor learning concepts (i.e., practice parameters, feedback, stages of learning, task analysis, environmental conditions) should be incorporated into balance training. Box 16-3 provides examples of balance exercises and progressions to address identified deficits in static, dynamic, anticipatory, and reactive balance control as well as problems involving sensory organization, functional performance, and safety.

BOX 16-3 Postural Stability Exercises and Interventions

Static balance control

To promote static balance control, the patient can start by maintaining a standing posture on a firm surface. More challenging activities include practice in the tandem and single-leg stance, lunge, and squat positions. Progress these activities by standing on soft surfaces (e.g., foam, sand, and grass), narrowing the base of support, moving the head, or closing the eyes. Add a secondary task (i.e., catching ball or mental calculations) to further increase the level of difficulty.

Dynamic balance control

To promote dynamic balance control, interventions may involve the following:

- Maintain equal weight distribution and upright trunk postural alignment while standing on a soft surface (e.g., carpeting, foam, wobble boards). Progress the activities by superimposing movements such as shifting the body weight, rotating the trunk, rotating the head side-to-side or up and down.
- Perform standing bends and squats on firm surface. Progress to narrow base of support, eyes closed, soft surface, reaching to touch floor.
- Transitions into and out of chair or on and off floor. Progress to without arm support, eyes closed.
- March in place with eyes open on a firm surface. Progress to marching with eyes closed, on soft surfaces, and with head turns.
- Walk and turn suddenly or walk in a circle while gradually decreasing the circumference of the circle, first in one direction and then in another.

Anticipatory balance control

To practice anticipatory balance control the patient can perform the following:

- Reach in all directions to touch or grasp objects, catch a ball, or kick a ball.
- Bend and pick up objects off of lower surfaces.
- Perform step-up and down exercises or lunges in multiple directions.
- Maneuver through an obstacle course.

Reactive balance control

To train reactive balance control the patient can perform the following activities:

- Work to gradually increase the amount of sway in standing in different directions while on a firm stable surface.
- Practice forward walking with abrupt stops. Progress to backward walking.
- To emphasize training of the *ankle strategy*, practice swaying while standing on one leg with the trunk erect.
- To emphasize training of the *hip strategy*, walk on lines drawn on the floor, perform tandem stance, perform single-leg stance with trunk bending, or stand on a rocker balance board.
- To emphasize the *stepping strategy*, practice stepping up onto a stool or curb or over progressively larger obstacles (i.e., electric cord, shoe, phone book) or practice stepping with legs crossed in front or behind the other leg (e.g., weaving or braiding).
- To increase the challenge during these activities, add anticipated and unanticipated external forces. For example, have the patient lift boxes that are identical in appearance but of different weights, throw and catch balls of different weights and sizes.

Sensory organization

Many of the activities previously described can be utilized while varying the reliance on specific sensory systems.

- To reduce or destabilize the *visual inputs*, have the patient close the eyes or practice in low lighting or darkness, or move the eyes and head together during the balance activity.
- To decrease reliance on *somatosensory cues*, patients can narrow the BOS, stand on a soft surface, or stand on an unstable surface (i.e., rocker or incline board).

Examples of these types of activities might include the following:

- Walking backward, side-stepping, and braiding performed with the eyes closed.
- Walking while watching a ball being tossed from one hand to the other.
- Walking with head and eye movements.
- Standing or marching in place on foam performed first with eyes open and later with eyes closed.
- Walking across an exercise mat or mattress in the dark.

Balance during functional activities

Clinicians should focus on activities similar to the activity limitations identified in the evaluation. For example, if reaching is limited, then the patient should work on activities such as reaching for a glass in the cupboard, reaching behind (as putting arm in a sleeve), or catching a ball off center. Having the patient perform two or more tasks simultaneously increases the level of task complexity. Practicing recreational activities that the patient enjoys, such as golf, increases motivation for practice while challenging balance control.

Safety during gait, locomotion, or balance

To emphasize safety, clinicians should have the patient practice postural sway activities within the person's actual stability limits and progress dynamic activities with emphasis on promoting function. If balance deficits cannot be changed, environmental modifications (e.g., better lighting, installation of grab bars, removal of throw rugs), assistive devices, and increased family or external support may be required to ensure safety.

CASE B, PART II

Based on Mr. Huffman's diagnosis of right UVH and the results of his physical therapy examination, the therapist developed an individualized vestibular rehabilitation program for Mr. Huffman that included progressive gaze stabilization exercises and static and dynamic balance exercises.

Gaze stability exercises included horizontal and vertical head movements, performed while the patient moved his head as quickly as possible, while keeping a stationary target in focus. These exercises were performed with near and far targets four to five times a day. Static and dynamic balance exercises were performed on compliant surfaces (carpeting, foam) with varied foot positions. Visual input was altered by having Mr. Huffman close his eyes or wear blurry glasses to obscure his vision. He rated his dizziness at the beginning and end of each session, using a VAS to determine correct exercise intensity. The physical therapist periodically provided education about his diagnosis, the course of treatment, and prognosis. After completing seven 1-hour treatments, spaced 1-week apart, Mr. Huffman reported 0/10 dizziness and scored a 5% on the DHI, indicating minimal perception of handicap from dizziness. With the exception of the DHI, the majority of vestibular outcome measures do not have established clinically meaningful difference values (MCID). Since the MCID values for the DHI is 18 points, Mr. Huffman's change of 35 points may be considered clinically important.[40] He had a normal score on the mCTSIB and a score of 24/24 on the DGI. Over a long walkway, he easily stayed inside a 12-inch wide path. Mr. Huffman's gaze stability was within normal limits, with a change in visual acuity from 20/20 to 20/30 on the DVA test. He scored "independent" on the VD-ADL and was able to resume his previous activities and roles and responsibilities without symptoms.

Bilateral Vestibular Hypofunction

General physical therapy goals for individuals with BVH and expected outcomes are to (1) improve the patient's gaze stability, (2) decrease the patient's complaints of disequilibrium and oscillopsia with head motions, (3) improve static and dynamic postural stability, during functional tasks, and (4) prevent physical deconditioning by engaging in a walking program. Mechanisms of recovery of gaze stability in BVH are central preprogramming of eye movements and modifications in saccadic and smooth pursuit eye movements.[94] A study that examined recovery of postural stability in patients with bilateral vestibular deficits over a 2-year period found that patients initially rely on visual inputs as a substitute for loss of vestibular inputs, but over time, they become more dependent on somatosensory inputs to maintain balance.[94] Several studies support the use of a vestibular rehabilitation exercise program to decrease subjective complaints, improve visual acuity during head movement, and improve postural stability during functional activities.[95-99] Recovery for individuals with bilateral vestibular deficits is slower than for unilateral lesions and may take up to 2 years.[94] Certain activities will always be limited, such as walking in low-vision conditions or over uneven surfaces, night driving, and sports that involve quick movements of the head.[94,100]

For patients with BVH who have some remaining function, gaze stability exercises can be similar to the X1 paradigm exercises used for people with UVH. Some individuals with BVH do not tolerate the X2 paradigm exercises due to excessive retinal slip, but those with asymmetrical BVH may tolerate and benefit from the exercise. Patients with very low or no peripheral vestibular function will benefit from the sequenced eye and head movement and imaginary target exercises (see earlier section) that substitute smooth pursuit and saccadic eye movements to stabilize gaze. Additional substitution strategies to improve eye stabilization include performing eye movements without head motion (i.e., stop and stand still while reading signs) and with head movement while focusing on a distant object (i.e., walk in open spaces while focusing the eyes on a distant object).

Balance exercises for individuals with BVH should enhance the substitution of visual and somatosensory information to improve postural stability and develop compensatory strategies that can be used in situations where balance is highly stressed.[94] People with BVH are at high risk of falls, and therefore, clinicians must be careful that balance exercises are performed safely. Balance exercises that vary the reliance on specific sensory systems similar to those for individuals with UVH may be beneficial. Compensatory strategies that can be taught to prevent falls are (1) using night lights if they get out of bed at night, (2) using lights that come on automatically, (3) having emergency lighting inside and outside of the house in case of power failure, and (4) learning how to safely move around places with busy visual environments such as shopping malls and grocery stores.[94] Some individuals with BVH may require the use of an assistive device when walking at night, on uneven surfaces, and in busy environments.

Patients with BVH may become physically deconditioned due to decreased activity levels, resulting from a fear of falling or increased dizziness from movement.[94] Therefore, it is very important to get individuals with BVH on a walking program, preferably daily. This program should be progressed to challenge patients by having them walk over different surfaces (e.g., carpeting, foam, grass, sand) and in different environments (e.g., mall, grocery store). Exercises in a pool may be advantageous, as the buoyancy of the water may allow the person with BVH to move without fear of falling to the ground. Patient should be educated on the importance of maintaining daily activity after vestibular rehabilitation ends.

Central Vestibular Disorders

General physical therapy goals and expected outcomes for patients with central vestibular disorders include (1) demonstration of appropriate fall prevention strategies and precautions for safe functioning in daily life, (2) demonstration of appropriate selection of compensatory strategies for gaze stability, and (3) prevention of physical deconditioning by engaging in a walking program. Recovery from central lesions is often prolonged (≥ 6 months) and may be incomplete because areas of the central nervous system that are likely responsible for adaptive mechanisms may be damaged by the initial lesion.

Physical therapy interventions for individuals with central vestibular lesions will depend on the location of the lesion and the patient's signs and symptoms. Treatment of people with lesions of the vestibular nuclei will probably be similar to treatment for a person with UVH. Treatment of patients with complaints of dizziness may respond to gaze stability and/or habituation exercises. However, clinicians are cautioned not to be too aggressive with these exercises to avoid excessive aggravation of the patient's symptoms. Gait and balance exercises that promote integration of somatosensory, visual, and vestibular inputs are often effective with these patients.

● CEREBELLAR DISORDERS

CASE C, PART I

Mrs. Falstaff is a 52-year-old homemaker who has experienced progressive balance problems, for the last 3 years, and several episodes of spontaneous vertigo, lasting for a few seconds while walking. She was referred to physical therapy for balance and gait training and fall prevention with a genetically confirmed diagnosis of spinocerebellar atrophy type 6 (SCA 6). Her subjective history reveals that she has fallen five times in the last 6 months, all of which occurred in her home while walking, and once sustained an ankle sprain, while descending stairs, that required medical care. She uses a cane, when walking in the community, but at home, prefers to use walls and furniture to navigate in her house. Her father, sister, and two brothers all have the same condition. The result of a recent head MRI indicates cerebellar atrophy. The physical therapist's examination findings include dysarthric speech and cerebellar ataxia in the lower extremities. Her Scale for the Assessment and Rating of Ataxia (SARA) score was 28/40 and her performance on the TUG was 25 seconds with use of a cane. Her mCTSIB results showed an impaired ability to maintain balance when her vision was removed or standing on foam (i.e., Conditions 2–4). She rated herself as 30% on the ABC Scale.

Anatomy and Physiology of the Cerebellum

For a discussion of the anatomy and physiology of the normal cerebellum and its role in control of movements, readers are referred to Chapter 5.

Disorders of the Cerebellum

Due to the cerebellum's critical role in coordinating and adapting movements, damage to the cerebellum often results in disabling **ataxia**, defined as the loss of muscle coordination without apparent weakness. Cerebellar ataxia results from a variety of acquired and hereditary causes as described in Table 16-10. Strokes that involve any of the three arteries that supply blood to the cerebellum (e.g., superior, anterior inferior, and posterior inferior cerebellar arteries; refer to Chapter 10) can result in cerebellar damage. The cerebellum is also sensitive to toxins, including heavy metals, solvents, and alcohol. Chronic alcoholism causes cerebellar atrophy primarily in the anterior superior vermis.[101] Medications that can cause cerebellar ataxia are certain antiepileptic drugs (e.g., carbamazepine [Tegretol], phenytoin [Dilantin]), lithium salts (Eskalith, Lithobid), certain cancer chemotherapeutic drugs, cyclosporine (Gengraf, Neoral, Sandimmune), and the antibiotic metronidazole (Flagyl). Tumors in the posterior fossa, in or near the cerebellum, occur more frequently in children than in adults.[102] Multiple sclerosis is the most common nonhereditary cause of cerebellar damage.[103] Chiari and other congenital malformations cause damaging pressure and mechanical deformation of the cerebellum (see Chapter 18). Studies in animals and individuals with TBI demonstrate that the cerebellum is often damaged in traumatic brain injuries, even when the initial mechanical forces are directed at the cerebral cortex (see Chapter 11).[104,105]

Of the hereditary causes of cerebellar damage, the highest prevalence is Friedreich's ataxia, followed by the spinocerebellar ataxias.[103] **Friedreich's ataxia** (also called FA or FRDA) is an autosomal recessive inherited disease that causes progressive damage to the spinal cord (dorsal columns, corticospinal and spinocerebellar tracts), dorsal root ganglia, cerebellum, and cranial nerves

TABLE 16-10	Selected Causes of Cerebellar Damage[102,103]
ACQUIRED CAUSES	**HEREDITARY CAUSES**

• Stroke (ischemic, hemorrhagic)
• Toxicity (alcohol, heavy metals [mercury, lead, thallium], medications, organic solvents [toluene, benzene], phencyclidine [PCP])
• Tumor (primary cerebellar tumor, metastatic disease)
• Immune-mediated (multiple sclerosis, celiac disease, vasculitis [Behcet's disease, lupus], paraneoplastic cerebellar degeneration)
• Congenital and developmental (Chiari malformation, agenesis, hypoplasias [Joubert syndrome, Dandy–Walker cyst], dysplasias)
• Infection (cerebellitis, abscess)
• Metabolic (hypothyroidism, acute thiamine [B1] deficiency, chronic vitamin B_{12} and E deficiencies)
• Trauma
• Degenerative nonhereditary diseases (multiple system atrophy [MSA], idiopathic late-onset cerebellar ataxia [ILOCA])
	Autosomal recessive:
	  • Friedreich's ataxia (FA)
	  • Early onset cerebellar ataxia (EOCA)
	  • Ataxia telangiectasia
	Autosomal dominant:
	  • Spinocerebellar ataxias (SCAs)
	  • Episodic ataxias (EAs)
	  • Dentato-rubral-pallidoluysian atrophy (DRPLA)
	  • Gerstmann–Straussler–Scheinker (GSS) disease
	X-linked disorders:
	  • Mitochondrial disease
	  • Fragile X-associated tremor/ataxia syndrome

VII, X, and XII, causing progressive limb and gait ataxia, dysarthria, loss of proprioception and vibration sensations, absent tendon reflexes, abnormal eye movements, and upper motor neuron signs. Other symptoms that often accompany FA are hypertrophic cardiomyopathy, diabetes, scoliosis, pes cavus, and restless leg syndrome. Symptoms typically begin between the ages of 5 and 15 years, and generally patients lose the ability to transfer and walk without assistance between 10 and 15 years after disease onset.[102] **Spinocerebellar ataxias** (SCAs) are a group of over 35 distinct autosomal dominant hereditary diseases, which are named by numbers (e.g., SCA1, SCA2).[102] Depending on the genetic abnormality, cerebellar damage may occur alone or may be combined with extracerebellar damage. Onset is usually during the third or fourth decade of life, and progression is usually slow, which means that children of affected parents will likely not know until they are adults whether they are affected. Related autosomal dominant inherited diseases that are more rare are the **episodic ataxias** (EAs), characterized by recurrent, discrete episodes of vertigo, ataxia, and often migraine headaches and nausea, lasting minutes to hours that are provoked by stress, excitement, or exercise.[102] Some of the EAs are effectively treated with aminopyridines (3,4-diaminopyridine [3,4-DAP] and 4-aminopyridine [4-AP]) and acetazolamide (Diamox).[102,106]

Clinical Manifestations of Cerebellar Damage

Ataxia is the primary sign of cerebellar damage, which can be used to describe uncoordinated gait (**gait ataxia**) or uncoordinated arm and leg movements (**limb ataxia**). Cerebellar ataxia worsens with movements of multiple joints and with quick movements. Table 16-11 shows the common signs and symptoms of cerebellar dysfunction.

Limb Movements

Limb movements, in cerebellar disease, are characterized by dysmetria, dyssynergia, dysdiadochokinesia, movement decomposition, and rebound. **Dysmetria** is an inaccuracy of

TABLE 16-11	Signs and Symptoms of Cerebellar Damage		
SYMPTOM/SIGN	**AREA OF CEREBELLAR DAMAGE**	**FUNCTIONAL MANIFESTATION**	**EXAMINATION FINDINGS**
Limb ataxia • Dysmetria • Dyssynergia • Dysdiadochokinesia • Decomposition • Rebound	Lateral cerebellum, deep cerebellar nuclei (globose, emboliform, part of dentate nuclei)	Uncoordinated movement of ipsilateral arm and/or leg	Impaired FTN* and HTS** • Impaired rapid alternating movements • Slow, effortful fine finger movements • Impaired limb rebound
Tremor	Cerebellar efferent pathways to the red nucleus and inferior olivary nucleus, deep cerebellar nuclei	• Postural tremor • Kinetic tremor • Intention tremor (<5 Hz)	• Side-to-side tremor of out-stretched arms or tremor when standing still • End-point tremor on FTN or HTS test
Hypotonia	Vermis, flocculonodular lobe	Decreased ability to maintain a steady force	• Ipsilateral hypotonia of limbs • Pendular deep tendon reflexes
Balance and gait dysfunction	Anterior lobe, vermis, fastigial nucleus	• Wide-based stance • Uncoordinated gait • Difficulty with stopping or turning • Frequent falls	• Impaired sharpened Romberg test • Impaired spatiotemporal/ kinematic gait parameters • Unsteady tandem gait • Impaired stopping and turning
Oculomotor dysfunction	Flocculonodular lobe, vermis, fastigial nucleus	• Oscillopsia • Blurred or double vision	• Nystagmus • Impaired slow pursuit • Impaired shift of gaze/saccades • Impaired VOR cancellation
Speech impairments	Rostral paravermal region of the anterior lobes	• Dysarthria • Slurred speech	• Impaired articulation and prosody • May be slow, hesitant, or accentuate some syllables
Cognitive and psychiatric impairments	Bilateral posterior lobes (cognitive), vermis (emotional)	• Memory problems, difficulty functioning at work or in home • Impaired communication skills • Personality changes	• Impaired executive functions • Impaired visuospatial function • Agrammatism, dysprosodia • Blunted affect or disinhibited, inappropriate behavior

*FTN, finger-to-nose.
**HTS, heel-to-shin.

movement in which the desired target is either under-reached (hypometria) or over-reached (hypermetria). Dysmetria is generally worse with multi-joint compared to single-joint limb movements, and slow movements tend to produce hypometria while fast movements produce hypermetria.[107] **Dyssynergia** describes uncoordinated multi-joint movements, where movements of specific segments are not properly sequenced or of the appropriate amplitude or direction. Dysmetria and dyssynergia appear to be related and are thought to be due to a deficit in predicting and accounting for the dynamics of the limbs.[107] **Dysdiadochokinesia** refers to an impaired ability to perform rapid alternating movements (e.g. supination-pronation). Patients with cerebellar dysfunction typically demonstrate excessive slowness with inconsistency in the rate and range of alternating movements, which worsen as the movement continues.[108] **Movement decomposition** refers to the breakdown of a movement sequence or multi-joint movement into separate movements that are simpler to perform than the combined movement. A well-known example of this is that patients with cerebellar damage, when asked to reach for an object in front and above the resting arm, will often flex the shoulder first and then, while holding the shoulder fixed, extend the elbow.[107] This produces a slower and more curved path of the finger to the target, compared to the faster and straight line path of healthy individuals. Movement decomposition may be a compensatory strategy for dealing with impaired multi-joint movements.[107] **Rebound** refers to an inability to rapidly and sufficiently stop movement of a body part after strong isometric resistance of the body part is suddenly removed. Healthy individuals are able to quickly halt the movement, while patients with cerebellar damage show considerable movement in the direction opposite to the applied resistance. This phenomenon is thought to be caused by delayed cessation of the agonist muscles and/or delayed activation of the antagonist muscles.

Tremor

Tremors caused by cerebellar damage are called **action tremors**, meaning that they are elicited during muscle activation and not when the person is at rest. Action tremors are further classified as **postural** or **kinetic** tremors. Postural tremors are seen in muscles that are maintaining a static position against gravity, while kinetic tremors are observed in muscles that are producing an active voluntary movement. Kinetic tremors typically occur at low frequencies below 5 Hz.[109] **Intention tremor** is a specific type of kinetic tremor that is observed as an increase in tremor amplitude that occurs in the terminal portion of visually guided movements toward a target. It occurs because the person is using visual feedback to make corrective movements to reach the target; an intention tremor is diminished or absent, if vision is removed.[103] **Titubation** is a specific type of postural tremor characterized by slow-frequency oscillations (about 3 Hz) of the head or trunk.[110] The cause of cerebellar tremors is not well understood but proposed mechanisms are (1) an inability to anticipate movements with excessive reliance on sensory feedback (i.e., vision, proprioception) and (2) central influences involving pathways connecting the dentate nucleus, red nucleus, and inferior olivary nucleus.[103,109]

Hypotonia and Muscle Force Generation

Hypotonia, in individuals with cerebellar damage, usually manifests as a decrease in extensor tone necessary to keep the body upright against gravity. Pendular deep tendon reflexes (e.g., leg swings more than four times in response to briskly tapping the quadriceps tendon) and inability to check forearm movement in the rebound test have been attributed to hypotonia but may have other explanations.[109] Hypotonia may be due to decreased excitatory inputs to the vestibulospinal and reticulospinal tracts from the cerebellar vermis and flocculonodular lobe, as individuals with severe cerebellar hypoplasias, affecting the vermis, such as Joubert syndrome, have greater degrees of hypotonia.[111] Notably, hypotonia usually does not interfere with physical function in individuals with cerebellar damage.[112]

Although cerebellar damage does not typically cause loss of functional motor strength, many patients experience problems with sustaining a steady force with their hands, which they may refer to as weakness. A reduced rate of force generation (power) as well as variability in maintaining a constant level of force have been reported in individuals with cerebellar damage.[113,114] These deficits in force generation may affect performance of precision manipulative hand tasks.

Balance and Gait Dysfunction

Individuals with cerebellar damage demonstrate impaired static, dynamic, reactive, and anticipatory balance control. Increased postural sway is typically observed in quiet stance, with some variations in sway frequency, amplitude, and direction depending on the site of the lesion.[115,116] Individuals with cerebellar damage, isolated to the anterior lobe, show increased postural sway, which is high-frequency, low amplitude, and mainly in the anterior–posterior direction. They also exhibit postural tremor and increased movements of the head, trunk, and legs and tend to improve their stability with visual feedback. In contrast, individuals with isolated damage to the flocculonodular lobe tend to exhibit low-frequency, high-amplitude sway without a preferred direction and without associated head, trunk, and leg movements. These individuals do not improve performance with visual feedback. Individuals with lateral cerebellar lesions tend to have slight or even no postural instability.

In response to an unexpected perturbation of the support surface, individuals with cerebellar damage show hypermetric responses, characterized by abnormally large and prolonged muscle activity and greater surface-reactive torque responses that cause them to overshoot the initial posture during the balance recovery phase.[117] This seems to indicate an inability to set the correct size (or gain) of the response.[103] However, similar to healthy individuals, people with cerebellar damage are able to decrease the size of their postural responses with repeated trials of a predictable perturbation and can change their response magnitude appropriately to an expected change in the size of a perturbation, although the overall size of the responses remain increased compared to normal.[118,119] Lack of anticipatory postural adjustments (APAs) results in imbalance during self-generated movements, as for example not leaning forward prior to standing on the toes resulting in the person falling backwards.

Gait ataxia in individuals with cerebellar dysfunction is characterized by reduced speed, prolonged time in double stance, abnormal interlimb coordination, and increased variability in stride lengths and kinematics of the hip, knee, and ankle joints, although their base of support may not be increased as commonly presumed.[120-122] Balance deficits have a direct and marked impact on walking, as individuals with cerebellar damage and significant imbalance typically demonstrate the classic features of gait ataxia, while those with cerebellar damage and significant leg coordination deficits but slight to no balance deficits typically have few gait abnormalities.[123] Gait variability (i.e., coefficient of variation in stride time), during slow walking, is associated with a history of falls in individuals with cerebellar ataxia.[124] During walking, individuals with cerebellar ataxia have great difficulty in stopping abruptly and adopt a multistep stopping strategy to compensate for their inability to control the upper body and to generate appropriate braking forces in the lower extremities to stop the progression of the body in the forward direction.[125] Some patients with cerebellar ataxia occasionally stop abruptly with feet parallel instead of one foot forward in relation to the other, which is never seen in control subjects.[125] They also have difficulty performing large turns and adopt compensatory strategies such as enlarging the base of support, shortening step length, increasing the number of steps, and using multiple steps to turn rather than a "spin-turn" strategy.[126,127] Deficits in balance and walking may contribute to the reported high incidence of falls in cerebellar ataxia.[128]

Oculomotor Dysfunction

Since normal oculomotor function relies heavily on the cerebellum for adaptive control, it is not surprising that cerebellar damage can significantly affect eye movements.[103] Smooth pursuit eye movements are slowed, requiring catch-up saccades to keep the eyes fixated on the moving target.[129] The speed of saccadic eye movements is normal in cerebellar disease, but the accuracy is impaired so that both hypometric or hypermetric saccades are seen.[129] VOR cancellation may be diminished or absent.[129,130] There is also reduced velocity of divergent eye movements, which affects the ability to shift gaze from targets close and far away.[103] Numerous types of nystagmus can be seen with cerebellar damage, but the most common form is gaze-evoked nystagmus, elicited near the end ranges of lateral and/or vertical gaze.[129,130] Gaze-evoked nystagmus results in the inability to maintain an eccentric position of gaze. Individuals with significant oculomotor dysfunction should be referred to a vestibular specialist.

Speech Impairments

The speech deficit of individuals with cerebellar dysfunction is **ataxic dysarthria**. The most consistent impairments are found for articulation (pronunciation of speech sounds) and prosody (patterns of stress and intonation of speech). The speech is described as scanning in nature, consisting of hesitations, accentuations of some syllables, the addition of pauses or omission of appropriate pauses, and, in some cases, slurring of syllables.[131] Speech intelligibility may be decreased with problems in distinguishing the difference between plosives (e.g., [p], [t], [k]) at the end of words.[132]

Impaired Motor Learning

Motor learning may be impaired in individuals with cerebellar damage. The cerebellum is very important for motor skill learning through repeated practice of a motor behavior and using error information from one trial to improve performance on the next trial. It is also important for **motor adaptation**, a form of motor learning that involves modification of an already well learned motor skill in response to altered conditions (e.g., adaptation to prism glasses or walking on a split-belt treadmill), which is also an error-driven process. Studies suggest that the type of error that drives cerebellar-dependent learning of reaching is a sensory prediction error (i.e., "How far am I from where I initially predicted that I would be?") rather than a target-referenced error (i.e., "How far am I from the desired target?").[133,134] Similarly, studies have shown that individuals with cerebellar damage have difficulty learning both simple and complex motor behaviors, including recovery from a balance disturbance,[135] walking in a new pattern,[136] or adjusting arm movements for reaching.[137] Thus, clinicians should be aware that individuals with cerebellar damage may take longer to acquire motor skills and adapt motor behaviors and may not ever attain full recovery.

Cognitive and Psychiatric Impairments

Evidence suggests that cerebellar damage can result in a cerebellar-cognitive affective syndrome that consists of executive dysfunctions (i.e., impairments in planning, set-shifting, verbal fluency, abstract reasoning, and working memory), impaired visuospatial functions (organization and memory), mild language difficulties (i.e., agrammatism [inability to construct a grammatical sentence] and dysprosodia [impaired speech intonation patterns]), and personality changes (i.e., blunting of affect, disinhibition, and inappropriate behavior).[138] Certain cerebellar ataxias are associated with neuropsychiatric symptoms such as distractibility, hyperactivity, compulsive obsessive behavior, anxiety, depression, aggression, hallucinations, lack of empathy, and avoidant behavior.[139]

● MEDICAL MANAGEMENT OF CEREBELLAR DAMAGE

There are no curative interventions for people with cerebellar damage. Pharmacological interventions to date have had limited success in reducing symptoms or slowing or stopping disease progression. Individuals with ataxia and degenerative cerebellar disorders are often prescribed vitamin E, coenzyme Q10, acetazolamide (Diamox), 4-aminopyridine (Ampyra), amantadine hydrochloride (Symmetrel), and buspirone chlorhydrate (Buspar), but the effectiveness of these drugs is questionable.[139,140] The mainstays of treatment for people with degenerative cerebellar ataxias are physical therapy, occupational therapy, and speech therapy.[98,102]

● PHYSICAL THERAPY EXAMINATION

Examination of the patient with cerebellar damage includes assessment of limb movement coordination, tremor, balance and gait. These tests would be performed in addition to a systems review and standard neurological assessment that includes evaluation of somatosensation (including cutaneous sensation and proprioception), pain, passive muscle tone, range of motion, muscle strength, muscle endurance, and posture to identify concurrent impairments that might affect the patient's prognosis and treatment (refer to Chapter 9 – Neurologic Evaluation).

Limb Movements

Dysmetria, dyssynergia, and movement decomposition are typically tested with the finger-to-nose (FTN) and heel-to shin (HTS) tests. The FTN test asks the patient to repeatedly touch the tip of his/her nose and then the tip of the clinician's nose or fnger. The HTS test is performed by having the patient bring the heel of the tested leg to the opposite knee and sliding it in a straight line down the anterior aspect of the tibia to the ankle, while keeping the foot nearly vertical. The clinician assesses for movement decomposition, movement speed, variability in the spatial path, and over/undershooting of the target.[103] Dysdiadochokinesia is typically tested by asking the patient to (1) supinate and pronate the forearm or (2) tap the hand or foot. The clinician assesses the rate and amplitude of movement on these tests, which should be performed (1) on both sides to make comparisons, (2) at slow and fast speeds to determine severity of ataxia, (3) with and without vision to determine if vision improves movement quality, and (4) multiple times on the same limb to observe variability in movements (i.e., hypometric on some, hypermetric on others). It is also important to give the patient the proper amount of head and trunk support so that balance deficits do not affect limb movements and to ensure that the patient does not have visual or other oculomotor impairments that would prevent accurate location of a target. Rebound is tested by asking the patient to flex the elbow against the clinician's hand and then the clinician abruptly removes the resistance and assesses the patient's ability to stop the sudden flexion.[129]

Tremor

Postural tremor is tested by asking the patient to stand in place or with the arms out in front of the body with palms facing down. Kinetic tremor can be tested during nontarget directed movements (forearm pronation/supination, hand and foot tapping) or during targeted movements such as the FTN or HTS tests. Intention tremor can be tested by repeating targeted movements with eyes closed; a decrease or disappearance of the tremor with eyes closed compared to eyes open indicates an intention tremor. The clinician assesses tremor amplitude and frequency during these tasks. Tremor may also be observed by asking the patient to write something.[103]

Balance and Gait

Examination of balance and gait for individuals with cerebellar damage is performed in the same manner as for individuals with other neurological diagnoses and so is not described in detail here (see Chapter 9 – Neurologic Evaluation). Documentation of level of assistance needed, movement quality, including severity and frequency of specific features of ataxia (e.g., postural tremor or titubation, movement decomposition, rebound), and time taken to perform functional tasks is useful for treatment planning and tracking patient progress.

Standardized Clinical Scales

The best studied and validated standardized rating scales for quantifying the severity of cerebellar ataxia are the International Cooperative Ataxia Rating Scale (ICARS) and the SARA.[141] The ICARS is a semi-quantitative 100-point scale that measures a person's ability to perform 19 specific activities and movements, divided into four categories: posture and gait, limb movements, speech, and oculomotor function.[142] The higher the score, the worse is the patient's performance. The SARA has eight items, yielding a total score of 0 (no ataxia) to 40 (most severe ataxia) and rates quality of movement during gait, stance, sitting, speech, finger movement, and limb coordination functions.[143] Although the SARA was initially developed and tested for the quantification of ataxia due to spinocerebellar atrophy, it has proven validity in the evaluation of ataxia with other diagnoses.[141] The BARS (Brief Ataxia Rating Scale) is a shorter modified version of ICARS that consists of five items that evaluate walking capacity, decomposition, using the HTS and FTN tests, and dysmetria, dysarthria, and abnormalities of ocular pursuit.[138] Higher scores, on the 30-point scale, indicate worse performance. Use of these scales provides the therapist with an objective and quantifiable measure to demonstrate severity of ataxia and to track progress of therapy. Using a Delphi survey, a panel of experts recommended the SARA, BBS, and TUG Test for the assessment of balance in people with cerebellar ataxia.[144] A systematic review of the psychometric properties of balance measures of cerebellar ataxia found that the posture and gait subcomponent of ICARS demonstrates strong psychometric properties with acceptable clinical utility.[145]

● PHYSICAL THERAPY TREATMENT

Recovery of motor function in individuals with cerebellar damage depends on the cause, extent, and site of the damage as well as numerous other factors such as damage to other brain regions, coexisting medical conditions, and age. Prognosis for recovery may be better for individuals with ataxia, following stroke, neurosurgery, trauma, or MS because only specific areas of the cerebellum are affected, leaving intact regions that might be able to compensate for the damaged parts. In contrast, the prognosis for individuals with degenerative cerebellar diseases may be worse due to the progressive nature and widespread effects of these diseases on all areas of the cerebellum. One study showed that people with damage to the deep cerebellar nuclei did not recover as completely as those with damage isolated to the cerebellar cortex and white matter.[146]

General physical therapy goals and expected outcomes for individuals with cerebellar ataxia include to: (1) improve static and dynamic postural stability during functional tasks, (2) develop appropriate fall prevention strategies and precautions for safe functioning in daily life, and (3) prevent physical deconditioning by engaging in aerobic exercise and/or resistance training.[147] Marquer et al.[147] performed a systematic review of the literature on the efficacy of rehabilitation in treating cerebellar ataxia and found a total of 15 studies, 3 of which were randomized controlled trials, and the remaining were case studies. The fact that there were so few studies, featuring a multitude of different patient populations (MS, stroke, TBI, cerebellar degeneration) makes it difficult for clinicians to make evidence-based decisions about the most effective interventions for their patients. Therefore, only a summary of the major findings is provided to assist clinicians with their decision-making.

Treatment of Body Structure/Function Impairments

Depending on the patient's individual body structure or function impairments, interventions such as stretching of tight hip flexors, hamstrings, quadriceps, and ankle plantarflexors or strengthening of pelvic and lower extremity musculature may be needed.[148] If the patient is experiencing vertigo, nystagmus, or oculomotor symptoms, he/she may benefit from gaze stability exercises for the VOR and habituation exercises (as described earlier in this chapter).[148] Individuals with cerebellar ataxia expend more energy and require greater concentration levels to perform their daily activities than nondisabled individuals, which may result in excessive fatigue. Integration of aerobic exercise (i.e., walking, stationary cycling, swimming and aquatic exercise, arm ergometry) and submaximal resistance exercise to improve cardiovascular endurance and reduce muscle fatigue is recommended for the majority of individuals with cerebellar ataxia.

Gait and Balance Interventions

Most of the intervention studies for cerebellar ataxia to date emphasize intensive static and dynamic balance exercises and coordination exercises to improve stability, particularly during gait.[147] For specific exercises to improve coordination and motor control of the extremities, see Chapter 13 – Multiple Sclerosis. Initially, the exercises are performed using vision to assist in controlling the movement and progressed to working on movement without the aid of vision. Examples of static and dynamic balance exercises that are commonly prescribed can be found in Box 16-2 and Table 16-12. Gait training over ground as well as on treadmills (with or without body weight support) has had some success is single case studies and one randomized controlled trial.[149-151] Individuals with progressive ataxia due to cerebellar degeneration, who participated in a 4-week physical therapist-directed intensive coordinative training program, focused on static and dynamic balance exercises and walking, followed by performance of an HEP of similar exercises for an additional 4 weeks, had significant improvements in ICARS, SARA, and BBS scores and in gait speed, step length, and lateral trunk sway measures that were sustained 8 weeks after the intervention (see Table 16-12).[152] With all balance and gait activities, it is essential that patients are sufficiently challenged to drive compensatory neuroplasticity in the central nervous system.[153]

TABLE 16-12	Exercises for Cerebellar Ataxia[152]
EXERCISE TYPE	**VARIATIONS**
Static balance activities	Single limb stance Quadruped weight shift – lift one arm, lift one leg, lift one arm and the opposite leg
Dynamic balance	
Kneeling	• Alternately put one foot in front and then the other (1/2 kneeling position) • Alternately put one foot to the side and then the other • Alternately come to standing, using a ½ kneel position and return to kneeling
Standing	• Swing arms • Step in each direction – front, side, back • Braiding stepping • Stair climbing • Overground walking on different surfaces
Whole body movements	
Quadruped	• Raise one arm and the opposite leg; flex them to touch elbow and knee under the trunk and then extend (repeat multiple times then complete with opposite arm and leg)
Kneeling	• Crouch to floor, bending knees, arms and trunk; then extend back up into a kneeling position • Move into side-sitting to one side, return to kneeling and then to side-sitting on the opposite side
Fall prevention activities	
Standing	• Therapist disturbs balance in forward, backward, and lateral positions • Toe touches – bends to touch toes and returns to upright; therapist may introduce a balance displacement • Repeatedly move to quadruped from standing and return to upright; therapist may introduce a balance displacement • When pushed in upright, patient practices flexing forward to the floor
Walking	• Therapist provides balance displacement while the patient is walking
Trunk and shoulder mobility	• From prone lying, push up into extended arms position to stretch upper back • Spine rotation: supine lying – bend knees and alternately rotate the knees to the right and left side • Flexion of the shoulder: supine lying – lift the arms in the direction of the head

Compensatory Strategies

Ataxia can be difficult to treat and individuals with cerebellar lesions often rely on compensatory techniques, including (1) the use of vision to guide movement, (2) weighted utensils and the weighting of the limbs to increase proprioceptive awareness, and (3) the use of assistive devices, such as a rollator walker, to maximize function and minimize fall risk.[154-156] Canes and standard walkers may be difficult to use, if ataxia is present in the upper extremities, as the individual may not be able to coordinate the use of the assistive device.

CASE C, PART II

Based on Mrs. Falstaff's diagnosis of SCA 6 and her physical therapy examination findings, the physical therapist instructed Mrs. Falstaff in exercises for balance and gait that were updated weekly. Balance retraining was performed with varying sensory conditions (i.e., standing with eyes open and then closed, on firm surface and then on foam). The patient practiced standing in a modified single-leg stance position (i.e., patient placed her foot on an egg carton and maintained her balance without crushing the egg carton) with eyes open and then closed, with and without a handhold, and eventually stepping, while alternating foot placement on the egg carton. Gait training initially included walking forward, backward, and sideways on level surfaces with a cane. Later, walking under a variety of challenges was progressed, including (1) while making head turns slowly side-to-side, (2) through an obstacle course that required stepping over small objects, (3) walking over uneven surfaces (foam mat, grass), and (4) walking up and down slight inclines. She was instructed in a HEP that included lower extremity coordination and balance exercises, including tandem stance, marching in place, sit-to-stand, sideways and backward walking with stand-by assistance from her husband. After completing nine 1-hour sessions spaced 1-week apart, Mrs. Falstaff scored a 10/40 on the SARA and completed the TUG in 12.5 seconds. She was able to maintain her balance on the mCTSIB in all conditions except for Condition 4 (standing on the foam with eyes closed). Her ABC Scale score was 75%. The patient was instructed to continue a home program that included a walking program and balance exercises. At a 2-week follow-up appointment, the patient reported that she was able to perform all of her daily activities with no episodes of dizziness and did not need further therapy.

REFERENCES

1. Agrawal Y, Carey JP, Della Santina CC, Schubert MC, Minor LB. Disorders of balance and vestibular function in US adults. *Arch Intern Med.* 2009;169(10):938-944.

2. Hobeika CP. Equilibrium and balance in the elderly. *Ear Nose Throat J.* 1999;78(8):558-565.

3. Grimby A, Rosenhall U. Health-related quality of life and dizziness in old age. *Gerontology.* 1995;41(5):286-298.

4. Strupp M, Brandt T. Diagnosis and treatment of vertigo and dizziness. *Dtsch Arztebl Int.* 2008;105(10):173-180.

5. Megna J. The differential diagnosis of dizziness in the older adult. In: Hardage J, ed. *Topics in Geriatrics. Volume 6, Issue 3. An Independent Study Course Designed for Individual Continuing Education.* Alexandria, VA: Geriatric Section, American Physical Therapy Association; 2010.

6. Curthoys IA, Halmagyi GM. Vestibular compensation-recovery after unilateral vestibular loss. In: Herdman SJ, Clendaniel RA, eds. *Vestibular Rehabilitation.* 4th ed. Philadelphia, PA: F.A. Davis Company; 2014:121-150.

7. Fetter M. Vestibular system disorders. In: Herdman SJ, Clendaniel RA, eds. *Vestibular Rehabilitation.* 4th ed. Philadelphia, PA: F.A. Davis Company; 2014:50-58.

8. Thompson TL, Amadee R. Vertigo: a review of common peripheral and central vestibular disorders. *Ochsner J.* 2009;9(1):20-26.

9. Strupp M, Zingler VC, Arbusow V, et al. Methylprednisolone, valacyclovir, or the combination for vestibular neuritis. *NEJM.* 2004;351:354-361.

10. Gill-Body KM. Current Concepts in the Management of Individuals With Vestibular Dysfunction. 1st ed. Monograph published by the American Physical Therapy Association, Alexandria, VA.

11. Fife TD, Iverson DJ, Lempert T, et al. Practice parameter: therapies for benign paroxysmal positional vertigo (an evidence-based review): report of the Quality Standards Subcommittee of the American Academy of Neurology. *Neurology.* 2008;70:2067-2074.

12. Shaia WT, Zappia JJ, Bojrab DI, LaRouere ML, Sargent EW, Diaz RC. Success of posterior semicircular canal occlusion and application of the Dizziness Handicap Inventory. *Otolaryngol Head Neck Surg.* 2006;134(3):424-430.

13. Lacour M, van de Heyning PH, Novotny M, Tighilet B. Betahistine in the treatment of Meniere's disease. *Neuropsychiatr Dis Treat.* 2007;3(4) 429-440.

14. Grad A, Baloh RW. Vertigo of vascular origin. Clinical and electronystagmographic features in 84 cases. *Arch Neurol.* 1989;46:281-284.

15. Cooke DL. Central vestibular disorders. *Neurol Rep.* 1996;20:22-29.

16. Berman JM, Fredrickson JM. Vertigo after head injury – a five year follow-up. *J Otolaryngol.* 1978;7(3):237-245.

17. MacGregor EA, Brandes J, Eikermann A Migraine prevalence and treatment patterns: the global Migraine and Zolmitriptan Evaluation survey. *Headache.* 2003;43(1):19-26.

18. Stewart WF, Shechter A, Rasmussen BK. Migraine prevalence: a review of population-based studies. *Neurology.* 1994;44(suppl 4): S17-S23.

19. Dieterich M. Central vestibular disorders. *J Neurol.* 2007;254:559-568.

20. Radtke A, von Brevern M, Neuhauser H, Hottenrott T, Lempert T. Vestibular migraine: long-term follow-up of clinical symptoms and vestibulo-cochlear findings. *Neurology.* 2012;79(15):1607-1614.

21. Furman JM, Whitney SL. Central causes of dizziness. *Phys Ther.* 2000;80(2):179-187.

22. Wrisley DM, Whitney SL, Furman JM. Vestibular rehabilitation outcomes in patients with a history of migraine. *Otol Neurotol.* 2002;23(4):483-487.

23. Murdin L, Davies RA, Bronstein AM. Vertigo as a migraine trigger. *Neurology.* 2009;73(8):638-642.

24. Brainard A, Gresham C. Prevention and treatment of motion sickness. *Am Fam Physician.* 2014;90(1):41-46.

25. Shupak A, Gordon CR. Motion sickness: advances in pathogenesis, prediction, prevention, and treatment. *Aviat Space Environ Med.* 2006;77(12):1213-1223.

26. Rine RM, Schubert MC, Balkany TJ. Visual-vestibular habituation and balance training for motion sickness. *Phys Ther.* 1999;79:949-957.

27. Clendaniel, RA, Landel R. Physical therapy management of cervicogenic dizziness. In: Herdman SJ, Clendaniel RA, eds. *Vestibular Rehabilitation.* 4th ed. Philadelphia, PA: F.A. Davis Company; 2014:590-609.

28. Wrisley DM, Sparto PJ, Whitney SL, Furman JM. Cervicogenic dizziness: a review of diagnosis and treatment. *J Orthop Sports Phys Ther.* 2000;30(12):755-766.

29. Schubert MC. Vestibular function tests. In: Herdman SJ, Clendaniel RA, eds. *Vestibular Rehabilitation.* 4th ed. Philadelphia, PA: F.A. Davis Company; 2014:178-194.

30. Fife TD, Tusa RJ, Furman JM. Assessment: vestibular testing techniques in adults and children: report of the Therapeutics and Technology Assessment Subcommittee of the American Academy of Neurology. *Neurology.* 2000;55:1431-1441.

31. Slattery EL, Sinks BC, Goebel JA. Vestibular tests for rehabilitation: applications and interpretation. *Neurorehabilitation.* 2011;29:143-151.

32. Dieterich M, Brandt T. Ocular torsion and tilt of subjective visual vertical are sensitive brainstem signs. *Ann Neurol.* 1993;33(3):292-299.

33. Min KK, Jong S, Kim MJ, Cho CH, Cha HE, Lee JH. Clinical use of subjective visual horizontal and vertical in patients of unilateral vestibular neuritis. *Otol Neurotol.* 2007;28(4):520-525.

34. Baier B, Dieterich M. Ocular tilt reaction: a clinical sign of cerebellar infarctions? *Neurology.* 2009;72(6):572-573.

35. Schneider R, Leigh RJ. Pharmacological and optical methods to treat vestibular disorders and nystagmus. In: Herdman SJ, Clendaniel RA, eds. *Vestibular Rehabilitation.* 4th ed. Philadelphia, PA: F.A. Davis Company; 2014:250-265.

36. Schwartz R, Longwell P. Treatment of vertigo. *Am Fam Physician.* 2005;71(6):1115-1122.

37. Powell LE, Myers AM. The Activities-specific Balance Confidence (ABC) Scale. *J Gerontol A Biol Sci Med Sci.* 1995;50:28-34.

38. Whitney SL, Herdman SJ. Physical therapy assessment of vestibular hypofunction. In: Herdman SJ, Clendaniel RA, eds. *Vestibular Rehabilitation.* 4th ed. Philadelphia, PA: F.A. Davis Company; 2014:359-393.

39. Cohen HS, Kimball KT. Development of the vestibular disorders activities of daily living scale. *Arch Otolaryngol Head Neck Surg.* 2000;126:881-887.

40. Jacobson GP, Newman CW. The development of the Dizziness Handicap Inventory. *Arch Otolaryngol Head Neck Surg.* 1990;116(4):424-427.

41. Jacobson GP, Newman CW, Hunter L, Balzer GK. Balance function test correlates of the Dizziness Handicap Inventory. *J Am Acad Audiol.* 1991;2(4):253-260.

42. Coward JL, Wrisley DM, Walker M, Strasnick B, Jacobson JT. Efficacy of vestibular rehabilitation. *Otolaryngol Head Neck Surg.* 1998;118(1):49-54.

43. Morris AE, Lutman ME, Yardley L. Measuring outcome from vestibular rehabilitation, part II: refinement and validation of a new self report measure. *Int J Audiol.* 2009;48(1):24-37.

44. Côté P, Kreitz BG, Cassidy JD, Thiel H. The validity of the extension-rotation test as a clinical screening procedure before neck manipulation: a secondary analysis. *J Manipulative Physiol Ther.* 1996;19(3):159-164.

45. Clendaniel R. The effects of habituation and gaze-stability exercises in the treatment of unilateral vestibular hypofunction – preliminary results. *J Neurol Phys Ther.* 2010;34(2):111-116.

46. Jeffcoat B, Shelukhin A, Fong A, Mustain W, Zhou W. Alexander's law revisited. *J Neurophysiol.* 2008;100(1):154-159.

47. Dieterich M, Brandt T. Vestibular lesions of the central vestibular pathways. In: Herdman SJ, Clendaniel RA, eds. *Vestibular Rehabilitation.* 4th ed. Philadelphia, PA: F.A. Davis Company; 2014:59-84.

48. Schubert MC, Tusa RJ, Grine LE, Herdman SJ. Optimizing the sensitivity of the head thrust test for identifying vestibular hypofunction. *Phys Ther.* 2004;84(2):151-158.

49. Smith-Wheelock M, Shepard NT, Telian SA. Physical therapy program for vestibular rehabilitation. *Am J Otol.* 1991;12:218-225.

50. Telian SA, Shepard NT. Update on vestibular rehabilitation therapy. *Otolaryngol Clin North Am.* 1996;29(2):359-371.

51. Akin FW, Davenport MJ. Validity and reliability of the Motion Sensitivity Test. *J Rehabil Res Dev.* 2003;40(5):415-421.

52. Seung-Han L, Kim JS. Benign paroxysmal positional vertigo. *J Clin Neurol.* 2010;6:51-63.

53. Herdman SJ, Hoder JM. Physical therapy management of benign paroxysmal positional vertigo. In: Herdman SJ, Clendaniel RA, eds. *Vestibular Rehabilitation.* 4th ed. Philadelphia, PA: F.A. Davis Company; 2014:324-354.

54. Newton RA. Review of tests of standing balance abilities. *Brain Inj.* 1989;3:335-343.

55. Vellas BJ, Wayne SJ, Romero L, Baumgartner RN, Rubenstein LZ, Garry PJ. One-leg balance is an important predictor of injurious falls in older persons. *J Am Geriatr Soc.* 1997;45(6):735-738.

56. Whitney SL, Wrisley DM, Marchetti GF, Gee MA, Redfern MS, Furman JM. Clinical measurement of sit-to-stand performance in people with balance disorders: validity of data for the five-times-sit-to-stand test. *Phys Ther.* 2005(10):1034-1045.

57. Fukuda T. The stepping test: two phases of the labyrinthine reflex. *Acta Otolaryngol.* 1959;50(2):95-108.

58. Honaker JA, Shepard NT. Performance of Fukuda Stepping Test as a function of the severity of caloric weakness in chronic dizzy patients. *J Am Acad Audiol.* 2012;23(8):616-622.

59. Duncan PW, Weiner DK, Chandler J, Studenski S. Functional reach: a new clinical measure of balance. *J Gerontol.* 1990;45(6):M192-M197.

60. Newton RA. Validity of the multi-directional reach test: a practical measure for limits of stability in older adults. *J Gerontol A Biol Sci Med Sci.* 2001;56(4):M248-M252.

61. Munhoz RP, Li JY, Kurtinecz M, et al. Evaluation of the pull test technique in assessing postural instability in Parkinson's disease. *Neurology.* 2004;62(1):125-127.

62. Rose DJ. *FallProof! A comprehensive balance and mobility program.* Champaign, IL: Human Kinetics; 2003.

63. Wolfson LI, Whipple R, Amerman P, Kleinberg A. Stressing the postural response. A quantitative method for testing balance. *J Am Geriatr Soc.* 1986;34(12):845-850.

64. Shumway-Cook A, Horak FB. Assessing the influence of sensory interaction of balance. Suggestion from the field. *Phys Ther.* 1986;66(10):1548-1550.

65. Nashner LM. Sensory neuromuscular and biomechanical contributions to human balance. In Duncan PW, ed. *Balance Proceedings of the APTA Forum.* Alexandria, VA: American Physical Therapy Association; 1990.

66. Keshner EA, Galgon AK. Postural abnormalities in vestibular disorders. In: Herdman SJ, Clendaniel RA, eds. *Vestibular Rehabilitation.* 4th ed. Philadelphia, PA: F.A. Davis Company; 2014:85-109.

67. Giray M, Kirazli Y, Karapolat H, Celebisoy N, Bilgen C, Kirazli T. Short-term effects of vestibular rehabilitation in patients with chronic unilateral vestibular dysfunction: a randomized controlled study. *Arch Phys Med Rehabil.* 2009;90(8):1325-1331.

68. Horak FB, Nashner LM. Central programming of postural movements: adaption to altered support surface configurations. *J Neurophysiol.* 1986;55:1369-1381.

69. Horak FB, Nashner LM, Diener HC. Postural strategies associated with somatosensory and vestibular loss. *Exp Brain Res.* 1990;82(1):167-177.

70. Tinetti ME. Performance-oriented assessment of mobility problems in elderly patients. *J Am Geriatr Soc.* 1986;34(2):119-126.

71. Podsiadlo D, Richardson S. The timed "Up & Go": a test of basic functional mobility for frail elderly persons. *J Am Geriatr Soc.* 1991;39(2):142-148.

72. Berg KO, Wood-Dauphinee SL, Williams JI, Maki B. Measuring balance in the elderly: validation of an instrument. *Can J Public Health.* 1992;83(suppl 2):S7-S11.

73. Whitney SL, Hudak MT, Marchetti GF. The dynamic gait index relates to self-reported fall history in individuals with vestibular dysfunction. *J Vestib Res.* 2000;10(2):99-105.

74. Wrisley DM, Marchetti GF, Kuharsky DK, Whitney SL. Reliability, internal consistency, and validity of data obtained with the functional gait assessment. *Phys Ther.* 2004;84(10):906-918.

75. Nunez RA, Cass SP, Furman JM. Short and long-term outcomes of canalith repositioning for benign paroxysmal positional vertigo. *Arch Otolaryngol Head Neck Surg.* 2000;122:647-652.

76. Sakaida M, Takeuchi K, Ishinaga H, Adachi M, Majima Y. Long-term outcome of benign paroxysmal positional vertigo. *Neurology.* 2003;60(9):1532-1534.

77. Brandt T, Daroff RB. Physical therapy for benign paroxysmal positional vertigo. *Arch Otolaryngol.* 1980;106:484-485.

78. Kim JS, Oh SY, Lee SH, et al. Randomized clinical trial for geotropic horizontal canal benign paroxysmal positional vertigo. *Neurology.* 2012;79(7):700-707.

79. Mandalà M, Pepponi E, Santoro GP, et al. Double-blind randomized trial on the efficacy of the Gufoni maneuver for treatment of lateral canal BPPV. *Laryngoscope.* 2013;123(7):1782-1786.

80. Casani AP, Vannucci G, Fattori B, Berrettinin S. The treatment of horizontal canal positional vertigo: our experience in 66 cases. *Laryngoscope.* 2002;112:172-178.

81. Vannucchi P, Giannoni B, Pagnini P. Treatment of horizontal semicircular canal benign paroxysmal positional vertigo. *J Vestib Res.* 1997;7:1-6.

82. Massoud EAS, Ireland DJ. Post-treatment instructions in the nonsurgical management of benign paroxysmal positional vertigo. *J Otolaryngol.* 1996;25:121-125.

83. Nuti D, Nati C, Passali D. Treatment of benign paroxysmal positional vertigo: no need for postmaneuver restrictions. *Otol Heal Neck Surg.* 2000;122:440-444.

84. Herdman SJ, Whitney SL. Physical therapy treatment of vestibular hypofunction. In: Herdman SJ, Clendaniel RA, eds. *Vestibular Rehabilitation.* 4th ed. Philadelphia, PA: F.A. Davis Company; 2014:394-431.

85. Hillier SL, Hollohan V. Vestibular rehabilitation for unilateral peripheral vestibular dysfunction. *Cochrane Database Syst Rev.* 2007;(4):CD005397.

86. Hillier SL, McDonnell M. Vestibular rehabilitation for unilateral peripheral vestibular dysfunction. *Cochrane Database Syst Rev.* 2011;(2):CD005397.

87. Tee LH, Chee NWC. Vestibular rehabilitation therapy for the dizzy patient. *Ann Acad Med Singapore.* 2005;34:289-294.

88. Cawthorne T. The physiological basis for head exercises. *J Chart Soc Physiother.* 1944;30:106.

89. Cooksey FS. Rehabilitation in vestibular injuries. *Proc Royal Soc Med.* 1946;39:273-278.

90. Norre ME, De Weerdt W. Treatment of vertigo based on habituation. 1. Physio-pathological basis. *J Laryngol Otol.* 1980;94:689-696.

91. Dix MR. The rationale and technique of head exercises in the treatment of vertigo. *Acta Otorhinolaryngol Belg.* 1979;33:370-384.

92. Shepard NT, Telian SA, Smith-Wheelock M. Habituation and balance retraining therapy. *Neurol Clin.* 1990;5:459-475.

93. Clendaniel R. The effects of habituation and gaze-stability exercises in the treatment of unilateral vestibular hypofunction: preliminary results. *J Neurol Phys Ther.* 2010;34(2):111-116.

94. Herdman SJ, Clendaniel RA. Physical therapy management of bilateral vestibular hypofunction and loss. In: Herdman SJ, Clendaniel RA, eds. *Vestibular Rehabilitation.* 4th ed. Philadelphia, PA: F.A. Davis Company; 2014:432-456.

95. Krebs DE, Gill-Body KM, Riley PO, Parker SW. Double-blind, placebo-controlled trial of rehabilitation for bilateral vestibular hypofunction: preliminary report. *Otolaryngol Head Neck Surg.* 1993;109(4):735-741.

96. Brown KE, Whitney SL, Wrisley DM, Furman JM. Physical therapy outcomes for persons with bilateral vestibular loss. *Laryngoscope.* 2001;111:1812-1817.

97. Krebs DE, Gill-Body KM, Parker SW, Ramirez JV, Wernick-Robinson M. Vestibular rehabilitation: useful but not universally so. *Otolaryngol Head Neck Surg.* 2003;128(2):240-250.

98. Patten C, Horak FB, Krebs DE. Head and body center of gravity control strategies: adaptations following vestibular rehabilitation. *Acta Otolaryngol.* 2003;123(1):32-40.

99. Herdman SJ, Hall CD, Schubert MC, Das VE, Tusa RJ. Recovery of dynamic visual acuity in bilateral vestibular hypofunction. *Arch Otolaryngol Head Neck Surg.* 2007;133(4):383-389.

100. Cohen HS, Wells J, Kimball KT, Owsley C. Driving disability and dizziness. *J Safety Res.* 2003;34(4):361-369.

101. Sullivan EV, Rose J, Pfefferbaum A. Effect of vision, touch and stance on cerebellar vermian-related sway and tremor: a quantitative physiological and MRI study. *Cereb Cortex.* 2006;16:1077-1086.

102. Mancuso M, Orsucci D, Siciliano G, Bonuccelli U. The genetics of ataxia: through the labyrinth of the Minotaur, looking for Aridne's thread. *J Neurol.* 2014;261(suppl 2):S528-S541.

103. Marsden J, Harris C. Cerebellar ataxia: pathophysiology and rehabilitation. *Clin Rehabil.* 2011;25:195-216.

104. Park E, Ai J, Baker AJ. Cerebellar injury: clinical relevance and potential in traumatic brain injury research. *Prog Brain Res.* 2007;161:327-338.

105. Potts MB, Adwanikar H, Noble-Haeusslein LJ. Models of traumatic cerebellar injury. *Cerebellum.* 2009;8(3):211-221.

106. Strupp M, Kalla R, Glasauer S, Wagner J, Hüfner K, Jahn K, Brandt T. Aminopyridines for the treatment of cerebellar and ocular motor disorders. *Prog Brain Res.* 2008;171:535-541.

107. Bastian AJ, Martin TA, Keating JG, Thach WT. Cerebellar ataxia: abnormal control of interaction torques across multiple joints. *J Neurophysiol.* 1996;76:492-509.

108. Holmes G. The cerebellum of man. *Brain.* 1939;62:1-30.

109. Javalkar V, Khan M, Davis DE. Clinical manifestations of cerebellar disease. *Neurol Clin.* 2014;32:871-879.

110. Deuschl G, Bain P, Brin M. Consensus statement of the Movement Disorder Society on Tremor. Ad Hoc Scientific Committee. *Mov Disord.* 1998;13(suppl 3):2-23.

111. Chance PF, Cavalier L, Satran D, et al. Clinical nosologic and genetic aspects of Joubert and related syndromes. *J Child Neurol.* 1999;14:660-666.

112. Diener HC, Dichgans J. Pathophysiology of cerebellar ataxia. *Mov Disord.* 1992;7:95-109.

113. Boose A, Dichgans J, Topka H. Deficits in phasic muscle force generation explain insufficient compensation for interaction torque in cerebellar patients. *Neurosci Lett.* 1999;261:53-56.

114. Mai N, Diener H-C, Dichgans J. On the role of feedback in maintaining constant grip force in patients with cerebellar disease. *Neurosci Lett.* 1989;99:340-344.

115. Mauritz KH, Dichgans J, Hufschmidt A. Quantitative analysis of stance in late cortical cerebellar atrophy of the anterior lobe and other forms of cerebellar ataxia. *Brain.* 1979;102:461-482.

116. Diener HC, Dichgans J, Bacher M, Gompf B. Quantification of postural sway in normals and patients with cerebellar diseases. *Electroencephalogr Clin Neurophysiol.* 1984;57:134-142.

117. Horak FB, Diener HC. Cerebellar control of postural scaling and central set in stance. *J Neurophysiol.* 1994;72:479-493.

118. Mummel P, Timmann D, Krause UW, et al. Postural responses to changing task conditions in patients with cerebellar lesions. *J Neurol Neurosurg Psychiatry.* 1998;65:734-742.

119. Schwabe A, Drepper J, Maschke M, Diener H-C, Timmann D. The role of the human cerebellum in short- and long-term habituation of postural responses. *Gait Posture.* 2004;19:16-23.

120. Palliyath S, Hallett M, Thomas SL, Lebiedowska MK. Gait in patients with cerebellar ataxia. *Mov Disord.* 1998;13:958-964.

121. Earhart GM, Bastian AJ. Selection and coordination of human locomotor forms following cerebellar damage. *J Neurophysiol.* 2001;85:759-769.

122. Seidel B, Krebs DE. Base of support is not wider in chronic ataxic and unsteady patients. *J Rehabil Med.* 2002;34:288-292.

123. Morton SM, Bastian AJ. Relative contributions of balance and voluntary leg-coordination deficits to cerebellar gait ataxia. *J Neurophysiol.* 2003;89:1844-1856.

124. Schniepp R, Wuehr M, Schlick C, et al. Increased gait variability is associated with the history of falls in patients with cerebellar ataxia. *J Neurol.* 2014;261(1):213-223.

125. Serrao M, Conte C, Casali C, et al. Sudden stopping in patients with cerebellar ataxia. *Cerebellum.* 2013;12(5):607-616.

126. Mari S, Serrao M, Casali C, et al. Turning strategies in patients with cerebellar ataxia. *Exp Brain Res.* 2012;222(1-2):65-75.

127. Serrao M, Mari S, Conte C, et al. Strategies adopted by cerebellar ataxia patients to perform U-turns. *Cerebellum.* 2013;12(4):460-468.

128. van der Warrenberg BP, Steijens JA, Muneke M, Kremer PB, Bloem BR. Falls in degenerative cerebellar ataxias. *Mov Disord.* 2005;20:497-500.

129. Javalkar V, Khan M, Davis DE. Clinical manifestations of cerebellar disease. *Neurol Clin.* 2014;32:871-879.

130. Lewis RF, Zee DS. Ocular motor disorders associated with cerebellar lesions: pathophysiology and topical localization. *Rev Neurol (Paris)*. 1993;149(11):665-677.

131. Urban PP. Speech motor deficits in cerebellar infarctions. *Brain Lang*. 2013;127(3):323-326.

132. Blaney B, Hewlett N. Dysarthria and Friedreich's ataxia: what can intelligibility assessment tell us? *Int J Lang Commun Disord*. 2007;42:19-37.

133. Tseng YW, Diedrichsen J, Krakauer JW, et al. Sensory prediction errors drive cerebellum-dependent adaptation of reaching. *J Neurophysiol*. 2007;98:54-62.

134. Shadmehr R, Smith MA, Krakauer JW. Error correction, sensory prediction, and adaptation in motor control. *Ann Rev Neurosci*. 2010;33:89-108.

135. Timmann D, Horak FB. Perturbed step initiation in cerebellar subjects. 1. Modifications of postural responses. *Exp Brain Res*. 1998;119:73-84.

136. Earhart GM, Fletcher WA, Horak FB, et al. Does the cerebellum play a role in podokinetic adaptation? *Exp Brain Res*. 2002;146:538-542.

137. Smith MA, Shadmehr R. Intact ability to learn internal models of arm dynamics in Huntington's disease but not cerebellar degeneration. *J Neurophysiol*. 2005;93:2809-2821.

138. Schmahmann JD, Sherman JC. The cerebellar cognitive affective syndrome. *Brain*. 1998;121(pt 4):561-579.

139. Marmolino D, Manto M. Past, present, and future therapeutics for cerebellar ataxias. *Curr Neuropharmacol*. 2010;8:41-61.

140. Trujillo-Martin MM, Serrano-Aguilar P, Monton-Alvarez F, Carrillo-Fumero R. Effectiveness and safety of treatments for degenerative ataxias: a systematic review. *Mov Disord*. 2009;24(8):1111-1124.

141. Saute JA, Donis KC, Serrano-Munuera C, et al.; Iberoamerican Multidisciplinary Network for the Study of Movement Disorders (RIBERMOV) Study Group. Ataxia rating scales – psychometric profiles, natural history and their application in clinical trials. *Cerebellum*. 2012;11(2):488-504.

142. Trouillas P, Takayanagi T, Hallett M, et al. International Cooperative Ataxia Rating Scale for pharmacological assessment of the cerebellar syndrome. The Ataxia Neuropharmacology Committee of the World Federation of Neurology. *J Neurol Sci*. 1997;145:205-211.

143. Schmitz-Hübsch T, du Montcel ST, Baliko L, et al. Scale for the assessment and rating of ataxia: development of a new clinical scale. *Neurology*. 2006;66:1717-1720.

144. Winser SJ, Smith C, Hale LA, Claydon LS, Whitney SL. Balance outcome measures in cerebellar ataxia: a Delphi survey. *Disabil Rehabil*. 2015;37(2):165-170.

145. Winser SJ, Smith C, Hale LA, Claydon LS, Whitney SL, Mehta P. Systematic review of the psychometric properties of balance measures for cerebellar ataxia. *Clin Rehabil*. 2015;29(1):69-79.

146. Schoch B, Dimitrova A, Gizewski ER, Timmann D. Functional localization in the human cerebellum based on voxelwise statistical analysis: a study of 90 patients. *Neuroimage*. 2006;30(1):36-51.

147. Marquer A, Barbieri G, Perennou D. The assessment and treatment of postural disorders in cerebellar ataxia: a systematic review. *Ann Phys Rehabil Med*. 2014;57:67-78.

148. Gill-Body KM, Popat RA, Parker SW, Krebs DE. Rehabilitation of balance in two patients with cerebellar dysfunction. *Phys Ther*. 1997;77:534-552.

149. Cernak K, Stevens V, Price R, Shumway-Cook A. Locomotor training using body-weight support on a treadmill in conjunction with ongoing physical therapy in a child with severe cerebellar ataxia. *Phys Ther*. 2008;88:88-97.

150. Vaz DV, Schettino Rde C, Rolla de Castro TR, et al. Treadmill training for ataxic patients: a single-subject experimental design. *Clin Rehabil*. 2008;22:234-241.

151. Miyai I, Ito M, Hattori N, et al. Cerebellar ataxia rehabilitation trial in degenerative cerebellar diseases. *Neurorehabil Neural Repair*. 2012;(5):515-522.

152. Ilg W, Synofzik M, Brötz D, et al. Intensive coordinative training improves motor performance in degenerative cerebellar disease. *Neurology*. 2009;73:1823-1830.

153. Kleim JA, Barbay S, Nudo RJ. Functional reorganization of the rat motor cortex following motor skill learning. *J Neurophysiol*. 1998;80:3321-3325.

154. Bateni H, Maki BE. Assistive devices for balance and mobility: benefits, demands, and adverse consequences. *Arch Phys Med Rehabil*. 2005;86:134-145.

155. Gibson-Horn C. Balance-based torso-weighting in a patient with ataxia and multiple sclerosis: a case report. *JNPT*. 2008;32:139-146.

156. Widener GL, Allen DD, Gibson-Horn C. Randomized clinical trial of balance-based torso weighting for improving upright mobility in people with multiple sclerosis. *Neurorehabil Neural Repair*. 2009;23:784-791.

Review Questions

1. **A sensation of motion which is associated with various vestibular disorders in which the person experiences a sensation that he/she is spinning or the person's surroundings are spinning is called:**

   A. Lightheadedness

   B. Oscillopsia

   C. Disequilibrium

   D. Vertigo

2. **Benign paroxysmal positional vertigo is most commonly caused by particles in the:**

   A. Utricle

   B. Saccule

   C. Posterior semicircular canal

   D. Anterior semicircular canal

3. **Horizontal semicircular canal BPPV can be identified with the:**

   A. Dix–Hallpike test

   B. Roll test

   C. Rotational chair test

   D. Sidelying test

4. **Dysdiadochokinesia refers to the inability to:**

   A. Perform coordinated multi-joint movements

   B. Perform rapid alternating movements

   C. Perform tandem gait

   D. Control the distance or speed of a movement

5. **An early symptom of a vestibular schwannoma (acoustic neuroma) is:**

   A. Gait ataxia

   B. Impaired eye movements

   C. Hearing loss

   D. Facial numbness

6. **The most prominent symptom of bilateral vestibular loss is:**

   A. Nystagmus

   B. Vertigo

   C. Nausea

   D. Postural imbalance

7. **Ménière's disease is caused by:**
   A. Increased endolymphatic pressure within the ear
   B. An inflammation of the membranous labyrinth
   C. Leakage of perilymph into the middle ear
   D. An inflammation of the vestibular nerve

8. **The ocular vestibular-evoked myogenic potential (VEMP) test is used to evaluate the function of the:**
   A. Horizontal semicircular canals
   B. Saccule
   C. Utricle
   D. Saccule and utricle

9. **The best exercise to improve gaze stability in an individual with bilateral vestibular loss with no peripheral vestibular function is the:**
   A. X1 paradigm exercise
   B. X2 paradigm exercise
   C. Sequenced eye and head movement exercise
   D. Brandt–Daroff exercise

10. **When evaluating a patient with residual balance deficits from vestibular neuritis, you observe that the patient bends her hips and trunk when she experiences a small perturbation or weight shifts while standing on a firm surface. The exercise intervention that would retrain the patient to use a more normal balance strategy under these conditions is:**
    A. Tandem standing or walking
    B. Balancing on a narrow beam or line
    C. Standing on one leg
    D. Small forward and backward sways

11. **A person with an acute right unilateral vestibular nerve function loss will likely experience:**
    A. Spontaneous right-beating nystagmus and loss of balance to the left side with head rotations to the right
    B. Spontaneous right-beating nystagmus and loss of balance to the right side with head rotations to the right
    C. Spontaneous left-beating nystagmus and loss of balance to the left side with head rotations to the left.
    D. Spontaneous left-beating nystagmus and loss of balance to the right side with head rotations to the right.

12. **The treatment of choice for a patient with posterior semicircular canal canalithiasis BPPV is the:**
    A. Liberatory (Semont) maneuver
    B. Brandt–Daroff exercises
    C. Canal repositioning (Epley) maneuver
    D. Bar-B-Que roll maneuver

13. **A patient who presents with spontaneous down-beating nystagmus that does not change with visual fixation most likely has:**
    A. Ménière's disease
    B. Bilateral vestibular nerve function loss
    C. Unilateral vestibular nerve hypofunction
    D. Central vestibular dysfunction

14. **The most common hereditary cerebellar disease is:**
    A. Spinocerebellar atrophy
    B. Friedreich's ataxia
    C. Episodic ataxia
    D. Ataxia telangiectasia

15. **A patient with cerebellar damage who has difficulty performing rapid forearm supination and pronation is demonstrating:**
    A. Dyssynergia
    B. Dysmetria
    C. Dysdiadochokinesia
    D. Rebound

16. **When performing the finger-to-nose test you note that a patient with cerebellar damage exhibits a tremor as his finger approaches a target. This tremor is called:**
    A. Intention tremor
    B. Postural tremor
    C. Essential tremor
    D. Titubation

17. **Spinocerebellar ataxias:**
    A. Typically have their onset in childhood
    B. Typically have a rapid progression
    C. Are a group of over 35 diseases
    D. Are autosomal recessive inherited diseases

18. **Individuals with vestibular dysfunction or loss are likely to have difficulty maintaining their balance in which of the following Sensory Organization Test conditions:**
    A. Conditions 3, 4, 5
    B. Conditions 3,6
    C. Conditions 3, 4, 5, 6
    D. Conditions 5, 6

Answers

1. D	2. C	3. B	4. B	5. C
6. D	7. A	8. C	9. C	10. D
11. D	12. C	13. D	14. B	15. C
16. A	17. C	18. D		

Age-Related Neurologic Changes

17

Deborah A. Kegelmeyer and Deborah S. Nichols-Larsen

Age is a very high price to pay for maturity.

Tom Stoppard

Experience is a wonderful thing – it enables you to recognize a mistake when you make it again.

Source Unknown

OBJECTIVES

1) Distinguish the aging process from pathologic conditions of aging

2) Differentiate the epidemiology and pathophysiology of conditions that produce dementia

3) Identify and discuss optimal treatment options for older adults and those with dementia to maximize function

The nervous system, including the autonomic, central, and peripheral components, along with our muscles and special senses experience changes with aging. Combined, these changes lead to declines in executive function and memory, sensory transmission and processing, motor performance such as slowing of movement, and impaired coordination, balance, and gait as compared to young adults.[1] Coordination is most impaired in bimanual and multi-joint movements. Balance impairment can be noted in increased postural sway and diminished dynamic balance, and gait is slower and impacted by cognitive, motor, and sensory system changes. Of the special senses, vision is most impacted by aging, yet, we also experience a decline in our ability to smell, taste, and hear as we age.

CASE A, PART I

Carol Schmidt is a 67-year-old female who has begun to experience some slowing of movement and difficulty with her tennis game. She has noted that she is slower to get to the ball and cannot make some of the trickier shots that she was able to make just a few years ago. Mrs. Schmidt's mother, Adele Weiss, is 90 years old and moves quite slowly with a stooped posture and is no longer able to run or to safely ambulate in low light conditions. She has fallen twice in the last year and no longer leaves her home other than to shop and go to religious services with her daughter. In addition, both women complain of being forgetful and needing to make shopping lists. Adele recently told Carol that she is having more difficulty bathing and cooking.

The nervous system experiences declines at a rate of 1% per year, starting at age 30.[2] Not all changes in function can be attributed to aging, and it is important for therapists to have an understanding of normal age-related changes versus pathologies, as behaviors that fall outside of what is considered to be the range of normal function should be assessed and treated. An understanding of the aging brain is necessary for successful examination and treatment of individuals with age-related decline in function.

CASE A, PART II

Mrs. Schmidt (Carol) would be expected to have changes in motor control, as compared to when she was younger, but is expected to continue to be able to function in normal daily activities. She would also be expected to function better than her 90-year-old mother. Adele is in the "old–old" age group and is expected to move slower than her daughter and to have difficulty with high level balance activities.

● TYPICAL NEUROMUSCULAR CHANGE WITH AGING

Changes in the Brain with Aging

Brain volume declines have been noted in gray matter, subcortical structures, and white matter with advancing age. For example, the gray matter cortical mantle is thinner in older adults with the greatest age-related differences in gray matter volume occurring in the prefrontal and orbitofrontal cortices, areas critical for executive function and memory.[3] The parietal cortex also shows more age differences in gray matter volume than either the temporal or occipital regions. Motor control is not only dependent on these areas but is also more dependent on these areas in the elderly than in young adults. Subcortical structures, including the cerebellum and basal ganglia, also exhibit reduced volume with aging. The cerebellum is important for movement timing and coordination, while the caudate nucleus of the basal ganglia is involved in skill acquisition, specifically motor planning.

Brain volume changes are not just the result of loss of gray matter (neuron cell bodies) but also loss of white matter (axonal projections). Declines in white matter volume begin later but

TABLE 17-1   Age-Related Changes in the Brain[4-6]

AREAS OF DECLINE	FUNCTIONAL IMPACT
Gray matter	
Cortical mantle	Deficits in memory, attention, perceptual awareness, thought, language, and consciousness
Prefrontal cortex	Disrupted learning, memory, problem solving, and planning
Orbitofrontal cortices	Decreased taste and smell, reward value of taste and smell; impaired learning and reversal of stimulus-reinforcement associations
Parietal cortex	Poorer body scheme, attention, and perception
Hippocampus	Declining memory, especially for recent memory
Thalamus	Impaired sensory perception and regulation of motor functions
Basal ganglia	Disrupted motor planning, limb movement, and skill acquisition
Cerebellum	Poorer coordination and movement timing
White matter	
Myelin	Slower or impaired stimulus conduction
Corpus callosum	Disrupted interhemispheric communication and decline in bimanual skills

continue at a more accelerated rate than gray matter changes.[4] Specifically, the corpus callosum, the largest white matter bundle, exhibits changes that may, in part, be due to deterioration of the myelin in multiple fiber bundles.[5] Changes in the corpus callosum significantly impact the efficiency of interhemispheric communication that is critical for bimanual coordination (Table 17-1). Similarly, there is a decrease in myelin in the gracilis fasciculus and an associated decrement in vibration threshold, indicating that fibers conveying proprioception are most affected by aging, which may contribute to balance deficits due to the loss of long latency postural reactions.[6] Fortunately, some brain areas do not exhibit age-related changes, including the cingulate gyrus (influential in linking behavioral outcomes to motivation) and the occipital cortex (vision).[7]

CASE A, PART III

Tennis requires fast coordinated movements that are highly dependent on sensory feedback and integration. Based on a rate of loss of 1% per year, Carol has likely lost 30% of her

brain volume in the frontal and parietal lobes as well as the cerebellum and basal ganglia, which would be expected to slow her tennis game and lead to more missed shots. In addition, she may be having more difficulty with tennis due to changes in the corpus callosum that are impacting her bimanual skills. Her mother, Adele, has experienced up to 60% decline in some areas, explaining her slower walking speed and making it impossible for her to run or play tennis as her daughter can.

Neurotransmitters

Cognitive decline is correlated with decreased levels of critical neurotransmitters, including acetylcholine, serotonin, norepinephrine, and dopamine. Acetylcholine declines are noted in the hippocampus and associated with changes in memory function, while age-related decreases in dopamine are associated with declines in frontal lobe function, including executive function and working memory. Motor declines are correlated with altered serotonin transmission and reduction in norepinephrine. Alterations in serotonin with age have also been correlated with declines in activity level and diminished balance in mice.[8] Norepinephrine levels decrease in the cerebellum and are related to diminished motor learning with age. The dopaminergic system has the broadest impact on motor function and is the most widely studied system. When compared to young adults, older adults exhibit a decrease in the absolute level of dopamine, the number of receptors, and transporter proteins responsible for moving the neurotransmitter across the cell membrane.[1] Based on declines in dopamine, the aging brain is on "the preclinical continuum of Parkinson's disease."[9] Ultimately, loss of dopamine is closely linked to impairments in gait, balance, and fine motor control.

CASE A, PART IV

Adele is exhibiting changes in her gait that are likely due to the loss of dopamine and changes in her basal ganglia and cerebellum.

Peripheral Nervous System

With aging, there is also degeneration of components of the peripheral nervous system. These changes lead to slowing of neural conduction of both motor and sensory information. Components of the peripheral nervous system known to degenerate are the anterior horn cells (alpha motor neurons), neuromuscular junctions, and dorsal root ganglia along with a reduction in the density of myelinated fibers in the spinal nerve roots. Further, there is a reduction in myelinated fibers in the fasciculus gracilis that is more apparent at rostral levels, indicating that, with increasing age, there is distal degeneration of afferent fibers. This likely contributes to diminished sensation in the feet and the potential for falling in older adults. Aging also leads to a progressive loss of cells and fibers in the sympathetic outflow tract, with an estimated loss of 8% of preganglionic cell bodies per decade in the mid-thoracic region.[6] These fibers contribute to autonomic regulation of blood vessel dilation/constriction, heart rate, and ultimately blood pressure, so one consequence of aging of the sympathetic nervous system may be hypertension (HTN); this is particularly evident in those that increase their body mass as they age.[10]

Distally, there is axonal degeneration and greater internodal length variability with shorter internodes more prevalent, suggesting a process of denervation and then regeneration. The capacity for axonal regeneration and reinnervation is maintained throughout life but tends to be slower and less effective with aging.[11] This pattern of degeneration and reinnervation also leads to changes in the muscle (see Box 17-1). Interestingly, there is also a decrease in the number of neurons per muscle fiber, leading to **fiber grouping**, a consequence of denervation and subsequent reinnervation. The result of this pattern of changes is likely an increased recruitment of motor units for a given task in older adults with increased effort required for any given functional task.[12] Yet, neural changes do not entirely account for changes in muscle function with aging.

CASE A, PART V

Both Carol and Adele are likely to say that it takes more effort to do their daily activities than it did when they were in their 30s and 40s; both are probably using more muscle tissue to do the same amount of work due to fiber grouping. However, Adele has likely lost significant muscle mass and has limited muscle elasticity. Notably, continued tennis playing may delay muscle changes for Carol, and strength training could help Adele recapture some of the strength loss that she's experiencing.

In general, normal age-related changes in the nervous system lead to small declines in the sensory and motor systems, including all three systems related to balance: the visual, vestibular, and somatosensory systems. These age-related declines result in slowing of movement and difficulty in situations that require faster responses or a higher level of sensory–motor integration. Overall, individuals experiencing healthy aging remain able to engage in typical daily activities such as transferring on and off of furniture, walking in their home, walking outside and in crowded environments, and balancing during functional activities. In the old–old, such as Adele, we would expect to see slowing of function and an inability to engage in high-level motor activities such as balancing on a moving surface or negotiating an unfamiliar area in low light. Any loss of function beyond this would potentially be beyond normal age-related changes and may be due to a treatable pathology. Adele's restriction of movement to her home and difficulty with bathing and cooking indicate a need for her to undergo an evaluation for problems beyond normal age-related changes.

BOX 17-1   Muscle Changes with Aging[13-15]

There are many changes in muscle, associated with aging, including a loss of muscle mass and fiber number (**sarcopenia**), loss of strength and elasticity, and an increase in adipose tissue between muscle fibers. The loss in muscle mass seems to particularly result from a decrease in Type II muscle fiber mass, while Type I fibers seem to maintain their size better with only a mild decline in size in older adults; thus, **strength** may only marginally decline while **power** (quick maximal contraction) declines to a much greater degree. Changes in fiber type ratio and innervation may contribute to this decrement in power by slowing the velocity of the muscle contraction. Old–old adults have fewer Type II fibers (fast twitch) with a secondary increase in the relative proportion of slow twitch to fast twitch fibers. More Type I fibers may result from the reinnervation of denervated Type II fibers by neurons that typically control Type I fibers. Of interest is the accumulation of adipose tissue between muscle fibers (not within them), which may contribute to the changing power of muscle contractions. Additionally, the elasticity of muscle is diminished with aging, resulting in increased muscle stiffness that actually may contribute to maintained strength. Another contributor to muscle loss with aging may be the subclinical occurrence of inflammation, noted in the elderly that may result in the metabolic breakdown of muscle (**catabolism**).

Motor Function

Healthy aging leads to slowing of movement, declines in bimanual and multi-joint coordination, and declines in balance as compared to young adults. Changes in muscles and joints also contribute to these changes. Gait becomes slower with smaller steps, a wider base of support, decrease in the swing to stance ratio (more time in double stance), initial contact in a flat footed posture and decreased rotation leading to a stiff, one-dimensional gait. These factors lead to an increase in the work of walking. Fine motor movements of the upper extremities are also impacted by the aging process, specifically fine motor movements of the fingers for tasks like writing. Activities that require multi-joint movements, such as dressing, and those that require simultaneous use of both upper extremities in a coordinated fashion (bimanual movement), such as stirring food in a held bowl, are also impacted by changes in the aging nervous system.[1]

Negative (Maladaptive) Plasticity of Aging

The **negative plasticity model of aging** states that, during normal aging, individuals undergo physical, behavioral, and environmental changes that promote negative plastic changes. In aging, sensory inputs become degraded, and thus, the sensation transmitted to the central nervous system is diminished, inaccurate, or not transmitted at all. Ultimately, this leads to a decline in CNS processing and inaccurate output from the cognitive and motor systems. Over time, neural systems change, based on these erroneous inputs, inducing negative plasticity changes in the brain and resulting in even greater impairments of function. Once this cycle of events begins, it induces a cascade of negative

TABLE 17-2 Factors of Negative Plasticity[16]

FACTORS	DESCRIPTION
Reduced schedules of activity	The level of engagement in cognitively demanding activities is lessened.
Noisy processing	Sensory input from all systems is degraded as a result of deterioration of peripheral sensory organs. Degraded sensory inputs lead to difficulty in accurately responding to relevant stimuli with increased likelihood of responding to irrelevant stimuli. These adaptive changes slow the speed of information processing.
Weakened neuromodulation	The metabolism, connectivity, and eventually, structure of neuromodulatory control systems, which regulate learning and plasticity in adults, become degraded. In aggregate, this degradation weakens the brain's control over its own plasticity, lowering learning rates and trapping the brain in potentially inappropriate or unhelpful patterns of activation.
Negative learning	As reduced schedules of activity, noisy processing, and weakened neuromodulatory control interact to make novel or demanding activities more challenging to perform, individuals naturally adapt their behaviors in ways that can reinforce negative aspects of the sensory input and motor output. For example, as it becomes harder to hear in a crowded environment, an older adult might ask the speaker to talk louder (increasing signal distortion along with loudness), find it more frustrating to have such conversations (decreasing neuromodulatory responses required to maintain high brain function), or simply choose to have fewer of such interactions (further reducing involvement in higher level brain activity).

interactions, resulting in worsening cognitive and motor function. Four interrelated and mutually reinforcing factors have been identified as central to this process: (1) reduced schedules of activity, (2) noisy processing, (3) weakened neuromodulatory control, and (4) negative learning[16] (see Table 17-2).

CASE A, PART VI

Adele's withdrawal into her home and diminished involvement in activities outside of the home are an example of *reduced levels of activity*. It is likely that she is experiencing *noisy processing* due to declines in vision (see Box 17-2), somatosensation, cerebellar and vestibular function. Noisy inputs from blurry vision and poor somatosensory feedback make it difficult for her to maintain safe balance in situations where the surface is soft or uneven with even greater difficulty in low lighting, bright lighting with a glare, or darkness. Adele experiences fewer situations in which these systems have to interact in a complex manner (*leading to weakened neuromodulatory control*) and due to neural plasticity the system remodels in response to this situation (*negative learning*). This remodeling leads to degradation of movement that is labeled negative plasticity.

Theoretically, age-related changes due to negative plasticity should be somewhat reversible with skilled training that promotes positive plasticity. Amelioration of negative plasticity has been reported, using training methods that ensure optimization of sensory inputs and intense cognitive task practice, characterized by many repetitions over 8–10 weeks, and resulting in improved memory.[16]

BOX 17-2 Changes in Vision, Hearing, Taste and Smell with Aging

Vision: Changes in visual function with aging may be noted as early as age 40 but include a variety of changes within the visual system; some are natural consequences of aging while others are pathologic changes. (1) **Presbyopia:** To accommodate to close vision, the ciliary muscles of the eye contract and pull the lens into a more rounded shape; the ability of the lens to be stretched in this way diminishes in the fifth and sixth decades, resulting in the loss of accommodation ability, and thereby, the development of presbyopia (poor near vision) that requires reading glasses for correction in almost all older adults.[17] (2) **Cataracts:** The lens of the eye is made up of proteins that over time can be destabilized by decades of ultraviolet light and chemical exposure; other pathologic conditions, especially diabetes, can further destabilize these proteins, leading to aggregation within the lens such that there are areas of protein aggregates and areas of sparse proteins. This disrupts refraction and creates poor visual acuity and light sensitivity.[17] (3) **Degeneration of the Vitreous Body:** The vitreous body fills the interior of the eye, providing architectural support for the shape of the eye; however, with aging, there can be some level of degradation of this gelatinous structure. Such loss places the aging adult at risk for **retinal detachment**.[17] (4) **Retinal Ganglion Cell Loss:** With aging, there can be up to a 30% loss of rods in the retina, yet there is almost no loss of cones; this loss of rods is related to the diminished "night" vision that older adults display. Despite the stability of absolute cone number, the density of cells in the central retina, where most cones are located, decreases by up to 15% as the overall size of the retina expands with age. Plus, the number of axons within the optic nerve decreases by up to 40% secondary to weakened mitochondrial activity; axons require a high level of metabolic support to produce action potentials, and thus, can be lost when that support becomes diminished with aging. These changes in combination contribute to the diminishing visual ability of older adults.[17] (5) **Glaucoma:** Although some loss of retinal ganglion cells is part of aging, glaucoma is a pathological loss of these cells and their axonal projections that ultimately results in blindness; these pathologic changes may stem from the diminished mitochondrial activity, noted above, triggering a cascade of cell death in extreme conditions. Signs of glaucoma include increased intraocular pressure and decreased blood flow to the retina.[18] (6) **Macular Degeneration (MD):** The macula is the central part of the retina, and a combination of genetic, environmental, and aging factors, along with the presence of heart disease, HTN, and diabetes, can result in its degeneration in older adults; this degeneration may be related to cholesterol metabolism abnormalities. In some, this degeneration is also accompanied by abnormal blood vessel proliferation (**wet MD**) while in others, there is no change in blood vessels (**dry**). Dry MD is more common and less severe than wet MD.[19]

Hearing: Older adults experience changes in the eardrum that disrupt the conduction of high tones; however, this does not impact overall hearing. Yet, **presbycusis** is a disruption of hearing that occurs equally in both ears in up to 30% of aging adults; however, there are at least four causes of this disorder: (1) **Sensory** – damage to hair cells in the organ of Corti disrupts high frequency hearing, similar to that described for normal aging, yet hearing for speech remains intact; (2) **Neural** – loss of cochlear neurons impedes hearing in the speech frequencies and thereby, impairs speech discrimination; (3) **Strial/metabolic** – the vascular support to the endolymph in the stria vascularis; atrophy of the stria results in a general loss of hearing (all frequencies); (4) **Conductive** – increased stiffness of the basal cochlea results in loss of low frequencies but doesn't impede speech discrimination. In addition, some presbycusis seems to result from a mix of these four types, and yet changes in other structures not encompassed by these four types may result from vascular changes or metabolic disorders such as diabetes with secondary hearing loss. Central processing of hearing may also be affected by aging, including slowing of neuronal conduction, loss of axons within the cochlear nerves, and cellular changes in the cochlear and olivary nuclei.[20]

Taste and Smell: Similar to the loss of brain tissue with aging, there is a concomitant loss of olfactory receptors of 10% each decade; thus by age 80, 75% of adults have an impaired sense of smell. Similarly, there seems to be a loss of taste buds with aging, most specifically in the epiglottis. However, there is wide variability in the number of taste buds between individuals, so the loss of these receptors may differentially affect taste ability in older adults, depending on their density at younger ages. Nonetheless, loss of taste and smell receptors contributes to the decrease in appetite (**aging anorexia**) experienced by many older adults; some decrease in appetite is expected due to a decrease in activity level plus there are other changes in GI function that contribute to the noted weight loss. However, for some adults, this decrease in appetite can result in dangerous weight loss, malnutrition, poorer overall health, and a diminished ability to combat illness.[21]

● CHANGE IN COGNITIVE FUNCTION

Teaching and Learning with Aging

CASE B, PART I

Mr. Thomas retired at age 65 and spent several years travelling and actively involved on several community-based committees. He is now 70 years old and feels like his "mind is slipping." He received a flyer in the mail offering free college courses to seniors and is considering signing up for a course on astronomy and one on using tablet computers. *What are the benefits of these classes for Mr. Thomas?* Coursework will provide mental stimulation and novel inputs that will help to keep him engaged and lead to maintenance of his cognitive functions.

Aging adults undergo changes that lead to slowing of processing and increased difficulty with skills related to *fluid intelligence*. Overall intelligence does not decline and *crystallized intelligence* improves or remains unchanged (see Box 17-3).[22] To accommodate for changes in fluid intelligence and maximize maintained crystallized intelligence, a class for older adults should provide examples and relate new concepts to previously well-learned information.

CASE B, PART II

For example, the instructor in the tablet computer course could relate functions of the computer to that of a typewriter. It is likely that individuals in Mr. Thomas' generation spent many years using a typewriter and are familiar with how one works; therefore, they could use this crystallized knowledge as a building block for new learning. Yet, novel concepts such as Wi-Fi and the internet that don't easily connect with any prior crystallized concepts will be more challenging for the older adult to learn.

Changes in cognitive function vary across individuals, differentially impacting the spectrum of cognitive functions, including attention, working memory, memory, perception, and higher level cognitive functions; however, changes may be interrelated or additive. Further, some areas of function are more likely to decline than others; for example, older adults may have difficulty with divided attention or attention switching but do well on sustained attention[23] (Table 17-3). Working memory is like computer RAM; it relates to the amount of information that the brain can process at any given time, and it decreases with age. Older adults also have increasing difficulty processing multiple information elements at the same time. Interestingly, while most older adults have good long-term memory, they typically remember the essence of the event but not all of the context or details of it.

BOX 17-3   Fluid versus Crystallized Intelligence[22]

FACTORS OF GENERAL INTELLIGENCE	DEFINITION	AGE-RELATED CHANGE
Crystallized	The ability to use skills, knowledge, and experience. It does not equate to memory, but relies on accessing information from long-term memory. It is demonstrated largely through one's vocabulary and general knowledge.	This improves somewhat with age, as experiences tend to expand one's knowledge
Fluid	The ability to analyze novel problems, identify patterns and relationships that underpin these problems, and the extrapolation of these using logic.	Peaks in adolescence and begins to decline progressively beginning around age 30 or 40

CASE B, PART III

To accommodate for these age-related changes in working memory, information within classes for older adults should be presented in smaller units; the instructor should speak more slowly than usual and pause after each group of facts to allow increased time for processing. In addition, the room should be quiet and set up with a microphone and speaker to ensure that everyone can hear; also, materials should be presented in large print of at least 14 font. Repeating information allows the older learner a second chance to process the information and improves retention and learning. Box 17-4 presents strategies to use when teaching older adults. Despite all of these challenges, the elderly are typically very motivated learners, and new learning may be effective in preventing or ameliorating the negative plasticity of aging.

BOX 17-4   Strategies to Use When Teaching Older Adults

- Connect new information to prior knowledge
- Utilize collaborative learning
- Allow learning to be self-paced
- Slow down
- Encourage elderly to use anticipation and self-cueing
- Use aids to compensate for sensory changes (decreased vision and hearing)

TABLE 17-3   Areas of Cognitive Function and the Impact of Aging[23]

AREA OF COGNITIVE FUNCTION	DESCRIPTION	IMPACT OF AGING
Basic cognitive function		
Perception	The process of becoming aware of something through the senses such as vision, hearing, and somatosensation. Highly integrated with cognition.	Reduced in older adults. Has a large impact on other cognitive functions and so should be thoroughly assessed. Frequently when declines in vision and hearing are accounted for, there are no longer age-related differences in cognitive functioning
Attention: Some form of attention is involved in all other cognitive domains except when the task has become automatic.		
Selective	Ability to attend to a stimuli while disregarding irrelevant stimuli	Maintained ability to concentrate and select relevant stimuli
Divided/Switching	Processing two or more sources of information at the same time requires dividing attention and the ability to switch smoothly between the information sources. It is assessed through dual task performance outcome measures.	Significant impairments on tasks that require dividing or switching attention among multiple tasks.

(continued)

TABLE 17-3	**Areas of Cognitive Function and the Impact of Aging[23]** (*Continued*)	
AREA OF COGNITIVE FUNCTION	**DESCRIPTION**	**IMPACT OF AGING**
Working memory: The system that involves the manipulation of information that is currently being maintained in focal attention.		
Attentional resources	There is a limitation in the resources available for attention-related tasks	Older adults demonstrate significant deficits in tasks that involve use of working memory such as active manipulation, reorganization, or integration of the contents of working memory. Attentional resources are reduced and speed of processing is significantly slower. Research results are mixed on whether inhibitory control is lacking.
Speed of processing	The speed with which information is manipulated, stored, or retrieved (processed)	
Inhibitory control	The ability to suppress irrelevant information in working memory	
Long-term memory: Stored information that is no longer present in or being manipulated in an active state.		
Episodic	Memory for personally experienced events that occurred in a particular place and time	Aging has the largest impact on episodic memory. Older adults believe that their long-term memory is better than their short-term memory but they have difficulty remembering the context or source of information like where or when they saw or did something or whether they actually did something or just thought about it. **Semantic memory is largely preserved.** Older adults have normal acquisition and retention of skills. Implicit memory remains intact. Prospective memory can be successfully augmented through the use of calendars and lists. When no such tool is available, deficits become noticeable.
Semantic	General knowledge about the world (factual information)	
Autobiographical	Memory for one's personal past	
Procedural	Knowledge of skills and procedures like driving a car	
Implicit	Refers to a change in behavior that occurs as a result of prior experience without conscious memory or recollection of that experience (the method for learning skills)	
Prospective	Remembering to do things in the future like a doctor's appointment.	
Higher level cognitive functions		
Speech and language	Ability to produce and understand speech and language, including written language.	Largely intact in older adults; may even improve with aging
Decision making	The thought process of selecting a logical choice from the available options.	There is little research but studies to date show that older adults come to the same decisions as young adults but reach them in a different way. Older adults tend to rely on prior knowledge and less on new information while younger adults consider more alternatives in coming to a conclusion. Older adults also rely more heavily on expert opinion.
Executive control	A multicomponent construct consisting of a range of different processes that are involved in the planning, organization, coordination, implementation, and evaluation of nonroutine activities. Depends heavily on the prefrontal cortex.	Declines in executive control are noted in aging and correlate with findings of neuroimaging studies showing volume and function decline in the prefrontal brain regions.

● DEMENTIA

Dementia is a chronic or persistent disorder of the mental processes, caused by brain disease or injury, and marked by changes in memory, personality, and reasoning. It is a common disorder involving 6% of those over age 65 and 50% of those over age 85 with one out of three families having a parent affected. The annual cost of managing dementia is more than $100 billion in the United States alone.[24,25]

In order to be classified as having dementia, an individual must demonstrate deficits in at least three of the following spheres of mental activity: (1) language, (2) memory, (3) visuospatial skills, (4) emotion, or (5) cognition (abstraction, calculation, judgment, and executive function).[26]

Some forms of dementia are amenable to treatment and can be slowed or even reversed; for this reason, it is very important that patients get a diagnostic workup to identify any reversible causes of dementia (Box 17-5) so that individualized treatment specific to the cause can be initiated. Note that the most common cause of treatable dementia is depression, which can be screened by the therapist, and is amenable to treatment. The **PHQ-2** (Box 17-6), a two-question depression screen, is a simple, fast, and easy tool to screen for depression and should be used in physical therapy practice.[27]

Dementia versus Delirium

Dementia can be confused with delirium, which is a transient condition with a rapid onset and fluctuating symptoms that include poor maintained and shifting attention to external stimuli and disorganized thinking, manifested by rambling and incoherent speech. Two significant differences between dementia and delirium are (1) the acute onset of delirium and (2) consciousness is affected in delirium and not in dementia (Table 17-4).[28] Delirium is typically caused by a severe stressor to the system such as surgery, anesthesia, or disease with *post-anesthetic delirium* most common. When working with an elderly individual who has undergone a recent trauma or significant change in health status, therapists should assess for cognitive impairment but remember that the impairment may be delirium. If cognitive impairment is due to delirium, then the individual's prognosis will be significantly better due to its temporary and time limited status. In older individuals, delirium can last up to 12 months. Notably, individuals with dementia are likely to have delirium in times of stress, and so, health care professionals need to be aware

---

BOX 17-6   PHQ-2 Depression Screen[27]

OVER THE LAST 2 WEEKS, HOW OFTEN HAVE YOU BEEN BOTHERED BY ANY OF THE FOLLOWING PROBLEMS?	NOT AT ALL	SEVERAL DAYS	MORE THAN HALF THE DAYS	NEARLY EVERY DAY
	0	1	2	3
1. Little interest or pleasure in doing things?	☐	☐	☐	☐
2. Feeling down, depressed, or hopeless?	☐	☐	☐	☐

A score of 3 or more indicates a positive screen for depressive symptoms.

---

that both conditions may be present during illness and after injury or surgery. In those with dementia, a larger percentage of individuals (39%) had delirium 6 months post discharge, from an acute illness or surgery, than those without dementia (9%).[29]

CASE C, PART I

Mrs. Ludwig is 72 years old with an uncomplicated medical history. She recently lost her husband and moved from the home in which they had lived for 40 years to a condominium on a single level, where she lives alone. She was seen by her family physician for complaints of back pain and referred for therapy. On initial evaluation, she is quiet and answers questions with single-word responses. She presents with unkempt hair and her shoes do not match. She states that she has to get up at night to go to the bathroom and feels that her gait is unsteady. On her second visit, the therapist asks her to demonstrate the three home exercises she was prescribed, but Mrs. Ludwig does not remember two of the three exercises. The therapist is concerned that Mrs. Ludwig may have dementia due to her unkempt hair, mismatched shoes, single-word answers, and poor memory for her exercise program.

Causes of Dementia

The most common form of dementia is Alzheimer's disease, accounting for 50–60% of all cases of dementia. The next most common cause is vascular dementia, 20% of all cases. Yet there

---

BOX 17-5   Reversible Causes of Dementia

Depression (most common) – 4.5%

Overuse or misuse of certain medications

Normal pressure hydrocephalus – 1.6%

Metabolic including B12 deficiency – 1.5%

Hypothyroidism

Neoplasm – 1.5%

Infections – 0.6%

AIDS

TABLE 17-4 | **Differentiating Dementia from Delirium and Depression**[29]

	DEMENTIA	DELIRIUM	DEPRESSION
Onset	Insidious	Acute	Acute
Conscious state	Impaired very late	Variable consciousness	Unusual
Mood	Stable	Highly variable	Depressed with diurnal variation
Duration	Long term	Short (days)	Short (weeks)
Cognitive features	Reduced short > long-term memory	Short attention span	Reduced short- and long-term memory
Sleep/Wake cycle	Day/Night reversible	Hour to hour variation	Hypersomnia or insomnia
Psychomotor changes	Late	Marked	–
Associated features	–	Medical conditions – medications	Past history

are many causes of dementia, associated with different diseases (Table 17-5) that damage the nervous system through different pathologic processes. In this section, we will discuss the most common causes.

TABLE 17-5 | **Causes of Dementia**

Neurogenerative disorders	AD (43% of all cases) Parkinson's disease Lewy body dementia Frontotemporal dementia (Pick's disease) Huntington's disease
Cerebrovascular disorders	Vascular dementia (20%) Vasculitis Subarachnoid hemorrhage
Toxic/Metabolic encephalopathies	Endocrine gland disorders Drugs (e.g., anesthetics, antibiotics, antidepressants, antivirals, chemotherapeutic) Alcohol Carbon monoxide poisoning Industrial agent Heavy metals
Prion associated disorders	Creutzfeldt–Jakob disease
Neurogenetic disorders	Down syndrome Myotonic dystrophy Spinocerebellar ataxias Wilson disease
Infectious disorders	Meningitis Encephalitis Neurosyphilis
Miscellaneous	Depression Posttraumatic dementia Demyelinating MS Neoplasm Normal pressure hydrocephalus

CASE C, PART II

Which conditions may be the cause of Mrs. Ludwig's poor cognitive functioning?

While from this information it is too early to know definitively, for a patient with Mrs. Ludwig's presentation and uncomplicated medical history, the most likely causes would be depression, Alzheimer's, normal pressure hydrocephalus, thyroid disease, or Parkinson's disease.

How should the therapist assess Mrs. Ludwig in light of these concerns?

Mrs. Ludwig is at risk for depression due to the major life changes she has experienced in the recent past. The PHQ-2 would be a simple tool that the therapist could use to screen for depression, and if positive, refer Mrs. Ludwig to her physician to follow up on this finding.

Neurogenic Causes of Dementia

Alzheimer's disease (AD) accounts for about half of all dementia cases. It is more common in women and in those who have first-degree relatives with the disease or a history of head trauma. Memory and cognitive problems associated with AD have a very slow, insidious onset between 40 and 90 years of age, most commonly after age 65. The intellectual decline eventually results in lasting changes in personality and the inability to perform activities of daily living (Box 17-7); this decline can be characterized by three descriptive stages (Box 17-8).

Alzheimer's disease is associated with multiple changes in the central nervous system, including a decrease in the overall number of synapses, the formation of amyloid plaques and neurofibrillary tangles, angiopathy, and ultimately brain atrophy that is symmetric and widespread, including loss of cortex and white matter with secondary ventricular enlargement. **Amyloid plaques**, also called **senile plaques**, are comprised of abnormally folded proteins that aggregate together with some neuritic components. Notably, many older adults without AD exhibit

---

BOX 17-7   Clinical Features of AD[30]

- Apraxia – impaired ability to do previously learned motor activities despite intact motor function
- Agnosia – failure to recognize or identify objects despite intact sensory function
- Memory loss – initially short-term memory with progression to include long-term memory
- Visuospatial impairment – diminished ability to identify stimuli and their location
- Concreteness – recognize concrete concepts but not abstract concepts or words
- Motor function – preserved motor function except in later stages

---

BOX 17-8   Three Stages of Alzheimer's Disease[31]

Early – Problems retaining new information and forgetfulness, social withdrawal, and may stop participating in activities and hobbies they formerly loved. Moody, time disoriented, and exhibit poor judgment.

Intermediate – Behavioral and personality changes, parkinsonism and psychotic symptoms are most evident. They begin to exhibit changes in gait, wandering starts, and confusion of day and night appears. Late in this stage there may be excessive wandering behavior, and they forget how to eat. Weight loss is a problem. The individual requires care in this stage.

Late – Loss of most functional abilities. Incontinence, loss of ability to walk, and the individual is at risk for contracture and development of decubiti, anorexia, and illogical thinking.

---

amyloid plaques, those with AD have a much higher number of plaques. Similarly, **neurofibrillary tangles** are aggregates of a protein, called tau, that are found in the cytoplasm of neurons (cell body and axons) and the extracellular space; tau is an elongated structure, and in neurofibrillary tangles, as the name suggests, they wind around each other to produce a tangled bundle. Neurofibrillary tangles are also present in other neurologic conditions so are not unique to AD. The angiopathy of AD is referred to as **cerebral amyloid angiopathy** and is characterized by amyloid material replacing the smooth muscle cells of the capillaries, arterioles, and sometimes larger arteries within the cerebral cortex but may also occur in the subarachnoid space and cerebellum. This change in the wall of these small vessels places them at risk for hemorrhage. Of note, AD and cerebrovascular disease are often found together; when this occurs, it is called mixed dementia. Interestingly, it has been shown that effective, early treatment of HTN can protect against cognitive decline.[32]

Lewy body dementia (LBD) is the presence of dementia with relative *sparing of memory*; other symptoms include gait and balance dysfunction, prominent *hallucinations and delusions* with *sensitivity to antipsychotics*, and *fluctuations in attention* and

cognition. Individuals with LBD are more impaired than those with AD on attention tests but continue to have fluctuations in cognition even in late stages. Yet, cognitive tests by themselves do not differentiate AD and LBD. Neuropsychiatric problems or symptoms are more common in LBD leading to entry into health care often within psychiatric centers. In one-third of cases, **visual hallucinations** are a presenting symptom. Depressive symptoms are also more common in LBD than AD. The hallmark **sensitivity to antipsychotic medications**, found in LBD, is due to the extrapyramidal syndrome features that are present in LBD. Gait and balance disorders are the same as those seen in Parkinson's disease (PD); therefore individuals with LBD may also be initially diagnosed as having PD. In addition, individuals with LBD show more rapid motor deterioration than those with AD.[33]

Lewy body dementia is part of a group of disorders, including PD, associated with an abnormal accumulation of a protein (**alpha-synuclein or α-Syn**) in the presynaptic terminals of neurons. This protein's normal function is to regulate neurotransmitter release and modulate synaptic function. However, in LBD, α-Syn aggregates into clusters, called Lewy bodies, in the axon terminals, becoming toxic, damaging the synaptic membrane and axonal mitochondria, and disrupting neuronal function, especially in dopaminergic and cholinergic neurons. Ultimately, there is a loss of synapses and neuronal death. The motor deficits mirror those of PD, yet there are also some similarities to AD, including the presence of amyloid plaques (common) and neurofibrillary tangles (less common). However, unlike AD, there is little brain atrophy with LBD.[34]

Frontotemporal dementias (FTD) are a group of disorders with a basic degenerative pattern of the frontal and temporal lobes, including behavioral variant frontotemporal dementia (bvFTD or Pick disease) and primary progressive aphasias (nonfluent-agrammatic and semantic). The more common form is Pick disease, which is characterized by mild to moderate frontal lobe atrophy with temporal lobe sparing early and degeneration later, often localized to the right hemisphere, a mean age of onset of 45–70 years and duration of 3–17 years. Compared to AD these patients are less disoriented but have more difficulty with problem solving. Short-term memory and the ability to negotiate in the environment (visuospatial ability) are relatively spared until later in the disease course. Speech is involved early, as it is in AD, as well as changes in personality and behavior, including disinhibition. Hypochondriasis, schizophrenia, obsessive–compulsive disorder, depression and anxiety can be so severe that these individuals may end up in a psychiatric emergency room or being treated for these psychiatric problems long before the diagnosis of dementia is made.

Similar to the other dementias already discussed (AD, LBD), FTDs result from protein anomalies of tau protein, transactive response DNA binding protein 43 (TDP-43), or sarcoma protein. The psychiatric symptoms, in FTD, stem from early degeneration of the paralimbic cortex in the ventromedial cortex along with the anterior cingulate and insular cortex. About 15% of FTD cases will also present with motor neuron disease and 20% with parkinsonism that can be distinguished from PD by the lack of rigidity in the arms, absence of a resting tremor, and presences of supranuclear palsy.[35]

Vascular Dementia (VaD)

The second most common form of dementia is VaD. Like many of the dementias, VaD encompasses a group of disorders, including multi-infarct, strategic infarct, and subcortical ischemic vascular dementia. VaD is associated with three common blood vessel disorders: atherosclerosis (ATS), small vessel disease (SVD), or cerebral amyloid angiopathy (CAA), which are described in Box 17-9. VaD is common in those with a history of diabetes and/or HTN; interestingly, HTN has been associated with hypoperfusion of the brain and diminished cortex thickness that may also contribute to the development of dementia.[36] **Multi-infarct dementia**, consistent with its name, results from a number of small infarcts (lacunar or micro) in concert with or without larger infarcts that can result from ATS, SVD, or CAA, although ATS seems to play a greater role. **Strategic infarct dementia** is induced by ischemia of vessels within regions that are critical for cognitive and memory function (e.g., hippocampus, thalamic paramedian nuclei, subiculum). Vascular damage, primarily from ATS, within the smaller penetrating blood vessels of the cortical white matter, can result in axonal demyelination and destruction of critical projecting neurons; this is known as **subcortical ischemic vascular dementia**.[36]

Because the lesions in VaD are typically small and functional deficits begin to appear when the burden of lesions is high enough to create significant tissue loss, progression is usually in a step-wise fashion rather than linear. Unlike AD, vascular dementia may be accompanied by early gait disturbances, frequent falls, and personality changes. Because subcortical areas are more at risk for perfusion problems, individuals with VaD may be apathetic and depressed but are less likely to be agitated

or psychotic as compared to those with AD. See Table 17-6 for a comparison of the most common dementias.

Normal Pressure Hydrocephalus

Normal pressure hydrocephalus (NPH) is associated with enlargement of the ventricles without an increase in intracranial pressure or interstitial edema; this enlargement creates ischemia of the deep white matter such that the myelinated fibers appear pale. Ultimately, there is tissue atrophy and dementia. NPH seems to result from a disturbance in the outflow of cerebrospinal fluid into the subarachnoid space (see Chapter 18 for a review of CSF flow). There is some indication that NPH occurs in individuals that may have had infantile external hydrocephalus, a condition of poor CSF absorption in young infants secondary to immature arachnoid granulations that resolves. One hypothesis is that this condition triggers an alternate CSF flow pathway that transfers the fluid into the interstitial space and then via small channels (aquaporin-4 channels) within the linings of veins into the venous system. However, with aging, this secondary system is disrupted, resulting in NPH.[37]

Normal pressure hydrocephalus creates both motor disturbances and dementia; however, it is one of the few causes of dementia that is treatable. With therapists' roles in assessing gait and mobility, they are often the first to pick up on the pattern of symptoms associated with normal pressure hydrocephalus. NPH usually presents with progressive mental impairment, problems with walking, and impaired bladder control. Gait is typically slow and shuffling, and the bladder control issues are more prevalent at night. This leaves these individual at high risk for falling, and often first presenting to the health care system after suffering an injury from a fall. NPH has symptoms much like Alzheimer's and Parkinson diseases so is often misdiagnosed or unrecognized. When NPH is caught early, at the point of gait disruption without significant mental deterioration, shunting (as described in Chapter 18) is often effective in preventing further deterioration and may allow recovery of motor ability.

BOX 17-9   Vessel Disorders Associated with VaD[36]

Atherosclerosis (ATS) is the build-up of lipids, typically cholesterol, and proteins into plaques within the walls of larger arteries, weakening the arterial wall and creating the potential for rupture and hemorrhage, manifested as a stroke. However, pieces of these plaques can also break off and cause downstream blockage and ischemia within smaller vessels (smaller often subclinical infarcts).

Small vessel disease (SVD), as the name implies, is a disorder of smaller vessels that can be similar to that of ATS in larger vessels, characterized by a hardening of the arterial wall and hypoperfusion of the surrounding tissue. Alternatively, arteriosclerosis is associated with a thickening of small vessel walls that impedes blood flow and can result in **lacunar** (small) or even smaller **micro** infarcts. SVD is typically localized to the basal ganglia early but expands into the white matter, thalamus, and cerebellum over time.

Cerebral amyloid angiopathy (CAA) results from amyloid β-protein deposits within the smooth muscle of blood vessels that eventually lead to blockage or rupture of the vessel. This occurs first in the small vessels within the pial and arachnoid maters that provide collateral circulation to the brain's surface but eventually occurs in vessels to deeper structures (hippocampus, amygdala) and finally within the basal ganglia, thalamus, and brainstem.

CASE C, PART III

Mrs. Ludwig is exhibiting symptoms that are consistent with both AD and NPH. For this reason a cognitive screen such as the Folstein Mini-Mental Status Examination (MMSE) or the Montreal Cognitive Assessment (MoCA) should be administered with referral to the physician, if she scores in the at-risk range on the screening assessment.

Additionally, Mrs. Ludwig could have thyroid disease or PD. The therapist would be able to screen for these disorders through a complete systems review including skin, hair, and weight changes, as changes in these systems are consistent with thyroid disorders. A thorough assessment of tone, gait, and motor skills would identify if the motor symptoms of PD such as rigidity, hypokinesia, and bradykinesia are present.

TABLE 17-6	Distinguishing Features of the Common Dementias					
	MEMORY	**LANGUAGE**	**EXECUTIVE FUNCTION**	**VISUOSPATIAL**	**BEHAVIOR**	**MOTOR SYMPTOMS**
AD	Early, short-term loss > long term	Poor word list generation	Preceded by memory loss	Early topographic disorientation	Socially inappropriate, late agitation	Apraxia, agnosia, mid stage develop shuffling gait
Vascular	Variable	Aphasia if cortex involved	Variable	Variable	Apathy or depression	Focal findings: mild bradykinesia if basal ganglia involved
LBD	Fluctuating alertness, memory spared	Slower	Impaired	Impaired	Hallucinations, bizarre delusions	Rigidity, bradykinesia, hypokinesia (parkinsonian gait)
FTD	Decreased concentration > short-term memory loss	Unrestrained but empty. Aphasia may precede dementia	Early decline	Spared	Early disinhibition, hypochondriasis, affective disorders, mania	Lack of coordination, rigidity, and may feel weak

Medical Management of Dementia

Evaluation and Diagnosis of Dementia

The physician will screen for depression and do blood tests to identify signs of reversible causes of dementia (e.g., medication issues, infection, hypothyroidism, B12 deficiency), including testing serum electrolytes, serum glucose, urea, nitrogen, and creatinine, B12 level, liver function tests, thyroid function tests. For reversible dementias, the specific remedy should be administered as soon as possible in order to reverse damage, if possible, and stop progression of damage. Imaging remains somewhat controversial; however, for NPH, imaging is critical for diagnosis to look for enlargement of the ventricles. In individuals with AD, imaging changes are typically not evident early in the disease, don't dictate the care provided, or affect the outcome of that care. Patients with non-AD dementias are likely to have findings on CT or MRI; therefore, the use of imaging is recommended in patients with less common dementia presentations such as onset before age 60, focal signs or symptoms, or the presence of early gait disturbance.

Intervention

Anyone diagnosed with dementia should receive family, caregiver, and patient education at the time of diagnosis. Treatment for AD includes the use of cholinesterase inhibitors which help postpone the onset of symptoms. Studies have shown that individuals who use NSAIDs have a 23% lower risk of developing AD than those who never use NSAIDs. Despite these findings, studies using NSAIDs to treat individuals with AD have demonstrated no positive benefit from the use of NSAIDs to slow progression of AD. Vascular dementia is managed through aggressive treatment of cardiovascular risk factors. Treatment of LBD can be challenging. Anti-parkinsonian agents may reduce extrapyramidal symptoms but, in general, are not as efficacious as they are in those with PD. NPH, as mentioned earlier, is treated with shunting.

Aggressive behaviors can be a common symptom in individuals with dementia and lead to challenges in caregiving. The use of restraints should be avoided as they increase agitation and can lead to injuries and even death. Behavioral management techniques are quite effective if implemented correctly and consistently (Box 17-10) and should help therapists deal with individuals with aggressive behavior as well. If behavioral and non-pharmacological management fail, physicians may use antipsychotic medications. These medications are only used if the patient is a danger to himself or others.

Physical Therapy Management of the Patient with Dementia

Screening

Signs or symptoms that would suggest dementia in a client include superficial answers to probing questions, inappropriate dress or hygiene, and inability to remember therapy from previous sessions. In at-risk individuals or someone that demonstrates signs or symptoms of dementia, the therapist should administer a cognitive screening exam such as the MMSE or the MoCA. Prior to assessing for cognitive function, first

---

BOX 17-10   Behavioral Management Techniques

- Stay calm and exemplify calm behavior
- Reassure and acknowledge their feelings
- Listen to what they are saying
- Maintain eye contact
- Simplify your instructions and if possible the environment
- Try to distract them
- Explain what you are about to do
- Reorient without arguing or demanding that they understand
- Slow down
- Avoid change in caregivers and the environment in which they live
- Encourage familiarity with consistent caregivers
- Use touch to connect with the person but do not use it to restrain or control them
- Educate and support family
- Respect individuals integrity and encourage independence

CASE C, PART IV

Mrs. Ludwig undergoes a thorough assessment and the therapist communicates with the physician regarding the new concerns related to cognition. Therapy can move forward with treatment for Mrs. Ludwig's back pain. Treatment for the back pain is modified to account for cognitive issues such as ensuring Mrs. Ludwig has written directions, maintaining a consistent structure and exercise program, and keeping all instructions simple.

---

ensure that the individual has adequate vision and hearing to understand instructions. The MMSE is the most common neurocognitive test. This is a screening tool that allows the clinician to identify potential cognitive issues but does not diagnose dementia or the type of dementia. The MMSE measures concentration, memory, visuospatial, and basic language. The MMSE is influenced by the person's culture and educational background but is the most commonly utilized test in the United States. It does not include any assessment of executive function. An individual scoring <24 on the MMSE should be referred to a physician as having a positive screen for cognitive impairment. The Clock Task is a means of assessing executive function and is commonly administered in conjunction with the MMSE; this is a simple test where the individual is asked to (1) draw the face of a clock with the numbers on it and (2) place the hands of the clock at a specified time (11:10 or 1:45). Patients with impaired executive function have difficulty performing complex tasks such as the clock task. They can perform the elements of the task but cannot put it all together to accomplish the entire task. Problems with executive function are found in the old–old, those with dementia, and individuals with diabetes, AIDS, or uncontrolled HTN. The MoCA is a 30-point test that can be administered in 10 minutes with a cutoff score for cognitive impairment of 26. The sensitivity and specificity of the MoCA for detecting early cognitive impairment were 100% and 87% respectively, compared with 78% and 100% for the MMSE. Since the MoCA assesses multiple cognitive domains, it may be a useful cognitive screening tool for several neurological diseases that affect younger populations, such as PD, vascular cognitive impairment, Huntington's disease, brain metastasis, primary brain tumors (including high- and low-grade gliomas), multiple sclerosis, and other conditions, such as traumatic brain injury, depression, schizophrenia, and heart failure.[38]

Motor Learning in Dementia

Individuals with dementia have deficits in areas related to memory, mood, and executive function but do not necessarily have damage in the areas related to motor learning. In fact, individuals with dementia can learn motor skills. **Remember, procedural learning uses different areas of the brain than semantic learning and does not require explicit knowledge of how a task is done** (see Chapter 7). However, in individuals with dementia, random practice offers no benefit and may impede learning, while blocked massed practice results in learning even when the individual has no explicit recall of the practice or learning. Blocked-variable practice has also been investigated in individuals with AD but resulted in no appreciable learning. It appears that patients with AD can acquire a motor skill, demonstrate intact implicit memory and learning, but no explicit memory or learning. Therefore, they are able to learn motor skills even though they do not remember having practiced the skill and could not describe what they are about to do. Motor learning is possible because the subcortical structures (e.g., cerebellum, basal ganglia), involved in skill acquisition, are not as affected by AD as the cortex and hippocampus. There is supposition that individuals with AD fail to develop a motor schema, which is associated with storage of the sensation of the movement, the context in which it occurred, the movement parameters, and the knowledge of the results; the inability to form a motor schema is likely due to involvement of the cortex and hippocampus such that some aspects of the schema are not encoded, limiting the transfer of newly learned skills to novel situations. Thus, physical therapy should be effective if the motor skill is practiced in the environment in which the skill will be performed.[39]

Physical Therapy for Individuals with Dementia

Individuals with dementia should receive therapy for any musculoskeletal disorders such as sprains, fractures, or joint replacements just as a non-impaired patient would. Therapy will be managed according to the guiding principles of implicit learning, using a high number of repetitions and low variability, and allowing few errors during learning.[40] The goals and timing of therapy should also be modified to fit the abilities of the client with dementia. In some situations, the most appropriate therapy may be training the individual to use a Rollator walker to improve safety. This can be initiated by the physical therapist and then continued by caregivers. Therefore, an appropriate care plan would be for therapy to see the client two to three times to determine appropriate assistive device and then train caregivers to continue with the plan. Alternatively, an individual with dementia who is falling when walking and transferring, while using a Rollator, may require more therapy sessions than the individual without dementia, in order to provide an adequate quantity of massed practice of each skill in which falls are occurring.

Interestingly, there have been a number of studies that have evaluated the impact of exercise on cognitive function and self-care in individuals with dementia, most frequently those with AD. In a recent Cochrane review, it was reported that exercise programs could improve cognitive function and ADLs in those with dementia; however, current trials are quite heterogeneous in the type of exercise used (balance activities, walking, specific tasks [throwing], strength training), the duration (2 weeks–12 months), the frequency (2–5 times/week), and the session duration (20–75 minutes), so specific guidelines for exercise programs have not been established.[41]

Fitness and the Role of Exercise in Preventing Dementia

Aerobic exercise has a focused benefit on both neurogenesis and angiogenesis in the hippocampus with increased synaptic plasticity, facilitating the integration of hippocampal neurons into existing brain networks. In one study of individuals at high risk for developing AD, those who were more physically active exhibited less hippocampal atrophy over an 18-month period than those who were inactive. However, the protective effects of physical activity were not observed in individuals who were at low risk for developing AD, indicating that the benefits of exercise may be dependent on the individual's genetic or physiologic makeup. The type of exercise is important as benefits vary by type of exercise. **Brain-derived neurotrophic factor** (BDNF) is important as it supports the survival of existing neurons and the growth of new neurons, while insulin-like growth factor 1 (IGF-1) supports neurogenesis, angiogenesis, and neural plasticity, especially after brain injury. Aerobic exercise upregulates BDNF while resistance exercise upregulates both BDNF and IGF-1. There is overwhelming evidence that BDNF is an important factor in exercise-induced improvement in brain function and cognition, yet the impact of age is not yet known.[42]

The evidence suggests that aerobic exercise benefits cognitive performance, brain function, and brain structure. Aerobic training in late life preferentially benefits executive functions, including multitasking, planning, and inhibition of extraneous information. All of these functions are performed in the prefrontal cortex. Animal models indicate that exercise brings about structural integrity improvement (neurogenesis and angiogenesis) and increased production of neurochemicals that promote growth, differentiation, survival, and repair of brain cells. Since improvement in function is often seen without apparent neurogenesis, it may not play an important role in improvement of functional performance. Thus, **angiogenesis** may underlie the improvement in function found in these studies. Yet, two studies have shown aerobic training related

increases in hippocampal angiogenesis in young but not aged mice, raising the question as to whether or not the benefits can be achieved in an aged system.[43]

Epidemiologic and prospective studies support the role of aerobic fitness in healthy cognitive brain function and in delaying the onset of dementia. Studies in humans, to date, have primarily been retrospective, and so, their conclusions are limited. They indicate that individuals who are more active in middle age have a lower likelihood of cognitive decline or dementia in old age. In addition, these studies do not tell us specifically what led to the protection from cognitive decline.

Resistance exercise has also been investigated as a means to protect cognitive function, but the findings to date have been equivocal. Protocols with positive benefit used 50–80% of a single repetition maximum lift and led to improvements in memory, when training was progressive and lasted more than 6 months.[43] Another study showed improved selective attention and conflict resolution after 1 year of one or two times weekly resistance training. Given the differences across studies it is possible that aerobic training will be more effective for some individuals, resistance training for others, and a combination of both for yet others.[43]

Despite positive findings related to exercise and cognition it is still unknown whether the benefits of exercise can be achieved in aged individuals, the type of exercise that is best, or how to improve specific areas of cognitive function. Additionally the majority of studies have been conducted in individuals experiencing healthy aging. Benefits of exercise to slow or prevent diseases like AD remain equivocal, needing more definitive study. Overall, exercise that is structured, individualized, higher intensity, longer duration, and multicomponent shows the most promise for preserving cognitive performance.[44]

REFERENCES

1. Seidler RD, Bernard JA, Burutolu TB, et al. Motor control and aging: links to age-related brain structural, functional, and biochemical effects. *Neurosci Biobehav Rev.* 2010;34(5):721-733.

2. Schut LJ. Motor system changes in the aging brain: what is normal and what is not. *Geriatrics.* 1998;53(S1):S16-S19.

3. Salat DH, Buckner RL, Snyder AZ, Greve DN, Desikan RSR, Busa E, Morris JC, Dale AM, Fischl B. Thinning of the cerebral cortex in aging. *Cereb Cortex.* 2004;14(7):721-730.

4. Courchesne E, Chisum HJ, Townsend J, Cowles A, Covington J, Egaas B. Normal brain development and aging: quantitative analysis at in vivo MR imaging in healthy volunteers. *Radiology.* 2000;216:672-682.

5. Ota M, Obata T, Akine Y, Ito H, Ikehira H, Asada T, Suhara T. Age-related degeneration of corpus callosum measured with diffusion tensor imaging. *NeuroImage.* 2006;31:1445-1452.

6. Wickremaratchi MM, Llewelyn JG. Effects of ageing on touch. *Postgrad Med J.* 2006;82:301-304.

7. Ding B, Ling HW, Zhang Y, Huang J, Zhang H, Wang T, Yan FH. Pattern of cerebral hyperperfusion in Alzheimer's disease and amnestic mild cognitive impairment using voxel-based analysis of 3D arterial spin-labeling imaging: initial experience. *Clin Interv Aging.* 2014;9:493-500.

8. Sibille E, Su J, Leman S, et al. Lack of serotonin1B receptor expression leads to age-related motor dysfunction, early onset of brain molecular aging and reduced longevity. *Mol Psychiatry.* 2007;12(11):1042-1056.

9. Romero DH, Stelmach GE. Changes in postural control with aging and Parkinson's disease. *IEEE Eng Med Biol Mag.* 2003;22(2):27-31.

10. Taylor JA, Tan CO. BP regulation VI: elevated sympathetic outflow with human aging: hypertensive or homeostatic? *Eur J Appl Physiol.* 2014;114:511-519.

11. Peters A, Sethares C. Is there remyelination during aging of the primate central nervous system? *J Comp Neurol.* 2003;460:238-254.

12. Deschenes MR. Motor unit and neuromuscular junction remodeling with aging. *Curr Aging Sci.* 2011;4(3):209-220.

13. Nilwik R, Snijders T, Leenders M, Groen BBL, van Kranenburg J, Verdijk LB, van Loon LJC. The decline in skeletal muscle mass with aging is mainly attributed to a reduction in type II muscle fiber size. *Exp Gerontol.* 2013;48:492-498.

14. Frontera WR, Zayas AR, Rodrigues N. Aging of human muscle: understanding sarcopenia at the single muscle cell level. *Phys Med Rehabil Clin N Am.* 2012;23(1):201-207.

15. Henwood TR, Rick S, Taaffe DR. Strength versus muscle power-specific resistance training in community-dwelling older adults. *J Gerontol.* 2008;63A(1):83-91.

16. Mahncke HW1, Bronstone A, Merzenich MM. Brain plasticity and functional losses in the aged: scientific bases for a novel intervention. *Prog Brain Res.* 2006;157:81-109.

17. Petrash JM. Aging and age-related diseases of the ocular lens and vitreous body. *Invest Ophthalmol Vis Sci.* 2013;54:ORSF54-ORSF59.

18. Wang Y, Xu K, Zhang H, Zhao J, Zhu X, Wang Y, Wu R. Retinal ganglion cell death is triggered by paraptosis via reactive oxygen species production: a brief literature review presenting a novel hypothesis in glaucoma pathology. *Mol Med Rep.* 2014;10:1179-1183.

19. Sharma K, Sharma NK, Anand A. Why AMD is a disease of ageing and not of development: mechanisms and insights. *Front Aging Neurosci.* 2014;6(151):1-11.

20. Lee KY. Pathophysiology of age-related hearing loss. *Korean J Audiol.* 2013;17:45-49.

21. Bhutto A, Morley JE. The clinical significance of gastrointestinal changes with aging. *Curr Opin Clin Nutr Metab Care.* 2008;11:651-660.

22. Beir ME, Ackerman PL. Age, ability, and the role of prior knowledge on the acquisition of new domain knowledge: promising results in a real-world learning environment. *Psychol Aging.* 2005;20(2):341-355.

23. Glisky E. Chapter 1: Changes in cognitive function in human aging. In: Riddle DR, ed. *Brain Aging: Models, Methods, and Mechanisms. Frontiers in Neuroscience.* Boca Raton, FL: CRC Press; 2007.

24. Available at: http://www.alz.org/downloads/facts_figures_2012.pdf

25. Available at: http://www.ninds.nih.gov/disorders/dementias/dementia.htm

26. Cummings JL, Benson DF. *Dementia: a clinical approach.* 2nd ed. Boston, MA: Butterworth-Heinemann; 1992.

27. Kroenke K, Spitzer RL, Williams JBW. The Patient Health Questionnaire-2: validity of a two-item depression screener. *Med Care.* 2003;41:1284-1292.

28. Downing LJ, Caprio TV, Lyness JM. Geriatric psychiatry review: differential diagnosis and treatment of the 3Ds – delirium, dementia, and depression. *Curr Psychiatry Rep.* 2013;15(365):1-10.

29. McCusker J, Cole M, Dendukuri N, Han L, Belzile E. The course of delirium in older medical inpatients. *J Gen Intern Med.* 2003;18(9):696-704.

30. Jacobs DH, Adair JC, Williamson DJ, Na DL, Gold M, et al. Apraxia and motor-skill acquisition in Alzheimer's disease are dissociable. *Neuropsychologia.* 1999;37:875-880.

31. Souder E, Chastain J, Williams RD. Dementia in the new millennium. *Medsurg Nurs.* 2002;11(2):61-69.

32. Vinters HV. Emerging concepts in Alzheimer's disease. *Ann Rev Pathol: Mech Dis.* 2014;16(57):291-319.

33. Vicioso BA. Dementia: when is it not Alzheimer's disease? *Am J Med Sci.* 2002;324(2):84-95.

34. Overk CR, Masliah E. Pathogenesis of synaptic degeneration in Alzheimer's disease and Lewy body disease. *Biochem Pharmacol.* 2014;88:508-516.

35. Karageorglou E, Miller BL. Frontotemporal lobar degeneration: a clinical approach. *Semin Neurol.* 2014;34:189-201.

36. Thal DR, Grinberg LT, Attems J. Vascular dementia: different forms of vessel disorders contribute to the development of dementia in the elderly brain. *Exp Gerontol.* 2012;47(11):816-824.

37. Bradley WG. CSF flow in the brain in the context of normal pressure hydrocephalus. *Am J Neuroradiol.* 2015 (epub ahead of print 10.3174/ajnr.A4124).

38. Oudman E, Postma A, Van der Stigchel S, Appelhof B, Wijnia JW, Nijboer TCW. The Montreal Cognitive Assessment (MoCA) is superior to the Mini Mental State Examination (MMSE) in detection of Korsakoff's syndrome. *Clin Neuropsychol.* 2014;28(7):1123-1132.

39. Dick MB, Hsieh S, Dick-Muehlke C, Davis DS, Cotman CW. The variability of practice hypothesis in motor learning: Does it apply to Alzheimer's disease? *Brain Cogn.* 2000;44:470-489.

40. White L, Ford MP, Brown CJ, Peel C, Triebel KL. Facilitating the use of implicit memory and learning in the physical therapy management of individuals with Alzheimer disease: a case series. *J Geriatr Phys Ther.* 2014;37:35-44.

41. Forbes D, Thiessen EJ, Blake CM, Forbes SC, Forbes S. Exercise programs for people with dementia (review). *Cochrane Database Syst Rev.* 2013;12:Art No.:CD006489 (doi:10.1002/14651858.CD006489.pub3)

42. Smith JC, Nielson KA, Woodard JL, et al. Physical activity reduces hippocampal atrophy in elders at genetic risk for Alzheimer's disease. *Front Aging Neurosci.* 2014;6:61.

43. Voss MW, Nagamatsu LS, Liu-Ambrose T, Kramer AF. Exercise, brain, and cognition across the life span. *J Appl Physiol.* 2011;111:1505-1513.

44. Kirk-Sanchez NJ, McGough EL. Physical exercise and cognitive performance in the elderly: current perspectives. *Clin Interv Aging.* 2014;9:51-62.

Review Questions

1. **The greatest age-related differences in gray matter occur in which area of the brain?**

   A. Prefrontal cortex

   B. Motor cortex

   C. Occipital cortex

   D. Sensory cortex

2. **Juggling is a bimanual task and these bimanual skills would be expected to decline with aging due to changes in which area of the brain?**

   A. Cingulate gyrus

   B. Corpus callosum

   C. Hippocampus

   D. Occipital cortex

3. **Decreased levels of which of the following neurotransmitters has been correlated with declines in activity level in an animal model?**

   A. Acetylcholine

   B. Dopamine

   C. Norepinephrine

   D. Serotonin

4. In aging it is noted that muscle fiber conversion to a slow twitch type occurs. This is proposed to be at least in part due to:

   A. Degeneration of the dorsal root ganglion

   B. Denervation followed by regeneration of distal axons

   C. Loss of preganglionic cell bodies in the sympathetic outflow tract

   D. Reduction in myelinated fibers in the fasciculus gracilis

5. Mrs. Smith who is 90 years old is unable to leave her home without assistance due to difficulty ambulating on uneven surfaces and an inability to step up or down from curbs. These functional losses would be considered normal age-related declines associated with aging. True or False.

   A. True

   B. False

6. Mr. Thomas who is 70 years old goes to his local gym and lifts weights four times a week. He does not participate in any aerobic exercises. This exercise program could provide which of the following benefits to Mr. Thomas:

   A. Upregulation of BDNF

   B. Less atrophy of the cerebellum

   C. Reversal of fiber type conversion in exercised muscles

   D. None of the above, only aerobic exercise improves neurologic function

7. According to the negative plasticity model typical age-related changes in somatosensation can lead to which of the following?

   A. Reduction in motor output

   B. Impaired or wrong sensory input

   C. Increasing complexity of sensory input

   D. An inability of the nervous system to remodel with age

8. Therapy for impaired balance can limit or reverse negative plasticity in aging individuals by?

   A. Reducing sensory inputs during activity such as limiting feedback

   B. Providing a balance program with progressively more difficult activities

   C. Instructing the person to avoid walking on uneven surfaces

   D. Providing an assistive device for use during all mobility

9. Typical age-related changes in gait include which of the following?

   A. Increased cadence

   B. Decreased swing to stance ratio

   C. Increased rotation of the trunk

   D. Landing on the toes at initial contact

10. Which of the following is an example of crystallized intelligence? Mr. Smith

    A. Relates a story to his grandchild about battle strategies he used in WWII and how they are similar to ones being used currently

    B. Announces he knows how a recent battle could have been won and describes a strategy that is a modification of one he used in WWII

    C. Announces that he has come up with a novel battle strategy that should be used in a current war zone

    D. Calculates the number of bombs dropped in a recent battle based on his knowledge of the number of bombs per plane and his count of planes from news reel footage.

11. Aging impacts attention in which of the following ways?

    A. Reduces ability to select relevant stimuli to focus on

    B. Decreases concentration

    C. Impairs ability to divide attention

    D. Impairs ability to reorganize information

12. Aging has the largest impact on which type of memory?

    A. Episodic

    B. Implicit

    C. Procedural

    D. Semantic

13. Which of the following is considered a higher level cognitive function?

    A. Attention

    B. Memory

    C. Speech and language

    D. Speed of processing

14. The most common cause of treatable or reversible dementia is?

    A. Alzheimer's disease

    B. Depression

    C. Normal pressure hydrocephalus

    D. Alcoholism

15. Delirium is different from dementia in that in delirium

    A. Consciousness is not affected

    B. Onset is acute

    C. There is impairment in attention

    D. The person has insomnia

16. Changes in gait first occur in which stage of Alzheimer's disease?

    A. Early

    B. Intermediate

    C. Late

17. Mr. Thomas has decreased concentration, impaired memory, and his wife complains that he has become very flirtatious and has begun to approach young women and tell them they are beautiful. She states that he has always been a shy and reserved person. Based on this description which form of dementia does Mr. Thomas most likely have?

    A. Alzheimer's

    B. Frontotemporal dementia

    C. Lewy body dementia

    D. Vascular dementia

18. True or False. The Mini Mental Status Exam includes an assessment of executive function

    A. True

    B. False

19. Mrs. Ludwig is taught to scoot to the edge of the chair and lean forward when transferring sit to stand. She is able to perform this skill when in the dining room with no cueing. When asked to tell her daughter about her therapy she does not remember the therapist or ever being in therapy. Which of the following statements is true about Mrs. Ludwig's learning?

    A. She has not learned how to transfer

    B. She has explicitly learned transfer skills

    C. She exhibits implicit learning of the transfer skills

    D. She has impaired motor learning and should not receive therapy

20. When working with Mrs. Ludwig who has Alzheimer's disease Mrs. Ludwig becomes agitated and starts yelling "get off of the boat." The therapist should respond in what manner?

    A. Ask the PT assistant to take over as a change in caregiver may help calm her down

    B. Avoid eye contact while explaining that everything is okay

    C. Place both hands on Mrs. Ludwig's shoulders and apply firm downward pressure

    D. Say "I understand you are upset, do you need to get up?" based on what Mrs. Ludwig is shouting

Answers

1. A	**2.** B	**3.** D	**4.** B	**5.** B
6. A	**7.** B	**8.** B	**9.** B	**10.** A
11. C	**12.** A	**13.** C	**14.** B	**15.** B
16. B	**17.** B	**18.** B	**19.** C	**20.** D

Neural Tube Disorders and Hydrocephalus

18

Jill C. Heathcock and Deborah S. Nichols-Larsen

OBJECTIVES

1) Distinguish the epidemiology and pathophysiology of neural tube defects

2) Identify the common sensorimotor deficits and associated comorbidities of myelomeningocele

3) Identify and help physical therapists choose optimal treatment interventions for children with myelomeningocele

CASE A, PART I

Dylan is a 15-year-old male with myelomeningocele. His birth history includes myelomeningocele identification from an ultrasound at 20 weeks of gestation. He was born via scheduled C-section at 38 weeks gestational age. He had postnatal surgery to close the lesion 24 hours later, and during surgery, the highest lesion level identified was L1/L2; he had a second surgery to implant a ventriculo-peritoneal shunt at 3 weeks of age. He wore a Pavlik harness for his first 6 months of life for bilateral hip dysplasia. He has had multiple episodes of physical therapy care throughout his lifetime. Dylan does not ambulate, but wore braces up to the age of 6 to facilitate standing and home ambulation with a walker. Currently, he is s/p spinal fusion for scoliosis and has restrictions, including no flexion of his trunk and no pushing or pulling with his arms; he has been fitted with a thoracolumbosacral orthosis (TLSO) to prevent trunk flexion during recovery. Dylan is unable to push or pull with his legs. His ankle ROM is lacking 5 degrees bilaterally and 20+ degrees of hip flexion contractures were corrected as part of his scoliosis surgery. In the past year, he has also had an increased weight gain of 30 pounds, and now weighs 150. Dylan will be starting high school in 2 months. He is currently in a manual wheelchair that he has had for 2 years. His current chair is too small, and he cannot propel it with the restrictions from the surgery. Right now his mom pushes him in the manual chair, and in school, a student peer is pushing him from one class to another.

● INTRODUCTION

To understand Dylan, we will start with a discussion of neural tube defects, including spina bifida and myelomeningocele. In clinical practice, the terms spina bifida and myelomeningocele are often used interchangeably; however, they actually refer to related congenital defects. Spina bifida is a defect of closure of the spinous processes of the spinal column; in the case of myelomeningocele, this spinal column defect is associated with a neural tube defect that results in protrusion of neural and spinal tissue outside the spinal column, typically within a dural sac, with secondary nerve damage and paresis below the level of the protrusion. Neural tube defects are not limited to the spinal

FIGURE 18-1 Illustration of meylomeningocele and Arnold–Chiari defects. The spinal defect (myelomeningocele) typically presents in the thoracolumbar spine as a bulging sac with neural and meningeal contents; the associated Arnold–Chiari malformation is illustrated at the craniocervical flexure with the cerebellum herniating down into the foramen magnum.

cord region but can actually occur in any region of the tube, and therefore, can include damage to the brain, brainstem, and spinal cord. In most cases, ultrasounds, taken of the fetus in utero, can visualize the defect and protrusion of spinal elements.

Neural Tube Defects

Neural Tube defects are a consequence of some disruption of the developing nervous system, resulting in very serious congenital defects. These defects happen, during **Neurulation** (see Box 18-1) within 3–4 weeks of conception. During this early

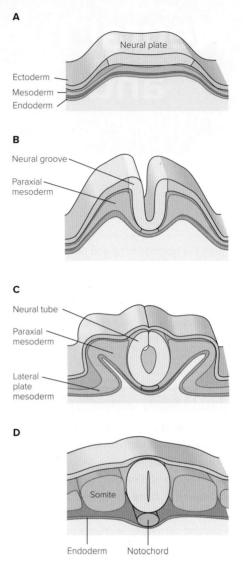

FIGURE 18-2 Neural tube development. (Reproduced with permission from Kandel ER, Schwartz JH, Jessell TM, Siegelbaum SA, Hudspeth AJ. *Principles of Neural Science*, 5th ED, New York, NY: McGraw-Hill; 2013. Figure 52-1 A-D Illustrations Only, p. 1166.)

BOX 18-1	Development of the Nervous System (Neurulation)

To understand neural tube defects, one must first understand a little about embryonic development. Within a few days of fertilization, the embryo is defined by three layers of tissue: the **endoderm** (inner layer) that will form into most of the internal organs; the **mesoderm** (middle layer) that will form into muscle and connective tissue as well as the cardiovascular system; and the **ectoderm** (outer layer) that forms the skin and nervous system. Within the ectoderm, the nervous system forms out of the centralized portion, known as the **neural plate**. The neural plate, over time, folds in on itself (invagination) to first create the **neural groove** that then comes together at the dorsal aspect to form the **neural tube** (Figure 18-2). Some of the neural crest cells remain outside of the neural tube and form the dorsal root and sympathetic ganglia of the nervous system. Once the tube is formed, cell proliferation occurs unequally along the tube such that a series of vesicles emerge along with bending of the tube to allow its expansion within the confines of the developing fetus. Early on, three vesicles emerge at the rostral aspect of the tube, referred to as the (1) **Prosencephalon** – the most rostral portion that will become the cerebral hemispheres; (2) **Mesencephalon** or middle portion that will become the midbrain; and (3) **Rhombencephalon** – the most caudal vesicle that will become the pons, cerebellum, and medulla, see Figure 18-3A. Further cell proliferation results in a five-vesicle structure (Figure 18-3B) that will ultimately expand into the mature brain areas. The prosencephalon will expand into the telencephalon that will become the cerebral hemispheres as well as the **diencephalon**, which will ultimately form the neural portion of the eyes (retina, lens) and the hypothalamus, thalamus, epithalamus, and subthalamus; the **mesencephalon** remains a singular structure that will mature into the midbrain. The rhombencephalon diverges into two vesicles: the **metencephalon** that forms the pons and cerebellum and the **myelencephalon** that forms the medulla. The myelencephalon is contiguous with the remaining neural tube that will form the spinal cord. As the vesicle structures emerge, the tube begins to flex in on itself to afford space for further expansion with first two flexures: one between the mesencephalon and rhombencephalon (**cephalic flexure**) and the other between the rhombencephalon and the remaining neural tube (**cervical flexure**). The five-vesicle structure exhibits a third flexure between the metencephalon and myelencephalon known as the **pontine flexure** (Figure 18-3C). The central opening of the neural tube develops into the ventricles, cerebral aqueduct, and spinal canal, containing the cerebrospinal fluid.

---

time period, the development of the fetus is primitive but crucial because these structures later grow and become the central nervous system (CNS). The closure of the neural tube first happens in the middle of the tube around day 21 of embryonic development, and then, it continues to close in both cephalic and caudal directions simultaneously (Figure 18-4). Please remember that neurulation happens extremely early in embryotic development, so the expecting mother may not know she is pregnant or may have just missed a menstruel cycle.

The location, size, and contents of the neural tube defect are important for, not only life and viability, but also for prediction of future disability. The location, which later becomes called a lesion, is where the neural tube defect happens and can occur in the cranial or spinal cord portions of the neural tube; however, it does not happen in the middle of the tube because that part closes first. The size is how big the lesion is or how much of the vertebral column it spans, ranging from very small to very large.

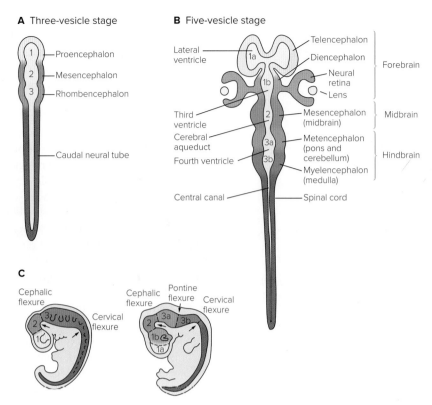

FIGURE 18-3 Neural vesicle development. (Reproduced with permission from Kandel ER, Schwartz JH, Jessell TM, Siegelbaum SA, Hudspeth AJ. *Principles of Neural Science*, 5th ED, New York, NY: McGraw-Hill; 2013. Figure 52-2, Parts A,B, & D Only, p. 1167.)

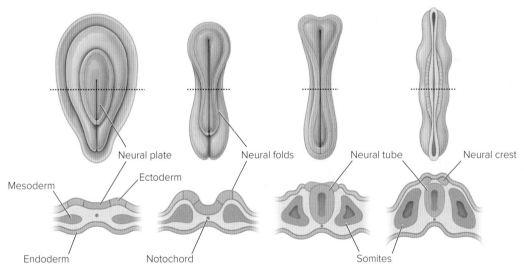

FIGURE 18-4 Neural tube closure. The closure of the neural tube begins in the center and proceeds both rostrally and caudally.

The length and position of the open segment (lack of closure of the neural tube) dictates its severity. The contents are what are inside the sac and can include components of the brain, skull, spinal cord, peripheral nerves, meninges, and cerebral spinal fluid or any combination of these.

Lesions of the Cranial Neural Tube

There are three main types of cranial neural tube defects, associated with a failure of closure of the rostral neural tube. **Anencephaly** is an absence of all or most of the brain without closure or covering of the skull. These infants often don't survive gestation, but if they do, die within the first few hours of birth. **Hydranencephaly** is an absence of the cerebral hemispheres or cerebral cortex, often replaced with cerebral spinal fluid. The skull and meninges may or may not be intact. If the skull and meninges are intact, and in the absence of in utero imaging, the defect may not be apparent at birth, and in some cases, may not be diagnosed for months. Typically, the cerebellum and brainstem are formed, so reflexes, such as sucking and swallowing, and spontaneous arm and leg movements can be present.

FIGURE 18-5 Illustration of encephalocele. A. Arrow marks the point of the neural tube where a failure of closure likely results in an encephalocele defect. **B.** As development continues, the encephalocele will present as a bulging sac at the site of the cranial defect with meningeal and neural contents within the sac.

Hydranencephaly is very rare at less than 1 in 200,000 live births, yet infants with hydranencephaly can live years; some have been known to live into their 30s. As the child ages, there is typically irritability, feeding difficulties, and significant motor delay and often seizures and breathing problems, some require tracheostomy and ventilation. An **encephalocele** is a smaller skull defect with partial protrusion of the brain, typically in the frontal or occipital regions (Figure 18-5). Occipital encephaloceles are more common in North America, while frontal lesions (facial area) are more common in Asia. Surgical repair to close this lesion is required. Encephalocele is also rare at 1.4 per 10,000 live births.[1] If there is brain tissue in the sac, then the damage is more severe and can be life threatening. If there is no brain tissue in the sac, even large cysts can be removed; brain damage in this case is focal with resulting neurological impairment based on brain-injury location. If the contents of the sac do not include brain tissue, then the repair and prognosis are generally good but dependent on the location of the defect. Hydrocephalus is a frequent comorbidity of encephalocele.[1]

Lesions at the Spinal Levels

Neural tube defects are much more common at the spinal level with the lower thoracic and lumbar levels most common. As a reminder, there are 7 cervical vertebra, 12 thoracic vertebra, 5 lumbar vertebra, and 5 fused sacral vertebra. Each vertebral body is different in shape and size based on the location. The bony spinal column offers a lot of protection to the spinal cord. The lamina forms and covers the spinal canal, where the spinal cord is located, with facet joints that articulate with the vertebra above and below. During development, each vertebra forms in a similar fashion to the neural tube, bending in on itself and coming together at the back into the spinous process. With *Spina bifida and neural tube defects, the lamina and spinous process are absent or malformed.* **Spinal dysraphism**, also historically

referred to as spina bifida, is a defect of the closure of the spinous process or processes at some level of the spinal column. **Spinal dysraphism occulta** or **spina bifida occulta** is the mildest and most common form, present in 10–20% of healthy babies. In this case, there is no lamina or spinous process but the spinal cord, meninges, and cerebral spinal fluid are contained in the spinal canal. There is skin covering the defect and there may be a dimple, a small patch of hair, changes in pigment or a small fatty lump over the missing spinous process. Typically, this kind of defect does not cause any neurologic problem, and most people do not know they have it. However, there is a higher incidence of spinal cord tethering with spinal dysraphism occulta where the spinal cord is attached (tethered) to the surrounding tissue. Spinal cord tethering gets increasingly more serious as children get older because their growth can cause damage to the cord as the tethering pulls on the spinal cord as the spinal column grows. Notably, cord growth is slower and to a lesser degree than the spinal column; thus, growth induces stretching, and thereby damage, to the cord.

A **meningocele** is where there is no lamina or spinous process, the spinal cord is still contained within the spinal canal, and there is a protrusion of the meninges and cerebral spinal fluid outside of the spinal canal. Meningocele is rare, but it is possible for the membrane or cyst to be surgically removed with little to no damage of any neural pathways. **Myelomeningocele** is where there is no lamina or spinous process and the protruding sac contains components of the spinal cord, meninges, and cerebral spinal fluid outside of the spinal canal. It is the most severe form of neural tube defect associated with spina bifida, and this means that during fetal development, the spinal cord is outside of the body in a closed or open sac. If the sac is closed, meaning covered with skin, then the contents within have some protection. The sac can be long and thin, resembling a tail or finger, or round and wide as in Figure 18-6. The sac can also be open where there are tissues and nerves exposed to amniotic fluid in utero and exposed to anything in the environment after birth. As such, infants with open lesions are at a greater risk for serious infections. Myelomeningocele is the most common form of neural tube defect with spina bifida. Because of this prevalence, these two terms, myelomeningocele and spina bifida are often used interchangeably; however, it is important to remember that they are actually separate conditions. With both meningoceles and myelomeningoceles, there is a visible defect on the baby.

Myelomeningocele (MMC)

CASE A, PART II

In our case, Dylan presented in utero with an MMC at L1/L2, meaning the sac was between the first and second lumbar vertebra, which is a very common location for these lesions. He was diagnosed in utero via ultrasound and presented at birth or soon after with several common comorbidities (Arnold–Chiari malformation [A–CM], hydrocephalus, and hip dislocation). In the following discussion, we will examine how diagnosis of MMC occurs, the functional presentation of MMC, and the comorbidities associated with this defect.

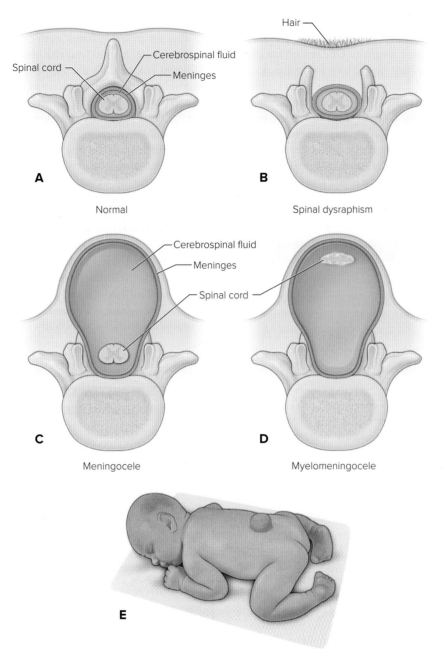

FIGURE 18-6 Spina bifida defects. A. Normal spinous process and vertebra. **B.** Spinal dysraphism occulta (failure of spinous process closure without protrusion of the spinal canal contents) with hair patch on skin above. **C.** Meningocele – fluid filled sac of meninges protrudes through the spinal defect with spinal cord contained in the spinal canal. **D.** Myelomeningocele – spinal cord components within the meningeal sac protrude through the spinal defect. **E.** Appearance of myelomeningocele defect on infant at birth.

Since MMC is the most common form of spina bifida and requires extensive physical therapy management, we will focus much of this chapter on this disorder. The term spina bifida is often used by the rehabilitation community as synonymous with MMC, but we will try to distinguish the two for clarity in the following discussion.

Location

The location of the lesion in patients with MMC is typically in the thoracic, lumbar, or sacral level of the spine and rarely in the cervical spine; this is also true of meningoceles and spina bifida occulta. Motor and sensory deficits include paralysis and loss of sensation, including touch, pain, temperature, and proprioception, below the lesion level. Bowel, bladder, and sexual dysfunction are similar to patients with spinal cord injury.

Causes

The specific cause(s) of neural tube defects is (are) unknown, yet nutrition and genetics seem to play a critical role in the disruption of development that produces neural tube defects. Folic acid and other vitamins are extremely important during the development of the neural tube. There are several public health campaigns aimed at getting women to start taking 400 mcg of folic acid supplement every day when planning a pregnancy and not just after they become pregnant. One reason for starting supplementation early is that neural tube formation occurs very early after conception.[2] There also appears to be a genetic component to the development of MMC. For example, if one sibling or the mother has spina bifida or there has been a previous pregnancy with a neural tube defect, then the risks of spina bifida increase, thus, suggesting a genetic influence. Overall, it is thought that a combination of nutritional, environmental, and genetic factors contribute to spina bifida and its associated neural tube defects.

Incidence

CASE A, PART III

In our case, Dylan's defect was diagnosed by fetal ultrasound at 20 weeks; ultrasound at this time point is common and often identifies this defect, during the second trimester of fetal development.

MMC is the second most common congenital birth defect with an incidence of 0.2–3 per 1000 live births. It is a life-long disability. Expectant mothers also frequently undergo a simple blood test for developmental disorders in their second trimester; the presence of alpha-fetoprotein in the blood is a sign that a neural tube defect may exist and is accurate 70–80% of the time. Mothers that test positive will typically undergo additional ultrasounds to look for the defect. Amniocentesis (an invasive test that takes amniotic fluid from inside the uterus with a needle) can also detect alpha-fetoprotein. However, ultrasound is the most common method of identification and is most often completed between 18 and 21 weeks of gestation.[3] Due to folic acid supplementation and improved nutrition during early pregnancy, the rates of MMC have been decreasing and are thought to be stabilizing.[2]

Surgical Management

Surgical management is necessary for protection and prevention of further injury of the spinal cord and peripheral nerves. This is a surgical repair of the lesion but without repair of the damaged neural tissue. Presently, once the spinal cord and peripheral nerves are damaged, there is no surgical fix. The goal of surgery is to put the neural tissue back in the spinal column, protect it from future damage, and guard against infection. Surgery can happen at two time periods: postnatally and prenatally.[4] Prenatal surgery means they do the surgery to close the spinal column of the fetus in utero. Here they make an incision in the uterus, position the baby so the lesion of the spinal defect is exposed, put the neural contents back in and sew both fetus and mother back up. This kind of surgical procedure is relatively new; the outcomes were first published in 2011. Postnatal surgery is very similar for baby as the goal is closure of the defect. There has been a randomized controlled trial looking at prenatal and postnatal surgical outcomes. In this trial, the prenatal surgery group had a decreased need for shunting for hydrocephalus, better motor outcomes, but also increased maternal and fetal risk, including preterm birth with additional risk of CNS damage. Even with the higher rate of preterm birth, the motor outcomes were better for this group compared to the postnatal surgery group.[4] Most of the time, spina bifida is identified in utero, and a C-section is scheduled to avoid any trauma to the skin or membranes around the sac and lesion that might occur with a vaginal delivery. Remarkably, fetuses with unknown spina bifida have been delivered vaginally without rupture of the sac or membrane. The surgery to close the lesion is typically done 24–48 hours after birth. After surgery, the primary goals are aimed at healing and protection of the surgical site. The role of the PT following surgery includes examination of the skin, position changes to avoid skin breakdown and pressure sores, evaluation of bowel and bladder function, providing the appropriate environment for feeding, and monitoring of growth and development. Throughout childhood, the PT has a large role in age appropriate activities and mobility.

BOX 18-2   **Surgical Closure of the Lesion**

Repair of the myelomeningocele lesion involves further extension of the skin opening to allow sufficient room to work and eventually sufficient skin to pull over the opening. Some neural elements that are caught in the sac itself may need to be sacrificed. Other neural contents that can be saved are enclosed in the dura mater, which may require augmentation with paravertebral muscles or fascia, and the dura closed. These elements (paravertebral muscles and fascia) are also used to provide some additional protection over the dural closure, and then, the skin is closed. An extensive scar will be left; notably, the spinal column defect is typically not repaired but rather soft tissue is used to cover the opening to protect the spinal cord.

FIGURE 18-7 Postsurgical repair scarring: The need to pull skin over the space occupied by the myelomeningocele typically results in a large scar that further expands as the child grows. (Used with permission of Jill C. Heathcock, MPT, PhD, The Ohio State University.)

Common Sensorimotor Characteristics in Myelomeningocele

The location and structure of damage are important for understanding common sensorimotor characteristics of MMC. Infants, children, and adults with MMC often show both upper and lower motor neuron signs, similar to what has been described in Chapter 12 for spinal cord injuries. Upper motor neuron (UMN) signs are observed when there is damage to the UMNs within the cortex or their projections (axons) within the brainstem, corticospinal tracts, or spinal cord. UMN signs are specific to the descending motor pathways in MMC. Cerebral palsy (Chapter 19) is a common pediatric UMN disorder, and stroke is a common UMN adult disorder. Common ways to assess UMN and LMN signs are to examine muscle tone, reflexes, and involuntary movements. In children with UMN signs, you will see increased tone (hypertonia), spasticity, and often clonus as well as poor muscle control and synergistic movements (see Table 18-1 for descriptions). Patients with MMC often have bilateral but asymmetrical lesions due to the nature of the defect, similar to patients with traumatic spinal cord injuries. This means that one leg might have more or different function than the other leg. In terms of muscle development, there is always disuse atrophy and incomplete muscle development with UMN and LMN lesions. Patients with MMC will have a different developmental trajectory than infants with typical development, and they will not show the same types of antigravity movements, such as kicking, that effect their muscle growth and development over time. Disuse atrophy is typically widespread across all antigravity muscles below the lesion. Voluntary movements with UMN injuries are very difficult, ranging from impaired to absent.

Lower motor neuron signs result from damage to specific locations and structures including cranial nerves and nuclei, parts of the spinal cord including anterior horn cells (alpha motor neurons) and spinal roots, and any peripheral nerve damage (nerve that innervates skeletal muscle). Peripheral nerve damage often comes in the form of pulling, stretching,

TABLE 18-1	Signs of Upper and Lower Motor Neuron Damage	
UMN signs	Hypertonia	Increased muscle tone
	Spasticity	Velocity-dependent resistance to passive stretch such that a quick stretch elicits more resistance and a slow stretch less resistance.
	Hyperreflexia	Hyper-responsive monosynaptic stretch reflexes (brisk), elicited by a tendon tap.
	Clonus	Repetitive muscle contraction in response to a quick stretch. This is most common with a quick stretch of the gastrocnemius, elicited by quickly moving the foot into dorsiflexion. The number of beats of extension can be counted as an indication of severity
	Babinski sign	An upward movement of the hallux and splaying of the toes in response to a stroke (heel to toe) on the sole of the foot. This is a normal response in children under 4–6 months and abnormal after that. A negative sign in a mature child/adult is a downward movement of the hallux with minimal or absent toe movement.
	Autonomic reflexes	With the loss of UMN control of brainstem centers, an increase in blood pressure, heart rate, and sweating is often seen.
	Synergistic movement	Movement in flexor or extensor patterns that make voluntary control difficult (e.g., when flexing the elbow, the wrist and fingers also flex; when extending the elbow, the hand opens).
	Muscle weakness (paresis)/poor force generation	UMN's activate alpha motor neurons in the spinal cord, so damage to them results in difficulty in activating muscles and resultant diminished force generation
LMN signs	Flaccid paralysis	A loss of active muscle control and reflex activity due to damage of alpha motor neurons in the spinal cord or cranial nerve nuclei
	Hypotonia	Decreased muscle tone, often associated with increased joint laxity
	Areflexia	Absent reflex activity due to loss of alpha motor neurons or Ia afferents in the spinal cord
	Hyporeflexia	Diminished reflex activity due to partial damage to the alpha motor neurons, Ia afferents, or both
	Fasciculations	Small involuntary muscle twitches of skeletal muscle associated with denervation of the muscle

or tearing of any part of the nerve(s) that connect(s) the spinal cord to a specific muscle. One of the most common pediatric injuries that cause LMN signs is brachial plexus palsy, an injury that occurs during birth (See Chapter 15). A hallmark of LMN injury is flaccid paralysis and areflexia, but partial innervation hypotonia and hyporeflexia may be present (see Table 18-1 for definitions). Also, fasciculations are common; such small and occasional muscle twitches are common in a typical population, but those from LMN injury are more frequent and measurably different on EMG. Weakness and paralysis is segmental and focal, based on the lesion site, and is often asymmetrical with one side more affected than the other, or one side is affected and the other side unaffected. Complications to the muscle and to muscle development include neurogenic atrophy, since the affected muscles may have never received appropriate nerve signals; this results in immediate and severe focal wasting, ultimately leading to current and future disuse and further atrophy. Voluntary movements with LMN injuries are very difficult and are described as weak or absent.

Notably, LMN signs are common in muscles innervated at the level of the spinal cord defect; UMN signs will be present at levels below the defect where the spinal reflexes remain intact in the absence of supraspinal control.

Comorbidities Associated with Myelomeningocele/Spina Bifida

Latex Allergies

Infants with spina bifida are at high risk for developing latex allergies.[5] This is something that everyone on the health care team, especially the physical therapist, needs to know. Repeated exposure to latex is the primary reason for an increased risk of the allergy. Infants with spina bifida are exposed to latex during the initial surgical procedure to close the spinal column, frequently have other surgeries (orthopedic, shunt implants for hydrocephalus), and have frequent bladder catheterizations. Notably, gloves, balloons, and balls all can have latex in them. The symptoms of latex allergies include skin rashes, common nasal signs like sneezing, itching and a runny nose, and more serious signs like difficulty breathing, confusion, wheezing, and anaphylaxis, which can be life threatening. Therefore, it is important to limit the number of exposures to latex. In many pediatric physical therapy clinics, all the equipment, including the gloves, are latex free. To avoid repeated exposures, parents will be instructed by their physician to ask and require that all equipment used during rehabilitation be latex free.

Associated Brain Abnormalities

Hydrocephalus and A–CM are two complications associated with MMC that can affect the brain and cause additional CNS problems. Both can occur in the absence of spina bifida but are common comorbidities of this disorder.

Hydrocephalus is an accumulation of cerebral spinal fluid in the ventricles leading to increased intracranial pressure. This pressure and accumulation of fluid pushes out and compresses the brain, causing damage to brain structures and disrupting brain development. Hydrocephalus can be congenital (present at birth) or acquired after an event, typically an injury to the

> ### CASE A, PART IV
>
> **What brain malformation might we expect in Dylan?*
> - He has an A–CM and a history of hydrocephalus. He has had one shunt placement when he was an infant.
> ***Is this typical?*
> Yes; here we discuss these two common comorbidities of MMC and their relationship to each other.

brain such as hemorrhage or a complication from a tumor (see Box 18-4). Overall hydrocephalus affects 1–2 out of 1000 live births. Signs and symptoms of hydrocephalus include a bulging fontanelle and scalp veins, behavioral changes, high-pitched cries, seizures, vomiting, and changes in appetite. **Fontanelles** (also spelled fontanels) are the "soft spot" on newborns' heads where the cranial sutures have not yet come together or fused. Patients with hydrocephalus typically have a large head due to fluid accumulation. Hydrocephalus may cause additional deficits in learning and memory, hearing loss, headaches, and impaired vision due to compression of brain tissue as the ventricles expand; deficits are related to the degree and location of tissue compression.[6,7]

The treatment for hydrocephalus, with or without MMC, historically has been shunting. A shunt is a tube that is placed with one end typically in one of the lateral ventricles of the brain (can also be placed in the subarachnoid space), threaded down the neck just behind the ear, and terminates in the abdominal cavity (ventriculo-peritoneal), atrium of the heart (ventriculo-atrial), or pleural cavity (ventriculo-pleural), allowing the excess fluid to drain. The fluid is then reabsorbed back into the body. The shunt can be visible and palpable on the side of the infants' head

FIGURE 18-8 Illustration of shunting for hydrocephalus.
This is a radiograph illustration of a ventriculoperitoneal shunt, extending from the lateral ventricle to the peritoneum. The red arrow is pointing to the shunt valve, which is translucent. (Reproduced with permission from Shah BR, Lucchesi M, Amodio J, Silverberg M (Eds). *Atlas of Pediatric Medicine*, 2ED. New York, NY: McGraw-Hill; 2013. Fig 13.54: Photo contributor: John Amodio, MD)

The brain is supported structurally and chemically via the ventricular system and the cerebrospinal fluid (CSF) that circulates within it. The **ventricular system** is a series of ventricles and their connecting passages (Figure 18-9). The largest of the ventricles are the **lateral ventricles** within the cerebral hemispheres; these connect to the **third ventricle**, which is centered between the two thalamic nuclei, via the **intraventricular foramina**. The third ventricle connects to the **fourth ventricle** in the brainstem via the **cerebral aqueduct**. The fourth ventricle is contiguous with the central canal of the spinal cord; it also connects to the subarachnoid space through two foramina (Magendie and Luschka). This allows CSF to flow through the subarachnoid space that lies between the arachnoid and pia maters and provides some cushioning of the brain within the cranial cavity. Further, the subarachnoid space continues within the spinal canal between its arachnoid and pia mater linings, allowing fluid to move down the cord, pooling in the lumbar cistern, and back up the ventral side of the cord. From the cerebral subarachnoid space, CSF is absorbed through a specialized network of valves, called the **arachnoid villi**, into the venous sinuses, primarily the superior sagittal sinus, allowing it to enter the venous blood flow as it returns to the heart. CSF is produced in the **choroid plexuses**, located within the ventricles. CSF serves many functions, including providing a cushion for the brain and spinal cord from their bony enclosures as well as from external blows to the head, serving as a source of nutrients for the surrounding brain tissue, and absorbing metabolic waste from those brain tissues (Figure 18-10).

behind the ear and typically includes a small valve or pump that can be externally massaged to prevent blockages; usually, two segments of tubing are used with one segment running from the lateral ventricle to the junction behind the ear (proximal segment) and the second (distil segment) running from this junction to the point of fluid distribution (abdomen, heart). This allows replacement of the lower portion as the child grows without disruption of the proximal segment. There is a relatively high rate of shunt failure or malfunctioning with most children requiring some repair within 5 years of initial placement, so there must be ongoing neurosurgical follow-up to make sure the shunt stays in place, especially during growth and development, and to make sure there are no blockages. Monitoring of behavioral signs of shunt failure is necessary across all health care professions and caregivers. Hydrocephalus and shunt placements have several implications for PT, including knowledge of the signs of shunt failure, which mimic the signs of increased intracranial pressure discussed above, and its counterpart – over drainage that results in a depression of the fontanel with associated dizziness and headache. These are both treated as medical emergencies. Education of caregivers to recognize the signs of shunt failure is critical as is routine shunt follow up with a physician. Severe neck flexion should be avoided in all patients with a shunt as it can cause a kink in the tubing or a separation of the shunt at the junction behind the ear. Common signs of shunt problems include: (1) a change in motor status, tone (e.g. increased spasticity) or postural control; (2) nausea or vomiting; or (3) behavioral change, such as irritability, or more subtle poorer school performance.

Although motor deficits in children with hydrocephalus but not MMC are typically mild, **hydrocephalus with MMC can exaggerate already compromised gait, transfers, and postural**

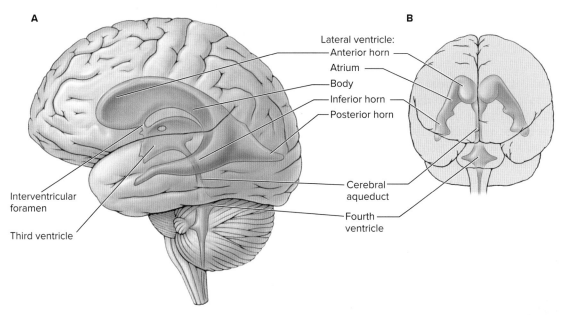

FIGURE 18-9 Ventricular system. A. Lateral (sagittal view) depicting ventricular system. **B.** Frontal section, depicting ventricular system. (Reproduced with permission from Martin JH (Ed). *Neuroanatomy Text and Atlas*, 4th Ed. New York, NY: McGraw-Hill; 2012. Fig 1-13A&B, pg 23.)

① CSF is produced by the choroid plexus in the ventricles.

② CSF flows from the third ventricle through the cerebral aqueduct into the fourth ventricle.

③ CSF in the fourth ventricle flows into the subarachnoid space by passing through the paired lateral apertures or the single median aperture, and into the central canal of the spinal cord.

④ As the CSF flows through the subarachnoid space, it removes waste products and provides buoyancy to support the brain.

⑤ Excess CSF flows into the arachnoid villi, then drains into the dural venous sinuses. Pressure allows the CSF to be released into the blood without permitting any venous blood to enter the subarachnoid space. The greater pressure on the CSF in the subarachnoid space ensures that CSF moves into the venous sinuses.

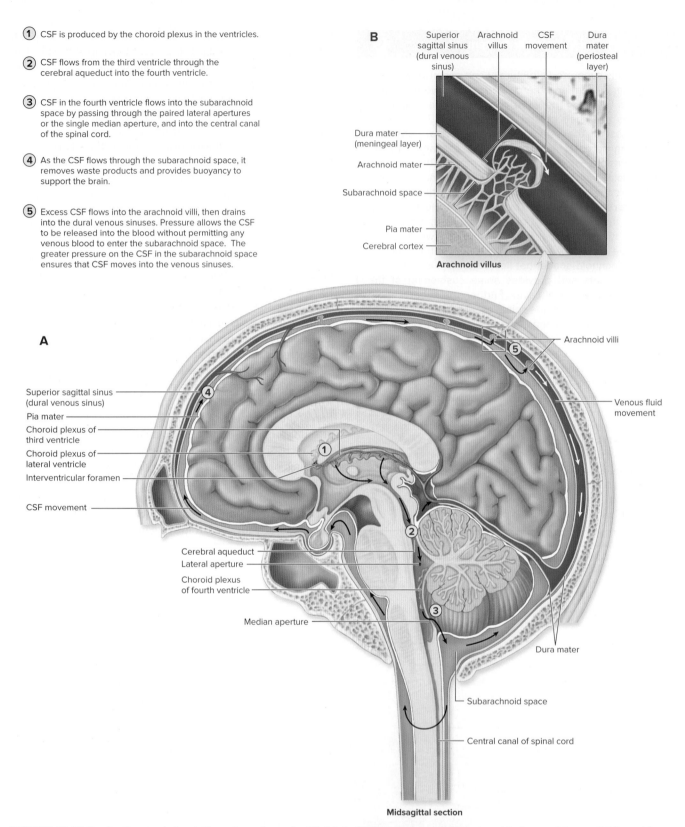

FIGURE 18-10 Production and circulation of cerebrospinal fluid. A. CSF is produced in the choroid plexus of the ventricles and circulates from the lateral ventricles (not pictured) to the third and fourth ventricles and within the central spinal canal; fluid then moves into the subarachnoid space of the brain and spinal canal, providing a compliant cushion for these structures. **B.** Small portals within the arachnoid mater (arachnoid villi) allow the CSF to move from the subarachnoid space to the superior sagittal sinus as well as other dural sinuses. (Reproduced with permission from McKinley M, O'Laughlin VD. *Human Anatomy*. 3rd Ed, New York, NY: McGraw-Hill; 2012, Fig. 15.8A&B, P. 453.)

Although MMC-associated hydrocephalus is the most common type of hydrocephalus, it can occur in the absence of MMC. Hydrocephalus without MMC occurs due to either (1) obstruction of the CSF pathway secondary to malformation (noncommunicating hydrocephalus) or blockage (obstructive hydrocephalus) or (2) overproduction or decreased absorption of CSF, known both as communicating or non-obstructive hydrocephalus. Overproduction is most commonly associated with a benign tumor (papilloma) within the choroid plexus, while diminished absorption is typically related to abnormal function within the subarachnoid villi, often associated with subarachnoid hemorrhage. Post-hemorrhagic hydrocephalus is a common consequence of prematurity.[8]

Regardless of the cause of hydrocephalus, expansion of the ventricles due to excessive CSF, produces both stretching of white matter and compression of the adjacent brain tissue; further, disruption of CSF flow may interrupt the nutritional support to the brain or removal of metabolic waste typically provided by CSF, resulting in additional compromise to brain tissue. In infants, prior to fontanel closure, ventricular expansion is accompanied by expansion of the cranium. **Prior to the implementation of surgical shunting, children with congenital hydrocephalus experienced extreme enlargement of the cranium until eventually death ensued; this may still occur in 3rd world countries**. Now, surgical implantation of a shunt is done very early, sometimes in utero, to minimize the ventricular expansion and secondary brain tissue damage, and thus, maximizes brain preservation and neurologic function. Many children with congenital hydrocephalus live normal lives without any or with very mild complications. However, hydrocephalus may be associated with diminished intelligence (lower IQ scores on testing) and greater incidence of nonverbal learning disabilities[7]; the cause of these cognitive disabilities is likely multifaceted with disrupted early brain development as well as damage from surgical implantation of the shunt contributing factors. Motor characteristics of hydrocephalus include poor fine motor skills such as handwriting with minimal effect on gross motor skills; however, early development may be delayed due to the enlarged head.

abnormalities. Balance and coordination are often poor in children with hydrocephalus, especially in infancy, as they have a larger head, elevating their center of gravity further. Early postural training may include necessary activities like strengthening of the neck muscles. After the shunt is placed, patients with hydrocephalus can participate in almost any activity (including sports) that is based on their level of function; gymnastics with its many somersaults and severe neck flexion positions and contact sports, such as football and soccer, should be avoided due to the likelihood of shunt damage. The PT should avoid positions and interventions that increase intracranial pressure, such as inversion (head lower than trunk).

For patients with MMC, the hydrocephalus is commonly associated with an **A–CM**. An A–CM is the displacement of the brainstem and cerebellar tonsils inferiorly beyond the foramen magnum and subsequent disruption of the flow of cerebral spinal fluid within the cerebral aqueduct or fourth ventricle, referred to as obstructive hydrocephalus (Figure 18-11). There are four levels of A–CM with Level I being the least severe and Level IV being the most severe. Level II is associated with MMC, and almost all children with MMC have a Level-II A–CM. With growth and development, the cerebellum can become more involved and children can display motor skill impairments that are typical of cerebellar involvement such as poor predictive motor control and ataxic gait. Symptoms of cranial nerve disruption can also emerge with further compression of the brainstem where these nerves originate.

In Dylan's case, as with many children, the hydrocephalus was not apparent at birth and manifested in the first weeks of life. This delayed presentation has led to much speculation that closure of the spinal defect plays a role in its development. Since hydrocephalus in MMC is almost always associated with the A–CM, additional speculation focused on compression of structures in the brainstem as a contributing factor in the development of hydrocephalus; a more recent hypothesis is that leakage of CSF through the spinal defect creates more room in the foramen magnum, allowing the A–CM, which in turn, creates the hydrocephalus. Notably, A–CM blocks the outlets for the 4th ventricle, impeding CSF flow into the subarachnoid space. It is likely that this combination of factors contributes to the development of hydrocephalus in most children with MMC.

FIGURE 18-11 Arnold–Chiari malformation. A. Typical brain image with brainstem and cerebellum above the foramen magnum. **B.** Arnold–Chiari malformation with elongation of cerebellum into foramen magnum (type 1); in type II, which is common in MMC, there is further subluxation of the cerebellum and brainstem into the spinal canal. (Reproduced with permission from Carney PR, & Geyer JD (Eds). *Pediatric Practice Neurology.* New York, NY: McGraw-Hill; 2010. Figure 8-3 Parts B&C Only.)

In Dylan's case, immediate shunting upon identification of hydrocephalus was the common course of treatment 13 years ago. Dylan has normal intelligence but has been diagnosed with a visual learning disability, so he has his books on tape and takes his tests orally. Currently, with folic acid supplementation and the increasing use of prenatal MMC repair, the occurrence of A–CM and hydrocephalus in MMC is decreasing. Further, shunting is often delayed to determine the relative progressiveness of the hydrocephalus with only about 50% of infants having early shunt insertion currently; recent findings suggest that the hydrocephalus may spontaneously arrest, and thus, early shunting may not be necessary. Infection, post-shunting in children with MMC, is also much higher than for hydrocephalus alone, so waiting to determine absolute need is becoming the preferred management method; these challenging medical decisions are based on infection and surgical risk, pressure on periventricular white matter, and severity of the hydrocephalus. Also, there is an increasing use of shunts within the 3rd ventricle that can be inserted endoscopically rather than placement in the lateral ventricle.[9]

Since infancy and childhood are rapid periods of growth and development, changes associated with growth should be a consideration for the PT. With **Arnold–Chiari (A–C) malformations**, pressure on the brainstem, spinal cord, or cerebellum can be exaggerated with growth, causing increased pressure of CSF within the spinal cord. One of the signs of increased A–CM compression can be weakness in the upper extremities. Any changes in sensorimotor status should be taken seriously. Characteristics of cerebellar involvement may also increase with growth. Major growth-related changes to the A–CM may require surgery that opens up the spinal canal in the cervical region. **Spinal cord tethering** occurs when the spinal cord adheres to the spinal column, thought to be due to scarring at the site of the lesion closure, and is a common condition in patients with MMC; when the children grow, there can be additional pulling that can produce serious damage to the spinal cord that may require a surgical release.

Orthopedic Complications of Myelomeningocele

Orthopedic complications of MMC are common. Causes include (1) abnormal positioning in utero due to diminished muscle activity and movement; (2) asymmetrical muscle pull at the trunk and many lower extremity joints; and (3) poor or absent antigravity movement, specifically hip and knee extension, resulting in excessive flexor muscle activity that is exacerbated by time spent in flexed postures (e.g., sitting). It is critical to remember that the neurologic compromise to the spinal components, associated with MMC, is almost always asymmetric, and thus, results in normal or partial innervation of some muscles while others exhibit flaccid (at the level of lower motor neuron injury) or spastic (below the level of the lesion) paralysis. This asymmetry of muscle pull has an exaggerated effect in the young child, compared to his adult spinal cord injured counterpart, because it is occurring during development with no period of normal innervation. Notably, infants with MMC have limited extensor muscle activity that in combination with

the baby's flexed posture in late stage gestation contributes to positional changes in bone and joint alignment. Additionally, the baby may have limited mobility after birth, compounding these positional changes.[10]

Club foot, hip dysplasia, and **scoliosis** are three orthopedic complications commonly associated with MMC. Both club foot and hip dysplasia are often apparent at delivery; scoliosis is more likely to develop over childhood as the child grows.

Club Foot

A patient can have club foot without MMC, and the overall incidence of club foot is 1 in 1000 live births. Of those who have club foot, 50% are bilateral, and males are twice as likely as females to have club foot. A family history and maternal smoking increases the risk of club foot by twentyfold. Club foot is typically congenital and can be (1) teratologic – due to an underlying disorder that effects boney growth and position such as arthrogryposis; (2) positional – secondary to a poor position in utero; and (3) syndromatic – having a co-occurrence with other syndromes such as Down syndrome or spina bifida.[11] In club foot, the patients' foot is severely deformed due to the misalignment of the bones, ligaments, and muscles. There are four general characteristics of club foot: forefoot <u>C</u>avus and <u>A</u>dduction, heal <u>V</u>arus and <u>E</u>quinus, making the mnemonic device CAVE (Figure 18-12). With unilateral clubfoot, the affected limb may be shorter with a thinner calf and shorter foot. There is a muscle imbalance with the lateral muscles more stretched and the medial muscles tight. Common motor characteristics are focused around gait abnormalities where PT can have a large role in evaluation and treatment.

Midfoot adducted and supinated

Ankle plantarflexed

Heel inverted and internally rotated

FIGURE 18-12 Club foot deformity. (Reproduced with permission from Skinner HB & McMahon PJ (Eds): *Current Diagnosis & Treatment in Orthopedics*, 5th ed. New York, NY: McGraw-Hill; 2014. Fig 10-15.)

Common gait abnormalities, associated with clubfoot, include decreased dorsiflexion, foot drop, in-toeing, decreased plantarflexion strength, and compensatory increases in knee hyperextension and hip external rotation. Range of motion at the foot and ankle is very important in patients with club foot with or without MMC. Contractures of the Achilles tendon can be the most common and most limiting. In addition, without any correction of the clubfoot deformity, the lateral surface of the ankle becomes the weight-bearing surface, making walking difficult, if not impossible. Implications for PT include awareness of any precautions, early treatment, and promotion of motor development within the context of spina bifida. Infants with idiopathic club foot (and not MMC) scored worse on motor skill development on scales at 12 and 18 months of age. These ages represent a time period when motor skills include pulling-to-stand and walking that demand more of the foot and ankle. So, infants with club foot are at risk for motor delay even in the absence of MMC. The first goal of treatment for club foot is correction of the deformity. The most common method for treating clubfoot is the Ponsetti method, which consists of serial casting, followed often by surgical lengthening of the Achilles tendon and subsequent bracing with a foot abduction brace.[11] Clubfoot is present in 50–90% of children with MMC at birth,[12] since they almost always have limited and/or asymmetric muscle activity at the foot/ankle, and thereby, are more at risk for abnormal posturing during gestation.

Developmental Dysplasia of the Hip

Developmental dysplasia of the hip (DDH) is a condition that ranges in severity from mild ligamentous laxity in the hip, to mild changes in the development of the hip joint (acetabulum, femur, or both) with or without subluxation (partial dislocation), to complete dislocation that cannot be manually reduced (head of femur relocated into the acetabulum). It is diagnosed in 1–1.5 per 1000 live births in otherwise typically developing infants, but is quite common in children with MMC. During typical development, as infants achieve weight-bearing postures, the acetabulum increases in depth and the femoral head develops a spherical shape; these two changes create a stable hip joint. Risk factors for DDH include female sex, as 80% of patients with hip dysplasia are girls, Native American descent, and a breach position in utero. When the acetabulum and/or femoral head demonstrate abnormal development, subluxation or dislocation is more likely. In some cases of DDH, the femoral head remains dislocated and a secondary, or artificial joint, develops as weight is born, pushing the femur into a higher point on the posterior pelvis. Neither hip dysplasia nor dislocation is thought to be painful in infancy, but both are associated with pain in older children and adults.[13]

Signs of DDH (Figure 18-13): If the hip is subluxed or dislocated, the infant may display uneven skin folds on the thigh, limited abduction, and a longer affected limb. Limited hip abduction in the affected limb with a discrepancy of greater than 10 degrees is the most reliable clinical measure in childhood, indicating the child needs to be referred. There are two additional clinical tests for young infants that can be performed easily. The Ortolani sign is performed by flexing the

FIGURE 18-13 Early signs of developmental dysplasia of the hip. A. An adducted LE with uneven skin folds. **B.** Posterior uneven skin folds. **C.** Limited abduction. **D.** Pistoning of the hip with upward pull on the hip. **E.** Subluxation or dislocation with external rotation. **F.** Reseating of the hip with adduction. (Reproduced with permission from Skinner HB & McMahon PJ (Eds): *Current Diagnosis & Treatment in Orthopedics*, 5th ed. New York, NY: McGraw-Hill; 2014. Fig 10-4.)

infants' hips to 90 degrees and abducting the hip looking for a palpable and audible click, indicating that the femoral head is moving back into the acetabulum; however, some children will demonstrate a click due to ligaments moving over the greater trochanter, so this may result in a false positive. The Barlow sign is more aggressive, flexing the hip to 90 degrees and then adducting the hip, which, in an unstable hip, will allow the femoral head to dislocate from the acetabulum; again, some children with DDH will not dislocate with this test and may be missed. Motor milestones may be delayed in children with DDH, especially upright activities. Early detection is the key for effective management of DDH. Infants who are identified after 9 months of age have a higher prevalence of surgical reduction of the hip than those identified earlier. Although hip abduction differences and the Ortolani and Barlow signs are the most common and effective clinical tests, they have questionable reliability, so imaging is the only definitive test for DDH.

Treatment for DDH: The most common treatment for DDH is the Pavlik Harness (Figure 18-14), which forces the hips into a flexed and abducted position to achieve acetabular and femoral head development. The Pavlik harness has success rates between 85 and 95%. Infants with DDH should not be positioned in

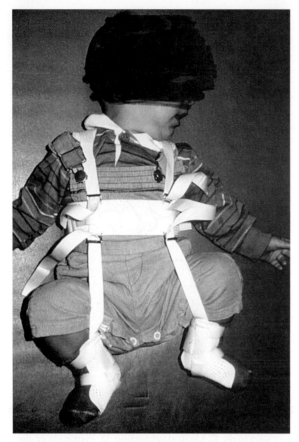

FIGURE 18-14 Pavlik harness treatment of DDH. The harness is optimal for infants prior to 6 months of age and is worn 24 hours/day for up to 12 weeks, and then, at night for another 4–6 weeks. (Reproduced with permission from Skinner HB & McMahon PJ (Eds): *Current Diagnosis & Treatment in Orthopedics*, 5th ed. New York, NY: McGraw-Hill; 2014. Fig 10-6.)

CASE A, PART VI

Dylan was treated with a Pavlik harness to correct his bilateral DDH; in children with MMC, that never achieve independent standing, it is more difficult to treat DDH, since weight-bearing is essential for normal acetabulum and femoral head development. In addition, it is likely that Dylan would have spastic paralysis of his hip flexors and adductors, since his lesion level is at L1/L2, and these muscles are innervated at L2–4. Spasticity of the hip flexors and adductors often can contribute to hip dislocation, especially when inadequate development of the acetabulum and femoral head are present. Yet, neural damage may be greater than the level of apparent spinal damage, so flaccid paralysis is also a possibility. Often, some degree of DDH persists in children with MMC despite early treatment, and if not painful, is left untreated in the older child. Even though children with this level of injury have limited potential for ambulation, standing is important to help combat hip flexion contractures, associated with prolonged sitting, and to assist development of the hip joint. An orthotic that supports the hips, knees, and ankles is essential for allowing standing. Ambulation may be achieved by a swing to or through gait (see description in Part IX), initially with a walker. However, few children with an L1/L2 lesion will walk beyond early childhood due to the high energy cost of this type of ambulation.

---

extreme hip extension or adduction, and sidelying should be avoided during sleeping because of the adducted position of the top leg. Parent education will be important for avoiding these positions. If untreated, complications include arthritis, pain, and difficulty with ambulation.[13,14]

DDH is very common in children with MMC because either (1) there is an absence of any activity at the hip, and therefore, limited muscle pull to keep the head of the femur in the acetabulum or (2) there is an asymmetrical muscle pull such that the hip flexors and adductors remain innervated while hip extensors and abductors are not (L3/L4 level of activity), resulting in a pulling of the femoral head out of the shallow acetabulum. Both of these conditions are exacerbated by delayed weight-bearing; thus, early PT treatment should focus on weight-bearing postures (quadruped, standing). For infants with MMC and club foot or DDH, the timing of interventions can also create a very complicated picture, further limiting early weight-bearing. Surgical healing, after correction of each orthopedic condition, in combination with the need to develop motor skills need to be carefully considered when creating an appropriate treatment plan.

Scoliosis

Scoliosis is a curvature and possible rotation of the spine that can occur in typically developing children but is also quite common in neuromuscular disorders such as cerebral palsy, muscular dystrophy, and MMC due to asymmetrical muscle activity in the trunk or differences in leg length in ambulating children. The Adam's forward bend test is the most common screening measure for scoliosis, where the child bends forward from a standing position and a rib hump is prominent on one side but not the other (Figure 18-15).

Idiopathic scoliosis has no known cause and can be diagnosed at any age, occurring in .5–5% of the general population. Curves of 10 degrees or less are considered minor and affect females and males almost equally (1.4 females:1 male). Curves of greater than 20 degrees affect females almost 7 times more frequently than males. Congenital scoliosis is caused by vertebral abnormalities that are already formed at birth but do not induce a scoliosis until childhood or adolescence under periods of rapid bone growth.[15] Characteristics of scoliosis depend on whether it is (1) **structural**, meaning the curve is fixed and inflexible and is typically caused by abnormal vertebrae; or (2) **nonstructural**, meaning the curve corrects completely or partially with lateral bending and is commonly caused by positioning, muscle asymmetry, weakness, or neuropathy. In upright postures (standing or sitting), the height of the iliac crest

FIGURE 18-15 Presentation of S-curve scoliosis. A. Adam's forward bend test illuminates a prominent rib bump on the right consistent with a right thoracic concavity. B. Right lower shoulder and raised left hip are visually apparent in this right thoracic, left lumbar S-curve. (Reproduced with permission from Rudolph CD, Rudolph AM, Lister GE, First LR, Gershon AA (Eds). *Rudolph's Pediatrics*, 22ed. New York, NY: McGraw-Hill; 2011. Fig 216-5 and 216-4.)

and shoulders may be unequal with scoliosis of any etiology (Figure 18-15B). Frequently, scoliosis presents as an S-shaped deformity with a primary (largest) curve and secondary curve that compensates for the primary curve (see Table 18-2 for the Lenke classification of scoliosis). Terminology focuses on the convexity of the curves, structural versus nonstructural nature, and location (e.g., right primary thoracic structural curve and left secondary nonstructural lumbar curve). Motor characteristics include difficulty breathing due to the small intercostal space on the concave side of the curve and a large intercostal space on the convex side, weakness of the surrounding spinal musculature, and possible delays in motor milestone acquisition and other domains of development. The physical therapist has a role in the evaluation of scoliosis, and in patients with spina bifida, needs to be aware that it is a common co-occurrence. There is an overall poorer prognosis, if the vertebral growth plate is affected, which may occur in MMC. For children with curves greater than 40 degrees with vertebral rotation, spinal fusion is typically required for correction. Inpatient physical therapy after this surgery will include activities such as bed mobility (without rotation), lower extremity strengthening, orthoses, and parent and patient education on precautions and short- and long-term limitations. For children with curves between 20 and 40 degrees the focus is on maintaining activity and spinal stabilization exercises while wearing a brace, sometimes up to 23 hours per day. Many of these children go on to have spinal fusion surgery, if their curve progresses to 40 degrees or is preventing them from maintaining a functional sitting position.[16] Figure 18-16 illustrates how scoliosis curves are measured.

TABLE 18-2	Lenke Classification of Scoliosis[17]
LENKE CLASSIFICATION	**DESCRIPTION**
Lenke 1	Single structural thoracic curve with either a nonstructural compensation above (upper thoracic) or below (lumbar); correction of the thoracic curve results in spontaneous correction of the lumbar curve
Lenke 2 – Double thoracic curve	Two structural thoracic curves – the primary is typically midthoracic with a secondary upper thoracic curve; a nonstructural lumbar compensatory curve may also exist
Lenke 3 – Double major curves	A primary thoracic structural curve with a secondary lumbar structural curve; a nonstructural proximal thoracic compensatory curve is also present
Lenke 4 – Triple major curves	A midthoracic primary structural curve with both a proximal and lumbar secondary structural curves
Lenke 5 – Primary thoracolumbar or lumbar curve	A primary structural thoracolumbar or lumbar curve with a secondary thoracic nonstructural compensation
Lenke 6 – Thoracolumbar/ lumbar/thoracic curves	A primary structural lumbar curve with a structural thoracic secondary curve

CASE A, PART VII

Scoliosis correction is typically done in the teenage years, when growth is complete or almost complete. Surgery entails realigning the involved vertebrae and then fusing them together; this can partially correct the curve and then prevent further deformity. Small bone grafts are inserted between the vertebrae, which will then fuse with the vertebrae to create a solid bony structure; this procedure will change the mobility of the spine and stop all future growth in the area of the fusion, so that is why surgery is done when growth is nearly complete. Often metal rods are also inserted to prevent movement during the healing process. In Dylan's case, his fusion was accompanied by hip flexor tendon releases (cutting of the tendon, typically in a diagonal and then reattaching the ends to allow increased length). His limitations in moving (avoidance of lifting, pushing his chair, twisting, etc.) will be in place for the first 3 months or so after surgery; then, he will gradually be able to return to his normal level of activity, although often with some diminished trunk mobility.

FIGURE 18-16 Scoliosis measurement: The angle of the curve is measured on an anterior-posterior radiographic image by identifying the top point of the curve (where it begins to realign) and the bottom point (where it begins to reverse itself); a line is drawn parallel to each of these points and then perpendicular lines are drawn into the curve till they intersect. This provides a measureable angle of 59 degrees for the primary curve in this image; the secondary curve measures 38 degrees (lines of measurement not shown). (Reproduced with permission from Rudolph CD, Rudolph AM, Lister GE, First LR, Gershon AA (Eds). *Rudolph's Pediatrics*, 22ed. New York, NY: McGraw-Hill; 2011. Fig 216-6.)

● PHYSICAL THERAPY MANAGEMENT

There are 2500–6000 babies born each year with MMC. Lesions are primarily in the lumbar and sacral regions, yet rarer cervical and thoracic lesions do occur. In terms of **general motor skill development**, we know that most children with MMC do not sit or crawl until 1–2 years of age and often do not walk or even pull-to-stand until they are 3 years of age or older. Many children and adolescents with MMC use wheelchairs as their primary form of mobility even if, as young children, they took some steps. Some of this is a shifting in goals by the child as they prefer to keep up with their peers in school and be more independent from their parents. Since MMC is a lifelong disability, there are implications for bone and muscle health at all ages. As a group, patients with MMC have higher rates of obesity, poor fitness, and poor levels of independence.

Movement Potential in MMC

Kicking behavior: Ultrasound observations indicate that fetuses with MMC move their legs and kick at the same rates as fetuses without MMC.[18] So, in utero, in a crowded and gravity-free environment, they move in equal amounts to typically developing infants. In addition, mothers of babies with and without MMC have done subjective kick counts and report similar amounts of movement and activity. Kicking behaviors in infancy are well studied, and there is a developmental progression of kicking that can be monitored and tracked. In terms of frequency, we know that older babies kick less than younger babies. In terms of pattern, babies start off by kicking in an alternating pattern; then as they get older, they start to show more single leg kicks, and as they get even older, they show more parallel kicks.[19] Since patients with MMC most commonly have thoracic, lumbar, and sacral lesions, PTs are most concerned about the sensorimotor function of the trunk and legs. There are a handful of studies that have quantified the leg movements of young infants with MMC. Infants who are 4–6 months of age with MMC show less movement and less variability in kicking patterns than typically developing infants[20]; yet, they can and do change their kicking frequency, based on their position, and they kick the most when in supine and in an open space. Physical therapists can use this information to modify the environment to improve the number of kicking repetitions as a strengthening exercise. Infants who are 1–6 months of age with MMC also show a shorter kicking duration, meaning their kicks do not last as long, with fewer movements and more asymmetry than infants with typical development.[21]

Ambulation: There are some predictors of ambulation ability based on lesion level with better prognosis for functional ambulation associated with lower lesion levels (Table 18-3). Bracing is a necessary component to facilitate ambulation, and most children will also need crutches or a walker to achieve ambulation except for L5/sacral lesions that may ambulate with only minor bracing and no walking aid. Lesions above L1 result in absent lower extremity muscle function, and thereby, children with lesions at this level will require complete support of the hip, knee, and ankle to stand. Common abbreviations for orthotics use the first letter of each joint supported, such as a KAFO for the knee-ankle-foot orthosis. Lower lesions are associated with greater muscle control and less need for bracing. Table 18-3 examines muscle activity and bracing needs for children with lumbar and sacral lesions.

This can be thought of as a guideline for prediction of ambulation status. Other published rates of ambulation include even more general characteristics. Twenty percent of patients with high lumbar lesions achieve some walking most often using a hip strategy. Eighty percent of patients with low lumbar lesions walk, likely because of the additional knee and ankle control. Ninety percent of patients with sacral lesions walk with sensorimotor function in the hip, knee, and ankle.[24,25] It is also very common for younger children to ambulate to some degree but give it up as they get older despite motor function that would enable them to ambulate; this results from both the increased energy cost in moving a larger body mass and the need to move more quickly to keep up with peers. Each patient with MMC

TABLE 18-3	Ambulatory Potential based on Lesion Level[22,23]		
LESION LEVEL	**EXPECTED MUSCLE FUNCTION**	**WALKING POTENTIAL**	**BRACING OPTIONS/ ASSISTIVE DEVICES**
L1 or above	No lower extremity muscle function; trunk function normal	Poor walking potential but may ambulate some within their household at young ages	Trunk-hip-knee-ankle-foot (THKAFO) orthosis or HKAFO with walker/crutches
L2	Possible hip flexion but no other lower extremity muscle function	Some household ambulation but will use a wheelchair for most settings and at older ages	Hip-knee-ankle-foot (HKAFO) or reciprocal gait orthosis (RGO) with walker/crutches
L3	Good to normal hip flexion and antigravity knee extension likely	Household ambulation likely but will use a wheelchair for community/school ambulation and often at older ages	Knee-ankle-foot (KAFO) or ankle-foot (AFO) orthosis with crutches
L4	Good to normal hip flexion and knee extension plus antigravity dorsiflexion	Household or community ambulation; may convert to wheelchair at older ages	Ankle-foot (AFO) orthosis with crutches
L5	Good to normal dorsiflexion plus good eversion/inversion and some plantarflexion, knee flexion and hip extension (usually poor)	Community ambulation	AFO or supramalleolar orthosis, no crutches
S1	Antigravity hip extension and abduction and knee flexion plus some plantarflexion	Community ambulation	No orthotics
S2	Good to normal function at hip, knee and ankle, missing some toe and foot muscle control		

is unique and so is their functional status. Since the lesions are typically asymmetrical and incomplete, this results in unique functional features for each child. The exact level of lesion may be very important for a surgeon and much less important for the rehabilitation team. Some MMC clinics do not use lesion levels in the chart because it is not always accurate in describing the client's current level of performance. Functional abilities are charted directly instead of lesion level as that is more meaningful information to the rehabilitation team.

Orthotics

Orthotic prescription focuses on achieving joint alignment while not impeding function; it is important to not over brace, or in other words, to allow functional muscles to be active, even if they are only partially innervated. The joints of the orthotic should align with the anatomical joints, and orthotics should be comfortable, as easy to don and doff as possible, and as cosmetic as possible. Orthotics are typically made of thermoplastics that can be molded to the child's extremity (Table 18-4).

Role of the Physical Therapist

As a lifelong disability, patients with MMC will have multiple episodes of physical therapy throughout their lifespan. The role of the pediatric physical therapist is to provide training and skills necessary for functional independence to the best extent possible. This typically focuses on the achievement of

early motor milestones, especially in infants and young children, as well as enhancing independent mobility (ambulation or wheelchair use) and maximizing stability to facilitate play, social development, learning, language, etc. Treatment will vary depending on the sensorimotor characteristics of the child and the treatment setting.

Episodes of physical therapy can happen in a variety of care settings.

CASE A, PART VIII

In the NICU, Dylan was seen by the PT in the first days after his surgery. [If surgery is delayed, treatment may be initiated day 1 or 2 and then resume after surgery.] Initially, Dylan's treatment focused on positioning and handling techniques, promoting overall range of motion as well as protection of the spinal surgical site. Early education of the parents on how to handle Dylan facilitated early bonding. Once the shunt was placed in week 3, Dylan's parents were also educated on shunt protection (positions to be avoided) and signs of shunt dysfunction (this is typically done by the nursing or medical staff but should be emphasized by the PT). Dylan initially presented with excessive range of motion at the hips, so although early treatment focuses on promoting range of motion, excessive hip extension and adduction were avoided to prevent hip subluxation or dislocation. Dylan's parents were also instructed to avoid tight swaddling of Dylan to avoid forcing his legs into an extended and adducted position; again, this can lead to further hip instability and subluxation/dislocation. In Dylan's case, his DDH was treated with a Pavlik harness that was fitted at about 1 month of age, after his initial surgeries to correct the lesion and implant the shunt were completed. In many children, the Pavlik harness may be fitted even earlier, if DDH is identified at birth. Pain management, providing an environment of developmental care to promote growth and development, and comprehensive parent education are key elements of NICU care for the infant with MMC.

From birth to 3 years of age, Dylan received early intervention services first in his home, and then, twice per week as part of an early intervention infant program. Home-based services are common for EI before 3 years of age. Therapy, at this age, focused on maintaining/promoting normal range of motion and preventing contractures of the lower extremities; evaluating and teaching body awareness (e.g. exploring feet with hands); promoting positional and milestone development in supine, prone, sitting and standing; promoting head and truck control and reaching, including object exploration; evaluating sensory dysfunction and developing sensory-precautions (e.g., bath water temperature, getting toes stuck in cribs or toys; see Box 18-5); enhancing sensory input for kicking and stepping development; promoting weight-bearing and independent mobility; learning of cause and effect relationships; avoiding learned disuse; and parent education on all of the above.

TABLE 18-4	Orthotic Options for Children with MMC
ORTHOTIC	**DESCRIPTION OF FIT AND USE**
Foot orthotic	Shoe insert that is fitted to support the arch of the foot and minimize pronation/supination
Supramalleolar	Fits around malleoli to stabilize forefoot (adduction/abduction), midfoot (pronation), and/or hindfoot (valgus/varus) while allowing dorsiflexion/plantarflexion.
Ankle-foot (AFO)	Typically fit to just below the knee to provide ankle stability with straps at the ankle and/or upper aspect
(1) Solid/Rigid	Blocks dorsiflexion and plantarflexion; controls foot (forefoot, midfoot, hindfoot) as needed
(2) Hinged/Articulating	Hinge at ankle between upper and foot segments; blocks plantarflexion with free or assisted dorsiflexion
(3) Floor reaction	An AFO with an anterior rigid, padded shell on the upper shin to control excessive dorsiflexion and assist knee extension at midstance
(4) Dynamic	Thinner material allows more flexibility; wraps around foot; resists plantarflexion and assists dorsiflexion; stabilizes foot
Knee-ankle-foot (KAFO)*	Typically constructed of a thermoplastic sleeve at the mid-thigh, with velcro strap(s) closure and a supporting metal frame both medial and lateral, connecting to an AFO. A drop lock at the knee joint allows the device to bend while sitting and then the lock to "drop" into place when the child assumes standing. In reality, the child typically locks the knee before pulling to stand and unlocks it after returning to sit.
Hip-knee-ankle-foot (HKAFO)*	Adds a pelvic band and hip joint to the KAFO. Locks at the hip joint will prevent hip flexion and extension, requiring both legs to move in unison (swing to or swing through gait).
Trunk-hip-knee-ankle-foot* (THKAFO)	An additional thoracic support, added to the HAFO, provides trunk support to the child with limited abdominal/spinal muscle activity.
Reciprocating gait (RGO)*	An HKAFO constructed with a cable connection between the two leg components to facilitate hip flexion on the unweighted leg and extension on the weight-bearing leg, creating an alternating or reciprocal gait pattern. Unweighting is typically achieved by lateral trunk bending, and hip extension is further enhanced by shoulder retraction and back extension on the side of the stance leg. For those with some hip flexion, an RGO will assist hip flexion while maintaining extension in the stance leg.
Parapodium*	A rigid THKAFO support (standing frame) that can allow some forward movement in a swing-to or swing-through manner. Typically have joints at the hip and knee to allow sitting when locks are disengaged.
Swivel walker*	A parapodium attached to a swivel base that achieves forward propulsion through alternating trunk rotation.

*All of these devices will require upper extremity assistance through the use of an assistive device, typically a walker initially and then crutches.

CASE A, PART IX

Given Dylan's lesion level, what type of orthotic would you likely recommend for Dylan as a toddler?

If you said an HKAFO or RGO, you're right; either of these would be appropriate for Dylan.

With an L1/L2 lesion, Dylan has only minimal hip flexion. When he was 2, he was fitted with an HKAFO and was able to walk short distances within his home first with a standard walker and then with forearm crutches, using a swing-to gait pattern, which refers to moving both crutches forward and then swinging both legs simultaneously toward the point of crutch placement; typically, the toes stay slightly behind the crutches. In older children, this may progress to a swing-through pattern, where the legs move past the crutches; this more advanced method requires considerable arm strength and balance; Dylan never achieved a swing-through pattern. Early therapy focused on strengthening his arms for not only ambulation but for wheelchair mobility, using lift-ups, wheelbarrow walking, and throwing activities with and without wrist cuff weights. By the age of 3, he was able to get in and out of his wheelchair and keep up with his friends easily in the wheelchair. To get into his low wheelchair, he would pull up into a kneeling position and then pull to a supported standing position, pulling on the wheelchair arms, and then rotate to sit down. As he aged, he could push up into the chair from the floor by aligning himself with his back to the chair and placing both hands on the seat and performing a lift-up into the chair. As he grew, it became more and more energy intensive to walk even short distances; by the time he was 6, he primarily used a manual chair for both in-house and community mobility as this allowed him the speed and independence to keep up with his family and peers. Since his family had a two-story house, he managed the stairs by sitting and performing an arm lift up to pull himself backwards up the stairs. Scooting down the stairs was fun but resulted in several instances of ischial sores until he learned to slowly go down the stairs, lifting up, and slowly dropping down to the next stair. His family was able to purchase a ranch-style home when he was 5 to eliminate the need to go up and down stairs. If this hadn't been possible, there are some seated stair lifts that might have been needed to facilitate stair ascent/descent as he aged.

BOX 18-5   Sensory Loss in the Lower Extremities Requires Special Attention

With MMC, there is a partial or complete loss of somatosensory function in the legs. This requires constant attention and vigilance to assure that the child does not injure themselves while moving or especially that the parents not injure the child unknowingly. For example, when putting on shoes, toes can become curled within the shoe; typically developing children will fuss if this happens, and the parents are alerted to the discomfort. Children with insensate feet will not fuss, and thus, can get pressure sores on their feet from getting a toe curled under the foot within a shoe. Similarly, ill-fitting shoes can create pressure sores that the child will not feel; even clothing can cause problems if too tight or it becomes wrinkled underneath the child. Frequent repositioning and parent attention can minimize the likelihood of pressure problems.

One of the more common problems that arise occurs as the child begins moving; creeping or crawling on rough surfaces can abrade the knees, shins, or toes without the child knowing it, so protection of these areas is critical as the child starts moving. Shoes or at least socks should always be worn; long pants can protect the legs, or knee pads can be worn. Additionally, there needs to be constant vigilance with bath time. Parents must always check water temperature carefully so that the child is not placed in water that is too hot. Older children also need to be well educated in the dangers of getting into a tub without checking the water temperature with their hand. Much like the patient with a spinal cord injury, children with MMC need pressure relief so that they don't maintain a given position for too long. Typically developing children move constantly; however, children with MMC may demonstrate much less lower extremity movement, especially with high lumbar or thoracic lesions. Thus, parents must be instructed to vary the positioning of the infant so that pressure ulcers do not develop (every 4 hours at a minimum); using a pressure mattress cover (sheepskin or gel) can also be useful in preventing ulcer development in infants. As the child ages, they should be instructed in pressure relief at frequent intervals, at least every 15–20 minutes, if they are sitting in a wheelchair. The use of appropriate seating cushions will also help prevent ulcer development. Finally, a frequent cause of pressure sores for children with MMC are ill-fitting braces; it is critical that braces be frequently evaluated to assure a good fit in a growing child. It is quite common that the child enters a growth spurt and quickly the brace begins to rub in a given area. On removal of any brace, parents should be instructed to look for red spots; if these do not dissipate in 5–10 minutes, the brace needs to be adjusted.

For children with MMC and associated hydrocephalus, early treatment must focus on developing head control, which is complicated by a slightly enlarged head and diminished lower extremity muscle activity that is needed to weight down the lower half of the body as the head is lifted. Trunk strengthening is also a focus of early treatment, since in the presence of lower extremity paresis, the trunk must work harder for the child to sit and achieve standing. Like other children with developmental disabilities, treatment also focuses on achieving developmental milestones. Table 18-5 presents ideas of early treatment activities for children with MMC.

Overlapping with early intervention and continuing throughout the lifespan, PTs will see patients of any age with MMC in an outpatient or school setting with similar objectives to those listed for the infant. PTs address milestone delay, develop functional training interventions, and provide adaptive equipment

TABLE 18-5	Treatment Activities for Infants with MMC
TARGETED MOVEMENT	**ACTIVITY**
Upright head control	Babies first learn to hold their head upright, while being held, before any other position. Encouraging head control in sitting, while the trunk is well supported, can be done with the child sitting on the therapist's or parent's lap with the head and trunk against the trunk of the holder or with support at the shoulders and the child sitting away from the holder's trunk. Moving a toy in the visual field of the child will encourage head turning and lifting away from the support, especially if the toy is moved in a slow vertical motion (up-down). Also, tilting the child in each direction while encouraging him/her to look at a toy or another person, will encourage the head to be held upright. As some control is achieved, increasing the speed and range of toy movement or the degree of tilt will stimulate increased head control. These same activities will encourage trunk control with support at the lower trunk or hip. Also, working on prone and supine head control will facilitate upright head control.
Prone head lifting	Placing the child prone on a wedge or Thera-Ball so that head lifting can be done in a partial gravity-eliminated position will allow the child to develop neck extensor strength initially. Over time, the incline of the wedge or the position of the child on the ball can be adjusted to require more chin tucking while holding the head horizontal. An interesting toy should be used to stimulate head lifting.
	Parents can work on this by having their child lay on their belly across their lap. Placing one of their feet on a stool will help create an incline so that the child can work with gravity partially eliminated. Placing a toy for the child to look at on the floor, slightly in front of the child will encourage head lifting. As the child gains strength, decreasing the incline and moving the toy higher onto a chair or eventually a table will stimulate head lifting toward 90 degrees.
Supine head lifting	Similar to prone head lifting activities, a wedge or ball is a good way to work on supine head lifting by having the child move toward upright from an angled position; this will strengthen the neck flexors. Decreasing the incline as the child gains strength, will make this more challenging until the child is able to be pulled to sitting with the chin tucked.
	Parents can work on this by sitting on the floor in a partially reclined position with their back against the wall or a piece of furniture, their hips and knees flexed and their feet flat on the floor. The infant can then be placed on their lap with their head and trunk against their parent's thighs. Encouraging the child to look at a toy on the parents stomach or just come to an upright position, without losing control of the head, will encourage neck flexor strength. Parents can support the child by holding the child's hands or as strength is gained, supporting the child's upper trunk and eventually the hips.
Rolling – prone to supine	For many children with MMC, rolling is done entirely with the head and upper body, since leg movement may be minimal. Encouraging the child to look at a toy from a prone prop position and reaching with the hand in the direction of the roll will encourage rolling. Assistance from the therapist or parent can be done at the hip, first to assist, and then to resist the roll to further strengthen the trunk. Starting from a side-lying position will allow the child to strengthen the trunk initially, with the therapist resisting the roll at the hip and/or shoulder; also, using a wedge such that the child rolls "downhill" can make this easier early on.
Rolling – supine to prone	Similar to the prone to supine roll, children with MMC will roll supine to prone with minimal LE movement. Strong neck flexion will need to be achieved prior to successful rolling in this direction. Encouraging reaching for a toy across the body in the direction of the roll will facilitate this movement. Assisting lower extremity movement and trunk rotation is typically required early, but in children with hip flexor innervation, this motion should be encouraged as the child rolls. The side-lying and wedge methods, listed for prone–supine will also work for supine to prone.
Sitting	Sitting is a challenge for many children with MMC, since LE activity is typically needed to anchor the child while in sitting. However, most children will achieve some degree of independent sitting on the floor but may require some arm support, if their lesion is in the thoracic trunk. Lots of reaching with decreasing amounts of trunk and hip support are critical to develop sitting balance. Having the child straddle a roll or sit on a Thera-Ball with support at the lower trunk or hip can be good methods for working on sitting with reaching or weight shift activities. Tilting the roll or ball with encouragement to return to upright will strengthen the trunk and develop balance (provide verbal encouragement to return to upright; focus the child on the muscles that need to be working by touching or tapping them). Reaching to the side, the floor, and across midline will strengthen critical trunk muscles; support will need to be provided at the lower trunk and then the hip for most children to be successful in this activity.

(Continued)

TABLE 18-5	**Treatment Activities for Infants with MMC** (*Continued*)
TARGETED MOVEMENT	**ACTIVITY**
Abdominal strengthening	Assisted sit-ups, performed with the knees bent and holding the therapist's or parent's hands, can be an early way to begin abdominal strengthening, allowing the child to use some UE pull along with the abdominals. Slowly returning to supine (roll-down) will require eccentric abdominal activity, further strengthening the abdominals. Over time, decreasing and then eliminating the UE assistance should occur until none is provided. An incline can also be used to decrease the effect of gravity while performing a sit-up or roll-down to work on abdominal strengthening. Some support at the legs may need to be provided, since hip extension may be absent.
Upper extremity weight-bearing	Initial weight-bearing on the arms is critical for future functional movement. (1) For the infant, this can be done over a small roll or rolled towel to facilitate prone-propping. (2) For the older child, a larger roll may be used. Reaching for toys will facilitate weight shift and strengthen each arm while bearing weight on one and reaching with the other. (3) Once weight-bearing is achieved, having the child walk on their hands with support at their hip, a "wheelbarrow walk," will continue to strengthen the arms. (4) Performing "lift ups" (lifting the bottom off the support surface by pushing with the arms, while sitting) from a chair with arms or on the floor with the hands first on large block so that the elbows are flexed initially are also good ways to strengthen the arms, which will be critical in walking and wheelchair use.
Lower extremity weight-bearing/ strengthening	Lower extremity innervation and muscle strength will be determinants of the focus of physical therapy for children with MMC. Although most children with MMC will require some bracing for standing/walking, early therapy should include LE weight-bearing in a variety of positions with support from the therapist as appropriate. Strengthening of muscles will be critical to maximizing function in upright postures. (1) Weight-bearing in quadruped can be facilitated over a roll initially with the hands on the floor and therapist support at the hips; rocking forward and back or side to side will increase strength and stability over time; reaching for toys will also require weight-shifting to improve stability and trunk strength. (2) Kneeling or half-kneeling are great postures to strengthen the hips in those with some muscle function in the gluteal muscles; kneeling will also facilitate trunk muscle activity and upper extremity weight-bearing; reaching in these positions will strengthen trunk muscles and develop balance. For children with limited LE muscle activity, kneeling may still be appropriate to create some weight-bearing on the LE and especially the hips; however, this will require therapist control of the hips and considerable UE support by the child. (3) Weight bearing in sitting astride a roll or in a low chair is also a good position for LE strengthening. Coming to standing and controlled return to sitting from standing will further strengthen the quadriceps as well as hip muscles, if innervated. For those with limited quad strength, pulling up with the arms will be required. (4) "Push-aways" are a simple way to strengthen the quads and potentially the gluts in young children. For this activity, the therapist holds the child's heels in their hands with the child supine and the therapist sitting and facing the child. Bend the knees to the chest and then have the child "push away" the therapist by straightening their legs. (5) Kicking a ball, with or without ankle weights, in sitting is another fun way to strengthen the quads for standing. (6) Squatting from standing and returning to standing is a great quad strengthening activity with or without UE support for the child with some quad strength; (7) Bridging in a supine position will increase gluteal strength in those with some innervation of these muscles; this can easily be a fun play activity with a car or ball to roll "under the bridge." (8) Early standing with appropriate bracing should be initiated when head and trunk control are sufficient; the use of appropriate assistive devices (e.g., wheeled walker, crutches) or other support (furniture, walls, therapist/parent hands) will likely be required. (9) Recent evidence suggests that body-weight supported treadmill training or weight-supported walkers may facilitate early weight-bearing activities with the potential to elicit walking at an earlier age.

for mobility and transfers. For toddler and preschool ages, the PT may begin to have a large role in: (1) identifying appropriate assistive devices (including canes, walkers, manual wheelchairs, power wheelchairs, standers, and orthotic devices); (2) enhancing independent mobility and transfers; (3) beginning a standing program; and (4) providing the means for early social interactions with peers. Orthotic devices are very common for children with MMC; as listed in Table 18-6, orthotic device choice is predicated on lesion level with bracing providing support at joints with absent or minimal muscle function.

In **school-based settings**, PTs will see children with MMC to help with educational progress, including classroom mobility. This will include working closely with the teacher(s) and other support service providers (e.g., adaptive physical educators, occupational therapists) to adapt the classroom to meet the needs of the child, which may include assuring wider separation of desks to allow wheelchair access, encouraging longer transition times to afford the child sufficient time to move from one class to another, adaptation of bathroom facilities to allow catheterization (see Box 18-6 for information on bowel and bladder function), and education of the teacher on how to integrate a child with MMC into the classroom. For some children, a standing podium may be incorporated into some classroom activities to afford some time out of their wheelchair each day. Notably, children with MMC have a higher incidence of learning disabilities and lower cognitive scores than the general population, likely related to hydrocephalus, yet many children with MMC have no learning disabilities and typical intelligence.

CASE A, PART X

Dylan has been seen episodically over his school years to maximize function and assure maximum independence in the school setting, especially to help him transition from one school building to another as he progressed. In preschool and kindergarten, treatment focused on strengthening, ambulation, and wheelchair mobility in the classroom. However, by first grade, PT focused most on wheelchair mobility, including over ground propulsion (uneven surfaces such as ramps, gravel, and grass), wheelies to go over uneven surfaces, reaching for objects from his chair (laterally, overhead, and on the floor), and managing the cafeteria (carrying a tray and manipulating his chair). As he grew, continued UE strengthening was a focus along with transfers for toileting and moving to other surfaces (floor, bed, etc.) as well as wheelies for larger obstacles and righting the wheelchair if it tipped over (see Chapter 12 for wheelchair activities for the spinal cord patient). Following his scoliosis and tendon-lengthening surgery, his school-based therapist implemented a program to maximize the hip range of motion gained from the surgery; this involved getting Dylan out of his chair once per day to stretch his hip flexors for 5–10 minutes by lying prone and to evaluate his ability to propel his wheelchair with his limited mobility or to use powered mobility in the school setting (the school has been fortunate to have a number of chairs donated from other children as they were outgrown).

BOX 18-6 Bowel and Bladder Management for Children with Myelomeningocele

Bowel and bladder management is a critical component of any program for patients with MMC, since they have disrupted bowel and bladder innervation. Often, there is a catheterization program for bladder voiding and a bowel program that may include dietary and pharmaceutical management as well as rectal stimulation. Bowel and bladder programs are taught to children so that they can be as independent as possible with toileting and not reliant on an adult for assistance as they age. Poor bladder management can cause back up into the kidneys, which can cause kidney damage. It is very important to be aware that patients with MMC are at an increased risk for obesity, sedentary behavior, and decreased physical fitness. This can be cyclical as they have a disability that prevents typical use of the lower extremities in a way that might promote physical fitness. Fitness should be addressed in all settings and at all ages.

The physical therapist may be involved in training chair–commode transfers in the home and the school setting to facilitate bowel/bladder management.

In **acute or inpatient rehabilitation settings**, the PT will see patients with MMC periodically throughout their lifespan for additional postsurgical (e.g., spinal fusion for scoliosis, other orthopedic surgery) or other rehabilitation needs. Evaluation and training for new orthotics, assistive devices, and wheelchairs are also critical as the child ages to determine the best choice(s) and then train the child on appropriate use.

CASE A, PART XI

For Dylan, he was seen postoperatively to discuss movement limitations and to educate the family on transfer techniques, since he wasn't able to perform a push-up necessary for a chair to bed transfer. The parents were taught to perform a standing pivot transfer from the bed to the wheelchair and back.

Functional training, strengthening, electrical stimulation, exercise training, and motor skill training have been shown to be effective in improving impairments and function in children with MMC. Interestingly, there is very little research on the effectiveness of aquatic PT for these children. Preventative techniques to avoid contractures, arthritis, skin breakdown (with pressure relief), and pain are all necessary components of a PT regimen. For example, pressure relief by tilting the wheelchair or doing an upper extremity sitting-pushup is prescribed every 15–20 minutes as are daily full body skin checks with a mirror. Exercise regimes or physical therapy to maintain function and prevent decline of current status is also important.

Adults with MMC also have decreased levels of fitness, decreased activity levels, and increased rates of obesity. It is important to have comprehensive health programs that include nutrition and individual or group fitness for patients at all ages to maximize their health. Bone health should also be emphasized, since weight-bearing is necessary for bone development and maintenance. It should be noted that these types of programs are not very common, but this is an area of potential growth in practice for PTs interested in maximizing function in adults with MMC.

Wheelchair Prescription

In many clinics and school settings, the PTs are responsible for deciding the type of wheelchair, including the seating and frame, for a child with MMC. Team evaluations and decision-making are common and typically include an equipment provider(s), a third-party payer representative, and the medical team. The PT is part of this team, evaluating the patient, problem-solving, and providing recommendations for design, purchase, and maintenance of wheelchairs as well as other adaptive equipment (Table 18-6). Toddlers and young children need to be able to navigate their environment on their own, so choosing the right mobility device involves a balance between safety and the importance of independent mobility for child development. Choosing the type of wheelchair and

accessory components is very much a team activity with a lot of caregiver input. Most wheelchairs are customized to fit the size and unique sensorimotor, orthopedic, and functional abilities to meet the daily activities of each child. Yet, assuring appropriate positioning of the child by manipulating or adding features to a wheelchair due to changes in age, growth, development, functional status, orthotic conditions, etc. is commonplace.

The process from assessment of the patient to ordering a wheelchair and ultimately receipt of the wheelchair by the patient can take a lot of time. Demonstration chairs are often available from vendors or housed in clinics for patients to try out. Sometimes demonstration that patients have the ability to safely operate a wheelchair, especially with powered mobility, is required to justify the chair choice to third-party payers and sometimes the family. One critical aspect of wheelchair choice is the cognitive maturity of the child, including ability to understand the demands of a mobility device and impulse control, which is necessary to assure safety (e.g., slowing the chair in the presence of other children). Demonstration wheelchairs offer the opportunity to consult with the child and caregivers about what will work best for them with consideration of their ability to transport the chair and manage it in the home. Asking about the current equipment the family uses may give the PT an idea about what is working and what is needed. Ordering any kind of

TABLE 18-6	Wheelchair Measurements
MEASUREMENT	**RATIONALE**
Seat to top of head Seat to occiput Seat to top of shoulder Seat to inferior angle of scapula	These measurements allow a determination of the height of the back of the chair and head rest, if needed. A head rest should hit at the occiput and support the head to its top. Most children with MMC will not need a head rest to maintain head control, but young children will have one to support their head for comfort or the back of the chair will go up to the top of the head to provide support when tired. For older children with limited trunk control but good head control, the chair back will typically end at the top of the shoulder; however, for teenagers and those with good trunk control, the back will end at the inferior angle of the scapula.
Seat to elbow	This measurement determines the height of the arm rest.
Seat to iliac crest	If a pelvic support is needed, this measurement will determine the height of the support. It can also identify pelvic obliquity (asymmetry) that may be addressed with the seat cushion to align the pelvis.
Chest width	If lateral trunk support is required, this will determine the width of the lateral supports. A measurement from the seat to the axilla will also be needed to determine the maximum height of the support, with 1–2 inches subtracted to prevent rubbing.
Chest depth	For children with limited trunk control, a chest harness may be needed, and this measurement will help determine the strap length. For transportation on a school bus, young children are required to have a chest harness.
Hip width – measure at widest point	Determines seat width; the seat should be at least 2 inches wider than this measurement to prevent pressure on the hips and allow a coat to be worn. Most pediatric chairs allow for the seat width to increase several inches over the life of the chair (the frame has the ability to expand) with or without replacement of the seat itself.
Thigh length (sacrum to popliteal fossa)	Determines seat depth; subtract 2 inches to prevent rubbing of the back of the leg by the seat. Similar to seat width, pediatric chair frames allow expansion of seat depth of several inches.
Knee to heel	Determines foot rest position; must allow 2 inches above the ground to allow clearance over uneven surfaces. Footrests are also typically adjustable to allow leg growth over the 5-year period.
Foot length	Determines foot rest depth

assistive equipment that the child or caregiver does not like will often result in that equipment being unused.

Part of the wheelchair evaluation will include a comprehensive medical history with emphasis on anything that might impact seating requirements or restrictions, including surgical history, orthopedic conditions, and respiratory or cardiac impairments. A new wheelchair is typically prescribed every 5 years, so the chair needs to have the ability to grow with the child and the potential for adapting to changes in the child's functioning over that time period; in some respects, this forces the PT to make "best guesses" of the future needs of the child. Despite our best efforts, children will sometimes change in unpredictable ways, including unexpected weight gain, surgery, or a change in function before the 5-year timeframe has passed, and the therapist and family will need to negotiate with the third-party payer for consideration of an early wheelchair replacement request.

A thorough evaluation of seating and postures, accounting for any deformities and ROM deficits, can be completed by the PT, including measurements as outlined in Table 18-6. Measurements are ideally taken in a seated position, typically a chair, if the patient has adequate postural and trunk control.

● WHEELCHAIR COMPONENTS

Considerations for wheelchairs for all children in need of one will include selection of appropriate components: (1) base (manual or powered); (2) frame; and (3) seating system as well as assessment of the environments, in which the child will function (home, school, other) and the activities, in which the child will participate, including for the older child, sporting activities.

Bases

The type of base, either powered or manual, should be determined first. Most children with MMC have adequate ROM and strength in their upper extremities to independently propel a manual wheelchair. After some training and daily use, young toddlers can be expert navigators of a manual wheelchair at home and in the community. Manual wheelchairs give children with MMC early functional mobility, the ability to keep up with age-matched peers, and a way to quickly explore their environment. The best choice for many young toddlers is an ultra-lightweight, rigid-frame chair that is low to the floor and can have a handle for parental control (Figure 18-17).[26] This will afford the child easier transfers into and out of the chair from the floor as well as put them at the eye-level of their peers. Many preschoolers are able to manipulate their wheelchairs through complex environments and, by early school age, to perform a wheelie to clear a low curb. If, and when, a power chair is needed, it is important to note that power bases are larger, heavier, and do not collapse as easily as manual bases, so consideration should also be given to maneuverability in the home and the ability of the family to transport the chair. Some children have declining function over their lifetime and might eventually need a power chair. Both manual and power bases are somewhat adaptable for different seating systems, accessories, and features. Accessories

FIGURE 18-17 Manual wheelchair for toddler (see video of use). This ultralight manual wheelchair is consistent with that described for Dylan, including a leg rest to support the whole lower extremity, a handle for the caregiver to control the chair. (Used with permission of Jill C. Heathcock, MPT, PhD, The Ohio State University).

include arm rests, foot rests, tilt or recline positioning, type of wheels and tires, hand rims, and brakes. Considerations for manual versus powered WCs include (1) whether the child or caregiver will be moving the chair; (2) the ability to self-propel, understand safety, and control impulsivity; (3) UE strength, overall endurance, and transfer abilities/potential; (4) cognition and vision; and (5) any restrictions on mobility (e.g., orthopedic limitations similar to Dylan's).

CASE A, PART XI

By the time Dylan was 2 years old he had a custom-made manual wheelchair with a leg rest to support his entire lower extremities. The leg rest could bend to 90 degrees so as he got older and longer his legs could be in a flexed position at the knee and accessory foot rests added to the frame. The handle allowed his caregivers to maneuver the wheelchair in a similar manner as a stroller and provided safety support when needed, while allowing Dylan the ability to independently explore and participate in his environment at a speed equal to his peers. He used a reverse rolling walker with HKFOs for short distances at home and for lower extremity weight-bearing and upright ambulation training and exercise. Dylan continued to use standard light-frame manual wheelchairs as his primary form of independent mobility until the scoliosis surgery.

Frames

Frames can be rigid or folding. Folding frames allow for the WC to be collapsed and stored or transported in a small car trunk. Rigid frames cannot be folded but do allow for easy removal of the tires for storage and transport. Frames for WCs can be of many materials, including stainless steel, aluminum, and titanium. Traditional stainless steel frames are heavier than newer lightweight frames that are made out of titanium or composite material.

Seating Systems

A seating system should create a functional sitting position that assures comfort, baseline pressure relief, adequate trunk support, and good postural alignment. The latter is especially important in children with thoracic lesions as they are likely to develop kyphosis, scoliosis, or both due to asymmetric trunk muscle activity. Scoliosis or pelvic obliquities can be observed in sitting posture and will result in asymmetrical seat to top of shoulder and seat to iliac crest measurements. Seat cushions vary greatly in firmness and pressure relief capacity, ranging from those made with air to those made of a hard foam. A balance is needed to minimize the shear force (friction across the skin as the body moves on the seat), created by the seating material, with the need to find the best position for the child to maximize function while also protecting boney prominences and avoid pressure ulcers. For example, some positions, such as a reclined position, increase the potential for shear that needs to be offset by a higher friction seating material; however, this will make it more likely for movement to create excessive shear. The PT should obtain a history of skin integrity to determine cushion selection. If needed, pressure mapping systems are now available to accurately identify points of increased pressure where additional padding may be needed.

Notably, PTs should also provide patient and caregiver education on the type and timing of pressure relief for children with poor sensation in their buttocks/legs. Standard practices for pressure relief for older children include independent WC push-ups where the child uses the armrests to lift their lower body off the seat by pushing up with their arms; frequent weight shifts by leaning all the way forward and leaning side to side; having a caregiver tilt the chair back with proper body mechanics; and manually changing the position of the legs to unweight one side. With power chairs the reclining or tilt in space features can be used for pressure relief. Tilt-in-space frames retain the seat to back angle but the seat orientation to the ground changes. A tilt of between 25 and 65 degrees has been shown to provide pressure relief in adults. Reclining chairs allow the back of the chair to change in relation to the seat, which affords pressure relief but increases the shear imposed on the skin. Most seating systems are aligned in a 90-90-90 alignment, representing the hip, knee, and ankle angles.

Other options for seating systems include back height, headrest, lateral and pelvic supports, belt system, and foot rest. Tall seat backs are common for children with low tone, poor sitting balance, and poor trunk control. A head rest can be included as an accessory if the patient child also has poor head control. A head rest is needed for head support during tilting or reclining in a power chair. A mid seat back height, just below the scapula, allows freedom of the shoulders for propulsion as well as sports activities. Young toddlers with MMC, who have lower level lesions and have adequate hip control, may use a standing WC that looks similar to Figure 18-17 but with a platform to stand with support at the knees and hips instead of a seat. Lap belts are necessary for young children, and chest harnesses are needed for those with poor trunk control or very young children, if they are transported in a school bus. Additional lateral supports may also be needed for the child with poor trunk control.

Environmental Factors

Final determination of the appropriate wheelchair system should include assessment of the home and school environments as well as the family's ability to manage the device. Assessment of the child's current home environment is critical to wheelchair selection, including the size and type of vehicle that is owned by the family and its capacity to transport a wheelchair, as well as the entry to the home to determine whether there are stairs to manage. Some third-party payers will require that a ramp is in place or currently being built before they will approve an order for a wheelchair. Home visits to evaluate individual needs are often conducted by a therapist and equipment provider. Smaller manual chairs for younger toddlers and children can be folded to fit in a small trunk and are lightweight, allowing for them to be carried up stairs, and thus eliminating the need for a ramp, since young children with or without impaired mobility are commonly carried into the home. Community needs including daycare, school, work, medical appointments, religious services, adaptive sports, and other unique considerations will also inform decision-making wheelchair specifications.

***Is Dylan a candidate for power mobility?*

There is not a simple answer to this question. First, his chair is only 2 years old, and his third-party payer typically only funds a new chair every 5 years; however, it may be possible to request consideration due to his change in status – recent weight gain and spinal fusion. As his PT, you would need to carefully document his change in status and evaluate his capacity to use a power chair, including whether he has any spatial perceptual deficits, associated with his visual learning disability. It is likely that he would be able to learn to control a power chair; however, if the limitations to his UE and trunk mobility are temporary, it will likely be better for him to continue to use a manual chair to maximize his physical activity and potentially reverse the weight gain. However, his family may also need to obtain a lift to assist with transfers to avoid injuring themselves, if he continues to grow. Aging with MMC is often associated with weight gain, resulting in a decrease in functional status. Fitness programs should be developed to minimize this problem in older children and adults with MMC. Increased risk of cardiovascular problems may occur in adults with MMC due to decreased mobility, resulting in a sedentary lifestyle. It is important to have comprehensive health programs that include nutrition counseling and individual or group fitness for patients at all ages to maximize their health.

Bone health should also be emphasized, since weight-bearing is necessary for normal bone development and maintenance; adults with MMC are at risk for osteoporosis and bone fractures, especially if they aren't walking.

COMPARISON TO SPINAL CORD INJURY

As mentioned earlier, there are some parallels between spinal cord injury and MMC. For example, in both, the spinal cord and neural tissue is damaged such that sensorimotor function is lost below the lesion level. The level gives necessary initial information about what kind of function a patient may have. Patients with SCI and MMC demonstrate a combination of UMN and LMS signs, and asymmetrical function is often present though the injury is typically bilateral. However, function and treatments are very different. For patients with a traumatic SCI, rehabilitation is *relearning* a skill that was already present, like walking. For infants with MMC, rehabilitation is the teaching of new skills such as the *emergence* of walking in a baby or child who has never walked before.

REFERENCES

1. Rowland CA, Correa A, Cragan JD, Alverson CJ. Are encephaloceles neural tube defects? *Pediatrics*. 2006;118(3):916-923.

2. Williams LJ, Rasmussen SA, Flores A, Kirby RS, Edmonds LD. Decline in the prevalence of spina bifida and anencephaly by race/ethnicity: 1995-2002. *Pediatrics*. 2005;116(3):580-586.

3. Trudell AS, Obido AO. Diagnosis of spina bifida on ultrasound: always termination? *Best Pract Res Clin Obstet Gynaecol*. 2014;28:367-377.

4. Bebbington MW, Danzer E, Johnson MP, Adzick NS. Open fetal surgery for myelomeningocele. *Prenat Diagn*. 2011;31(7):689-694.

5. Boettcher M, Goettler S, Exchenburg G, Kracht T, Kunkel P, Von der Wense A, Reinshagen K. Prenatal latex sensitization in patients with spina bifida: a pilot study. *J Neurosurg Pediatrics*. 2014;13:291-294.

6. Del Bigio MR. Neuropathology and structural changes in hydrocephalus. *Dev Disabil Res Rev*. 2010;16:16-22.

7. Dalen K, Bruroy S, Wentzel-Larsen T, Laegreid LM. Intelligence in children with hydrocephalus, aged 4-15 years: a population-based, controlled study. *Neuropediatrics*. 2008;39:146-150.

8. Oi S, Inagaki T, Shinoda M, Takahashi S, Ono S, Date I, Nomura S, Miwa T, Araki T, Ito S, Uchikado H, Takemoto O, Shirane R, Nishimoto H, Tashior Y, Matsumura A, COE-Fetal and Congenital Hydrocephalus Top 10 Japan Study Group. Guideline for management and treatment of fetal and congenital hydrocephalus: center of excellence-fetal and congenital hydrocephalus top 10 Japan guideline 2011. *Childs Nerv Syst*. 2011;27:1563-1579.

9. Tamburrini G, Frassanito P, Iakovaki K, Pignotti F, Rendeli C, Murolo D, Di Rocco C. Myelomeningocele: the management of associated hydrocephalus. *Childs Nerv Syst*. 2013;29:1569-1579.

10. Swank M, Dias L. Myelomeningocele: a review of the orthopaedic aspects of 206 patients treated from birth with no selection criteria. *Dev Med Child Neurol*. 1992;34(12):1047-1052.

11. Gibbons PJ, Gray K. Update on clubfoot. *J Paediatr Child Health*. 2013;49:E434-E437.

12. Swaroop VT, Dias L. Orthopaedic management of spina bifida-part II: foot and ankle deformities. *J Child Orthop*. 2011;5:403-414.

13. Holroyd B, Wedge J. Developmental dysplasia of the hip. *Orthop Trauma*. 2009;32(3): 162-168.

14. Dezateux C, Rosendahl K. Developmental dysplasia of the hip. *Lancet*. 2007;369:1541-1552.

15. Konieczny MR, Senyurt H, Krauspe R. Epidemiology of adolescent idiopathic scoliosis. *J Child Orthop*. 2013;7:3-9.

16. Negrini S, Donzelli S, Lusini M, Minnella S, Zaina F. The effectiveness of combined bracing and exercise in adolescent idiopathic scoliosis based on SRS and SOSORT criteria: a prospective study. *BMC Musculoskelet Disord*. 2014;15(1):263.

17. Hoashi JS, Cahill PJ, Bennett JT, Samdani AF. Adolescent scoliosis classification and treatment. *Neurosurg Clin N Am*. 2013;24:173-183.

18. Korenromp MJ, van Gool JD, Bruinese HW, Kriek R. Early fetal leg movements in myelomeningocele. *Lancet*. 1986;1(8486):917-918.

19. Kamm K, Thelen E, Jensen JL. A dynamical systems approach to motor development. *Phys Ther*. 1990;70(12):763-775.

20. Chapman D. Context effects on the spontaneous leg movements of infants with spina bifida. *Pediatr Phys Ther*. 2002;14(2):62-73.

21. Rademacher N, Black DP, Ulrich BD. Early spontaneous leg movements in infants born with and without myelomeningocele. *Pediatr Phys Ther*. 2008;20(2):137-145.

22. Seitzberg A, Lind M, Biering-Sorensen F. Ambulation in adults with myelomeningocele. Is it possible to predict the level of ambulation in early life? *Childs Nerv Syst*. 2008;24:231-237.

23. Bartonek A, Saraste H. Factors influencing ambulation in myelomeningocele: a cross-sectional study. *Dev Med Child Neurol*. 2001;43:253-260.

24. Findley TW, Agre JC, Habeck RV, Schmalz R, Birkebak RR, McNally MC. Ambulation in the adolescent with myelomeningocele. I: Early childhood predictors. *Arch Phys Med Rehabil*. 1987;68(8):518-522.

25. Pauly M, Cremer R. Levels of mobility in children and adolescents with spina bifida – clinical parameters predicting mobility and maintenance of these skills. *Eur J Pediatr Surg*. 2013;23:110-114.

26. Meiser MJ, McEwen IR. Lightweight and ultralight wheelchairs: propulsion and preferences of two young children with spina bifida. *Pediatr Phys Ther*. 2007;19:245-253.

Review Questions

1. The form of spina bifida in which part of the spinal cord and nerves protrude through an incompletely closed spine is:

   A. Acute spinal defect

   B. Meningocele

   C. Myelomeningocele

   D. Spina bifida occulta

2. A baby is born with a small sac at the occiput of the cranium, filled with fluid and a small amount of neural tissue; this defect would correctly be called a/an:

   A. Anencephaly

   B. Encephalocele

   C. Hydrocele

   D. Meningocele

3. **Which of the following regarding spina bifida is accurate:**
   A. Myelomeningocele is the least severe form.
   B. The bony deformity involves malformation of the transverse process of the vertebral body.
   C. The most common location is within the cervical spine.
   D. Folic acid deficiency may contribute to spina bifida

4. **The most appropriate orthosis for a child with myelomeningocele who has medial and lateral knee instability, has inadequate toe clearance during gait, has quad strength of 2, and is a household ambulator with limited community ambulation is:**
   A. HKAFO
   B. KAFO
   C. SMA
   D. TKAFO

5. **When a PT positions the infant in supine with hips flexed to 90 degrees and abducts one hip, causing the head of the femur to move posteriorly, the PT is using the**
   A. Clunk test to determine hip symmetry
   B. Ober test to determine iliotibial band tightness
   C. Galeazzi sign to determine differences in thigh length
   D. Ortolani sign to identify hip dislocation

6. **You're evaluating an infant with a myelomeningocele defect that has 4/5 ileopsoas and quad strength and 3/5 anterior tibialis strength. It is likely that this child's lesion is at level:**
   A. L3
   B. L4
   C. L5
   D. S1

7. **Children with myelomeningocele typically have**
   A. **A mixture of lower motor neuron and upper motor neuron dysfunction**
   B. A high likelihood of having mental retardation
   C. Normal bowel and bladder function
   D. A high probability of improvement in ambulation skills through the teenage years

8. **Which of the following is most commonly associated with myelomeningocele?**
   A. Intraventricular hemorrhage
   B. Congenital brain malformation involving the brainstem and foramen magnum
   C. Spasticity below the level of the spinal lesion
   D. Intact sensation below the level of the lesion

9. **The neural tube is created by what process**
   A. Diaschisis
   B. Formulation
   C. Neurolation
   D. Tubalgation

10. **Spina bifida is most commonly detected in utero by**
    A. Amniocentesis
    B. Blood tests
    C. Decreased fetal kicking movements
    D. Ultrasound

11. **Children with lesions above L1 are typically**
    A. Household and limited community ambulators
    B. Household ambulators or non-walkers
    C. Unrestricted ambulators
    D. Community ambulators with assistive devices

12. **A child presents with a 45-degree right thoracic and 25-degree left lumbar scoliosis. The best treatment for this child would be:**
    A. Abdominal and back strengthening exercises
    B. Bracing
    C. Lateral wheelchair trunk supports
    D. Spinal fusion surgery

13. **The following is a common complication of spina bifida**
    A. Brachial plexus palsy
    B. Club foot
    C. Peanut allergy
    D. Male gender

14. **When ordering a wheelchair, the seat depth should be determined as:**
    A. Greater trochanter to popliteal fossa plus 2 inches
    B. Greater trochanter to medial femoral condyle minus 2 inches
    C. Sacrum to popliteal fossa minus 2 inches
    D. Sacrum to medial femoral condyle plus 2 inches

15. **Which of the following activities, described in this chapter, can be used primarily to strengthen the arms in toddlers, preparing them to use their arms for ambulation and transfers?**
    A. Assisted sit-ups
    B. Bridging
    C. Push aways
    D. Wheelbarrow walking

Answers

1. C	2. B	3. D	4. B	5. D
6. B	7. A	8. B	9. C	10. D
11. B	12. D	13. B	14. C	15. D

Cerebral Palsy 19

Jill C. Heathcock and Deborah S. Nichols-Larsen

CASE A, PART I

Alejandro Lobo was born at 30 weeks gestation with a birth weight of 1.75kg, length of 43cm, and head circumference of 29cm. He spent 7 weeks in the Neonatal Intensive Care Unit (NICU). On day of life 25, he had an ultrasound, which revealed a grade IV periventricular hemorrhage (PVL). He was born to Carmen and Paul Lobo and has an older sister Carla (2 years old, when he was born). Carmen is a physical education teacher at a local high school and Paul is a software developer.

OBJECTIVES

1) Understand the pathophysiology of cerebral palsy

2) Identify the common risk factors for cerebral palsy

3) Identify the typical characteristics of cerebral palsy

4) Identify common classification systems of cerebral palsy

5) Identify and choose optimal treatment interventions for children with cerebral palsy post-stroke

PATHOPHYSIOLOGY

What Is Cerebral Palsy?

Cerebral palsy (CP) is a term that describes a collection of disorders of posture and movement that result from a defect or anomaly of the developing brain and is one of the top diagnoses of childhood disability, affecting 1–2.5 out of every 1000 live births. CP is nonprogressive, which means that there was an event (or discrete series of events) that caused damage to the brain by disrupting typical brain structure and function, but the brain damage does not worsen over time. Similar to brain injury in adults, CP presents with a disturbance of motor function but also may be accompanied by sensory dysfunction, cognitive impairments, language delay/dysfunction as well as medical disorders such as epilepsy and malnutrition. Although the lesion is nonprogressive, the presentation of CP may change as the child goes through developmental stages, and secondary musculoskeletal conditions are common as the child grows. An estimated 800,000 people in the United States have CP, and more than 450,000 are children less than 18 years of age.[1]

ETIOLOGY

CP may occur when there is an interruption of blood flow or damage to the brain during the fetal, perinatal, or neonatal periods, resulting in a permanent lesion with diverse consequences, depending on the location, severity, and time of insult. It should be noted that brain injury, during fetal development and early infancy, may not be immediately obvious, and therefore, the exact cause or timing of the insult may not be known. These events are typically single or a discrete series and not active at the time of diagnosis. Risk factors and the incidence of certain types of brain lesions are known, but the cause is often unknown. Injury to the developing brain results in changes to otherwise predictable brain formation, growth, and maturation, as described in Chapters 8 and 18. However, it should be noted that CP can occur in those without known risk factors or obvious causes and is, then, referred to as idiopathic (without known cause). Notably, the causative brain injury for CP can occur during gestation, in the perinatal period (during labor, delivery, or shortly after delivery) or in the early developmental period. The etiology of these injuries is heterogeneous, but the most common known causes will be discussed here. Notably, prematurity is one of the most common risk factors for CP; Box 19-1 describes the impact of prematurity on brain development and its association with CP.

CASE A, PART II

Alejandro was born at 33 weeks gestation and weighed 1.75kg or 1750g. Thus, he would be categorized as preterm with low birth weight. His IVH was a grade IV, indicating that there was blood in the ventricle and the adjacent tissue. Physical therapy for Alejandro began in the NICU, which is common practice for preterm infants. Within the NICU, physical therapy treatment focused on positioning to promote physiological flexion; facilitating auto-regulation of autonomic functions, behavioral state, and sensorimotor responses; and assisting parents in the handling of their tiny son. Preterm infants do not experience the close confines of the latter part of gestation, so they present without the physiological flexion induced by that confinement; in fact, they may seem hypotonic at birth with limited antigravity movement. Thus, positioning of Alejandro focused on flexed postures to encourage increased flexor tone, especially sidelying, where he was able to begin bringing his hands together and toward his mouth to self-comfort. To facilitate autonomic autoregulation, he was swaddled after any medical procedure and when resting/sleeping, and his parents were encouraged to provide slow, gentle, calming massage or containment, when he was in his isolette, and to hold him against their skin (kangaroo care). These techniques lowered his respiration rate, heart rate, and blood pressure. As is true for many preterm infants, Alejandro demonstrated a stressful reaction to the many noises in the NICU and to all medical care (increased blood pressure, heart rate, and muted crying); therefore, he was protected from the environmental noise in a quieter area of the NICU, handling was provided in concentration to allow longer periods between episodes, and then, gradually he was reintroduced to sounds and light, as his responses normalized, to prepare him to go home. Notably, changes in heart rate or respiration rate are often the primary signs of distress rather than crying in preterm infants, so these need to be carefully monitored by the physical therapist, while working in the NICU.[3]

BOX 19-1   Encephalopathy of Prematurity

Babies born prior to the 37th week of gestation are considered premature, or preterm, but are further differentiated into **preterm** (32–37 weeks), **very preterm** (28–32 weeks), and **extremely preterm** (<28 weeks). They can be further differentiated into **low birth weight** (<2500 g), **very low birth weight** (<1500 g), and **extremely low birth weight** (<1000 g). *It should be noted that babies with intrauterine growth restriction (see congenital anomalies in the next section) are also classified via these categories.* With improvements in the care for preterm infants, most are surviving; however, the incidence of neurologic impairment (CP, intellectual disability, learning disability) continues to be relatively high with up to 50% displaying some level of neurologic deficit. Not surprisingly, the incidence and severity of neurologic insult increases as the degree of prematurity increases (lower gestational age). The term used for neurologic injury secondary to prematurity is **encephalopathy of prematurity (EoP)**. However, there is not a singular cause of EoP.

A primary cause of EoP is **periventricular leukomalacia** (PVL), which is linked to hypoxia/ischemia and inflammation. Inflammation is a secondary consequence of a hypoxic/ischemic incident but can also occur in association with a systemic infection. Preterm infants, especially extremely preterm babies, are at significant risk of bacterial infection (bacteremia) that can result in sepsis, meningitis, and/or necrotizing enterocolitis (see section at the end of this box). As described in Chapter 8, neurons are produced in the area surrounding the ventricles (subventricular zone – SVZ) and then migrate to their final destination within the brain; similarly the oligodendrocytes that produce central myelin begin as stem cells within the SVZ, yet myelination occurs much later in gestational development than neuronal migration. In fact, myelination is initiated in the last trimester of pregnancy and continues through the second year of life. Thus, myelination is just beginning in babies born very preterm or extremely preterm. Inflammation secondary to hypoxia/ischemia or systemic infection brings microglia to the SVZ that apparently attack the pre-oligodendrocyte cells, creating a lesion in the SVZ with subsequent loss of neuronal myelination and thereby neurologic deficits.

Why is the premature brain at risk for hypoxia/ischemia? First, the blood vessels within the brain are still developing in the preterm infant, and thus, are at risk for hemorrhage or an ischemic incident. Second, the preterm infant lacks the capability to **autoregulate blood flow**, which is a necessary function to assure blood flow to the brain. For example, if the infant experiences an infection in another body system, blood may be diverted from the brain to meet the needs of the other system, resulting in brain hypoxia/ischemia, or if the infant is highly stressed, the blood pressure in these immature vessels may exceed the vessel capacity, resulting in hemorrhage. At particular risk for hemorrhage are the vessels in the endothelial lining of the ventricles; a hemorrhage in this area is referred to as an **intraventricular hemorrhage – IVH** and is graded from level I (most mild) to IV (most severe); the most common place for IVH is in the frontal and parietal regions, making damage to the sensorimotor regions likely. Similar to PVL, hemorrhages in this area disrupt the development of oligodendrocytes and subsequent myelination of neurons, leading to neuronal death. However, the effect of IVH is typically more focal than that of PVL.[2]

IVH grades:

I: bleeding is confined to the germinal layer of the endothelium

II: bleeding into the ventricle(s) without enlargement of the ventricle

III: bleeding into the ventricle(s) with enlargement of the ventricle

IV: bleeding into the ventricle and adjacent brain tissue

Notably, both PVL and IVH can be detected by ultrasound.

Necrotizing enterocolitis (NEC) is a condition of the bowel, characterized by death of the mucosal lining of the intestines and disruption of bowel function. While this can occur in full-term infants, it is much more common in preterm babies. When present, the intestine is susceptible to intestinal perforation, which can quickly generate into peritonitis and sepsis. It is a common cause of death in preterm infants and is linked to neurologic insults, secondary to inflammation.

Congenital Abnormalities

CP can originate from a disruption of development, during embryogenesis, resulting in brain malformation. Potential causative factors can be maternal medical conditions (e.g., seizure disorder, heart disease, thyroid disorder) or substance use (drugs, alcohol, or smoking), infections (see section below), placental insufficiency or thrombosis (clotting) of the placenta or umbilical cord. Placental insufficiency can generate ongoing hypoxia in early gestation and also impede umbilical glucose passage, resulting in impaired nutrition of the developing fetus; these two things can result in a condition known as intrauterine growth retardation (IUGR) that impedes overall growth of the fetus, including brain development.[4] Notably, multiple births are at greater risk for IUGR, and therefore, CP. There are also other reasons for the increased incidence of CP in pregnancies with multiple babies, including the likelihood of premature birth (Box 19-1). Maternal metabolic disorders (e.g., diabetes), ingestion of toxins, and rare genetic syndromes are also known contributors to neurological disorders in childhood, including CP.[4]

Perinatal asphyxia refers to a disruption of oxygen, resulting in a period of anoxia to the developing brain, that takes place during later fetal development (2nd and 3rd trimesters), labor, delivery, or the neonatal period. An estimated 75% of CP cases result from an anoxic event. Notably, the vasculature of the fetal brain is very fragile, putting it at risk for an infarction or hemorrhage. The most common area of injury is the middle cerebral artery (MCA), which supplies blood to portions of the frontal, parietal, and temporal lobes. This means that a large proportion of brain tissue is at risk, if there is an infarction of the MCA (see Chapter 10 for information on the MCA). Asphyxia can result from abnormalities of the placenta or thrombosis of the placenta or umbilical cord; however, there are many other causative events. During labor and delivery there is a possibility of the umbilical cord wrapping around the infant's neck and impeding respiration, during the initial moments of extrauterine life. Also, neonates may excrete their first bowel movement (**meconium** – a dark pasty stool) during labor, allowing aspiration of the substance by the baby that impedes breathing upon delivery. **Placental previa** refers to an abnormal attachment of the placenta to the uterine wall such that it partially or completely covers the cervix; it may be associated with abnormal bleeding, during the pregnancy, especially in the last trimester, and thus, diminishes oxygenation for the baby in the latter stages of gestation. Also, **placental abruption**, which refers to premature detachment of the placenta from the uterine wall, can also be a source of fetal hypoxia in utero and prematurity. Since partial abruption can occur fairly early (2nd to 3rd trimester), it can result in a period of prolonged hypoxia prior to delivery and, thereby, significant brain damage in the developing baby. Notably, abruption is also a cause for premature delivery. Occasionally, the umbilical cord comes out of the vaginal canal before the head of the baby, referred to as **umbilical cord prolapse**; this is a medical emergency because of the immediate threat of cutting off the oxygen and blood supply to the fetus as well as the likelihood of abruption and subsequent maternal hemorrhage. **Pre-eclampsia**, which is also a maternal condition of pregnancy, is characterized by hypertension and proteinuria (protein in the urine) secondary to kidney dysfunction and can result in fetal growth restriction, premature birth, and placental abruption. The progression of pre-eclampsia to **eclampsia** is a life-threatening situation for both mother and baby; in eclampsia, the mother can experience convulsions, coma, and potentially death. The baby's life is also in jeopardy, since oxygenation

can be disrupted, with the risk of CP or other developmental disorder likely, if the baby survives.[5]

Infection is a common cause of CP in both the natal and postnatal time frames. For the fetus, immune function is dependent on the maternal immune system. Some pathogens can cross the placenta and cause infection. Maternal illnesses can be unsafe for a fetus, causing spontaneous abortion or major developmental disorders (including CP), while others have no effect. Maternal infections that have known neurological consequences to the fetus include (1) **rubella** (measles), which is linked to deafness, eye abnormalities, congenital heart defects, developmental delay, learning disabilities, and CP; (2) **cytomegalovirus (CMV)**, which causes intrauterine growth restriction and enlarged brain tissue with subsequent CP and/or other developmental problems; and (3) **toxoplasmosis**, which is transmitted by exposure to infected cat feces and causes hydrocephalus and encephalitis that can lead to CP.[5]

Perinatal Birth Trauma can cause a lack of oxygen to the brain that can result in a brain injury and subsequent CP. **Obstructed labor** is when the fetus cannot fit out of the vaginal canal, typically from **cephalo-pelvic incompatibility** (the baby's head is too big for the mother's pelvis), resulting in too much and repeated force on the skull of the fetus as the mother attempts to push the baby out. The use of forceps to assist the baby's passage through the birth canal can, in rare instances, result in cranial trauma, leading to CP; thus, they are used only when the mother is exhausted or the baby is in distress to assist in delivery.

Postnatal Causes of CP

A CP diagnosis is typically given to children that acquire brain injury in the first 3 years of life. Causes of such brain damage include (1) metabolic encephalopathy, (2) primary infections such as meningitis or malaria, or (3) trauma such as shaken baby syndrome or infantile stroke. Metabolic encephalopathy can result from disrupted kidney or liver function, toxicity from an ingested or inhaled toxin (including alcohol or drug toxicity, which can be transmitted through breast milk), or subsequent to electrolyte disturbance, associated with an acute illness (e.g., diarrhea with a high fever).

● RISK FACTORS

Although CP is not apparent at birth, there are many factors associated with an increased risk of CP. These factors are correlational, meaning there is an association, but they are not causal. Maternal risk factors have been extensively studied; paternal risk factors have been relatively ignored. In earlier sections, we have described maternal conditions that place one at risk for having a child with CP; these include substance abuse and medical conditions (seizure disorder, diabetes, thyroid disorders, cardiopulmonary disorders, including hypertension); in addition, women who have a history of delayed menstruation; prior miscarriage, preterm birth, or an existing child with a motor deficit; or are of advanced age are at greater risk for having a baby with CP and other developmental disorders (e.g., Down syndrome). Similarly, there is some suggestion that advanced paternal age can be a contributing factor. Preterm birth is also associated with an increased risk of CP (see Box 19-1) as is low birth weight, which can be an indication of IUGR, as discussed previously, low placental weight, which is a sign of placental insufficiency with secondary IUGR, and low APGAR scores, which are an indication of fetal distress at birth (see Box 19-2). During the newborn period, the occurrence of seizures, sepsis, or respiratory distress can disrupt oxygenation and/or brain development, resulting in brain damage and, ultimately, CP.[4]

DIAGNOSIS

Despite the precipitating injury typically occurring in the perinatal period, CP is commonly not diagnosed until 18 months–2 years of age, when there is an obvious absence of major motor milestones (e.g., creeping and walking) and the presence of abnormal muscle tone. Children with greater severity or often those with hemiplegia may be diagnosed earlier. Those with greater severity often have associated eating problems, limited head control, and more severe muscle tone abnormalities such as hypotonia or spasticity that make diagnosis at an earlier age easier. Those with hemiplegia have an obvious disparity in limb movement, alerting observant parents and pediatricians to the limited use of one arm and leg. However, many physicians take a "wait and see" approach to the diagnosis in an attempt to avoid

inappropriate labeling of the child, providing a "developmental delay" label initially and waiting to see if early intervention will resolve the delay. Over the first 2 years of life, abnormalities of tone and delayed motor skill acquisition become more apparent, making the diagnosis clear. From a medical perspective the diagnosis is based on the clinical presentation, requiring a combination of abnormal tone, altered deep tendon reflexes (e.g., Achilles tendon reflex), delayed motor development, and postural instability.[7,8] Neuroimaging is rarely ordered or required for the diagnosis; however, when imaging is conducted, often a localized lesion, apparent brain malformation, or periventricular leukomalacia (see Box 19-2) can be visualized. There have been some advances in early prediction of CP in at-risk populations, especially preterm birth, with general movement analysis. In brief, full term infants demonstrate what are called writhing movements from birth to 9 weeks but begin to transition to fidgety movements at about 7 weeks, continuing these until up to 20 weeks, when purposeful movements are initiated. Altered writhing movements, called cramped synchronized, at one month and abnormal general movements in the fidgety period are predictive of CP.[9]

BOX 19-2 Neonatal Assessment – APGAR

At delivery all newborns undergo a quick assessment, known as the APGAR to determine their overall well-being upon delivery; each is assessed at 1 and 5 minutes on each of the following:

A – appearance (skin color): pink all over = 2, pink body with blue extremities = 1, blue = 0;

P – pulse: normal rate (>100 beats/min) = 2, slow (<100 beats/min) = 1, no pulse = 0

G – grimace (response to mild pinch): strong cry, extremity withdrawal or facial grimace = 2, milder response (weak cry, little movement) = 1, no response = 0

A – activity (muscle tone): actively moving = 2, some flexion of limbs = 1, no movement = 0

R – respiration (airway): strong cry = 2, weak cry or respiratory effort = 1, no breathing = 0

Obviously, a perfect score is 10, but since the birth process is fairly traumatic to a baby, many will score below that level, especially in terms of color as many babies have a blue hue in the first minutes after birth, but will be fine. In fact, APGAR scores of 7–10 are considered normal; scores of 4–6 are of some concern, especially if they don't improve at the 5-minute assessment; scores of 0–3 indicate a need for immediate resuscitation and place the baby at risk for subsequent developmental problems. Infants with low APGAR scores are much more likely to have CP than those that score in the normal range.[6]

CASE A, PART III

Alejandro was followed in a high-risk clinic for the first year of his life. One month after discharge from the NICU, he was diagnosed with myoclonic seizures that appeared like startle reactions without a precipitating stimulus and was given sodium valproate (see Table 19-4). At his 5-month visit, the physical therapist noted that he had increased tone in his legs and always kicked with both legs simultaneously (no alternating kicks) with associated movements in the trunk and arms. The physician and the therapist diagnosed "possible CP" and referred him to an early intervention program. In the EI program, he received PT 2–3 times per week within the class environment to facilitate the development of motor milestones. He rolled in both directions by 8 months, pushed into quadruped by 11, and back into w-sitting by his first birthday. Therapy, at this time, was directed at increasing his ability to sit in different positions (ring, tailor), reaching and weight-shift in quadruped to stimulate creeping, and standing activities (see later section on treatment).

Classification

Functional classification is descriptive of the way the child performs common functional motor activities. The most common, evidence-based, and helpful way to classify and predict future motor function of children with CP is the Gross Motor Function Classification System (GMFCS), which is a five-level system that categorizes children with CP, based on the motor function and limitation in daily motor abilities, based on the Gross Motor Function Measure (see Box 19-3). Classification levels are based on independent motor function and the use of

---

BOX 19-3 | **Gross Motor Function Measure**

The Gross Motor Function Measure (GMFM) is an assessment tool for children ages 5 months–16 years with CP that was used to develop the GMFCS levels. There are two versions of the GMFM, the GMFM-88 and GMFM-66, with the number corresponding to the number of items on the tool. All 66 items on the GMFM-66 are on the GMFM-88, so if the -88 is tested in the clinic, both -88 and -66 scores can be easily calculated. The GMFM is standardized and has five dimensions of gross motor function: (1) lying and rolling; (2) crawling and kneeling; (3) sitting; (4) standing; and (5) walking, running, and jumping. GMFCS levels have been plotted from GMFM-66 scores over time (age) to demonstrate when children show 90% of their maximal expected motor function. It is important to note that there is a plateau and/or decline in motor function for all levels after age 8, indicating the likelihood that children will not acquire new skills after this age and may lose skills, often secondary to increasing body size, greater influence of tone, and acquired orthopedic conditions that in insolation or combination make moving more difficult.[10]

---

assistive technology for mobility. They create meaningful comparisons for research studies, can guide treatment goal setting, and allow for accurate counseling, planning, and education for families and children with CP. Lower levels, starting with level I, indicate better motor function and fewer functional limitations. Broadly, children classified as GMFCS level I walk independently and have few motor impairments or limitations in daily life. Their impairments may not be noticeable until they perform high-level motor skills like advanced sports or skills that require precise coordination and timing (e.g., kicking a ball, climbing, riding a bike). Higher levels, ending with level V, indicate more severe limitations in motor function, limited independence, and use of assistive devices or powered mobility. Children with GMFCS level V have little to no antigravity movements or voluntary motor control and are dependent on a caregiver for all aspects of care. They are transported by a caregiver or use a power chair with lots of postural support (see Box 19-4 for additional details).[8]

BOX 19-4 | **GMFCS Levels**[8]

- Level I – Walks and runs independently in all settings but may be slower or less coordinated than peers
- Level II – Walks independently but has limitations in running, with uneven surfaces and stairs (may require hand rail or 2 step/tread pattern)
- Level III – Walks with an assistive device in most settings and/or uses a manual wheelchair
- Level IV – Limited standing and walking ability, often with assistance; primarily uses power wheelchair
- Level V – Very limited mobility; reliant on caregiver support for movement and wheelchair propulsion; may use powered mobility

---

GMFCS levels are further clarified by age with separate descriptions for levels I–V in the following age ranges: less than 2, between 2 and 4, 4–6, 6–12, and 12–18. GMFSC levels are quite stable overtime, meaning that once classified, 73% of children remain in the same GMFCS level over time. Children in levels I and V are most likely to be reclassified, and children under 6 are most likely to be reclassified in a lower (higher functioning) level. All information on the GMFCS levels and descriptions of each level can be found on the CanChild web page,[11] with free and meaningful assessment tools and descriptions of motor function for children with CP at different ages.

Severity of Functional Impairment

The categories of mild, moderate, and severe are used to quickly and easily communicate general levels of impairment when specific details are not needed. In general, **Mild** means that the child can move and complete daily activities without assistance and may have limitations with higher-level motor skills such as sports or activities that require more advanced coordination. **Moderate** means that the child will need some assistance from a caregiver and/or adaptive equipment including braces, mobility aids, or technology in order to participate in daily activities. **Severe** means that the child cannot move very well independently, will need a wheelchair to move or be transported, and will need assistance from a caregiver for most or all daily activities. GMFCS levels are used when detail about functional status and prediction are necessary.

Typography (Body Area(s) Affected)

The categories of quadriplegia, diplegia, hemiplegia, and triplegia are used to describe the extremities affected by abnormal tone and movement impairment. **Quadriplegia** means all four limbs and the trunk/head are affected, often the arms more than the legs. Typically, those with quadriplegia are more disabled than those in the other typography groups and are more likely to have associated conditions. **Diplegia** means both lower extremities are affected and the upper extremities are not affected or affected to a lesser degree than the lower extremities; the trunk and neck muscles are typically not impaired or only mildly impaired. **Hemiplegia** means that one side of the body, an ipsilateral upper and lower extremity are affected; in some, there is also an asymmetry of trunk involvement on the same side as the extremities. (*Much recent research suggests that the "non-affected" side in hemiplegia also has some changes in function though much more mild than the "affected" side, so terms like paretic and nonparetic are often used to distinguish the more involved side from the lesser involved side*). These typography categories are illustrated in Figure 19-1. **Triplegia** is a term that is occasionally used when all four extremities are affected, but one extremity has much more function in comparison to the other three; the head and trunk are also affected. Movements of children with triplegia are initiated with the highest functioning extremity.

Type (Predominate Motor/Muscle Tone Characteristic)

The categories of spastic, dyskinetic, ataxic, and hypotonic are used to describe the primary motor characteristics of CP, including tone and accessory or involuntary movements. It should be noted that, since CP occurs in the developing brain, widespread

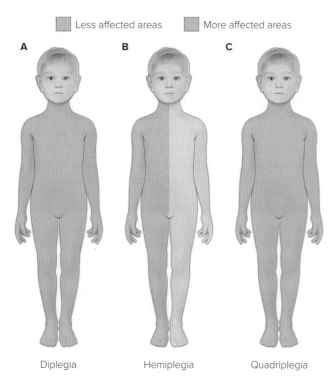

Less affected areas   More affected areas

A   B   C

Diplegia   Hemiplegia   Quadriplegia

FIGURE 19-1 Representation of typography. A. Diplegia – greater involvement of the legs than arms and trunk.
B. Hemiplegia – greater involvement of the contralateral arm and leg with little trunk involvement and very mild ipsilateral involvement from the side of the lesion. **C.** Quadriplegia – all four extremities are involved (arms often more than legs and trunk).

brain damage may result rather than the focal damage discussed with stroke; thus, it is possible for CP to present with "mixed" types of muscle tone variations that may impact different body parts, be influenced by body position, or may present differently in infancy than at older ages. Up to 10% of children with CP will present with mixed muscle tone. Some information on prevalence of motor characteristic and area of the brain implicated for the types of CP are discussed in Box 19-5.

Integration of topography, type, and severity classifications provides a comprehensive description of a child's presentation. However, the characteristics may change over time or children may present with mixed types, so this language can lead to confusion for families and medical professionals. GMFCS levels are the most widely used and reliable way to classify individual children with CP and group children with CP in research studies.

BOX 19-5   Motor Characteristics in Cerebral Palsy[12,13]

Spastic – Spastic CP is characterized by hypertonia (spasticity) and hyperreflexia of deep tendon reflexes (DTRs). *Remember, spasticity is a velocity-dependent resistance to passive stretch that can be measured with the modified Ashworth Scale (see Chapter 9 for details).* Spastic CP is associated with damage to the cerebral cortex and pyramidal

tracts. Damage to these areas also results in poor force generation in muscles and often an imbalance of muscle activity at joints. As is found with spasticity in adult conditions, the muscles typically affected in children are the UE flexors at all joints with the shoulder internal rotators and the hip flexors and adductors, the hamstrings at the knee, and the plantarflexors at the ankle. Children with spastic diplegia will have much less spasticity in their UE than LE but in these same muscle groups where present (some or all UE muscles may have normal tone). Children with spastic CP account for 80–90% of children with CP with quadriplegia most common (35%) then hemiplegia (31%), diplegia (21%), and triplegia (2%); therefore, the remaining types are sometimes grouped together as non-spastic CP.

Dyskinetic – Disruption of the basal ganglia and its connections to the motor cortex produces abnormal involuntary movements, associated with difficulty in movement coordination, and accounts for 7–15% of children with CP. This can present in multiple variations of movement that are distinguished by the speed and appearance of the involuntary movements. **Athetosis** is characterized by slow writhing (worm-like) movements that typically impact the distil portion of the limbs more than the proximal joints. **Chorea** is characterized by more rapid involuntary movements that can involve any part of the body (face, limbs, trunk). **Choreoathetosis** represents a combination of athetosis and chorea, in which both distil athetoid movements and proximal chorea movements occur. **Ballismus**, as the name suggests, involves quick jerky movements of the entire extremity as though the limb is "blasting" through the air, involving the proximal joints primarily. **Dystonia** is characterized by sustained co-contractions of muscles, leading to maintained postures often with twisting of the trunk or limbs and resulting from disrupted inhibition as a motion is initiated; these postures may be quite uncomfortable to the child, yet they will have difficulty moving out of the posture.

Ataxic* – Ataxic CP is characterized by difficulty with coordination, balance, and initiating movement, resulting from damage of the cerebellum; like adults with cerebellar dysfunction, children with ataxic CP have trouble with co-contraction of muscles, so their movements are characterized by over- and under-shooting of targets, swaying in a maintained posture, and a wide-based stance in weight-bearing postures and when walking to provide stability. Notably, children with ataxic CP also display mild to moderate hypotonia as the cerebellum contributes to the generation of resting muscle tone. In children with ataxic CP, DTRs are normal. Also, an **intention tremor** is common; with this type of tremor, the oscillation of the extremity increases during a directed movement (e.g., reaching).

Hypotonic/Atonic* – Hypotonic CP is characterized by low muscle tone and decreased deep tendon reflexes and is thought to result from widespread brain damage most commonly in early fetal development. However, it should be noted that some children will present as hypotonic early in infancy but at later ages will present with dyskinetic, ataxic, or mixed CP.

Mixed – Refers to a combination of the motor presentations of more than one of the above groups, often dyskinesia with spasticity.

*Children with ataxic or hypotonic CP account for <5% of children with CP.

At age 3, Alejandro presents with hypertonia and hyperreflexia in all four extremities (legs much greater than arms) and 5 degrees of hip and knee flexion contracture of both legs. He sits on the floor by "w-sitting," can creep on hands and knees without reciprocal leg movements, moving first both arms and then both legs, and takes steps in his preschool class room using a reverse walker. No cognitive, learning, or language delays have been noted. He lives in a two-story house with one bathroom on the second floor; he is still carried up and down the stairs.

Alejandro is presenting with moderate spastic diplegia with a GMFCS of III. Since he is 3, with spasticity and hyperreflexia of both arms and legs (mild in the arms and moderate in the legs), and limited walking at age 3, he has a moderate level of involvement. The combination of hypertonia and hyperreflexia is consistent with spasticity, and the presentation of greater involvement of the legs versus the arms meets the distribution (topography) of diplegia. He is beginning to ambulate with a reverse walker, so is not independent in his ambulation (GMFCS levels I and II), thus, placing him in GMFCS III. He is using a stroller still for community ambulation but may be a candidate for a manual wheelchair soon.

MOTOR PATTERNS OF CHILDREN WITH CEREBRAL PALSY

As should be evident from the preceding discussion, CP is a highly heterogeneous disorder, yet pediatric physical therapists can expect some common movement patterns in children with this disorder, depending on type of tone and its distribution and severity. General findings are that motor development will be delayed due to nervous system damage, abnormal tone and strength in major muscle groups, and potentially, the presence of other conditions such as orthopedic deformities and cognitive impairment (discussed later in this chapter). In addition, the disruption in neural maturation that results from early brain damage can also disrupt the integration of primitive reflexes and delayed development of mature protective, postural, and equilibrium reactions (see Chapter 9 for description of each of these).

Head Control

Many children with CP will present with delayed development of head control. Surprisingly, both children with hypertonia and hypotonia, including those that will develop ataxia, have poor antigravity neck strength and poor co-contraction of the neck muscles necessary for upright head control, yet they often can momentarily lift their heads in prone, using their neck extensors but can't maintain it upright, since they lack co-contraction. When pulled to sit, they will demonstrate poor neck flexion (Figure 19-2), but those with spasticity will appear to have a strong arm pull that is not truly "strong," since it is generated by spasticity. Not surprisingly, children with hemiplegia tend to develop

FIGURE 19-2 Head lag in cerebral palsy. Many children with cerebral palsy of all types will show early head lag when pulled to sit; as they age the LE and UE may show increased tone (spasticity) pulling the arms and legs into flexion but the head may still lag behind the shoulders. (Reproduced with permission from Carney PR, & Geyer JD (Eds). *Pediatric Practice: Neurology.* New York, NY: McGraw-Hill; 2010. Figure 11-1, Part A Only.)

head control much like their typical peers; those with diplegia may have a delay but will usually attain good head control.

Rolling

Quadriplegia: Children with spastic or dystonic quadriplegia are not only delayed in their rolling, but if they are able to roll, will typically use a log roll, since they have difficulty dissociating the upper trunk from the lower trunk and the arms from the legs. In other words, they tend to move in patterns of total flexion or total extension. Also, they are often influenced by a persisting ATNR, which pulls their skull side extremities into flexion, making it difficult for them to incorporate these limbs into the roll. So, when rolling prone to supine, they will extend their head and trunk, turn their head, and appear to "fall" into supine with little involvement of the extremities (they may push up with hands if able); this may be facilitated by the presence of the STNR, which triggers UE extension when the head is lifted and the ATNR, which will trigger some skull-side UE flexion as the head is turned. When rolling supine to prone, which is often quite delayed, if achieved at all, children with spastic quadriplegia or dystonia tend to assume a complete flexion pattern (head, trunk, legs), often leading with the legs, which may be less involved, and using the body on body reaction and much effort to move to prone. In those with limited neck flexor strength, the head doesn't contribute much to the roll. In addition, it is common for the arm, over which they are rolling, to be "caught" underneath them, and they may not have the ability to shift their weight to free it. For children with ataxia or hypotonia, rolling requires achieving sufficient antigravity strength to move out of supine or prone, and many will not be able to do so. However, those that do, lead with their strongest body part – head, arm, or leg, facilitated by the body on body reaction. Those at GMFCS level V often do not roll without assistance but those at level IV and above commonly achieve rolling.

Diplegia: Since head control is typically good to normal in those with diplegia, children with this type of CP tend to roll close to the 6–8 month mark but may exhibit some of the total flexion/extension of their peers with quadriplegia, depending on the degree of tone expressed. Most will lead with their head and arms with little leg contribution; for many, the legs will be strongly extended, when rolling. They may also log roll longer than their typical peers but often will acquire a segmental roll, at least of the head and upper trunk, if not the legs. *Hemiplegia*: For children with hemiplegia, they may initially only roll in one direction toward or over their paretic side (supine to prone – will reach across their trunk with their non-paretic arm and leg and roll over their paretic side; prone to supine – will reach back with their non-paretic arm and leg and roll over their paretic side). Eventually, they will be able to roll in both directions, using a segmental roll.

Sitting

For children at GMFCS levels V, sitting is not achieved without external support or assistance. For those at GMFCS level IV, sitting will be delayed, but most will be able to sit, when placed into the position, but may not be able to assume the position; most will also require upper extremity support, of at least one arm, to maintain upright and will be delayed in developing protective or equilibrium reactions or may not develop them. Spasticity in their hamstrings may result in a posterior pelvic tilt that pulls them backward and makes sitting difficult; positions that diminish the effect of this spasticity (e.g., ring or tailor sitting) will be easier for them to maintain but harder to assume. Children that can achieve sitting independently, especially those at GMFCS level III, often push back from prone or quadruped and assume a w-sitting position (bottom between heels) with an anterior pelvic tilt. Although this position strains the hips, which may already be at risk for hip dysplasia (see Table 19-1), it is easier to access than any other sitting posture and provides a wide base of support for those with poorer trunk control, so it is common for children with all types of CP except hemiplegia to prefer w-sitting, even those with dyskinetic or ataxic presentations. Overtime, many develop more flexibility in sitting with the ability to assume other sitting positions and acquire protective and equilibrium reactions to free their arms for play. Children at GMFCS I and II will easily assume sitting, many initially in a "w" position, but will be able to move into and out of sitting easily, developing appropriate protective and equilibrium reactions. Those with hemiplegia tend to ring or side-sit initially with weight on the non-paretic arm; however, they typically are independent sitters with more flexibility than their peers with quadriplegic or diplegic presentations.

Crawling/Creeping

For clarification, crawling is used to describe movement on the belly that involves reciprocal and alternating movement of the arms and legs; in contrast, creeping is that same movement pattern in quadruped (all fours). Laymen usually call the latter crawling, so it may help the novice to think of this as belly crawling and quadruped creeping. Children at GMFCS levels V do not achieve either of these movement patterns. Those at level IV may achieve crawling but rarely creeping, and they tend to move with limited dissociation of limbs (total flexion, followed by total extension) Those at level III, especially those with spasticity, will also use a bilateral symmetrical UE/LE pattern and achieve both crawling and creeping (often called bunny hopping); the STNR may facilitate this pattern (*head extension leading to UE extension and LE flexion forward; head flexion with UE flexion and LE extension to propel them forward*). Some children mature into an alternating pattern; children with diplegia may alternate with their arms but not their legs, depending on severity. Children at levels I and II will achieve mature crawling and creeping, sometimes with mild asymmetry of movement. *Note: children with hemiplegia may not crawl or creep due to their asymmetric presentation; it is not uncommon for these children to scoot in sitting, pulling and pushing with their non-paretic arm and leg, respectively.*

Standing and Walking

Children at GMFCS level V do not stand or walk but may benefit from supported standing activities. Those at level IV will usually be able to achieve standing with assistance and may walk in a limited fashion with assistive devices and caregiver assistance, especially when turning; in contrast, those at level III can typically walk around their house or classroom with assistive devices but will use a wheelchair for community mobility, the playground, or longer distances within their school. By definition, those at levels I and II are independent community ambulators, differing most in the higher level skills that they acquire (e.g., running, skipping, ball manipulation) with those in level I performing more activities with mild incoordination and those at level II typically not achieving jumping and running. Children with spasticity, whether diplegic or quadriplegic, tend to have similar LE presentation of their spastic limbs when standing and walking, if these are achieved (see Figure 19-3): (1) **crouched gait** includes hip and knee flexion (crouching), internal rotation with adduction of the hip (genu valgum), and excessive dorsiflexion, usually with pes planus, during stance; (2) a **stiff knee gait** is also common with LE spasticity; in this variation, there is less knee and hip flexion, than in crouched gait, with equinus at the ankle and either valgus (pronation) or varus (supination) of the forefoot. During swing, children with a stiff knee gait will have difficulty clearing their toes, due to limited limb flexion at all joints and may exhibit scissoring of the legs due to excessive adductor tone. This stiff knee pattern is also common in hemiplegia but manifests in one leg only. In some children with spasticity, the presenting gait pattern occurs with an equinus deformity at the ankle and compensatory recurvatum at the knee (see Table 19-1). All of these spastic gait patterns are characterized by a shortened stride length, shortened single limb stance phase, and increased energy expenditure during gait. Children with ataxia will walk with a wide-base and often stiff LE (limited flexion) to maximize stability, if they achieve walking. For many children with all types of CP, the UE are commonly held in a high guard position for much longer than is typical in development, unless used for managing an assistive device, and may demonstrate increased tone, even in the level I or II child with spasticity, when speed or difficulty is increased (e.g., running, kicking).

Many children with spasticity will initially pull to stand without assuming a half-kneeling posture, as a typical child would, relying on the arms to do much of the work with little LE contribution until almost upright; this is especially true of the child with diplegia. Children at level III usually continue to require the UE to pull to stand and are unstable in attempts to squat to the floor or retrieve an object and return to stand without holding on to a support.

TABLE 19-1	Orthopedic Conditions Associated with Cerebral Palsy	
JOINT	**CONDITION**	**DESCRIPTION**
Trunk	Scoliosis	Asymmetry of muscle tone and strength in the trunk muscles can result in abnormal rotation and scoliosis of the trunk. Scoliosis is most common in those with spastic quadriplegia or dystonia.
	Kyphosis	Asymmetry between trunk flexors and extensors as well as posturing can result in a kyphotic deformity; this may also occur in combination with scoliosis.
Hip/thigh[14]	Hip dysplasia	Spasticity of the hip flexors, adductors, and internal rotators in association with elongated and weak hip extensors can allow the femoral head to be pulled in the direction of the spastic muscles. In addition, delayed standing can limit the deepening of the acetabulum that should occur. Together, these factors place the hip at risk for subluxation or dislocation. Sitting postures, especially w-sitting with the buttocks between the heels, further place the hip at risk. HD occurs in up to 30% of children with spasticity and 50% of those with quadriplegic spasticity. HD can also occur in the non-spastic forms of CP due to poor or asymmetrical muscle control at the hip, delayed or absent standing, and a reliance on abnormal postures (e.g., w-sitting).
	Femoral anteversion	Tight adductors and internal rotators can place an abnormal pull on the distil femur that over time increases the natural amount of femoral anteversion; this may contribute to other LE abnormalities.
Knee[15]	Flexion contracture	Spasticity of the hamstrings occurs in all forms of spastic CP; for those that spend most of their time in a wheelchair or seated position, significant shortening of the hamstrings with decreasing extensor strength at the knee can occur.
	Genu varum	With femoral anteversion, secondary to adductor and internal rotation spasticity/shortening, the knee is pulled medially and there is a lateral compensation of the lower leg. This contributes to a crouched gait along with hamstring spasticity/shortening, weak quadriceps and hip extensors, and equinovarus in the foot.
	Genu recurvatum	Knee recurvatum is most common in children with an equinus deformity at the ankle due to gastrocnemius spasticity or hamstrings that are too long (often after lengthening or dorsal rhizotomy) or too weak to oppose the gastroc spasticity; the pull of the gastrocnemius on the distil femur draws it posterior during stance as the proximal femur advances forward, resulting in hyperextension at the knee (recurvatum).
Ankle/ foot[16]	Equinus	Spasticity of the gastrocnemius plus weak dorsiflexors can result in a plantar flexion deformity with secondary decrease in dorsiflexion and resultant gait abnormalities.
	Equinovalgus	Equinus of the ankle in association with eversion and pronation of the foot results from shortening of the gastroc and peroneal muscles; weight is born on the medial aspect of the foot.
	Equinovarus	Equinus of the ankle with inversion of the foot due to spasticity of the gastroc/soleus, flexor digitorum and hallucis, and posterior tibialis with weakness of the opposing muscles. This is the most common foot deformity in CP.
Shoulder[17]	Shoulder dysplasia	Spasticity of the internal rotators and adductors and secondary tightness of the joint capsule can pull the humeral head from the socket, resulting in subluxation or dislocation.
	Adductor contractures	Spasticity in the pectoralis major, teres major, and latissimus dorsi can occur, limiting abduction.
Elbow[17]	Flexor contractures	Spasticity of the biceps brachi and brachioradialis is common with the arm held in flexion at the elbow and loss of ROM over time.
Forearm[17]	Pronation contracture	Spasticity in the pronator teres and quadratus with weak supinators can lead to a contracture. Usually occurs with an elbow flexion contracture
Wrist[17]	Contracture	Spasticity in the flexor muscle(s) – flexor carpi ulnaris and radialis with weak wrist extensors can occur, especially in those with severe spasticity, limiting hand use.
Hand[17]	Swan-neck deformity	This is a deformity of hyperflexion of the distil IP joint with hyperextension of the proximal IP joint due to spasticity in the finger flexors and slippage of the extensor tendon laterally within its sheath.
	Thumb in palm	Spasticity of the thumb adductors with weakness in thumb abduction can lead to an adducted thumb within the flexed fingers; this severely limits hand function.

FIGURE 19-3 Crouched versus stiff knee gait. A. Crouched gait – hip and knee flexion with femoral anteversion, tibial torsion, and equinus with pes planus. **B.** Stiff knee gait – knee extension with some scissoring of the legs during ambulation and equinovarus.

Children with hypotonia and/or ataxia perform functional movements by using a small (less than available) ROM, often hold stationary postures without adequate muscular activation (referred to as "hanging on ligaments"), move less and seem to move from one static posture to another with poor

CASE A, PART V

Alejandro is demonstrating the stereotypical movement patterns of a child with spastic diplegia. He bunny-hops when he's creeping, walks with a crouched gait, w-sits, and lacks variation in his patterns of movement. This refers to his inability to use multiple movement patterns. For most typically developing children, they can sit in almost any position and walk slow, fast, on toes, backward, etc. For children with CP, they are often "locked" into moving in one way (e.g., bunny hopping). Therapy is focused on increasing their repertoire of movements so that they have greater independence in their environments.

For Alejandro (AJ), a typical treatment session might look like this: First, the therapist might do some gentle rocking on a ball to lower his tone while performing some gentle

ROM of his LE. Then, with AJ sitting on the ball and the therapist stabilizing his pelvis, she encourages reaching in a variety of directions to elicit trunk rotation and strengthen the trunk muscles, as she stabilizes AJ on top of the ball. Bringing him down off the ball into a standing position with feet flat, the ball can now be pushed into the wall so that it bounces back, while AJ works on stance. Reaching in this position is also done to further work on balance and trunk rotation. Squatting to the floor is a nice way to strengthen the quads and gluts, which are key muscles to oppose the spasticity of the hamstrings and hip flexors. For most children, reaching through their legs to a toy behind their heels (a 4-inch ball works nicely) will encourage a squat with the feet flat and knees apart; this avoids the child coming up on their toes with knees together, which is the common way children with spasticity squat. It is critical that the therapist be able to identify tasks, such as this, that encourage more typical movement patterns rather than strengthening the synergistic patterns and the tone. Toward the end of the session, the therapist focuses on gait training, using an obstacle course with objects of various heights in an alternating ladder formation for AJ to step over, an incline to walk up, and many turns for him to negotiate. Stepping over obstacles stimulates a longer step with the "stepping foot" and induces increased single limb stance contralaterally. Obstacles and inclines can stimulate dorsiflexor activation to clear the obstacle and make it up the incline. Since dorsiflexors are typically weak and toe-walking common, these are good activities to encourage an improved gait pattern. Also, moving into and out of a variety of sitting postures should be addressed so that AJ has a greater repertoire for play and increased hip mobility; he may be able to move into side-sitting or tailor-sitting more easily by rotating as he pushes back from quadruped to assume these positions. However, in many children, their tight internal rotators and adductors make these positions quite difficult to assume and uncomfortable to maintain; it may be better for AJ to sit in a low chair rather than w-sit to protect his hips. As should be evident, therapists must be creative, making the tasks fun, yet finding ways to facilitate more normal movement patterns.

Home tasks could include (1) long sitting or prone propping to provide passive stretch to his hamstrings and hip flexors, while watching TV or coloring; (2) stair climbing with assistance for quad strengthening; (3) half-kneeling for play to decrease reliance on bilateral symmetrical movement; (4) standing catch and throw with his sister, while a parent provides stability at the waist to increase standing balance and trunk rotation; and (5) kicking a ball, while standing with his walker, to increase single limb stance, dorsiflexion of the kicking leg, and balance. All of these can easily be built into the everyday activities of the family.

stability during the movement. They often have kyphosis and lordosis, which puts them at risk for trunk deformities, including scoliosis, and contractures and dislocations of the limbs. Although children with hypotonia often begin with excessive ROM, they repeatedly use only a part of it and frequently have contractures secondary to this limited posturing.

Upper Extremity Function

Characteristics of upper extremity impairment in children with CP include (1) posturing in shoulder adduction and internal rotation, elbow flexion, forearm pronation, and flexion of the wrist and fingers, including thumb adduction and flexion (thumb in the palm); (2) spasticity in the muscles contributing to this posture; (3) weakness of both spastic muscles and their antagonists; (4) secondary loss of range of motion (contractures); (5) loss of sensation and proprioception; and (6) diminished dexterity and isolated finger motion. The position of the elbow in flexion with forearm pronation puts the radial head in a position of risk for subluxation or dislocation. Contractures of the UE are common due to limited mobility and spasticity. For children with milder presentation, there is still diminished grip force, poor grip precision (inability to adjust to size and shape of the object), and reliance on more immature grasp methods.[17] While UE function may be primarily addressed by occupational therapists, the physical therapist should understand UE movement and reaching patterns and incorporate them into: (1) reaching while addressing trunk control and balance, (2) weight-bearing on the UE while working on creeping, pulling to stand and standing, (3) strengthening of the UE through weight-bearing and play activities, and (4) more typical movement patterns (e.g. arm swing during gait).

● ASSOCIATED CONDITIONS OF CEREBRAL PALSY

Orthopedic

Children with CP often either have insufficient muscle tone to support joint integrity or an imbalance of muscle tone and strength around joints that can result in soft tissue lengthening on one side and shortening on the other side. Such differences in muscle activity around joints can create instability and the potential for deformity over time. Further, delays in weight-bearing, especially standing, can affect bone health and joint maturation, especially at the hip where the acetabulum deepens with weight-bearing. Table 19-1 outlines common orthopedic deformities associated with CP.

Intellectual Developmental Disability/Epilepsy

The term intellectual developmental disability (IDD) has replaced the use of mental retardation to describe individuals with deficits in cognitive function (reasoning, judgment, symbol use, memory, processing speed for acquiring new information) and adaptive behavior, which refers to the skills necessary to function in an age and culturally/environmentally appropriate manner, including social skills and behavioral management, that manifests during the developmental period (birth to age 18). This change in terminology reflects an increased emphasis on the limitations in adaptive behavior and a decreased reliance on IQ testing, in part, stemming from the problems inherent in IQ testing that may be biased against certain socioeconomic or racial/ethnic groups as well as those with motor or communication disorders where testing can be difficult.[18]

However, the categorization of children with IDD into levels of severity (mild, moderate, severe, and profound) persists and allows easier communication between health professionals, yet the primary criterion for these levels is IQ, based on a test with a mean of 100 and an SD of 15, with a deficit of 2 SD below the mean defining IDD (<70). Similarly, tests of adaptive behavior allow corresponding categorization with a focus on conceptual skills (ability to learn concepts), practical skills (ability to learn daily living skills, including work-related skills), and social skills. Table 19-2 provides descriptions of these categories of IDD with IQ level and adaptive behavior potential.

Approximately 45% of children with CP have IDD, and when epilepsy is also present, the incidence increases to nearly 80%. This concomitant occurrence of IDD and epilepsy with CP should not be surprising given that each can individually be caused by damage to the developing brain, and therefore, can also be induced collectively by a single incident.[19]

TABLE 19-2	**IDD Categories[18]**	
LEVEL	**IQ RANGE**	**ADAPTIVE BEHAVIOR ABILITY/POTENTIAL**
Mild	69–56	Develop communication and social skills. Slow academic progress to 4th/5th grade level (unable to manage abstract concepts) by adulthood with mild limitations in coordination and higher-level motor skills; typically able to live independently, manage simple finances, and work in unskilled jobs.
Moderate	55–40	Slow acquisition of language, social, and motor skills with some difficulty in all areas at adulthood but acquire independent self-care abilities; academic progress to 2nd grade level (simple reading and math); may live in the community with supervision and work a repetitive manual job.
Severe	39–21	Considerable limitations in acquisition of language, motor, and social skills; academic focus is on teaching practical and social skills; will require assistance/supervision with self-care; may work in supervised environment; will not live independently.
Profound	<20	Minimal practical skill acquisition, including mobility; will require assistance with most self-care skills.

Epilepsy (seizure disorder) is a condition of repetitive seizures in the absence of active disease; this is an important distinction, since seizures can occur in the presence of acute illness/disease, such as encephalitis, but will resolve once the disease has been treated unless brain damage occurs as a result of the disease. A **seizure** is an abnormal discharge of neurons in the brain, associated with motor, sensory, autonomic, emotional, or cognitive symptoms, dependent on the area of the brain affected. Damage to the brain can leave scar tissue that irritates surrounding intact tissue, thereby, inducing the abnormal activation that creates the seizure. Thus, seizures present in a variety of ways (see Table 19-3) that are differentiated, in part, as: (1) generalized, referring to involvement of both hemispheres with a loss of consciousness, or (2) partial, indicating localization to one hemisphere and that some degree of consciousness remains intact. In the typically developing child population, epilepsy occurs in less than .4–1% of the population; in children with developmental disabilities, this incidence increases to 30–50%, and in children with CP it may be as high as 62%.[19] Children with quadriplegia or hemiplegia are much more likely to develop epilepsy than those with diplegia; additionally, epilepsy in children with CP is often more difficult to treat (refractory), requiring several medications to control the seizure activity. Uncontrolled seizures can lead to additional brain damage and in some instances, death secondary to a condition known as **status epilepticus**, where a prolonged seizure state persists (longer than 5 minutes) that places the child in a medically unstable condition, associated with diminished oxygen to the brain and multiple system decline, including dysfunction in the cardiopulmonary system.

Sensory Dysfunction

Concomitant disruption of vision is common in CP with up to 70% of children experiencing some change in their **visual system**; most commonly, this presents as poor visual acuity but the causative pathology is different than diminished acuity in their peers. Additionally, more severe changes can include blindness, retinopathy (especially in children with prematurity), and strabismus. Strabismus refers to poor coordination of the extraocular muscles, resulting in poor synchronization of eye movement and disruption of binocular vision. **Hearing loss** can also occur in children with CP but is much less common than visual deficits. **Vestibular dysfunction** can also occur with over or under responsiveness to vestibular input possible. Taste and smell are typically maintained.

Deficits in **somatosensory function** are also common, presenting similarly to that described in Chapter 10 for stroke, including diminished touch perception, tactile discrimination abilities, and proprioception/kinesthesia. Somatosensory dysfunction is more common in hemiplegia and quadriplegia than diplegia.[19]

Language/Communication Disorders

As was described in Chapter 10 for stroke, language disorders are common in children with CP and present similarly to the adult presentation. There seems to be a greater potential for plasticity in children, especially in those with hemiplegia, that allows for fairly normal speech development even with left hemisphere damage, likely resulting from the potential of the right hemisphere to control language when the left is damaged early. Notably, the most common language disorder in CP is dysarthria, resulting from disrupted control of the oral muscles. The severity of language impairment correlates with the severity of the motor impairment, so those with severe spastic quadriplegia are most affected while those with diplegia are rarely affected. When IDD is also present, this will further impact the ability of the child to develop speech such that those with profound IDD rarely have functional speech. Yet, there are children with severe CP presentation that have limited speech without IDD; for these children, a communication device may unlock their world by allowing them to communicate through a synthesized voice or written word (see section on assistive technology).

TABLE 19-3	Seizure Classifications[20]
SEIZURE TYPE	**DESCRIPTION**
Generalized	Loss of consciousness due to involvement of both cerebral hemispheres
Tonic-clonic (grand mal)	A period of tonic (maintained) muscle co-contraction, followed by repetitive alternating muscle contractions of flexors and extensors (clonic phase).
Absence (petit mal)	Brief loss of consciousness (<10 seconds) associated with staring and loss of responsiveness that may go unnoticed by the child. Atypical absence seizures may have clonic, atonic, or stereotypic movements (e.g., swallowing, chewing, blinking) and last up to 20 seconds.
Myoclonic	Quick generalized muscle contraction similar in appearance to a startle response but without a precipitating stimulus.
Tonic	Generalized and maintained muscle contraction (identical to tonic phase of tonic-clonic) without a clonic phase.
Atonic	Generalized loss of muscle activity, resulting in complete collapse of the body (drops to floor)
Partial	Focal seizure without loss of consciousness, characterized by symptoms linked to the area of the brain in which the seizure occurs (e.g., sensory, motor, autonomic (changes in blood pressure, sweating, nausea), or emotion (fear, anxiety). Can progress to generalized seizure, commonly tonic-clonic.
Complex partial	Characterized by a variety of complex motor behaviors, such as chewing, picking at clothes, walking in circles with some disruption of awareness (not a complete loss of consciousness)

MEDICAL MANAGEMENT OF THE CHILD WITH CP

The management of the child with CP is dependent on presentation and comorbidities; since each child will present uniquely, treatment needs to be directed at the specific needs of the child. For both medical and therapeutic management, the focus is on maximizing function and preventing secondary complications. From the discussion of this condition in previous sections, it should be apparent that medical management of the child with CP can include surgery for orthopedic conditions; pharmaceutical management of seizures, spasticity, or other conditions; prevention of secondary conditions, including orthopedic deformities; and maximizing growth and development through adequate nutritional management.

Management of Seizures

The primary treatment for seizures is pharmacological; unfortunately, antiseizure medications have a variety of side effects, including sedation/somnolence/lethargy, dyscoordination, poor attention, hyperactivity/agitation, irritability and aggression (see Table 19-4 for common medications, usage, and side effects). When combined with CP and IDD, these medications may significantly impact the child's ability to function, so treatment focuses on achieving the best seizure control while minimizing side effects to maximize function. In many instances, more than one drug is required to provide effective seizure control; obviously this may have an additive effect for the side effects as well. On rare occasions, surgery is indicated for the treatment of severe and refractory seizures. This may involve ablation of the seizure-generating neurons in focal epilepsy or severing of the corpus callosum in those with generalized seizures to stop the progression of the seizure activity from one hemisphere to the other. Of course, surgical intervention of this sort has its own set of consequences that will also impact the child's function.

Management of Spasticity

In children with spasticity, medical management is aimed at limiting the impact of spasticity on range of motion and movement, preventing orthopedic deformities, and minimizing pain, if present. Multiple **oral medications** can be used to decrease spasticity systemically, but they all have side effects that may compromise function, most commonly sedation. Further, many children with CP "rely" on their spasticity to achieve posture and movement; thus, they may experience a decrease in function when using an oral medication. Common oral medications are gamma aminobutyric acid (GABA) agonists (e.g., baclofen, diazepam, gabapentin, tiagabine), adrenergic agonists (tizanidine), and calcium channel blockers (sodium dantrolene). For children with severe spasticity or dystonia, **intrathecal baclofen** may be used to allow better positioning, hygiene, and mobility. This involves surgical placement of a catheter into the epidural lumbar space with a pump that is subcutaneous (just below the skin surface), which allows it to be refilled via injection. Although the effect of intrathecal baclofen can be widespread, including LE, UE, and trunk, it avoids the central effects, including sedation. For children with focal spasticity that is limiting mobility of single joints or a few joints, injections of **botulinum toxin** (Botox) may be effective in diminishing spasticity for up to 3 months so that therapy can focus on improving motor control and strength within the muscles to avoid surgery. Often Botox injections are accompanied by splinting (orthotics) to maintain improved range of motion, following the injection. The long-term effects of Botox injections is equivocal, since the spasticity will return as the effect of the injection wears off; however, with intensive physical therapy, long-term effects have been reported.[21] In some cases, surgery is required to increase range of motion and prevent further joint deformity (see surgical management in the next section). Of note, there is a surgical procedure that is focused on decreasing the spasticity itself, called a **selective dorsal rhizotomy**. In this procedure, the dorsal root afferents of the lumbar spine that are contributing to LE spasticity and hyperreflexia are lesioned; this is a tedious process that includes electrical stimulation to identify appropriate nerve roots to be sectioned and to preserve nerve roots that are least involved in the spasticity to maintain function. Following the surgery, intensive physical therapy is provided to work on strengthening, reeducation of muscles, and increasing mobility (6 weeks of daily therapy, 6 hours per day). This procedure is particularly effective for children with spastic diplegia at GMFCS levels II and III, reportedly, decreasing the need for orthopedic surgeries, enhancing the development of gross motor skills, and delaying the typical plateau of those skills.[22]

TABLE 19-4	Common Antiepileptic Medications[20]	
DRUG	**USES**	**SIDE EFFECTS**
Phenytoin (Dilantin)	Partial or generalized	Unsteadiness, ataxia, sedation, attention deficits, disrupted problem solving
Carbamazepine (Tegretol)	Partial	Disrupted sleep, irritability, attention deficit
Phenobarbital	Partial or generalized	Hyperactivity, lethargy, sleep disruption, memory impairment, attention deficit
Valproic acid (Depakene/Depakote)	Absence, tonic-clonic, myoclonic	Sedation, minimal cognitive side effects
Lamotrigine (Lamictal)	Partial, complex partial, generalized	Minimal side effects; tremor, changes in balance, fatigue, hair loss
Ethosuximide	Absence	Psychosis
Gabapentin	Partial (usually a secondary drug)	Somnolence, hyperactivity, aggression

Orthopedic Management

The first step in orthopedic management should be to prevent a deformity from developing through positioning, movement, orthotics, and stretching. In some cases, **serial casting** is used; this technique casts the body part at an end of range position for a week or so; then, the cast is removed and reapplied at the new end of range position, gradually increasing the length of the soft tissue and increasing range of motion. The goals of surgery are often different, depending on the functional level of the child: for those at higher GMFCS levels (II and III) the goal is improved function (ambulation or hand use); for those at lower GMFCS levels (IV and V), the goal is typically to minimize pain and/or improve hygiene care by the care providers. For the most part, surgery is not considered unless there is a fixed deformity, subluxation/dislocation, or significant impedance to mobility. Orthopedic surgeries can be categorized into four types: (1) lengthening of the tendon (tendonotomy) to improve range of motion; (2) transfer of a tendon to improve muscle balance at a joint (e.g., changing a spastic flexor carpi ulnaris to an extensor muscle by reattaching it to the dorsum of the wrist); (3) osteotomy (cutting the bone) to shorten, lengthen, or change the rotation of a bone to improve alignment (e.g., derotation osteotomy of the femur to correct excessive anteversion); and (4) fusion (arthrodesis) to fix the joint in an improved alignment (e.g., spinal arthrodesis for scoliosis).[23] Tendonotomies (lengthening) are typically done by cutting the tendon in a Z pattern (see Figure 19-4), which allows the two ends of the Z to be stitched together,

thereby, lengthening the tendon. Following surgery, splinting or casting are used in combination with therapy to maintain the new length, strengthen the lengthened and opposing muscles, and promote joint mobility. Notably, these procedures may be done in combination to achieve maximum results; for example, a femoral derotation osteotomy may be done in conjunction with an adductor lengthening to prevent reoccurrence. However, since growth can negate results, it is often recommended that the child be at least school age before such surgery is done to avoid reoccurrence and the need for subsequent surgeries.

Nutritional Management

Approximately 85% of children with CP will have oropharyngeal dysphagia (disrupted motor control for eating) that can have nutritional, growth, or respiratory consequences, most commonly aspiration of food, resulting in pneumonia or other respiratory consequence.[24] Dysphagia is most common in lower functioning children (GMFCS III–V). Additionally, these same children may suffer from **gastroesophageal reflux**, which refers to regurgitation of stomach contents to the esophagus, secondary to dysfunction of the lower esophageal sphincter. Stomach acids can erode the esophagus, causing pain and further eating avoidance. Due to the many challenges in eating, many children with CP have very poor food consumption and are at risk for malnutrition that can further impede brain development and overall health. Initial treatment for feeding difficulty is to adjust the feeding process to make eating easier; this includes improved positioning, use of adaptive feeding methods (e.g., nipples with smaller holes, adaptive utensils for self-feeding), and alteration of foods to make eating easier (e.g., thickening of liquids to decrease aspiration). Some children are very picky eaters, which can affect the nutrients ingested, also impacting growth and development. **Nutritional supplements** may be prescribed to address imbalances, including increasing the caloric content of foods consumed. Of note, children with CP typically require up to 70% more calories than their typically developing peers due to the energy costs of moving and/or wheelchair propulsion.[25] For some children, these methods are insufficient, and they require surgical intervention to assure nutritional intake; the most common is surgical implantation of a tube into the stomach (**percutaneous endoscopic gastrostomy** [PEG]),

Achilles tendon

FIGURE 19-4 Z-plasty. To lengthen the Achilles tendon, a Z-incision is made in the tendon (above cut left to right) and then the two ends of the "Z" are sutured together to allow lengthening of the tendon.

CASE A, PART VI

Alejandro, like most children with diplegia, has no apparent language or intellectual delays; although he is still young to be certain that he won't display any learning disabilities. He has outgrown his seizures and is no longer taking medication. He is developing hip and knee flexion tightness that needs to be carefully managed. He may be a candidate for botox injections in these muscles to temporarily block spasticity, while a range of motion and strengthening program is implemented to improve knee and hip extension. At some point, he may also be a candidate for a selective dorsal rhizotomy, but typically, this is done when the child is 5–6 years of age.

which allows thick liquids to be pushed directly into the stomach, bypassing the mouth and esophagus.[24] For many children, this may also require an anti-reflux procedure that prevents further leakage of stomach contents into the esophagus.

PHYSICAL THERAPY MANAGEMENT

Treatment of the child with CP is aimed at maximizing function, increasing the variety of movements available to the child, and preventing secondary complications, especially orthopedic deformities. Similar to the treatment of adults with neurologic disorders, treatment of children is based on the growing body of evidence related to motor control and neuroplasticity, more specifically, what is needed to induce change in the nervous system (see Chapter 8). The basic tenets of inducing motor learning and plasticity are (1) plasticity requires intensity of practice that challenges the current level of function and thereby the nervous system, including numerous repetitions at the maximum ability of the individual; (2) practice needs to be task specific (e.g., to improve walking, the child should be walking); (3) practice of the whole activity is preferable to practicing part of the activity (e.g., although single limb stance is part of gait, practicing single limb stance may not improve stance during gait); (4) practice that requires problem solving and variability is critical to learning and ultimately transferring the skill to new situations; (5) feedback should provide knowledge of performance (how the movement "looked") and results (success/failure) in limited amounts (more initially with less as the skill is acquired); and (6) feedback from the therapist should be weaned as the child becomes able to rely on his own sensory feedback (how the movement feels). Handling the child to facilitate a movement should also be considered a form of feedback that limits the degrees of freedom available to the child and changes his own sensory experience of the movement; thus, like verbal feedback it should be used as little as necessary, greater initially with weaning as each new skill is learned. In addition, therapy needs to be fun and interactive between therapist and the child but should also be focused on the family (family-centered), directed toward mutually developed goals, and in consideration of the family structure, culture, and daily activities. Therapists should be cognizant that they will spend, at best, a few hours per week with a child while the caregivers will spend up to 100 waking hours with their child per week. Thus, for therapy to be effective, the families must be able to implement components of the therapy in the home, yet this should not be overwhelming nor interfere with their function as a family. Similarly, teachers should be part of the therapy program for the child, implementing components within the school day of the child to maximize effectiveness.

Managing the Effects of Abnormal Muscle Tone

Although abnormal tone should not be a primary focus of treatment, it often impacts treatment, and therefore, requires attention. For example, in the child with spasticity, tone will increase when the child gets excited, so treatment in a quiet environment may be preferable initially, when focused on a new skill. Yet, as the skill is learned, the child must manage their enthusiasm and, thereby, tone, to function in the many environments that he might experience. There are techniques to increase tone in those with hypotonia and lower tone in spasticity/dystonia that may allow the child to move against gravity or move out of synergistic patterns temporarily. Techniques that may increase tone are bouncing on a ball/bolster, swinging, or joint compression (either manual or through weight-bearing); in contrast, slow rocking on a ball or bolster, passive rotation of the extremity or trunk, and active movements outside of synergistic patterns can diminish tone. However, it should be clear that these are transitory changes that can allow the child to move more easily momentarily but do not change the physiological causes of abnormal tone. So, it is important to strengthen antagonists and create movement opportunities that challenge the child's motor control system to generate new patterns of movement, breaking through synergistic patterns.

For children with significant spasticity or dystonia, the family should be instructed in range of motion exercises early to help prevent loss of motion and potential deformity; simple motions that can be done during diaper changes, bath time, and dressing (e.g., rocking into abduction, leg extension with dorsiflexion) will be easier for them to remember than a complex routine that takes a lot of time. Emphasis should be on LE extension, abduction, external rotation, and dorsiflexion as well as UE extension, abduction, external rotation, and supination. Making these a part of the caregivers' daily play time with the child will assure that they are completed. Also, positioning of the child to minimize the effects of spasticity is also critical: (1) maintaining abduction during sitting (ring or tailor positions) or while being carried (e.g., straddling the parent's hip); (2) early standing to achieve hip and knee extension with feet flat; and (3) trunk and head support in sitting and when transporting for children with poor control to prevent scoliosis or kyphosis. These positioning suggestions are also important for children with dyskinetic, ataxic, or hypotonic CP. While children with ataxia and hypotonia have greater freedom of movement than the child with spasticity or dystonia, they also have diminished antigravity movement and stability so that they spend long periods of time in a single position (e.g., supported sitting), resulting in the potential for scoliosis or other orthopedic problems. Muscles will shorten if the legs are always flexed and abducted, whether spastic or hypotonic; thus, positioning is a critical component of preventative and therapeutic intervention for all children with CP. Notably, instructing the family in appropriate handling and carrying methods will also help them contend with a child that is difficult to handle.

Strengthening

Interestingly, weakness and poor force generation are common elements of CP regardless of type and varies with the GMFCS level with those at level I demonstrating the best strength and those at level V the worst; thus, strengthening is an important part of treatment. However, the best method and expected results remain elusive with insufficient evidence to determine best practices. As is described for the child with myelomeningocele in Chapter 18, encouraging antigravity movement is the initial method for developing strength in neck and trunk muscles and hip extensors in infants and young children with CP via the same activities described in Table 18-3. Additionally, use of weight-bearing postures and functional activities (e.g., squatting and returning to stand; pushing away from the wall when rolled forward on a ball; maneuvering a scooter board with the hands) can further increase strength in children with CP. In many children, weight-training with free weights or resistive exercise equipment can improve strength (e.g., quadriceps strength); however, it may not translate into improved function (e.g., knee extension during gait), yet has been found to improve gait speed even in the absence of improved kinematics.[26]

Novel Treatment Approaches

Much research is now devoted to identifying best practices to maximize function in children with CP, including treadmill training, robotic training, gaming, aquatic therapy, and hippotherapy. Each has demonstrated some degree of success. These approaches are all focused on increasing the intensity and variability of practice to achieve improved function and variability of movement. **Treadmill training with partial body-weight support** may facilitate earlier walking and allows the therapist to facilitate LE position and weight-shift, while not worrying about the child falling. Further, it can stimulate increase gait speed that may improve aerobic capacity in older children.[23] Similarly, partial body-weight support can also be achieved with mobile systems that allow over ground walking that may facilitate better transfer of gait changes to the standard environment. Also, **biofeedback-assisted gait training** that provides visual and auditory feedback in response to movement (e.g., walking on a treadmill) has also been found to improve gait speed, step length, and single limb support.[27] **Robotic-assisted therapy** is being used for both gait training and arm training in children with CP. Robots can facilitate intense practice (many repetitions) with assistance or resistance that is task specific; this can be reaching or grasping with the arm/hand or step and dorsiflexion assistance for gait.[28,29] Concerns for robotic therapy have suggested that, like handling, it changes the sensory perception of a movement and diminishes the feedback and feed-forward mechanisms critical for voluntary movement; research to date remains equivocal as to whether robotic-assisted therapy produces greater functional improvement than intense practice. Similar to robotics, **gaming** is being incorporated into therapy sessions and home programs, using interactive systems, such as the Nintendo Wii™, to improve weight-shift and balance as well as UE and LE movements outside of synergistic patterns; initial results suggest that this type of program has potential for increasing balance and gait parameters[30] as well as UE use.[31] **Constraint-induced Movement Therapy (CIMT)**, which has been used primarily for children with hemiplegia to increase use of the paretic UE, was initially designed as a treatment method for stroke but has been found to increase use of the paretic arm in children with hemiplegic CP. In this treatment paradigm, the non-paretic arm is typically splinted or casted, but gloves/mittens have been used, for several weeks (2–10, depending on the study) while intense therapy is focused on reaching, grasping, and manipulation activities with the paretic hand. CIMT has been attempted with a broad age range of children

(2–18) and some of the variability in outcomes may result from this variability in age. Yet, almost all studies have shown UE improvement to some degree with this treatment. As more research is done, it will be important to examine its use with even younger children as they are developing reach and grasp skills.[32] **Hippotherapy** is a form of treatment where a therapist uses a horse as a therapeutic tool to stimulate the visual, vestibular, and proprioceptive systems of the child; the therapist and aide(s) guide the horse's movements to challenge the child's posture and develop improved stability; this differs from therapeutic riding, where the focus is on teaching the child to ride a horse but the intent is also to improve balance and coordination. Hippotherapy has been studied much more than therapeutic riding and found to improve gross motor function, posture in standing and sitting, trunk strength, and reaching skills to a greater extent than standard treatment alone.[33] Another interesting treatment approach for children with CP is **aquatic therapy**, in which movement in water is used to improve mobility. Water is a supportive medium for children with CP as it provide buoyancy, decreasing the effect of gravity and allowing children with challenged balance to move easier while in it. Most aquatic therapy is done in warm water that helps to lower spasticity; then, skills that might not be possible on land can be attempted, such as single limb stance, walking without an assistive device, squatting, jumping, or hopping. As skills are developed in the water, they can, then, be attempted on land. The fun environment of the pool may keep the child engaged, while the buoyant setting allows a greater number of repetitions to be completed. Aquatic therapy has been found to improve gross motor skills but not to change overall spasticity measures.[34]

Assistive Technology

The function of children with CP can be enhanced with a large variety of assistive technology that includes mobility devices (e.g., crutches, walkers, wheelchairs, orthotics), adaptive equipment for activities of daily living (feeding, bathing, toileting), positioning equipment (standers, seating systems), communication devices, and environmental controls. With the expanding computer technology, the field of assistive technology is expanding exponentially so that it is quite challenging for the therapist to keep up with the changes.

Mobility Devices

In Chapter 18, we discussed orthotics, ambulation devices, and wheelchair fitting for the child with MMC; many of these same devices are also commonly used for children with CP. In the case of CP, the decision about what devices should be used is more complex in many ways than for the child with MMC, since tone is highly variable and the head, trunk, and arms are also commonly involved. While children with CP don't have the insensate issues that children with MMC have, they do require seating systems that provide appropriate support and protect from pressure ulcers, since often they are less mobile than their MMC peers.

Orthotics

The goals of orthotic prescription often differ for children at higher and lower GMFCS levels. Orthotics for those at GMFCS levels II and III aim primarily to increase function, especially gait, and prevent deformity while those for children at GMFCS

FIGURE 19-5 Solid versus articulating AFO. A. A single molded AFO with forefoot, ankle, and calf straps. **B.** An articulating AFO with plantarflexion stop.

levels IV and V aim principally at preventing deformity, especially scoliosis and hip dislocation.

The most common orthotic for ambulating children with CP is an AFO (Figure 19-5), to control the common equinovarus position of the foot that impedes the swing phase of gait as the toe drags and to assist with achieving heel strike. The child's ankle function and tone will determine the kind of AFO that is preferable: articulating or non-articulating (solid or flexible). A **non-articulating AFO** is a single piece (no ankle joint) that is typically fit with the foot at a 90-degree angle with the calf. The thickness of the material allows for degrees of flexibility or rigidity. When the AFO is rigid, it will help the child achieve heel strike but limits push-off, since plantarflexion is blocked. Flexible AFOs allow some degree of plantarflexion for push-off and can assist dorsiflexion after toe off, as the elastic (spring) nature of the material pushes the foot into dorsiflexion to assist during swing and heel strike; for children, with mild spasticity this is appropriate, but for children with moderate to severe spasticity, it may elicit strong plantarflexion or clonus, which defeats the purpose of the AFO, and therefore, should be avoided. Also, it is important for the therapist to evaluate the effect of the AFO on knee position. **Articulating AFOs** have a joint at the ankle and are constructed of two pieces. This allows active or active-assisted dorsiflexion via a spring mechanism but can block or limit plantarflexion. Either type of AFO can also assist with blocking knee hyperextension via a slightly forward positioning of the calf component; however, knee flexion often is not changed with either type of AFO.[35]

Adaptive Seating Systems/Wheelchairs

The goal for adaptive seating for children with CP is to maximize function by providing appropriate postural support that allows the best upper extremity use, controls abnormal tone, prevents deformity, and, in the case of wheelchairs, allows the most freedom of movement whether self-propelled or caregiver-propelled. Seating choices are dependent on the individual child's presentation (tone, deformities, and motor abilities), family situation, and growth potential. Thus, choosing a system for a child requires a comprehensive assessment and some trial and error with potential systems prior to purchase.

In Chapter 18, we discussed the general components of wheelchairs (bases, frames, seating systems) and measurements taken to determine the appropriate chair size and features. For children with CP, the combination of abnormal tone (e.g., spasticity or hypotonia), abnormal movements (e.g., dystonia, chorea, athetosis), and limited trunk control makes finding the right seating system and wheelchair challenging yet critical, especially for those at GMFCS levels IV and V. For example, the orientation of the chair in space has received much consideration. An **anterior tilted chair** (see Figure 19-6), typically 5 degrees forward from upright, may facilitate an anterior pelvic tilt and encourage trunk extension with improved UE function in some children. However, in others, especially those with poor head control, a **posterior tilt** may be advantageous to facilitate improved head positioning and minimize LE extensor patterns; a posterior tilt is often used with a wedge seat to increase hip flexion to further diminish excessive extensor tone. Although this may improve head control and trunk posture, it may also put the child at increased risk for hip flexion contractures. A **head rest** may be essential to provide postural support for a child with poor head control, yet it may also stimulate an extensor thrust (full body extension triggered by pressure on the back of the head) unless positioned carefully; different positions may need to be evaluated to minimize the tendency to thrust into extension and to maximize the most upright head position possible. **Straps** or **harnessing** may be used to provide trunk support, maintain head position, and position the feet flat on the footrest. A **three-point lateral control system** can be used to support the trunk and minimize or prevent scoliosis; this system uses a pad at the hip and upper trunk just below the axilla on one side and a mid-thoracic pad on the other to align the trunk. An **abduction device** is often used to break-up adductor tone and help position the legs in a position of abduction and

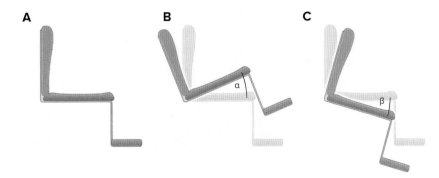

FIGURE 19-6 Seating orientation. A. A standard 90-90-90 seat representation that positions the hip, knee, and ankle at 90 degrees. **B.** A posterior tilt chair with additional hip flexion can be effective in controlling severe spasticity or dystonia yet limits active head motion. **C.** An anterior tilt chair can encourage an anterior pelvic tilt and an upright posture.

mild external rotation; this has been found to improve trunk control and UE function. Similarly, **saddle-style** or **bolster seats** have been used in a number of commercially available systems to maintain hip abduction with some degree of external rotation and hip and knee flexion (usually ≥90 degrees) to break up tone, create an anterior pelvic tilt, and thereby, facilitate postural stability and afford better upper extremity function. A **contour seat** or **seating system** (back, seat, lateral support) may be best for children and adults with CP that have complex postural control needs, including scoliosis, kyphosis, or hip dysplasia; a contour system is individually fit to the child through a molding process (there are several commercially available) that creates a seat that conforms to the body. Additional external hardware can also be attached to provide maximal support, as needed. A contour seat can often be removed from the chair for sitting on the floor or a standard chair at a table as well as within a wheelchair frame[36] (Figure 19-7 shows a wheelchair that has been adapted for a child with dystonia at GMFCS level V).

One of the first decisions to be made in choosing a wheelchair is whether it can be propelled by the child, either manually or via electric power, or will be pushed by the caregiver. Children, as young as 1–3 years of age, can propel a manual chair or learn to operate a power chair. Providing a wheelchair early allows independent exploration of the child's environment and is expected to improve social interactions and ultimately cognitive development. There are also many choices of control devices for power chairs that accommodate the limited motor abilities of some children with CP. However, the child must have sufficient cognitive and perceptual motor skills to comprehend cause and effect, problem solve their position relative to where they want to go, understand how the wheelchair functions, and be able to plan their movement within complex environments. This requires the ability to maintain attention and diligently scan the environment for obstacles. Control systems for power chairs include joysticks, switches, touch pads, head systems, mouth controls (e.g., sip and puff), and voice controls. Within each of these categories are numerous selections,

allowing control of the wheelchair with a finger, fingers, or the hand; the chin, mouth or head; or even the knee or foot. Thus, determining the best control device also requires trial and error with a variety of devices to find the best one. Fortunately, most wheelchair vendors will be able to outfit many devices to a given chair so that the right one can be determined.

Part of the decision of what type of wheelchair is appropriate for a given child includes an analysis of the home and school/work environments as well as the family's or for older adolescents/adults, the individual's ability to transport the chair. There needs to be a ramp into the home to allow entrance and exit; the household needs to have appropriate doorway clearance and minimal clutter to allow movement of the chair through the rooms. If the bedrooms are on an upper floor, there may need to be a home modification to allow the older child to have a bedroom on the main floor; young children may be easily carried upstairs, but this may be quite difficult for older children as they grow. A power chair requires a lift and van for transportation; yet even a manual chair that is fitted with many components may not be easily collapsible for transport in the trunk of a standard car, so a van or minivan may be required. Thus, physical therapists will play an important role in home assessment and the choice of the best wheelchair option for the child and family.

Ambulation Devices

Most children with CP that have ambulation potential, especially those at GMFCS levels III and IV, will initially walk with an assistive device; some children, who will eventually reach level II, may initially walk with a device but will progress to independence over time. For most, the first device will be a wheeled walker, typically a **posterior walker** (Figure 19-8); this type of walker places the walker frame behind the child with the grips at the side to encourage a more upright posture. Although anterior walkers are available for children, they can encourage a forward lean and flexed posture, so posterior walkers are more often the first device of choice. Progression to **forearm crutches**

FIGURE 19-7 Power wheelchair for child with dyskinetic cerebral palsy. A. Head array allows control of the wheelchair by touch of cheek/head. **B.** Upper arm trough helps to control dystonic motions. **C.** Lateral trunk support to assist upright posture. **D.** Shoulder support pads to maintain shoulder contract with chair back. **E.** Abduction pommel maintains hip abduction. **F.** Footstraps on a rigid footplate maintain foot position. Note the seat is posteriorly tilted to assist with tone management.

FIGURE 19-8 Posterior walker – the reverse walker encourages a more upright posture and is easier for the child to control than the standard anterior walker that can be pushed too far ahead of the child, resulting in forward falling.

is common as children gain upright stability, affording them the ability to maneuver on uneven terrains and stairs, and they will continue to be used through adulthood for those at GMFCS level III. For those at level IV, a wheeled walker may always be used, and in some cases, they will walk as children but not as adults.

Positioning Devices

For children with a more severe level of disability, especially those at GMFCS level V, many devices are available to assist with positioning to increase weight-bearing and provide stability in a variety of postures for pressure release, deformity prevention, and assistance with activities of daily living. There are a variety of **standers** that provide maximal support for the child, who is unable to stand on their own; standers often come with a tray or can be placed at a table or counter to allow the child to play while standing. Some power wheelchairs can also transform into a stander to afford the child time in standing to offset the hours spent in sitting. Early standing is thought to assist with LE bone development, prevent hip and knee flexion contractures, and enhance social interaction with peers, even in children at GMFCS level V, who do not have ambulation potential. **Sidelyers**, as the name suggests, assist in positioning a child in sidelying, which often allows the child more freedom of UE motion, including bringing the hands together for play, without excessive tone interference. There are also a variety of toileting and bathing devices to provide support for these activities, allowing greater independence for the child or adult with CP or assistance for their caregiver. As the child with severe disability ages, the family may need a **lifting device** to allow easier transitions from bed to wheelchair and for bathing and toileting. There are also a variety of lifts available.

Communication, Play, and Environmental Control Devices

For children with limited mobility, technology is making an incredible difference in their ability to communicate and interact with their environment. Computer technology is creating ever-expanding opportunities for the child and adult with severe mobility limitations. **Communication devices** can be a simple array of pictures, attached to a wheelchair tray, depicting common needs (e.g., foods, drink, family photos) to a complex computerized system that allows the child to indicate complex concepts or complete school work through a synthesized voice or onscreen writing. Like wheelchairs, these devices can be activated by touch of an individual finger, the entire hand, the head, or even eye movement. Note, many children with severe mobility impairment do not have intellectual deficits or have mild deficits, so these devices are opening up the world to them. For young children, many common toys can be modified with switches that enable the child with limited mobility to activate them; similarly, computer programs and video game systems can be modified so that small movements or voice activation are effective means for the child to control the program or game. Likewise, **environmental control systems** allow voice or switch activation of lights, computers, televisions, sounds systems, and almost any electric device. With the expansion of computer capabilities, it will be interesting to see what the next decade brings to the field of assistive technology and devices to assist those with disabilities to communicate and control their environments.

CASE A, PART VII

Alejandro was fitted with an articulating AFO with a plantarflexion block to help him achieve better heel strike and dorsiflexion during swing. Although he currently walks with a posterior walker, eventually, he will be a candidate for forearm crutches. Treadmill training might also be effective in improving his step length and speed of ambulation.

● SUMMARY

As this chapter indicates, CP is a heterogeneous condition, presenting with a myriad of needs for the physical therapist and the rest of the school-based and rehabilitation-focused team members to address. As a lifelong condition, it requires treatment across the lifespan to assure the best outcome for the child and eventually the adult to function in their many environments (school, play, work, home, community). For children with severe disability, this also includes helping the family to manage the child and potentially the adult within the home. A growing area of need is to assist the adolescent's or young adult's transition to independence outside the family home. With such transitions, assessment of the new home and/or workplace with appropriate modifications may allow the adult with CP to function independently or with some care assistance in an independent living situation.

REFERENCES

1. Cerebral Palsy Organization. Available at: http://cerebralpalsy.org/about-cerebral-palsy/prevalence-and-incidence/. Accessed November 13, 2014.

2. Ortinau C, Neil J. The neuroanatomy of prematurity: normal brain development and the impact of preterm birth. *Clin Anat.* 2014. doi:10.1002/ca.22430 (epub).

3. McManus BM, Chambliss JH, Rapport MJ. Application of the NICU practice guidelines to treat an infant in a level III NICU. *Pediatr Phys Ther.* 2013;25:204-213.

4. Halliday HL. Neonatal management of long-term sequelae. *Best Pract Res Clin Obstet Gynaecol.* 2009;23:871-880.

5. Reddihough DS, Collins KJ. The epidemiology and causes of cerebral palsy. *Aust J Physiother.* 2003;49:7-12.

6. Phalen AG, Kirkby S, Dysart K. The 5 minute Apgar score: survival and short-term outcomes of extremely low-birth-weight infants. *J Perinatal Neonatal Nurs.* 2012;26(6):166-171.

7. O'Shea TM. Diagnosis, treatment and prevention of cerebral palsy in near-term/term infants. *Clin Obstet Gynaecol.* 2008;51(4):816-828.

8. Palisano R, Rosenbaum P, Walter S, Russell D, Wood E, Galuppi B. Development and reliability of a system to classify gross motor function in children with cerebral palsy. *Dev Med Child Neurol.* 1997;39(4):214-223.

9. Brogna C, Romeo DM, Cervesi C, Scrofani L, Romeo MG, Mercuri E, Guzzetta. Prognostic value of the qualitative assessments of general movements in late-preterm infants. *Early Human Development.* 2013;89:1063-1066.

10. Hanna SE, Bartlett DJ, Rivard LM, Russell DJ. Reference curves for the gross motor function measure: percentiles for clinical description and tracking over time among children with cerebral palsy. *Phys Ther.* 2008;88:596-607.

11. CanChild GMFSC Levels. Available at: http://www.canchild.ca/en/measures/gmfcs.asp. Accessed November 13, 2014.

12. Shevell M, Dagenais L, Hall N. The relationship of cerebral palsy subtype and functional motor impairment: a population-based study. *Dev med Child Neurol.* 2009;51:872-877.

13. Himmelmann K, Hagberg G, Wiklund LM, Eek MN, Uvebrant P. Sykinetic cerebral palsy: a population-based study of children born between 1991 and 1998. *Dev Med Child Neurol.* 2007;49:246-251.

14. Valencia FG. Management of hip deformities in cerebral palsy. *Orthop Clin N Am.* 2013;41:549-559.

15. Young JL, Rodda J, Selber P, Rutz E, Graham HK. Management of the knee in spastic diplegia: what is the dose? *Orthop Clin N Am.* 2010;41:561-577.

16. Davids JR. The foot and ankle in cerebral palsy. *Orthop Clin N Am.* 2010;41:579-593.

17. Koman LA. Sarlikiotis T, Smith BP. Surgery of the upper extremity in cerebral palsy. *Orthop Clin N Am.* 2010;41:519-529.

18. Katz G, Lazeano-Ponce E. Intellectual disability: definition, etiological factors, classification, diagnosis, treatment and prognosis. *Salud Publica Mex.* 2008;50(S2):5132-5141.

19. Odding E, Roebroeck ME, Stam HJ. The epidemiology of cerebral palsy: incidence, impairments and risk factors. *Dis Rehabil.* 2006;28(4):183-191.

20. Depositario-Cabacar DFT, Zelleke TG. Treatment of epilepsy in children with developmental disabilities. *Dev Disabil Res Rev.* 2010;16:239-247.

21. Papavasiliou AS. Management of motor problems in cerebral palsy: a critical update for the clinician. *Eur J Paediatr Neurol.* 2009;13:387-396.

22. Dudley RR, Parolin M, Gagnon B, et al. Long-term functional benefits of selective dorsal rhizotomy for spastic cerebral palsy. *J Neurosurg Pediatr.* 2013;12:142-150.

23. Damiano DL, Alter KE, Chamber H. New clinical and research trends in lower extremity management for ambulatory children with cerebral palsy. *Phys Med Rehabil Clin N Am.* 2009;20(3):469-491.

24. Benfer KA, Weir KA, Bell KL, Ware RS, Davies PSW, Boyd RN. Oropharyngeal dysphagia in preschool children with cerebral palsy: oral phase impairments. *Res Dev Disabil.* 2014;35:3469-3481.

25. Kuperminc MN, Gottrand F, Samson-Fang L, Arvedson J, Bell K, Craig GM, Sullivan PB. Nutritional management of children with cerebral palsy: a practical guide. *Eur J Clin Nutr.* 2013;67:521-523.

26. Damiano DL, Arnold AS, Steele KM, Delp SL. Can strength training predictably improve gait kinematics? A pilot study on the effects of hip and knee extensor strengthening on lower-extremity alignment in cerebral palsy. *Phys Ther.* 2010;90:269-279.

27. Gharib NMM, El-Maksoud GMA, Rezk-Allah SS. Efficacy of gait trainer as an adjunct to traditional physical therapy on walking performance in hemiparetic cerebral palsied children: a randomized controlled trial. *Clin Rehabil.* 2011;25(10):924-934.

28. Chen YP, Howard AM. Effects of robotic therapy on upper-extremity function in children with cerebral palsy: a systematic review. *Dev Neurorehabil.* 2014;1–8. doi:10.3109/17518423.2014.899648.

29. Druzbicki M, Rusek W, Snela S, et al. Functional effects of robotic-assisted locomotor treadmill therapy in children with cerebral palsy. *J Rehabil Med.* 2013;45:358-363.

30. Tarakci D, Ozdincler AR, Tarakci E, Tutuncuoglu F, Ozmen M. Wii-based balance therapy to improve balance function of children with cerebral palsy: a pilot study. *J Phys Ther Sci.* 2013;25:1123-1127.

31. Winkels DGM, Kottink AIR, Temmink RAJ, Nijlant FMM, Buurke JH. Wii™-habilitation of upper extremity function in children with cerebral palsy. An explorative study. *Dev Neurorehabil.* 2013;16(1):44-51.

32. Chen YP, Pope S, Tyler D, Warren GL. Effectiveness of constraint-induced movement therapy on upper-extremity function in children with cerebral palsy: a systematic review and meta-analysis of randomized controlled trials. *Clin Rehabil.* 2014;28(10):939-953.

33. Silkwood-Sherer DJ, Killian CB, Long TM, Martin KS. Hippotherapy – an intervention to habilitate balance deficits in children with movement disorders: a clinical trial. *Phys Ther.* 2012;92:707-717.

34. Lai CJ, Liu WY, Yang TF, Chen CL, Wu CY, Chan RC. Pediatric aquatic therapy on motor function and enjoyment in children diagnosed with cerebral palsy of various motor severities. *J Child Neurol.* 2014. doi:10.1177/0883073814535491.

35. Chisholm AE, Perry SD. Ankle-foot orthotic management in neuromuscular disorders: recommendations for future research. *Dis Rehabil Assist Technol.* 2012;7(6):437-449.

36. Chung J, Evans J, Lee C, Lee J, Rabbani Y, Roxborough L, Harris SR. Effectiveness of adaptive seating on sitting posture and postural control in children with cerebral palsy. *Pediatr Phys Ther.* 2008;20:303-317.

Review Questions

1. **Which of the following best describe the condition of cerebral palsy?**

   A. The initial lesion may progress as the child ages

   B. It always involves a motor impairment

   C. All children diagnosed with cerebral palsy have an apparent lesion on MRI

   D. The type of tone a child has will be constant over his/her lifetime

2. **A lesion in the germinal region of the developing brain that damages pre-oligodendrocytes is known as:**

   A. Intraventricular hemorrhage

   B. Necrotizing enterocolitis

   C. Neonatal stroke

   D. Periventricular leukomalacia

3. **A grade III intraventricular hemorrhage includes which area(s)?**
   A. Endothelial layer only
   B. Endothelial layer plus ventricle
   C. Endothelial layer, ventricle, and brain tissue
   D. Endothelial layer, ventricle, brain tissue, and cortex

4. **A child presents with spasticity in all four extremities, but her arms are more affected than her legs. This child is presenting with:**
   A. Spastic diplegia
   B. Spastic hemiplegia
   C. Spastic quadriplegia
   D. Spastic triplegia

5. **A swan neck deformity involves which body part?**
   A. Ankle
   B. Finger
   C. Knee
   D. Trunk

6. **A child you are working with stares off into space while chewing and picking at her clothes. This is most likely what type of seizure?**
   A. Atonic
   B. Complex partial
   C. Myoclonic
   D. Tonic-clonic

7. **An adolescent with IDD is learning to work at the grocery store, bagging groceries, is able to read street and bus signs to travel to and from the store, and has a few friends from high school with whom he likes to watch football games. This teenager is demonstrating what level of IDD?**
   A. Mild
   B. Moderate
   C. Severe
   D. Profound

8. **Your 7-year-old patient with diplegia walks with equin-ovarus, minimal knee flexion with recurvatum during stance, and frequently tripping when walking. She is demonstrating what gait pattern?**
   A. Ataxic gait
   B. Crouched gait
   C. Stiff-knee gait
   D. Scissor gait

9. **Which of the following comorbidities occur in children with CP at the highest incidence rate?**
   A. Epilepsy
   B. IDD
   C. Sensory dysfunction
   D. Malnutrition

10. **A 4-year-old is walking with forearm crutches independently for all home and community activities except trips to the mall, zoo, or park. This child would likely be classified at which GMFCS level?**
    A. Level I
    B. Level II
    C. Level III
    D. Level IV
    E. Level V

11. **A child has severe spasticity in both UE and LE that is impeding his parents' ability to bath and toilet him. The best spasticity management would most likely be?**
    A. Botulinum toxin injections
    B. Intrathecal baclofen
    C. Surgical lengthening of all flexor tendons
    D. Oral gabapentin

12. **A 3-year-old child at GMFCS level IV with no IDD but severe dystonia, right hip dislocation, and emerging scoliosis would be a candidate for what type of wheelchair?**
    A. A manual chair for self-propulsion
    B. A manual chair for caregiver propulsion
    C. A power chair with an anterior-tilted seat
    D. A power chair with a contour seat

13. **Therapy in the NICU is focused on which of the following?**
    A. Facilitating acquisition of developmental milestones
    B. Facilitating self-regulation
    C. Inhibiting abnormal tone
    D. Maximizing stimulation

14. **The "P" in APGAR stands for which of the following?**
    A. Airway
    B. Heart rate
    C. Color
    D. Respiration
    E. Muscle activity

15. **Which emerging treatment method for children with CP is not focused on increasing postural control and gait?**
    A. Aquatic therapy
    B. CIMT
    C. Hippotherapy
    D. Robotic therapy

16. **A condition of pregnancy characterized by hypertension and proteinuria is?**
    A. Prolapsed umbilical
    B. Placenta abruption
    C. Placental previa
    D. Pre-eclampsia

Answers

1. B	**2.** D	**3.** B	**4.** C	**5.** B
6. B	**7.** B	**8.** C	**9.** C	**10.** C
11. B	**12.** D	**13.** B	**14.** B	**15.** B
16. D				

Developmental Disabilities

20

Deborah S. Nichols-Larsen and Jill C. Heathcock

OBJECTIVES

1) Differentiate the pathophysiology of common developmental disorders

2) Distinguish the diagnostic criteria of common developmental disorders

3) Compare the treatment needs of children with common developmental disorders from those discussed for children with cerebral palsy

● INTRODUCTION

The term "developmental disorder" or "developmental disability" refers to any injury or disease that occurs prior to the age of 18 and disrupts the acquisition of typical developmental milestones, including motor, cognitive, language, and psychosocial skills.[1] Thus, this term includes a vast number of disorders; however, in this chapter, we are going to focus on those disorders commonly seen by physical therapists. We have separated out the two most common developmental disorders in their own chapters – cerebral palsy and myelomeningocele; however, it should be remembered that these are also developmental disorders.

As the time of onset (birth–18 years) indicates, developmental disabilities can occur throughout childhood and adolescence. However, many are present at birth (**congenital**), occurring **prenatally** (prior to birth) or **perinatally** (during or close to the time of birth). Others occur **postnatally**, often the result of trauma or disease processes that impact the nervous system (e.g., meningitis). In this chapter, we will focus on those that are congenital; it should be noted that many congenital disorders are not diagnosed until much later in the developmental period. Causes of congenital disorders may be known (genetic – chromosomal anomaly or inherited, birth trauma, environmental exposure) or unknown (e.g., developmental coordination disorder), yet their presentations may be quite similar or highly unique. This chapter will focus on the common and unique elements of these disorders.

CASE A, PART I

Pauli Sabat is a 40-month-old little girl of Latino heritage, whose parents immigrated to the United States from Argentina a year before her birth, initially on student visas but now on work visas; both are college educated – Dr. Sabat as a PhD in physics and Mrs. Sabat as a computer scientist. They have scheduled an appointment at a diagnostic clinic for children with developmental disorders. They report that Pauli is not keeping up with the other kids at daycare; she doesn't run, doesn't catch or throw a ball like her peers, continues to walk up and down stairs with a two-step/stair pattern, while holding the railing, and tends to be easily distracted, rushing from one toy to another without spending more than 30 seconds with any one of them. She also has limited verbal language skills, mostly repeating syllables of words that she hears but not really initiating speech; she does say mama and papa appropriately but infrequently. Although she is being raised in a bilingual home, her parents report that her speech development is much slower than her two older siblings. However, she does seem to understand what is said to her, following directions like "come here" but inconsistently, both in English and Spanish. She feeds herself but prefers her fingers to utensils and is a very picky eater, eating pancakes, hot dogs, chicken nuggets, tater tots, and apples (peels removed) but no other foods. She can dress herself except for shoes and socks but is also very picky about the texture of the clothes that she wears, becoming very agitated in rough textures and requiring that all tags be removed from her clothing. She is not an affectionate child, rarely giving hugs as her siblings do, yet she is hardly ever fussy either. She tends to amuse herself with toys and still takes a 2-hour afternoon nap, while sleeping 10 hours at night, typically without waking. She is not toilet trained and has refused all attempts to do so. She also resists having her teeth brushed but will chew on the toothbrush; her hair is cut short because she hates to have it brushed or any type of barrette or band in it. Although she has received some medical care over the last 3 years, they have moved twice as a result of Mr. Sabat's change in work – first completing his doctorate, then a post-doc, and finally a faculty position. Thus, her developmental profile is incomplete, based on limited follow-up with medical providers.

● MEDICAL DIAGNOSIS

The diagnosis of a given developmental disorder often begins with a diagnostic workup that will include a detailed family and pregnancy history, a comprehensive developmental assessment and potentially laboratory, imaging, and genetic testing; although the physician will likely initiate the assessment with a comprehensive morphometric, neurologic, and physical examination; other professionals (physical therapist, occupational therapist, speech and language pathologist, and developmental psychologist) are typically involved in this comprehensive assessment. In the case of Pauli, she appears to have a global developmental delay (significant delay in two or more areas – motor, language, intellectual). Normally, this diagnosis is based on a delay of ≥2.0 standard deviations (SD) on a standardized test in each of these areas, so confirmation of this will occur via appropriate testing.[2]

CASE A, PART II

Pauli's parents report an uncomplicated pregnancy and full term delivery. This was their third pregnancy and live birth. Mrs. Sabat received prenatal care at the University student clinic with one ultrasound at 15 weeks with no abnormalities noted; the delivery was vaginal after an 8-hour labor. The perinatal period was uncomplicated, and mother and baby were discharged home after 42 hours. Mrs. S reports that Pauli was a fussy baby, who didn't nurse like her other children (Lilliana – age 5 and Simon – age 7) and was primarily fed with a bottle, which worked much better. Pauli was slow to transition to soft foods; although she ate cereal fairly well, if quite thick, she did not progress to fruits and vegetables easily and has never eaten rice or pasta. Once her first eight teeth had erupted (approximately 13 months), she transitioned to solid foods, primarily those listed earlier. She will also eat snack foods, such as crackers and goldfish crackers as well as some plain hard cookies. Although Pauli began verbalizing as the other two children had, Mrs. S reports that she is more likely to grunt or point to make her needs known; her verbal speech consists of mama, papa, ball, up, down, and no. For the most part, she has been healthy except for 2–3 ear infections per year and has never required hospitalization. She rolled over at 6 months, sat and pulled to stand at 12 months, and began walking at 17 months. She uses both hands for play, not demonstrating any hand preference, scribbles when given a crayon, takes apart many of her toys, demonstrating good dexterity, but doesn't complete puzzles or put shapes in a shape-sorter.

The other two children in the household are in kindergarten and second grade, both achieving at or above age level in their schoolwork, despite moving to the United States just a few years ago, and participating in many extra-curricular activities, including soccer, piano lessons, karate, and swimming. They are bilingual, speaking Spanish in the home and English at school and with friends. Neither has any health issue and their developmental history is unremarkable.

Physical Examination

The physical examination will typically begin with growth measurements: height, weight, and head circumferences. Growth tables are available to plot these measures across gender and age. Many children with developmental disabilities are small for age, which may relate to feeding or eating issues, such as displayed by Pauli, or growth differences may be part of a more complex pathology, such as Down syndrome. Similarly, extreme differences in head circumference (2 or more SD from the mean for age and gender) can be indicative of specific developmental syndromes or disorders. **Microcephaly** refers to a small head circumference in association with normal growth of other facial features, while **macrocephaly** refers to a larger than normal head circumference. Each of these is more than just a difference in cranium size, including an underlying difference in brain development. Additionally, the physical examination should look for any other **dysmorphic feature**, which is an asymmetry or abnormality of a body structure that can be as simple as having one ear lower than the other or much more complex, such as the characteristic look of a child with Down syndrome; again, many developmental disabilities are associated with specific dysmorphic features, especially the many genetic syndromes that result in a specific array of features. So, the physical examination looks for asymmetries in the face and body structure as well as general range of motion. Furthermore, a neurologic examination (as described in Chapter 9) should be conducted to assess reflexes, muscle tone, strength, and age specific motor, language and cognition skills. From a medical standpoint, this is typically a brief screening with subsequent referral to physical and/or occupational therapy, if delay is noted. In children with speech delay, a comprehensive hearing and speech evaluation should be conducted to assure adequate hearing to support speech perception and language development as well as to document any language delay; this should be conducted by an audiologist and speech/language pathologist, respectively.

CASE A, PART III

Pauli measures at the 15th—20th percentile for height, weight, and head circumference, so although generally small for age, she is at the 40th percentile of weight for height and is neither micro nor macrocephalic. She is mildly hypotonic with normal tendon reflexes and slight joint hypermobility (typically associated with hypotonia), including moderate pes planus (flat feet). At the physician's office, she did not respond to commands to walk forward or backward, stand on one foot, or jump, so she was referred to both physical and occupational therapy for further assessment (see Box 20-1). Due to her language delay, she was evaluated first by an audiologist, who found her responses to be inconsistent, although she startled to louder sounds, indicating some degree of hearing, but tended to ignore directions and softer sounds. The speech/language pathologist identified a significant language delay (see Table 20-1 for typical language milestones); based on the table, her language skills are at the 9–12 month level.

BOX 20-1 Methods of Genetic Inheritance

Our attributes (e.g., hair color, eye color, height, and body type) are the result of genetic inheritance. At conception, the chromosomes of the mother join with those of the father, resulting in gene pairing; it is this pairing that decides how the traits of our parents will be expressed (or not). Traits can be either dominant or recessive. For a dominant trait, only one allele (gene component that carries the trait) is necessary to express the trait (e.g., brown eyes); for a recessive trait, both genes must carry the trait in order for it to be expressed (e.g., blue eyes). In this example (eye color), if both parents have blue eyes, their children will all have blue eyes; however, as is depicted in Figure 20-1, when parents both have brown eyes or one has blue and the other brown, their children's eye color can be either brown or blue, depending on which genes are contained within the egg and sperm at conception. If two parents both have both alleles for brown eyes (BB), then all of their children will have brown eyes (the reverse of "A" in Figure 20-1). Traits carried on the X or Y gene are considered sex-linked; all others are considered autosomal.

Genetically inherited disorders can also be inherited through dominant or recessive transmission. With recessive inheritance, both parents must carry the genetic defect for the child to manifest the disorder; with dominant inheritance, the parent would also manifest the disease but often to a lesser degree than the child. Notably, there are many genetic disorders associated with the X chromosome. *Remember that girls have two X chromosomes, but boys have an X and a Y chromosome.* So, if a dominant defect is carried on one of the mother's X chromosomes and not the father's, 50% of the children (both boys and girls) will have the disorder (20-2A). However, if the defect is carried on the father's X chromosome and not the mother's, all of his daughters will have the disease, and none of his sons will have the disease (20-2B). If the mother has a recessive mutation on the X chromosome, she will not manifest the disease but serves as a carrier, transmitting the defect to 50% of her daughters, who will also be carriers, and 50% of her sons, who will manifest the disorder (20-2C).

TABLE 20-1	Language Milestones Birth–4 Years[3,4]
AGE	**LANGUAGE SKILL**
Language production	
0–2 months	Cries
2–4 months	Vocalizations other than crying, beginning with vowel sounds such as "oo" and "aa" Responds to heard vocalization with sounds of their own
4–9 months	Babbling – playing with sounds, eliminate sounds not heard in their native language; mama, dada without meaning; laughs
9–12 months	First words – typically mama, dada; imitates sounds; waves for bye and hello
12–15 months	Single words to express sentences (at least 3 words with meaning), expanding vocabulary; animal sounds
15–18 months	Vocabulary increased to 6–10 words
18–24 months	Rapid vocabulary expansion; two-word sentences initiated (noun + verb; e.g., dada away); naming pictures initiated
24–30 months	400-word vocabulary, 50% of production is understandable; two-word sentences initiated; begins imitating words heard
30–36 months	Beginning use of adjectives (big, little); understandability increases to 100%; 700+ words; sentence length of 3–5 words
3–4 years	Naming of colors, defining of words begins; sentence length increases to 5–8 words; begins asking questions
4–5 years	Clearly understandable by others
Language reception	
0–2 months	Responds to loud noises with startle or awakening.
2–4 months	Responds to familiar voice by calming.
4–6 months	Turns to sounds/voice; begin to distinguish sounds, especially mother's voice
6–9 months	Change vocalizations to those that are heard
9–12 months	Respond to simple words (bye-bye, no, food items); follows a one-step command; knows name; begins to point to named picture

(Continued)

TABLE 20-1	Language Milestones Birth–4 Years[3,4] (*Continued*)
AGE	**LANGUAGE SKILL**
12–18 months	Begin to follow commands and point to body parts
18–24 months	Expanding identification of body parts and understanding of words and commands
24–30 months	Can point to at least 6 body parts; listens to short story (5–10 minutes)
30–36 months	Begins to follow two-step commands (e.g., get the toy and bring it to me)
3–4 years	Begins to answer questions (e.g., who, where)
4–5 years	Shows understanding of longer stories (>short stories)

Laboratory Testing

Genetic Testing

Genetic testing is not always done for children with developmental delay, especially when the cause is known (e.g., infantile stroke) but can help to rule out or diagnose potential causes of a global delay. Genetic disorders can be **inherited** from one or both parents or the product of a genetic mutation, also referred to as an **acquired mutation**. Acquired genetic mutations that occur during gestation, typically occur at the point of conception or very soon afterward. If they occur at conception, every cell in the body will have the mutation; if they occur at a later point, only a portion of the body's cells will have the mutation and the presentation of the disorder will typically be milder than a defect that happens at conception. A genetic mutation is a disruption in the DNA sequence that occurs as cells are rapidly multiplying. *Remember that in typical cell mitosis, the two strands of DNA separate and then are duplicated, making two complete DNA strands that become part of the **offspring cells**, which in turn, will duplicate the DNA strands and produce additional offspring cells.*

Mutations occur from four basic errors: (1) translocation – the gene or portion of the DNA chain replicates in a different location than normal; (2) duplication – when the DNA strands initially separate, one chromosome pair fails to separate and the resultant cells have three of a given chromosome; (3) deletion – loss of a part of the DNA strand; or (4) inversion – a gene or fragment of the strand breaks off and then reattaches in a reverse (upside down) orientation.

For children with an obvious genetic defect (e.g., Down syndrome), for which there is a specific genetic test, a karyotyping analysis is done to confirm the presence of the abnormal or mutated gene and determine the percentage of cells with the mutation. Box 20-2 outlines the genetic manifestations of Down syndrome. When there is a global delay without an obvious genetic disorder, a chromosomal microarray (CMA) may be ordered. This type of analysis looks for duplications and deletions within the DNA strands, which can identify inherited conditions or acquired mutations.[5] For those with a normal CMA analysis, additional genetic

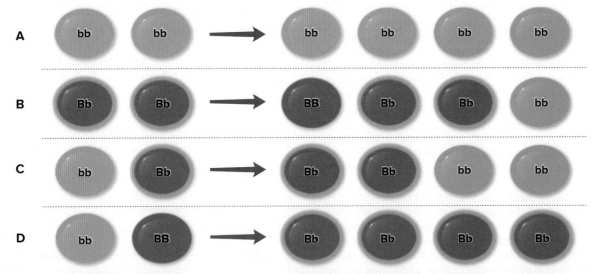

FIGURE 20-1 Genetic inheritance (potential trait expression with possible allele pairings). B = dominant gene for brown eyes; b = recessive gene for blue eyes. **A.** Two blue-eyed parents each have two genes for blue eyes (bb), so they will have all blue-eyed children (it is possible that both parents could have two genes for brown eyes (BB + BB), and then, similarly, all of their children will have brown eyes). **B.** Two brown-eyed parents with one gene for brown eyes (B) and one for blue eyes (b), depicted by the blue circle around the brown, have a 50/50 chance of contributing either the brown or blue-eyed gene to the embryo, and thus, there is a 75/25 chance that the child will have brown (BB or Bb) or blue eyes (bb). **C.** When there is one brown eyed parent with both a blue and brown allele (Bb) and one blue eyed parent (bb), the blue-eyed parent will always contribute a blue-eyed gene, but the brown-eyed parent has a 50/50 chance of contributing a brown or blue-eyed gene, resulting in only a 50% chance that the child will have brown eyes (Bb). **D.** A blue-eyed parent and a brown-eyed parent with both genes for brown eyes (BB), will always have brown-eyed children, but they will all carry a blue-eyed gene (Bb). (Used with permission of Deborah S. Nichols Larsen, PT, PhD. The Ohio State University.)

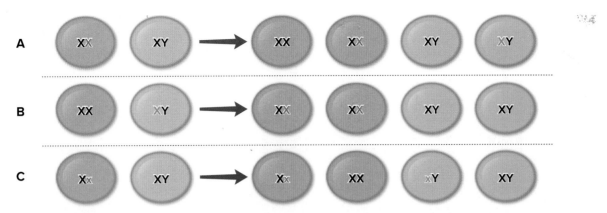

FIGURE 20-2 X-linked Inheritance. A) Trait manifested in mother as a dominant gene; all children have a 50% chance of inheriting the trait; **B)** Dominant trait carried by father on the X chromosome will be manifested in all daughters. **C)** When a recessive trait is carried by mother, 50% of the daughters will be carriers and 50% of the sons will have the disorder. X = normal X chromosome; X = trait carrying; left side of diagram: pink oval = mother's genes; blue oval = father's genes. Right side of diagram = genetic possibilities for offspring (pink = girls; blue = boys). (Used with permission of Deborah S. Nichols Larsen, PT, PhD. The Ohio State University.)

BOX 20-2	Genetic Causes of Down Syndrome

A good example of the variability in acquired genetic mutations can be seen in Down syndrome (DS), which is caused by an additional 21st chromosome. In the most common presentation, **Trisomy 21**, which accounts for 90+% of children with this disorder, there is duplication at conception of the 21st chromosome in either the egg or sperm at fertilization, resulting in a third 21st chromosome in all cells of the body. However, in some children, this duplication happens at some time after conception, resulting in three 21st chromosomes in only a portion of the child's cells; this type of DS is referred to as **Mosaic Trisomy 21**, accounting for about 2% of children with DS. Finally, for some children (less than 5%), the extra 21st chromosome (or a fragment of it) attaches at a different point in the DNA strand (**translocation**), commonly on the 14th chromosome. It should be noted that in a small percentage of children with translocation DS, the chromosomal mutation will be present in some cells of a parent, and thus, it is an **inherited mutation**. We will discuss the presentation of children with DS later in this chapter, but it should be noted that those with mosaicism or translocation will typically manifest the characteristics of the syndrome to a lesser degree than children with Trisomy 21.

buildup in the blood or urine. The genetic defects for many of these disorders have been identified. One example of this type of disorder, as listed in Table 20-2, is Phenylketonuria (PKU), for which all newborns in the United States are screened prior to going home from the hospital. Table 20-3 outlines these groups of disorders that have variable presentations and outcomes; some are treatable (e.g., PKU) but others are still lethal (e.g., Tay–Sachs).

Imaging

Imaging of infants and young children is rarely done as part of the diagnostic process, although many disorders have characteristic (e.g., Down syndrome) or definitive findings (e.g., cerebral palsy), when imaging is done; magnetic resonance imaging (MRI) has been found to be the preferred method of imaging over computerized tomography (CT). Most imaging requires sedation in young children and, therefore, is not done unless imaging is needed for analysis of an obvious anomaly (e.g., orthopedic malformation). Recent success in conducting MRI imaging in sleeping infants without sedative medication holds promise for increased use of this modality to evaluate neurologic lesions in young children.

testing may be done, including gene panels that examine specific genes, or X chromosome analysis because of the number of disorders associated with X chromosome abnormalities (e.g., Fragile X syndrome, Rett syndrome).[6] Table 20-2 describes common developmental disorders that are known to have a genetic mutation or inherited transmission that may be seen by a physical therapist.

Metabolic Testing

There are a group of disorders that result from what is known as inborn errors in metabolism, which stem from a disruption in the metabolism of amino acids (e.g., creatine), carbohydrates, or lipids, usually due to a single gene anomaly that disrupts the encoding of an enzyme that is necessary to metabolize a given substrate. Blood testing or urinalysis will identify metabolite

---

CASE A, PART IV

Pauli's chromosomal array did not identify any genetic mutations nor did a secondary X chromosome analysis. Her metabolic tests were also normal. No imaging was ordered. Thus, Pauli's medical diagnosis for the time being will remain idiopathic global developmental delay, which means the cause is unknown. This is not an uncommon diagnosis, especially for children at a relatively young age (<4) with signs of mild to moderate global delay. Continued observation by the family physician and potentially a referral to a pediatric neurologist or physiatrist may occur. However, some diagnoses (e.g., autism spectrum disorders) become more evident as the child ages.

TABLE 20-2 Common Developmental Disorders with a Genetic Cause

GENETIC DISORDER	GENETIC ABNORMALITY	PRESENTATION	DIAGNOSIS	MEDICAL MANAGEMENT
Angelman syndrome[7]	Deletion of a gene (UBE3A) on the 15th chromosome, typically from the father, allowing overexpression of the maternal 15th chromosome[7]	Severe intellectual disability; global developmental delay with limited speech development; balance problems/ataxia; seizure disorder with abnormal EEG; hyperactivity, dysmorphic features (microcephaly, jaw protrusion, protruding tongue, teeth wide-spaced, deep set eyes), hypopigmentation, sleep pattern disruption, happy disposition with arm/hand flapping[8]	Clinical presentation of global delay with limited speech, dysmorphic features, and unusually happy disposition. Genetic testing to identify the chromosomal anomaly.[8]	Pharmacological seizure management; treatment of associated disorders (gastrointestinal reflux, surgery to correct strabismus; surgical correction of associated orthopedic problems – scoliosis, plantarflexor shortening)[9]
Becker Muscular Dystrophy[10]	Mutation of the DMD gene on the X chromosome, which is critical for the development of dystrophin (a protein that anchors muscle fibers to the extracellular matrix), resulting in an abnormal form of dystrophin; occurs only in boys.	Progressive muscle weakness (proximal greater than distil), beginning in late childhood (age 10). Calf hypertrophy as in Duchenne but ambulate until late teens or early adulthood	Elevated creatine kinase; abnormal dystrophin in muscle biopsy; genetic analysis of the DMD gene	Similar to Duchenne MD but without corticosteroid treatment.
Charcot–Marie–Tooth disease[11]	Multiple genetic anomalies, some with autosomal dominant inheritance and others X-linked or autosomal recessive inheritance, with up to 40 genes involved	Most common progressive peripheral demyelinating neuropathy of both sensory and motor nerves (motor more impaired than sensory) with loss of reflexes, beginning distally, with variable onset (infancy–adulthood) and presentation. Pes cavus deformity is common, caused by loss of intrinsic foot muscle function.	Genetic testing	Surgical correction of orthopedic deformities; pharmacologic management of pain.
Cri-du-chat[12]	Deletion of the short-arm of chromosome 5	High-pitched "cat like" cry with facial dysmorphic features (broad nose, epicanthal folds, small jaw, microcephaly); small for age (weight more than height); severe mental retardation with global developmental delay and behavioral problems (hyperactivity, self-injurious or aggressive behavior, stereotypic behavior); hypotonia; potential organ malformations (heart, kidneys)	Initial diagnosis is often based on observation of the dysmorphic features and the cry with secondary karyotype genetic testing.	No specific medical management; only developmental support.

Disorder	Genetics	Pathophysiology	Diagnosis	Management
Cystic Fibrosis[13]	Autosomal inheritance of a mutation on chromosome 7, resulting in a deficiency of the transmembrane conductance regulator protein (CFTR) that functions to control permeability of the chloride ion channel.	Thickening of secretions in the lungs, intestines, pancreas, and gall bladder associated with chronic infections and nutritional issues.	Newborn screening for a pancreatic enzyme (immunoreactive trypsinogen); DNA testing; sweat test for elevated chloride ($\geq$60 mmole/L)	Maintaining airways through postural drainage/percussion/chest compression; use of bronchodilators; frequent culturing for infections with early or prophylactic treatment; anti-inflammatory drug treatment; new CFTR modulating drugs to target chloride channel function.
Down syndrome	Mutation of chromosome 21 with duplication at conception (Trisomy 21) or later in cell proliferation (Mosaic Trisomy 21) or translocation (most frequently onto chromosome 14). Increased prevalence with maternal age.	Abnormal brain development, mental retardation, hypotonia with joint laxity, dysmorphic features (epicanthal folds, small mouth that allows tongue to protrude, single palmar crease, short/curved little finger, low set ears), potential for cardiac, GI, or other organ malformations, with aging, Alzheimer's disease is common.[14]	Screening – Maternal blood test for elevated human chorionic gonadotropin and pregnancy-associated plasma protein-A with ultrasound to measure Nuchal Translucency (measures the amount of fluid at the upper cervical spine), which is greater with DS. Subsequent amniocentesis and karyotyping if DS is suspected. Diagnosis after birth includes observation of dysmorphic features and karyotyping.[15]	Well child care with attention to potential comorbidities and specific treatment for those present: (1) Auditory – otitis media, conductive hearing loss (2) Visual – congenital cataracts, strabismus, nystagmus, glaucoma (3) Oral – feeding issues, speech delay (4) Congenital heart defects (5) Endocrine – diabetes, hypo or hyperthyroidism (6) Hematologic – leukemia (7) Neurologic – seizures, mental retardation, autism, developmental delay (8) Orthopedic – joint laxity, atlanto-occipital instability (9) Dermatology – folliculitis, hyperkeratosis, seborrhea[14]
Duchenne Muscular Dystrophy[10]	Mutation of the DMD gene on the X chromosome, resulting in a complete absence of functional dystrophin in affected boys	Progressive muscle weakness (proximal more than distil) in early childhood (ages 2–5) with toe walking and muscle pseudohypertrophy (loss of muscle with fat replacement) early, followed by loss of ambulation ability (late childhood) and progressive respiratory and cardiac compromise, leading to death in late adolescence/early adulthood	Elevated creatine kinase; absent dystrophin in muscle biopsy; genetic analysis of the DMD gene	Corticosteroid treatment to support muscle function with management of the side effects of this treatment (weight gain, osteoporosis, cataracts, delayed sexual maturity); gene therapy; pharmacologic management of associated cardiomyopathy; respiratory exercises and support (ventilators); managing orthopedic changes (e.g., scoliosis) with potential surgery or bracing. Surgery needs to be carefully considered due to potential respiratory compromise.

(Continued)

TABLE 20-2 Common Developmental Disorders with a Genetic Cause *(Continued)*

GENETIC DISORDER	GENETIC ABNORMALITY	PRESENTATION	DIAGNOSIS	MEDICAL MANAGEMENT
Fragile X syndrome	Disruption of a gene, named the Fragile X Mental Retardation gene 1 (FMR1) that is critical to the development of an RNA binding protein necessary for neuronal development, specifically dendrite formation. X-chromosome linked with many adults (much more frequent in women) carrying an incomplete defect (permutation) without notable symptoms.[16]	Milder but more frequent presentation in girls than boys. Intellectual disability, global delay, hyperactivity and attention deficits with autistic symptoms, frequently seizures and sleep disturbances, facial dysmorphic features. Carriers may demonstrate hyperactivity, attention deficit, learning disabilities, and behavioral problems.[16]	Observation of developmental delay with subsequent X chromosomal analysis[16]	New focus on pharmacologic management, targeting GABA and glutamate receptors (antagonists), to control seizures, psychiatric, and behavioral symptoms.[17]
Niemann–Pick disease[18]	An autosomal inherited disorder of the NPC1 on chromosome 18 or NPC2 gene on chromosome 14 that disrupts lysosomal lipid storage (cholesterol, sphingomyelin, glycolipids) with secondary buildup in tissues.	Variable onset from infancy to adulthood with liver, spleen, and nervous system abnormalities, including vertical supranuclear palsy, and later respiratory failure. Early infantile onset (2 months–2 years) – enlarged liver/spleen, initial hypotonia that progresses to spasticity, motor delay and eventual loss of motor skills, intention tremor; typically die by age 5. Childhood onset (2–6 years) – ataxia, clumsiness, dysarthria, dysphagia, intention tremor, intellectual disability, vertical supranuclear palsy. Seizures and dystonia are also common. Survive to ages 7–12.	Delayed motor development and an enlarged liver/spleen are early signs in infants and children. Skin or liver biopsy plus serum analysis for abnormal cholesterol measures, followed by NPC1 and NPC2 sequencing.	Symptom specific (e.g., seizure medications to control seizures); recently, pharmacological administration of iminosaccaride inhibitors (e.g., miglustat) have had some success.
Prader–Willi syndrome	Deletion of multiple genes on the 15th chromosome, typically from the maternal contribution, allowing the paternal 15th chromosomal contribution to be overexpressed[7]	Initial failure to thrive, followed by excessive eating (hyperphagia) in childhood; global developmental delay; mental retardation or learning disabilities; behavioral problems, impaired psychosocial development; abnormal sleep patterns; hypogonadism with disrupted sexual maturation. Symptoms are related to hypothalamus malfunction.[19]	DNA methylation testing.[19]	Pharmacologic management with human growth hormone and sex steroid treatments. Behavioral treatment to control diet and provide a feeling of food security.[20]

Condition	Etiology	Description	Diagnosis	Treatment
Phenyl-ketonuria (PKU)[21]	Autosomal recessive inheritance of a mutation of the phenylalanine hydroxylase (PAH) gene, resulting in an absence of PAH, which is a key enzyme necessary for neurotransmitter production	Without treatment, severe mental retardation occurs; however, with neonatal diagnosis and implementation of standard treatment, children develop normally but poor bone density due to limited protein consumption is common. Diet lapses can result in deterioration of brain function.	Neonatal blood screening for elevated phenylalanine levels	Diet low in phenylalanine, which is found in many foods, especially proteins, and amino acid supplementation for brain development and neurotransmitter maintenance.
Rett syndrome[22]	X-linked chromosomal mutation of the gene that encodes methyl-CpG binding protein, resulting in disrupted synapse formation within neural networks, primarily in boys in infancy; occasionally, males with XXY genotype survive with similar presentation to girls plus Klinefelter's syndrome.	Normal development up to 18 months with subsequent loss of neural function, resulting in intellectual disability, loss of motor skills, seizure onset and autistic behaviors (hand-wringing, poor communication).	Observed loss of motor and communication skills with slowing head circumference growth and emergence of stereotypical movements (hand wringing). Genetic testing for the MECP2 gene mutation confirms the diagnosis in most girls.	Symptomatic (e.g., pharmacologic seizure management; orthopedic management of scoliosis that can develop)
Spinal Muscular Atrophy[23]	Deletion or mutation of the SMN1 gene, resulting in loss of the SMN (survival motor neuron) protein with ultimate loss of alpha motor neurons throughout the spinal cord and resultant loss of muscle fibers; inherited through autosomal recessive inheritance	Type I – present at birth, limited antigravity movement with no acquisition of motor milestones, life expectancy <2 years (leading genetic cause of infant death) Type II – diagnosis in first 18 months of life with progressive muscle weakness, will sit but not walk, life expectancy to teenage/early adulthood Type III – diagnosed after 18 months, walk independently with later progressive muscle weakness, life expectancy is near normal Type IV – diagnosed at adulthood, normal life expectancy	Genetic analysis to confirm the SMN1 mutation.	Symptomatic – respiratory support (oxygen, ventilator); nutrition support (feeding tubes); selection of adaptive equipment to maximize function and adapt the home for caregiving. Focus is on developing gene therapies to increase SMN protein.
Trisomy 18 (Edwards syndrome)	Genetic mutation at conception, resulting in three 18th chromosomes[24]	Multiple organ defects, especially congenital heart defects (many types) and dysmorphic features (e.g., skull malformations, finger anomalies); 75% mortality in first year of life with severe global developmental delay in survivors, some of whom have lived into their 20s.[24]	Physical appearance typically identifies the condition that is confirmed by karyotyping.[24]	Surgical correction of organ defects (CHD); respiratory support; assisted feeding (gastrointestinal tubes); in some cases, only palliative care is provided.[25]
Wilson's disease[26]	Mutations of the ATP7B gene, resulting in disruption of copper metabolism, with autosomal recessive inheritance	Buildup of copper in tissues with brain and liver most vulnerable, resulting in progressive neural and liver damage.	Difficult diagnosis, often delayed until symptoms present, which can be as early as 4 but as late as 20+; no effective infant screening. Blood and urine tests for copper, confirmed by DNA testing are diagnostic.	Copper chelating agents plus zinc salts to decrease copper absorption from the gastrointestinal system, which can stabilize or result in improvements in symptoms.

TABLE 20-3 | **Inborn Errors of Metabolism**

INBORN ERROR	DESCRIPTION/PRESENTATION	DIAGNOSIS/TREATMENT
Lysosomal storage disorders[27] • Autosomal recessive inheritance or X-linked inheritance • Examples: Hunter syndrome, Turner syndrome, Danon disease, Fabry disease, Niemann–Pick, Tay–Sachs	Variable, often neurologic with global developmental delay, ataxia, seizures, some variants have dysmorphic features; at older ages, strokes, neuropathies, and extrapyramidal symptoms may present. Liver and spleen enlargement due to accumulation of un-metabolized macromolecules. Tay–Sachs and other GM2 gangliosidosis disorders are neurodegenerative, characterized by loss of motor skills (head control, sitting), increasing hypotonia and exaggerated startle.[28]	Brain imaging, skeletal x-rays for abnormalities, and ultrasound for liver enlargement Symptomatic treatment (e.g., antiepileptics for seizures); enzyme replacement therapy or hematopoietic stem cell transplantation. No effective treatment for GM2 gangliosidosis disorders (Tay Sachs), which are ultimately lethal before age 5.[27,28]
Sterol synthesis disorders[29] • Disruption in cholesterol storage/metabolism • Examples: Smith–Lemli–Opitz syndrome, Antley–Bixler syndrome, CK syndrome	Cholesterol is critical for neuronal cell membrane and myelin formation and derived from sterols (precursors). Presentation is highly variable but can include dysmorphic features (cleft palate, microcephaly, limb anomalies), GI symptoms, congenital heart defects, global developmental delay with motor and speech delays, sleep disturbances, self-injurious behaviors, tactile hypersensitivity, autistic behaviors	Blood or urine analysis for specific markers; skin analysis for some disorders. No effective medical treatment.
Creatine deficiency disorders[30] • Autosomal recessive	Disruption in the metabolism of creatine, which is necessary to support cellular energy, especially in the brain and muscles. Mild to severe global delay, behavioral problems, and seizures.	Abnormal creatine in urine (high/low). Enzymatic assays, followed by genetic testing, is diagnostic. Treatment is focused on creatine supplementation or creatine precursor supplementation

PHYSICAL THERAPY ASSESSMENT

To evaluate Pauli, there are many standardized tests that can be used with the Bayley Scales of Infant and Toddler Development[31] and the Peabody Developmental Motor Scales[32] the most commonly used. Since the Bayley is aimed at children 0–3½ years of age and given Pauli's current age (40 months), the therapist has chosen to use the Peabody, which will allow documentation of her motor skills through age 5 (or longer given a motor delay). For most developmental scales, the evaluator determines a basal level (the last level at which the child completes all items) and then a ceiling level (the first level at which the child doesn't pass any item). Then, there is a process for converting these raw scores into a standard score, typically a z-score, which indicates the difference from the mean (SD).

CASE A, PART V

Pauli's PDMS assessment indicated a basal level of 13 months and a ceiling level of 19–20 months for the gross motor subscales. This gave her a z-score of −3.53, which places her 3.5 SD from her age-matched peers and in the bottom percentile for children her age.[32] From this assessment, Pauli should be receiving physical therapy as part of an early intervention

(EI) program. Goals for therapy should focus on (1) increasing strength to improve stability for single limb stance activities (stair climbing, kicking a ball); (2) improving locomotion skills such as stair climbing, negotiating obstacles and complex environments, walking backward or on a line, and running; and (3) object manipulation skills – throwing, catching, and kicking. A challenge for the therapist will be getting Pauli to follow directions and interact with the therapist for play skills such as throwing and kicking. Working with the educational team, the physical therapist should include behavioral management techniques to promote desired behaviors and minimize unwanted behaviors. Some group play activities will be beneficial to facilitate peer engagement and social skills such as turn taking.

COMMON DEVELOPMENTAL DISABILITIES

Down Syndrome

As mentioned earlier in the chapter, Down syndrome (DS) is one of the most common developmental disabilities; it results from a genetic mutation during conception or soon after, resulting in either three 21st chromosomes (Trisomy 21 or Mosaic Trisomy 21) or a translocation of the 21st chromosome, typically to the 14th chromosome. The occurrence of DS increases as maternal age increases with those 35–40 at greater risk. Currently, most expectant mothers undergo a screening process to diagnose DS, other potential trisomies (e.g., Trisomy 18), and neural tube disorders (e.g., myelomeningocele), during the first trimester of pregnancy. Markers for DS include serum biomarkers (free β-hCG, pregnancy associated plasma protein-A [PAPP-A]) and ultrasound examination of *Nuchal Translucency*, which measures an area of fluid buildup in the cervical spine between the cervical spine and the skin that is increased in children with DS as well as those with Trisomy 18.[15]

Intellectual Disability in DS

DS is the most common cause of **intellectual disability** (ID) in children, yet the degree of ID varies considerably in children with DS. Most children have a moderate level of ID (>70%) but some have a mild (7%) or severe (7%) level of ID. Interestingly, 7% of children with DS have normal intelligence. The ID in DS is characterized by poor short-term verbal and long-term explicit memory (facts, episodic) but good visuo-spatial short-term and implicit (procedural) long-term memory. Further, the ID interacts with language development to result in a delay in language skills. Children with DS also often demonstrate behavioral problems (attention deficit, hyperactivity, autistic features).[33]

Dysmorphic Features of DS

There are multiple features of DS that may be present in children with a DS diagnosis (Figure 20-3; not all children have all of these): (1) hypotonia – low muscle tone with joint hypermobility (often the first thing noted at birth); (2) epicanthal folds – an extra fold of skin on the upper eyelid between the nose and the eyebrow; (3) flat nasal bridge; (4) short or curved 5th fingers; (5) single palmar crease; (6) low set ears with a folded meatus; (7) gap between the great toe and the 2nd toe; (8) high palate and small oral cavity with hypotonia of the tongue, leading to a protruding tongue. Some of these, commonly hypotonia and epicanthal folds, are obvious at birth; others become more evident as the child ages.[14]

Organ Anomalies

In addition to the dysmorphic features listed above, there is an increased incidence of congenital organ anomalies in children with DS. Most common are **congenital heart defects** (ventricular septal defects, atrioventricular canal defects), which occur in approximately 50% of children with DS, so all children will undergo an electrocardiogram to screen for a defect in the first days of life. Also common are **gastrointestinal defects**, such as atresia of the esophagus or duodenum, tracheoesophageal fistulas, pyloric stenosis, Hirschsprung's disease or Meckel's diverticulum, and gastroesophageal reflux. Diagnosis of these disorders may require a GI series (barium enema with CT scan; barium swallow), and treatment requires immediate surgical correction. Eating problems are also common due to gastroesophageal reflux and oral musculature hypotonia, which may necessitate special feeding measures such as thickening of liquids and

FIGURE 20-3 Dysmorphic features of Down syndrome. A. This little girl demonstrates the common epicanthal folds, flat nasal bridge, low set ears, and lax oral musculature of Down syndrome. **B.** Single palmar crease associated with Down syndrome (note – this type of single crease is found in many children and adults without DS). (Part A: Reproduced with permission from Jorde LB, Carey JC, Bamshad MJ, White RL. *Medical Genetics.* St. Louis, MO: CV Mosby; 2000.)

evaluation of different nipple types for best feeding. Reflux is worrisome as aspiration may occur; with repeated aspiration, lung infections, such as pneumonia, may occur, so it is critical to find feeding methods that prevent aspiration and maximize nutrition.[14]

Brain Differences in DS

There has been considerable research into the causative brain changes that are responsible for many of the cognitive, learning, motor, and behavioral deficits found in DS. The brain, itself, is small in DS, especially the frontal and temporal lobes, including the hippocampus and surrounding areas, as well as the cerebellum. As discussed in Chapter 7, the temporal and frontal lobes are particularly critical to episodic memory and executive function, both of which are typically impaired with DS. The cerebellum has also been implicated in learning, especially motor learning, and muscle tone with damage typically resulting in hypotonia and postural control issues. Additionally, there are differences in neuronal function in those with DS, including decreased synaptic density and fewer dendritic spines, which ultimately may disrupt the neural circuits that support learning and memory. Neurogenesis (new neuron formation) is also diminished within the hippocampus in DS and thought to contribute to the cognitive deficits in DS.[34]

Orthopedic Problems in DS

The hypotonia, associated with DS, is accompanied by ligamentous laxity that can contribute to joint instability. Common areas for this are at the atlanto-occipital joint or the atlantoaxial joint of the cervical spine. The occiput of the skull connects with the first cervical vertebra (C1), also called the atlas, resting on the superior articulating processes of C1, and is connected by thick ligaments between the occiput and C1, allowing for much of our cervical flexion and extension as well as lateral bending; however, in DS, the laxity of these ligaments may result in dangerous instability at this joint. Similarly, the joint between C1 and C2, also called the axis, is characterized by a protruding odontoid process from C2 that projects up into C1. This arrangement allows rotation of C1 on C2, accounting for much of our cervical rotation ability. Again, laxity of ligaments at this joint can result in dangerous laxity; both of these conditions pose potential risk for spinal cord injury. Neurologic symptoms, pain, or observed excessive mobility warrant further assessment with radiographs (x-rays); for many children, the condition is mild, but it is recommended that they avoid excessive flexion (e.g., somersaults) and contact sports (e.g., soccer or football). In some cases, the laxity is more severe and requires posterior fusion of C1 and C2.[35]

Other Health Complications in DS

Ear, **nose**, and **throat problems** are common in DS in association with malformation of these structures. Infections are often frequent, including otitis media and pneumonia, and **hearing loss** may occur in association with repeated infection or malformation of the inner ear. A brainstem auditory evoked assessment can be used to evaluate the ability of the aural structures to transmit sound to the brain. This test involves measuring EEG (electroencephalography) responses to auditory stimulation and can be done in infants. Similarly, children with DS may have **missing or misshaped teeth** or **late tooth eruption** that may impact eating, especially transitioning to solid foods, or require orthodontics. Other conditions that occur at a higher frequency in children with DS than typically developing children are **thyroid disease**, **eye problems** (amblyopia, congenital cataracts, glaucoma, nystagmus, strabismus, and refraction errors – myopia, astigmatism), **epilepsy**, and **leukemia**. Notably, children with DS are also **smaller in stature** with shortened limbs than their typical peers; there are growth curves that have been developed specific to DS growth patterns for comparison. At older ages, **obesity** is often a problem, associated with decreased activity, so weight management and a healthy diet should be initiated early and maintained.[14]

Motor Development in DS

Children with DS tend to be quiet, sleepy babies with diminished antigravity movement, especially in supine, and less engagement with their environment. In general, they develop motor skills at a slower rate to their typical peers that is even more delayed in upright postures. Rolling and early weight-bearing and mobility in prone and quadruped tend to occur within 1–3 months of typically developing children (on average); however, independent sitting, pulling to stand, cruising, and walking can be delayed by many months, especially walking. It is not uncommon for children with DS to delay walking until nearly 3 years of age. There is likely an interaction between the ID and motor delay in children with DS; lack of interest in exploring the environment may delay motor behavior while delayed exploration may impede intellectual development.[36]

Infants with DS are typically seen in the NICU prior to discharge to home; this is a critical time for assessment for any orthopedic issue and to prepare the parents for handling the child, who is floppy and hard to hold. Once at home, **early physical therapy treatment** focuses on developing antigravity movement and acquisition of motor milestones. Most children with DS will be enrolled in EI services, so physical therapy will be provided in an EI environment. Families should be encouraged to establish a bright and engaging environment and to create opportunities for the child to play in prone, supine, and supported sitting to minimize the time spent sleeping, sitting in an infant seat, or lying quietly. Instruction in handling and positioning techniques is important to facilitate the development of antigravity movement, head control, rolling, and sitting. These techniques mirror those used with children with MMC and CP, as described in Chapters 18 and 19, respectively. Body-weight-supported treadmill training (BWSTT) has been found to be particularly effective in children with DS, facilitating earlier acquisition of independent walking and improving gait speed in older children.[37] Many children with DS have pes planus (flat feet) that may require some orthotic support – either a foot or supramalleolar orthotic.[38] Older children with DS benefit from therapy directed at improving upright postural control to assure safety, during play and school, including single limb stance for stair-climbing and adaptive physical education to improve play skills. Strength training has also been found to increase muscle strength and postural control and secondarily play skills.[39,40]

Aging with DS

Although some children with DS succumb to congenital heart defects or other organ malformations; with improved surgical management, the majority of children are living to adulthood (>88%), and many are living into their 60s. Thus, additional information relative to the aging of individuals with DS is pertinent to physical therapy practitioners. Notably, adults with DS demonstrate **accelerated aging** of many organ systems, including the brain. Adults with DS exhibit earlier aging of **the integumentary system** (wrinkles, graying, and hair loss), **earlier menopause** in women, advanced aging in the musculoskeletal system, resulting in early and widespread **osteoporosis**, increased occurrence of **cardiovascular problems** (atherosclerosis), and increased incidence of

Alzheimer's disease (AD). The latter (AD and DS) has received much attention as early reports predicted a 100% occurrence of AD in adults with DS. AD is associated with amyloid beta (Aβ) deposits in the extracellular areas of the brain; Aβ seems to be a catalyst for the development of the amyloid plaques and neurofibrillary tangles that are the characteristic anomalies of AD, ultimately resulting in neuronal death. Interestingly, the Aβ precursor gene has been localized to the 21st chromosome, which likely accounts for the exaggerated occurrence of AD in adults with DS. Notably, not all adults with DS develop AD, so other factors must contribute to the expression of AD in DS. Early symptoms of AD in adults with DS are often behavioral (aggression, change in sleep patterns, emotional outbursts), or in adults with seizures, increased seizure activity. Pharmacological treatments, typically used to treat AD, seem less effective in the DS population.[41] For physical therapists, it is important to note that exercise programs (aerobic and strengthening) have been found to offset many of the aging problems of adults with DS, including osteoporosis, obesity, cardiovascular fitness, and decreased muscle mass.[40]

BOX 20-3 | **Neuromuscular Degenerative Disorders (NMDs)**

Within Table 20-2, there are a number of NMDs, including the muscular dystrophies and spinal muscular atrophies. While these two groups of disorders have different pathologic etiologies, they all result in progressive loss of skeletal muscle and fatigue. For the physical therapist, the management of these conditions is similar, focusing on optimizing motor function, preventing deformities, specifically muscle contractures that result from limited mobility and maintained postures, and selecting appropriate adaptive equipment to facilitate function and mobility. Care providers should be instructed in range of motion and static stretching activities (maintained stretch at the end of the range) as well as proper positioning to minimize the risk for contractures and skeletal deformities (e.g., scoliosis) as soon as the child is diagnosed; appropriate seating should be an ongoing concern with the therapist helping the family choose options that will adapt as the child grows and loses muscle control.[42]

There is some evidence to suggest that low resistive or isometric exercise can help to maintain strength or improve strength in those with some NMDs, yet there is concern that overwork can cause muscle injury, especially in those with muscular dystrophy with the use of eccentric contractions in strengthening programs especially detrimental.[43] Strength training should target weak muscles as well as potential compensatory muscles, as muscle mass is lost in primary movers, to prolong function.[42] Aerobic exercise training, using a bicycle or upper extremity ergometer has been reported to increase aerobic capacity and strength without inducing muscle damage. In addition, strengthening of respiratory muscles may improve ventilation and delay the need for a ventilator in those with mild or moderate weakness; however, it is not effective for those with severe weakness.[43] Therapists can also help the children adapt their movement patterns to progressively changing muscle strength to assist them to maintain function; this takes creativity to identify stronger muscles and potential movement patterns

(e.g., side stepping up stairs to use both UE). The physical therapist also plays a critical role in determining when power mobility should be initiated, identifying other adaptive equipment needs (e.g., ambulation aids and lifting devices for transferring to and from the wheelchair, bed, toilet, or tub), and helping the family to adapt their home and the school to adapt the classroom to meet the needs of the child/adolescent.[42] Further, the physical therapist can contribute to the documentation of disease progression as well as treatment outcomes through careful recording of movement, strength, and range of motion (ROM). Since most developmental measures are inappropriate for the child with an NMD, therapists can use timed measures of coming to standing from the floor and a chair, walking 10 m, ascending and descending stairs, or more standard measures such as the Timed Up and Go test to document functional mobility changes. Also, careful manual muscle testing to regularly document muscle strength is important as is observation of the child's ability to maintain a muscle contraction and recruit agonists for sustained muscle activity; using a handheld dynamometer will improve the therapist's ability to objectively quantify muscle strength. Finally, frequent ROM measurement should be completed to identify developing contractures to target positioning and stretching activities.[42] It should be noted that in some cases contractures result from adaptation of movement that actually stabilizes the joint (e.g., the ankle) and overstretching can result in joint instability and loss of function, so the therapists must carefully evaluate the child's movements to determine how much stretching should be done. Again, static stretching that includes holding the stretch at the end of the ROM for 5–10 seconds or the use of night splints has been found to limit the progression of contractures.[42]

Developmental Coordination Disorder (DCD)

DCD is a disorder of fine and gross motor dyscoordination that affects new skill acquisition (motor learning and motor planning), activities of daily living, and participation in school and later work environments that affects up to 6% of school-aged children[44] and boys much more commonly than girls[45]; the motor deficit includes poor balance and postural control as well as disrupted visual-spatial and sensorimotor processing.[46] In addition, deficits in self-organization and time management skills are also common.[45] It is distinguished from other disorders, such as autism spectrum disorder and cerebral palsy, with its presentation of clumsiness, slow motor skill learning (both gross and fine motor) given the child's age and intellectual function, and absence of overt neurologic signs (spasticity, hyperreflexia, etc.).[45] Notably, soft neurologic signs may be present (wide-based gait, mild ataxia, ligamentous laxity). Although some children with DCD will present with intellectual deficits, this occurs in the same proportion as the general population and is not a diagnostic criterion; similarly, some children with DCD will also present with speech and language impairments, epilepsy, joint hypermobility, attention deficit/hyperactivity disorder (ADHD; see Box 20-4), or dyslexia.[47] In fact, up to 60% of children with DCD present with ADHD, reading deficits, and/or language impairment. The impact of DCD spreads into the educational and social participation for children and adolescents with academic performance

BOX 20-4	Attention Deficit/Hyperactivity Disorder (ADHD)[49]

ADHD is another developmental disorder found in up to 5% of children and characterized by poor attention, impulsiveness, and exaggerated activity levels; although many children outgrow this disorder in adolescence/early adulthood, 50% or so will continue to demonstrate problems as adults with an impact on employment and social interactions. There is a strong familial hereditary component to ADHD, yet the actual genetic abnormality has not been identified. While attention deficit can occur in the absence of hyperactivity, and vice versa, these two disorders commonly occur together. ADHD is associated with decreased brain volume, involving many areas of the brain, including the basal ganglia, anterior cingulate, inferior parietal lobule, cerebellum, and hippocampus, as well as a general thinning of the cortex. In addition, diffusion tensor imaging has found white matter irregularities, especially in the superior longitudinal fasciculus that connects the inferior parietal lobe with the lateral prefrontal cortex, a critical pathway for attention. The most common treatment for ADHD is psychostimulants (e.g., methylphenidate, which blocks the reuptake of norepinephrine and dopamine) or selective norepinephrine reuptake inhibitors (e.g., atomoxetine) that have their primary influence on prefrontal, basal ganglial, and cerebellar brain regions, involved in attention.

impeded by deficits in hand writing and organization; limitations in the acquisition of age appropriate motor skills impede social participation, which may be further disrupted by speech intelligibility deficits that are often present.[48]

Etiology of DCD

A definitive cause for DCD has not been found; however, there is some suggestion that it results from mild damage to multiple areas of the brain, rather than focal damage, with irregular activity noted on fMRI in the temporal, parietal, and frontal lobes as well as the cerebellum, and a general decrease in white matter within the internal capsule and periventricular areas. Not surprisingly, DCD is more common in children born preterm, who have experienced neonatal encephalopathy.[44] The cerebellum has received much attention related to DCD, based on its critical role in motor learning and movement coordination. Two theories have been proposed to explain the deficits of DCD: (1) a disruption in the ability to translate movements from a cognitive to an automatic phase or (2) a deficit in the internal representation of movement, which refers to the inability to compare the efference copy generated during motor planning to the execution of the movement in order to make a correction. Both of these theories emphasize the role of the cerebellum in this deficit; however, it is not felt that this is singularly a cerebellar problem. Interestingly, children with DCD show impaired anticipatory postural adjustments, requiring a reliance on feedback mechanisms for postural control that are ineffective for coordinated quick movements.[50]

Prognosis for Children with DCD

DCD is not just a pediatric disorder; rather, like so many developmental disabilities, it has a lifelong impact. Early diagnosis is associated with delayed motor skill acquisition and peer play. However, school-aged children demonstrate increasing difficulty with academic and social skills as well as emotional and behavioral concerns. Similar to their peers with DS, children with DCD are at risk for obesity and ultimately for cardiovascular conditions, resulting from decreased activity levels and community engagement. There are limited studies on adult outcomes for children with DCD, but it is expected that they will do best with employment opportunities that require limited motor skill.[51]

Treatment Approaches for DCD

Treatment recommendations for children with DCD include (1) process-focused approaches that address the impairments and functional limitations of DCD (e.g., balance, strength) and (2) task-focused paradigms that aim to improve motor planning and motor learning through task practice. In general, and not surprisingly, task-focused programs have been found to achieve greater improvements than process-focused programs.[52] One method that has been successful is the use of gaming, specifically the WiiFit™, which has been used to provide highly repetitive task practice that challenges postural control and interlimb coordination with improvements noted in those same areas as well as running speed and agility, after a 6-week training program, using the "Balancing Games."[50] However, in a comparison of WiiFit Balance training and task training, focused on common playground games (e.g., tag, ball activities), greater improvement occurred in the task training group for strength, aerobic, and anaerobic measures.[52] Thus, in planning treatment for children with DCD, therapists should keep in mind that a high level of repetition is likely required to improve motor performance, but task practice may be as good or better than gaming in achieving therapy goals.

Autism Spectrum Disorder

As mentioned earlier in the chapter, some signs of autism spectrum disorder (ASD) are not identified until 3 or 4 years of age. ASD is a common developmental disorder with a myriad of symptomatology, most concentrated in impairments in language, social-emotional, communication, and restrictive repetitive behaviors. As a spectrum disorder, the combinations of behavioral symptoms are varied such that no two children with ASD are the same. Current estimates of ASD are 1 in 68 children without racial or ethnic disproportions but with gender disproportions as there are five times more boys than girls diagnosed.[53] The cause of ASD is unknown but both genetic predisposition and environmental contributions have been implicated. A genetic component is suspected as siblings of children with a current ASD diagnosis have a 1/10 chance of an ASD diagnosis themselves.[54] In some cases, regressive symptoms are identified with a decline in language and social skills in the second or third year of life. Even so, a high percentage of parents report that they were concerned about their baby's development at 1 and 2 years of age. The prevalence of ASD is higher in children with Fragile X or tuberous sclerosis and with older parents. There is no cure or prenatal diagnostic tests for ASD, and accurate identification of abnormal symptoms in infancy and toddlerhood is difficult and infrequent. An ASD diagnosis is given by psychologists and psychiatrists using the DSMV criteria which include deficits in social communication and interaction, restrictive perseverative behavior, including repetitive motor movements, and sensory impairments that limit function. Severity levels are distinguished by the level of support needed. Children previously diagnosed with an autistic disorder, Asperger's disorder, or pervasive developmental disorder not otherwise specified under the DSM-IV criteria are now reclassified as ASD under the DSMV, but the former diagnostic categories are still used by many clinicians and lay persons. Intellectual disabilities and other language impairments frequently co-occur with ASD and require additional testing and separate diagnosis categorization. See Box 20-5 for common features of ASD.

BOX 20-5 | Common Features of ASD[55]

- Poor eye contact
- Lack of pointing or waving by 14 months
- Not responding to name by 12 months
- Few large smiles
- Language delay
- Self-stimulatory behaviors
- Delays or lack of pretend play and imagination
- Spinning body or objects repetitively
- Flapping hands and arms
- Rocking
- Echolalia – repeating what others have said
- Repeating phrases from television
- Narrow interests
- Perseverative movements and actions (repeating them over and over)
- Decreased social skills
- Inflexible routines
- Unusual sensory interests
- Difficulty initiating conversation
- Lack of understanding and use of gestures
- Wanting to be alone
- Decreased ability to describe feelings
- Poor emotional regulation
- Unusual reactions to new sensory information such as smell or taste
- Decreased ability to read facial expression
- Lack of understanding social cues
- Flat affect
- Using language in an unusual way
- Routine oriented
- Respond negatively to minor changes in routine
- Lack of the ability to direct another's attention to themselves or objects (joint attention)
- Difficulty with imitation
- Poor understanding of cause and effect

Brain Differences in ASD

There are over 100 research articles identifying brain abnormalities between adults and children with ASD and typical comparison groups, yet identifying one individual with ASD, based on brain imaging, such as MRI, is not currently possible. Children with ASD may have a larger head circumference as toddlers and the white matter of their brains is proportionally larger in some areas, especially the frontal cortex; there are also more white matter connections between areas in the same hemisphere of the brain than between hemispheres and a greater number of synapses in the brains of some people with ASD, and this is thought to come from a lack of pruning, during brain development (see Chapter 8 for a description of pruning).[56] Altered white matter connectivity, enlarged ventricles, and an underactive amygdala (when looking at facial expressions) have been noted.[57,58] Diffusion tensor imaging has identified decreased connectivity in three areas associated with emotions and social interactions: (1) the limbic system (cingulum bundle, uncinated fasciculus, mammillo-thalamic tract, and anterior thalamic projections); (2) the mirror neuron system that is involved in facial expression recognition with projections within the arcuate fasciculus, connecting the frontal, parietal, and temporal lobes; and (3) the face processing system that is responsible for face recognition as well as determination of the social implications of facial expression and involving areas of the occipital and temporal lobes with their interconnections. In young children, there seems to be an over-connectivity in many areas compared to their typical peers; while in older children, these same areas yield lower connectivity than their peers. Ultimately, neural changes may not be stable until late childhood or early adolescence.[59] Some of the same areas, associated with ASD symptomology, have also been identified as brain abnormalities in children with language impairment, ADHD, sensory processing disorder, and other developmental disabilities.

Epilepsy in ASD

Epilepsy is a common occurrence in ASD with one in four diagnosed children also having some seizure activity by adolescence. Factors associated with epilepsy are increasing age, lower cognitive ability (specifically lower IQ), more severe ASD, and developmental regression.[60] Abnormal brain structure and development is thought to be the likely reason for a high prevalence of epilepsy in ASD. An electroencephalogram (EEG) is a noninvasive measure of spontaneous brain activity that can be used to determine if a person is having seizures. Pharmacological management of seizures is necessary in most cases. As discussed in Chapter 19, antiepileptic medications have many associated side effects, including drowsiness, dizziness, fatigue, weakness, irritability, anxiety, and confusion, that can exacerbate the symptomology of ASD. Physical therapists should be aware of these side effects and may need to time treatment sessions to avoid periods of fatigue and weakness.

Developmental Differences in ASD

The five domains of child development – cognitive, language, social, motor, and emotional – are all described as atypical in children with ASD.

Cognitive Function in ASD. There is a large range of intelligence in children with ASD. Most children with ASD have an IQ <70%, indicating an ID. Yet, some people with ASD can have normal or above average intelligence or exhibit savant behaviors, typically in one area, like math or music. There are wide ranging reports of the prevalence of savant characteristics in people with ASD from 1 in 200[61] to 1 in 3.[62] While some adults live independently or with minimal support, supportive services are typically needed as people with ASD and ID age.

Language Development in ASD. A key feature of ASD is **delayed language**, both expressive and receptive, with children with ASD often not saying a first word until 2 or 3 years of age, and many children have no verbal skills. Sign language is often introduced as a means of communication. Interestingly, toddlers with ASD who were trained to use several simple signs for communication also increased the number of spoken words, suggesting that any successful communication is important in facilitating overall communication and that teaching sign language does not prohibit the development of verbal language. Delays and differences in the language skills of children with ASD also include difficulty understanding simple sentences or words, speaking with unusual intonations, repetition of words with no intent to communicate (echolalia), understating or using humor inappropriately, and the difficulty understanding abstract language and nonverbal cues – all contributing to difficulties in communication.[63] Children with ASD also frequently have visual and auditory processing disorders, meaning that their eye sight or hearing might be normal but they have disrupted visual or auditory processing that makes communication and learning difficult.

Socio-Emotional Development in ASD. Another feature of ASD is poor social skill development. Behaviors exhibited include a mismatch between facial expression, body language, gestures, and the environmental context as well as a lack of eye contact. Children with ASD often demonstrate a resistance to being touched, have difficulty understanding the perspective of others, and do not independently seek out social situations or express interest in what others are doing or experiencing. Children with ASD frequently have difficulty or cannot make friends with same-age peers. They avoid group situations and prefer spending time alone. Another feature of ASD is impairments in emotional development. Behaviors exhibited include (1) difficulty understanding facial expressions and the emotions of others – often described as a lack of empathy, (2) poor imitation of or use of facial expressions, (3) disrupted emotional control, and (4) inappropriate responsiveness to emotional situations.[59]

Motor Development in ASD. Impaired motor skill development is also a characteristic of ASD, although it is not part of the DSMV diagnostic criteria except for stereotypical repetitive movements. Interestingly, a high percentage of children with ASD qualify for supportive services such as physical therapy with delays on standardized testing for fine and/or gross motor skills. Due to the variability of normal motor development and the symptomatology of ASD, specific motor impairments are difficult to identify. However, children with ASD have been found to have a myriad of motor skill impairments, including hypotonia,

clumsiness, apraxia, and poor balance and postural control; delayed gross and fine motor skills; poor coordination in reaching and gait; difficulty with the learning of and execution of skilled movements (planning and refinement), performing movement sequences or rhythmic movements as well as poor ball skills; and impaired proprioception, strength, agility, and speed.[64] It is important to note that children with ASD often avoid new physical activities, placing them at higher risk for decreased endurance and resulting in less practice and exploration of new motor skills.

Since ASD is not typically diagnosed before 3 years of age, infants who go on to develop ASD are not frequently seen by physical therapists for ASD, but they could be referred to physical therapy for global developmental delay. Therapists should be aware of the early signs of ASD and the genetic predisposition in order to refer a family to appropriated health care professionals, if an ASD diagnosis is suspected in an infant or toddler. ASD screenings, using both parent surveys and clinical tools that are a combination of survey and clinical assessment, are routinely done at pediatrician's offices and can be incorporated into a physical therapy assessment, if needed. The Modified Checklist for Autism in Toddlers (M-CHAT)[65] is the most frequently used checklist for common features and behaviors that could be indicative of ASD, including social interaction, imaginative play, responses to sensory stimulation, and language and motor skills. This checklist is completed by a parent or caregiver and interpreted by a medical professional. EI (birth–3) may be available for children who are at risk for developmental disabilities, so some children with ASD may receive EI; however, since many children aren't diagnosed until 3, many will not receive EI services. Children with ASD commonly receive occupational therapy for sensory integration therapy (see description in Box 20-6), and Applied Behavioral Analysis (ABA) at home or school; ABA is an individualized program of one-on-one treatment to encourage positive behaviors (e.g., vocalizations, eye contact, modeling of facial expressions) while discouraging negative behaviors (e.g., hand flapping, aggression) in order to improve function and learning.[66] Treatment programs, for children with ASD who are receiving physical therapy, should incorporate behavioral modification techniques, including positive reinforcement for target behaviors (e.g., attention, eye gaze) and to minimize disruptive behaviors. There is a paucity of research to document effective physical therapy treatment approaches for children with autism. Hippotherapy has been reported to improve postural control as well as communication and adaptive behavior, facilitating participation and social interactions.[67] Common practices to improve impairment-specific deficits include using a metronome for timing and sequencing of motor skills and providing vestibular and proprioceptive feedback.

Sensory Differences in ASD

From poor visual and auditory integration to sensorimotor impairments, sensory differences are commonplace in children with ASD with greater than 90% of children demonstrating atypical reactivity to sensory stimulation, referred to as sensory integration disorder (SID); this prevalence has made SID a component of the DSMV diagnostic criteria for ASD. SID refers to over- or under-responsiveness to sensory stimulation, thought to result for impaired sensory processing, and can impact leaning,

---

BOX 20-6 Sensory Therapies for ASD

Sensory-focused treatments for ASD include both **sensory integration therapy** (SIT) and **sensory-based interventions** (SBI). SIT, developed by Ayres[69] focuses on activities that require the child to process sensory information within a motor task; consistent with motor learning strategies, SIT challenges the child at the "peak" of their skill level, using vestibular (e.g., swings), proprioceptive (e.g., bouncing on therapy balls or trampolines), and tactile challenges (e.g., reaching for objects in sand). SBIs apply either active or passive sensory stimulation to improve sensory processing, self-awareness, and self-regulation; techniques used include weight vests or therapeutic wrapping to increase proprioceptive awareness; massage to improve body awareness, responsiveness to touch or to calm the child; or auditory therapy to improve responsiveness to auditory stimuli. While there is fairly good evidence to support the use of SIT for children with ASD, there is limited evidence to support the use of SBI; however, this is likely due to the large variability in how it is applied and the methods for assessment.[68] Yet, the physical therapist, working with the child with ASD, may find some of these techniques helpful in their treatment strategies.

CASE A, PART VI

While Pauli does not have an ASD or ADHD diagnosis at this point, she does display many behaviors similar to those of these diagnoses. Therefore, physical therapy treatment should benefit from incorporating behavioral management techniques in her treatment program to improve her participation and diminish negative behaviors; working with the health care team or educational team and the family to develop strategies will be important to assure consistency across settings and maximize her outcomes. Further, her limited food choices and response to sensory stimuli (e.g., needing tags removed from clothes) suggest that she should be evaluated for sensory integration problems and potentially would benefit from a sensory integration treatment program as part of her occupational therapy treatment. Pauli is definitely a candidate for an educational program for children with developmental delays and a comprehensive treatment program; since she is almost 3, an IEP and preschool program should be identified. Like many young children with a global developmental delay, Pauli's condition does not fit into any definitive diagnostic category, and she will continue to be classified with a global developmental delay diagnosis. As she gets older, a more definitive diagnosis may be found, or she may continue with this diagnosis.

---

motor function, and independence. As a result of SID, children with ASD either seek out sensory stimulation (e.g., spinning themselves or objects) or avoid sensory stimulation (e.g., smell aversions that affect eating, hypersensitivity to clothing textures that impact what the child will wear) with the child also demonstrating stereotypic behaviors to calm or stimulate themselves to meet this "sensory need." It is thought that sensory input is not integrated or organized appropriately in the brain, based on the disruption of connectivity described earlier. As a result of over- and under-responsiveness sensory stimuli can be disproportionally distressing or comforting to children with ASD.[68]

Other Treatments of ASD Symptoms

Pharmacology and dietary management of ASD symptoms are commonplace. Atypical antipsychotic medications are often used, with risperidone (commercially known as Risperdal) the most frequently prescribed, which has been found to decrease hyperactivity, irritability, aggression, and stereotypical behaviors (e.g., hand flapping) while improving social interactions. Unlike typical antipsychotics, like haloperidol, risperidone has fewer and less severe side effects, including weight gain, dizziness, tiredness, fatigue, fever, and nausea. Children with autism also have common **gastrointestinal dysfunction**, including coeliac disease and inflammatory bowel disease, so diet is used in one in five children with ASD for management of GI conditions but also behavioral symptoms. Gluten-free (limiting wheat, barley, and rye products) and/or casein-free (limiting milk products) diets are the most commonly applied programs in ASD. The available evidence of their impact remains equivocal with some studies reporting improvements in communication, attention, motor coordination, and social skills with decreases in hyperactivity, stereotypical and self-injurious behaviors while others report no effect.[70]

REFERENCES

1. National Institute of Child Health and Human Development. Intellectual and Developmental Disabilities: condition information. Available at: http://www.nichd.nih.gov/health/topics/idds/conditioninfo/Pages/default.aspx. Accessed January 6, 2015.

2. Tirosch E, Jaffe M. Global developmental delay and mental retardation – a pediatric perspective. *Dev Disabil Res Rev*. 2011;17:85-92.

3. Lawrence R, Bateman N. 12 minute consultation: an evidence-based approach to the management of a child with speech and language delay. *Clin Otolaryngol*. 2013;38:148-153.

4. McLaughlin MR. Speech and language delay in children. *Am Fam Physician*. 2011;83(10):1183-1188.

5. Moeschler JB, Shevell M, and Committee on Genetics. Comprehensive evaluation of the child with intellectual disability or global developmental delays. *Pediatrics*. 2014;134;e903.

6. Flore LA, Milunsky JM. Updates in the genetic evaluation of the child with global developmental delay or intellectual disability. *Semin Pediatr Neurol*. 2012;19:173-180.

7. Nicholls RD. The impact of genomic imprinting for neurobehavioral and developmental disorders. *J Clin Invest*. 2000;105(4):413-418.

8. Duca DG, Craiu D, Boer M, et al. Diagnostic approach of Angelman syndrome. *J Clin Med*. 2013;8(4):321-327.

9. Buggenhout GV, Fryns JP. Angelman syndrome. *Eur J Hum Genet*. 2009;17:1367-1373.

10. Flanigan KM. Duchenne and Becker muscular dystrophies. *Neurol Clin*. 2014;32:671-688.

11. Vallat JM, Mathis S, Funalot B. The various Charcot-Marie-Tooth diseases. *Curr Opin Neurol*. 2013;26(5):473-480.

12. Mainardi PC. Cri du Chat syndrome. *Orphanet J Rare Dis*. 2006;1:33:1-9.

13. Martiniano SL, Hoppe JE, Sagel SD, Zemanick ET. Advances in the diagnosis and treatment of cystic fibrosis. *Adv Pediatr*. 2014;61:225-243.

14. Saenz RB. Primary care of infants and young children with Down syndrome. *Am Fam Physician*. 1999;59(2):381-390.

15. Spencer K. Screening for Down syndrome. *Scan J Clin Lab Invest*. 2014;74(S244):41-47.

16. Maurin T, Zongaro S, Bardoni B. Fragile X syndrome: from molecular pathology to therapy. *Neurosci Biobehav Rev*. 2014. Available at: http://dx.doi.org/10.1016/j.neubiorev.2014.01.006.

17. Gallagher A, Hallahan B. Fragile X-associated disorders: a clinical overview. *J Neurol*. 2012;259:401-413.

18. Vanier MT. Niemann-Pick disease type C. *Orphanet J Rare Dis*. 2010; 5(16):1-18.

19. Jin DK. Systematic review of the clinical and genetic aspects of Prader-Willi syndrome. *Korean J Pediatr*. 2011;54(2):55-63.

20. Emerick JE, Vogt KS. Endocrine manifestations and management of Prader-Willi syndrome. *Int J Pediatr Endocrinol*. 2013;14. Available at: http://www.ijpeonline.com/content/2013/1/14

21. Ney DM, Blank RD, Hansen KE. Advances in the nutritional and pharmacological management of phenylketonuria. *Curr Opin Clin Nutr Metab Care*. 2014;17:61-68.

22. Briggs A. Primary care of a child with Rett syndrome. *J Am Assoc Nurse Pract*. 2014;26:471-480.

23. Nurputra DK, Lai PS, Harahap NIF, et al. Spinal muscular atrophy: from gene discovery to clinical trials. *Ann Hum Genet*. 2013;77:43-463.

24. Rosa RFM, Rosa RCM, Zen PRG, Craziadio C, Paskulin GA. Trisomy 18: review of the clinical, etiologic, prognostic and ethical aspects. *Rev Paul Pediatr*. 2013;31(1):111-20.

25. Lorenz JM, Hardart GE. Evolving medical and surgical management of infants with trisomy 18. *Curr Opin Pediatr*. 2014;26:169-176.

26. Merle U, Schaefer M, Ferenci P, Stremmel W. Clinical presentation, diagnosis and long-term outcome of Wilson's disease: a cohort study. *Gut*. 2007;56:115-120.

27. Pastores GM. Neuropathic lysosomal storage disorders. *Neurol Clin*. 2013; 31(4):1051-1071.

28. Bley AE, Giannikopoulos OA, Hayden D, Kubilus K, Tifft CJ, Eichler FS. Natural history of infantile GM2 gangliosidosis. *Pediatrics*. 2011;128:e1233. doi:10.1542/peds.2011-0078.

29. Kanungo S, Soares N, He M, Steiner RD. Sterol metabolism disorders and neurodevelopment – an update. *Dev Disabil Res Rev*. 2013;17:197-210.

30. Stockler-Ipsiroglu S, van Karnebeek CDM. Cerebral creatine deficiencies: a group of treatable intellectual developmental disorders. *Semin Neurol*. 2014;34:350-356.

31. Bayley Scales of Infant and Toddler Development®, 3rd ed. Pearson. 2005. Available at: http://www.pearsonclinical.com/psychology/products/100000123/bayley-scales-of-infant-and-toddler-development-third-edition-bayley-iii.html.

32. Peabody Developmental Motor Scales. 2nd ed. Austin, TX: Pro-Ed. 2000.

33. Malak R, Kotwicka M, Krawczyk-Wasielewska A, Mojs E, Samborski W. Motor skills, cognitive development and balance functions of children with Down syndrome. *Annals Agric Environ Med*. 2013;20(4):803-806.

34. Lott IT, Dierssen M. Cognitive deficits and associated neurological complications in individuals with Down syndrome. *Lancet Neurol*. 2010;9:623-633.

35. Rosenbaum DM, Blumhagen JD, King HA. Atlantooccipital instability in Down syndrome. *AJR*. 1986;146:1268-1272.

36. Pereira K, Basso RP, Lindquist ARR, DaSilva LGP, Tudella E. Infants with Down syndrome: percentage and age for acquisition of gross motor skills. *Res Dev Disabil*. 2013;34:894-901.

37. Valentin-Gudiol M, Bagur-Calafat C, Girabent-Farres M, et al. Treadmill interventions with partial body weight support in children under six years of age at risk of neuromotor delay: a report of a Cochrane systematic review and meta-analysis. *Eur J Phys Rehabil Med*. 2013;49:67-91.

38. Looper J, Benjamin D, Nolan M, Schumm L. What to measure when determining orthotic needs in children with Down syndrome: a pilot study. *Pediatr Phys Ther*. 2012;24:313-319.

39. Shields N, Taylor NF, Wee E, Wollersheim D, O'Shea SD, Fernhall B. A community-based strength training programme increases muscle strength and physical activity in young people with Down syndrome: a randomized controlled trial. *Res Dev Disabil*. 2013;34:4385-4394.

40. Barnhart RC, Connolly B. Aging and Down syndrome: implications for physical therapy. *Phys Ther*. 2007;87:1399-1406.

41. Zigman WB. Atypical aging in Down syndrome. *Dev Disabil Res Rev*. 2013;18:51-67.

42. Johnson LB, JM, Abresch RT. Physical therapy evaluation and management in neuromuscular diseases. *Phys Med Rehabil Clin N Am*. 2012;23:633-651.

43. Abresch RT, Carter GT, Han JJ, McDonald CM. Exercise in neuromuscular diseases. *Phys Med Rehabil Clin N Am*. 2012;23:653-673.

44. Peters LHJ, Maathuis CGB, Hadders-Algra M. Neural correlates of developmental coordination disorder. *Dev Med Child Neurol*. 2013; 55(suppl 4):59-64.

45. Kirby A, Sugden D, Purcell C. Diagnosing developmental coordination disorders. *Arch Dis Child*. 2014;99:292-296.

46. Vaivre-Douret L. Developmental coordination disorders: state of art. *Clin Neurophysiol*. 2014;44:13-23.

47. Lingam R, Golding J, Jongmans MJ, Hunt LP, Ellis M, Emond A. The association between developmental coordination disorder and other developmental traits. *Pediatrics*. 2010;126:e1109-e1118.

48. Sylvestre A, Nadeau L, Charron L, Larose N, Lepage C. Social participation by children with developmental coordination disorder compared to their peers. *Disabil Rehabil*. 2013;35(21):1814-1820.

49. Friedman LA, Rapoport JL. Brain development in ADHD. *Curr Opin Neurobiol*. 2015;30:106-111.

50. Jelsma D, Geuze RH, Mombarg R, Smits-Engelsman BCM. The impact of Wii Fit intervention on dynamic balance control in children with probable developmental coordination disorder and balance problems. *Hum Mov Sci*. 2014;33:404-418.

51. Zwicker JG, Missiuna C, Harris SR, Boyd LA. Developmental coordination disorder: a review and update. *Eur J Paediatr Neurol*. 2012;16:573-581.

52. Ferguson GD, Jelsma D, Jelsma J, Smits-Engelsman BCM. The efficacy of two task-orientated interventions for children with developmental coordination disorder: neuromotor task training and Nintendo Wii Fit training. *Res Dev Disabil*. 2013;34:2449-2461.

53. Centers for Disease Control and Prevention. Autism Spectrum Disorder Research. Available at: http://www.cdc.gov/ncbddd/autism/research.html.

54. Constantino JN1, Zhang Y, Frazier T, Abbacchi AM, Law P. Sibling recurrence and the genetic epidemiology of autism. *Am J Psychiatry*. 2010;167(11):1349-1356.

55. Zwaigenbaum L, Bryson S, Garon N. Early identification of autism spectrum disorders. *Behav Brain Res*. 2013;251:133-146.

56. Schaer M, Ottet MC, Scariati E, Dukes D, Franchini M, Elie S, Glaser B. Decreased frontal gyrification correlates with altered connectivity in children with autism. *Front Hum Neurosci*. 2013;7:750. doi:10.3389/fnhum.2013.00750.

57. Waterhouse L, Fein D, Modahl C. Neurofunctional mechanisms in autism. *Psychol Rev*. 1996;103:457-489.

58. Wong TK, Fung PC, Chua SE, McAlonan GM. Abnormal spatiotemporal processing of emotional facial expressions in childhood autism: dipole source analysis of event-related potentials. *Eur J Neurosci*. 2008; 28(2):407-416.

59. Ameis SH, Catani M. Altered white matter connectivity as a neural substrate for social impairment in autism spectrum disorder. *Cortex*. 2015;62:158-181.

60. Viscidi EW1, Triche EW, Pescosolido MF, McLean RL, Joseph RM, Spence SJ, Morrow EM. Clinical characteristics of children with autism spectrum disorder and co-occurring epilepsy. *PLoS One*. 2013;8(7):e67797.

61. Hermelin B. *Bright Splinters of the Mind: A Personal Story of Research with Autistic Savants*. London: Jessica Kingsley Publishers; 2001.

62. Howlin P, Goode S, Hutton J, Rutter M. Savant skills in autism: psychometric approaches and parental reports. *Philos Trans R Soc Lond B Biol Sci*. 2009;364:1359-1367.

63. Mody M, Belliveau JW. Speech and language impairments in autism: insights from behavior and neuroimaging. *N Am J Med Sci*. 2013;5(3):157-161.

64. Hilton CL, Zhang Y, Whilte MR, Klohr CL, Constantino J. Motor impairment in sibling pairs concordant and discordant for autism spectrum disorders. *Autism*. 2012;16(4):430-441.

65. Robins DL, Fein D, Barton ML, Green JA. The Modified Checklist for Autism in Toddlers: an initial study investigating the early detection of autism and pervasive developmental disorders. *J Autism Dev Disord*. 2001;31(2):131-144.

66. Vismara LA, Rogers SJ. Behavioral treatments in autism spectrum disorder: what do we know? *Ann Rev Clin Psychol*. 2010;6:447-468.

67. Ajzenman HF, Standeven JW, Shurtleff TL. Effect of hippotherapy on motor control, adaptive behaviors, and participation in children with autism spectrum disorder: a pilot study. *AJOT*. 2013;67:653-663.

68. Case-Smith J, Weaver LL, Fristad MA. A systematic review of sensory processing interventions for children with autism spectrum disorders. *Autism*. 2014. doi:10.1177/1362361313517762.

69. Ayres AJ. *Sensory Integration and Learning Disorders*. Los Angeles, CA: Western Psychological Services; 1972.

70. Whiteley P, Shattock P, Knivsberg AM, et al. Gluten- and casein-free dietary intervention for autism spectrum conditions. *Front Hum Neurosci*. 2013;6(344). doi:10.3389/fnhum.2012.00344.

Review Questions

1. **Global delay is defined as:**
   A. Delay in 1 SD in 3 or more developmental areas
   B. Delay of 1 SD in 2 or more developmental areas
   C. Delay of 2 SD in 3 or more developmental areas
   D. Delay of 2 SD in 2 or more developmental areas

2. **A 12-month-old child is saying 7 words and can point to all of his facial features; this child would correctly be described as:**
   A. Mildly delayed (functioning within 3 months of age)
   B. On target for age
   C. Slightly advanced for his age

3. **If both parents are carriers of a recessive genetic trait, they will have**
   A. A 25% chance of having a child with that trait
   B. A 50% chance of having a child with that trait
   C. A 75% chance of having a child with that trait
   D. A 100% chance of having a child with that trait

4. **The most common genetic cause of Down syndrome is?**
   A. Trisomy 21
   B. Mosaic Trisomy 21
   C. Translocation

5. **Which of the following is an X-linked disorder?**
   A. Cri-du-chat
   B. Duchenne Muscular Dystrophy
   C. Niemann–Pick disease
   D. Spinal Muscular Atrophy

6. **Which developmental disorder can be ameliorated through diet?**
   A. Fragile X
   B. Phenylketonuria
   C. Rett syndrome
   D. Trisomy 18

7. **Tay–Sachs is associated with what type of inborn error of metabolism?**
   A. Creatine deficiency
   B. Lysosomal storage
   C. Sterol synthesis

8. **Which of the following correctly describes the intellectual abilities of children with Down syndrome?**
   A. All children with Down syndrome have an intellectual deficit
   B. Most children with Down syndrome have severe intellectual deficits
   C. Most children with Down syndrome have only a mild intellectual deficit
   D. Most children with Down syndrome have a moderate intellectual deficit

9. **Down syndrome is associated with many dysmorphic features, which of the following correctly describes one of these features?**
   A. Hypertonia
   B. An eyelid that has an extra fold of skin
   C. Longer 5th fingers
   D. Multiple palmar creases

10. **Which of the following correctly describes the brain anomalies with Down syndrome?**
    A. The brain is larger with deeper sulci
    B. Neurogenesis is prolonged in those with Down syndrome
    C. The cerebellum is smaller than expected with fewer synapses
    D. The dendrites of those with DS have a greater number of dendritic spines

11. **Physical therapy for the child with Down syndrome will commonly include which of the following?**
    A. Creation of a quiet environment to prevent overstimulation
    B. The use of hip-knee-ankle (HKAFO) orthotics to provide support for gait training
    C. Body-weight-supported treadmill training to stimulate independent ambulation
    D. Avoidance of resistive exercises to prevent muscle fatigue

12. **For neuromuscular disorders, like Becker Muscular Dystrophy, which of the following treatment methods should be avoided?**
    A. Concentric muscle strengthening
    B. Eccentric muscle strengthening
    C. Isometric muscle strengthening

13. **Developmental coordination disorder is thought to result from focal brain damage to the cerebellum?**
    A. True
    B. False

14. **Which of the following treatment methods is likely to have the best results for children with developmental coordination disorder?**
    A. Balance training
    B. Body-weight-supported treadmill training
    C. Strength training
    D. Task-specific training

15. **A motor delay is a diagnostic criterion for autism spectrum disorder?**
    A. True
    B. False

16. **Which of the following correctly describes the brain anomaly/anomalies associated with autism?**
    A. Mild microcephaly
    B. Thicker corpus callosum
    C. More synapses
    D. Hyperactive amygdala

17. **Which of the following statements about the motor behavior of children with ASD is correct?**
    A. Many children with ASD have difficulty with rhythmic or sequential movements
    B. Most children with ASD demonstrate typical motor development
    C. Toe-walking in ASD is the result of hypertonia of the gastrocnemius
    D. Despite many motor impairments, children with ASD excel at ball skills

18. **The sensory deficit(s) associated with ASD are correctly described by which of the following?**
    A. Atypical sensory receptor function
    B. Delayed sensory nerve conduction
    C. Impaired sensory processing

19. **Which of the following correctly describes Sensory Integrative Therapy for ASD?**
    A. Passive application of vibration or massage to hypersensitive body areas
    B. Wearing a weighted vest to increase body awareness
    C. Uses motor tasks with sensory challenges to improve sensory processing
    D. Includes auditory stimulation to address communication deficits

20. **Which food products are often limited in the dietary management of children with ASD?**
    A. Wheat, rye, barley, and milk products
    B. Wheat, rye, barley, and red meat
    C. Leafy vegetables and milk products
    D. Milk products and red meat

Answers

1. D	2. C	3. A	4. A	5. B
6. B	7. B	8. D	9. B	10. C
11. C	12. B	13. B	14. D	15. B
16. C	17. A	18. C	19. C	20. A

Appendix
Adult Outcome Measures by ICF Category and Diagnostic Group

	BODY STRUCTURE AND FUNCTION	ACTIVITY	PARTICIPATION
CVA	**Ashworth** Chedoke-McMaster Stroke Assessment Dynamometry Fugl-Meyer Assessment of Motor Performance NIH Stroke Scale Orpington Prognostic Scale Postural Assessment Scale for Stroke Patients Rivermead Motor Assessment Tardieu Spasticity Scale (Modified Tardieu)	**10 Meter Walk Test** (10MWT) 5 times sit to stand **6 Minute Walk Test** (6MWT) 9 Hole Peg Test Action Research Arm Test (ARAT) Activities-specific Balance Confidence Scale (ABC Scale) Arm Motor Ability Test **Berg Balance Scale** (BBS) **Functional Gait Assessment** (FGA) (Dynamic Gait Index-Revised) Functional Ambulation Categories **Functional Independence Measure** (FIM) Functional Reach Motor Activity Log **Timed Up and Go (TUG) Test** Trunk Impairment Scale Wolf Motor Function Test	Assessment of Life Habits EuroQoL Falls Efficacy Scale (FES) Goal Attainment Scale Modified Rankin Scale Stroke Adapted SIP-30 Stroke Impact Scale Stroke Rehabilitation Assessment of Movement MS Impact Scale (MSIS-29)
MS	Box and Blocks Test Disease Steps Dizziness Handicap Inventory Fatigue Scale for Motor and Cognitive Functions Functional Assessment of MS FIM Guy's Neurological Disability Scale Maximal Inspiratory and Expiratory Pressure Rivermead Mobility Index MS Functional Composite	12-Item MS Walking Scale **6MWT** 9-Hole Peg Test **ABC Scale** **BBS** **FGA** (Dynamic Gait Index-Revised) Four Square Step Test Functional Assessment of MS FIM Functional Reach Hauser Ambulation Index Modified Fatigue Impact Scale MS Functional Composite Timed 25 Foot Walk **TUG** with Cognitive and Manual Trunk Impairment Scale Visual Analog Scale (fatigue) VO_2 max and VO_2 peak	FIM Goal Attainment Scale Guy's Neurological Disability Scale Medical Outcome Study (SF-36) Short Form Health Survey of Medical outcome study (SF-36) Functional Assessment of MS MS Functional Composite MS International Quality of Life Questionnaire MS Quality of Life (MS-QoL 54) MS Quality of Life Inventory

(Continued)

	BODY STRUCTURE AND FUNCTION	ACTIVITY	PARTICIPATION
TBI	Agitated Behavior Scale Apathy Evaluation Scale **Ashworth Scale (Modified)** Cog-Log and O(rientation)-Log Coma Recovery Scale-Revised Disorders of Consciousness Scale Dizziness Handicap Inventory Global Fatigue Index Moss Attention Rating Scale Patient Health Questionnaire Rancho Levels of Cognitive Function	12-Item MS Walking Scale **6MWT** Cognitive Functions Action Research Arm Test Balance Error Scoring Scale Barthel Index **BBS** Community Balance and Mobility Scale **FIM** Functional Assessment Measure High Level Mobility Assessment	Disability Rating Scale Sydney Psychosocial Re integration Scale Quality of life after brain injury
SCI	Ashworth Scale (Modified) Bryce–Ragnarsson Pain Taxonomy Classification for Chronic Pain in SCI Donovan SCI Pain Classification Grasp and Release Test (GRT) Hand Held Myometry/ Myometry International Spinal Cord Injury Pain Classification (ISCIP) International Standards for Multidimensional Pain Inventory – SCI version Neurological Classification of Penn Spasm Frequency Scale, Spinal Cord Injury, ASIA Impairment Scale (AIS) Numeric Pain Rating Scale 6-Minute Arm Test (6-MAT) Spastic Reflexes (SCATS) Spinal Cord Assessment Tool for Spinal Cord Injury Spasticity Evaluation Tool (SCI-SET) Tardieu Scale, Modified Tardieu Scale Wheelchair Users Shoulder Pain Index (WUSPI)	10MWT 6MWT ARAT ABC Scale Balance Evaluations Systems Test (BESTest) **BBS** Capabilities of UE Functioning Instrument (CUE) FES **FGA** (Dynamic Gait Index-Revised) **FIM** Functional Reach Test (FRT)/Modified Graded and Redefined Assessment of Sensibility Strength and Prehension (GRASSP) High Level Mobility and Assessment Tool (HiMAT) Jebsen–Taylor Hand Function Test **TUG** Test Toronto Rehabilitation Institute Hand Function Test Wheelchair Skills Test Functional Tests for Persons who Self Propel a Manual Wheelchair (4FTPSMW) Quadriplegia Index of Function (QIF) and short form	Craig Handicap Assessment and Reporting Technique (CHART) Craig Hospital Inventory of Environmental Factors (CHIEF) Impact on Participation and Autonomy Questionnaire (IPA) Life Satisfaction Questionnaire (LISAT-9) Needs Assessment Checklist (NAC) Quality of Well Being Short Form 36 (SF-36) Sickness Impact Profile 68 (SIP 68) Participation Assessment with Physical Activity Recall Assessment for People with Spinal Cord Injury (PARA-SCI) Quality of Life Index, Spinal Cord Version (QLI-SCI, Ferrans and Powers) Recombined Tools-Objective (PART-O) Reintegration to Normal Living Index (RNL) Satisfaction with Life Scale (SWLS, Deiner Scale) Spinal Cord Injury Lifestyle Scale (SCILS) World Health Organization Quality of Life-BREF (WHOQOL-BREF)
PD	Montreal Cognitive Assessment MDS UPDRS Parkinson's Fatigue Scale	**10MWT** 5 times sit to stand **6MWT** 9-Hole Peg Test **ABC Scale** **FGA** (Dynamic Gait Index-Revised) Mini BESTest MDS UPDRS **Time Up and Go** Cognitive Freezing of Gait Questionnaire	Parkinson Disease Quality of Life 39 or 8 item (PDQ-8 or PDQ-39)

(Continued)

	BODY STRUCTURE AND FUNCTION	ACTIVITY	PARTICIPATION
Vestibular	Dix–Hallpike Dynamic Visual Acuity (Instrumented) Dynamic Visual Acuity (Non-Instrumented) Head Impulse Test Modified Clinical Test of Sensory Interaction on Balance (mCTSIB) Romberg Sensory Organization Test (NeuroCom) Sharpened Romberg Vertigo Symptom Scale (VSS) Visual Analogue Scale (VAS) Visual Vertigo Analogue Scale (VVAS)	**ABC Scale** Balance Evaluation Systems Test (BEST) **BBS** Four Square Step Test **FGA** (Dynamic Gait Index-Revised) Mini Balance Evaluation Systems Test (Mini BEST) **TUG** Test	Dizziness Handicap Inventory
Motor Neuron Disease	ALS Depression Inventory 12 **Ashworth Scale** (Modified) Beck Depression Inventory Hospital Anxiety and Depression Scale Verbal fluency VASVAS Maximal Inspiratory and Expiratory Pressure Fatigue Severity Scale (FSS)	**10MWT** 9-Hole Peg Test **BBS** Functional Reach Test **FIM** Performance Oriented Mobility Assessment (POMA) **TUG Test**	Schedule for Evaluation of Individual Quality of Life-Direct Weighting Sickness Impact Profile Short Form-36
ALS		ALS Functional Rating Scale-Revised Appel ALS Scale ALS Severity Scale Norris Scale	ALS Assessment Questionnaire 40 (ALSAQ-40; ALSAQ-5) ALS-Specific QOL Instrument
GBS		Inflammatory Neuropathy Cause and Treatment group ODSS, modified GBS Disability Scale, modified Rankin Scale	
Developmental Disorders in Children	Bayley Scales of Infant and Toddler Development (1 month–42 months) Peabody Developmental Motor Scales (PDMS) (birth–6 years) Gross Motor Function Measure (GMFM) (5 months–16 years with CP)	Bayley Scales of Infant and Toddler Development (1 month–42 months) PDMS (birth–5 years) GMFM (5 months–16 years with CP) Pediatric Evaluation of Disability Inventory (PEDI) (birth–20 years)	Caregiver Priority and Child Health Index of Life with Disabilities (1–13 years old) Child Health and Illness Profile (11–17 years old) Child Health Questionnaire (5–18 years old) School Function Assessment (SFA) (K–6th grade)

Bolded measures are potentially key measures to use in the neurologic population as they are recommended by multiple Neurology Section EDGE task force groups.

Details on the Neurology Section of the APTA's EDGE task force recommendations can be found at: http://www.neuropt.org/professional-resources/neurology-section-outcome-measures-recommendations

Detailed reviews of outcome measures cited here and others commonly used in therapy practice are available through RehabMeasures.org and include links to the actual instruments when available. Current website page address: http://www.rehabmeasures.org